Operative Oral and Maxillofacial Surgery

Operative Oral and Maxillofacial Surgery

SECOND EDITION

John D. Langdon Emeritus Professor of Oral and Maxillofacial Surgery, King's College London, UK

Mohan F. Patel Consultant Surgeon, Department of Oral and Maxillofacial Surgery, Royal Berkshire Hospital, Reading, UK

Robert A. Ord Professor, Department of Oral and Maxillofacial Surgery, Baltimore College of Dental Surgery, Baltimore, Maryland, USA

Peter A. Brennan Consultant Oral and Maxillofacial Surgeon, Honorary Professor of Surgery, Department of Oral and Maxillofacial Surgery, Queen Alexandra Hospital, Portsmouth, UK

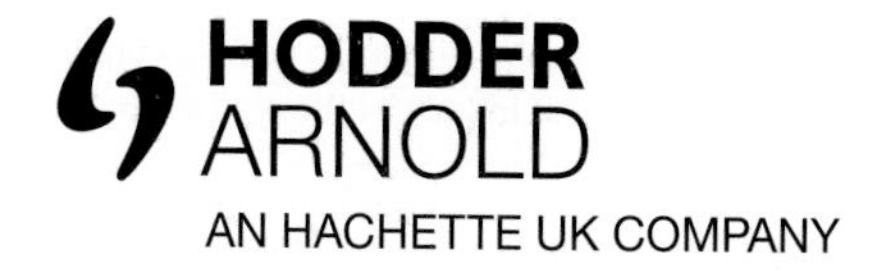

First published in Great Britain in 1998 by Chapman and Hall.
This second edition published in 2011 by
Hodder Arnold, an imprint of Hodder Education, an Hachette UK Company,
338 Euston Road, London NW1 3BH

http://www.hodderarnold.com

British Library Cataloguing in Publication Data
A catalogue record for this book is available from the British Library

Library of Congress Cataloging-in-Publication Data
A catalog record for this book is available from the Library of Congress

ISBN-13 978 0 340 945 896

1 2 3 4 5 6 7 8 9 10

Commissioning Editor: Gavin Jamieson
Project Editor: Francesca Naish
Production Controller: Joanna Walker
Cover Designer: Helen Townson
Index compiled by: Indexing Specialists (UK) Ltd.

Typeset in 10 on 12 pt Minion by Phoenix Photosetting, Chatham, Kent
Printed and bound in Italy by Printer Trento

What do you think about this book? Or any other Hodder Arnold title?
Please visit our website: www.hodderarnold.com

Dedication

To Paul, Jane, Sue and Rachel, and to colleagues and trainees: past, present and future.

Contents

PART THREE: SURGICAL TECHNIQUES

PART FOUR: MALIGNANT DISEASE OF THE MOUTH AND JAW

PART NINE: CLEFT LIP AND PALATE

PART TEN: CRANIOFACIAL SURGERY

PART ELEVEN: FACIAL AESTHETIC SURGERY

Contributors

Christopher M Avery
Maxillofacial Unit, Leicester Royal Infirmary, Leicester, UK

Ashraf F Ayoub
Professor and Honorary Consultant in Oral and Maxillofacial Surgery, Glasgow University Dental Hospital and School, Glasgow, UK

Andrew W Baker
John Radcliffe Hospital, Oxford, UK

Robert P Bentley
King's College Hospital, London, UK

Pradeep Bhandari
Department of Gastroenterology, Queen Alexandra Hospital, Portsmouth, UK

Greg Boyes-Varley
Morningside Medi-Clinic, Johannesburg, South Africa

Jaime Brahim
University of Maryland Dental School, Oral and Maxillofacial Surgery Department, Baltimore, Maryland, USA

Peter A Brennan
Department of Oral and Maxillofacial Surgery, Queen Alexandra Hospital, Portsmouth, UK

Andrew E Brown
Honorary Consultant, Queen Victoria Hospital, East Grinstead, UK

James S Brown
Regional Maxillofacial Unit, University Hospital Aintree, Liverpool, UK

Jacqui E Brown
KCL Dental Institute of Guy's, Kings's College and St Thomas' Hospitals, London, UK

Catherine Bryant
Department of Oral Surgery, King's College Hospital NHS Foundation Trust, London, UK

John F Caccamese Jr
Department of Oral and Maxillofacial Surgery, University of Maryland Medical Center and Kernan Hospital and Greater Baltimore Medical Center Cleft Teams, Baltimore, MD, USA

Luke Cascarini
North West Hospitals, London, UK

John Cawood
Spire Murrayfield Hospital, Wirral, UK

Luc Cesteleyn
Department of Maxillofacial Surgery, AZ St Lucas Gent, Belgium and University of Michigan, Ann Arbor, MI, USA

Domenick P Coletti
University of Maryland Dental School, Oral-Maxillofacial Surgery, Baltimore, MD, USA

Stephen EJ Connor
Neuroradiology Department, Kings College Hospital, London, UK

Bernard J Costello
Pediatric Oral and Maxillofacial Surgery, Children's Hospital of Pittsburgh, and Department of Oral and Maxillofacial Surgery, University of Pittsburgh, Pittsburgh, PA, USA

Roger Currie
Crosshouse Hospital, Kilmarnock, UK

Eric J Dierks
Oregon Health and Science University, Legacy Emanuel Hospital, Portland, OR, USA

George Dimitroulis
Department of Surgery, St Vincent's Hospital, University of Melbourne, Australia

André Eckardt
Department of Oral and Maxillofacial Surgery, Hanover Medical University, Hannover, Germany

Michael P Escudier
King's College London Dental Institute, London, UK

Madanagopalan Ethunandan
Maxillofacial Unit, St Richard's Hospital, Chichester, UK

Barrie Evans
Southampton University Hospitals NHS Trust, Southampton, UK

Rhodri Evans
Consultant Radiologist, Radiology Department
Morriston Hospital, Swansea, UK

Tirbod Fattahi
University of Florida – Jacksonville, Department of Surgery, Jacksonville, FL, USA

Stephen E Feinberg
Oral and Maxillofacial Surgery, University of Michigan, Ann Arbor, MI, USA

Tim Flood
Salisbury District Foundation Trust, Salisbury, UK

GE Ghali
Department of Oral and Maxillofacial Surgery, LSU Health Science Center, Shreveport, LA, USA

Susannah Green
Department of Gastroenterology, Queen Alexandra Hospital, Portsmouth, UK

Joseph Helman
University of Michigan Hospital, Ann Arbor, MI, USA

Robert Hensher
Kind Edward VII's Hospital, London, UK

Ian Holland
Southern General, Glasgow, UK

Colin Hopper
Consultant Oral and Maxillofacial Surgeon, University College London Hospitals, London, UK

Bruce B Horswell
Charleston Area Medical Center, Charleston, WV, USA

Dale Howes
Morningside Medi-Clinic, Johannesburg, South Africa

Christoph Huppa
South Thames Cleft Service, Guy's Hospital, London, UK

Ilanko Ilankovan
Poole General Hospital, Poole, UK

Kenji Izumi
Oral Anatomy, Niigata University, Niigata, Japan

Paul A Johnson
Royal Surrey County Hospital, Surrey, UK

Corazon Collantes Jose
Asian Hospital, Manila, Philippines

Leonard B Kaban
Harvard School of Dental Medicine, Massachusetts General Hospital, Boston, MA, USA

Eugene Keller
Mayo Clinic, Department of General Surgery, Rochester, MN, USA

Cyrus J Kerawala
Royal Marsden Hospital, London, UK

King Kim
Oral and Maxillofacial Surgery Program, Nova Southeastern University/Broward General Medical Center, Fort Lauderdale, FL, USA

Moni Kuriakose
Chief of Department of Surgical Oncology, Head of Department of Head Neck Surgery, Mazumdar Shaw Center & NH, Bangalore, India

Janice Lee
Oral and Maxillofacial Surgery, Department of Oral and Maxillofacial Surgery, UCSF, San Francisco, CA, USA

Dorothy Lang
Wessex Neurological Centre, Southampton University Hospitals NHS Trust, Southampton, UK

John D Langdon
King's College London, UK

Andrew Lyons
Guy's Hospital, London, UK

David W Macpherson
Maxillofacial Unit, St Richard's Hospital, Chichester, UK

E Antonio Mangubat
Southcentre Cosmetic Surgery, Seattle, Washington DC, USA

Chi Mao
Peking University School of Stomatology, Beijing, China

Brian Martin
Pediatric Dentistry, Children's Hospital of Pittsburgh, University of Pittsburgh, Pittsburgh, PA, USA

Joseph McCain
Nova Southeastern University/Broward General Medical Center, Fort Lauderdale, FL, USA

Mark McGurk
Dental Institute at Guy's, King's College and St Thomas' Hospitals, London, UK

Jeremy McMahon
Southern General, Glasgow, UK

Joe McManners
Forth Valley Royal Hospital, Larbert, UK

Matthias AW Merkx
Department of Oral and Maxillofacial Sugery, Radboud University, Nijmegen Medical Center, Nijmegen, The Netherlands

John S Millar
Wessex Neurological Centre, Southampton, UK

Suhail K Mithani
Plastic and Reconstructive Surgery, Johns Hopkins University School of Medicine, Baltimore, MD, USA

David M Montes
Department of Oral and Maxillofacial Surgery, LSU Health Science Center, Shreveport, LA, USA

George Obeid
Washington Hospital Center, Department of Oral-Maxillofacial Surgery, Washington, DC, USA

Rachel S Oeppen
Department of Radiology, Southampton University Hospitals NHS Trust, Southampton, UK

Robert A Ord
University of Maryland/Greenebaum Cancer Center, Baltimore, MD, USA

Maria E Papadaki
Harvard School of Dental Medicine, Massachusetts General Hospital, Boston, MA, USA

Mohan F Patel
Royal Berkshire Hospital Foundation Trust, Reading, UK

Chris Penfold
Glan Clwyd Hospital, Rhyl, UK

Xin Peng
Peking University School of Stomatology, Beijing, China

Michael Perry
School of Dentistry, Royal Group of Hospitals, Belfast, UK

CA Pratt
Maxillofacial Unit, St Richards Hospital, Chichester, UK

Krishna Shama Rao
Professor, President of Maaya Foundation and Clinical Director, Centre for Craniofacial Anomalies, University of Karnataka, India

Alexander D Rapidis
Eastman Dental Institute, University College London, University of London, UK and Department of Head and Neck Surgery, Greek Anticancer Institute, Saint Savvas Hospital, Athens, Greece

N Ravindranathan
Department of Maxillo Facial/Facial Plastic Surgery, RIPAS Hospital, Brunei, Darussalam

Eduardo D Rodriguez
Plastic and Reconstructive Surgery, University of Maryland School of Medicine, Baltimore, MD, USA

Henning Schliephake
Department of Oral Maxillofacial Surgery, University Medicine Göttingen, George Augusta University, Göttingen, Germany

Andrew J Sidebottom
Queens Medical Centre, Nottingham, UK

Miller H Smith
Oral and Maxillofacial Surgery, University of Michigan, Ann Arbor, MI, USA

Helen Spencer
Queen Alexandra Hospital, Portsmouth, UK

Leo Stassen
Maxillofacial Unit, St James' Hospital, Dublin, Eire

Paul JW Stoelinga
Former Head of Department of Oral and Maxillofacial Surgery, Radboud University, Medical Center, Nijmegen, The Netherlands

James Swift
University of Minnesota, Minneapolis, MN, USA

Andrew BG Tay
Department of Oral and Maxillofacial Surgery, National Dental Centre, Singapore

Nirav Pravin Trivedi
Consultant, Department of Head Neck Surgery, Mazumdar Shaw Cancer Center & NH, Bangalore, India

David A Walker
Hospital for Sick Children, Faculty of Dentistry, University of Toronto, Toronto, Canada

Gary Warburton
University of Maryland Medical Center, Baltimore, MD, USA

Peter Ward Booth
Honorary Consultant, Queen Victoria Hospital, East Grinstead, UK

Michael Williams
Eastbourne District General Hospital, Eastbourne, UK

Julia A Woolgar
University of Liverpool, Liverpool and Royal Liverpool and Broadgreen University Hospitals NHS Trust, Liverpool, UK

Guang-yan Yu
Peking University School of Stomatology, Beijing, China

John Zuniga
University of Texas Southwestern Medical Centre, Division of Oral and Maxillofacial Surgery, Department of Surgery, Dallas, TX, USA

Foreword

The book is beautifully produced with clear text and especially helpful, well-drawn diagrams, supplemented in some sections with photographs. At the end of each section is a box headed 'Tops Tips' which look to be extremely valuable and should save the surgeon and the patient from avoidable complications.

This is the second edition of a major text on Operative Oral and Maxillofacial Surgery. The subject is now enormous, extending from repair of trauma, cosmesis, and of course traditional management of infections and malignancy, with important and continuing advances in all these areas. In addition the editors have included major sections on dental and jaw surgery. The rapid advances in surgical techniques involve mastering of new materials and instruments and above all an extreme attention to detail. This book clarifies the approach that the surgeon should make to each operation and gives a well-illustrated exposition of the technique. However, as it is repeatedly emphasised in the text, complicated surgery requires many hours of intense apprenticeship and practice so as to provide patients with the best possible advice, management and operation.

As a surgeon but non-specialist in this area I cannot make authoritative comments but I am sure this volume, like its predecessor will be essential reading for specialist trainee surgeons and established practitioners, particularly valuable when their work leads them to transitional anatomical sites which may necessarily take them from their main stream of experience.

I can confidently expect that this edition, like its predecessor, will be an important and successfully contribution to maxillofacial surgery.

Sir Roy Calne FRS

Preface

It has been over 10 years since the first edition of *Operative Maxillofacial Surgery* was published. Although the book was primarily aimed at trainees and was intended to provide a step-by-step guide to learning and subsequently performing a surgical procedure, in practise it was also used by many established specialists. It was used as an operative text by almost all UK trainees approaching the exit FRCS examination, and it also sold widely throughout the world.

Since the original edition of the book was published, there have been many advances in surgical techniques. For example, in reconstructive surgery, perforator flaps have become widely accepted as an alterative to the workhorse radial forearm free flap, while techniques such as distraction osteogenesis are giving results that were not thought possible in the head and neck region twelve years ago when the first edition was being compiled. The demand for aesthetic facial surgery has grown enormously and this is now a recognised part of the specialty. Innovations in diagnosis have resulted in new imaging techniques and sentinel node biopsy.

One of the perceived criticisms of the original edition was that it did not contain operative images but exclusively relied on line diagrams to demonstrate the technique and associated surgical anatomy. While this may be useful for showing certain procedures, many surgeons like to see operative images of the actual technique, and preferably in colour! Many chapters now have operative pictures but due to production costs these have not been used universally throughout the book, and, where appropriate, diagrams drawn by a specialist artist using the original image have been included.

The title of the book now includes oral as well as maxillofacial surgery. Oral surgery in its widest sense is performed by both oral and maxillofacial surgeons, and specialists in oral surgery. Expertise in this area needs to be taught and maintained and it forms a core part of training and the practise of oral and maxillofacial surgery. We hope that these chapters will also be of interest to our oral surgery colleagues.

Throughout the book, some chapters have been re-worked and updated from the previous edition while the majority are entirely new and re-written chapters. The book represents a distillation of experience from well respected and recognised teachers across the breadth of the specialty. We have deliberately included a faculty of authors from across the globe. While many procedures in this book could be undertaken by other specialties, we have tried to recruit authors from our own specialty wherever possible.

Inevitably with a large project such as this and with the constant development of surgical techniques, it not possible to cover every last element of the specialty, and for this we apologise in advance.

John Langdon
Mohan Patel
Robert Ord
Peter Brennan

List of abbreviations used

ABC	airway, breathing and circulation
ACF	anterior cranial fossa
AGA	androgenetic alopecia
ALA	aminolaevulinic acid
ALARA	as low as is reasonably achievable
ALT	anterolateral thigh flap
AMSO	anterior maxillary segmental osteotomy
ANS	anterior nasal spine
AP	anterior posterior
ASA	anterior septal angle
ATLS	advanced trauma life support
AVM	arteriovenous malformations
BAHA	bone-anchored hearing aid
BCC	basal cell carcinomas
BMP	bone morphogenic proteins
BSSO	bilateral sagittal split osteotomy
CECT	contrast enhanced computed tomography
CLP	cleft lip and palate
CSA	circumflex scapular artery
CSF	cerebrospinal fluid
CST	cerebral sinus thrombosis
CT	computed tomography
CULLP	congenital unilateral lower lip palsy
DCIA	deep circumflex iliac artery
DMSO	dimethyl sulphoxide
DO	distraction osteogenesis
DSN	depressor septi nasi
ECA	external carotid artery
ECD	extracapsular dissection
ECS	extracapsular spread
EHL	extensor hallucis longus
ELISA	enzyme-linked immunosorbent assay
EM	electromagnetic
ENT	ear, nose and throat
EUA	examination under anaesthetic
EVPOME	*ex vivo* produced oral mucosa equivalent
FAMM	facial artery musculomucosal flaps
FHL	flexor hallucis longus
FISH	fluorescent *in situ* hybridization
FNAB	fine needle aspiration biopsy
FNAC	fine needle aspiration cytology
FUT	follicular unit transplantation
GCS	Glasgow Coma Scale
GI	gastrointestinal
HE	haematoxylin and eosin
HRS	hair restoration surgery
HSV	herpes simplex virus
HT	hair transplantation
ICP	intracranial pressure
IMF	intermaxillary fixation
IMRT	intensity-modulated radiotherapy
IPL	intensity pulse light
ITC	isolated tumour cells
LLAN	levator labii alaeque nasi
LLC	lower lateral cartilage
LM	lymphatic malformations
MCF	middle cranial fossa
MDT	multidisciplinary team
MMF	maxillomandibular fixation
MR	magnetic resonance
MRA	magnetic resonance angiography
MRND	modified radical neck dissection
MSCT	multislice computed tomography
MSS	medium septal system
MTA	mineral trioxide aggregate
NCA	nurse-controlled analgesia
NFA	nasofrontal angle
NICE	National Institute for Clinical Excellence
NOE	naso-orbital ethmoidal
NSAID	non-steroidal anti-inflammatory drug
OCS	orbital compartment syndrome
OFG	orofacial granulomatosis
OMFS	oral and maxillofacial surgery
OPG	orthopantomogram
ORIF	open reduction and internal fixation
PAS	periodic acid Schiff
PCR	polymerase chain reaction
PDT	photodynamic therapy
PEG	percutaneous endoscopic gastrotomy
PEJ	percutaneous endoscopic jejunostomy
PET	positron emission tomography
PF	posterior fossa
PMSO	posterior maxillary segmental osteotomy
PSA	posterior septal angle
PT	prothrombin
PTE	pulmonary thrombo-embolism
PTT	partial thromboplastin times
PVA	polyvinyl alcohol

RBH	retrobulbar haemorrhage
RED	rigid external distraction
RFFF	radial forearm free flap
RLN	recurrent laryngeal nerve
RND	radical neck dissection
ROOF	retro-orbicularis fat
RSTL	relaxed skin tension lines
SCC	squamous cell carcinoma
SCM	sternocleidomastiod muscle
SLS	selective laser sintering
SMAS	superficial muscoloaponeurotic system
SND	selective neck dissection
SOHND	supra-omohyoid neck dissection
SPECT	single photon emission computed tomography
SSTE	skin soft tissue envelope
STR	stereotactic radiosurgery
TCA	transverse cervical artery
TIG	tetanus immune globulin
TMF	temporalis muscle flap
TMJ	temporomandibular joint
TPFF	temporoparietal fascial flap
TUG	transverse gracilis
UGFNAB	ultrasound-guided fine needle aspiration biopsy
ULC	upper lateral cartilage
US	ultrasound
VA	vertebral arteries
VM	venous malformations
VPD	velopharyngeal dysfunction
VPI	velopharyngeal insufficiency

PART 1

DIAGNOSTIC INVESTIGATIONS

1.1

Imaging techniques, including computed tomography-guided biopsy and FDG-PET

STEPHEN E J CONNOR

INTRODUCTION

Maxillofacial imaging has evolved in parallel with the development of newer imaging technologies. Traditional plain radiography and dental imaging is now frequently supplemented by cross-sectional modalities, such as computed tomography (CT), magnetic resonance imaging (MRI) and ultrasound, together with functional imaging modalities, such as positron emission tomography (PET). It is important to be aware of the benefits and limitations of such imaging examinations such that they are applied to the appropriate clinical scenario.

RADIATION PROTECTION

Some imaging investigations use ionizing radiation which has the potential to result in biological damage. The aim of radiation protection is to provide a safe environment for the worker and patient. The Ionising Radiation (Medical Exposure) Regulations 2000 (IRMER) lay down basic measures required for protection against the harmful effects of medical radiation exposure. There are duties of the employer who provides a framework within exposures which take place, the operator who carries out the exposure, the practitioner who justifies the exposure and the referrer who requests the exposure. Key principles are that the examination should be of sufficient benefit to justify radiation exposure, that dose is optimized by the ALARA (as low as is reasonably achievable) principle and that dose limits should be recorded.

PLAIN RADIOGRAPHS

X-rays are produced by a point source and, after passing through the body part of interest, are detected by non-screen (dental radiography) or intensifying screen/film combinations (extraoral radiography). Selected facial radiographic views are listed in Table 1.1.1. Tomography refers to a technique whereby the x-ray source and film move during the exposure. The aim is to demonstrate only a section which is in focus, whereas structures outside this section are blurred. Applications include conventional dental panoramic tomography, tomograms of the temporomandibular joints and mandibular tomograms for implant planning.

Table 1.1.1 Radiographic views of the facial skeleton.

	Radiographic view	Comment
Mid and upper third	Occipito-frontal (OF) 15-20 (Caldwell view)	Used to visualize upper third of face
	OF 25 (modified Caldwell view)	Superior visualization of orbital floor relative to Caldwell view
	Occipito-mental (OM)	Used to visualize mid-third of the face
	OM 10	Less obscuration of maxillary antrum than an OM view
	OM 30	Superior view of malar arches and inferior orbital margins. Preferable to submentovertical (SMV) view
	Lateral	Supplementary for central midface injury
Lower third	Postero-anterior (PA) mandible	
	Lateral oblique	Replaces OPG if not available or impractical
	Reverse Townes	Better visualizes mandibular condyles
	Orthopantomogram (OPG)	

Digital radiography units (using digital receptors to intercept the x-ray beam rather than intensifying screens) are now replacing conventional units. This allows transmission of data to image processing and storage devices, as well as communications networks.

CONTRAST STUDIES

Contrast media may be introduced into a vessel, lumen or cavity in order to render it radio-opaque and hence radiographically visible. This may then be viewed in real time with fluoroscopic imaging or with serial radiographs. Contrast media used for this purpose include barium sulphate suspensions and non-ionic iodinated contrast agents. There is a small risk associated with the intravascular iodinated contrast agents which must be weighed against the potential benefits. Information which should be sought from the patient before contrast injection includes previous contrast reactions, asthma, renal problems, diabetes and metformin therapy.

Contrast studies with maxillofacial applications are:

1. **Angiography**: Conventional angiography is generally performed as a precursor to interventional radiological techniques. CT and MR angiography have largely replaced diagnostic applications in maxillofacial pathology. It remains appropriate for the planning of embolization of high flow vascular malformations and tumours (Figure 1.1.1) and for the evaluation of arterial injury (traumatic or tumour erosion). Angiographic catheters are generally introduced over a guidewire via a common femoral artery puncture. Small calibre microcatheters may be introduced into distal external carotid artery branches.
2. **Barium/contrast studies**: Barium swallows may be required to evaluate high dysphagia and pain. Rapid serial radiography or video recording may be used to assess the hypopharynx and upper oesophagus during deglutition (Figure 1.1.2). Barium may be combined with a gas-producing agent and an intravenous smooth muscle relaxant to produce double-contrast images of the lower oesophagus. If aspiration or tracheo-oesophageal fistulation is suspected, then a low osmolar iodinated contrast medium will be used.
3. **Sialogram**: Iodinated contrast medium may be introduced into the salivary duct ostium via a polythene catheter. Fluoroscopy or radiography is used including delayed images after administration of a sialagogue. This is compared with preprocedure control films.
4. **Sinogram/fistulogram**: A sinogram involves the insertion of a fine catheter into the orifice of a sinus and injection of contrast medium in order to delineate a sinus or fistula. If there is a complex tract then it may be combined with CT.
5. **Temporomandibular joint (TMJ) arthrogram**: Iodinated contrast medium is injected into the joint under fluoroscopic guidance and double-contrast studies may be achieved by contrast withdrawal and replacement with air.
6. **Dacrocystogram**: The nasolacrimal sac and duct may be cannulated and injected with contrast medium in patients with epiphora. The lacrimal drainage system may also be evaluated with CT and MRI following conjunctival application of contrast medium.
7. **Percutaneous venogram**: Percutaneous venography may be used as a precursor to sclerotherapy for the assessment of volume and venous run off in the setting of low flow venous malformations. A similar technique (lymphogram) is used for a lymphatic malformation. Ultrasound is used to guide the needle placement if the lesion is not clinically palpable.

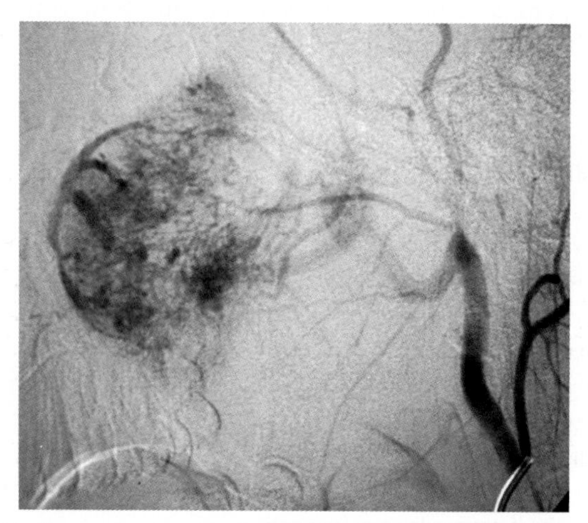

1.1.1 Lateral projection in the arterial phase of a common carotid angiogram demonstrates a vascular blush arising from the maxillary artery secondary to a juvenile angiofibroma.

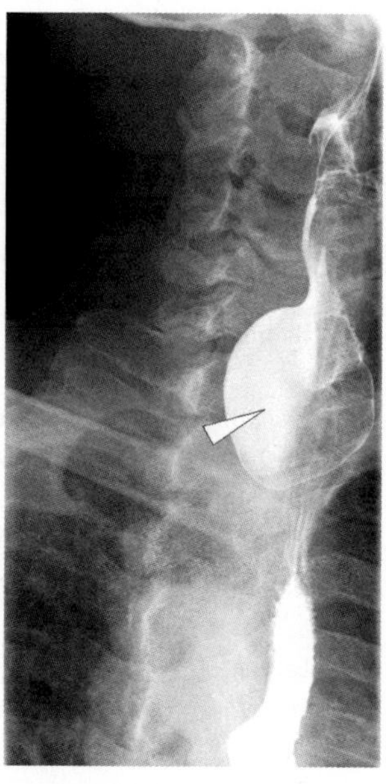

1.1.2 Oblique projection of a barium swallow demonstrates a pharyngeal pouch (white arrowhead).

COMPUTED TOMOGRAPHY

Computed tomography is an imaging modality which is rapid and widely available. A CT scanner consists of an x-ray tube which sends a fan of x-rays through the patient and the attenuation of the beam by the patient is detected. The process is repeated as the tube and detectors rotate and the patient is advanced through the scanner. The degree of x-ray absorption by each volume of tissue (voxel) is displayed as a pixel which is allocated a number (Hounsfield unit) (Table 1.1.2). This information may be digitally manipulated so as to best demonstrate the tissues of interest (e.g. by changing the range of numbers in the grey scale or window width or by using algorithms to alter the sharpness of the image). The same information may be used to provide multiplanar reformats or rendering of three-dimensional objects to facilitate visual assessment. Imaging of soft tissues generally requires the administration of iodinated contrast medium to enhance pathological tissues and help delineate vascular structures from other soft tissue, such as lymph nodes. The availability of CT fluoroscopy and in-room CT controls/monitors has improved the safety and efficacy of CT-guided biopsies of deep facial and skull base lesions (Figure 1.1.3).

Contemporary multislice computed tomography (MSCT) differs in that a number of slices (current scanners are typically 64 slice) are obtained per tube rotation. Multislice CT has the potential to scan standard volumes with shorter acquisition times so reducing movement artefact (e.g. due to swallowing) or the requirement for sedation and optimizing vascular opacification (e.g. for CT angiographic studies) (Figure 1.1.4). It also allows the scanning of larger volumes or the use of narrower section thickness so optimizing the three-dimensional dataset for post-processing and interactive 3D image-guided surgery. The large number of images generated by MSCT impacts on workstation performance and PACS archiving/networking. It also precludes traditional hard copy review with cine paging and reformatting on a workstation being required.

The benefits of CT (Table 1.1.3) should always be weighed against the risks of ionizing radiation exposure. Whilst imaging of soft tissues requires higher radiation doses and hence strong clinical justification (typical effective dose for brain CT is 2 mSv which is equivalent to 100 chest radiographs or ten months of natural background radiation),

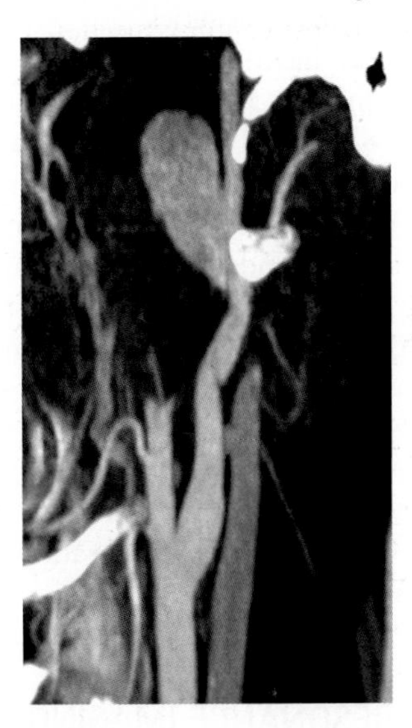

1.1.4 Lateral maximum intensity projection of a computed tomography (CT) angiogram demonstrates a post-traumatic pseudoaneurysm of the internal carotid artery.

Table 1.1.2 Hounsfield units (attenuation) of tissues.

	Typical Hounsfield units	Computed tomographic appearance
Air	−1000	Black
Fat	−50 to −100	
Water	0	
Soft tissue	+30–50	
Acute blood	+50–80	
Bone	+1000	White

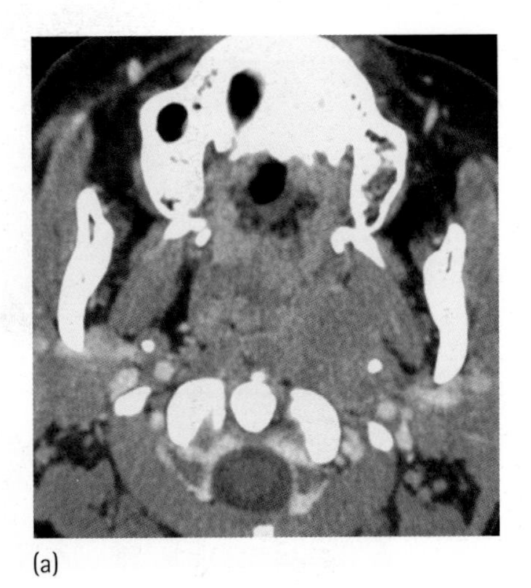

(a)

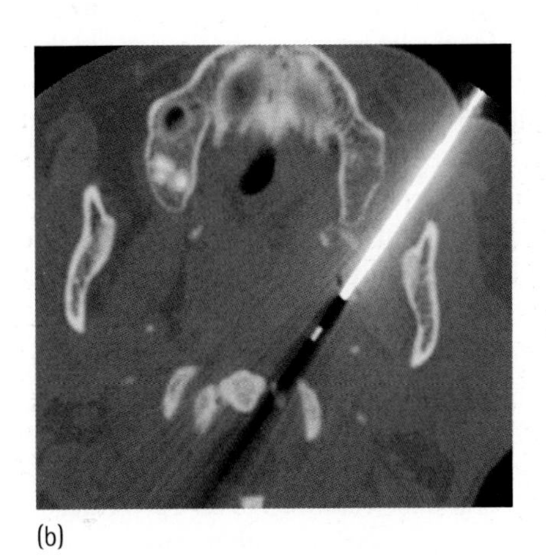

(b)

1.1.3 (a) Computed tomography (CT) displaced with soft tissue windows demonstrates a left retropharyngeal and parapharyngeal soft tissue mass. (b) CT displaced with bone windows delineates the core biopsy needle via a retromaxillary approach.

Table 1.1.3 Advantages and disadvantages of computed tomography (CT) and magnetic resonance imaging (MRI).

	CT	MRI
Advantages	Widely available	Does not require ionizing radiation
	Rapid so less prone to movement artefact	Usually less image distortion than CT from metallic foreign bodies
	Demonstrates cortical bone and calcification well	Delineates bone marrow pathology well (e.g. mandible/central skull base)
	May be combined with imaging of the lungs	Superior for skull base and intracranial imaging
	Excellent spatial resolution and 3D post-processing	Excellent contrast resolution with direct multiplanar imaging
Disadvantages	Ionizing radiation	Absolute contraindications preclude some patients
	May require iodinated contrast media (incidence of severe reactions is 0.04%)	Claustrophobia precludes some patients
		Time consuming and prone to motion artefact if patient breathless/unwell
		Expensive

low-dose imaging focused on bony detail (e.g. dental CT for implantology) may be performed with 0.2–0.3 mSv, whilst 3D cephalometric bone landmarks may be identified at doses approaching a radiographic series.

Cone beam CT has developed as a technique which provides high resolution 3D data at low radiation doses (e.g. equivalent to 2–8 OPGs). The equipment may resemble that of a conventional dental panoramic tomography unit (patient erect) or may mimic a conventional CT scanner (patient supine). A cylinder- or sphere-shaped volume of data is rapidly acquired with a single tube rotation. Some cone beam CT equipment is designed to simulate intraoral radiographs by imaging small volumes (e.g. two or three teeth) at high resolution, whilst other equipment is designed to image the whole maxillofacial region (e.g. 15-cm^3 spheres). The low tube currents utilized to reduce the radiation dose unfortunately preclude adequate imaging of soft tissue structures.

MAGNETIC RESONANCE IMAGING

Magnetic resonance imaging does not require ionizing radiation so should be preferred in cases where it would provide similar information to CT and both are available. Advantages and disadvantages relative to CT are shown in Table 1.1.3. There are some definite contraindications to the use of MRI, including metallic foreign bodies in the orbit, intracranial aneurysm clips, cardiac pacemakers and cochlear implants.

MRI signal is tissue dependent and is based on the behaviour of protons within that tissue when they are exposed to radiofrequency pulses within a magnetic field. Signal can be resolved into two components (T1 and T2). Selecting appropriate pulse sequences allows images to reflect the T1-weighted or T2-weighted characteristics of tissues. Most pathology results in increased water content relative to normal tissues and thus is shown as decreased signal on T1-w images and increased signal on T2-w images (Figure 1.1.5). There are various other tissues and substances which may be distinguished by differing MRI signal (Table 1.1.4). Pre- and post-gadolinium (contrast medium) sequences should be performed with T1-w. T1-w sequences may also be combined with fat saturation post-gadolinium, such that increased signal due to enhancement is not masked by that due to fat. Pathological lesions undergo variable enhancement and gadolinium is used to help characterize lesions. Normal structures that markedly enhance include mucosal linings and lymphoid tissue. The STIR (short time inversion recovery) sequence has been shown to be very sensitive to pathology which generally demonstrates increased signal. Multiplanar imaging (coronal and axial imaging as a minimum) is routinely performed with 4–5-mm section thickness.

Typical imaging sequences for a study of the face and neck would include: T1-w axial, T2-w axial, T1-w post-gadolinium axial, STIR coronal, T1 fat saturated post-gadolinium coronal images.

MR angiography may demonstrate flow in relation to a vessel lumen with or without the use of gadolinium. Other MRI techniques (such as spectroscopy, diffusion and perfusion imaging), higher field magnets (3 Tesla as opposed to standard 1.5 Tesla) and novel contrast agents, have been applied to the face and neck although clinical utility has not yet been established.

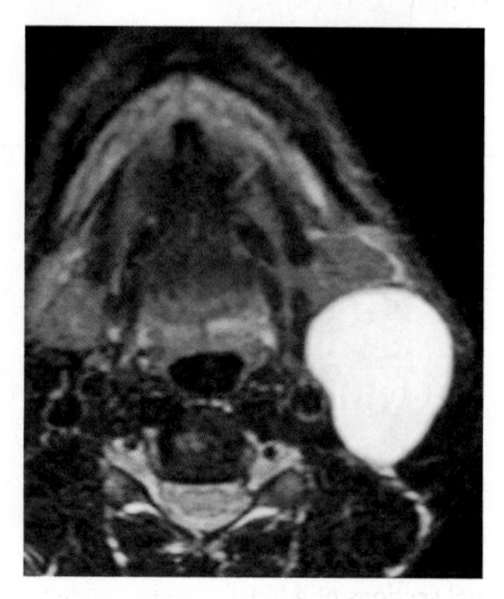

1.1.5 Axial T2-weighted fat saturated magnetic resonance (MR) image shows a T2 hyperintense left second branchial cleft cyst.

Table 1.1.4 Magnetic resonance imaging (MRI) characteristics of tissues relevant to face and neck MRI.

Signal	Substrate
High T1-w signal	Proteinaceous secretions, fat, gadolinium enhancement, subacute haemorrhage, slow flowing blood (e.g. veins)
Low T1-w signal	Most pathology (Note: Pathology generally intermediate to low T1-w signal)
High T2-w signal	Most pathology (Note: Cellular tumour is intermediate T2-w signal, whereas necrosis/cyst/inflammatory paranasal mucosal thickening is markedly increased T2-w signal)
Low T2-w signal	Mature fibrosis/scar, very dense proteinaceous secretions, acute haemorrhage
Signal void (very low T1-w and T2-w)	Cortical bone and dense calcification, air, fast flowing blood

POSITRON EMISSION TOMOGRAPHY AND OTHER RADIOISOTOPE IMAGING

Positron emission tomography differs from the previously mentioned anatomical techniques in that it provides functional imaging of metabolic activity. This has proved very useful in the setting of maxillofacial malignancy (Figure 1.1.6) with improved diagnostic accuracy relative to CT and MRI (see Table 1.1.10 p. 11). Most PET imaging studies of the head and neck use the short-lived radiotracer 18-fluorodeoxyglucose (^{18}FDG) which allows an examination of altered glucose metabolism as a marker of tumour activity. This unstable radioisotope releases a positron over a short distance after which it annihilates with an electron and emits the photons that are detected. This process of photon production implies a lower limit of spatial resolution (3–4 mm), so PET does not provide the same anatomical detail as CT or MRI. To improve the localization of pathology, PET images were initially co-registered with CT or MR images; however, techniques have now progressed such that functional and anatomical CT images (PET-CT) may be obtained on the same scanner.

It should be noted that the CT component of such PET-CT scanners may be performed without contrast medium and does not generally use the same parameters as diagnostic CT so is not a direct substitute. Multiple slices are obtained and multiplanar reformats are routine. A dedicated head and neck field of view may be followed by a separate half body study.

PET must be interpreted with an awareness of the limitations in detecting small volume (particularly <3–4 mm) disease, including superficial mucosal lesions, lymph node micrometastases and necrotic lymph nodes. Some tumours, such as salivary gland tumours, are not ^{18}FDG avid. Some centres use an objective measure of FDG uptake (standardized uptake value (SUV)) to help distinguish a malignant lesion. There are also pitfalls due to false-positive findings resulting from normal tracer distribution (e.g. salivary and thyroid gland, muscle activity and Waldeyer's ring) and inflammatory tissue (e.g. lymph nodes, early stages post-tumour treatment and healing bone).

Other radioisotopes used in the investigation of maxillofacial disease include:

1 ^{99m}Tc-MDP for the evaluation of bone disease (e.g. condylar hyperplasia, degree of activity in fibro-osseous lesions, bone metastases, bone invasion by tumour, osteomyelitis, integrity of blood supply in radionecrosis or vascularized grafts).

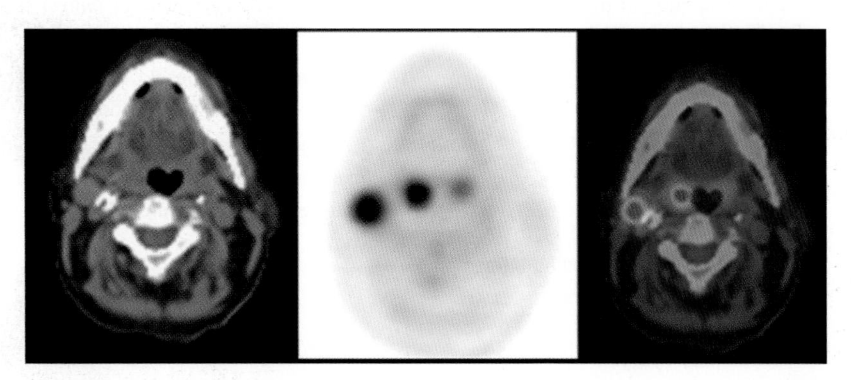

1.1.6 Axial sections of a PET-CT study: computed tomography (CT) (left), positron emission tomography (PET) (middle), fused PET-CT (right). Patient presented with a right level 2 lymph node and an unknown primary tumour. ^{18}FDG uptake is demonstrated within the lymph node and related to a right tonsilla fossa primary carcinoma. Note the physiological uptake within the left-sided tonsillar tissue.

2 ^{111}Indium-labelled and ^{99m}Tc-HMPAO-labelled leukocytes together with ^{67}Ga-gallium citrate for the diagnosis and localization of infection or inflammation in soft tissues.
3 ^{99m}Tc-pertechnetate for dynamic salivary gland imaging or to detect ectopic thyroid tissue.

IMAGING IN DIFFERENT CLINICAL SCENARIOS

Tables 1.1.5–1.1.16 and Figures 1.1.7–1.1.14 provide information on imaging in different clinical scenarios.

Table 1.1.5 Imaging of craniofacial malformations and craniosynostosis.

Imaging modality	Imaging issues	Comment
Radiography: OPG, cephalometry, skull series		Isolated sagittal, metopic or unilateral coronal synostosis may be confirmed with radiography
Low dose CT 3D data (cranial or craniofacial) with post-processing	Define foci of sutural synostosis for surgical planning 3D assessment of facial deformity and orofacial clefts	CT with post-processing is more definitive and superior for defining foci of sutural closure. Required for surgical planning and for assessment of complex craniofacial anomalies/petrous temporal bone anomalies 3D data set may be used for preoperative surgical stimulation with stereolithography or fused deposition modelling
Cranial CT/CTV/MRI	Detect intracranial malformations and venous stenosis in the setting of complex synostosis	

CT, computed tomography; CTV, computed tomography venogram; MRI, magnetic resonance imaging.

Table 1.1.6 Imaging of facial/craniofacial trauma.

Imaging modality	Imaging issues	Comment
Radiographs: Standard midfacial series is OM, OM 15/30 and lateral Standard mandibular series is OPG (lateral obliques if not available/impractical) and frontal	Screen for fractures and assess need for further CT	Most uncomplicated zygomatic, orbital and mandibular injuries may be evaluated with plain radiography alone
Low dose CT with 3D post processing Standard CT	Delineate extent and displacement of fractures Review key sites, e.g. displaced fractures of frontal sinus posterior wall	Always consider intracranial and cervical spine imaging in the early management of high energy facial injury CT is also required for suspected craniofacial injury or when there is orbital dysfunction (Figure 1.1.7), fractures are severe/comminuted or as a precursor to surgery Standard (non low dose) CT may be used to evaluate orbital or cranial soft tissue complications 3D data set post processing may be used for modeling of implants and to aid surgical planning in patients with complex fracture geometry (Figure 1.1.8)
MRI	Soft tissue (including intracranial) complications	
Others: ocular ultrasound, dacrocystography, sialography, CT cisternography	Soft tissue complications	Selected cases depending on clinical findings

CT, computed tomography; MRI, magnetic resonance imaging.

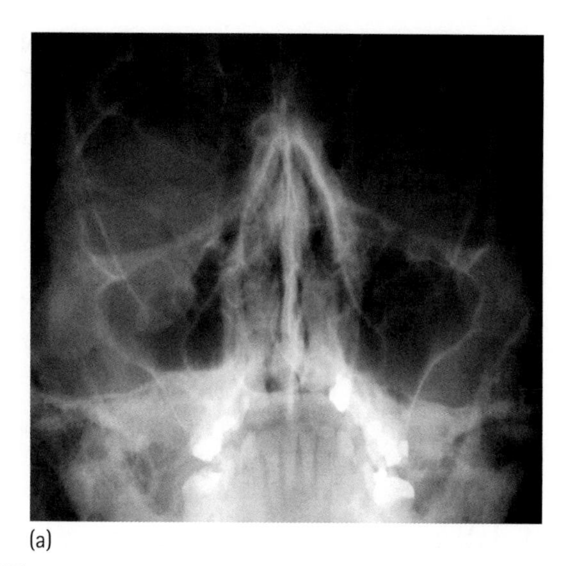

(a)

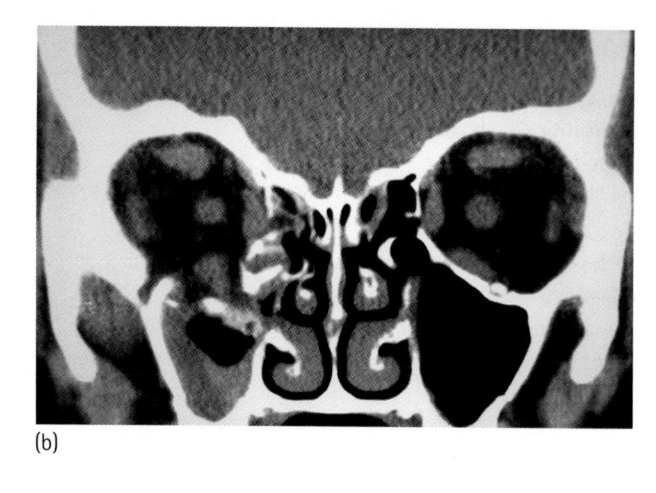

(b)

1.1.7 (a) OM view demonstrates a right orbital floor fracture with soft tissue prolapsing into the maxillary antrum and a fluid level. (b) Coronal computed tomography (CT) study in a different patient with an orbital floor fracture and persistent diplopia reveals prolapse of orbital fat and distortion of the inferior rectus muscle.

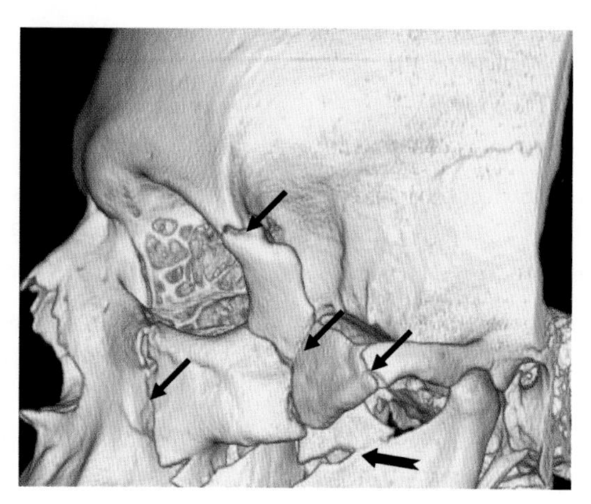

1.1.8 Volume rendered lateral projection of a three-dimensional computed tomography (CT) data set. There is a comminuted left zygomaticomaxillary fracture (arrows).

Table 1.1.7 Imaging of facial vascular malformations.

Imaging modality	Imaging issues	Comment
Ultrasound	Extent Characteristics of high or low flow vascular malformation/tumours	Ultrasound imaging of choice for assessing superficial lesions
MRI	See Ultrasound	MRI better for assessing deep extent and for further characterization of lesions
Conventional angiography ± embolization	Assess arterial feeders and extra/intracranial arterial connections prior to embolization	For assessment and potential embolization of high flow arteriovenous malformations/fistulae and tumours (alone or as precursor to surgery)
Percutaneous venography/ lymphography with sclerotherapy	Assess venous drainage and volume of malformation prior to sclerotherapy	For assessment and sclerotherapy (STS, alcohol) of low flow venous malformations and lymphangiomas

MRI, magnetic resonance imaging; STS, sodium tetradecyl sulphate.

Table 1.1.8 Imaging of facial and neck infection.

Imaging modality	Imaging issues	Comment
Radiographs		Radiographs to assess for dental disease
CT (contrast enhanced) Disease extent Vascular compromise Infection source	Distinguishing abscess from phlegmon	Contrast enhanced CT and gadolinium enhanced MRI equivalent for assessing phlegmon versus abscess (Figure 1.1.9) CT superior for assessing associated mandibular cortical erosion and salivary gland calculi
MRI (gadolinium enhanced)	See CT	See CT

CT, computed tomography; MRI, magnetic resonance imaging.

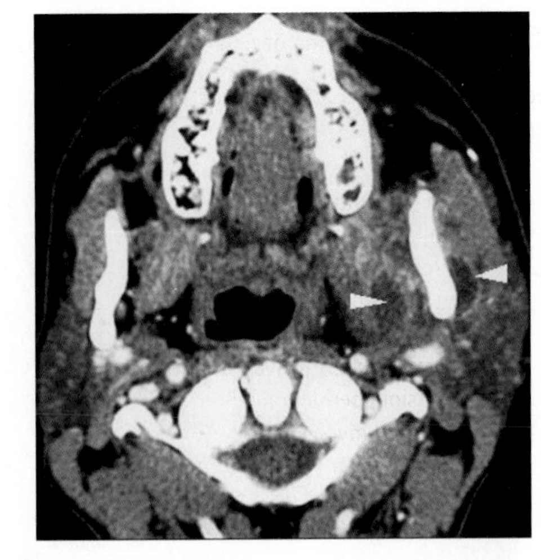

1.1.9 Axial contrast enhanced computed tomography (CT) section reveals ring enhancing abscesses (arrows) within the left masticator space including the left submasseteric region.

Table 1.1.9 Imaging of mandibular osteomyelitis.

Imaging modality	Imaging issues	Comment
Radiography	Confirm diagnosis and exclude other lesions	OPG helpful for assessing dentition and predisposing conditions such as fractures or systemic bone disease
	Response to treatment	Appropriate for follow up (Figure 1.1.10)
MRI (thin section)	MRI should be primary cross sectional imaging for acute and chronic osteomyelitis	Low T1-w with gadolinium enhancement and increased STIR signal corresponds to active infection in the medullary cavity
CT	CT superior for detecting the degree of cortical destruction, presence of sequestra and the degree of cortical removal that would be required (Figure 1.1.10)	Osteolysis in the acute phase with subsequent periosteal reaction
Radioisotope	May be used as an adjunct particularly prior to surgery Lacks the anatomical detail for surgical planning	Sclerosis sequestration in subacute/chronic osteomyelitis Multifocal disease

CT, computed tomography; MRI, magnetic resonance imaging; OPG, orthopantomogram.

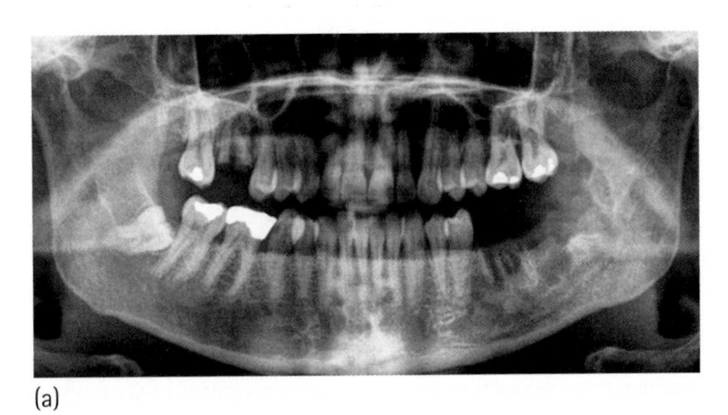

(a)

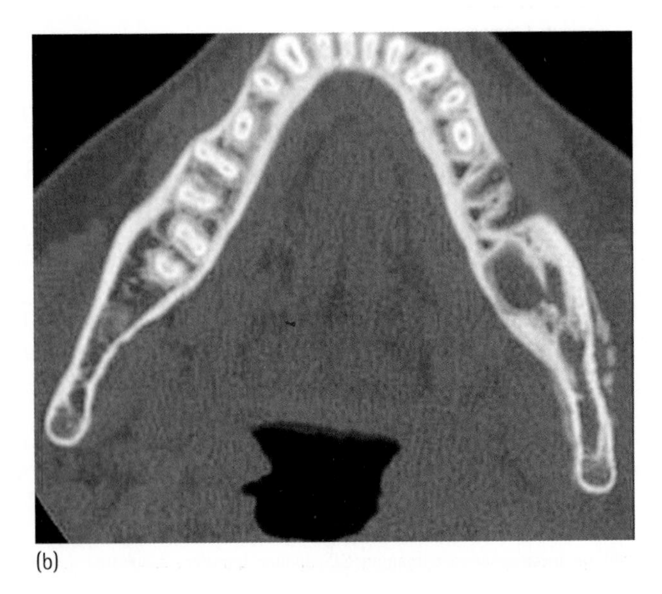

(b)

1.1.10 (a) Orthopantomogram (OPG) and (b) axial computed tomography (CT) section imaged on bony windows. There is medullary lysis, cortical irregularity and sequestration related to left subacute mandibular osteomyelitis.

Table 1.1.10 Imaging of maxillofacial malignancy.

Imaging modality	Imaging issues	Comment
CT (contrast enhanced)	Primary tumour extent Imaging detects submucosal extension to correlate with mucosal inspection Key issues depend on subsite and include bone invasion (e.g. mandible), neurovascular involvement, midline extension, perineural extension, orbital and skull base involvement Nodal metastases (especially if outside area of intended neck dissection or radiotherapy) Distant metastases or synchronous primary tumours	CT preferred: if CT chest also required; in very unwell or elderly patients; if MRI contraindications or if obscuring dental amalgam. Expect spurious changes if performed within 10–14 days of biopsy
MRI (gadolinium enhanced)	See CT	MRI preferred: for salivary gland tumours; any potential skull base or intracranial involvement (Figure 1.1.11); to attempt better definition of poorly defined primary lesion on CT; MR and CT complementary for paranasal sinuses tumours and mandibular invasion (CT initially preferred)
PET CT	See CT	1. In the setting of symptomatic recurrent disease: if suspicion of recurrence but biopsy negative; conventional (CT/MRI) assessment not fully delineated recurrence (due to scar tissue); occasionally before undergoing treatment with curative intent to exclude other synchronous primaries/metastases 2. Surveillance imaging: persistent primary/nodal disease post-chemo-radiotherapy; surveillance of primary tumour with high risk of recurrence 3. In the setting of an unknown primary tumour ideally prior to panendoscopy and biopsy 4. Rarely for assessment of primary or nodal disease for primary staging
Ultrasound	See CT	There are advantages of ultrasound (relative to MRI/CT) for nodal assessment Ultrasound uses additional criteria to detect smaller pathological nodes and may also be used to guide FNA Utility is guided by local expertise Particular scenarios in which ultrasound $\pm$ FNA may be required include indeterminate contralateral nodes in the N0 neck using CT/MRI
Chest, abdominal staging: CXR, CT, CT PET	See CT	CT chest (usually including upper abdomen) may be indicated depending on local protocols Particularly consider if N2 or N3, lower jugular nodes, advanced T stage, tongue base primary, locoregional recurrence, poorly differentiated histology or indeterminate CXR

CT, computed tomography; FNA, fine needle aspiration; MRI, magnetic resonance imaging; PET; positron emission tomography; OPG, orthopantomogram.

Table 1.1.11 Imaging of maxillofacial skeleton cysts and tumours.

Imaging modality	Imaging issues	Comment
Radiographs	Relationship to teeth	Radiographs ideal for showing relationship to and effect on dental structures`
CT	Internal density Extent within bone Relationship to mandibular canal Extraosseous extension	CT especially useful to detect cortical breakthrough (Figure 1.1.12)
MRI	See CT	MRI (with gadolinium) has potential to distinguish between cysts and benign tumours (Figure 1.1.12) Best delineates extraosseous extension (especially within the paranasal sinuses) Used for long-term follow up of maxillary lesions

CT, computed tomography; MRI, magnetic resonance imaging; OPG, orthopantomogram.

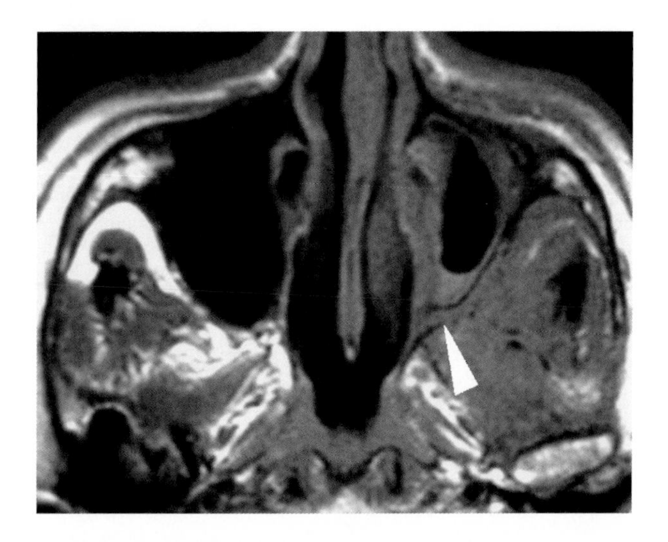

1.1.11 Axial T1-weighted magnetic resonance (MR) image demonstrates effacement of the fat planes around the left masticator space and extension into the pterygopalatine fossa (arrowhead) by an adenoid cystic carcinoma.

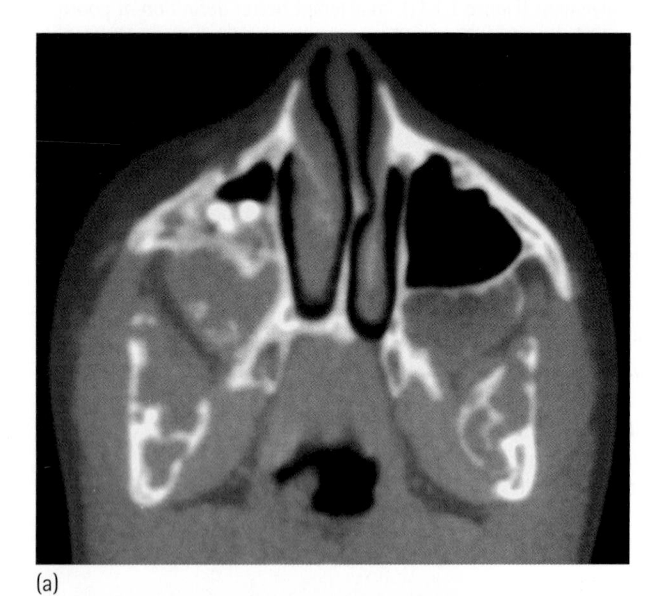

(a)

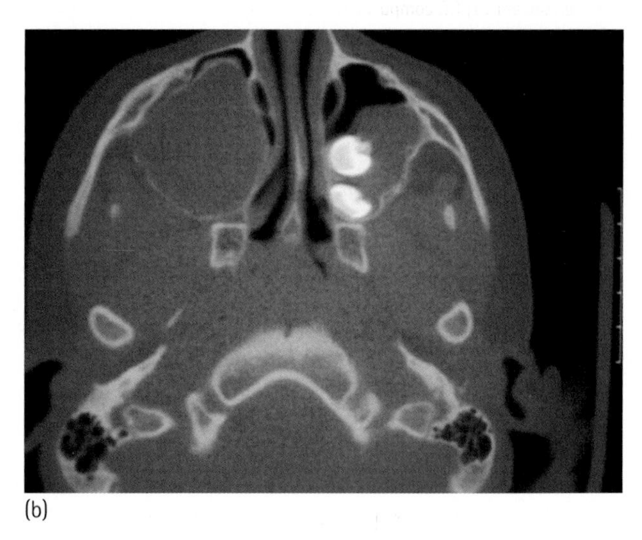

(b)

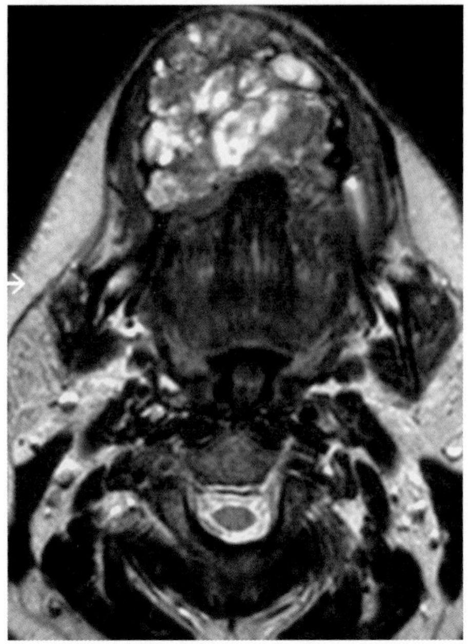

(c)

1.1.12 (a) Multiple expansile lucencies within the maxilla and mandible bilaterally are seen in this patient with cherubism. (b) Bilateral well-defined soft tissue opacities expand the maxillary antra (more markedly on the right) and displace left-sided teeth superiorly. Bilateral odontogenic keratocysts were discovered at operation. (c) T2-weighted axial magnetic resonance (MR) image demonstrates a complex (partially T2 hyperintense and isointense) ameloblastoma, involving the parasymphyseal mandible and displacing the extrinsic tongue muscles.

Table 1.1.12 Imaging for dental implantology.

Imaging modality	Imaging issues	Comment
Radiographs (intraoral peri-apicals and OPG)	Rule out adjacent bony pathology Where each implant should be inserted and at what angle Whether there is sufficient bone density and quantity Delineate sensitive anatomy, such as the mandibular canal	Radiography required for preliminary assessment
Tomography (linear or complex motion)	See Radiographs	Tomography or CT required for direct measurement of prospective implant site
CT with post processing software (e.g. Dentascan or SimPlant) and CBCT	See Radiographs	Tomography adequate for limited region and where there is no significant anatomical variation CT advantageous for multiple implants but increased radiation dose and cost

CBCT, cone beam CT; CT, computed tomography; OPG, orthopantomogram.

Table 1.1.13 Imaging for orthognathic surgery.

Imaging modality	Imaging issues	Comment
Radiographs (OPG and cephalometry)	Evaluation of skeleton and soft tissue patterns	Conventional approach is with radiographs
Low dose 3D CT and CBCT		CBCT and low-dose CT is being introduced for complex orthognathic cases 3D data sets and new 3D cephalometric landmarks will overcome the problems of magnification and distortion due to severe facial asymmetry

CBCT: cone beam CT; CT, computed tomography; OPG, orthopantomogram.

Table 1.1.14 Imaging for salivary gland pathology.

Imaging modality	Imaging issues	Comment
Ultrasound	Demonstrating calculi Diagnosing ductal obstruction (calculi and strictures) and demonstrating appearance of ductal system (e.g. in connective tissue disease) Demonstrating salivary gland parenchymal appearances Distinguishing salivary gland from perisalivary gland masses	Ultrasound is the primary imaging modality for most salivary gland disease and guides FNA
Sialography	See Ultrasound	Indicated if proximal extraglandular calculus demonstrated by ultrasound (as a precursor to potential radiological intervention for smaller calculi) In the presence of severe obstructive symptoms/sialadenitis (if no calculus demonstrated) in order to detect stricture
Radiographs	See Ultrasound	May be used if diagnosis of calculus unclear on ultrasound
MRI/MR sialography	See Ultrasound	MRI is ideal (and superior to CT) for assessing deep lobe of parotid masses (Figure 1.1.13), perineural extension of malignant tumours and recurrent tumours MR sialography is used in some centres to evaluate ductal disease
CT	See Ultrasound	Occasionally helpful if abscess suspected or if multiple calculi

CT, computed tomography; FNA, fine need aspiration; MRI, magnetic resonance imaging.

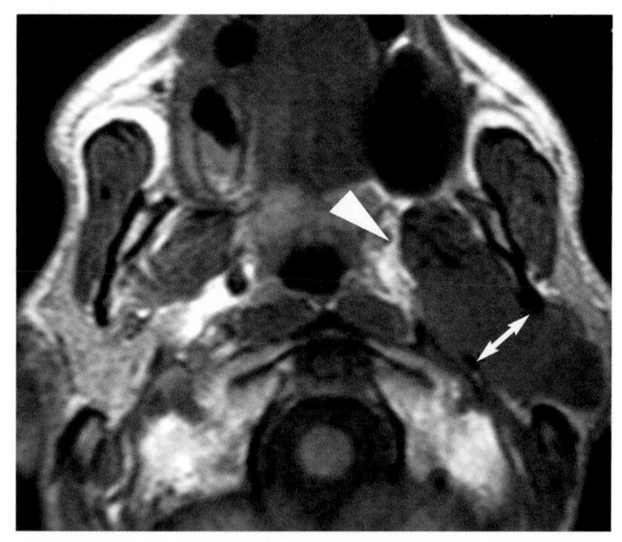

1.1.13 T1-weighted magnetic resonance (MR) image shows a parotid mass centred in the deep lobe. It widens the stylomandibular window (double-headed arrow) and displaces the parapharyngeal fat medially (arrowhead).

Table 1.1.15 Imaging of a face or neck mass.

Imaging modality	Imaging issues	Comment
Ultrasound	Cystic or solid lesion Location-common origins ?thyroid ?salivary gland ?nodal	Ultrasound is generally the first-line imaging investigation for a palpable mass and this will guide biopsy
CT	See Ultrasound	CT/MRI are supplementary in order to show deep extension, to identify additional lesions and for staging of malignancy CT-guided biopsy may be required for deep face and skull base lesions
MRI	See Ultrasound	See CT

Table 1.1.16 Imaging of temporomandibular joint pathology.

Imaging modality	Imaging issues	Comment
(Radiographs)	Detection of late bony changes	The majority of TMJ problems are soft tissue related The utility of radiography (generally OPG) is limited, although it may be used to demonstrate gross bony changes associated with the arthritides. Cone beam CT has a developing role
MRI (arthrography)	Position of the articular disc in the open and closed mouth positions	MRI (Figure 1.1.14) is non-invasive, so has gained greater acceptance than arthrography

MRI, magnetic resonance imaging; OPG, orthopantomogram; TMJ, temperomandibular joint.

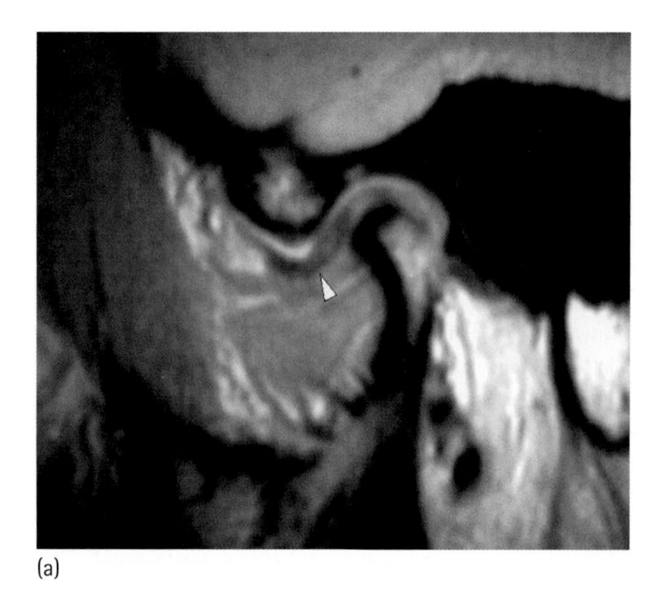

(a)

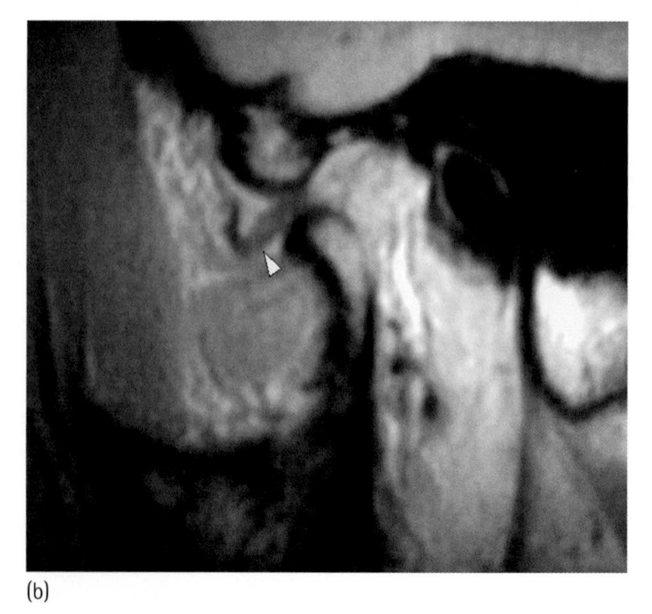

(b)

1.1.14 Oblique sagittal proton density weighted magnetic resonance (MR) images in (a) closed and (b) open mouth positions demonstrates a distorted anteriorly displaced meniscus (arrowheads) which does not reduce on mouth opening.

FURTHER READING

Ahuja AT, Evans RM, King AD, van Hasselt CA (eds). *Imaging in head and neck cancer.* London: Greenwich Medical Media, 2003.

Schoder H, Yeung HW. Positron emission imaging of head and neck cancer, including thyroid carcinoma. *Seminars in Nuclear Medicine* 2004; **34**: 180–97.

Waites E (ed.). *Essentials of dental radiography and radiology*, 4th edn. London: Churchill Livingstone, 2006.

Weber AL. Imaging of the mandible, maxilla and pharynx. *Neuroimaging Clinics of North America* 2003; 13: xiii–xiv.

Royal College of Radiologists Working Party. *Making the best use of clinical radiology services: Referral guidelines*, 6th edn. London: The Royal of College of Radiologists, 2003.

1.2

Ultrasound imaging, including ultrasound-guided biopsy

RACHEL S OEPPEN, RHODRI EVANS

INTRODUCTION

Ultrasound imaging does not require ionizing radiation and is a relatively inexpensive, non-invasive and readily available technique which is well tolerated by patients. It is particularly useful in examining superficial structures (less than 5 cm deep to the skin surface), where the use of a high frequency linear probe (7.5–12 MHz) produces high definition images in multiple imaging planes. The spatial resolution achieved by ultrasound surpasses that of either computed tomography (CT) or magnetic resonance imaging (MRI), and when combined with tissue sampling techniques (percutaneous fine needle aspiration (FNA) for cytology or core biopsy for histopathology), ultrasound is a highly specific diagnostic tool.

Clinicians who have detailed knowledge of the anatomy of the head and neck region may choose to learn how to use ultrasound as an adjunct to clinical examination and as an aid to biopsy techniques. This chapter aims to give an overview of the use of ultrasound in the neck with relevance to clinicians who either want to gain a greater understanding of the technique or who wish to begin to use ultrasound in their practice.

PRINCIPLES OF ULTRASOUND

An ultrasound image represents the reflection and scattering of ultrasound waves caused by variation in acoustic impedance by the various tissues being scanned. A detailed discussion of the physics involved is beyond the scope of this text, but essentially the ultrasound probe acts as both transmitter and receiver for sound waves. Images are generated by computerized analysis of the sound waves reflected back to the probe. The higher the frequency of the sound wave generated, the greater the resolution obtained, but there is a resultant fall off in penetration with higher frequencies. Typically, 8–12 MHz probes are used in assessment of the neck, giving improved resolution for superficial structures but with reduced penetration, i.e. a failure to generate images of deeper structures. This trade off is not usually a problem in the neck.

Air causes marked scattering of the ultrasound wave, hence gel is used as the interface between skin and probe to optimize the thoughput of the sound wave signal. Gas and bone represent a problem as far as ultrasound is concerned; gas will cause scatter which results in a 'white out', while bone and other calcified structures transmit little sound causing acoustic shadowing (black hole). In general, highly reflective tissues appear echogenic (white) on an ultrasound image, whereas structures with poor reflectivity (e.g. blood within the internal jugular vein (IJV)) will be hypo-echoic (black) on an ultrasound image. The high reflectivity of some tissues may be desirable (e.g. identification of a core biopsy needle with ultrasound) or undesirable (e.g. a calcified thyroid lamina which prevents assessment of the larynx).

Sadly for the uninitiated, not all hypo-echoic structures are cystic or fluid in composition. Solid structures in the neck that may appear typically hypo-echoic or 'pseudocystic' (i.e. black) include lymphoma, salivary pleomorphic adenomata, nerve sheath tumours and parathyroid adenomata. Conversely, some cysts do not abide by the rules of physics – a true cyst should be hypo-echoic or black on ultrasound, but the congenital cysts of the neck (e.g. branchial and thyroglossal duct cysts) often appear echogenic, i.e. pseudosolid in appearance.

Colour and power Doppler may be used to assess flow in normal vascular structures (e.g. assessment of carotid arteriopathy and venous thrombosis) and abnormal flow in pathological processes (e.g. hilar vessels in metastatic nodal disease). Colour flow Doppler is standard on most modern machines and can help the beginner to find vascular structures. A power Doppler function is useful for assessing flow patterns, such as the vascularity in lymph nodes (Figures 1.2.1 and 1.2.2).

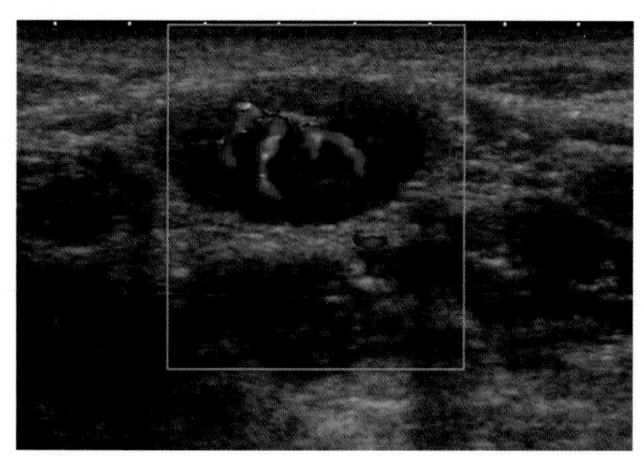

1.2.1 Normal hilar vessel seen on colour flow Doppler in a benign reactive node.

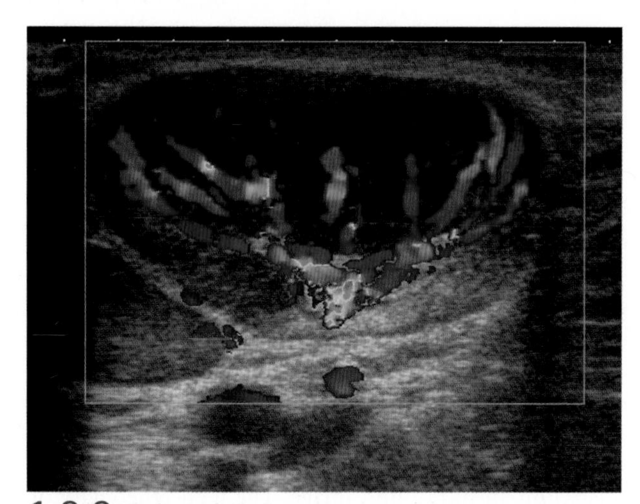

1.2.2 Exaggerated blood flow, seen on colour flow Doppler in a lymphoma node.

SCANNING POSITION AND BASIC TECHNIQUE

The operator will normally be positioned to the left of the patient, but for biopsies of the left cervical region, the recommended operator position is to the right of the patient. There must therefore be adequate space to allow a range of operator positions in relation to the patient.

The patient should be positioned with the neck extended, using a pillow behind the shoulders. This is sometimes difficult to achieve in patients with cervical spondylosis, in which case the procedure can be performed with the patient sitting or at 45 degrees. Comfort, both of the patient and operator, is essential.

The choice of where to start scanning will depend on the clinical scenario. For example, for a patient with a lipoma of the posterior triangle, a detailed assessment of both sides of the neck is not required, whereas a patient with a squamous cell carcinoma primary who is undergoing a staging scan of the neck needs a bilateral assessment of all the major lymph node territories in the neck.

INDICATIONS FOR HEAD AND NECK ULTRASOUND

The following indications will be considered:

- lymph node assessment
- salivary glands
- thyroid gland
- imaging lumps and bumps
- ultrasound-guided FNA and percutaneous core biopsy.

Lymph nodes

Sonographic criteria for lymph node assessment have been extensively described in the literature. Normal nodes have a well-defined ellipsoid or fusiform shape, with an intermediate to low reflectivity homogeneous cortex and highly reflective central hilus. Overall length is irrelevant, with normal cervical nodes frequently measuring 3 or 4 cm in maximum longitudinal (L) dimension. However, short axis (S) measurements should not normally exceed 10 mm. An S/L ratio greater than 0.5 implies a round node: the more rounded a node, the more likely it is to contain metastatic disease (Figure 1.2.3). However, in the submandibular and submental regions, normal nodes tend to be more rounded or reniform, and here shape alone should not be used as a predictor of malignancy. Intranodal vessels are visible with colour imaging, and in benign nodes are typically central or hilar in distribution.

Abnormal nodes display reduced reflectivity (i.e. tend to be hypo-echoic or 'black') with a tendency to lose the central echogenic hilus. Short axis measurements increase, giving a rounder rather than elongated shape. Vascularity may increase and have a disordered pattern. Peripheral or subcapsular vessels, in particular, are a strong sign of malignancy.

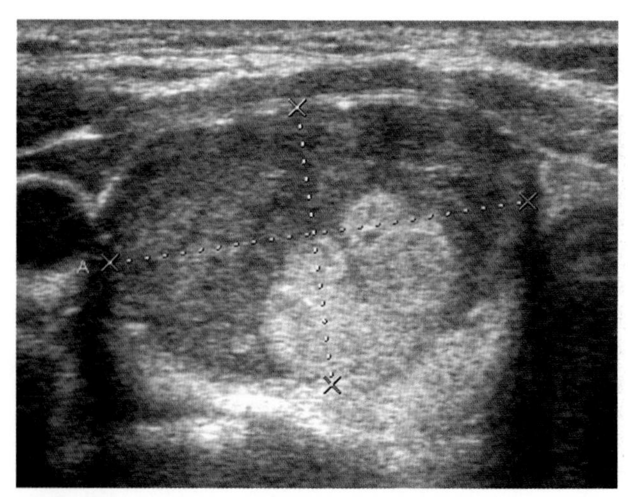

1.2.3 Node with greater than normal short/long ratio: a metastatic squamous cell carcinoma node.

Lymphomatous lymph nodes characteristically appear rounded, often retaining a central echogenic hilus and possess a homogenous, hypo-echoic (pseudocystic) cortex (Figure 1.2.4). Colour flow imaging often reveals plethoric hilar vascularity (i.e. an exaggerated benign flow pattern) (Figure 1.2.2). Identification of these characteristics should prompt the operator into carrying out a core biopsy or recommending excision biopsy, depending on local preference, to allow rapid diagnosis.

Salivary glands

The most common problems encountered include sialolithiasis, inflammatory conditions and tumours.

SUBMANDIBULAR GLAND

The normal submandibular glands are homogeneous echogenic (bright) structures lying inferolateral to the mylohyoid muscle in the submandibular space. Intraglandular ducts are visible as short defined hyperechoic lines, but Wharton's duct is only usually visualized when it is dilated. Lymph nodes in the submandibular space are exclusively extraglandular.

PAROTID GLAND

The parotid gland lies in the parotid space which is the most lateral space in the nasopharyngeal area, extending from the external auditory canal superiorly to the level of the angle of the mandible inferiorly. The gland is arbitrarily divided into superficial and deep lobes by the facial nerve, but this structure cannot be identified with ultrasound. The retromandibular vein passes superiorly through the parotid and can be used as a landmark for dividing the parotid into superficial and deep lobes, i.e. as a predictor of likely proximity of a mass to, and involvement of, the facial nerve. The external carotid artery passes through the gland deep to the retromandibular vein. Intra- and extraglandular nodes are seen in the parotid space. Stenson's duct may be visualized as bright parallel echogenic lines, 3 mm in diameter within the superficial lobe.

SIALOLITHIASIS

Intraglandular calculi are easier to identify than ductal stones. Frank duct dilatation (Figure 1.2.5) or sialectasis may be seen and ultrasound will also demonstrate the complications of calculi, abscess formation and sialocele.

Ultrasound cannot definitively exclude calculi, if there is a strong clinical suggestion of salivary duct obstruction and ultrasound examination is negative, sialography will be required in order to exclude a stone/stricture.

INFLAMMATION

Acute salivary gland inflammation occurs in response to suppurative sialadenitis and viral infection. Inflammation causes gland hypertrophy and hypo-echogenicity, i.e. the salivary glands lose their normal bright echotexture. Ultrasound can be used to exclude abscess formation and may demonstrate hyper-reflective microbubbles of gas in suppurative sialadenitis, which usually affects a single gland, along with reactive nodes. In the case of abscess formation in acute suppurative sialadenitis, ultrasound-guided percutaneous drainage combined with antibiotic therapy may avoid surgical intervention.

There are two chronic salivary gland conditions which cause a distinctive 'leopard skin' or 'currant cake' appearance, namely juvenile chronic sialadenitis and Sjogren's syndrome. The distribution of the changes allows a distinction between the two conditions. In Sjogren's disease, the changes are classically bilateral, affecting parotid and submandibular glands, whereas in juvenile chronic sialadenitis there is unlilateral change. The classical findings of Sjogren's disease on ultrasound obviate the need for sialography.

The association of Sjogren's disease with lymphoma needs to be recognized and if a hypo-echoic mass is seen within an affected salivary gland, lymphoma must be considered.

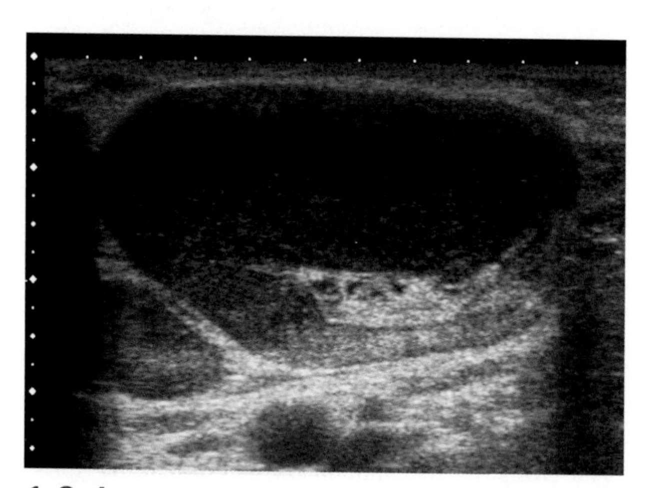

1.2.4 Rounded, homogenous, hypo-echoic (pseudocystic) cortex of lymphoma.

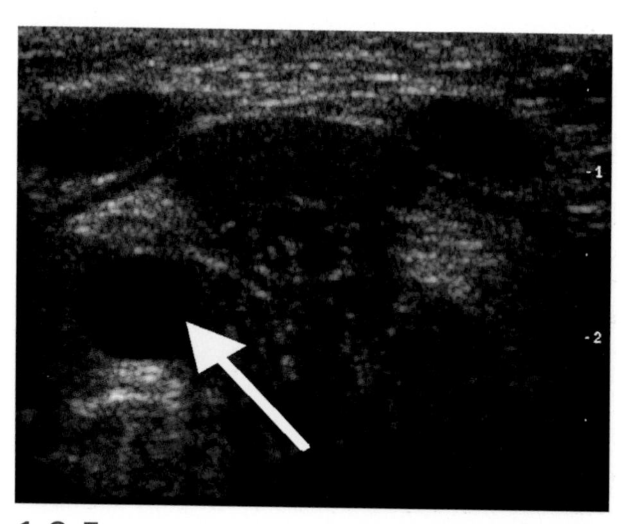

1.2.5 Dilated submandibular duct (arrowed), typical of ductal stone.

TUMOURS

Approximately 80 per cent of salivary tumours are benign, 80 per cent occurring within the parotid with 80 percent of these being pleomorphic adenomata. The vast majority of parotid tumours lie within the superficial portion of the gland, allowing easy assessment with ultrasound. However, in the case of large or deep masses, the deep extent of a lesion can be difficult to assess (necessitating CT or MRI). Ultrasound cannot always predict whether salivary gland lesions are benign or malignant (although irregularity, abnormal vascularity and the presence of enlarged or suspicious nodes aids accuracy), and is usually used in conjunction with fine needle sampling. The smaller the salivary gland, the more likely that any tumour detected will be malignant, i.e. a tumour in the sublingual gland has a far higher likelihood of malignancy compared to a mass in the parotid gland.

Pleomorphic adenoma

This accounts for 80 per cent of parotid tumours, arising in the superficial gland in 90 per cent of cases and typically occurs in females over 40 years of age. On ultrasound, pleomorphic adenoma has the appearance of a well-defined, hypo-echoic homogeneous solid mass (pseudocystic) with a lobulated border and internal vascularity and may display posterior acoustic enhancement. Smaller adjacent daughter tumours are often identified. Cervical lymphadenopathy is not usually seen.

Warthin's tumour (adenolymphoma)

Warthin's tumour commonly occurs in the elderly male (>50 years) as a lump in the parotid tail, sometimes bilaterally (15 per cent) and is rarely seen in the submandibular gland. It arises from heterotopic salivary gland tissue in parotid lymph nodes. On ultrasound, a Warthin's tumour is usually well circumscribed and measures less than 3 cm in size. It typically contains heterogeneous cystic and solid areas, or appears pseudocystic with through transmission of sound (posterior acoustic enhancement) (Figure 1.2.6).

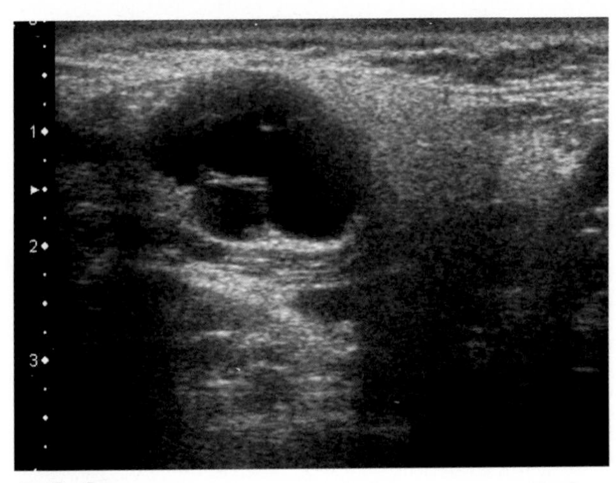

1.2.6 Warthins tumour of the parotid showing cystic change and acoustic enhancement.

Other malignant salivary gland tumours (muco-epidermoid, adenoid cystic and acinic cell carcinomas) occur more frequently in the sublingual and submandibular glands than in the parotid glands. Features suggestive of malignancy include poor definition with heterogeneous echotexture, disorganized colour flow and the presence of associated nodes. Using these criteria, malignancy can be predicted in around 80 per cent of cases using ultrasound alone.

Thyroid

A detailed description of thyroid ultrasound is beyond the scope of this text, however thyroid disorders, including generalized gland enlargement and focal nodules, are relatively commonly encountered in clinical practice. In the one-stop clinic environment, thyroid nodules are likely to represent the second most common cause of symptomatic neck lumps, after lymph nodes. The increasing use of ultrasound means that the incidentally detected thyroid nodule is a significant problem; ultrasound will detect nodules in between 50 to 70 per cent of females over the age of 50 years. Although thyroid nodules are very common, thyroid cancer is extremely rare. As the thyroid gland is situated in a superficial location in the anterior neck, it is readily imaged with ultrasound, although retrosternal extension may require cross-sectional techniques (CT or MRI) for adequate visualization of caudal extent.

The normal thyroid is a vascular gland with a homogeneous hyperechoic texture. Adjacent structures, in particular the common carotid artery and internal jugular vein and deep cervical lymph nodes are clearly seen and are routinely examined, and tracheal deviation and retrosternal extension can be appreciated. In some centres, vocal cord mobility is also routinely assessed with ultrasound before surgery.

While some thyroid lesions have typical imaging features (e.g. papillary carcinoma), thyroid ultrasound is frequently combined with FNA to improve diagnostic accuracy.

PAPILLARY CARCINOMA

Papillary carcinoma accounts for 70–80 per cent of cases of thyroid malignancy. While papillary carcinoma may be multifocal at presentation, its typical appearance on ultrasound is as a solid hypoechoic mass. Punctate calcification is a variable finding, but when present is highly specific (Figure 1.2.7). Invasion of regional lymph nodes is common, and foci of microcalcification may also be detected in involved nodes.

THYROID NODULES

The typical benign thyroid nodule is usually heterogenous in echotexture, with a hypoechoic halo or perinodular rim. Cystic change is very common and may display the typical 'ring down' or 'comet tail' sign indicating colloid. Calcification is common: either peripheral eggshell or large

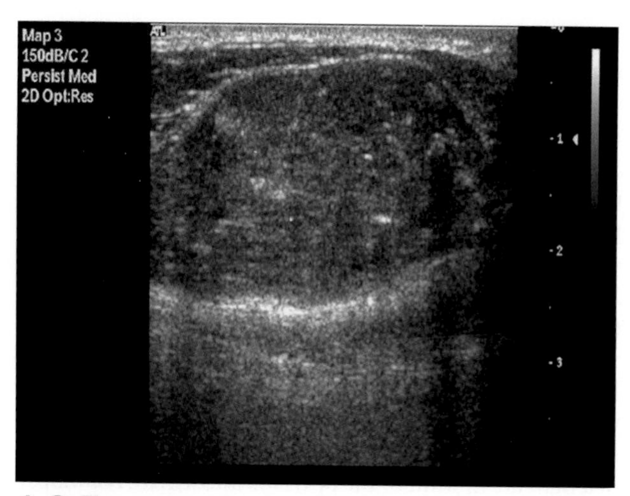

1.2.7 Punctate calcification, which when present is typical of papillary carcinoma.

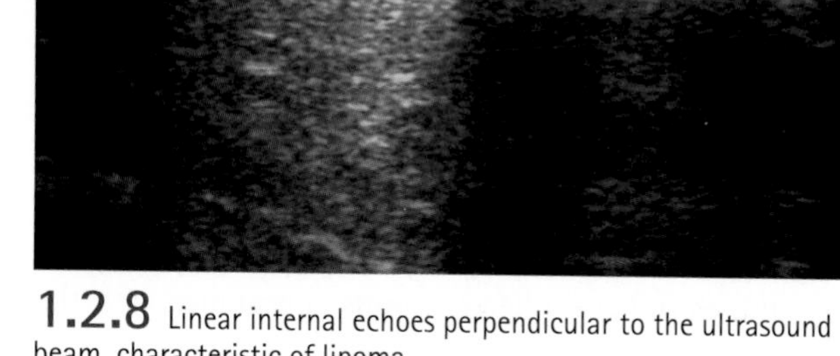

1.2.8 Linear internal echoes perpendicular to the ultrasound beam, characteristic of lipoma.

globular type calcification. Unfortunately, whether the nodule is solitary or part of a multinodular thyroid is not a predictor of malignancy. This myth is often perpetuated, but multiple large series have shown that the incidence of malignancy in solitary and multiple nodules is comparable.

A follicular lesion is a predominantly solid, hyperechoic, homogeneous nodule. Between 80 and 90 per cent of these lesions will turn out to be benign. However, differentiation between an invasive follicular carcinoma and a benign adenoma is not possible without histopathological examination of the entire lesion.

DIFFUSE THYROID DISEASE

We will consider just one diffuse thyroid disease as this may masquerade as a solitary nodule occasionally, namely Hashimoto's thyroiditis, which is the most common form of thyroiditis. This condition causes an enlargement of the gland in the acute phase with diffuse hypo-echogenicity which is typically patchy and starts in the anterior portion of the gland. In time, the whole of the gland is enlarged, hypo-echoic, contains echogenic striae and is usually hypervascular in the acute phase. With time the gland atrophies, loses its hypo-echoic appearance and its vascularity diminishes.

Miscellaneous lumps and bumps

LIPOMA

Lipomas are benign encapsulated subcutaneous lesions which are frequently encountered in the neck. Typical sonographic features include hyperechogenicity, linear internal echoes perpendicular to the ultrasound beam (Figure 1.2.8), compressibility and a lack of internal vascularity on colour flow or colour Doppler imaging. Intramuscular lipomas can mimic muscle and may be difficult to define with ultrasound.

HAEMANGIOMA

The head and neck is a relatively common site for haemangiomas. They are frequently seen in the masseter, trapezius and sternomastoid muscles. Haemangiomata may have large cavernous spaces and possess capillary and/or lymphatic elements. Phleboliths may be demonstrated within the lesion in 70 per cent of cases. In large or intramuscular haemangiomas, MRI is better at depicting the extent of the lesion.

BRANCHIAL CLEFT CYST

Most branchial cysts arise from the second branchial arch remnants and present as a mass at the angle of the mandible, often following an infection. The typical location is abutting the posterior aspect of the submandibular gland, lying lateral to the carotid vessels and immediately anterior to the anterior border of the sternomastoid. On ultrasound, these lesions may be cystic, but more commonly the presence of debris, haemorrhage or infection gives rise to a pseudosolid appearance and the cyst wall thickens in the presence of infection. It may be impossible to distinguish between a second branchial cleft cyst and a necrotic lymph node metastasis due to squamous cell carcinoma. Branchial cysts may extend between the carotid artery and lateral pharyngeal wall or have associated sinuses and these features are better demonstrated on MRI or CT than ultrasound.

THYROGLOSSAL DUCT CYST

Thyroglossal duct cysts can arise at any position along the course of the thyroglossal duct remnant, but the majority are related to the hyoid bone, with most occurring at the level of or inferior to the hyoid.

On ultrasound, thyroglossal duct cysts may appear cystic, heterogeneous or pseudosolid due to varying content of debris, haemorrhage or infection. Classically, they are embedded in the strap muscles, often 'splitting' the strap muscles. Malignant degeneration of the epithelial lining occurs rarely and any solid component which appears to contain microcalcification (i.e. suggestive of papillary carcinoma) should undergo sampling.

DERMOID CYST

Dermoids can be identified by their site, i.e. either midline or peri-orbital. In the peri-orbital region, they are typically (60 per cent) found in the upper outer quadrant of the orbit. These lesions arise from sequestration of the ectoderm from adjacent sutures, most commonly the frontozygomatic suture. Dermoid cysts arise from more than one germ cell layer and therefore will contain one or more dermal adnexal structures. Sebaceous glands, hair and fat are commonly found in dermoids, but they may also be purely cystic. They may therefore have a heterogenous appearance with the presence of fat manifesting as a fluid/fluid level or often as rounded echogenic masses within the cyst (representing sebaceous rests within the dermoid). The typical location for midline cysts is in the submental region either superficial or deep to mylohyoid.

ABSCESS

Infection in the submandibular region frequently arises from dental disease. Ultrasound can differentiate between infection with a fluid component (abscess) and cellulitis, and identify associated lymphadenopathy and venous thrombosis.

Ultrasound-guided fine needle aspiration and core biopsy

Ultrasound is a very useful adjunct in percutaneous sampling procedures, allowing direct visualization of the needle and structures to be avoided (such as vessels). A metallic needle is a reflective surface and if placed parallel or slightly oblique to the transducer surface the needle will be imaged as a very reflective or echogenic structure (Figure 1.2.9). Thus the needle must be in the plane of the ultrasound beam and as parallel to the probe surface as possible in order to optimally visualize it.

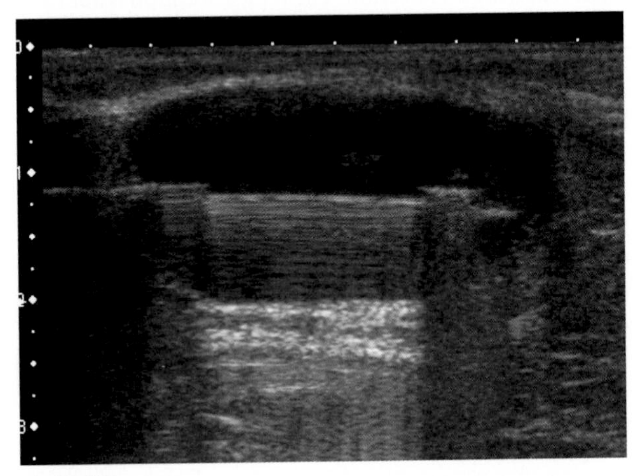

1.2.9 Ultrasound-guided fine needle aspiration showing reflective surface of the needle.

GENERAL TIPS: BIOPSY TECHNIQUES

It is essential that the patient and operator are comfortable when carrying out either FNA or core biopsy in the neck. Keeping the probe, needle, ultrasound monitor and patient in a tight arc in front of the operator is essential. For biopsy in a lesion in the left neck of a patient, the operator should move to the patient's left, allowing the probe, needle and monitor to lie in a comfortable parallel field of view. If necessary, for example for a lesion in the posterior triangle, the patient should lie on their side in order to allow easy access for a shallow approach.

Percutaneous biopsy is an outpatient procedure, but it is prudent to ask the patient to wait for 5–10 minutes post-biopsy, to check for possible haematoma.

Ultrasound guidance should allow a variety of sampling techniques to be performed, but if there is a good local cytology service, FNA under ultrasound control may be all that is required. However, where lymphoma is considered as a possible diagnosis, core biopsy undoubtedly has a superior role. Many centres are now able to diagnose and type lymphoma on core biopsy, using flow cytometry techniques, avoiding open biopsy and significantly reducing referral to treatment time.

For many conditions, e.g. squamous cell carcinoma lymph node metastases, FNA will be the initial sampling technique. Core biopsy may be reserved as a second-line test when cytology is unable to provide the answer. Some authors advocate the use of core biopsy as a universal first-line investigation, pointing out the fallibility of cytology for certain conditions. However, many others believe that squamous cell carcinoma can be seeded during percutaneous wide bore needle biopsy in the neck. The decision as to which technique to use for sampling neck masses will be influenced by local practice.

A skilled operator should be able to carry out FNA using aspiration and non-aspiration techniques, and if core biopsy can additionally be mastered then there will be few conditions in the head and neck that cannot be sampled under ultrasound control, allowing rapid diagnosis in patients who present with neck masses.

Top tips

- Echogenic or reflective structures are white (for example, bone, needle, calculi).
- Calcification causes complete reflection of ultrasound and an acoustic shadow beyond it.
- Hypo-echoic structures are black (for example, blood in the internal jugular vein).
- Fluid causes little or no reflectivity.
- Bone, gas and fat are echogenic.
- Congenital cysts are typically echogenic, but branchial cleft cysts, thyroglossal duct cyst, dermoid cysts are pseudocystic with some having solid elements.
- Some solid lesions may appear hypo-echoic (pseudo-cystic). These include salivary pleomorphic adenoma, parathyroid adenoma, nerve sheath tumours, lymphoma.
- When assessing nodes, the shape of nodes and blood flow is important.

FURTHER READING

Ahuja AT, Evans RM (eds). *Practical head and neck ultrasound.* London: Greenwich Medical Media, 2000.

Bruneton JN, Roux P, Caramella E *et al.* Ear, nose and throat cancer: Ultrasound diagnosis of metastasis to cervical lymph nodes. *Radiology* 1987; **152**: 771–3.

Van den Brekel M, Castelijns JA, Stel HV *et al.* Occult metastatic neck disease: Detection with US and US guided fine needle aspiration cytology. *Radiology* 1991; **180**: 457–61.

1.3

Surgical and other investigations

JULIA A WOOLGAR

INTRODUCTION

In many conditions, the formulation of a definitive treatment plan is based on accurate tissue diagnosis and, hence, biopsy and histopathology are fundamental to patient management. This chapter deals with practical aspects that are of direct concern to surgeons. In addition, practical aspects of other types of investigations, such as exfoliative cytology and microbiology, will be outlined.

SURGICAL BIOPSY

Surgical biopsy is removal and histopathological examination of a part (incisional biopsy) or the whole of a lesion (excisional biopsy) for diagnosis and treatment. Techniques/tools that may be used include:

- conventional scalpel
- cutting diathermy
- punch
- thick needle (core biopsy).

The choice of incisional versus excisional and technique depends on the indication for biopsy, the clinical diagnosis, the site, size and appearance of the lesion, and the ability to close the defect.

Punch biopsy

A punch biopsy is a simple, convenient method of obtaining a disc of mucosa of around 5 mm diameter and this is generally sufficient for histological confirmation of mucosal lesions in conditions such as lichen planus.

Thick needle (core) biopsy

This provides a core of tissue up to 2 mm diameter and 10 mm in length which is placed in fixative and processed as for a surgical biopsy. It is useful for inaccessible tumours and is more likely to result in a correct definitive diagnosis than fine needle aspiration cytology (FNAC). As with any small tissue sample, the core may not be representative of the lesion as a whole or may fail to show specific pathognomic features.

Core biopsy of a suspected parotid neoplasm in cases with an unhelpful FNAC is generally considered safe especially if narrow bore needles (less than 0.9 mm) are used. For example, reports show the risk of tumour seeding is extremely low and diagnostic accuracy in distinguishing non-neoplastic lesions, benign and malignant neoplasms is consistently greater than 97 per cent. Conventional incisional biopsy of parotid neoplasms should be avoided because of the risk of seeding in the incision wound (even in benign pleomorphic adenomas), facial nerve damage, facial scar and fistula development.

Excisional biopsy

INDICATIONS

- Simple mucosal and soft tissue lesions (clinically diagnosed as fibro-epithelial polyps, inflammatory epulides and mucocoeles, etc.) where excisional biopsy achieves diagnosis and cure simultaneously.
- Where the complete lesion can be removed without risk to important adjacent structures.

TECHNIQUE TIPS

- Infiltration of local anaesthetic should be into perilesional tissue, taking care to avoid distortion of the lesion.
- A traction suture through the lesion may help in stabilizing the surrounding tissue area.
- Care is needed to avoid crushing the tissue with tweezers.
- Any sutures used to control the specimen should be left in place to avoid possible misinterpretation of displaced surface epithelium.

- Following removal, mucosal specimens should be supported by placing the deep aspect on a piece of card in order to prevent distortion during fixation.
- Depending on the specimen, it may be necessary to label specific margins by using marker sutures or labelling a photograph or diagrammatic representation.
- Marker sutures should be tied securely, but not pulled tight, and should avoid areas of critical interest.
- Colour change following fixation may mask clinically obvious lesions and the pathology request form should include details on clinical appearance and size, as well as details on site and extent (including depth) of the biopsy.
- Diathermy damages the tissue periphery and may preclude histological assessment of the peripheral 1 mm of tissue, a factor that needs to be considered in biopsy of mucosal malignancies and premalignancies, both proven and potential.

Incisional biopsy

Incisional biopsy is indicated to determine the diagnosis before treatment – for larger lesions, lesions that are potentially malignant and lesions of uncertain nature.

The technique used involves removal of an ellipse of tissue, including both lesional and perilesional tissue.

Vesiculobullous/ulcerative lesions

Special care is needed in vesiculobullous/ulcerative lesions.

- Sloughs and necrotic areas should be avoided.
- Superficial biopsies often fragment and are unlikely to include vessels of sufficient thickness/calibre for assessment of possible vasculitis.
- The roof of a flaccid bulla is easily detached and manipulation of tissues before and after biopsy should be minimal.
- Tissue that may require direct immunofluorescent staining (such as demonstration of autoantibodies in pemphigus and pemphigoid) must not be placed in routine fixative solution. Special instructions should be sought from the pathologist before booking the biopsy procedure.

Labial gland biopsy

In investigation of xerostomia, after incising the mucosa, at least six glands should be removed. It is not usually necessary to include the surface mucosa overlying the glands.

Orofacial granulomatosis

In investigation of suspected orofacial granulomatosis (OFG) and related conditions, it is important to remove a good depth of tissue since granulomata are often more numerous within labial muscle rather than the lamina propria and superficial submucosa.

Oral cancer and precancer

Biopsy for histological assessment of leukoplakias, erythroplakias and erythroleukoplakias (speckled leukoplakias) requires careful planning. In many cases, the lesion is too large for excisional biopsy. In general, incisional biopsy should include areas of induration, erosion, erythroplakia and exophytic/papillary growth (Figure 1.3.1). It is helpful to include adjacent 'normal' mucosa if possible and several geographic biopsies (accompanied by a topographical diagram depicting their site) may be necessary in large lesions, especially when non-homogeneous.

Any biopsy for suspected mucosal squamous cell carcinoma must be sufficiently deep to include submucosal muscle, ideally at least 4 mm in thickness and 10×6 mm in surface area. Particular care is needed in lesions with an exophytic growth component and the request form should give accurate clinical details including the suspected clinical diagnosis. Superficial biopsies can be misleading since the architecture of the rete processes and interface between the epithelium and connective may not be accurately depicted and atypical cytological features may be confined to basal keratinocytes or even focal in distribution.

Assessment of proliferative verrucous leukoplakia, particularly the distinction between verrucous hyperplasia and verrucous carcinoma, is notoriously difficult to assess on incisional biopsy and the definitive diagnosis may be deferred or amended on assessment of the excision biopsy.

Inclusion of the deep advancing front in the diagnostic biopsy in conventional squamous cell carcinoma allows

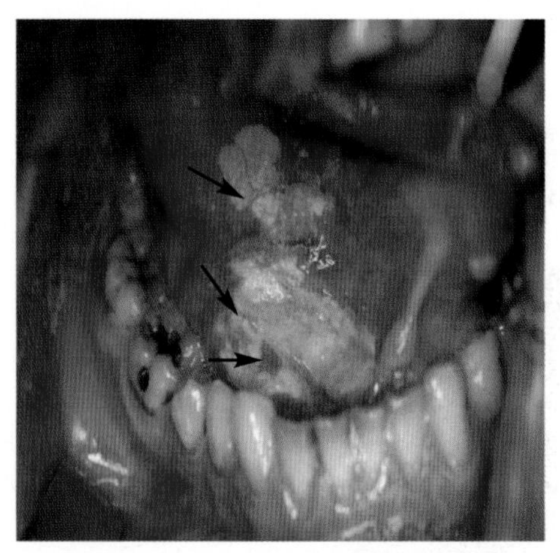

1.3.1 An extensive non-homogeneous leukoplakia of the floor of mouth/ventral tongue requires multiple incisional biopsies, selecting areas of erosion (bottom arrow), exophytic nodules (middle arrow) and thickening/induration (upper arrow). When possible, the biopsy ellipse should include the macroscopic edge of the lesion, including a narrow rim of macroscopically normal mucosa.

invasive front histological multifactorial malignancy grading. Table 1.3.1 outlines a system assessing five features on a four-point scale leading to a maximum of 20 points. The first three features relate to characteristics of the tumour keratinocytes, while the fourth and fifth relate to the epithelial–connective tissue interface (Figure 1.3.2). Several independent studies have shown that the total grading score is associated with overall survival (>16 indicating poor survival) and the pattern of tumour invasion (grades 3/4) is predictive of lymph node metastasis. Reproducibility of scoring is subject to inter- and intra-observer variation, but translation of descriptive histological terms to objective mathematical criteria suitable for morphometric evaluation seems promising. Also, molecular markers, once fully evaluated, may supplement the histological assessment.

The reliability of incisional biopsy of a clinically suspicious, potentially malignant or dysplastic lesion is questionable. A retrospective study comparing degree of dysplasia in biopsies and 101 definitive excision specimens found concordance in only 49 per cent of lesions, rising to 79 per cent when one degree up or down the scale of dysplasia was included. Underdiagnosis of the biopsy was made in 35 per cent of the lesions and overdiagnosis in 17 per cent. Eight per cent of lesions that on biopsy (taken on average ten months previously) showed no, slight or moderate dysplasia, harboured carcinomas and 50 per cent of these were clinically homogeneous. Poor reliability of incisional biopsy, possibly due to sampling errors, variation in reading degree of dysplasia, progression between biopsy and excision, and unimportance of histological appearances suggests that even 'non-dysplastic' lesions should be observed at three- to six-monthly intervals. Unimportance of histology seems, at least, partly responsible since the course of premalignant lesions after surgical removal is reportedly independent of their histological diagnosis.

Table 1.3.1 A system assessing five features on a four-point scale.

Morphologic feature	Score			
	1 point	2 points	3 points	4 points
Degree of keratinization	Heavily keratinized (>50% of cells)	Moderately keratinized (20–50% of cells)	Minimal keratinization (5–20% of cells)	No keratinization (<5% of cells)
Nuclear pleomorphism	Little (75% mature cells)	Moderate (50–70% mature cells)	Abundant (25–50% mature cells)	Extreme (<25% mature cells)
Number of mitoses (per high power field)	0–1	2–3	4–5	>5
Pattern of invasion	Pushing, well-delineated infiltrating borders	Infiltrating, solid cords, bands and/or strands	Small groups or cords of infiltrating cells	Marked and widespread cellular dissociation in small groups and/or in single cells ($n < 15$)
Host lymphocytic response	Marked	Moderate	Slight	None

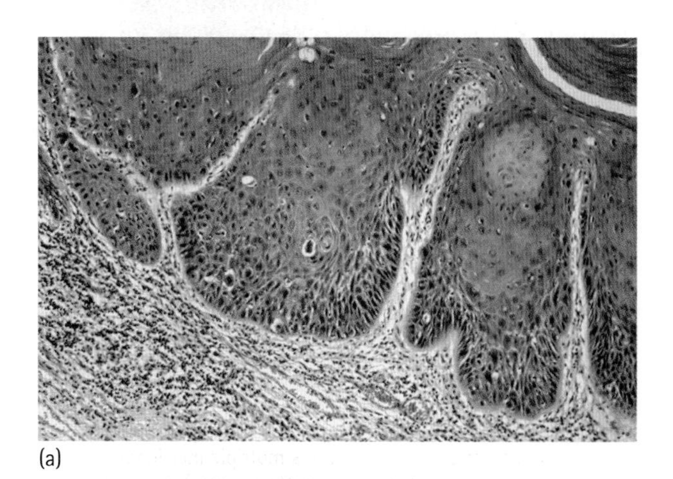
(a)

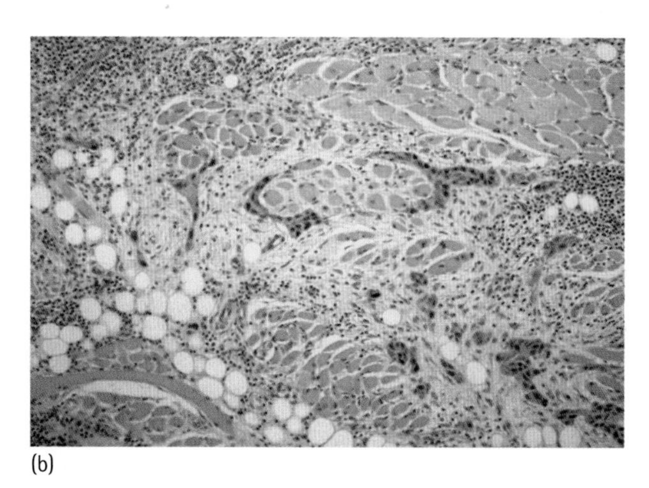
(b)

1.3.2 Invasive front histological multifactorial malignancy grading, pattern of invasion and host lymphocytic response. (a) A well-delineated advancing front composed of broad bands of tumour keratinocytes (score 1 point). The host lymphocyte response is moderate (score 2 points). (b) An ill-defined advancing front with tiny tumours islands and individual cells widely dispersed within muscle (score 4 points). The host lymphocytic response is slight (score 3 points).

Vital (*in vivo*) staining

Vital staining with aqueous solution of 1 per cent aqueous tolonium chloride (toluidine blue) is widely advocated as an aid in the clinical detection of oral epithelial dysplasia/early carcinoma. The dye binds to nucleic acids and is not a specific test. When applied to clinically suspicious lesions, the sensitivity was reported to be 77 per cent and the specificity 67 per cent. The technique is less reliable when used indiscriminately on white lesions and ulcers with a high false-positive rate. In addition, the dye is mutagenic leading to concerns about its safety, particularly when advocated as a general screening test. Nevertheless, the technique can be of value in deciding the site of biopsy in an extensive lesion, identification of synchronous/metachronous carcinomas, localization of superficial tumour borders during presurgical planning and in deciding whether to intervene with surgery or chemoprevention. In addition, a recent study showed that toluidine blue staining can identify those high-risk primary oral premalignant lesions with poor outcome even in lesions with low-grade or no dysplasia. The same study showed that the stain is preferentially retained by premalignant lesions with clinical features associated with risk (site, size and appearance), histologically severe dysplasia and high-risk molecular patterns as assessed by microsatellite analysis. Although there has been a resurgence of interest in toluidine blue in recent years, it should be regarded as an adjunct to clinical diagnosis rather than an accurate test.

Biopsy of soft tissue lesions within bone

Curettage is generally used for biopsy of tissue within an anatomical or pathological cavity or fistula, and in some conditions the procedure constitutes treatment. The soft tissues are scraped out with an appropriately shaped curette. All the tissue fragments must be submitted for pathology, including any bone spicules.

The precise diagnosis of odontogenic cysts depends on their relationship to teeth and radiographic details should be submitted on the request form. When feasible, teeth should be submitted with the soft tissue *in situ*. In order for thin sections to be cut, specimens containing teeth and bone need to be softened by immersion in acid following their macroscopic assessment in the laboratory. This delays the diagnosis by days or weeks depending on specimen size and composition.

Pathology request form

The request form should include the following:

- patient identification including surname, forename(s), address, sex, date of birth and unit number (always check the accuracy, legibility and completeness of preprinted stickers)
- name, address and contact details of requesting consultant/surgeon in charge
- details of previous oral/maxillofacial biopsies, including laboratory reference numbers
- nature of the specimen (skin lesion, mucosal biopsy, bony sequestra, etc.)
- date and time of biopsy procedure
- any specific risks of infection (including hepatitis, HIV)
- history of current condition (date of onset, duration, location, associated local factors, investigations so far, treatment already received)
- relevant medical history, including current and recent medication
- clinical description of the lesion (site, size, colour, surface ulceration, texture, mobility, induration, etc.)
- clinical diagnosis or differential diagnosis
- if applicable/relevant, state that the patient has consented for surplus material to be used for research/teaching
- type of request: urgent/non-urgent and date of follow-up appointment
- name, signature and contact details of surgeon responsible for the biopsy/request form.

Routine histological assessment of fixed tissue samples

High quality histological sections are dependent on adequate fixation of tissue samples. Depending on specimen size, 6–8 hours of immersion in a formaldehyde-based fixative is minimum, with 24 hours considered ideal. The volume of fixative solution should be at least ten times the volume of tissue. Specimens placed in saline and alcohols are often useless for histological assessment and biopsy should be delayed if adequate fixative is unavailable. When special investigations such as electron microscopy are required, the pathologist should advise on the special fixatives that are needed.

Laboratory processing involves dehydration of the fixed specimen by immersion in a series of solvents followed by impregnation with paraffin wax. The wax block supports the tissue which is mounted on a microtome for section cutting. Four microns thick sections are floated onto glass slides and after removal of the wax by solvents, stained. The routine process, from placing the specimen in fixative to pathological assessment, takes around 24 hours.

Intra-operative assessment of biopsy tissue

The aim is to provide accurate diagnostic information that will determine or alter the course of surgical treatment. The major indications are:

- diagnosis and assessment of the extent of malignant disease/status of surgical resection margins
- if previous biopsies or FNAC were unsuccessful or equivocal
- fresh material is necessary for special procedures including cultures and molecular studies and it is helpful

if the pathologist can check adequacy of tissue sample intra-operatively.

Techniques for intra-operative assessment include:

- frozen sections
- crush preparations, smears, touch preparations
- gross examination.

FROZEN SECTION TECHNIQUE

This allows histological assessment of a stained slide within 15 minutes of biopsy taking.

- Care is needed in planning the site and size of the specimen – generally, only small tissue pieces (<10 mm) freeze and cut well.
- Specimens should be delivered to the pathologist as quickly as possible, fresh (that is, not placed in fixative solution) but kept moist by a saline-soaked gauze.
- If possible, there should be face-to-face discussion of the correct specimen orientation and identification of specific areas of interest or concern.
- The fresh tissue is quickly frozen (to –70°C), usually by immersion in liquid nitrogen.
- The tissue is thus supported by ice crystals and thin sections are cut on a refrigerated microtome and stained.
- Sampling errors can be reduced by thorough examination of the most critical areas of the specimen. After discussion of the case, the pathologist should ensure that multiple levels (ribbons) are mounted and also that all remaining frozen tissue is fixed and processed routinely. This allows the routine slides to be checked to confirm or refute the frozen section report.

The appearances in frozen sections differ from those in fixed material (for example, the sections are usually thicker) and freezing artefacts due to poor technique can distort the cellular image further. Hence, a definite diagnosis may not be possible on the frozen sections, but the pathological process can be correctly determined in most cases. The overall accuracy of frozen section diagnosis depends on the tissue, pathological process and precision of diagnostic category. Diagnosis of malignant versus benign/reactive can be achieved with 98 per cent accuracy in most tissue types.

Limitations of surgical biopsy and histopathological assessment

Histological assessment of surgical biopsies remains the mainstay of diagnosis in oral and maxillofacial conditions. Even in conditions such as aphthous ulceration in which biopsy is generally unhelpful, it can exclude other possible causes. Inaccuracies can arise in both clinic and laboratory and include:

- errors in specimen labelling and submission of inaccurate clinical details on the pathology request form
- sampling errors at all stages from selection of biopsy site to laboratory trimming of the specimen to inadequate histological sectioning
- limitations inherent to the pathological assessment processes
- technical errors resulting in suboptimal stained slides (it is the pathologist's responsibility to correct technical problems as they arise)
- failure of the pathologist to notice critical histological features
- pathologist's misinterpretation of histological features
- miscommunication such as inadequacies in the written histopathology report
- secretarial/clerical errors.

EXFOLIATIVE CYTOLOGY AND BRUSH BIOPSY

Exfoliative cytology, examination of cells scraped from the surface of a lesion, is a quick, simple method of sampling surface cells without the need for local anaesthetic. It is widely used for detecting candidal hyphae, virally damaged keratinocytes and acantholytic keratinocytes of pemphigus (Figure 1.3.3). The area is scraped with a flat plastic

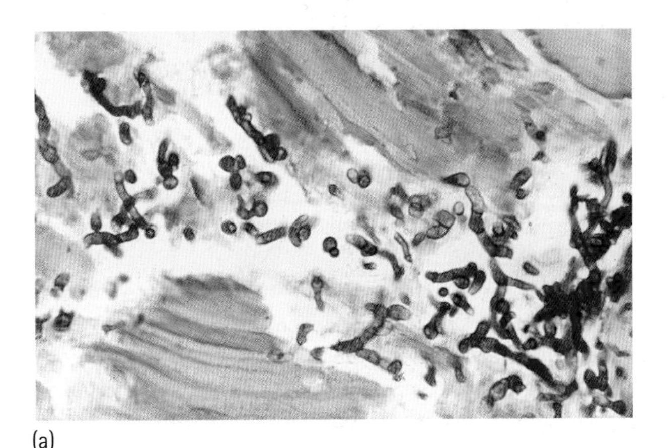
(a)

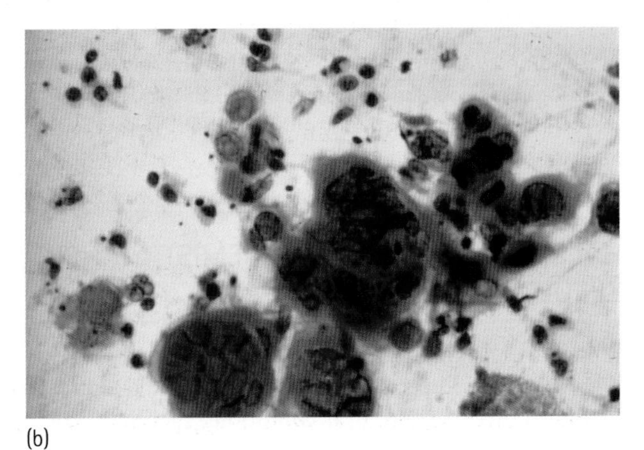
(b)

1.3.3 Exfoliative cytology. (a) Candidal hyphae are readily detected in a smear stained with periodic acid Schiff (PAS). (b) Virally damaged cells are evident in the fluid and cells of vesicles and ulcers in herpetic stomatitis.

instrument or dry tongue spatula and exfoliated cells are transferred to clean labelled microscope slides. Air-dried slides are used for Giemsa staining and alcohol-fixed slides for Papanicoloau staining. Special staining techniques, including immunohistochemistry, can be applied to the cellular smears to improve diagnostic specificity. The surface scrape provides no information on deeper tissues and, hence, is unreliable for diagnosing cancer by simple cytology.

The brush biopsy, vigorous abrasion with a stiff bristle brush, collects cells from the surface and subsurface layers of a lesion and is a simple, convenient way of obtaining DNA samples. To ensure the sample is sufficiently deep, the brush should be rotated in one spot until bleeding occurs. The cells are transferred from brush to a microscope slide. For optimum accuracy, cellular assessment involves a range of techniques, such as scanning by an image analyser, measurement of nuclear DNA content and molecular analyses, such as loss of heterozygosity and microsatellite instability. Overall, the literature suggests the brush biopsy may provide a reliable diagnostic sample once the assessment techniques have been more fully evaluated.

MICROBIOLOGY

A wide range of techniques can be used to aid diagnosis:

- Exfoliate cytology and smears (see above) for rapid confirmation of acute pseudomembraneous candidosis (thrush), acute ulcerative gingivitis and herpetic stomatitis.
- Culture and sensitivity of pus organisms. The sample should be taken before giving an antibiotic.
- Swab and enzyme-linked immunosorbent assay (ELISA) for virus detection.
- Molecular biological tests, such as polymerase chain reaction (PCR) and florescent *in situ* hybridization (FISH) for rapid identification of bacteria and viruses. PCR identification of mycobacterium, for example, takes around 48 hours and is more sensitive and specific at differentiating different types of mycobacteria than traditional culture and sensitivity tests.

Fresh samples are necessary, or at least preferable, for most microbiological and molecular tests and the microbiologist or pathologist should provide guidance on the exact nature and preservation of the sample.

HAEMATOLOGY, CLINICAL CHEMISTRY AND SEROLOGY

Blood investigations are essential for the diagnosis of blood dyscrasias and defects of haemostasis, and helpful in investigations of other oral conditions such as chronic candidosis, sore tongue and aphthous ulceration. Blood must be placed in the appropriate tube since some anticoagulants are incompatible with certain tests and the request form should include sufficient clinical detail to permit the haematologist or clinical chemist to check that appropriate tests have been ordered and to interpret the results. In difficult cases, advice should be sought prior to taking the blood sample.

Top tips

- Plan the biopsy type and the tools/techniques used, and the precise site(s) with due consideration of the purpose of the biopsy, the clinical features of the lesion and the clinical differential diagnosis.
- Small, superficial and crushed tissue samples may be non-diagnostic. Consider both the surface area and depth of the biopsy specimen. Tissue shrinks (on average 30 per cent) during fixation and processing for routine histological assessment.
- For routine histological assessment, the biopsy specimen should be placed immediately in a formaldehyde-based fixative (at least 10× the volume of tissue).
- Consult the pathologist before taking the biopsy when special investigations are required. Fresh tissue samples are necessary for immunofluorescent staining, and most microbiological/molecular techniques.
- Always check the accuracy and completeness of the information on the pathology request form and the specimen pot label.

FURTHER READING

Bankfalvi A, Piffko J. Prognostic and predictive factors in oral cancer: The role of the invasive front. *Journal of Oral Pathology and Medicine* 2000; **29**: 291–8.

Batsakis JG, Suarez P, El Naggar EK. Proliferative verrucous leukoplakia and its related lesions. *Oral Oncology* 1999; **35**: 354–9.

Bryne M, Boysen M, Alfsen CG *et al.* The invasive front of carcinomas. The most important area for tumour prognostication? *Anticancer Research* 1998; **18**: 4757–64.

Holmstrup P, Vedtofke P, Reibel J, Stoltze K. Oral premalignant lesions: Is a biopsy reliable? *Journal of Oral Pathology and Medicine* 2007; **36**: 262–6.

Kesse KW, Manjaly G, Violaris N, Howlett DC. Ultrasound guided biopsy in the evaluation of focal lesions and diffuse swelling of the parotid gland. *British Journal of Oral and Maxillofacial Surgery* 2002; **40**: 384–8.

Marcepoil R, Usson Y. Methods for the study of cellular sociology: Veroni diagrams and parametrisation of the spatial relationships. *Journal of Theoretical Biology* 1992; **154**: 359–69.

Mehrotra R, Gupta A, Singh M, Ibrahim R. Application of cytology and molecular biology in diagnosing premalignant or malignant oral lesions. *Molecular Cancer* 2006; **5**: 11–20.

Missmann M, Jank S, Laimer K, Gassner R. A reason for the use of toluidine blue staining in the presurgical management of patients with oral squamous cell carcinomas. *Oral Surgery, Oral Medicine, Oral Pathology, Oral Radiology, Endodontics* 2006; **102**: 741–3.

Odell EW, Jani P, Sherriff M *et al.* The prognostic value of individual histologic grading parameters in small lingual squamous cell carcinomas. The importance of pattern of invasion. *Cancer* 1994; **74**: 789–94.

Onofre MA, Sposto MR, Navarro CM. Reliability of toluidine blue application in the detection of oral epithelial dysplasia and *in situ* and invasive squamous cell carcinomas. *Oral Surgery, Oral Medicine, Oral Pathology, Oral Radiology, Endodontics* 2001; **91**: 535–40.

Sawair FA, Irwin CR, Gordon DJ. Invasive front grading: Reliability and usefulness in the management of oral squamous cell carcinoma. *Journal of Oral Pathology and Medicine* 2003; **32**: 1–9.

Zhang L, Williams M, Poh C *et al.* Toluidine blue staining identifies high-risk primary oral premalignant lesions with poor outcome. *Cancer Research* 2005; **65**: 8017–21.

1.4

Fine needle aspiration biopsy

MATTHIAS AW MERKX

INTRODUCTION

Prognosis and treatment of patients with an oral/oropharyngeal carcinoma are strongly determined by lymph node status. Therefore, optimal evaluation of the existence of lymph node metastasis is extremely important. Palpation of the neck alone is not specific and sensitive enough. Radiological evaluation of lymph node metastases is improved by new techniques, such as ultrasound-guided fine needle aspiration biopsy (UGFNAB), spiral computed tomography (CT) scans, magnetic resonance (MR) scans and positron emission tomography (PET) scans. Although these new techniques are more sensitive and specific, it is still difficult to demonstrate small (micro) metastases.

PRINCIPLES

Transmitting an electric current through a piezo-electric crystal in the transducer produces ultrasound (US). This current causes a vibration of the crystal, giving rise to high frequency sound waves, which are above the human auditory range. For diagnostic purposes in the head and neck region 5, 7.5 and 10 MHz transducers are used.

The sound waves penetrate the tissues to be examined and are reflected at interfaces of structures with different acoustic impedance. The greater the difference between the impedance of the involved tissues, the stronger will be the returned echo. The echo is picked up by the transducer, transferred into an electric current and displayed on a screen.

ULTRASOUND FINE NEEDLE ASPIRATION BIOPSY

Technique

Conventional fine needle aspiration biopsy (FNAB) of superficial, palpable masses has been successfully used for more than 40 years. In the head and neck region, FNAB provides an alternative to premature open biopsy of masses in the neck, which is especially ill advised in cases of neck nodes in patients with occult squamous cell carcinomas of the upper aerodigestive tract. The risk of tumour seeding in the tract of the needle is negligible. In a considerable number of cases, however, unsatisfactory aspirates vary from 2 to 14 per cent. Aspiration of material adjacent to the mass accounts for the majority of non-diagnostic biopsies.

With continuous advance of imaging techniques, e.g. ultrasound, the sensitivity for the detection of neck lesions is gradually increasing: lesions with a diameter of 5 mm or more can now be visualized. These non-palpable lesions cannot be examined by conventional FNAB, but require aspiration under ultrasound guidance.

Both the amount of unsatisfactory aspirations with conventional FNAB and the increasing number of neck lesions detected by ultrasound has led to the development of a technique for ultrasound-guided fine needle aspiration biopsy. During UGFNAB, a normal transducer is used, without an adapter for the needle. A 0.6-mm needle mounted on a Cameco needle-holder is used. For very small and/or mobile lesions, a butterfly needle is used instead. The latter needle allows subtler manoeuvring and is therefore a valuable alternative for the needle holder.

Once a mass is visualized it is centred on the monitor, by placing it right under the middle of the transducer. When the lesion is displayed in this way, it is, when necessary, fixed to surrounding tissues by applying gentle pressure with the transducer. While the sonographer provides optimal imaging, a co-worker introduces the needle into the overlying skin. Depending on the depth of the structures to be examined, the angle between needle and skin can be varied (Figure 1.4.1).

Once the tip of the needle is inside the lesion, it is recognized as a bright, echogenic structure and the plunger of the syringe is retracted, creating a negative pressure in the needle lumen (Figure 1.4.2). While a constant vacuum in maintained, the needle is moved back and forth under

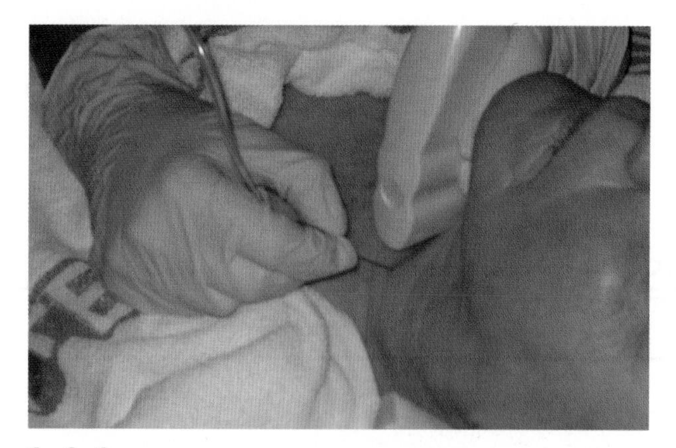

1.4.1 Clinical setting for ultrasound-guided fine needle aspiration biopsy (UGFNAB). Once the tip of the needle is inside the lesion, the plunger of the syringe is retracted, creating a negative pressure in the needle lumen.

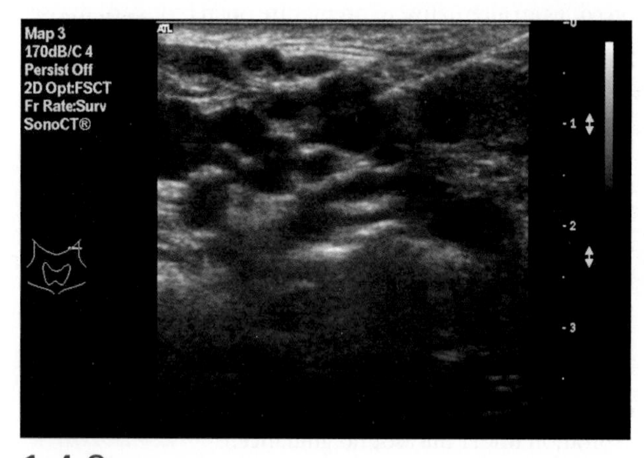

1.4.2 Ultrasound section parallel to the mandible showing the tip of the needle (bright echogenic structure) inside a submandibular lymph node.

ultrasound control, and the lesion is sampled in different areas. Subsequently, the negative pressure is slowly reduced and the needle is withdrawn.

The visibility of the tip reduces the danger of damage to surrounding tissues and ensures that the material is obtained from the lesion to be examined. With ultrasound examination, necrotic or cystic areas are distinguishable from solid areas, allowing selective cytologic examination of different parts of a lesion.

Guidelines for UGFNAB

With the introduction of ultrasound in combination with guided cytology, a new method was introduced with a high sensitivity as well as specificity. The sensitivity of a N_0 neck varies between 25 and 75 per cent, depending on the patient population and the experience of the physician performing the ultrasound. The specificity is up to 100 per cent. Having a minimal transversal diameter of a lymph node, there is evidence of an increased change of regional metastasizing in case of enlargement of a lymph node. For optimal sensitivity the largest and/or most suspect (round, irregular) node in the first level has to be aspirated. For optimal sensitivity, nodes larger than 4 mm in the subdigastric region and 3 mm in other regions have to be aspirated. In case multiple nodes are suspect, at least nodes in the first levels have to be aspirated. With UGFNAB it is possible, depending on the patient population and the experience of the physician, to detect 25–75 per cent of occult metastasis in a clinical negative neck.

Evaluating the lymph nodes of the neck in case of an oral or oropharyngeal tumour, levels I–VI on both sides have to be imaged. Ultrasound evaluation is performed with a 7.7 or 10 MHz linear array transducer. In a clinical negative neck by palpation, bilateral evaluation is necessary. In case of a clinical unilateral metastasis, the contralateral side has to be evaluated as well. In the event of bilateral positive neck by palpation, UGFNAB has no additional clinical value.

The physician who performs the US and FNAB needs to know the clinical parameters and the radiological characteristics of the primary tumour. In the event that the cytological results show 'insufficient material', the evaluation has to be repeated, depending on the co-operation of the patient and the clinical relevance.

For imaging the retropharyngeal lymph nodes, US is not suitable. Because primary tumours, metastasizing to these nodes also need CT and/or MR imaging, these techniques are the first choice of imaging. In the event of large lymph nodes, it is necessary to determine the relation with the carotid artery. The most important question is the invasion of this artery by tumour and if so, to what extent. In these cases, CT and/or MR imaging with contrast is more specific.

Top tips

- UGFNAB has a higher sensitivity and specificity for detecting lymph node metastases in case of an oral/oropharyngeal carcinoma than palpation. In a clinical negative neck, 25–75 per cent of the occult metastases can be traced by this technique.
- The experience of the physician has a positive influence on the sensitivity of this technique.
- To detect occult lymph nodes in an oral/oropharyngeal carcinoma in level I–VI UGFNAB is the preferred technique. For imaging retropharyngeal lymph nodes, ultrasound is not suitable.

FURTHER READING

Baatenburg de Jong RJ, Knecht P, Verwoerd CD. Reduction of the number of neck treatments in patients with head and neck cancer. *Cancer* 1993; **71**: 2312–18.

Baatenburg de Jong RJ, Rongen RJ. Ultrasound examination of the head and neck. Thesis, Erasmus University Rotterdam, The Netherlands 1990: 11–25.

Castelijns JA, Van den Brekel MW. Imaging of lymphadenopathy in the neck. *European Radiology* 2002; **12**: 727–38.

Curtin HD, Ishwaran H, Mancuso AA et al. Comparison of CT and MRI imaging in staging of neck metastases. *Radiology* 1998; **207**: 123–30.

Hodder SC, Evans RM, Patton DW, Silvester KC. Ultrasound and fine needle aspiration cytology in the staging of neck lymph nodes in oral squamous cell carcinoma. *British Journal of Oral and Maxillofacial Surgery* 2000; **38**: 430–36.

Leslie A, Fyfe E, Guest P *et al.* Staging of squamous cell carcinoma of the oral cavity and oropharynx: A comparison of MRI and CT in T- and N-staging. *Journal of Computer Assisted Tomography* 1999; **23**: 43–9.

Nieuwenhuis EJ, Castelijns JA, Pijpers R *et al.* Wait-and-see policy for the N0 neck in early-stage oral and oropharyngeal squamous cell carcinoma using ultrasonography-guided cytology: Is there a role for identification of the sentinel node? *Head and Neck* 2002; **24**: 282–9.

Stuckensen T, Kovacs AF, Adams S, Baum RP. Staging of the neck in patients with oral cavity squamous cell carcinomas: A prospective comparison of PET, ultrasound, CT and MRI. *Journal of Craniomaxillofacial Surgery* 2000; **28**: 319–24.

Takes RP, Knegt P, Manni JJ *et al.* Regional metastasis in head and neck squamous cell carcinoma: Revised value of US with US-guided FNAB. *Radiology* 1996; **198**: 819–23.

Takes RP, Righi P, Meeuwis CA *et al.* The value of ultrasound with ultrasound-guided fine-needle aspiration biopsy compared to computed tomography in the detection of regional metastases in the clinically negative neck. *International Journal of Radiation Oncology, Biology, Physics* 1998; **40**: 1027–35.

Tandon S, Shahal R, Benton JC *et al.* Fine needle aspiration cytology in a regional head and neck centre: comparison with a systematic review and meta analysis. *Head and neck* 2008; **10**: 1246–52.

Van den Brekel MW, Castelijn JA, Stel HV *et al.* Modern imaging techniques and ultrasound-guided aspiration guided cytology for the assessment of neck node metastases: A prospective comparative study. *European Archives of Otorhinolaryngology* 1993; **250**: 11–17.

1.5

Three-dimensional imaging

ASHRAF F AYOUB

INTRODUCTION

In the last decade, three-dimensional imaging has evolved greatly and found applications throughout the broad spectrum of oral and maxillofacial surgery. In three-dimensional imaging, a set of anatomical data is captured using diagnostic imaging equipment; it is then processed by a computer and displayed on a 2D monitor to give the illusion of the depth perception, which causes the image to appear in three dimensions.

FUNDAMENTAL 3D CONCEPTS

Before discussing the various techniques which are available for the diagnosis and planning of oral and maxillofacial surgery, some basic concepts of 3D imaging need to be clarified. In two dimensional (2D, photographs, radiographs) there are two axes (vertical and horizontal), while the Cartesian co-ordinate system in three-dimensional imaging consists of the x-axis (or the transverse dimension), y-axis (or the vertical dimension) and the z-axis (the anteroposterior dimension depth axis). The x, y and z coordinates define the orientation in which multidimensional data are represented in three-dimensional space (Figure 1.5.1).

Three-dimensional imaging of the craniofacial skeleton is classified into three main categories:

1 Slice imaging: The object is sliced into layers, the x and y dimensions are measured directly from the sliced surface and the z dimension is measured by tallying the number of slices in the area of interest. An example of this modality is a set of computed tomography (CT) axial data, producing reconstructed images.
2 Projective imaging: The object is simply imaged from different views simultaneously or in rapid succession. Basic mathematical calculation triangulation is applied on the views to produce a stereoscopic image. Laser scanning and stereophotogrammetry depends on this method of measurement, which is considered a 2.5 D-mode of visualization.
3 Volume imaging, holography or varifocal mirrors are the classic application of this method for 3D capture.

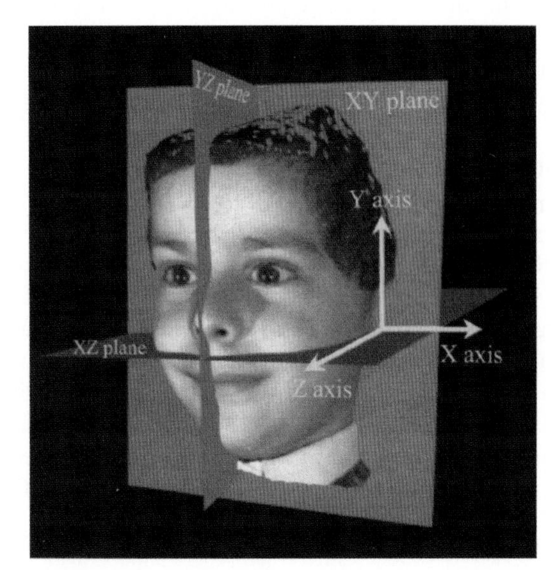

1.5.1 The X, Y and Z coordinate system, which is used in 3D medical imaging. Permission obtained from the copyright holder of this figure, Maney Publishing, which was published in the *Brit J Orthod* 2004; **31**: 62–70.

THREE-DIMENSIONAL IMAGING OF THE FACE

Three three-dimensional techniques have been used in an attempt to capture facial topography and to meet the shortcomings of conventional 2D (photograph or radiograph) methods. These include 3D cephalometery, morpho-analysis, laser scanning, 3D computerized tomographic scanning, stereolithography, 3D ultrasonography, 3D facial morphometry and Moiré topography.

Three-dimensional cephalometery

Three-dimensional cephalometry is based on manual techniques for developing three-dimensional co-ordinate data from two bi-orthogonal head films, i.e. lateral and anteroposterior radiographs. There are difficulties associated with this technique in locating the same landmarks accurately. There is also lack of soft tissue contour assessment.

Morpho-analysis

In the early 1970s, it was claimed that morpho-analysis was the method for obtaining three-dimensional records using photographs, radiographs and a study model of the patient. This would help analysis of the dentofacial morphology in three dimensions. The equipment, however, is extremely elaborate and expensive, and the technique is time consuming and not very practical for everyday use.

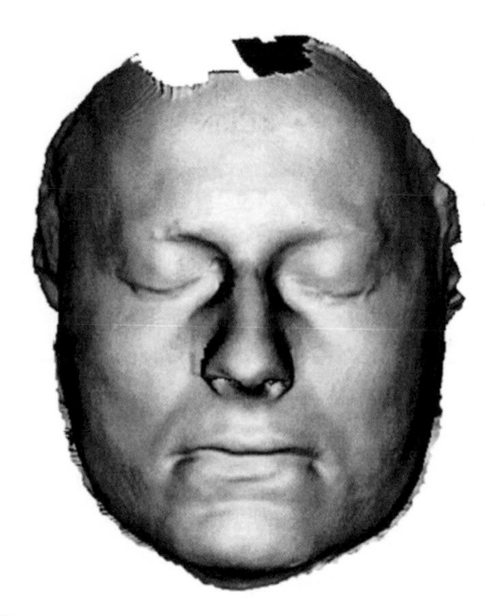

1.5.2 An example of three-dimensional facial image scanned by laser.

Computed tomography-assisted three-dimensional imaging

In the mid-1980s, CT-assisted 3D imaging and modelling of the skull structures was introduced for use in maxillofacial surgery. The technique provided comprehensive information on the skeleton of the face; however, it did expose the patient to a high radiation dose and there was a limited resolution of the facial soft tissue due to slice spacing, which could be 5 mm or more. In addition, the presence of artefacts created by metal objects, such as dental restorations and fixed orthodontic appliances, could cause problems.

Three-dimensional laser scanning

Laser scanning techniques provided a less invasive method for capturing the maxillofacial region in three dimensions. A laser beam was scanned onto the patient's face, and its reflection was recorded to build a three-dimensional model of the face. It was a less invasive method for capturing the maxillofacial region in three dimensions; however, it took about 8–10 seconds, the patient's eyes needed to be closed during scanning for their protection, and the soft tissue surface texture was not captured by this method (Figure 1.5.2).

Moiré topography technique

Moiré topography uses a grid projection during exposure which results in standardized contour lines on the face (Figure 1.5.3). It delivers three-dimensional information based on the contour fringes and fringe intervals. Any move or change in head position produces a large change in fringe pattern.

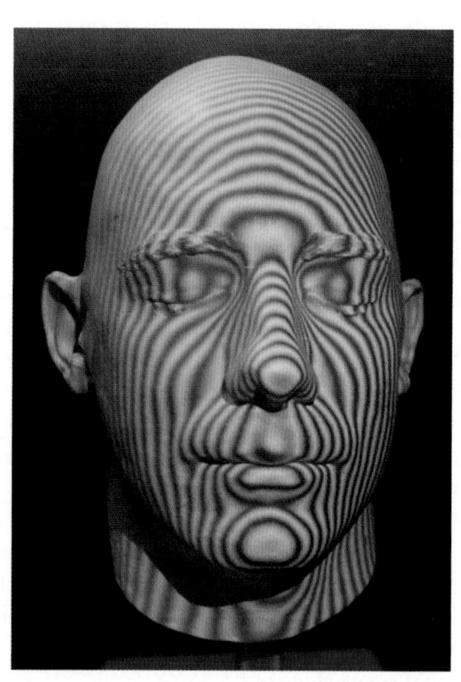

1.5.3 Contour line of Moiré fringe technique

Three-dimensional ultrasonography

This technique delivers a reflection picture which is transformed into digital information. Ultrasonographic waves do not visualize bone or pass through air, which acts as an absolute barrier during both emission and reflection, therefore a specific contact probe is required to generate a three-dimensional base. The procedure is time consuming and necessitates a very co-operative patient and a skilful operator.

Structured light technique

In the structured light technique, the scene is illuminated by a light pattern, but only a single source of energy is required. The position of the illuminated points in the captured image compared to their position on the light protection plane provides the information needed to extract the three-dimensional coordinates on the imaged optic. However, to obtain a high density model, the face needs to be illuminated several times with random patterns of light. This increases the capture time and the possibility of head movement. Additionally, the use of one camera provides a limited capture of the face.

Another variant of this technique has been reported. The system consists of two cameras and one projector. A colour-coded light pattern is projected onto the face before each image is acquired. The displacement of the pattern enables the software to compute an accurate three-dimensional model. Another image is acquired without any accompanying light pattern, to be used for texture mapping. Three acquisitions are needed, one from the front and one from each side, to cover the face. In a further step, the three stereo images are mathematically linked together using customized specific software to produce the three-dimensional facial image.

Stereophotogrammetry

Photogrammetry is defined as the science or art of obtaining reliable measurements by means of photographs. Stereophotogrammetry refers to the special case where two cameras are configured as a stereo pair and are then used to recover the three-dimensional distance to features on the surface of the face by means of triangulation (Figure 1.5.4). The incorporation of recent technology and computer science in stereophotogrammetry has given it the ability to process complex algorithms in order to convert simple photographs into three-dimensional measurements of facial changes. Full automation of the stereophotogrammetry process was described in 2000, when commercially available stereophotogrammetry equipment became widely available for hospital use, but did not require specialist operators. The fast capture time of 50 ms and the high resolution cameras allowed a high quality capture of facial features and more consistent identification of anthropometric landmarks. Therefore, this contemporary digital stereophotogrammetry offered fast capture and avoided the need for a textured light to capture the patient's face with a high resolution of the available cameras. This specification made the technique more appropriate for imaging children and infants, as well as adults. The longer the exposure or the data capture time, the more unreliable or blurred the image data became. This has important implications if measurement of the face to submillimetre accuracy is required.

HOW STEREOPHOTOGRAMMETRY WORKS

The stereo pair of cameras capture two images: for each point imaged in the left camera, the corresponding point in the right camera is determined. This is facilitated by the use of textured illumination or high resolution cameras. The output of this process is x and y co-ordinates 'disparity maps' of each pixel on the face (Figure 1.5.4a,b). The geometry of the camera set up is known from earlier calibration processes. This allows the third dimension (z co-ordinate) of each pixel to be calculated. The system then creates a photorealistic rendered model that can be viewed from any direction (Figure 1.5.5). Each model is measured in an analysis tool, where the operator can manipulate the model from any point of view through the use of magnification, translation and rotation functions (Figure 1.5.6).

APPLICATIONS OF THREE-DIMENSIONAL IMAGING FOR THE FACE

Assessment of outcome following surgical repair of cleft lip and palate

The role of surgical intervention for the repair of cleft lip and palate is restoration of normal facial morphology and normal function. Examination of a subtissue profile of individuals does not provide information on the three-dimensional nature of any asymmetric residual deformity. Three-dimensional imaging is essential for quantifying the magnitude of the anomaly (Figure 1.5.7a,b) and for comparing it with the non-cleft cases and then for measuring change following surgical repair.

Stereophotogrammetry fulfils the criteria for a fast capture time, 1 ms, and it would not expose children to harmful radiation. Published data using this technique have shown that patients undergoing surgical repair of cleft deformity were significantly different from controls. The alar base of the cleft side was displaced more laterally, inferiorly and inwards. It was clear that the nostrils were asymmetric with clear deviation of the columella towards the unaffected side (Figure 1.5.8a,b). The alar base width was significantly larger in surgically managed cleft cases, compared with non-cleft cases. The unilateral cleft lip and palate cases were more asymmetric than the unilateral cleft lip cases. It has been reported previously that there was no correlation between the magnitude or the severity of the cleft deformity and the residual nasolabial asymmetry.

Analysis of the dental arch in three dimensions provides valuable information on the development of the maxillary dental arch which is directly related to that of the nasomaxillary complex. Different methods have been used to capture the dental arch in three dimensions for a comprehensive assessment, these include laser scanning and CT imaging. Published data confirm that the maxillary arch dimensions differ significantly between the unilateral cleft lip and unilateral cleft lip and palate group, and the non-cleft cases.

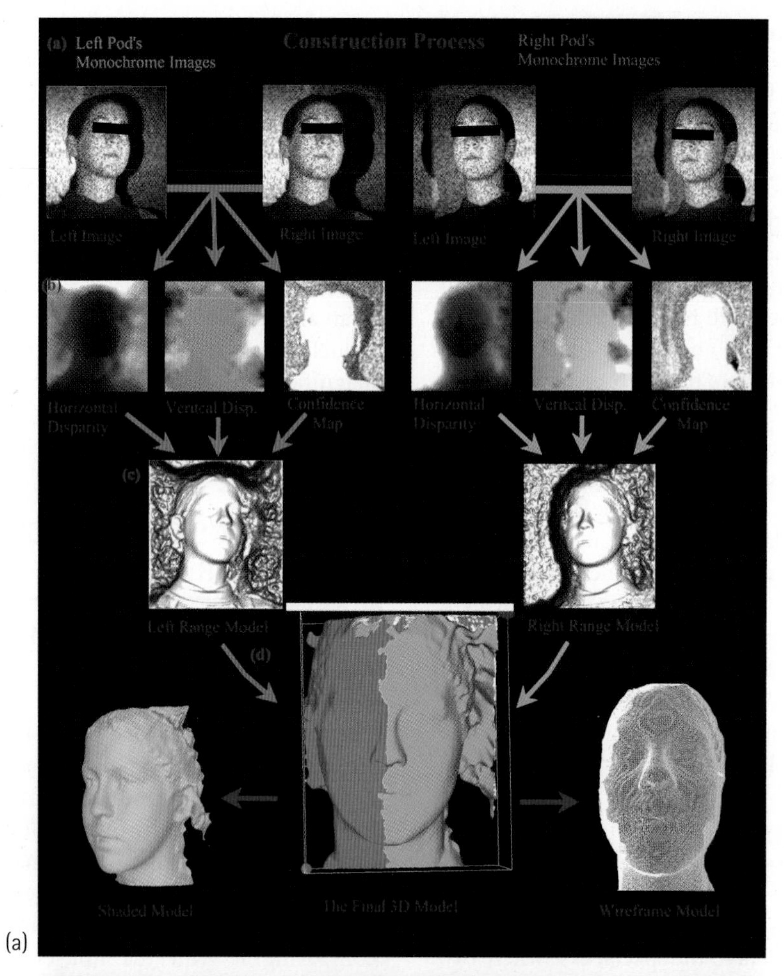

(a)

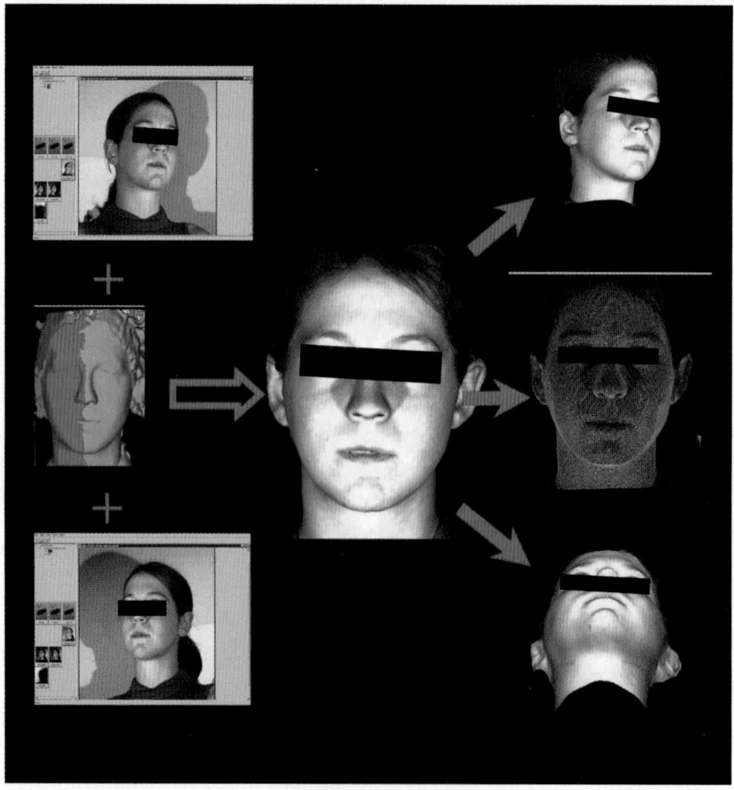

(b)

1.5.4 (a) Illustration of build up of the 3D facial image using stereophotogrammetry. The images captured by each pair of stereo cameras are used to build up a half side of the face. (b) The merging of the right and left halves of the face to build a photorealistic 3D facial model.

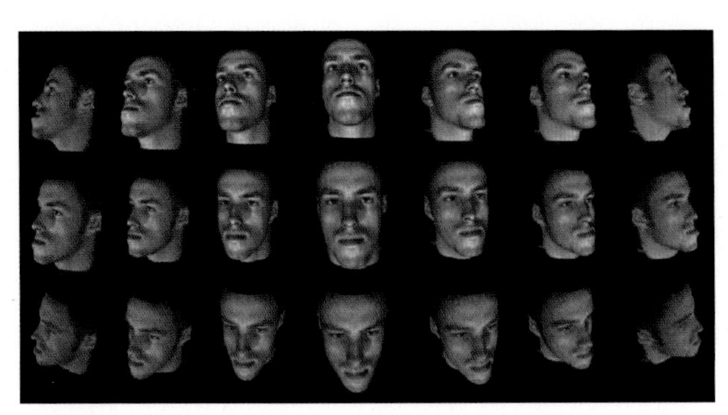

1.5.5 An example of 3D facial model recorded by stereophotogrammetry which can be manipulated and viewed from different positions. Permission obtained from the copyright holder of this figure, Maney Publishing, which was published in the *Brit J Orthod* 2004; **31**: 62–70.

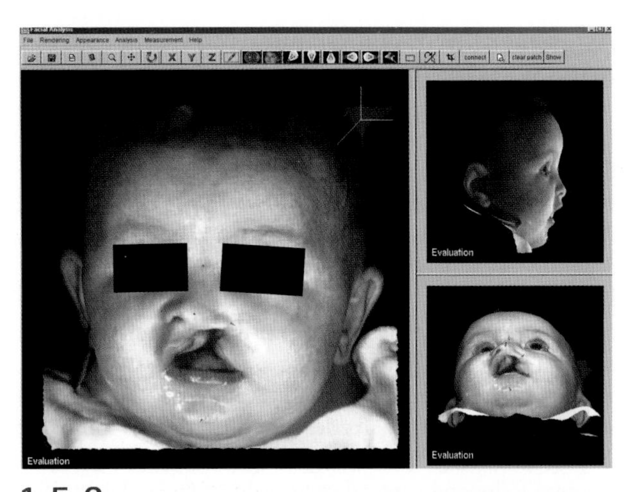

1.5.6 The facial analysis tool which views the 3D image in three different windows simultaneously to facilitate digitization of landmarks and facial measurements.

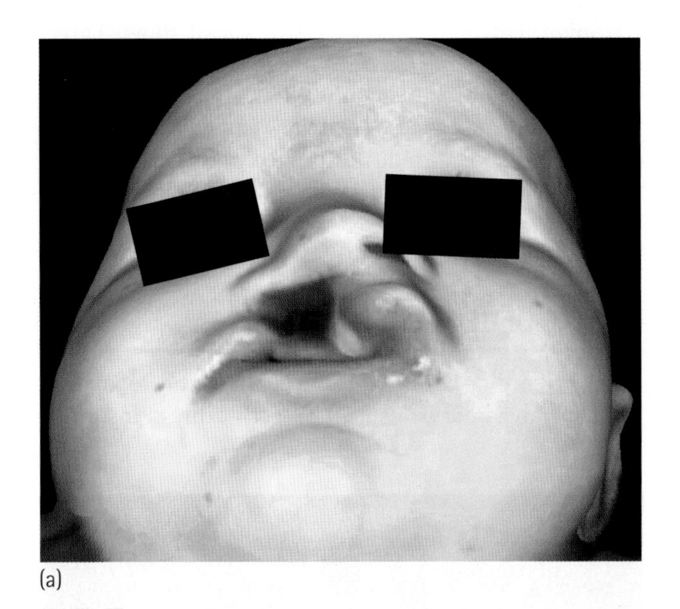

(a)

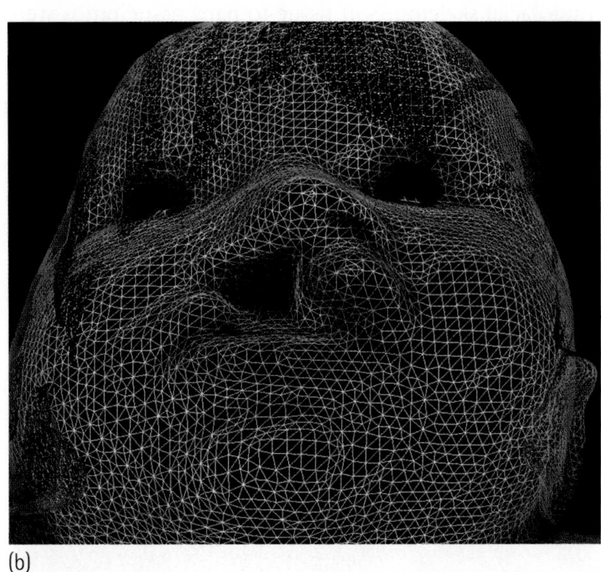

(b)

1.5.7 (a) The 3D image of a case of unilateral cleft lip and palate for pre-operative assessment of the deformity. (b) 3D wire mesh on the top of the 3D image of the same case to illustrate the 3D nature of cleft deformity.

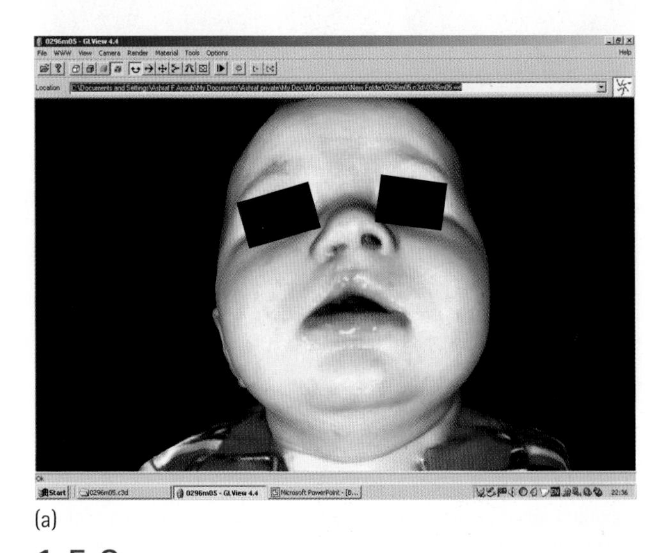

(a)

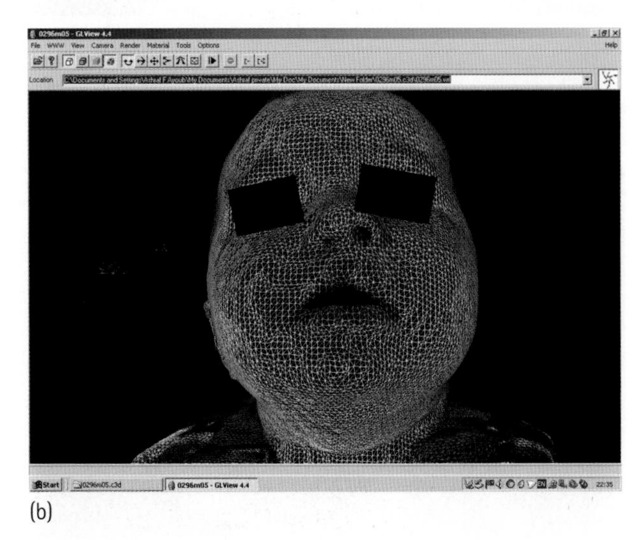

(b)

1.5.8 (a) 3D image following cleft repair showing the asymmetric appearance of the alar base. (b) 3D wire mesh superimposed on the 3D image to illustrate the magnitude of residual deformities following cleft repair.

Assessment of facial changes following orthognathic surgery

Despite the fact that deformity of the facial skeleton is three-dimensional in nature, diagnosis of these has been made principally using 2D records (photographs and radiographs). Three-dimensional virtual models provide an accurate reproduction of facial deformity. These images can be manipulated on the screen which allows comprehensive assessment of both the pre-operative deformity and the surgical outcome (Figure 1.5.9).

Using stereophotogrammetry, linear, angular and volumetric measurements describe the changes following orthognathic surgery. Laser scanning has been used to assess changes following surgical correction of facial deformities and three-dimensional CT scanning has been used to assess skeletal changes following corrective surgery of the craniofacial skeleton. Soft tissue to hard tissue ratios were calculated and a colour scale was used to identify the post-operative changes. This study, for the first time, provided important information about the three-dimensional nature of soft tissue changes following the underlying bony movements. These changes have been used to produce the first generation of three-dimensional prediction software. No doubt, in the future, this could be used as the *de facto* standard for evaluating soft tissue deformities and for planning orthognathic surgery in all three dimensions. Improving the accuracy of superimposition of 3D facial data on the underlying 3D skeletal data (Figure 1.5.10a,b) would effectively provide accurate prediction planning and also facilitate the understanding of the complex relationship between soft and hard tissues in craniofacial morphology.

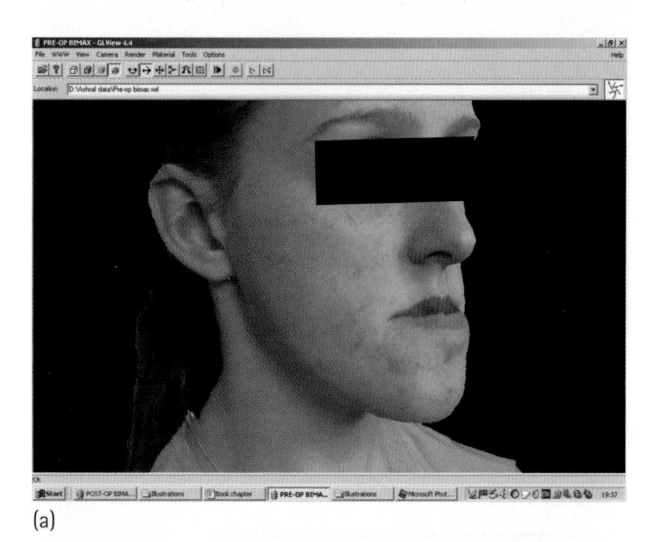

(a)

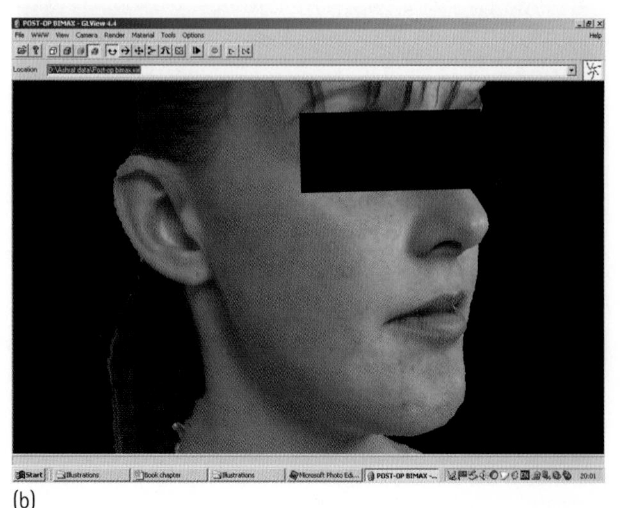

(b)

Assessment of facial injuries

Surgical access to the inferior orbital rim or orbital floor may be achieved through the lower eyelid, either through the skin (transcutaneous) or conjunctiva (transconjunctival). These approaches may be associated with complications including ectropion, entropion and excessive scleral show. Three-dimensional imaging has been utilized to capture the eyes (Figure 1.5.11a,b), measure the effect of incision types on eyelid position and assess scleral show following orbital floor exploration. The morbidity associated with transcutaneous incision was greater in comparison with transconjunctival approach.

FUTURE DEVELOPMENT

Adding recording of time, the fourth dimension, to imaging will allow dynamic assessment of facial expressions which

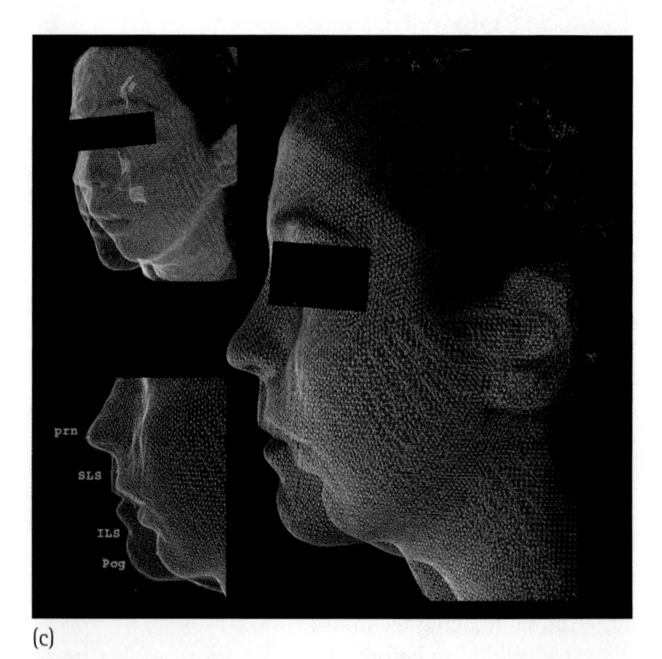

(c)

1.5.9 (a,b) 3D facial appearance before and after Le Fort I maxillary advancement and mandibular set back osteotomy for correction of facial deformities. (c) 3D images are superimposed to demonstrate the magnitude of improvement of facial appearance following mandibular advancement.

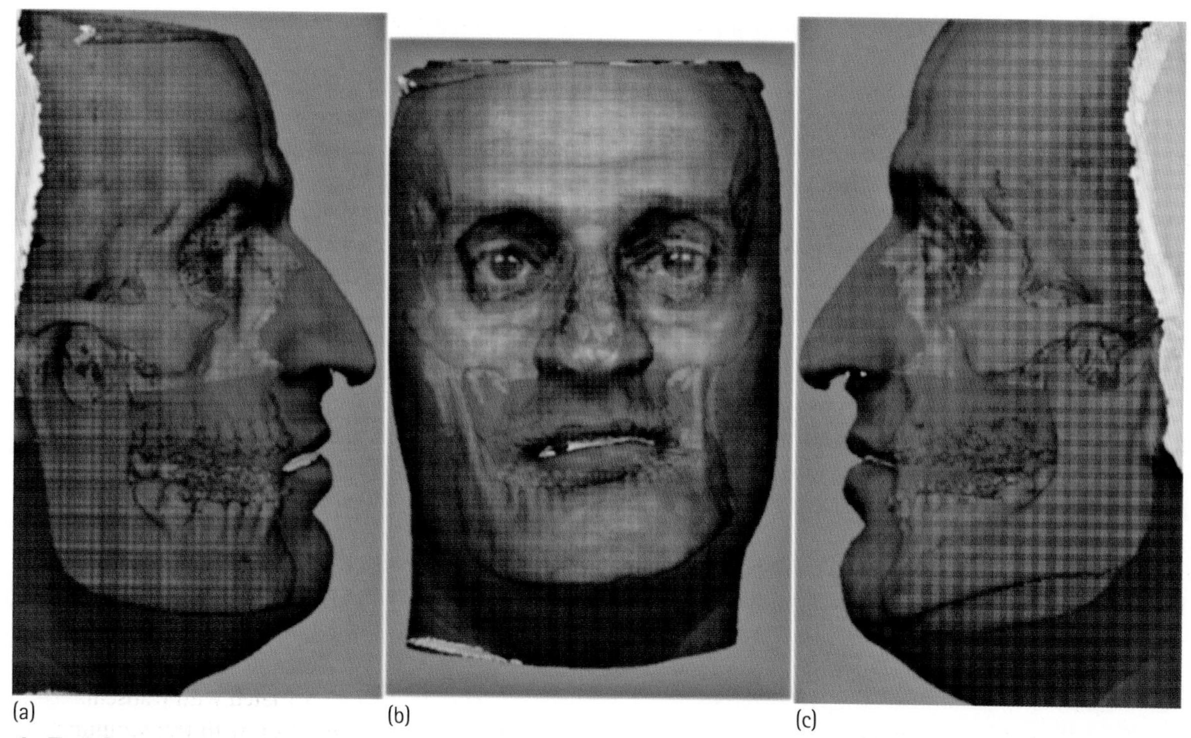

(a) (b) (c)

1.5.10 (a,b,c) Demonstration of superimposition of the 3D soft tissue of the face on the underlying 3D skeletal structure.

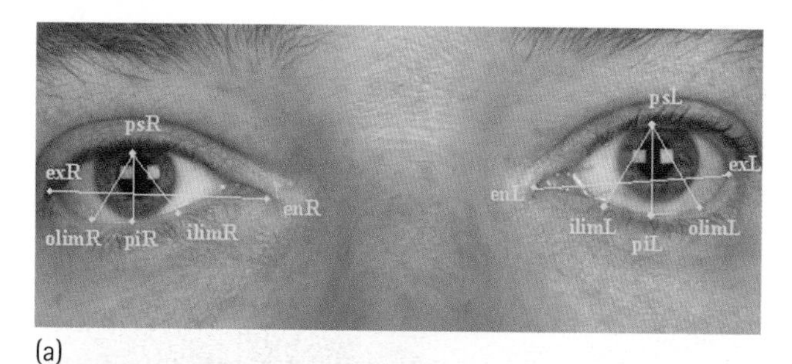

(a)

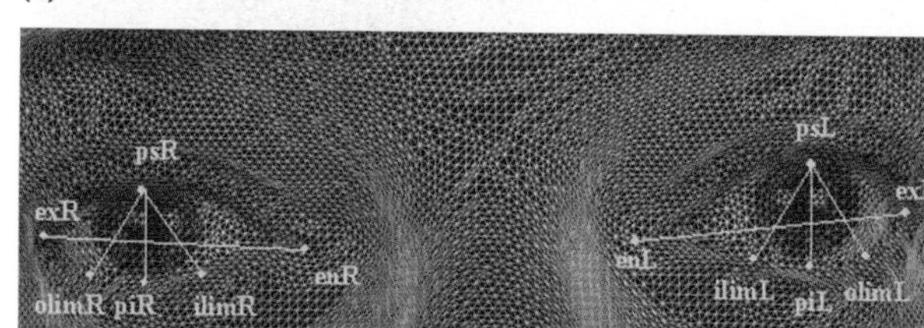

(b)

1.5.11 (a,b) Changes of the lower lip position following lower eyelid surgery to explore the orbital floor, with an increase of scleral shown on the left side.

would be valuable for measuring facial paralysis and animation following cleft lip repair. At present, four-dimensional imaging techniques are complex and require extensive validation before they can be applied in clinical situations.

Top tips

- Three-dimensional imaging overcomes the problem associated with two-dimensional imaging which are the projection and superimposition of the geometric and magnification errors.
- CT scanning, laser imaging, and stereophotogrammetry are the most common methods of imaging the maxillofacial region.
- Three-dimensional imaging is essential for the objective analysis of congenital, acquired and traumatic deformities of the face.

FURTHER READING

Ayoub AF, Xiao Y, Khambay B *et al.* Towards building a photo-realistic virtual human face for craniomaxillofacial diagnosis and treatment planning. *International Journal of Oral and Maxillofacial Surgery* 2007; **36**: 423–8.

Bell JC, Raugher JF, Dittmann W *et al.* Stereolithography in oral and maxillofacial operation planning. *International Journal of Oral and Maxillofacial Surgery* 1995; **24**: 98–103.

Cawie T, Natsume N, Shibata H, Yamamoto T. Three dimensional analysis of facial morphology using Moiré strips. Part I Method. *International Journal of Oral and Maxillofacial Surgery* 1990; **19**: 356–8.

Curry S, Baumrind S, Carlson S *et al.* Integrated three dimensional craniofacial mapping at the Craniofacial Research Instrumentation Laboratory, University of Pacific. *Seminars in Orthodontics* 2001; **7**: 258–65.

Ferrario VF, Sforza C, Toggio CE *et al.* A three dimensional study of sexual dimorphism in the human face. *International Journal of Adult Orthodontics and Orthognathic Surgery* 1994; **9**: 303–10.

Garrahy A, Millett DG, Ayoub AF. Early assessment of dental arch development in repaired unilateral cleft and unilateral cleft lip and palate vs. controls. *Cleft Palate-Craniofacial Journal* 2005; **4**: 385–91.

Hajeer MY, Ayoub AF, Millett DT *et al.* Three dimensional imaging in orthognathic surgery: The clinical application of a new method. *International Journal of Adult Orthodontics and Orthognathic Surgery* 2002; **17**: 318–30.

Hell B. 3D sonography. *International Journal of Oral and Maxillofacial Surgery* 1995; **24**: 84–9.

Hood CA, Bock M, Hosey MT *et al.* Facial asymmetry - 3D assessment of infants with three cleft lip and palate. *International Journal of Paediatric Dentistry* 2003; **13**: 404–10.

Hood CA, Hosey MT, Bock M *et al.* Facial characterisation of infants with cleft lip and palate using a three dimensional capture technique. *Cleft Palate-Craniofacial Journal* 2004; **1**: 27–35.

McCance AM, Moss JP, Fright WR *et al.* Three dimensional imaging analysis of soft and hard tissue changes following bimaxillary orthognathic surgery in skeletal class III patients. *British Journal of Oral and Maxillofacial Surgery* 1992; **30**: 305–12.

McCance AM, Moss JP, Fright WR *et al.* 3-Dimensional soft tissue analyses of 16 skeletal class III patients following bimaxillary surgery. *British Journal of Oral and Maxillofacial Surgery* 1992; **30**: 221–32.

Nguyen CX, Nissanov J, Ozturk C *et al.* Three dimensional imaging of craniofacial complex. *Clinical Orthodontics and Research* 2000; **3**: 46–50.

Nunu YH, Bell S, McHugh S *et al.* 3D assessment of morbidity associated with lower eyelid incisions in orbital trauma. *International Journal of Oral and Maxillofacial Surgery* 2007; **36**: 680–86.

Rabey G. Craniofacial morph analysis. *Proceedings of the Royal Society of Medicine* 1971; **64**: 103–11.

PART 2

ORAL SURGERY

2.1

Tooth extraction

CATHERINE BRYANT

INTRODUCTION

The extraction or removal of a tooth from the alveolus is a very commonly performed procedure, despite the increasing trend for the preservation and retention of teeth throughout life. Dental extractions can usually be performed in a controlled and atraumatic manner following careful evaluation of the patient and the tooth to be removed. All patients benefit from the increased comfort and reduced recovery time afforded by limiting the extent of surgical trauma. The avoidance or minimization of bone removal during dental extractions and the use of luxators and periotomes facilitates this to a greater degree than is possible with conventional techniques.

There are many indications for tooth extraction including caries, periodontal disease, pulpal necrosis, pericoronitis and traumatic injury. In addition, extractions may be indicated prior to orthodontic or prosthodontic treatment and before radiotherapy or treatment with bisphosphonates which render subsequent extractions potentially hazardous.

An intra-alveolar or 'forceps' extraction is one in which a tooth is removed from the alveolus without the surgical creation of a pathway for its delivery. A transalveolar or 'surgical' extraction is one which requires a mucoperiosteal flap to be raised, allowing visualization of the tooth and invariably bone removal to facilitate its removal. This technique may be used electively where factors precluding forceps extraction are appreciated from the outset or when a tooth proves resistant to, or fractures during attempts to deliver it with forceps.

PRE-OPERATIVE EVALUATION AND PREPARATION FOR A DENTAL EXTRACTION

Most of the difficulties, unpleasantness and complications associated with dental extractions can be avoided with proper pre-operative assessment and planning. Assessment of a patient's general health, their level of anxiety about the procedure, the condition of the tooth for extraction and its radiographic appearance all contribute to this evaluation. Patients requiring special measures to be taken before or after the extraction can therefore be identified so that the associated risks may be minimized and the surgical outcome is optimal. All patients should therefore undergo well-planned procedures with appropriate pain and anxiety control.

Given a co-operative patient, the vast majority of dental extractions can be completed successfully under local anaesthetic. For those patients who are anxious or undergoing prolonged or unpleasant procedures, intravenous sedation with midazolam offers a safe and reliable adjunct, producing around 40 minutes of anxiolysis, sedation and amnesia. Since local anaesthetic techniques provide a similar window of pulpal anaesthesia, it is widely accepted that procedures predicted to take longer than this should be done in stages or under general anaesthesia. General anaesthesia is therefore rarely indicated for dental extractions. Its use should be restricted to patients unable to co-operate with treatment in any other way or where there is a degree of urgency to complete treatment, but the presence of acute infection precludes the achievement of effective local anaesthesia.

The preparation of a patient for a dental extraction must include an explanation of the proposed treatment and appropriate warnings about the associated sequelae. Administration of a pre-operative analgesic to utilize its pre-emptive effect and reduce pain experience post-operatively and mouth rinsing with chlorhexidine should also be considered.

The operator usually stands to extract teeth, although technique and positioning can be modified to allow patients to be treated supine. Patients undergoing extraction of maxillary teeth should be positioned with their mouth level with the operator's elbow and the dental chair reclined so that the upper arch lies at an angle of 60 degrees to the floor (Figure 2.1.1).

For the extraction of mandibular teeth, the chair should be lower and reclined slightly less so that the lower arch is parallel to the floor (Figure 2.1.2).

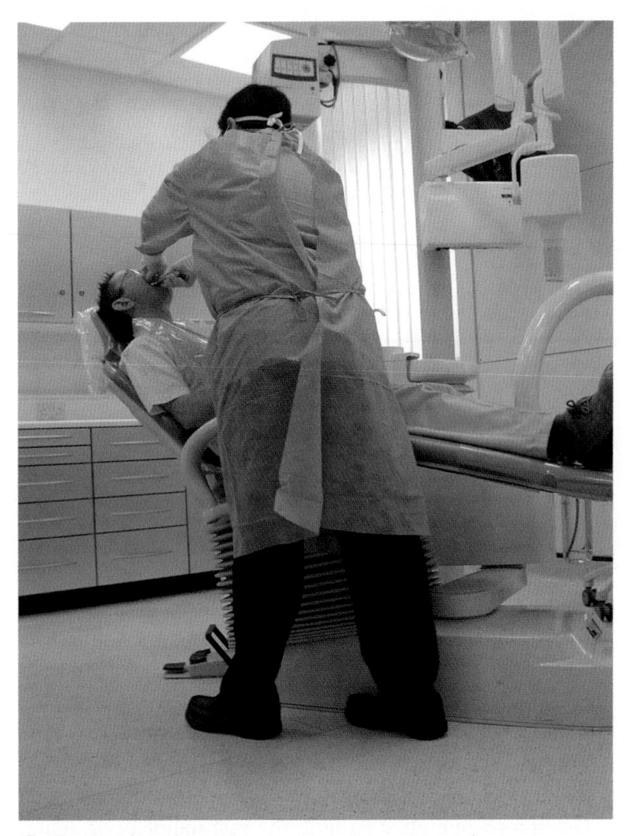

2.1.1 The positioning of a patient for the extraction of a maxillary tooth.

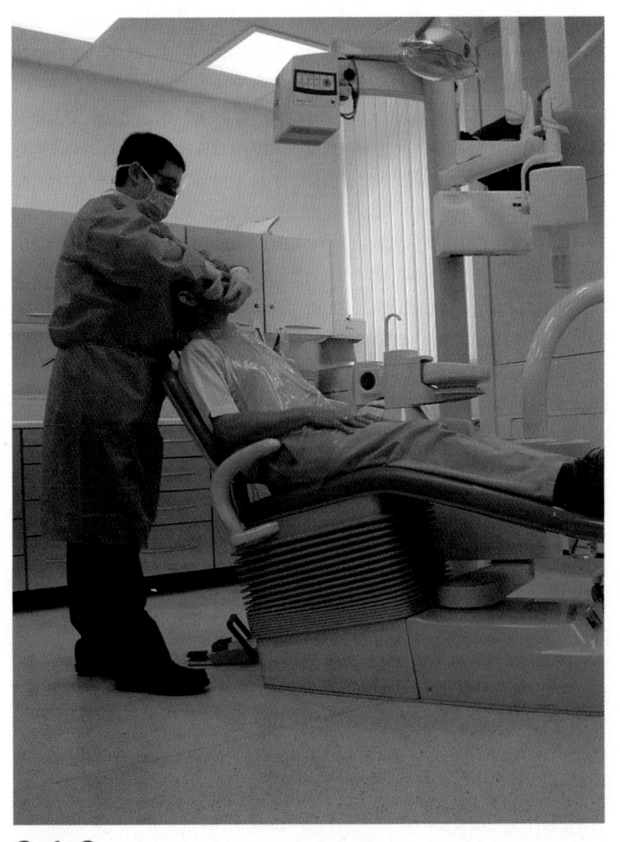

2.1.2 The positioning of a patient for the extraction of a mandibular tooth.

During routine extractions, the surgeon stands in front of the patient on the same side as his own dominant hand, except for mandibular extractions in the quadrant on the same side as his dominant hand. For these, the surgeon should stand behind the patient. When a surgical extraction is performed, the operator usually stands adjacent to the quadrant being treated to allow the best possible view and access.

INSTRUMENTS AND TECHNIQUES USED TO EXTRACT TEETH

An extraction may be successfully completed with the use of extraction forceps alone. Dental elevators are, however, often used to assist with the luxation of a tooth and the dilation of its socket prior to extraction with forceps, in addition to being essential to the removal of teeth and roots during surgical procedures. A range of new instruments, designed to remove teeth atraumatically prior to implant placement, have recently been introduced. These 'extraction systems' work by screwing a post into a retained root and pulling it out, as a cork from a bottle, by turning a screw connected to the root.

Extraction forceps

A wide variety of forceps is available with operator preference and the anatomy of the tooth being removed determining those selected for use. The pattern of mandibular extraction forceps in general use differs between the United Kingdom and the United States. In the USA, the blades of such forceps run in line with the handles, curving downwards to engage the buccal and lingual surfaces of a tooth. When in use, the handles enter the mouth from the front, are in line with the dental arch and are usually held with the palm of the hand facing upwards, the 'underhand technique'. In contrast, the mandibular forceps used in the UK have blades which run 'fore and aft' perpendicular to the handles, which cross the dental arch at right angles during an extraction. The principles of use are common to both. The operator must find the forceps comfortable to grip and the blades should fit closely around the tooth with the beaks engaging the radicular bifurcations (Figure 2.1.3).

When using forceps to extract a tooth, two movements are involved. The first severs the gingival and periodontal ligament attachment to the tooth. The blades should be positioned beneath the gingival margin on the buccal and lingual aspects of the tooth and then driven with increasing force in an apical direction. Thus they slide along the length of the root surface to their final position rather than gripping it from the outset. The placement of the forceps in the most apical position possible ensures that the mechanical efficiency of subsequent movements to extract the tooth is maximal and the risk of root fracture is minimized. The wedge shape of the blades also dilates the socket (Figure 2.1.4).

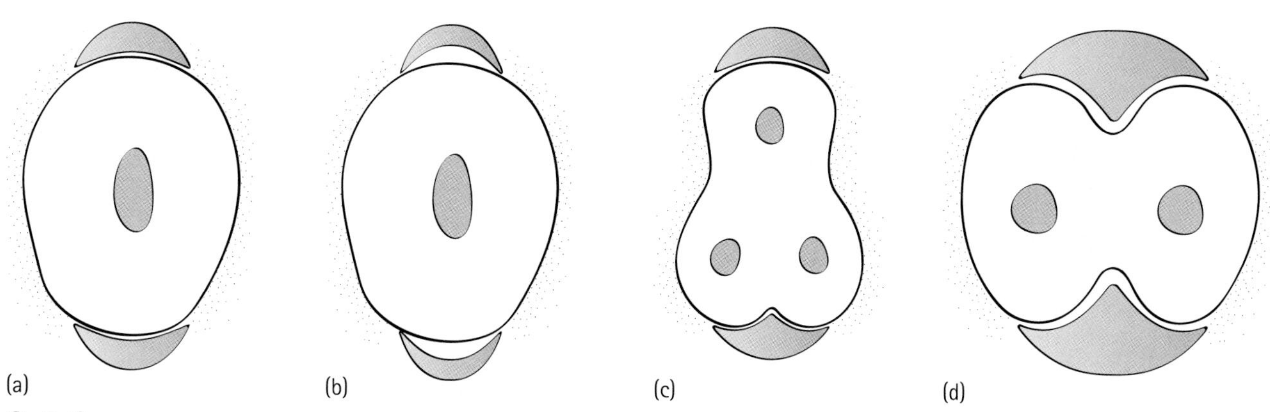

2.1.3 (a) Even distribution of force to tooth with closely adapted forceps; (b) blades which are too narrow distribute force unevenly. Molar forceps have beaks to engage the radicular maxillary (c) or mandibular (d) bifurcations.

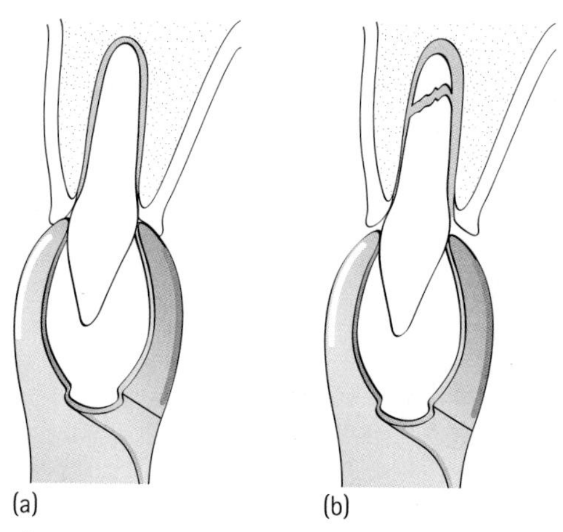

2.1.4 Failure to seat forceps apically results in a more coronal centre of rotation during the movements of the extraction. This increases the degree of movement of the root apex and predisposes to its fracture.

The second movement of forceps extraction removes the tooth from the alveolus. Whilst the apical position achieved in the first movement is maintained, the tooth should then be gripped firmly by the blades of the forceps and the tooth luxated in its bony socket. This allows the socket to dilate and the tooth to be lifted out. The movements involved should be slow and deliberate, allowing time for the alveolus to expand; their direction will be determined by the anatomy and position of the tooth being removed. Resistance to such forces should prompt consideration of a surgical approach.

Forceps technique

Forceps technique for maxillary teeth (incisors and canines) is depicted in Figure 2.1.5; for premolars, Figure 2.1.6; and for molars, Figure 2.1.7. The technique for mandibular teeth (incisors, canines and premolars) is depicted in Figure 2.1.8; for molars, Figures 2.1.9 and 2.1.10.

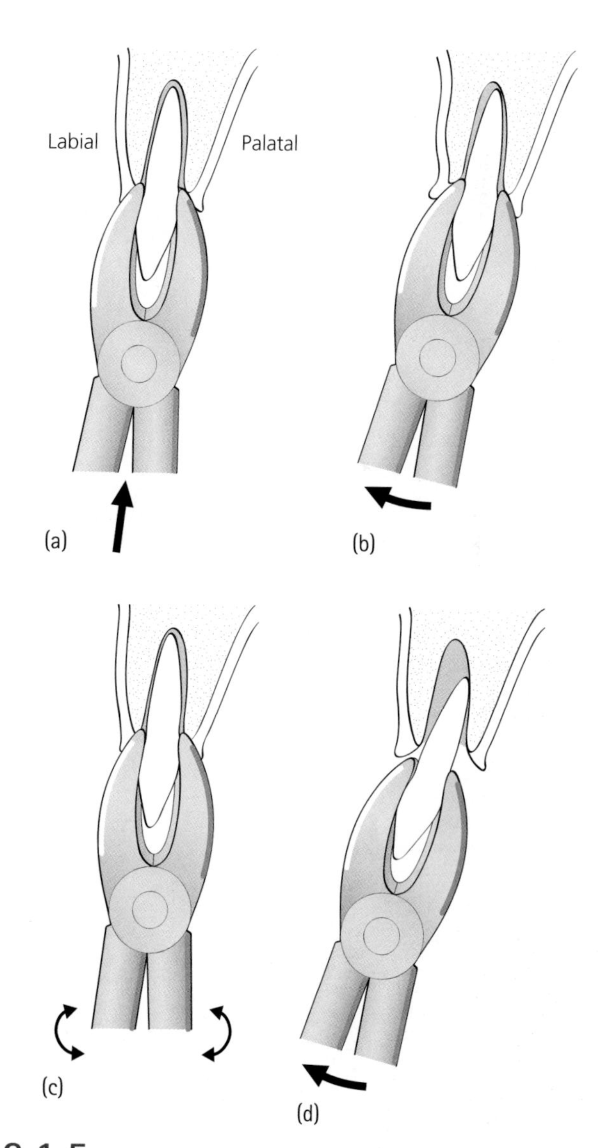

2.1.5 (a) Upper straight or universal forceps are seated as apically as possible. (b) Slow, steady labial movement followed by release then palatal movement is repeated with gradually increasing force. (c) Rotational movements may be introduced to completely sever the periodontal ligament fibres. (d) The tooth is delivered labially.

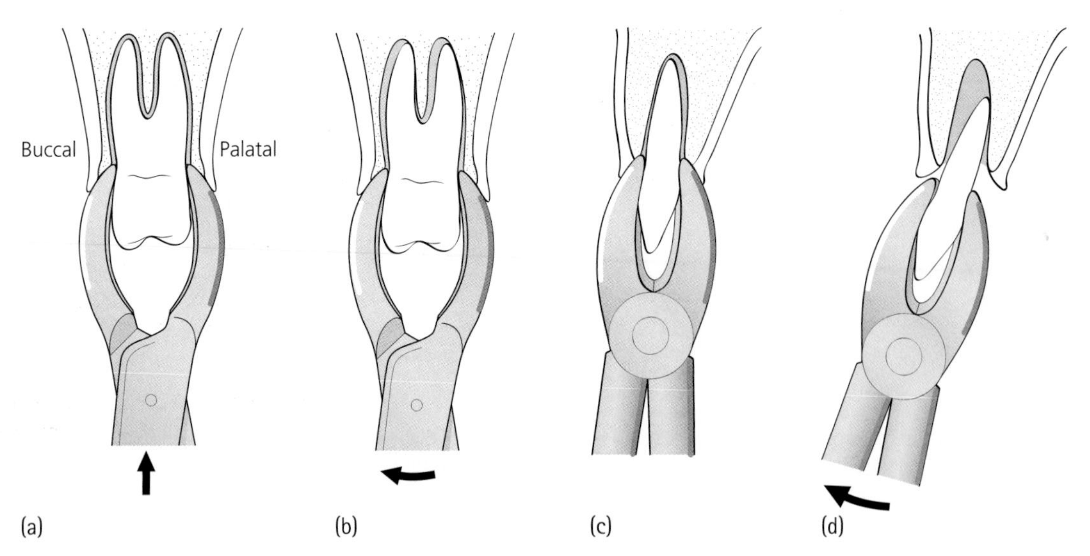

2.1.6 Prior to the application of forceps, the first premolar should be luxated to prevent fracture as this tooth is often two-rooted. (a) Upper premolar or universal forceps engage the tooth firmly and apically. (b) Buccal pressure is applied to the tooth. (c) Gentle palatal movements are introduced. (d) The tooth is delivered in a buccal direction, with additional tractional force to remove the tooth from its socket.

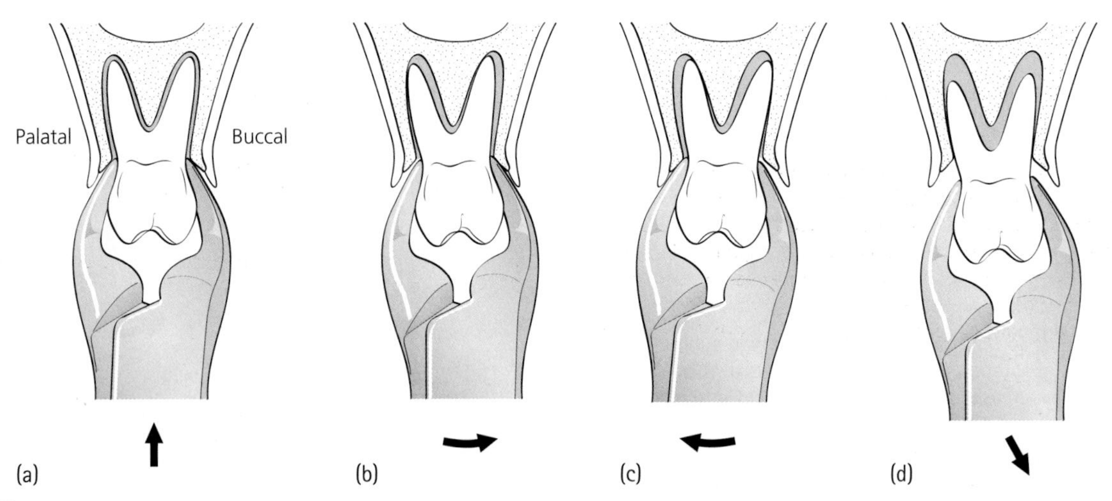

2.1.7 (a) Upper molar or anatomical forceps should be seated with their beaks engaging the buccal bifurcation. (b) The predominant movement is buccal and significant force may be required. (c) Palatal forces can be applied, although the palatal cortical plate is thick and unyielding. (d) Firm steady buccal pressure allows the socket to expand and the tooth is delivered in this direction.

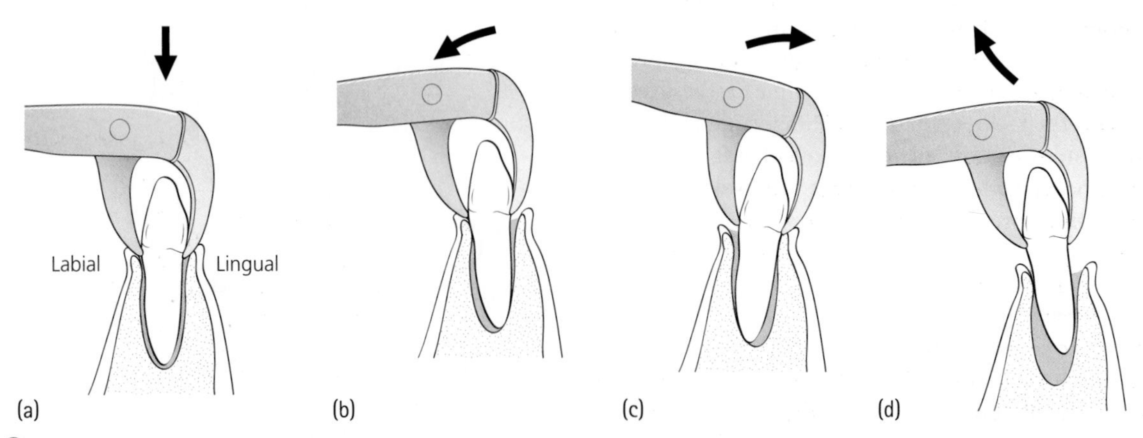

2.1.8 (a) These teeth with similar, single conical root morphology are removed with lower premolar or universal forceps which are positioned as far down the root surface as possible. (b) Force is applied labially and then lingually (c). Rotational movements are introduced until the tooth is finally delivered in a buccal-occlusal direction (d).

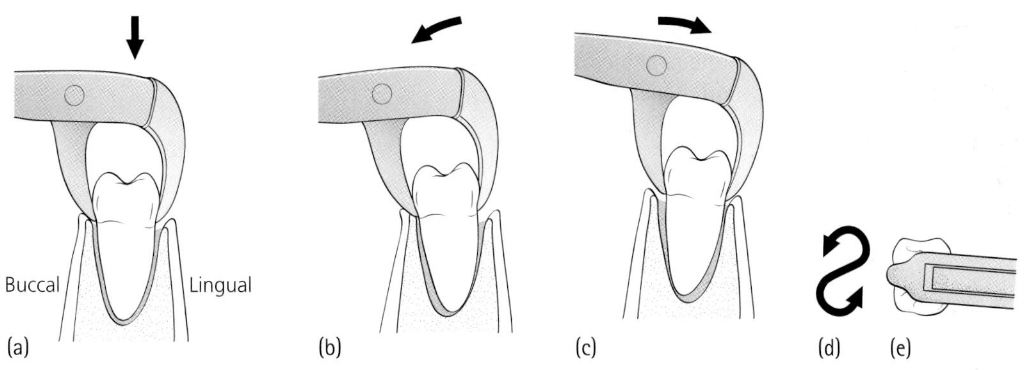

2.1.9 (a) Lower molar forceps are positioned with beaks engaging the bifurcation buccally and lingually. (b) Buccal and lingual (c) excursions are made, with increasing force as the tooth begins to become mobile. (d) A figure of eight movement independently dilates the mesial and distal sockets. (e) Tooth is delivered in a bucco-occlusal direction.

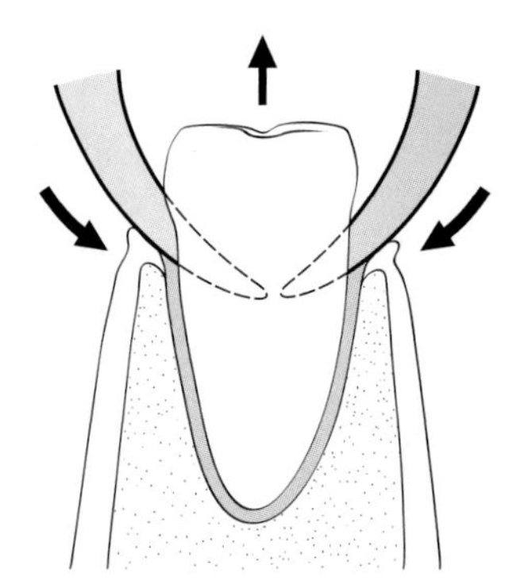

2.1.10 Where the crown of a mandibular molar is extensively destroyed, the use of Cow Horn forceps may allow an extraction to be completed routinely, thus a surgical procedure can be avoided. The sharp, curved buccal and lingual beaks are positioned between the mesial and distal roots. As the handles of the forceps are closed the beaks are squeezed further into the bifurcation and produce a tractional force which expels the tooth from its socket. Subsequent bucco-lingual movements allow the tooth to be lifted from its socket.

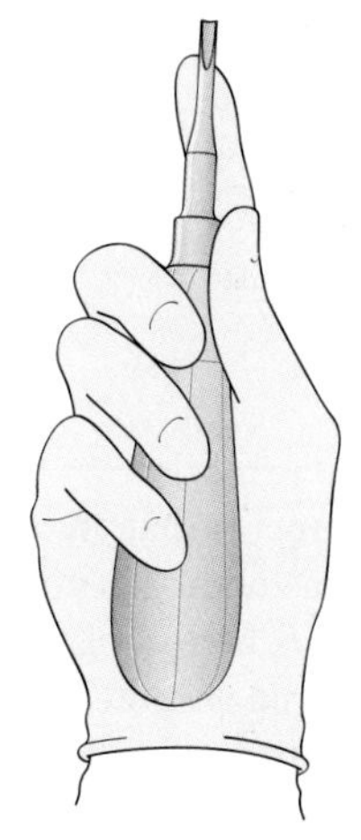

2.1.11 Operator's index finger is extended along the length of the elevator.

Dental elevators and their use

A wide variety of elevators is available. Although apparently very different in design, their common feature is their curved blades. The blades transmit forces, generated by rotating the handles around their long axis, to the surface of the tooth or root. This produces luxation and movement of the tooth away from the point of application, where the elevator contacts the tooth.

Forces may be applied perpendicular to the tooth with an elevator in the interdental space or along its long axis buccally. Since considerable force is applied to the tooth, the elevator must be prevented from slipping. While it is being used, the operator's index finger should therefore be extended along the length of the blade to act as a finger rest on adjacent hard tissues (Figure 2.1.11).

The curved blade of the elevator is placed on the root surface, thus lying between the tooth and the alveolar bone which acts as a fulcrum around which the elevator is turned.

Rotation of an elevator used in this way will produce a force which luxates the tooth and tends to displace it out of its socket (Figure 2.1.12a).

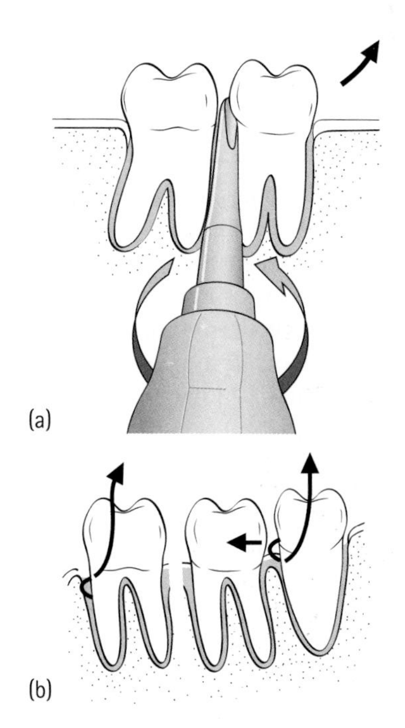

2.1.12 (a) The elevator produces a force which luxates the tooth, displacing it out of its socket. (b) An equal force will also be applied to the fulcrum.

An equal force will also be applied to the fulcrum, so it is important to ensure that this is alveolar bone capable of resisting such a force and not an adjacent tooth which may, as a result, become inadvertently loosened or displaced (Figure 2.1.12b).

Elevators must be used with caution when luxating teeth to avoid generating excessive and potentially damaging forces. Should a tooth resist attempts to luxate it, another solution should be sought.

Luxators

Luxators are sharp, fine, slightly flexible single-bladed instruments, not unlike Coupland's elevators in appearance. They are used to incise the soft tissue attachment of a tooth while sliding down the periodontal space to an apical position. Their subsequent rotation then luxates and promotes the displacement of the tooth, with a minimum of force and alveolar destruction.

Periotomes

Periotomes are instruments that are used to sever the soft tissue attachment of a tooth. They resemble fine straight elevators, but have sharp, narrow blades for cutting. Straight periotomes are used for single rooted teeth, while angled ones are appropriate for multirooted teeth. They are inserted into the periodontal space and with apical pressure are moved from the distal to the mesial aspect of a tooth or root, first buccally and then palatally. By severing the soft tissue attachment in this way, there is less need for vigorous manipulation of the tooth within its socket during the extraction. Alveolar expansion and destruction are therefore minimized.

NON-SURGICAL REMOVAL OF ROOTS

Where the crown of a tooth is largely absent, attempts can be made to remove it without a surgical procedure. Unpleasant post-operative sequelae, such as pain and swelling, will therefore be minimized. Using alveolar bone to act as a fulcrum to apply forces to the root, luxators or elevators may be used to displace roots from their sockets. Luxators are particularly effective in this situation.

- Single rooted teeth: The instrument should be inserted between the mesial and distal aspects of the root surface and alveolar bone. By rotating it, the root becomes mobilized ready for delivery by forceps or displaced out of the socket (Figure 2.1.13).
- Multirooted teeth: Where a multirooted molar with a destroyed crown must be removed, elevation alone may be fruitless and not result in delivery of the tooth. In this situation, the roots may be divided with the use of a water-cooled bur (Figure 2.1.14) or by rotating a straight elevator in the bifurcation (Figure 2.1.15). The separated roots are subsequently elevated or removed with forceps.

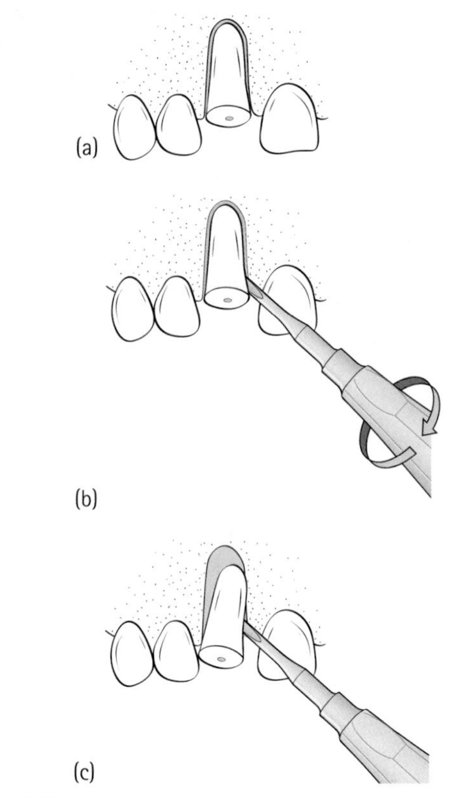

2.1.13 Elevation of a root.

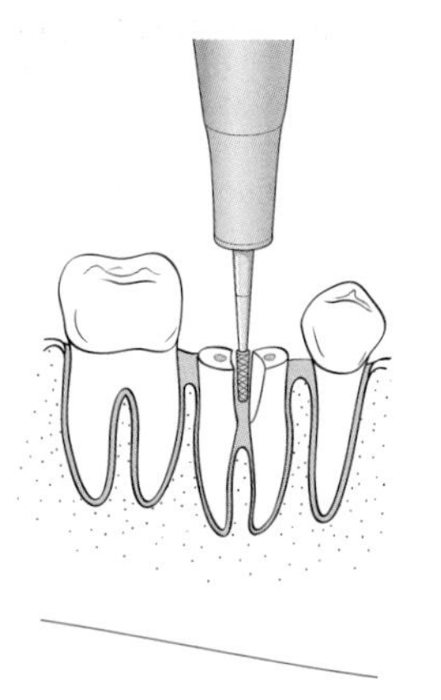

2.1.14 Division of a multirooted tooth with a bur.

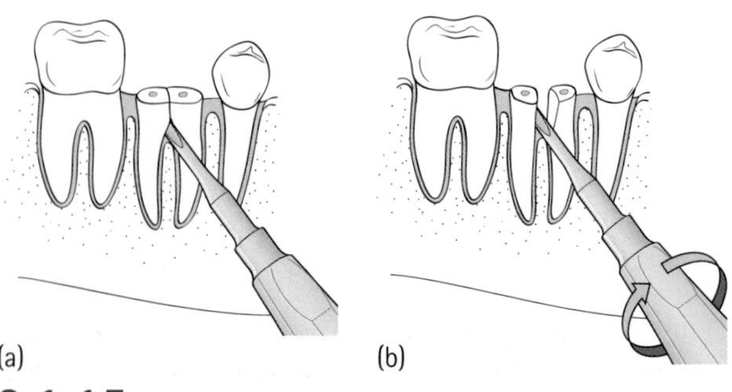

2.1.15 Division of a multirooted tooth using an elevator.

TRANSALVEOLAR, SURGICAL EXTRACTION

The surgical removal of teeth using a transalveolar approach utilizes the benefits of improved access and visibility afforded by raising a mucoperiosteal flap. The removal of alveolar bone and tooth division may also be necessary. Extensive coronal destruction, unusual root morphology, unfavourable root pattern, ankylosed or dilacerated roots are predictive of the need for a surgical extraction.

The aim of the surgical approach is to deliver a tooth or its remnants along a surgically created pathway. The first step involves the raising of a mucoperiosteal flap. An incision is made through the mucoperiosteum, allowing the site of surgery to be exposed. The incision defining the flap should be full thickness, placed over bone not planned for removal and distant from adjacent vital structures. A horizontal element around the gingival margin and vertical relieving incision buccally are usually indicated, with inclusion of the gingival papilla within the flap. Ensuring that the base of the flap is wider than the gingival aspect, careful manipulation and effective closure of the soft tissues optimizes the vitality and healing of the flap. Where visualization of the surgical site is still difficult, the provision of a further relieving incision to create a three-sided flap improves both this and surgical access (Figure 2.1.16).

Having exposed a tooth, the improved access and direct vision may allow it to be elevated or removed with forceps with no need for bone removal (Figure 2.1.17).

The removal of bone from around the tooth is, however, often necessary. Tungsten carbide-tipped round or fissure burs with water coolant are usually used. Creation of a bony gutter on the buccal aspect of a tooth reduces its support making it easier to displace, provides a point of application for elevators and exposes it sufficiently to facilitate its surgical division. Bone removal along the tooth's mesial–distal length should expose the root surface and produce a deep but narrow cut which may be engaged effectively by elevators (Figure 2.1.18).

A multirooted tooth may resist being elevated intact from the alveolus even after bone removal. It may have roots with no common path of withdrawal and surgical division is then indicated. This procedure allows the tooth to be removed in smaller constituent parts, bone is therefore preserved and the forces needed to complete the extraction are reduced. Maxillary molars have buccal roots which may be divided from the palatal root and each other if necessary (Figure 2.1.19). Mandibular molars may be divided with one bucco-lingual cut (Figure 2.1.20).

Where possible, the tooth should be divided following the exposure of its bifurcation with the use of a bur to cut from the bifurcation in an occlusal direction. This allows a greater degree of certainty that the roots will be effectively separated than when a cut is made from the occlusal surface towards the bifurcation. Decoronation prior to surgically dividing a tooth may further maximize the chance of successful section. It is often desirable to avoid cutting right through the root mass, instead the bur can be used to divide two thirds of the way through the tooth and then the remainder split by rotating a narrow, straight elevator within the cut.

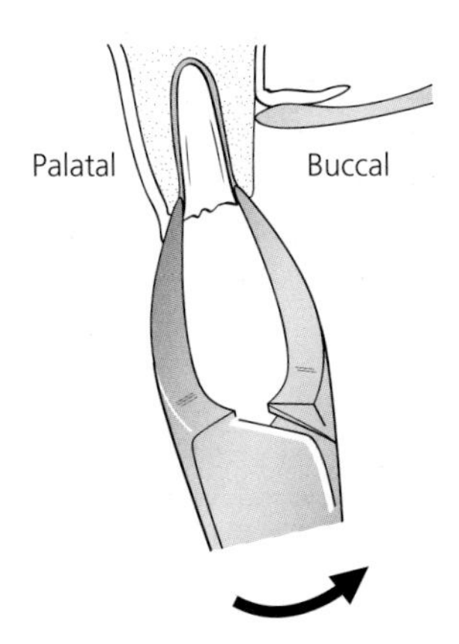

2.1.17 Removal of a root with forceps following the reflection of a mucoperiosteal flap.

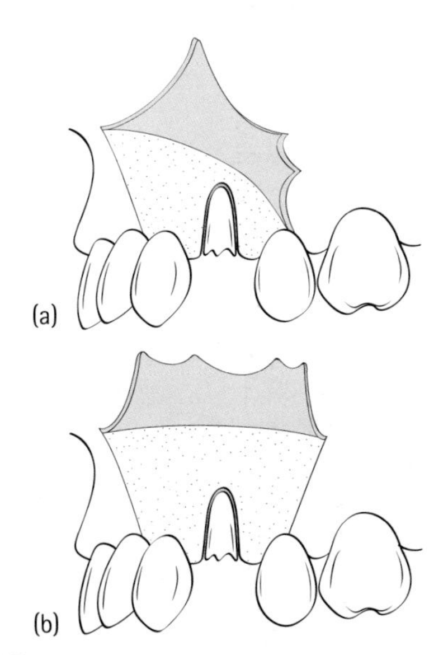

2.1.16 (a) A three-sided flap produced by a gingival and one relieving incision. (b) A further relieving incision creates a four-sided flap.

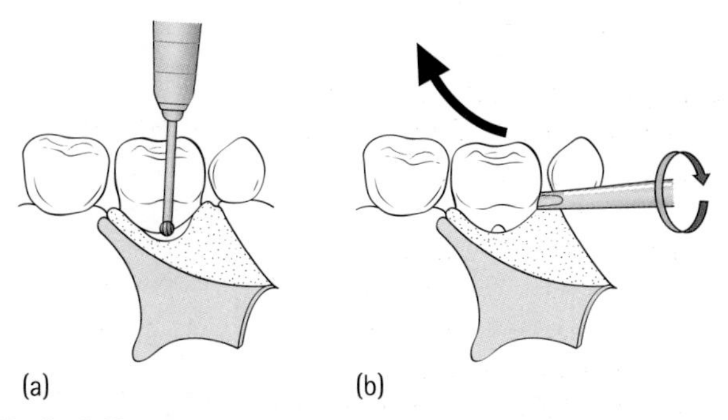

2.1.18 (a) Bone removal to expose the root surface and produce a gutter buccally. (b) Use of elevators at the point of application to displace a tooth.

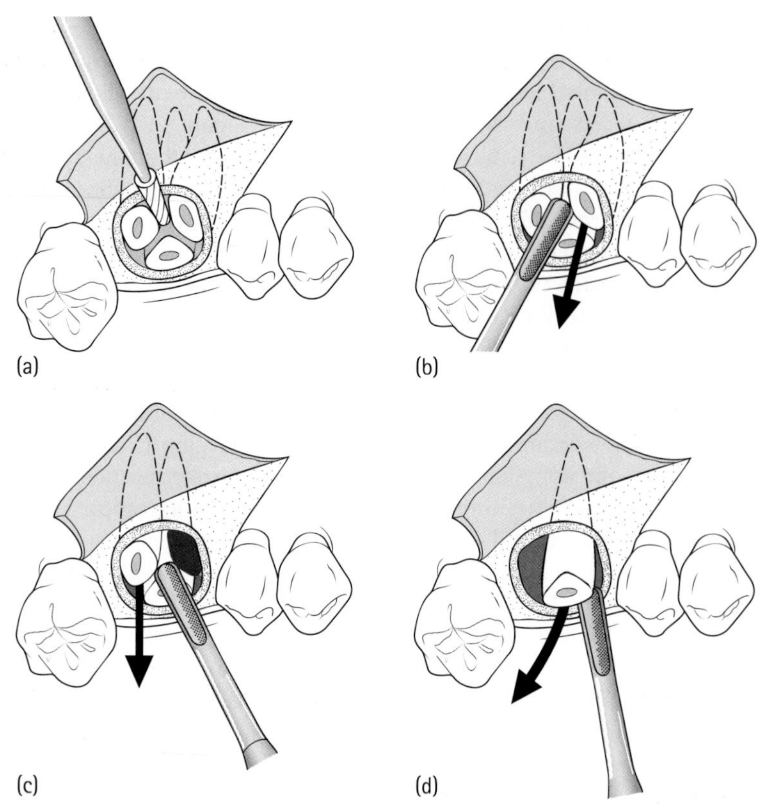

2.1.19 The division and elevation of the roots of a maxillary molar.

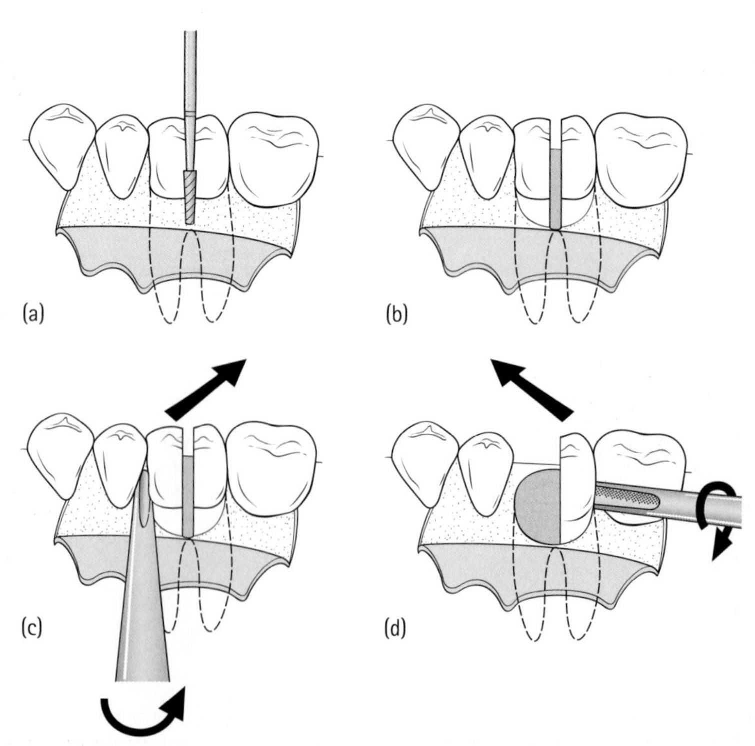

2.1.20 The division and elevation of the roots of a mandibular molar.

Such surgical division is usually sufficient to allow the tooth to be removed; however, in other cases the separated roots may still resist removal. Bone removal around each of them will then be necessary.

Following bone removal and tooth division, straight dental elevators of increasing size can be used to luxate and remove the tooth or its separated root fragments. Force should be applied mesially and buccally in the long axis of the tooth. Clinical experience brings with it the ability to generate, identify and use a point of application to its full advantage. An effective technique when applying a force to elevate a tooth is also essential.

The use of a sharp-ended Cryer's (east–west) elevator to remove a root of a multirooted tooth following extraction of an adjacent one is valuable. The sharp end is introduced to the depth of the socket generated by the removal of the first root and is used to engage the inter-radicular bone and remaining root. A rotational movement is produced as the handle is rotated, allowing the root to be removed (Figure 2.1.21).

Following the removal of a tooth or its constituent fragments, thorough debridement and closure of the surgical defect complete the procedure.

Where a tooth resists forceps extraction, despite the use of luxators and elevators, rather than progressing to a conventional surgical approach, buccal bone may be preserved if the tooth is sectioned, decoronated and inter-radicular bone removed without the raising of a mucoperiosteal flap. This avoids the creation of a defect in the buccal plate, but is not as predictable a technique as the conventional one. In experienced hands, however, it may offer the benefits of tissue preservation.

RETRIEVAL OF RETAINED ROOT TIPS

Where a small portion of a root is retained and resistant to removal with an elevator, curette, probe or root pick, an assessment of whether it may be left *in situ* should be made. If its removal is indicated, then a surgical procedure must be undertaken. The conventional technique of raising a buccal flap, removing bone to expose the root and deliver it may be utilized, however, this is a relatively destructive procedure. Alternatively, a more minimal technique where a soft tissue flap is raised but the bulk of the buccal plate is preserved may be preferred. This involves creating only a small fenestration in the buccal plate at the anticipated site of the retained root allowing an instrument to be inserted through it to displace the root coronally (Figure 2.1.22).

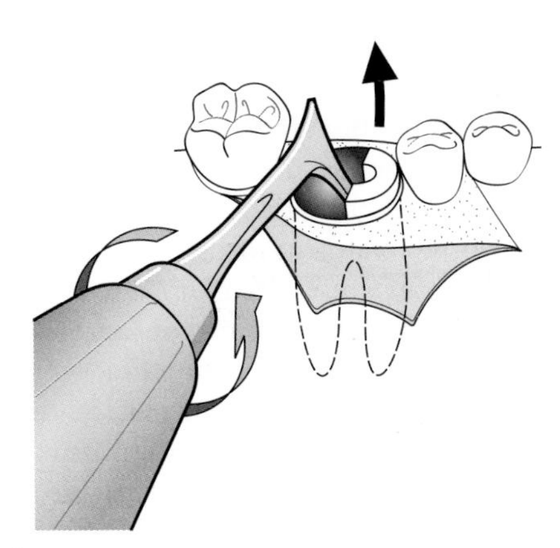

2.1.21 Use of a Cryer's elevator to engage and displace a retained root.

MULTIPLE EXTRACTIONS

The number of extractions that can be performed on one occasion is determined by the patient's co-operation, local anaesthetic dose and surgical difficulty. Maxillary extractions should be performed prior to those in the mandible to avoid debris from the former contaminating mandibular sockets. Posterior teeth should be removed prior to anterior ones in the same arch so that there is no obscuring of the view of the former by bleeding anteriorly. The use of papillary sutures to re-appose mucosal tissue allows better soft tissue healing and contour post-operatively, since the mucosa may gape even without the creation of surgical flaps.

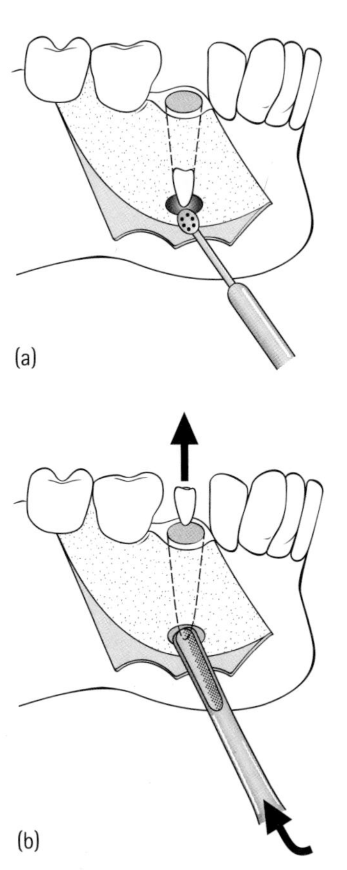

2.1.22 Retrieval of a retained root tip using a bone preserving technique.

DECIDUOUS EXTRACTIONS

The principles of extracting deciduous teeth are essentially the same as those for permanent teeth; however, there are some differences to consider. First, the unerupted permanent successor of the deciduous tooth being removed is likely to be in close proximity and as this erupts, the roots of the deciduous tooth become resorbed. Thus, the risk of inadvertently removing the developing permanent tooth with the deciduous tooth increases as the permanent tooth moves occlusally. It is, therefore, particularly important that smaller, deciduous, extraction forceps are applied to deciduous molar teeth either mesial or distal to but not within its bifurcation (Figure 2.1.23).

A second modification of technique is needed to reflect the fact that the roots of deciduous molars are divergent, relatively long and fragile. They are therefore prone to fracture during extraction resulting in retained fragments close to the developing crown of the successor. When this occurs, the remnants should be removed very carefully with the application of elevators to the mesial aspect of the mesial root and the distal aspect of the distal root only, thus avoiding the region of the bifurcation (Figure 2.1.24).

POST-EXTRACTION CARE

On completion of a dental extraction, the surgeon assumes responsibility for the patient's aftercare. Both verbal and written instructions should be given, explaining how the extraction site should be cared for, how to avoid precipitating bleeding and what to do should this occur. Responsible surgical practice requires the operator to prescribe suitable and effective post-operative analgesia for the patient as it is almost inevitable that pain will ensue.

The non-steroidal anti-inflammatory (NSAID) drugs have been shown to be highly effective in controlling acute pain following oral surgery. Of this group of drugs, ibuprofen is associated with the lowest incidence of side-effects and 400 mg controls this type of pain more effectively than 10 mg morphine i.m. Patients for whom the prescription of ibuprofen is contraindicated will benefit from a paracetamol containing analgesic.

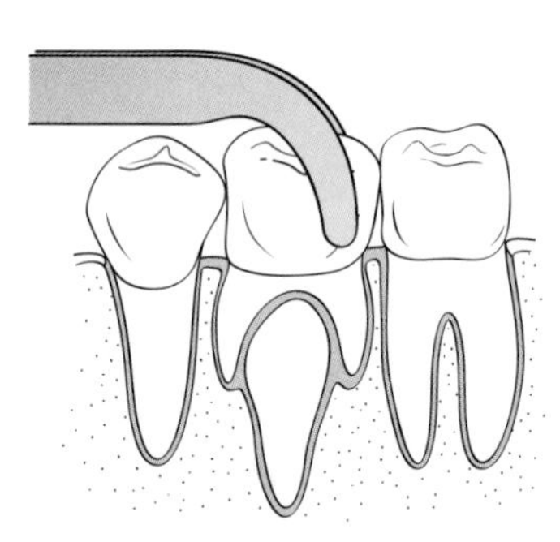

2.1.23 Application of forceps to a deciduous mandibular molar away from the bifurcation.

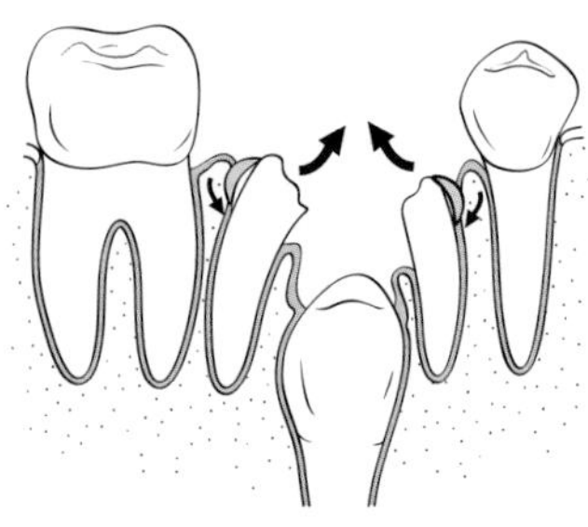

2.1.24 Elevation of the roots of a deciduous mandibular molar away from the bifurcation.

COMPLICATIONS

Careful pre-operative planning, an atraumatic surgical technique and attention to post-operative instructions will minimize the occurrence of complications following dental extraction. A patient must, however, be warned pre-operatively of those occurring commonly and sequelae such as pain, swelling and limited mouth opening should be expected. More significant complications are unusual, but include post-extraction haemorrhage and alveolar osteitis.

Under normal circumstances, following a dental extraction, a socket should stop bleeding in less than 10 minutes. When a patient presents with post-extraction haemorrhage, contributory systemic factors should be excluded. The mouth should then be cleaned thoroughly and the bleeding point identified (good illumination and suction will be required). Local pressure will usually control the bleeding; this can be aided by the insertion of a haemostatic agent, such as oxidized cellulose. Control of persistent haemorrhage may require the administration of local anaesthesia, placement of sutures, diathermy or ligation of vessels. Packing ribbon gauze, presoaked in Whitehead's varnish, into a socket usually achieves haemostasis when other means fail.

Alveolar osteitis (dry socket) is an acutely painful condition which can complicate dental extractions. It is characterized by the onset of pain 24–72 hours post-operatively. Examination reveals halitosis, erythema of surrounding soft tissues and an exposed bony socket from which the clot has been lost and which has often become filled with debris. Treatment involves debridement of the socket into which an antiseptic, obtundant dressing should be placed and the prescription of analgesia. Recent systematic reviews have examined the efficacy of therapeutic interventions undertaken to reduce the incidence of alveolar osteitis after oral surgery. These demonstrated that mouth washing with chlorhexidine pre-operatively and then for 7 days post-operatively has the most significant preventative effect, while antibiotic prescription does not appear to prevent its occurrence.

Top tips

- During an extraction, the proper positioning of the patient and operator ensures that both are comfortable and that the forces applied to the tooth are mechanically efficient.
- Attempts to remove a tooth using elevators and forceps when pre-operative evaluation suggests that a surgical procedure should be undertaken will be excessively traumatic and will prolong the procedure.
- The use of periotomes and luxators and the minimization of bone removal will preserve vital tissue and optimize outcome.
- When using an elevator, the blade must be positioned correctly between the root and alveolar bone and not between two teeth as this will mobilize and displace both.
- The generation of excessive force while using elevators or forceps should be avoided as this predisposes to the fracture of the tooth or alveolus.
- Mucoperiosteal flap design should provide optimal access and visualization of the surgical site, while limiting the extent of surgical trauma.
- Buccal bone removal to create a narrow gutter adjacent to a tooth reduces its bony support whilst preserving a ridge of buccal cortex, which then provides a fulcrum for the subsequent elevation of the tooth.
- Most complications result from inadequate pre-operative evaluation and poor surgical technique.

FURTHER READING

Fragiskos FD (ed.). *Oral surgery.* Heidelberg: Springer, 2007.

Gillbe GV, Moore JR. Extraction of erupted teeth and their roots. In: Moore JR (ed.), *Surgery of the mouth and jaws.* Oxford: Blackwell Scientific, 1985, 315–38.

Hedstrøm L, Sjøgren P. Effect estimates and methodological quality of randomised controlled trials about prevention of alveolar osteitis following tooth extraction: A systematic review. *Oral Surgery, Oral Medicine, Oral Pathology and Endodontology* 2007; **103**; 8–15.

Meechan JG (ed.). *Minor oral surgery in dental practice.* London: Quintessence, 2006.

Moore UJ (ed.). *Principles of oral and maxillofacial surgery,* 5th edn. Oxford: Blackwell Science, 2001.

Peterson LJ, Ellis E III, Hupp JR, Tucker MR (eds). *Contemporary oral and maxillofacial surgery,* 4th edn. St Louis, MO: Mosby, 2003.

Pedlar J. Extraction of teeth. In: Pedlar J, Frame JW (eds). *Oral and maxillofacial surgery. An objective-based textbook.* London: Churchill Livingstone, 2001, 27–47.

2.2

Removal of unerupted teeth

JAMES Q SWIFT

INTRODUCTION

Teeth that do not erupt to acceptable relationships with adjacent teeth or opposing teeth can be described as non-erupted, unerupted or partially erupted. When an individual presents for dental evaluation, it is incumbent on the oral health-care provider to determine the presence of a normal and full complement of 20 teeth in the child by approximately age five years, a varying number of teeth in the adolescent and young adult and a maximum of 32 teeth in the dental and skeletally mature adult, barring the presence of extra or supernumerary teeth which are relatively rare. The clinician must recognize that the absence of a normal complement of teeth may also be due to lack of tooth development. This occurs most often with third molars. There are, however, cases of hypodontia, oligodontia and anodontia where there are multiple teeth that do not develop. Any condition that results in fewer than the expected full complement of teeth visible in the oral cavity at any given age must be investigated to determine the reason and potential need for observation or partial or complete surgical removal. In general, it is accepted that a tooth that does not erupt into functional occlusion with absence of bacteriologic disease is pathology. This does not infer, however, that all unerupted teeth should be surgically or prophylactically removed.

ESTABLISHING A DIAGNOSIS

The surgeon must determine a differential diagnosis, rationale or reason as to why a tooth remains unerupted at an age where the eruption of the tooth should have occurred. In many situations, the unerupted tooth may be impacted or prevented from eruption by an obstacle, which could include an adjacent tooth or teeth, other adjacent normal anatomy, dense bone, fibrous connective tissue, cystic lesion or neoplasm. There may not be adequate arch space in the dental alveolus for a full complement of teeth to erupt. In other situations, there may not be an obvious reason for the uneruption of the tooth. Many clinicians would favour the diagnosis of ankylosis, a condition where there is direct contact of a calcified tooth surface with adjacent bone without an intervening periodontal ligament or dental follicle in the absence of other more obvious reasons for the lack of tooth eruption. A diagnosis of true ankylosis in most situations can be made with evaluation of imaging or radiographs.

DIAGNOSTIC IMAGING

Except in the case of the partially erupted tooth when a portion of the tooth is visible upon clinical examination, radiographic imaging is essential to determine the presence or absence of a tooth that is expected to be erupted. An orthopantomogram is an excellent screening image that will determine the presence and location of the unerupted tooth and will also reveal the proximity of the tooth to adjacent structures and anatomy. Peri-apical dental radiographs offer better resolution and image detail of the calcified structures but have a limited field of interest. In addition, peri-apical dental radiographs can be used in a 'shift shot' technique to try to determine palatal/lingual versus labial/buccal location of unerupted teeth in the dental alveolus. These images, however, are sometimes difficult to interpret.

The use of computed tomography (CT) with either direct images or reformatted images give additional information in alternative planes of space. Direct axial and coronal views will provide useful information as to the proximity of the unerupted tooth or teeth to adjacent anatomy and structures. Cone beam CT technology has resulted in more easily obtainable images in several viewing planes that allow the clinician to fully assess the unerupted tooth.

TREATMENT PLANNING

Once it is clinically determined that a tooth is present but unerupted, the surgeon must decide the benefits of removal compared to the risks associated with the difficulty of surgical removal, the surgical approach and the likelihood of potential complications. In some situations where the risks and potential complications are more frequent and/or severe than the benefit of tooth removal, a decision may be made to either remove a portion of the unerupted tooth, or to not attempt removal at all. If the surgeon and patient decide mutually that removal will not be performed based upon informed consent, there is an obligation to determine the need for continuous observation of a pathologic condition.

In general, the surgical approach with the least risk for complications is selected. An intra-oral approach is preferred in almost all situations as there is less risk for facial scarring and potential iatrogenic facial paralysis due to injury of the branches of the facial nerve. The least amount of disruption of normal maxillofacial tissues to obtain access to remove the unerupted tooth is the proper technique.

Consideration must be given to the clinical examination in hopes of determining the best surgical approach for removal. Complete palpation of the area of suspected unerupted tooth will give significant information as to the method of surgical approach. Any palpable tumescence will likely be the location of the erupted tooth. This technique is most useful in the anterior dentition.

Unerupted teeth lying in proximity to the branches of the second or third divisions of the trigeminal nerve harbour risk of partial or complete sensory deficit, and in some rare situations, dysesthesia. This risk is greatest with unerupted teeth approximating the inferior alveolar, lingual or mental nerve in the mandible.

Risk of mandibular fracture, either at the time of tooth removal or in the post-operative period, is of concern, especially in situations when a portion of the unerupted tooth contacts the inferior border of the mandible. The surgeon must be conscious of preserving as much normal tissue as possible to reduce the risk of fracture.

In the maxilla, there is risk of displacement of the unerupted tooth into the maxillary sinus or potential perforation into the maxillary sinus, which can result in a persistent opening that may require surgical closure if spontaneous closure and healing does not occur. There is also risk of tooth displacement into the nasal cavity in the anterior maxilla, which may result in persistent nasal oral communication requiring surgical closure.

There are also risks of damage to adjacent erupted functional teeth. Unerupted teeth located apical to erupted functional teeth may result in risk to tooth roots or preservation of tooth vitality with the surgical treatment. In some situations, consideration is given to removing teeth adjacent to the unerupted tooth to be removed for surgical access. Again, removing normal functional tissue for surgical access must be seriously considered before undertaking removal of an unerupted tooth that can be managed by observation or removed by an alternative route.

TECHNIQUE: GENERAL PRINCIPLES

When surgically removing unerupted teeth, the surgeon must remember to preserve as much normal tissue as possible for optimum dental health and function after healing. This requires attention to the preservation of soft tissues and in particular attached keratinized gingiva. This is especially important when approaching teeth in the anterior maxilla, as the tissues will be visible in a fully animated facial expression. The surgeon should also preserve alveolar bone as much as possible. This may require surgically dividing the unerupted tooth into many segments as opposed to removing bone to deliver the tooth in one or a few pieces. Surgical time is increased and technical prowess more demanding with this technique, but it will result in a better long-term outcome for the patient.

With preservation of tissues in mind, a major challenge to the removal of an unerupted tooth is a lack of visibility. Small incisions and limited exposure may result in longer and more challenging surgery. There should be a balance of adequate approach for visibility with preservation of normal tissues.

An additional rationale for the preservation of bone with surgical access is that if there is resultant loss of teeth in the dentition as result of removal of an unerupted tooth, reconstruction with a dental implant or implants is often the treatment of choice. Preservation of bone may allow future implant placement without the need for additional reconstructive regenerative surgical techniques and procedures, which can increase the cost and duration of the implant treatment.

INCISIONS

Maxilla

Incisions to develop and elevate flaps are dependent on the location and position of the unerupted tooth that is slated for removal. In the anterior maxilla between the first premolar teeth, named the 'aesthetic zone' as the facial soft tissues of the dental alveolus are many times visible with facial animation, there should be additional concern regarding tissue alterations, deficiency or scarring post-operatively. A sulcular incision around the cervical margins of the teeth allows the incision to be hidden and undetectable post-operatively. Vertical releasing incisions to increase exposure to the surgical site can be made distal to the canines and should extend from the mesial buccal or distobuccal line angles of the teeth to minimize loss of the dental papilla or formation of a double papilla, which can be unsightly.

An envelope flap technique without vertical releasing may be preferred, but will require a longer incision to obtain the same access as a flap with vertical release. This approach results in the least amount of detectable soft tissue scarring.

Muscosal incisions superior to the mucogingival junction may be made in the maxilla. Care must be given to avoid injury to the inferior orbital nerve in the canine/premolar area as it may result in sensory deficit to the upper lip. Mucosal incisions beyond the mucogingival junction in the posterior maxilla with perforation of the periosteum may result in the exposure of the buccal fat pad, which can result in limited visibility in this area.

If there is an unerupted tooth located to the palatal aspect of the maxilla, sulcular incisions can be used to expose the entire palate. Vertical releasing incisions may also be used. Vertical release in the maxillary second molar area could result in laceration of the greater palatine artery, which could result in profuse bleeding or flap necrosis. A vertical releasing incision in the anterior palatal midline should be avoided as it may disrupt the contents of the incisive canal.

Mandible

Sulcular and vertical releasing incisions can also be used with surgical approaches to the mandible. Long vertical releasing incisions or significant retraction force are contraindicated in the area of the mandibular premolar region as the mental nerve may be encountered which may result in sensory deficit and resultant anaesthesia or paraesthesia of the lower lip.

Surgical approaches to the posterior mandible in the area of the second and third molars must be performed with the utmost care and knowledge of the anatomic variability of the lingual nerve in relationship to the dental alveolus. Overzealous incision or excessive retraction can result in anaesthesia or paraesthesia of the tongue, which creates significant disability for most patients. There should never be lingual releasing incisions created in the posterior mandible.

Lingual approach to the mandible can again be obtained with sulcular incisions. Care must be given in the anterior lingual area so as to not disrupt the submandibular ducts and the lingual arteries.

In general in the mandible, a buccal or labial approach is preferred as the direct visibility is much greater that from the lingual approach. Preservation of papillae and concern about scarring is less important in the mandible as the tissues are not visible with normal facial animation or posture.

A combined buccal/labial and palatal/lingual approach is sometimes necessary for proper access.

OSTECTOMY AND REMOVAL

The surgeon should remove bone only as needed for visibility and removal of the tooth. Preservation of normal adjacent tissue is important. When deciding between sectioning of the tooth versus removal of more adjacent bone, the tooth should be sectioned.

A pretreatment plan for the sectioning of the tooth if necessary should be formulated with the use of the available imaging and the result of the clinical examination. In general, a portion of the unerupted tooth, which is most accessible, is removed first. This is usually the crown. With multirooted teeth, it may be necessary to remove the crown first and then remove each root individually.

Small root tip elevators or picks are useful to create space between the surface of the tooth and the adjacent bone. The surgeon must use delicate technique, as force may result in displacement of the remaining tooth segment(s) into an adjacent body cavity or space, such as the maxillary sinus, the nasal cavity, the submandibular space or the inferior alveolar nerve canal.

Coronectomy or removal of the crown of the unerupted tooth, with the intention of leaving tooth roots in place, is a technique that can be used if complete tooth removal presents high risk for severe complications. This technique should be considered, planned and discussed with the patient before it is attempted or undertaken.

With the use of rotary instrumentation, irrigation must also be used. Constant irrigation while drilling cleanses the burr for more efficient cutting, and will help to prevent overheating of adjacent bone that could result in necrosis and delayed healing.

AFTER REMOVAL OF THE TOOTH

After removal of the tooth, the socket should be examined for potential residual or unexpected root tips and residual soft tissue, including the dental follicle or remnants of it. If there is persistent ooze or bleeding from the site, topical haemostatic agents may be used.

If the unerupted tooth is located in the anterior maxilla or if there is a potential for implant reconstruction, preservation of the socket may be necessary. This can be done by inserting a graft or implant after the tooth removal. In general, however, if the residual bone is adequate and/or no implant reconstruction is planned, and there is no additional pathology that has resulted in resorption of a significant amount of bone, there is rarely a need for bone graft reconstruction following removal of unerupted teeth.

The tissue flaps are generally reapproximated and sutured. Post-operative course should be observed if there is expectation of complications.

2.3

Nerve injuries and repair

JOHN ZUNIGA, ANDREW BG TAY

PRINCIPLES AND JUSTIFICATION

Trigeminal nerve injuries may occur from third molar surgery, local anaesthetic injections, orthognathic surgery, maxillofacial trauma, implant surgery or pathology surgery, and most often involve the inferior alveolar nerve, the lingual nerve and the infraorbital nerve. Nerve repair is indicated where the nerve injury is significant (Sunderland IV or V degree injury), demonstrated either by direct visual inspection or by clinical neurosensory testing or adjunctive testing (i.e. magnetic resonance neurography, trigeminal nerve conduction, chemosensory testing, etc.). Repair should be carried out at the earliest opportunity under microscopic magnification by a trained microsurgeon. (Although no standard exists for training in microneurosurgery of the trigeminal nerve, suggested standards for training in microsurgery exist and include a minimum 40+ hours of didactic courses and laboratory experience including the successful anastomoses of ten arteries, ten veins and ten neural repairs. A trained microneurosurgeon should serve as first assistant to an experienced microneurosurgeon in at least three cases and then serve as primary surgeon in six cases.)

INDICATIONS

- Witnessed nerve injury from third molar surgery, orthognathic surgery (e.g. sagittal split osteotomy), implant surgery or mandibular or maxillary trauma.
- Non-witnessed nerve injury with persistent severe or complete sensory impairment for approximately three to six months from third molar surgery, orthognathic surgery (e.g. sagittal split osteotomy), implant surgery or mandibular or maxillary trauma.
- Chemical nerve injury (e.g. endodontic irrigation accident).
- Neuropathic pain.

PRE-OPERATIVE

Anaesthesia

The operation is performed under general anaesthesia with nasoendotracheal intubation. The throat is packed with moist ribbon gauze and the endotracheal tube secured. Microneurosurgery is difficult to perform under local anaesthesia owing to movements of the awake patient being magnified under the microscope, and requires a longer operating time than can be afforded by deep sedation.

OPERATION

Position of patient

The patient is laid supine on the operating table and turned to keep the anaesthetic machine at about the waist level of the patient. The patient should be positioned in a way to allow two surgeons to sit on either side of the patient's head with an operating microscope over the patient's head. The microsurgeons must be seated comfortably during the microsurgical phase of the procedure. Therefore, if the motor base of the operating table does not rotate free from the table, the patient should be positioned with the head at the foot end of the operating table. This affords the microsurgeons the freedom to sit with their legs under the operating table. The face around the mouth and the oral cavity is cleansed. A head drape is used. If a nerve graft site has been identified prior to surgery, the selected location is prepared and draped for access. An operating microscope with two operator eyepieces should be available; the microscope focal distance is set at 250 mm with the zoom at mid-range. The operator eyepieces should be adjusted to suit the surgeons and draped. If available, video camera feed from the operating microscope is useful for recording and allowing other team members to see the procedure. Microsurgery in the oral cavity requires longer microsurgical instruments, usually around 18 cm length and preferably of the bayonet design. Bipolar diathermy and two separate suction tubings should be available.

For lingual nerve surgery, the operating surgeon sits on the same side of the operation site. For inferior alveolar nerve or infraorbital nerve surgery, the surgeon sits on the opposite side as the operation. Local anaesthetic with epinephrine (adrenaline) is given as an inferior alveolar nerve block and infiltrated around the operative site.

Lingual nerve repair

ACCESS

The patient's head is kept central and a modified Dingman mouthgag is inserted to position the mouth open, using the tongue blade to keep the tongue from the operative site. Penny towels are used to prop up the Dingman handle (Figure 2.3.1). The modified Dingman should not be left in this position but removed, if there is a need to move away from the oral cavity for a time (e.g. to harvest a sural nerve graft) so as to avoid prolonged pressure and ulceration of the oral tissues.

An intraoral mucosal incision is made with a No. 15 Bard-Parker scalpel over the ascending ramus to the distal of the mandibular second molar. A buccal extension is made from the distal of the molar to the buccal sulcus, and a lingual extension is made to the lingual sulcus curving forward up to the mandibular first molar (Figure 2.3.2). The buccal and lingual mucosal flaps are raised supraperiosteally using a periosteal elevator and Metzenbaum curved dissecting scissors, and secured to the modified Dingman frame with 3/0 or 4/0 black silk sutures (Figure 2.3.3). Suction of the operative site is provided using a fine Frazier suction.

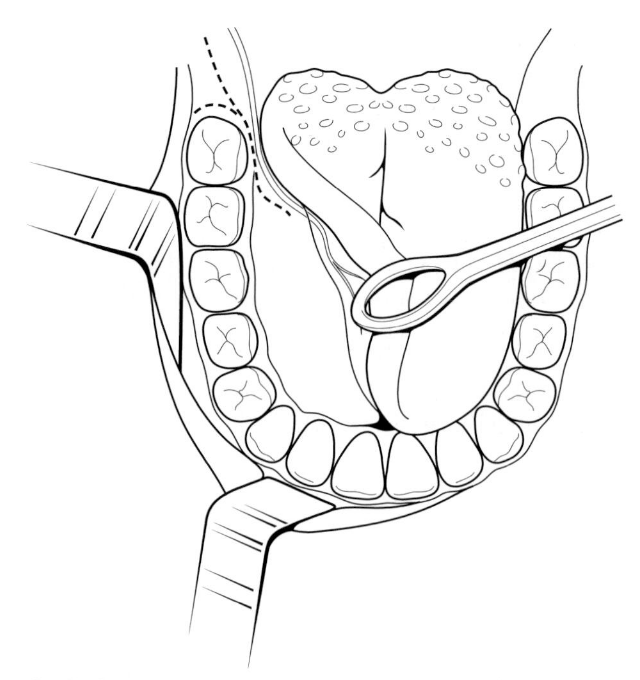

2.3.2 Supraperiosteal incision to access the lingual nerve.

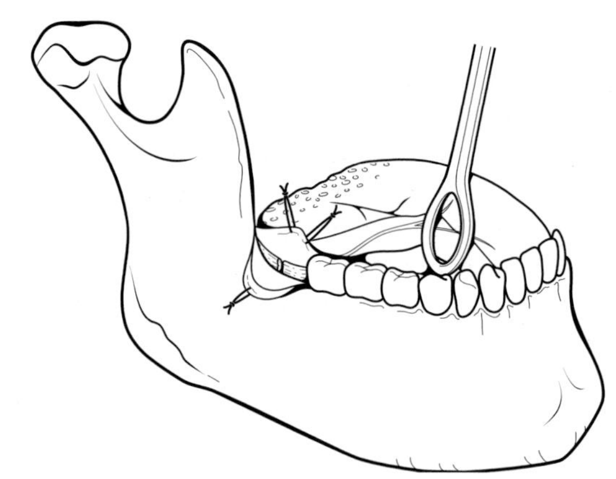

2.3.3 Supraperiosteal flaps are reflected and secured to the Dingman retractor for access to the lingual nerve.

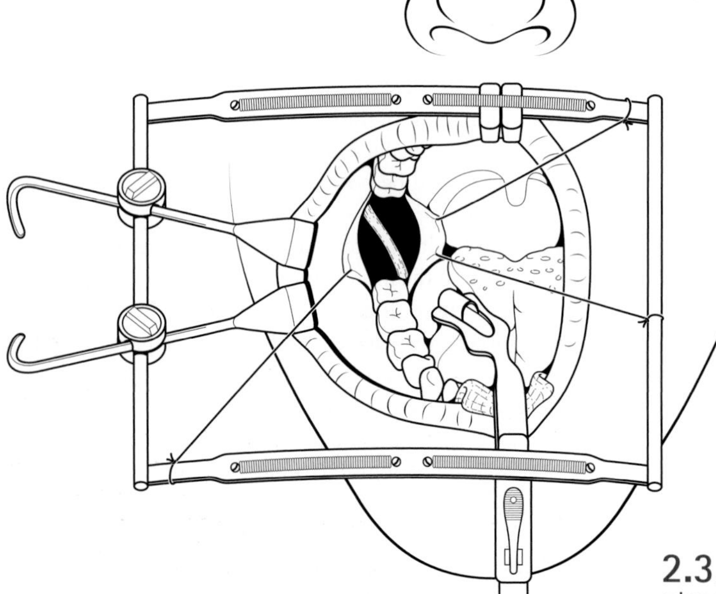

2.3.1 Modified Dingman retractor for lingual nerve microsurgical repair access.

PREPARATION

The operating microscope is brought into the operative field and positioned. The lingual nerve is located and exposed beginning at healthy nerve proximal and distal to the injury site; the lingual nerve is often found in a pouch of fat. The exposed proximal and distal nerve segments are carefully retracted with vessel loops, one proximal and one distal to the injury site (Figure 2.3.4). The injury site is often adherent to the lingual aspect of the mandible, and is released with careful microdissection using curved microscissors.

A modified background is placed beneath the released nerve. The background is made by sharply cutting the luer-lock end of the small gauge butterfly venipuncture system and then advancing this cut end through a tunnel created in a 1×1-inch neuropatty and then securing the tubing within the neuropatty with silk suture. The neuropatty is then placed beneath the nerve at the injury site, and the needle end of the modified butterfly venipuncture system is inserted into the lumen of an active suction tubing. The nerve is examined under microscopic magnification (25×). The injury may be a complete transection with a neuroma at the end of each nerve segment, or a partial transection with a neuroma in continuity. The neuroma is carefully excised with straight microscissors and the nerve ends trimmed to expose the fascicular surfaces with periodic irrigation with heparin-saline (Figure 2.3.5). A 6/0 or 7/0 monofilament suture is passed into the epineurium of each segment to the adjacent muscle and used to approximate the nerve segments together to facilitate repair without undue tension. If the nerve segments cannot be coapted without tension (approximately 1 cm or more of nerve gap), a nerve graft will be necessary.

MICROSUTURE

The trimmed nerve endings are coapted, using the vasa nervorum as a guide aligning the nerve segments. Using an 8/0 or 9/0 monofilament on a cutting needle, the first suture is placed at the 12 o'clock position; a longer strand is left. Further sutures are placed in similar manner at the 4 and 8 o'clock positions (Figure 2.3.6).

The nerve may be 'flipped over' holding the suture strands with microforceps. The intervening gaps in the coaptation site are closed with circumferential sutures placed at regular intervals around the nerve; usually six to eight sutures may be required.

The repaired nerve is examined and any excess suture is trimmed. The approximating suture and then the background are carefully removed.

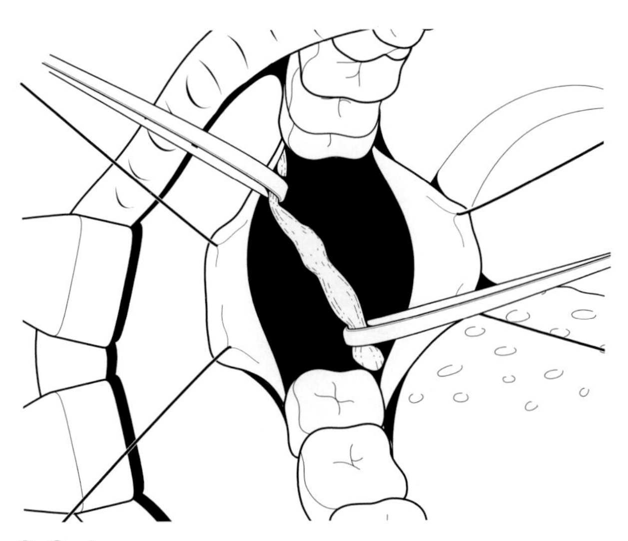

2.3.4 Retraction of proximal and distal LN with vessel loops to access LN injury site.

WOUND CLOSURE

The microscope is moved out of the operative field. The black silk sutures retracting the buccal and lingual mucosal flaps are released and removed. The operative site is irrigated

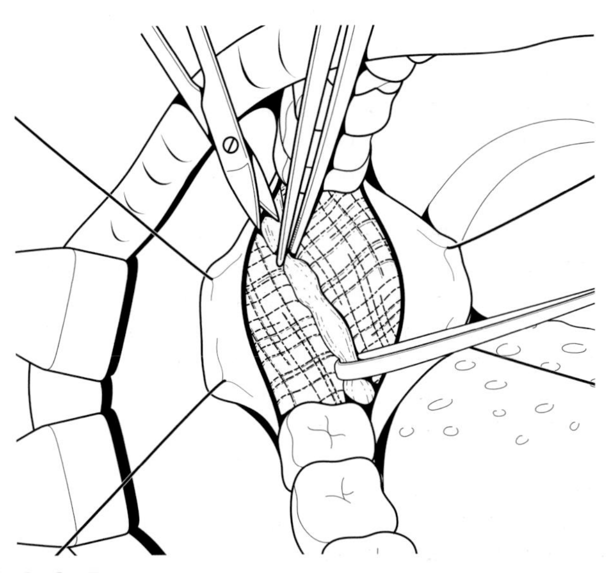

2.3.5 LN on modified background in preparation for repair.

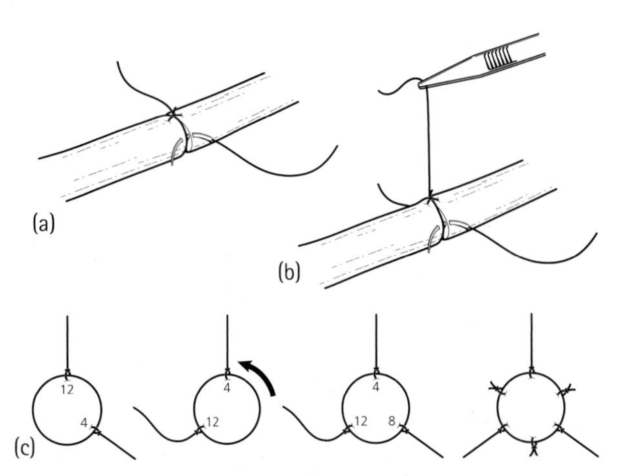

2.3.6 Microsuture sequence of neurorrhaphy. The first suture is placed at the 12 o'clock position, followed by the second suture at the 4 o'clock position (a). These sutures are left long to provide a holding point. The nerve is rotated to expose the underside surface, where the third suture is placed at the 8 o'clock position (b). The nerve repair is completed by placing other sutures in between the first three sutures (c, right).

with saline. The mucosal flaps are replaced and closed with 4/0 Vicryl interrupted sutures.

The modified Dingman mouth gag and then the throat pack is removed. The patient is reversed and extubated by the anaesthetist.

Inferior alveolar nerve repair

ACCESS

The patient's head may be turned to the side opposite the operation site. An incision is made just above the mandibular buccal sulcus from the midline of the lower lip posteriorly to the ascending ramus, using a No. 15 B-P scalpel. A subperiosteal flap is raised exposing the mandible from the alveolus to the inferior border, including the mental foramen, taking care to preserve the mental nerve.

A small round bur is used to create grooves radiating outwards from the mental foramen, then joined to form windows in the buccal cortical bone. The bone windows are carefully fractured with either a Coupland or Warwick–James elevator, taking care to avoid the mental nerve. Windows are created in a similar manner over the course of the inferior alveolar nerve from anterior to posterior, bearing in mind the downward and backward turn made by the nerve before it exits the mental foramen (Figure 2.3.7). The inferior alveolar nerve is exposed to 1 cm beyond the site of injury; the incisive branch is sharply divided with a scalpel and the inferior alveolar nerve is carefully dissected free from its bed (Figure 2.3.8).

PREPARATION

The operating microscope is brought into the operative field and positioned. The proximal and distal nerve segments are lifted from the mandibular bone with a nerve hook, and a modified neuropatty background is placed beneath the nerve segments. The nerve is examined under microscopic magnification. The injury may be a complete transection or a partial transection with a neuroma in continuity.

The neuroma is carefully excised with straight microscissors and the nerve ends trimmed to expose the fascicular surfaces with periodic irrigation with heparin-saline. If necessary, a 6/0 or 7/0 monofilament suture passed through the epineurium of each segment and used to approximate the nerve segments together to facilitate repair without undue tension. As the distal nerve is transposed towards the proximal, a nerve graft will usually not be necessary.

MICROSUTURE

The trimmed nerve endings are coapted, using the vasa nervorum as a guide aligning the nerve segments. Using an 8/0 or 9/0 monofilament on a cutting needle, the first suture is placed at the 12, 4 and 8 o'clock positions; a longer strand is left at each suture to facilitate further placement of sutures (Figure 2.3.6). The intervening gaps in the coaptation site are closed with circumferential sutures placed at regular intervals around the nerve; usually six to eight sutures may be required. The result is repositioning of the distal nerve segment so that the mental nerve is positioned posteriorly to the original foramen to avoid a nerve graft (Figure 2.3.9).

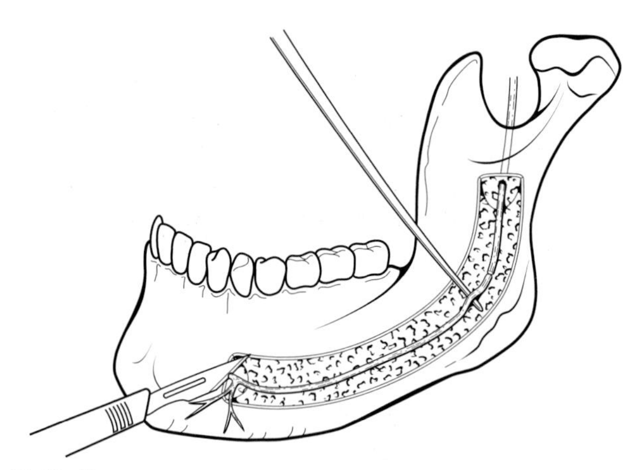

2.3.8 Incisive nerve division with a scalpel, lateralization of the inferior alveolar nerve and preparation of the nerve injury (nerve hook).

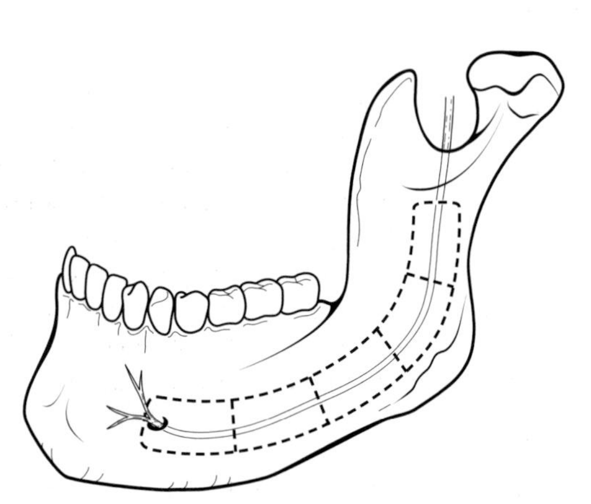

2.3.7 Lateral decortication to expose the inferior alveolar nerve.

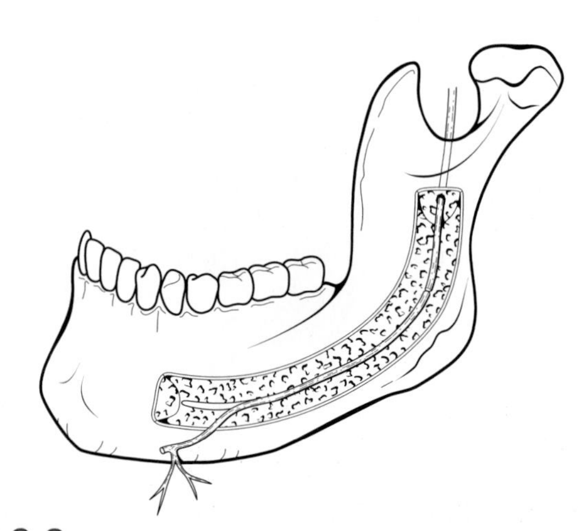

2.3.9 Transposition of the mental nerve posteriorly for completion of the inferior alveolar nerve repair.

The repaired nerve is examined and any excess suture is trimmed. The approximating suture and then the background are carefully removed. Gelfoam is sometimes placed around the nerve and the nerve is replaced in its bed.

WOUND CLOSURE

The microscope is moved out of the operative field. The operative site is irrigated with saline. The mucosal flap is replaced and closed with 4/0 Vicryl interrupted sutures.

The throat pack is removed and the patient is reversed and extubated by the anaesthetist.

Infraorbital nerve repair

ACCESS

Two approaches are used for microneurosurgical repair of the infraorbital nerve. A *cutaneous approach* is used when the site of injury is proximal to the infraorbital foramen. An *intraoral approach* is used when the site of the injury is close to or distal to the infraorbital foramen.

1. The globe is protected with a temporary tarsorrhaphy using 4/0 silk suture or a scleral shell. The subciliary incision line is drawn with a skin marker approximately 2 mm inferior to the eyelashes along the length of the lower eyelid. The incision may be extended laterally to 2 cm beyond the lateral canthus, curving inferio-laterally following a natural skin crease. The incision line is infiltrated with local anaesthetic with epinephrine. The subciliary incision is made with a No. 15 Bard–Parker scalpel to the subcutaneous layer, until the underlying orbicularis oculi muscle is visible. Sharp curved scissors are used for subcutaneous dissection for a few millimetres inferiorly toward the inferior orbital rim. Scissors are used to dissect through the orbicularis oculi muscle to the periosteum overlying the inferior orbital rim, reaching the plane between the muscle and septum orbitale. The skin–muscle flap of tissue is elevated from the lower eyelid and retracted inferiorly. The periosteum over the inferior orbital rim is incised with a No. 15 Bard–Parker scalpel a few millimetres below the edge of the rim. The periosteum is elevated with a periosteal elevator until the infraorbital foramen is reached, usually located 7–9 mm inferior to the inferior orbital rim.
2. An intraoral vestibular incision is made in the unattached mucosa of the maxillary vertibule from the midline to the zygomatic process. The nerve is exposed via a subperiosteal dissection. The infraorbital nerve immediately branches into up to ten branches at the foramen.

A small round bur is used to create a groove around the infraorbital foramen. The bone around the foramen is carefully removed with Rongeur forceps. The infraorbital canal is carefully unroofed exposing the infraorbital nerve until 1 cm beyond the injury site, and may reach the orbital floor (Figure 2.3.10).

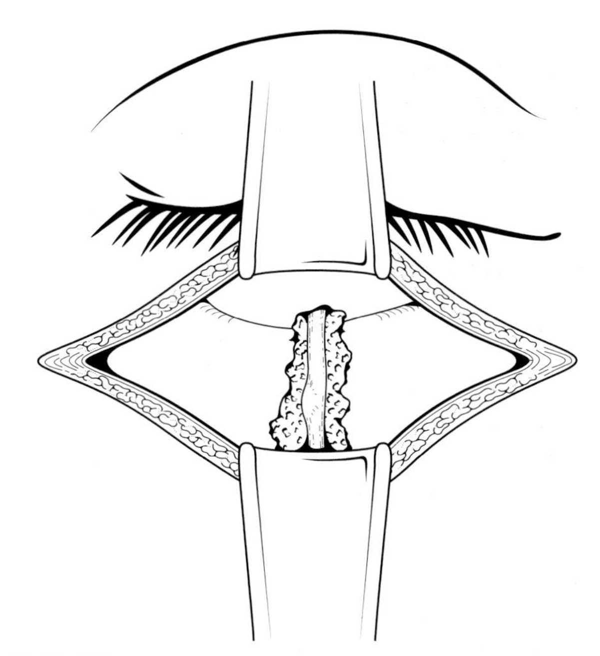

2.3.10 Transcutaneous approach to access injury of the infraorbital nerve.

PREPARATION

The operating microscope is brought into the operative field and positioned. The proximal and distal nerve segments are lifted from the bone with a nerve hook, and a modified neuropatty background is placed beneath the nerve segments. The nerve is examined under microscopic magnification. The injury may be a complete transection or a partial transection with a neuroma in continuity.

The neuroma is carefully excised with straight microscissors and the nerve ends trimmed to expose the fascicular surfaces with periodic irrigation with heparin-saline. An approximating suture using 6/0 or 7/0 monofilament is passed through the epineurium of each segment and used to approximate the nerve segments together to facilitate repair without undue tension.

MICROSUTURE

The trimmed nerve endings are coapted, using the vasa nervorum as a guide aligning the nerve segments. Using an 8/0 or 9/0 monofilament on a cutting needle, sutures are placed at the 12, 4 and 8 o'clock positions (Figure 2.3.6). Circumferential sutures are placed at regular intervals around the nerve; usually six to eight sutures may be required.

The repaired nerve is examined and any excess suture is trimmed. The approximating suture and then the background are carefully removed (Figure 2.3.11). Gelfoam may be placed around the nerve and the nerve is replaced in its bed.

WOUND CLOSURE

The microscope is moved out of the operative field. The operative site is irrigated with saline. The periosteum is closed with 4/0 silk sutures, and the skin–muscle flap is

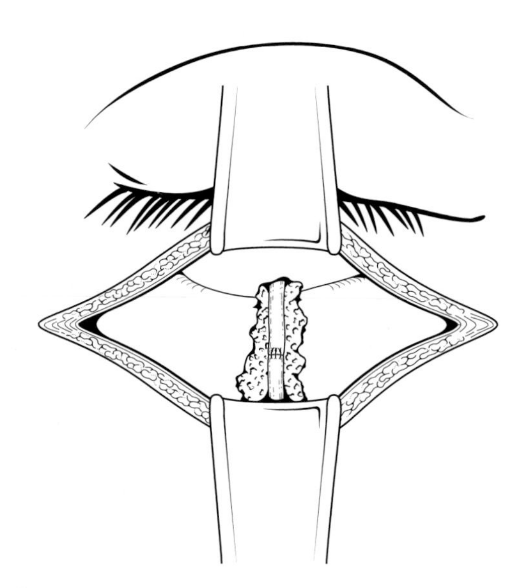

2.3.11 Infraorbital nerve microsuture repair *in situ.*

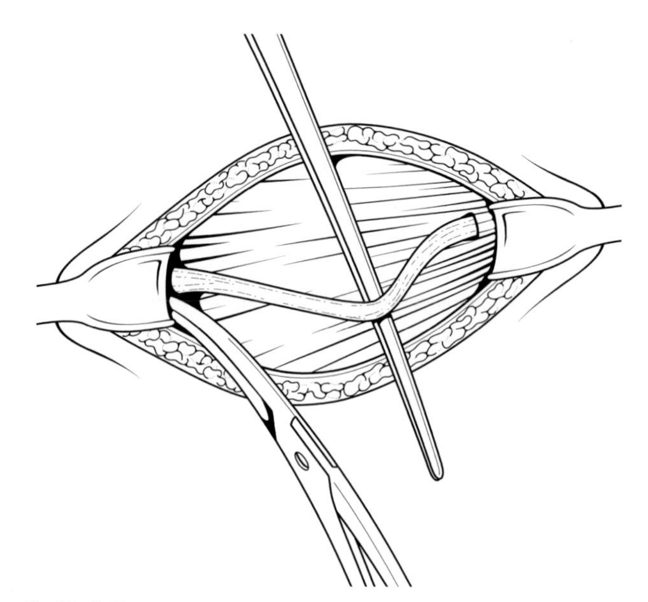

2.3.12 Sural nerve is lateralized.

replaced and closed with 4/0 silk interrupted sutures or a running 6/0 non-resorbable suture. The patient is reversed and extubated by the anaesthetist.

Sural nerve graft

The sural nerve remains the 'workhorse' of autogenous nerve graft applications in trigeminal nerve repair. Alternative autogenous nerve graft locations are the greater auricular and medial antebrachial cutaneous nerves. The sural nerve is easily harvested by a 2-cm curvilinear incision one finger breadth distal and superior to the lateral malleolus of the ankle. The sural nerve, the small saphenous vein and artery are within the subcutaneous tissues of the lateral leg and are superior to the fascia of the posterior tibialis muscle. The nerve is isolated from the vein and artery using vessel loops and dissected as far distally and proximally as possible (Figure 2.3.12). The most distal end is transected sharply and the sural nerve exteriorized to determine the length required for adequate grafting of the lingual or inferior alveolar nerve (Figure 2.3.13). If greater length is required, a second incision above and parallel to the first is made until the adequate length of nerve is obtained. At least 1 cm of proximal nerve is spared so that after harvesting, the proximal stump can be repositioned into the muscle to avoid painful neuroma formation. This is accomplished by creating a small 'trap door' access through the posterior tibialis fascia to expose the muscle and then suturing the proximal stump of the sural nerve against muscle using resorbable suture, closing the fascia over the stump and completing the skin closure (Figure 2.3.14). The wound is then dressed and supported with an elastic gauze bandage (Ace bandage). Non-weight bearing crutches are provided. The patient is instructed to change the bandage daily to avoid compression for 1 week. Non-weight bearing activity is enforced for 2 weeks after which sutures are removed.

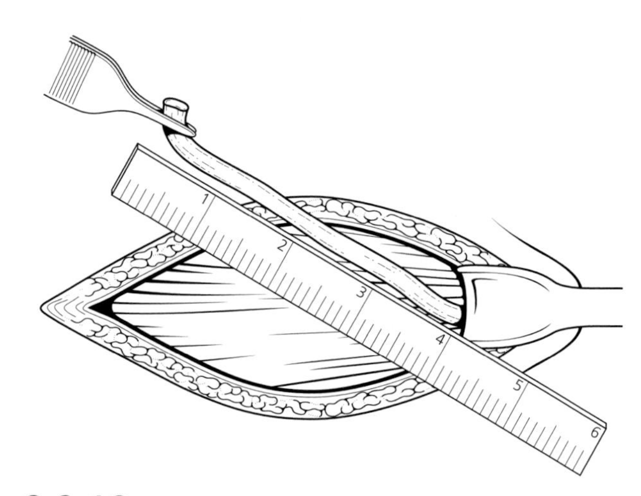

2.3.13 Sural nerve is exteriorized to determine its length.

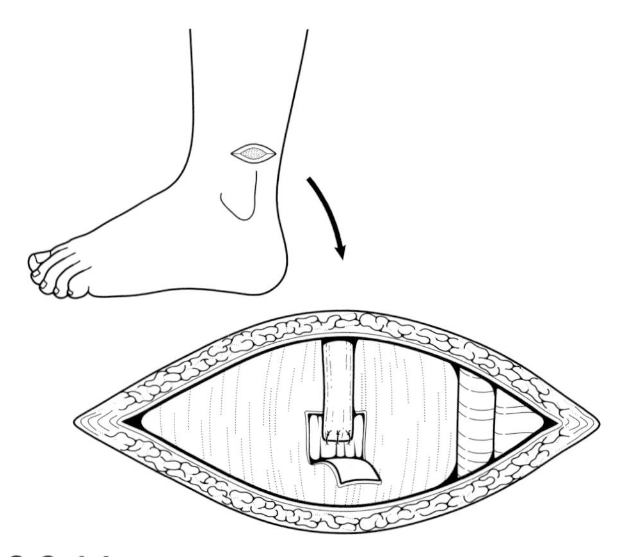

2.3.14 Sural nerve stump connected to muscle under fascial trapdoor.

POST-OPERATIVE CARE

A gauze pack may be placed over the operative site intraorally. The patient is transferred to the post-operative anaesthesia care unit and may either be allowed home or admitted to the ward overnight. Analgesia and chlorhexidine mouth rinse is prescribed; post-operative wound care instructions are provided. Adjunctive medication for neuropathic pain should be continued if these have been in use pre-operatively. The patient is followed up 7–10 days later and may be given instructions for sensory retraining which can begin immediately and continued for up to one year after surgery. Mandibular range of motion should be normal by one month. Clinical neurosensory testing can begin three months after surgery since the first statistical indicator of regeneration occurs no sooner than 6–8 weeks post-operatively in half the patients. Sensory regeneration should be complete by one year in the majority of patients so that discharge should occur after the one year follow-up time. Exceptions to this rule occur due to age, location of injury and degree of injury. Older patients, more distal injuries (mental nerve versus inferior alveolar nerve), complete transection injuries requiring nerve grafts are expected to reach maximum regeneration over longer times (beyond one year).

COMPLICATIONS

- Intraoperative bleeding
- Infection
- Pathologic fracture of the mandible
- Wound dehiscence
- Trismus
- Inability to locate one nerve segment
- Neuropathic pain
- Neuroma formation in nerve graft donor site.

Top tips

- Position the patient appropriately before commencing surgery so that the microsurgeons are comfortable throughout the procedure.
- Demagnetize the microsurgical instruments before surgery.
- Use an operating microscope that has two viewing ports and a video feed.
- Use a neuropatty with suction via a butterfly cannula as background.
- Irrigate the nerve repair site with heparin-saline during neurorrhaphy.

FURTHER READING

Epker BN, Gregg JM. Surgical management of maxillary nerve injuries. *Oral and Maxillofacial Surgery Clinics of North America* 1992; **2**: 439–45.

Gregg JM. Surgical management of lingual nerve injuries. *Oral and Maxillofacial Surgery Clinics of North America* 1992; **4**: 417–24.

LaBanc JP, Van Boven RW. Surgical management of inferior alveolar nerve injuries. *Oral and Maxillofacial Surgery Clinics of North America* 1992; **4**: 425–37.

Wolford LM. Autogenous nerve graft repairs of the trigeminal nerve. *Oral and Maxillofacial Surgery Clinics of North America* 1992; **4**: 459–63.

Zuniga JR, Essick GK. A contemporary approach to the clinical evaluation of trigeminal nerve injuries. *Oral and Maxillofacial Surgery Clinics of North America* 1992; **4**: 353–67.

2.4

Surgical endodontics

HELEN SPENCER

INTRODUCTION

Surgical endodontics aims to treat microbial infection of the tooth and peri-radicular tissues which persist following conventional orthograde treatment.

Surgical procedures include apical curettage, apicectomy (root end resection) usually in association with retrograde root filling, lateral perforation repair, root resection and hemisection. Root resection and hemisection will not be considered in detail, but the surgical principles are broadly similar.

The most frequently performed procedure is apicectomy with retrograde root filling following unsuccessful orthograde treatment.

It must be remembered that re-root treatment is the gold standard treatment in most cases and surgery should be considered only when more conservative treatment is not possible or appropriate (Table 2.4.1).

Presurgical assessment must ensure that retention of a surgically treated tooth is appropriate to the long-term dental health of the patient. The teeth listed for surgery should be restored with a successful coronal seal. Any extra-coronal restorations should not have a history of decementation. The vitality of adjacent non-endodontically treated teeth and mobility and periodontal pocketing of teeth in the surgical area may influence the outcome of surgery. Peri-apical radiographs must be available for teeth involved in surgery; they should be taken using a paralleling technique to enable root length determination. Panoral films may be necessary to demonstrate the extent of larger lesions.

The microbial invasion of most peri-radicular lesions can alter the clinical picture in a short period of time and these signs should be reassessed just prior to surgery.

SUCCESS RATES

Success rates have been shown to increase with recent advances in technique, including root-end resection without a bevel, the use of ultrasonics for root-end cavity preparation and the move away from amalgam as the restorative material of choice. Previously success rates of between 50 and 80 per cent were quoted, with highest success rates for upper anterior teeth. Full radiographic

Table 2.4.1 Indications and contraindications for surgery.

Indications/ contraindications	
Indications	Failed conventional orthograde treatment where repeat treatment is either not possible, appropriate or unsuccessful
	Canals unable to be instrumented fully by orthograde approach, for developmental or iatrogenic reasons
	Biopsy of peri-radicular lesion required
	Visualization of the root surface required (suspected root fracture)
	Root sectioning or amputation required
Contraindications	Anatomical, including root morphology, proximity to neurovascular bundle, access
	Subsequent successful and suitably aesthetic restoration not possible
	Periodontally compromised
	Unsuccessful surgery would compromise subsequent replacement
	Patient factors, including medical and social

healing is now being reported in more than 90 per cent of cases, with most studies suggesting over 80 per cent with full healing at one year. This improvement in initial outcome is likely to reduce the need for repeat surgery.

Unsuccessful apical surgery will reduce the volume of bone available for osseointegration. Repeat surgery may compromise or complicate future implant placement in the area.

PRE-OPERATIVELY

Provide chlorhexidene 2 per cent mouthwash to reduce the oral bacterial load. A pre-operative dose of non-steroidal analgesics can be provided for suitable patients. Some clinicians commence this regime 24 hours prior to surgery.

Magnification should be used to improve visualization of the lesion and root apex.

ANAESTHESIA

Whilst extensive lesions may require general anaesthesia, the majority of patients will be treated under local anaesthesia and will leave the surgery following a short recovery period. Regional local anaesthetic blocks, where possible, are to be recommended. The vasoconstriction provided by local infiltration in addition to either a regional block or general anaesthesia is advised for all patients. Topical benzocaine gel prior to lidocaine 2 per cent with epinephrine 1:80 000 will minimize the pain of administration of anaesthesia.

FLAP DESIGN

All the flaps described are full thickness mucoperiosteal, with the incision perpendicular to the mucosal surface in all areas other than the gingival sulcus where the scalpel is placed within the gingival crevice incising from the base of the pocket to the crest of the alveolar bone. Relieving incisions should not cross an eminence or divide a fraenal attachment as this will increase tension on the replaced flap (Figures 2.4.1 and 2.4.2)

The need to avoid the mental foramen and nerve will indicate the position of a relieving incision in the lower premolar and first molar region.

Flaps involving the gingival margin

The post-operative gingival recession is most relevant in the anterior region. An alteration to the emergence profile, especially in the presence of crown or bridge margins, may lead to failure of the apicectomy for aesthetic reasons.

For this reason, flaps which do not involve the gingival margin or gingival papilla are increasingly utilized (Table 2.4.2).

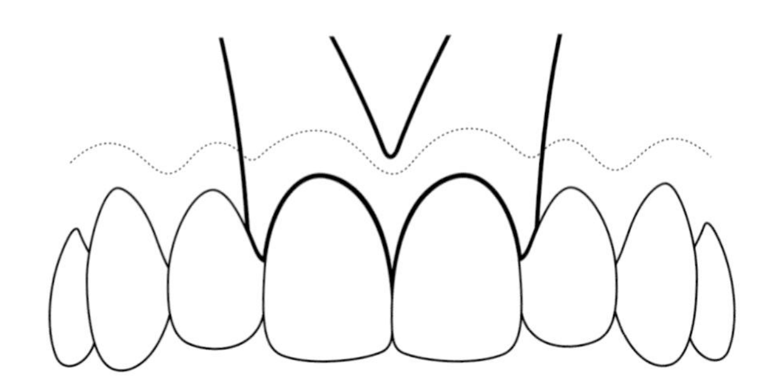

2.4.1 Three-sided flap (rectangular or rhomboid). Relieving incisions vertical, following orientation of vascular supply. Extend horizontally at least one tooth mesial or distal to the affected tooth providing a wide enough base to ensure adequate blood supply. When the upper central incisor is to be apicected, the flap should include the midline fraenum rather than dividing it vertically.

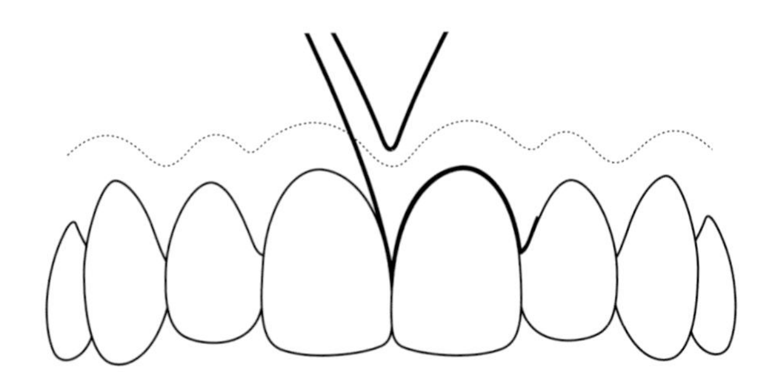

2.4.2 Two-sided or triangular flap. No distal relieving incision. Provides adequate access posteriorly and often sufficient anteriorly, especially if access to the apex is not required, e.g. lateral perforation repair. Can be extended to three-sided if greater access is found to be necessary. Again the fraenum or eminence should not be crossed with a relieving incision.

Table 2.4.2 Advantages and disadvantages of gingival margin flaps.

Advantages/ disadvantages	
Advantages	Excellent access, enabling visualization of full length of root/overlying bone
	Advantageous where lesion does not originate apically, or extends coronally beyond the area exposed by other designs of flap
	Good access for perforation repair, root resection and hemisection
	Horizontal element does not divide labial vessels, possibly improving visibility and reducing post-operative swelling
	Straightforward, uses technique routine in dentoalveolar surgery
Disadvantages	Gingival recession occurs post-operatively.

Flaps not involving the gingival margin

These include Luebke–Oschenbein (Figure 2.4.3), horizontal, vertical, semilunar and flaps utilizing microsurgical techniques, such as the papilla base incision.

This flap removes the risk of post-operative gingival recession, provides adequate access to the apex of the tooth and is easily replaced. The horizontal incision lies within the attached mucosa and follows the scalloped contour of the gingival margin. Literature suggests a minimum of 2 mm of attached mucosa coronally to the horizontal incision to minimize the risk of papillary necrosis, 4 mm is often more practical. Healing is compromised if periodontal bone loss extends apically or the lesion coronally beyond the horizontal incision. Placement of the vertical incision is as for gingival margin flaps. This flap was described as three sided, but may not require the second relieving incision. When treating a purely apical lesion and there is adequate height of unattached mucosa overlying the apex of the tooth, a similar flap may be raised wholly within the unattached mucosa. The slight increase in bleeding is minimized by infiltrating a vasoconstrictor containing local anaesthetic pre-operatively.

Other flaps not involving the gingival margin

Single horizontal and vertical incisions are used by some operators. The absence of a relieving incision minimizes access and for some small localized lesions this access may provide a successful result. The semilunar flap has the disadvantages of flaps without relieving incisions and its curvature can make retraction difficult and closure unpredictable and is not to be recommended.

Papilla base incisions and other microsurgical techniques are described in the recommended texts.

Procedure

Flaps are raised with fine periosteal elevators. In areas where the soft tissue of the lesion has perforated the bone, careful dissection is necessary to elevate the overlying mucosal flap without perforation.

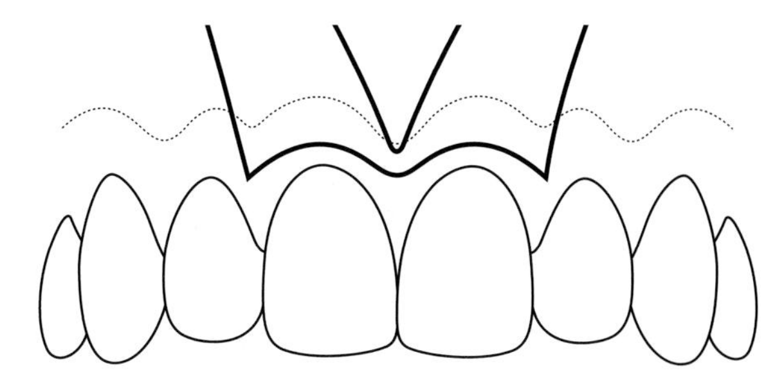

2.4.3 Luebke-Oschenbein flap.

Tissues should be retracted with an instrument such as a Cawood Minnesota retractor. This non-toothed retractor is wide enough to provide access and protect the labial soft tissues. If a lengthy procedure is expected, ensure that the flap does not desiccate. The author achieves this by placing saline-soaked gauze between the flap and retractor.

If there is no bone fenestration, the apex of the tooth is exposed by removal of bone using an irrigated round bur. The starting point may be identified by probing the bone surface with a sharp instrument to identify an area of thinning, and by estimating the length and alignment of the tooth from the pre-operative peri-apical radiograph. The true long axis may be disguised in a crowned tooth. From the initial point of entry, the bone window is increased to give sufficient access to perform the root-end resection and curette the soft tissue from the entirety of the defect. The position of the inferior alveolar canal and its upward curve to the mental foramen should be kept in mind during bone removal for apical surgery involving lower molar and premolar teeth.

The soft tissue is removed using curettes, dental excavators and gauze pellets. Similar gauze pellets may also be useful in removing the lesion from palatal mucosa where bony fenestration has occurred. It is not possible to determine clinically whether granulation tissue present is part of the destructive or reparative process, and it may be appropriate to retain tenacious granulation tissue rather than instrument the root surface of an adjacent tooth or remove more hard tissue to provide access. The soft tissue removed should be preserved for histological evaluation.

Root-end resection

The apex of the tooth is resected, using a straight bur, perpendicular to the long axis of the tooth to minimize the number of exposed dentinal tubules. Dentinal tubules allow communication between untreated contaminated areas of the root canal system and the peri-apical tissues. The level of the resection should be sufficient to remove the portion of the root canal system identified pre-operatively as potentially harbouring micro-organisms, usually 3–4 mm. It is not necessary to resect the root at the base of the cavity as this will expose a larger dentinal surface and reduce the remaining root length for restoration and stability. The orthograde root filling will usually be exposed by the resection. If mineral trioxide aggregate (MTA) has been used for the orthograde filling, no root-end preparation is necessary.

The root-end cavity is prepared using contra-angled surgical ultrasonic tips. These are preferred over rotary instruments as correctly angled cavity preparation is easier and there is a reduced risk of fractures forming within the retained tooth tissue. The preparation must encompass the width of the root canal system and have a minimum depth of 3 mm for adequate restoration (Figure 2.4.4).

The current retrograde filling materials of choice are MTA or modified zinc oxide eugenol cements (IRM, which includes polymethacrylate, or Super EBA, which includes

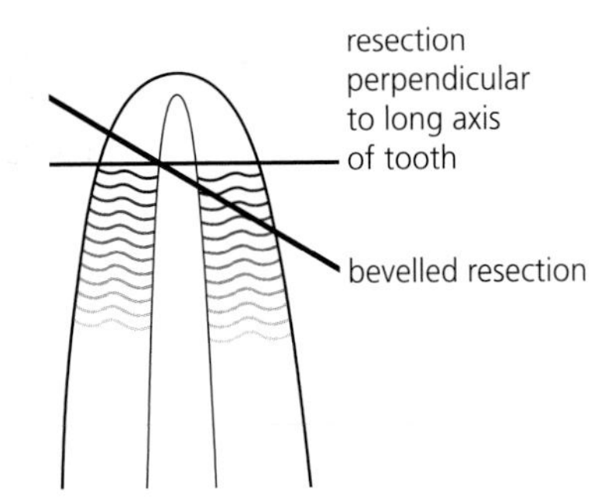

2.4.4 Root-end resection. Resection perpendicular to the long axis of the tooth.

ethoxybenzoic acid). These materials have been shown to be more successful than amalgam, which has the added disadvantage of tattooing adjacent soft tissues in some patients. Only MTA stimulates hard tissue deposition in direct contact with the filling material.

Some clinicians advocate the use of 0.5-inch ribbon gauze with or without a vasoconstrictor placed within the bony defect prior to placement of the retrograde filling to aid haemostasis and facilitate removal of excess filling material from the cavity.

The prepared cavity is dried with paper points and gauze pledgets or gentle air spray.

The filling material is mixed according to the manufacturers' instructions and placed into the prepared cavity using specially designed carriers, small pluggers and flat plastic instruments. Excess MTA is wiped away using damp cotton wool. The restoration should be adequately condensed and burnished for best results. The defect is irrigated to remove debris and the flap is repositioned and sutured. When early review is possible, 5/0 synthetic monofilament sutures are preferred. If this is not possible, vicryl rapide is recommended. Single interrupted sutures are used, however, and where a gingival margin flap has been raised, suspensory sutures can be placed.

Following suturing, pressure should be placed on to the flap using a moistened gauze pack. This pressure should be maintained for 5 minutes. This improves the adaptation of the flap and assists haemostasis.

Post-operatively

Antibiotics are not routinely prescribed; analgesia may be required for several post-operative days.

When possible, the patient should be reviewed 3–4 days later to remove sutures and take a peri-apical radiograph of the apicected tooth.

Subsequent reviews should note any pain or tenderness to percussion, buccal swelling or sinus, unexpected or increasing mobility, loss of vitality in adjacent teeth, presence of gingival recession.

Radiographically, the procedure is said to be successful with bony infilling of the peri-radicular defect and appearance equivalent to that of a normal periodontal ligament and lamina dura.

Complications

Once the flap is raised and the root is visualized, it may become apparent that the tooth is unrestorable. Likely causes include root fracture, palatal perforation, lateral canal inaccessible to surgery or root resorption. The tooth may be extracted immediately if a prosthetic replacement has been constructed pre-operatively in anticipation of this possible outcome or the patient accepts the aesthetic change.

Late complications are commonly due to failure to eliminate the causative micro-organisms resulting in continuation of the inflammatory and infective processes.

The possibility of aesthetic failure will have been discussed pre-operatively, in some cases gingival creep will improve the appearance of small defects over a period of months, but results cannot be predicted.

Top tips

- Ensure tooth has adequate coronal seal and is restorable post-operatively.
- Ensure best possible orthograde root filling is provided prior to considering surgical treatment.
- Reassess periodontal pocket depths prior to surgery.
- Consider a flap avoiding full gingival margin flap where the soft tissues and the access it would provide allows.
- Magnification.
- Prepare root-end cavity with ultrasonic instruments.
- Use mineral trioxide aggregate.
- Apply pressure for 5 minutes on completion of surgery.
- Remove sutures at 3–4 days.
- Avoid operating if there is a more appropriate conservative option.

FURTHER READING

Bernabe P, Holland R, Morandi R *et al.* Comparative study of MTA and other materials in retrofilling of pulpless dogs' teeth. *Brazilian Dental Journal* 2005; **16**: 149–55.

Carrotte P. Surgical Endodontics. *British Dental Journal* 2005; **198**: 71–9.

Chandler N, Koshy S. The changing role of the apicectomy operation in dentistry. *Journal of the Royal College of Surgeons of Edinburgh* 2002; **47**: 660–7.

Kim S, Kratchman S. Modern endodontic surgery concepts and practice. A review. *Journal of Endodontics* 2006; **32**: 601–23

Royal College of Surgeons of England. *Guidelines for surgical endodontics.* Faculty of Dental Surgery, Royal College of Surgeons of England, 2001.

Velvart P, Peters C. Soft tissue management in endodontic surgery. Journal of Endodontics 2005; **31**: 4–16.

2.5

Benign cysts of the face and jaws

JOSEPH HELMAN

BIOPSY OF SOFT AND HARD TISSUES

Principles and justifications

Biopsy of soft and hard tissues will allow histologic diagnosis of the cystic lesion allowing prediction of its clinical behaviour and the surgeon to proceed with later definitive treatment.

Indications

Any large lesion where the diagnosis of cyst versus a benign aggressive tumour must be established prior to definitive surgery.

Pre-operative

ANAESTHESIA

This office-based procedure can be performed under local anaesthesia or under conscious sedation. The goal is to make the patient comfortable and allow an appropriate sampling of the lesion for histopathologic evaluation.

Biopsy

FINE NEEDLE ASPIRATION

Cystic lesions located in soft tissues are palpated and stabilized. A sterile 18-gauge needle is inserted at the lesion's edge and advanced towards the centre of the lesion. Aspiration of the cystic content is collected and transferred to a slide for fixation and microscopic evaluation. Examination for protein content or cytokeratins may be useful in keratocystic odontogenic tumours.

PUNCH BIOPSY

The skin or mucosa is stretched perpendicular to the skin tension lines. The punch is pressed and twisted into the lesion to the hub, keeping in mind the anatomy of the area biopsied. The punch is removed. The specimen is gently grasped and using a sharp scalpel the specimen is freed from the base. The biopsy site can be closed with simple interrupted suture(s), Steri strips on skin or allowed to granulate if less than 4 mm in diameter.

EXCISIONAL AND INCISIONAL BIOPSIES

Soft tissue cysts, an elliptical incision utilizing a 3:1 ratio of length to width is made through skin and subcutaneous tissues. Blunt tissue dissection undermines the surrounding tissues to fully expose and deliver the cyst. Intra-bony lesions, sulcular or vestibular incision is made, a full thickness mucoperiosteal flap is raised and reflected. Using a large bore needle, the lesion is aspirated (to exclude a vascular lesion). A surgical bur is used to create a bony window to allow for an incisional biopsy to be harvested. An appropriate sample of the lesion is necessary for histopathologic evaluation.

ENUCLEATION AND CURETTAGE

Principles and justifications

Enucleation is removal of a lesion from bone with preservation of bone continuity. Curettage is removal of a lesion from bone with preservation of bone continuity by scraping due to absence of an intact capsule.

Indications

Enucleation and curettage is indicated for definitive treatment of benign cystic lesions that do not require resection.

Pre-operative

ANAESTHESIA

The procedure is performed under general endotracheal anaesthesia or i.v. conscious sedation. However, small lesions may be completed under local anaesthesia.

Operation

PATIENT POSITION

Under general endotracheal anaesthesia, the patient is positioned in a supine position with mild hyperextension of the neck. A shoulder roll is placed and the occiput is supported by a foam head ring. Under i.v. sedation, the patient is placed in a semi-supine position. Appropriate local anaesthetic blocks and infiltration is performed to establish anaesthesia and haemostasis.

PROCEDURE

A full thickness mucoperiosteal flap is then developed and reflected using a sulcular or vestibular incision. A bony window approximately one-third the overall diameter of the lesion is created using a round bur. Care is taken to leave the cystic lining intact. Once exposed, sinus curettes are used to reflect the cystic lining from the bony walls of the cavity. Once removed, curettes or molt instruments are used to curette the bony walls of the entire cavity being cognizant of the local anatomy. The area is then thoroughly irrigated with normal saline and primary closure achieved using a resorbable interrupted or running sutures.

PERIPHERAL OSTECTOMY AND RECONTOURING

Principles and justifications

The term 'peripheral ostectomy' has been used to describe an adjunctive surgical procedure following enucleation or curettage, in which the osseous walls of the defect are abraded with coarse surgical burs in an attempt to ensure that residual daughter cells and/or peripheral neoplastic tissue is removed. Recontouring is most often performed in situations where functional and aesthetic improvement is required.

Indications

Lesions with a high rate of recurrence following initial enucleation and curettage, such an keratocystic odontogenic tumour. Initial treatment in mature lesions that require recontouring as seen in fibrous dysplasia.

Pre-operative

ANAESTHESIA

The procedure may be performed under general anaesthesia, i.v. conscious sedation or local anaesthesia.

Operation

PATIENT POSITION

Under general endotracheal anaesthesia, the patient is positioned in a supine position with mild hyperextension of the neck. A shoulder roll is placed and the occiput is supported by a foam head ring. Under intravenous sedation, the patient is placed in a semi-supine position. Appropriate local anaesthetic blocks and infiltration is performed to establish anaesthesia and haemostasis.

PROCEDURE

A full thickness mucoperiosteal flap or vestibular incision is reflected in the surgical site. A large round bur or barrel bur may be used for bony reduction and recontouring of large hyperostosis. Intra-bony lesions may be exposed in a similar fashion to enucleation and curettage. A surgical bur is used to remove a small amount of cortical bone, usually less then 1 mm, from within the periphery of the lesion. Methylene blue dye may be used as an adjunct to aid in visualization of the removal of bone. The bony cavity is swabbed with methylene dye and surgical burs are used to remove all the colouration so as to minimize repeated bony removal within the same area. Once the ostectomy is complete, the area is thoroughly irrigated and primary closure achieved with resorbable sutures in a running or interrupted fashion.

For keratocystic odontogenic tumours a peripheral ostectomy has been advocated by applying Carnoy's solution to the bony cavity for a period of 3 minutes after enucleation and curettage. Since the solution is very caustic, it would be prudent to protect the surrounding tissues with a wet gauze and apply Carnoy's under general anaesthesia for additional safety. Due to restrictions in the use of chloroform (present in the original Carnoy's solution) by the Food and Drug Administration in the USA, a new formula has been utilized as follows:

30 cc absolute alcohol
10 cc glacial acetic acid
4 g ferric chloride.

DECOMPRESSION OR MARSUPIALIZATION

Principles and justifications

Leaving an open communication between the lumen of a cyst and the oral cavity allows for gradual decompression of the cyst, bone growth and potential preservation of teeth.

Indications

Decompression or marsupialization is indicated for the treatment of large odontogenic cysts and keratocystic odontogenic tumours (especially in children when the extension of the tumour may require the extraction of a significant number of teeth).

Pre-operative

ANAESTHESIA

The procedure can usually be performed under local anaesthesia. In specific situations in which patient collaboration is difficult to obtain, sedation or general anaesthesia may be indicated.

Operation

PROCEDURE

A mucosal incision is performed in the lateral aspect of the lesion, as close as possible to the alveolar ridge. A bony window is created with a rotatory instrument or with a rongeur. The cyst cavity could either be maintained open by means of a custom-made acrylic stent, or by packing the cavity with an iodoform gauze strip followed by a removable obturator. If the option of a stent is selected, the patient is instructed to irrigate the cavity at least once daily through the lumen of the tube.

The iodoform gauze strip may be removed once a week until epithelization of the fistula is completed (recommend one month) and then is replaced with an obturator to prevent accumulation of food and closure of the fistula.

Marsupialization is followed by enucleation after the resulting size of the cyst allows for preservation of dental structures and/or continuity of bone.

SURGICAL RESECTION WITH MARGINS OF MANDIBULAR LESIONS

Principles and justifications

Surgical resection with margins should be performed using conventional surgical and sound dissection techniques. Bony resection with 1.0- to 1.5-cm bony margins and anatomic barrier margins of one such uninvolved anatomic barrier are required for eradication.

Indications

Surgical resection with margins of mandibular lesions is indicated for aggressive benign tumours, aggressive 'cysts' of the jaws, e.g. recurrent keratocystic odontogenic tumour involving soft tissues and muscles.

Pre-operative

ANAESTHESIA

The operation is performed under general anaesthesia with either nasal (mandibular procedures) or oral (maxillary procedures) endotracheal intubation. Fibreoptic intubation may be necessary in rare cases depending on the size and location of the cyst.

Operation

PATIENT POSITION

The patient is placed in a supine position with mild hyperextension of the neck. A shoulder roll is placed and the occiput is supported by a foam head ring. The head is turned to the contralateral side to expose the ipsilateral neck and mandible. The patient is then prepped and draped in a sterile fashion.

INCISION AND DISSECTION

The inferior border of the mandible is palpated, marking the mandibular angle, antegonial notch and mandibular midline. A suitable skin crease approximately 2.0 cm is marked in an anterioposterior direction to provide adequate exposure to the mandible. A scalpel blade is used to incise skin and subcutaneous tissues sharply to the level of the platysma. Adequate caudal and cephalic underminding in the supraplatysmal plane aids in closure. An electrocautery bovie is used to incise the platysma and expose the underlying superficial layer of the deep cervical fascia. A subplatysma dissection is made in a cephalic direction elevating the skin, subcutaneous tissue and platysma superiorly to the level of the mandible. Next, the facial nerve is identified, freed and retracted superiorly. The facial artery and vein are identified using blunt dissection, ligated and divided. The inferior border of the mandible is then palpated and, using either electrocautery bovie or a scalpel, the periosteum is incised and reflected cephalic to the marginal gingiva using a periosteal elevator on the buccal and lingual aspects of the mandible. If the lesion perforates the cortices a supraperiosteal dissection is performed overlying the lesion and 1.0–1.5 cm anterior and posterior to the lesion.

RESECTION

If an inferior alveolar nerve is to be spared, a nerve lateralization procedure should be performed prior to resection. With the dissection complete, the lesion is now resected using a reciprocating saw under copious amounts of irrigation. The bony resection should include 1.0- to 1.5-cm of a bony margin and an uninvolved anatomic barrier. The resection should be started at the anterior aspect of the resection. The specimen is then sent to pathology. Marrow may be taken from the distal and proximal segments and sent to pathology for frozen sections.

Maxillary lesions should be resected with similar bony margins. The surgeon should consider a more aggressive approach on maxillary tumours due to the potential involvement of the orbit and base of the skull in case of recurrences.

RECONSTRUCTION

Primary or secondary reconstruction should ensue, but is beyond the scope of the limited discussion of this chapter.

CLOSURE

A three-layer closure of the tissues is performed after the placement of a suction drain. In the posterior aspect of the mandible, the masseteric sling is closed with interrupted resorbable suture. The superficial layer of the deep cervical fascia does not require definitive closure. The platysma is reapproximated and sutured with interrupted resorbable suture. Subcutaneous sutures are then placed followed by skin sutures.

Maxillectomy defects could be closed with obturators, local flaps or free tissue transfer.

Top tips

- Always aspirate before opening a suspected cystic lesion.
- Give strong consideration to biopsying a large lesion before proceeding with the excision or enucleation.
- Discuss extensively the need for patient compliance when a conservative treatment modality is implemented (i.e. marsupialization).
- Never underestimate the potential for recurrence in odontogenic keratocysts (keratocystic odontogenic tumours).
- Segmental resections should be performed after careful evaluation of all the available reconstructive options.
- Apply contemporary evidence-based medicine and critical thinking pathways to every recommendation of a treatment modality.

2.6

Basic implantology: An American perspective

JAIME BRAHIM

INTRODUCTION

The history of tooth replacement goes back to ancient civilization, but it was not until the work of Professor Branemark in Sweden in the early 1950s that biocompatibility of implants in experimental studies in animals was demonstrated. The depth of the scientific research specifically in titanium implants was the work of the group led by Per-Ingvar Branemark, an orthopaedic surgeon. His work defined osseointegration.

Osseointegration is the contact established between normal remodelled bone and an implant surface without the interposition of connective tissue with the normal bone component grown to within 100 to 200 A of the metallic surface and with the interface between the metal and the bone consisting of a titanium dioxide layer and a protein glycosaminoglycan. This definition of osseointegration has formed the basis for today's implantology science.

DIAGNOSIS AND TREATMENT PLANNING

The key to the success of implant treatment is collating appropriate information that will result in a well-performed and successful procedure. It is essential for the surgeon to understand the patient's chief complaint and why they want dental implants. Providing the patient with detailed information, including that about possible long-term complications, is equally important.

A good patient assessment plan should include:

- Medical, dental and social history: Review of the risks and benefits of the treatment plan should be discussed with the patient. Patients who are immunocompromised or smoke heavily should expect a lower success rate than other patients, for example.
- Clinical and oral examination of soft and hard tissues: This examination should include the condition of the mucous tissues, the condition of the remaining dentition and the quality and quantity of maxillary and mandibular bone.
- Radiographic examination: Intraoral peri-apical radiographs are very helpful in assessing the space between adjacent teeth and the direction of the adjacent roots. A three-dimensional computed tomography (CT) scan can demonstrate a cross-section that can provide the information about the different widths of the jaw, which in turn may help with the selection of the desired diameters of the implant (3–6 mm). CT scans can help identify anatomic structures, such as the mandibular canal and antrum.
- Articulated study casts: These provide essential information about the space between the adjacent teeth and the inter-arch space for the implant and restoration.
- Photographic records.
- Surgical plan.
- Template for surgery: A well-made template assists the operator in the correct placement of the dental implant. It is important that the template fits securely, and gives appropriated access to the drill to prepare the implant sites.
- Signed consent form: This ensures that the patient completely understands the surgical treatment and its complications.

ASSESSMENT OF BONE QUANTITY AND QUALITY

Every tooth extraction leads to remodelling of the alveolar bone and bone loss that is greater during the first three months. Remodelling is mostly complete after one year. Bone loss occurs in both the vertical and horizontal planes.

The surgeon should be able to asses bone quality and quantity. An elegant description is the one proposed by Leholm and Zarb (Figures 2.6.1 and 2.6.2).

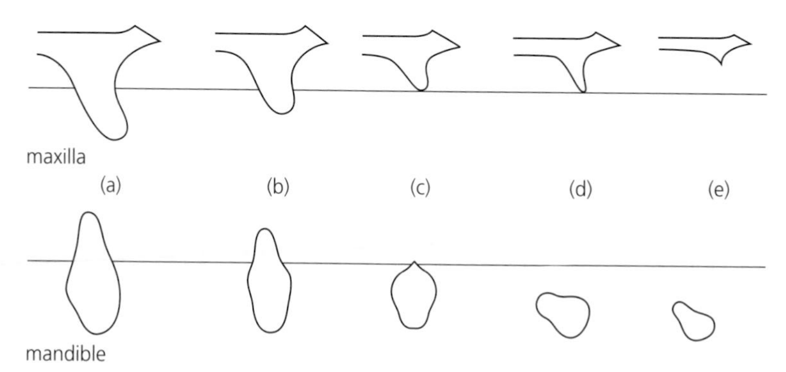

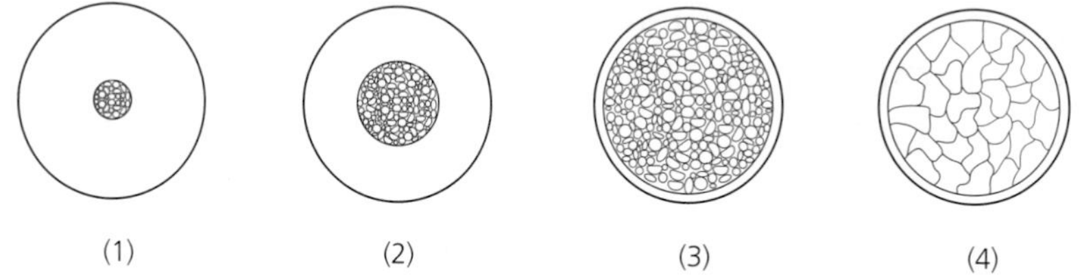

2.6.1 Lekholm and Zarb, degrees of resorption. (a) Most of the alveolar bone is present. (b) Moderate residual ridge resorption has occurred. (c) Advanced residual ridge resorption has occurred and only basal bone remains. (d) Some resorption of the basal bone has taken place. (e) Extreme resorption of the basal bone has taken place.

(1) (2) (3) (4)

2.6.2 Lekholm and Zarb bone quality classification. (1) Almost the entire jaw is comprised of homogenous compact bone. (2) A thick layer of compact bone surrounds a core of dense trabecular bone. (3) A thin layer of cortical bone surrounds a core of dense trabecular bone of favorable strength. (4) A thin layer of cortical bone surrounds a core of low-density trabecular bone.

ANATOMIC CONSIDERATIONS FOR DENTAL IMPLANTS

Maxilla

The maxillary bone is a hollow cuboid shape that houses the teeth, forms the roof of the oral cavity, forms the floor and contributes to the lateral wall and roof of the nasal cavity, houses the maxillary sinus, and contributes to the inferior rim and floor of the orbit. Two maxillary bones are joined in the midline to form the middle third of the face.

Performing implant surgery in the maxilla requires a detailed knowledge of the anatomical landmarks, such as the maxillary sinus, the nasal cavity, the nasopalatine canal, midline suture and cortical shell (especially when deficient). Appreciation of diminished vertical and horizontal dimensions is essential as well.

Mandible

The operator should be familiar with the effects of the loss of teeth, the effect and possible extent of the alveolar bone resorption, and also be familiar with the anatomical areas of the mandible, such as the body region, the exact location of the inferior alveolar nerve, the region of the symphysis, and of the mental nerve. Before exiting through the mental foramen, the mental nerve may form a loop that runs anterior and inferior to the foramen. This loop can extend from 1 to 7 mm. Generally, the mandibular canal runs from the mandibular foramen inferiorly and anteriorly, then runs horizontally and laterally most of the time just below the root apices of the molars. When placing implants in the area close to the inferior alveolar nerve, clearance of at least 2 mm from the most superior aspect should be allowed to prevent surgical trauma.

Knowledge of the concavities of the mandible, especially in the lingual region, is important to avoid any perforation while drilling that may produce significant bleeding from the sublingual vessels (Figure 2.6.3).

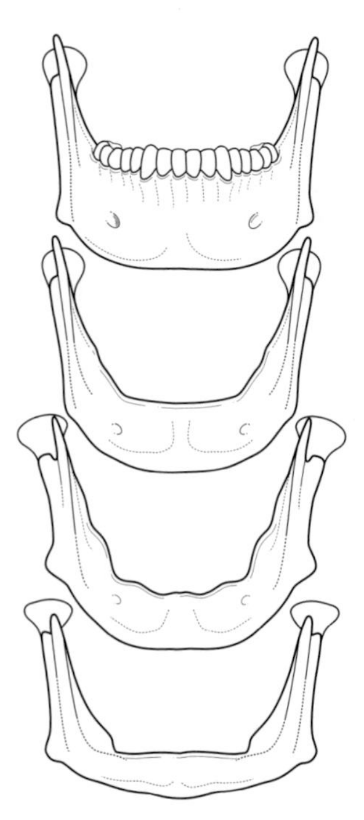

2.6.3 Different levels of mandibular resorption.

IMPORTANT ASPECTS TO INCREASE IMPLANT SURGICAL SUCCESS

1 Strict use of sterile technique, to minimize the risk of infection.
2 Oral rinsing with 0.2 per cent chlorehexidine prior to surgery.
3 Gentle surgical technique.
4 Light and intermittent drilling pressure (Figures 2.6.4 and 2.6.5).
5 Copious cooling irrigation.
6 Avoid contamination of implant surfaces with gloves, tubing, etc.
7 Well-trained staff.

SURGICAL PROCEDURES

Mandible

After administration of local anaesthetic and sedation as required, two different incision designs can be performed in the anterior mandible:

- *Crestal incision* is made when the mandible has adequate height and the muscle fibres are inserting below the alveolar crest. When the patient has healthy attached gingiva, a crestal incision provides good access to the labial and lingual regions (Figure 2.6.6).
- *Vestibular incision* is made for patients with poor attached gingiva or when the insertion of the muscle is high (Figure 2.6.7).

Both incisions must follow the principles of good incision design (adequate access and visibility to allow identification of important anatomical landmarks, such as mental foramina, incisal canal, etc., and a mucoperiosteal flap that provides good vascular supply). A careful blunt dissection is required to identify anatomical landmarks.

After the surgical template is positioned, a sterile pencil is used to mark the position of the implant in the bone.

After the flap is raised, with copious irrigation and a high speed (maximum 2000 rpm), the bone preparation can be initiated following the instructions of the different implant manufacturers. Most implant systems provide the surgeon with several drill sizes that will allow the gradual enlargement of the surgical site. The drilling should be done

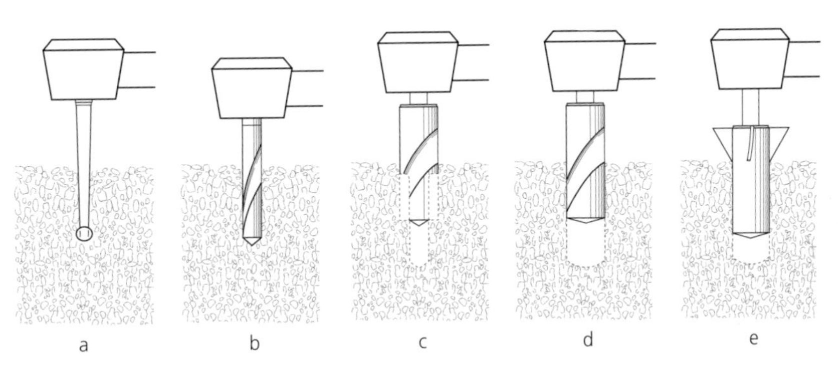

2.6.4 Steps in the preparation of implant osteotomy slides.

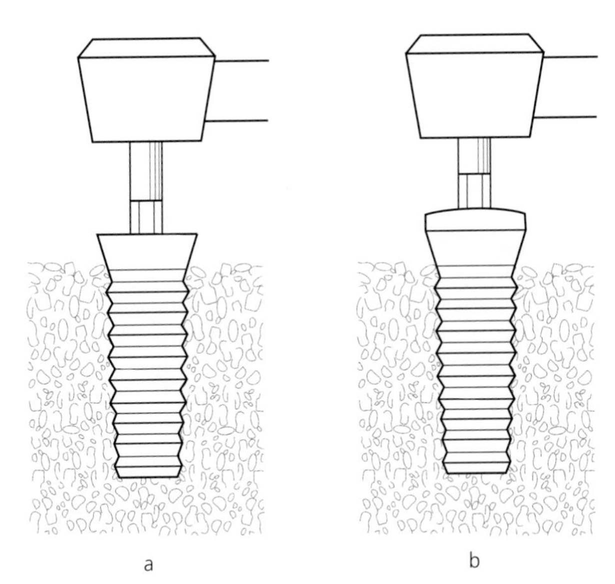

2.6.5 Implant insertion and cover screw placement.

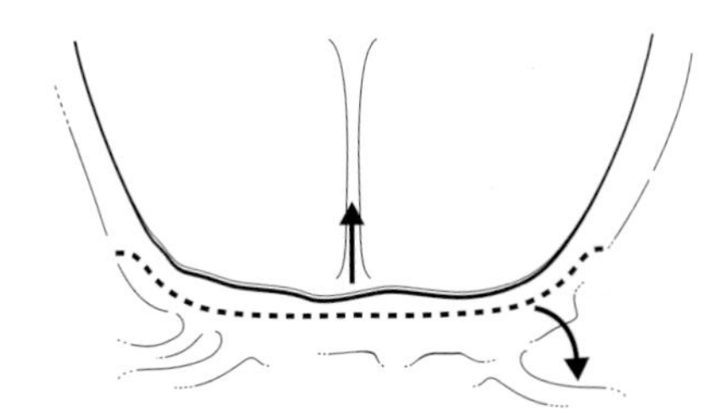

2.6.6 Crestal incision.

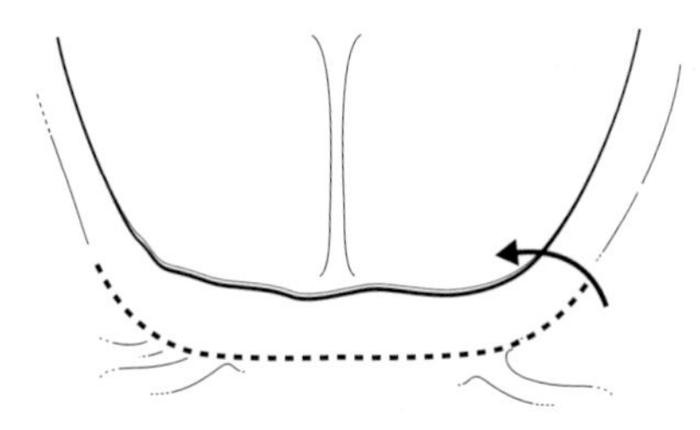

2.6.7 Vestibular incision.

with an intermittent technique, always having new sharp burs and copious irrigation.

When the osteotomy site is prepared, using a low speed of 15–20 rpm, the implant is placed, following which the healing abutment or cover screw is positioned. At the end of the procedure, the surgical area is irrigated and a primary closure is performed with 3/0 or 4/0, silk or vicryl sutures (Figures 2.6.8–2.6.14).

Maxilla

After administration of local anaesthetic and sedation as required, an incision that is slightly palatal to the alveolar crest is made. This incision design will allow the surgeon to visualize the palatal bone contours. After the flap is raised, the osteotomy of the implants sites is performed. In the maxillary arch it is sometimes possible to establish bicortical stability in the area of the sinus and nasal bone, being careful that only the apical tip of the implant engages the cortical plate. Then the healing abutment or cover screw is placed. At the end of the procedure, the surgical area is irrigated and a primary closure is performed with 3/0 or 4/0 silk or vicryl sutures.

POST-OPERATIVE CARE

- Antibiotics: The antibiotics should provide the maximum blood levels at the time of incision.

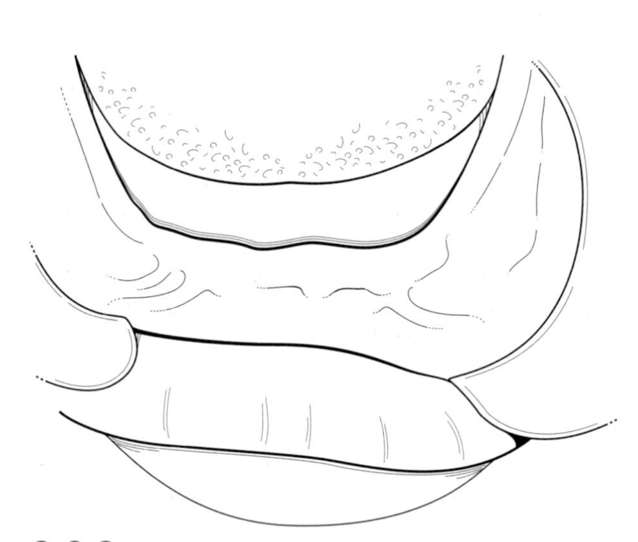

2.6.8 Pre-operative view of a mandible demonstrating a knife ridge.

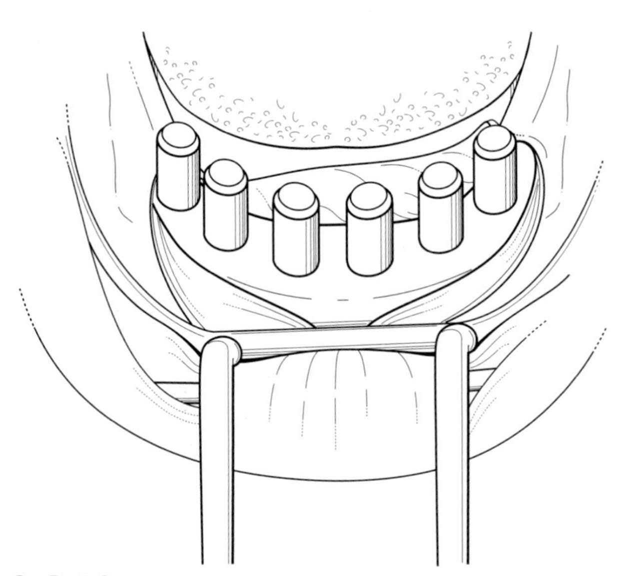

2.6.10 Clinical picture showing good parallelism of the abutment.

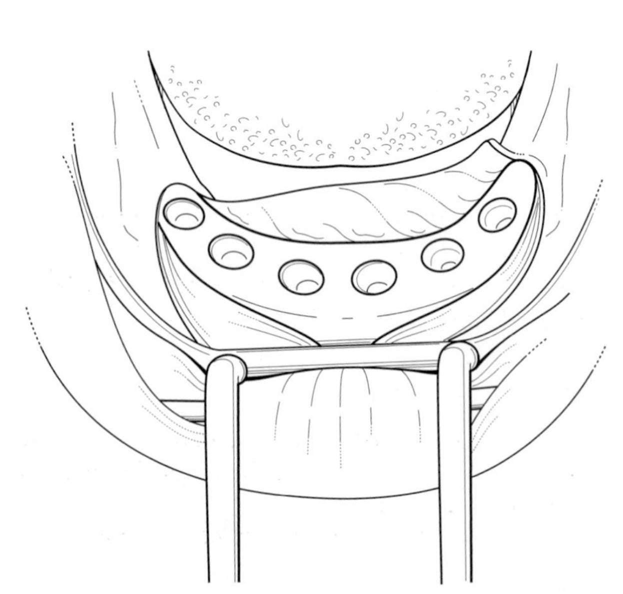

2.6.9 Final preparations of the implant sites showing a favorable distance from each other.

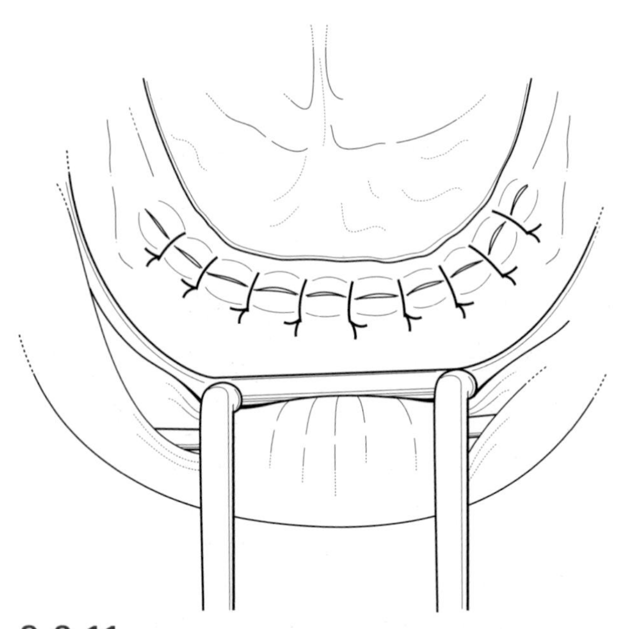

2.6.11 Primary closure of the incision using reabsorbable suture.

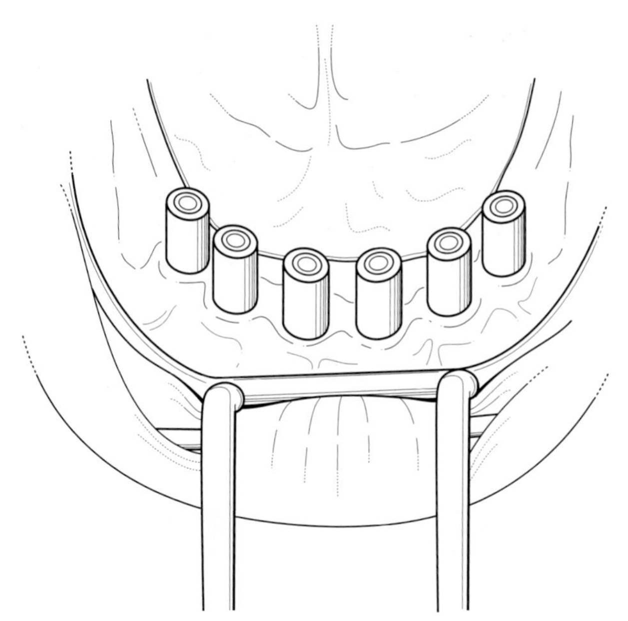

2.6.12 Note that abutments are parallel and ready for prosthetic rehabilitation.

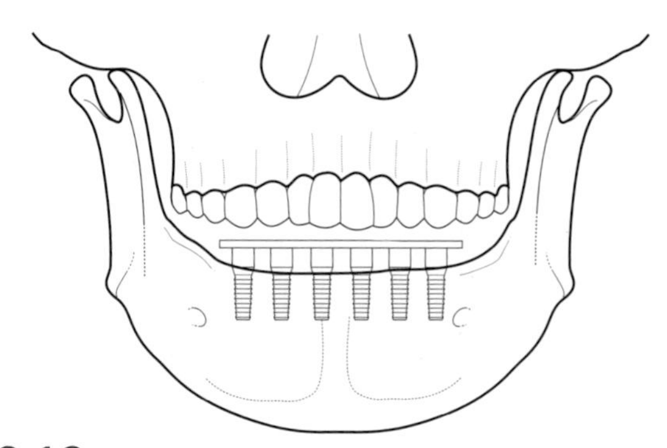

2.6.13 From view of integrated implants supporting mandibulary fixed-detachable prosthesis.

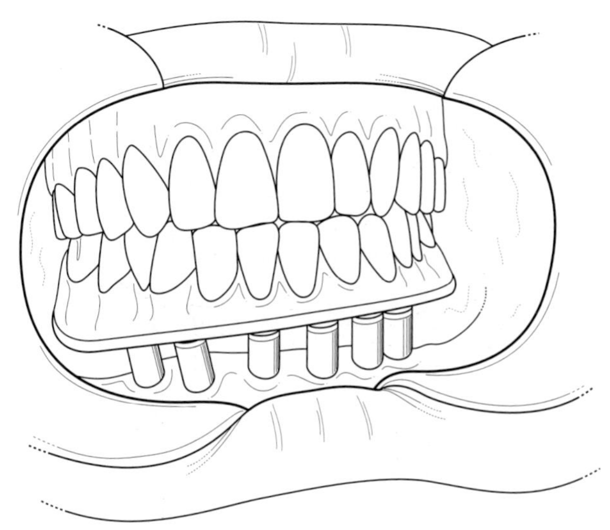

2.6.14 Three months after stage two implants have integrated and ready for implantborne and screw-retained prosthesis, the prosthesis is removable by the dentist.

- Analgesics: Patients usually only require ibuprofen 400 mg every 6 hours. If the implant procedure is more involved, a combination of an anti-inflammatory analgesic with codeine or paracetamol usually suffices.
- Oedema: Post-operative, mild oedema is sometimes present and generally settles uneventfully. Use of steroids intra-operatively and post-operatively can be considered for selected cases.
- Local care: Meticulous oral care with gentle rinses of 0.2 per cent chlorehexidine four times daily for 2 weeks, and gently brushing with a soft tooth brush, being careful with the operative site.
- Diet: A diet high in proteins and soft in texture that does not cause injury to the surgical sites should be advised.

SECOND-STAGE SURGERY

This is only performed if a two-stage technique has been selected with the implant not immediately loaded, but left to osseointegrate. During the second stage, the head of the implant body is exposed and the abutment is placed. Usually this procedure is carried out under local anaesthesia and the incision is made directly over the implant head and a small flap is raised, the cover screw removed and the appropriate healing abutment is secured on the implant. The flap is then repositioned and sutured.

POST-OPERATIVE CARE

Written post-surgical instructions for oral surgery should be given to the patient. If the patient is wearing dentures and a crestal incision was performed, wearing of dentures is acceptable during the healing period. If a vertical incision was performed, it is advisable for the patient not to wear the denture immediately. It is always necessary to examine the patient 1 week early for possible suture removal, irrigation and any denture adjustment.

BONE GRAFTING

Bone grafting can be performed at the time of surgery if the defects are small. The graft in these cases is usually taken from an intraoral site, such as:

- from the anterior mandible (chin)
- retromolar area of the mandible.

Bone can also be retrieved for the graft from the drilling site using a bone collector either from the suction line or from the drill bits (Figure 2.6.15).

Other areas to obtain autologous bone grafts are:

- iliac creast
- cranium
- tibia.

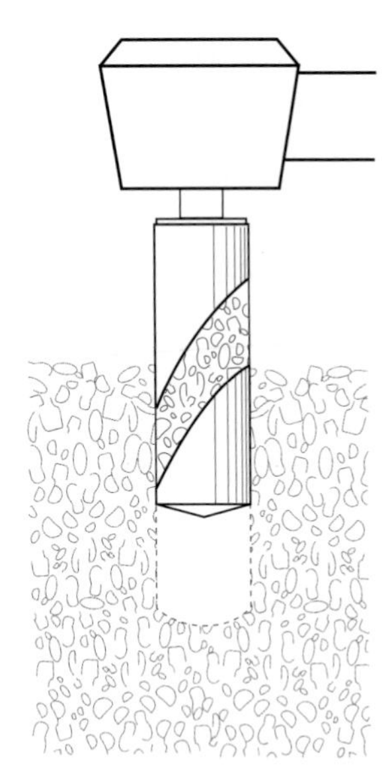

2.6.15 Bone bits trapped in the bur can be used as autologous graft.

Autografts are the preferred source of bone material due to the lack of antigenicity of the graft material. We also can use allografts which are generally obtained from a human cadaver, the clinical success of these grafts is well proven. The advantage of these grafts is that the patients will not have to undergo an additional surgical procedure to obtain the bone. Xenografts are the grafting from one species to another, e.g. bovine bone, and are useful when mixed with the patient's blood. Alloplastic grafts are synthetic bone substitute that may act as a framework for bone formation.

COMPLICATIONS

Stage-one surgery

- Haemorrhage during drilling. Most of the time, this occurs following perforation of the lingual cortex of the mandible. Sometimes bleeding can advance into the floor of the mouth, producing a threat to the patient's airway, necessitating emergency treatment.
- Implant mobility. Not being able to obtain stability is usually due to poor bone density or over preparation of the implant site.
- Exposed implants threads. The possible causes may be due to narrow crest.
- Paraesthesia. Trauma to the nerves in the area of the implant placement is the usual cause.
- Infection is unusual in implant surgery if a sterile technique is used.

Stage-two surgery

- Failure to integrate. Usually presenting as a painful and mobile implant. The reasons for this complication can be multifactorial. Poor clinical evaluation for surgical site, poor surgical technique, infection or lack of experience are the usual causes. The solution is removal of the implant.
- Difficulties placing the abutment. Possible causes include damage to internal features of the implant body during placement of the implant, and bone overgrowth during the healing process.

Top tips

- In order to preserve the interproximal dental papilla, it is important to have at least 3 mm between implants and 1.5 mm between natural tooth and implant.
- Ideally, the interarch distance should be greater than or equal to 7 mm. If this distance is greater than the 10-mm mesiodistal space, then single tooth implant is not recommended.
- Implants should be placed at a minimum of 2 mm from the inferior alveolar canal or below the maxillary sinus.
- Gentle surgical technique, light and intermittent drilling pressure and copious cooling irrigation are important factors to increase implant surgical success.
- The amount of bone needed both buccal and lingual to the implant (width) requires a minimum of 1 mm of cortical bone on the lingual and buccal.
- A good incision design should have good access and visibility to allow identification of important anatomical landmarks and have a good mucoperiosteal flap that provides good vascular supply.

FURTHER READING

Block MS. *Color atlas of dental implant surgery*, 2nd edn. Philadelphia: Elsevier, 2007.

Branemark P-I, Zarb GA, Albrektsson T. *Tissue-integrated prostheses. Osseointegration in clinical dentistry.* New Maldon: Quintessence, 1985.

Hobkirk JA, Watson RM, Lloyd JJ. Searson. *Introducing dental implants.* London: Churchill Livingstone, 2003.

Worthington P, Long BR, Rubenstein JE (eds). *Osseointegration in dentistry. An overview.* New Maldon: Quintessence, 2003.

2.7

Adjunctive office-based techniques for bone augmentation in oral implantology: An American perspective

GARY WARBURTON

GENERAL PRINCIPLES

Adequate bone stock is essential for successful implant placement. Deficient bone may arise due to the normal resorptive physiology of dentoalveolar bone in edentulous areas, or due to acquired defects following trauma or ablative surgery. Regardless of the underlying aetiology of the deficiency, there are numerous augmentation materials and techniques available if the bone volume is inadequate at the planned implant site. The selection of the appropriate augmentation material and technique is influenced by many factors, but the volume, location and morphology of the defect are primary determinants.

Classification of grafting materials

- Autogenous bone: Harvested from the patient.
- Allogenic: Typically harvested from cadavers.
- Xenogenic: Harvested from a different species (e.g. porcine or bovine).
- Alloplastic: Inert or synthetic materials.

These may be used individually or in combination to replace and/or regenerate deficient bone. Furthermore, they may be supplemented by biologically active materials such as platelet rich plasma and more recently with bone morphogenic proteins (BMP). Autogenous bone remains the gold standard graft material since it possesses osteogenic, osteoinductive and osteoconductive properties, whereas allografts have only osteoconductive and possibly inductive properties, and alloplasts are merely osteoconductive. This chapter will focus on autogenous augmentation techniques that can be performed in the office or outpatient clinic environment.

Selection of the appropriate donor site is determined by many factors including the volume and the type of bone required (cancellous or corticocancellous). Potential donor sites suitable for office or outpatient clinic bone harvesting include local sites in the maxilla and mandible, or remote sites such as proximal tibia. It should be recognized that mandibular and maxillary donor sites provide only a limited source of cancellous bone. It is reported that membranous bone grafts show less resorption than grafts harvested from endochondral bone. Although cancellous grafts vascularize more rapidly than cortical grafts, cortical grafts harvested from membranous bone vascularize more rapidly than endochondral bone grafts with a thicker cancellous component. Figure 2.7.1 shows the potential donor sites in the maxilla and mandible. Table 2.7.1 outlines the potential bone stock of different donor sites.

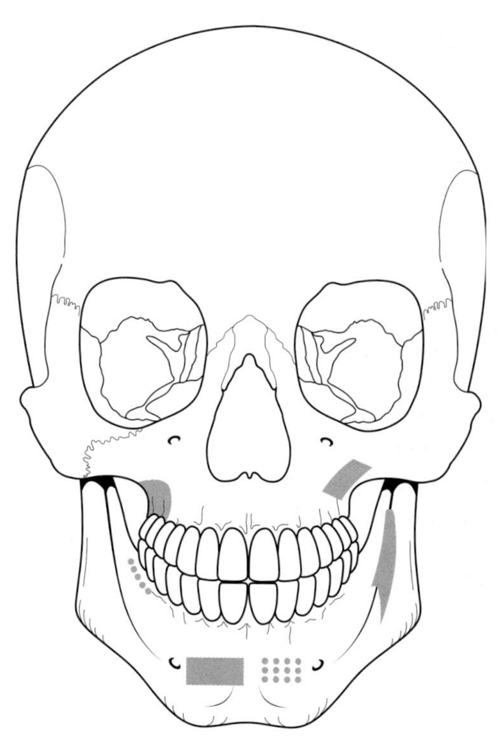

2.7.1 Donor sites in the maxilla and mandible.

Table 2.7.1 Potential donor sites in the maxilla and mandible.

Site	Potential bone volume (ml)
Cortical shavings from maxilla/mandible	2–5
Bony exostoses/tori	Variable
Suction-line bone traps	Variable
Mandibular symphysis	5
Mandibular ramus	5–10
Calvarial shavings	10–14
Proximal tibia	20–40
Anterior iliac crest	50
Posterior iliac crest	50–100

Instrumentation

The osteotomies allowing harvest of the autogenous graft from the donor site may be performed using traditional burs, saws, discs, trephines and osteotomes, or using recent technology, such as piezosurgery. Piezosurgery utilizes a range of working tips that oscillate at ultrasonic frequencies of around 10–60 Hz, thereby cutting bone while preserving soft tissue (nerves, sinus lining, blood vessels and mucosa). The reported advantages of piezosurgery over traditional rotary instruments are that there is no thermal injury or adjacent bone necrosis and the osteocytes remain viable at the osteotomy. Therefore, healing takes place more rapidly, with little or no inflammation and without the need for an osteoclastic phase. Moreover, the attachments can be used to scrape the bone surface, creating a collection of moist bone powder with viable osteocytes.

DONOR SITES

Proximal tibia

Drachter described tibial bone grafting of alveolar clefts in 1914, but it has regained popularity in the oral and maxillofacial surgery field in recent years. The cancellous bone of the proximal tibia can be harvested from a medial or lateral approach, and provides 20–40 ml of cancellous bone. Harvesting bone from this site can be performed in the office or outpatient clinic under intravenous sedation and local anaesthetic, with a low complication rate (1–2 per cent).

PREPARATION

Peri-operative antibiotic therapy and sterile technique are important. The donor leg should be slightly flexed at the knee with the aid of a popliteal fossa support bolster. The proximal tibia, tibial plateau and tibial tuberosity are palpated and Gerdy's tubercle is identified anteromedial to the proximal fibula syndesmosis.

MEDIAL APPROACH

The advantage of the medial approach is that no muscles are encountered and potentially incised, compared to the tibialis anterior in the lateral approach (Figure 2.7.2). Medially, at the level of the tibial tuberosity, there is only a thin layer of fascia and the insertion of the conjoined tendons of sartorius, gracilis and semitendinosus (the pes anserinus) between the subcutaneous tissues and the tibia (Figure 2.7.2). Therefore, this site may be less prone to complications.

Local anaesthetic (2 per cent lidocaine with 1:100 000 epinephrine may be mixed with 0.5 per cent bupivicaine) is injected. An oblique 1.5–2 cm skin incision is made centred between the tibial plateau, tibial tuberosity and the medial margin of the tibia with the distal limit at the tibial tuberosity (Figure 2.7.3). Blunt dissection is then used to reach the pes anserinus. At this point, there are two techniques available to access the cancellous bone within the proximal tibia (Figure 2.7.4). The first is an osteoplastic flap that is pedicled superiorly. Here a fissure bur or piezosurgery tip is used to create a three-sided osteotomy 1 × 1 cm in dimension, and the flap is greenstick fractured with an osteotome to allow its elevation and it is pedicled on the pes anserinus superiorly. The second technique is a cortical window, 1 cm in diameter which is removed after incising

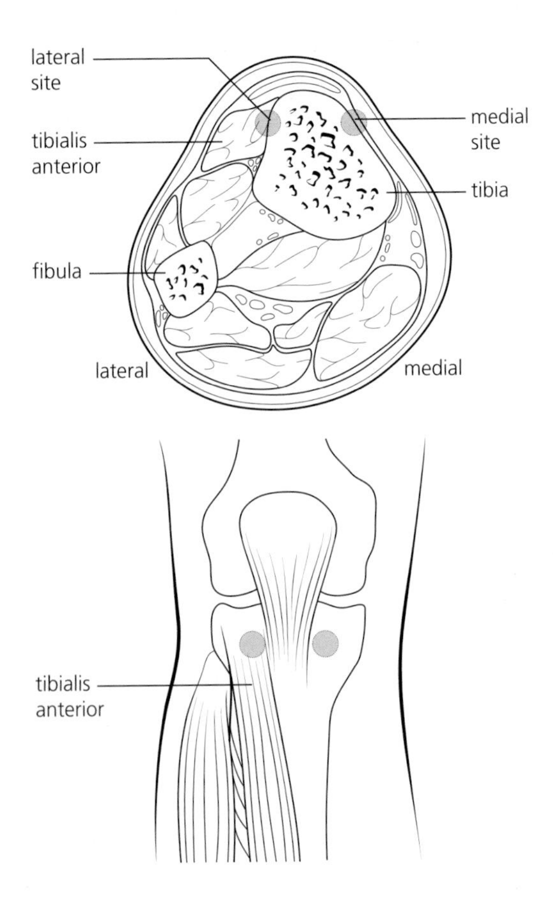

2.7.2 Sites for tibial bone harvest.

and elevating the periostium. This window may be subsequently replaced if only cancellous bone is required for the graft. Once the cancellous bone has been accessed, curettes are used to scoop out the spongy cancellous bone. Care must be taken not to violate the knee joint by perforating through the articular surface of the tibial plateau. This can be avoided by ensuring that the curettes are used without heading superiorly, thereby maintaining 1.5–2 cm of bone inferior to the tibial plateau. The harvested bone should be stored in saline. The bony cavity is irrigated, and if additional hemostasis is needed, microfibrillar soaked in thrombin may be placed in the cavity. The bony cap may then be replaced and stabilized with periostial sutures. The wound is then closed in layers and a pressure dressing applied.

LATERAL APPROACH

In the lateral approach, the iliotibial tract and the tibialis anterior are encountered and elevated. More laterally and deep to the tibialis anterior muscle lies the peroneal nerve; an important motor nerve of the leg.

Local anaesthetic (2 per cent lidocaine with 1:100 000 epinephrine may be mixed with 0.5 per cent bupivicaine) is injected over Gerdy's tubercle. An oblique 1.5–2 cm skin incision is made over Gerdy's tubercle and blunt dissection is used to reach the proximal tibia at the insertion of the iliotibial tract into Gerdy's tubercle (Figure 2.7.3). Here, an osteoplastic flap may be raised and pedicled on the periostium superiorly, or a 1-cm diameter cortical window may be removed. Once the cancellous cavity is accessed, the procedure continues as for the medial approach above.

POST-OPERATIVE MANAGEMENT

In addition to analgesics, many surgeons continue antibiotic therapy into the post-operative period for 5–7 days. Ice and elevation of the leg are helpful in reducing post-operative swelling for the first 24 hours. The patient may shower after 24 hours, but should avoid submersion of the incision in water for 7–10 days. The patient may bear weight on the donor leg immediately, but should be advised to avoid high impact loading, such as running or jumping, for 6 weeks.

COMPLICATIONS

Although the complication rate is low (1–2 per cent), the reported complications include bleeding, haematoma, infection and fracture of the tibial plateau. Fractures can be avoided by careful operative technique and post-operative care. Approximately 10 per cent of patients experience temporary paraesthesia of the skin distal to the incision in the distribution of infrapatellar branch of the saphenous nerve for the medial approach. Any gait disturbance and pain usually resolves within 2 weeks.

Mandibular symphysis

The mandibular symphysis presents a convenient donor site for corticocancellous bone due to its proximity to the recipient site. Although there is only a limited supply of cancellous bone in this region, there is adequate bone stock to augment up to 1.5–2 cm in length, 1 cm in height and 4–7 mm in thickness. Some reports suggest superior bone quality at the grafted site when the bone is harvested from

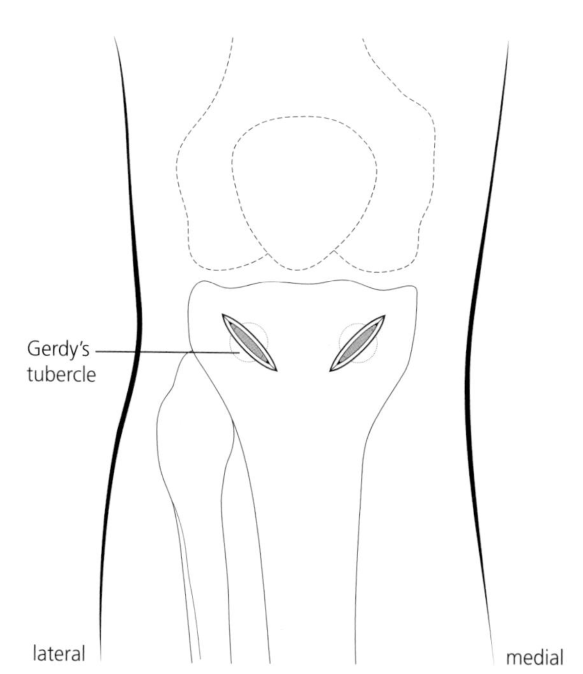

2.7.3 Access incisions for tibial bone harvest.

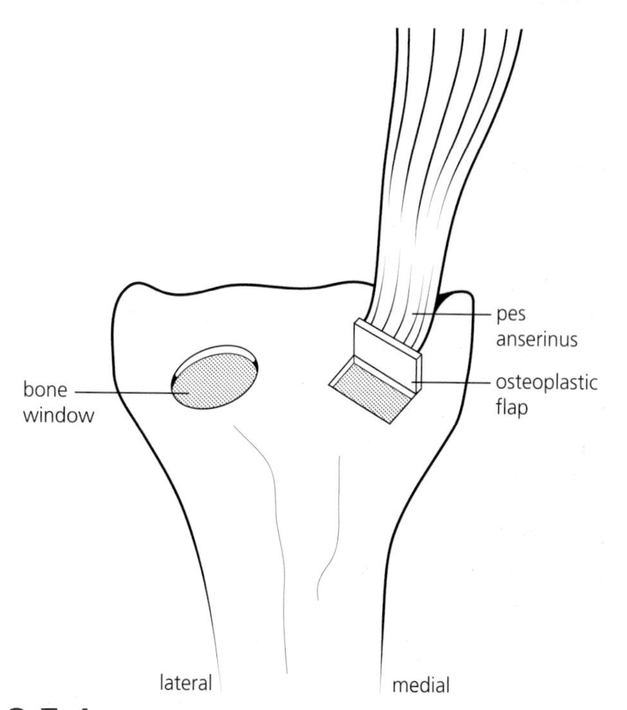

2.7.4 Access osteotomies for tibial bone harvest.

the symphysis compared to other sites, including the iliac crest.

PRE-OPERATIVE PREPARATION

Panoramic and lateral cephalometric radiographs are adequate to assess the volume of bone available within the anatomic constraints described later. Tomograms and computed tomography (CT) scans may add more information regarding bony undercuts and deficiencies. Local mouth preparation should include chlorhexidine mouth rinse pre-operatively. This procedure may be performed under intravenous sedation or local anaesthetic.

PROCEDURE

Local anaesthetic (2 per cent lidocaine with 1:100 000 epinephrine may be mixed with 0.5 per cent bupivicaine) is administered either as bilateral inferior alveolar and lingual nerve blocks, or as bilateral mental nerve blocks supplemented with labial and lingual infiltrations. Many surgeons use peri-operative antibiotic that is administered either enterally or parenterally before surgery. Access to the symphysis can be achieved either by a vestibular/labial incision or by a sulcular/crestal incision (Figure 2.7.5). A potential disadvantage of the sulcular incision is that it may result in bone resorption at the crest if the labial bone is thin and therefore reliant on the overlying periostium for its blood supply. In this situation, or when there is pre-existing marginal bone loss at the alveolar crest due to periodontal disease, a vestibular/labial approach is preferred.

For the vestibular/labial approach, a genioplasty incision is made in the vestibule or labial mucosa extending from canine to canine. The incision is carried through mucosa and submucosa until the bellies of the mentalis muscle is reached. These bellies may need to be divided depending on the level of the mentalis origin, to give access to the underlying symphyseal and parasymphyseal region of the mandible. The mentalis muscle is then detached from the anterior mandible using a periostial elevator or bovie electrocautery, and the soft tissues are elevated inferiorly down to the inferior border of the mandible. The required length of the bone graft dictates the lateral extension of the dissection. With larger corticocancellous blocks, it may be necessary to expose and identify the mental nerves. If a sulcular/crestal incision is made, it is necessary to create distal releasing incisions through the mucosa to allow adequate retraction of the flap as far inferiorly as the lower border of the mandible.

Once the anterior mandible is fully exposed down to the inferior border there are some important anatomic constraints that should be outlined prior to performing the osteotomies (Figure 2.7.6). The superior horizontal osteotomy should remain at least 5 mm inferior to the incisor and canine apices. The inferior horizontal osteotomy should maintain at least 5 mm of intact cortical bone at the inferior border. If the lateral osteotomies need to be placed close to the mental foramina for larger grafts, 5 mm of bone should remain anterior to the foramen to allow for the underlying mental nerve coursing anterior to the foramen before turning posteriorly to emerge through the foramen.

Bone may be harvested from the anterior mandible within these anatomic boundaries either using trephines to obtain multiple cores of corticocancellous bone (maintaining the integrity of the lingual cortex), or using small fissure burs, saws or piezosurgery tips to outline a block of corticocancellous bone. A midline vertical osteotomy may also be made to facilitate easy removal of two blocks of bone. The bone graft is then removed by completing the osteotomies with curved osteotomes. Small amounts of additional cancellous bone can be harvested up to the lingual cortical plate using curettes.

Once the bone is harvested, the bony defect may be filled with allogenic bone or collagen soaked in BMP (BMP-2 or BMP-7) and covered with a resorbable membrane. This

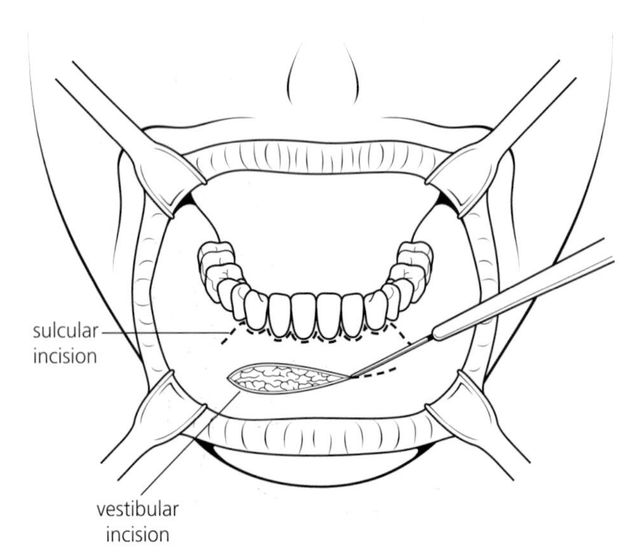

2.7.5 Access incisions for the mandibular symphysis.

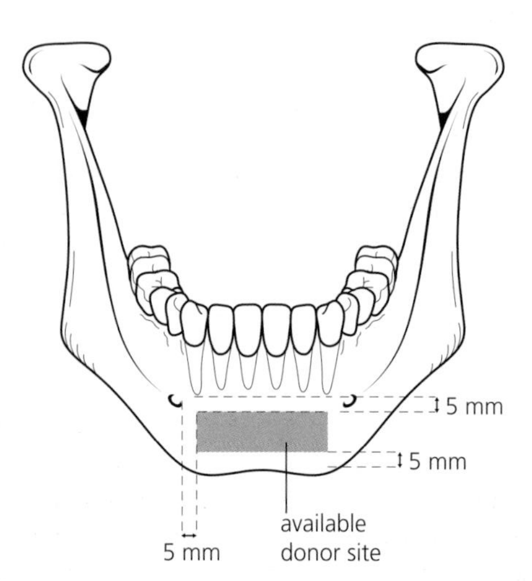

2.7.6 Mandibular symphysis donor site.

minimizes the bony defect after the healing phase compared to simply closing the soft tissues without grafting the donor site. The soft tissues are closed by resuspending the bellies of the mentalis muscles and closure of the mucosal incision with either non-resorbable or resorbable sutures.

POST-OPERATIVE MANAGEMENT

A genioplasty dressing may be applied to provide additional support during the initial healing phase. Appropriate analgesics (non-steroidal anti-inflammatory and narcotic) are prescribed and most surgeons continue antibiotic therapy (amoxicillin or clindamycin) for 5–7 days. The patient should use saline rinses after meals. After 48 hours, the patient should use chlorhexidine mouthwash for 2 weeks, in addition to saline rinses after meals. The diet should be restricted to a clear liquid diet for 24 hours and advanced to a soft mechanical diet for 2 weeks, to minimize the risk of wound dehiscence.

COMPLICATIONS

Possible complications include bleeding, haematoma, infection, wound dehiscence, nerve injury (mental nerve or its branches), incisor/canine tooth devitalization and mandible fracture. However, these complications can be minimized by careful surgical technique and post-operative care.

Mandibular ramus

The external oblique ridge of the mandibular ramus is another convenient site for bone harvest. A corticocancellous block of bone measuring up to 3 cm in length and 1 cm in height may be obtained from the ramus, although the thickness of bone is limited to approximately 4 mm due to the underlying inferior alveolar nerve. The actual size of the graft is determined by the dimensions of the ridge. This procedure may be performed under intravenous sedation or local anaesthetic.

PRE-OPERATIVE PREPARATION

Panoramic radiographs are adequate to assess the volume of bone available and the location of the inferior alveolar nerve. Tomograms and CT scans may add more information regarding bony undercuts, deficiencies and tooth root position. Local mouth preparation should include chlorhexidine mouth rinse pre-operatively and many surgeons use peri-operative antibiotic that is administered either enterally or parenterally before surgery.

PROCEDURE

Local anaesthetic (2 per cent lidocaine with 1:100 000 epinephrine may be mixed with 0.5 per cent bupivicaine) is administered either as inferior alveolar, lingual nerve and long buccal nerve blocks. The external oblique ridge is accessed through a linear mucosal incision starting at the level of the occlusal plane and extending down into the buccal vestibule as far forward as the first molar region. Alternatively, an incision starting on the external oblique ridge and extending crestally to the distal aspect of the last standing molar and then turning down into the vestibule as far forward as the first molar. Periostial elevators are used to elevate a buccal mucoperiostial flap, and also reflecting the lingual flap giving clear visualization of the superior ramus and external oblique ridge. The osteotomies may be created with burs, saws or piezosurgery tips. The posterior vertical osteotomy is made through the outer cortex perpendicular to the external oblique ridge at the level of the occlusal plane, or at a point of adequate thickness. The anterior vertical osteotomy is also made through the outer cortex. The distance between the posterior and anterior cut is determined by the desired graft length and may extend as far forward as the distal aspect of the first molar tooth. The height of these cuts corresponds to the height of the desired graft. The posterior and anterior osteotomies are then connected 3–4 mm medial to the outer cortex of the ridge. The depth of all these cuts is just through the cortical bone. The inferior connecting cuts are made with a No. 8 round bur or an angled piezosurgery tip. The inferior cut simply scores the cortex, enabling fracture along this line during subsequent luxation of the graft with osteotomes. Thin osteotomes are used to complete the osteotomies staying along the buccal cortical plate so as to avoid potential injury to the inferior alveolar nerve. Larger osteotomes are then used to free the block of bone (Figure 2.7.7). The surgeon should ensure that the inferior alveolar nerve is not tethered to the graft prior to removal. The bed of the osteotomy is then inspected and the inferior alveolar nerve may be visualized. Small amounts of cancellous bone may be removed with curettes while being mindful of the location of the nerve. The donor site is then irrigated and closed

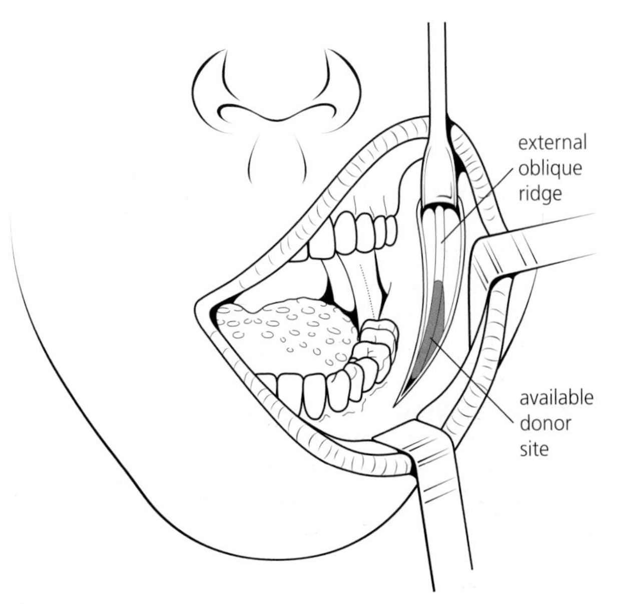

2.7.7 Mandibular ramus donor site.

using resorbable or non-resorbable suture with or without the use of haemostatic agents, such as microfibrillar soaked in thrombin. It is not usually necessary to graft the donor site since bony regeneration is adequate.

POST-OPERATIVE MANAGEMENT

An elasticated jaw bra-type dressing may be applied and the patient instructed to apply ice to the area for 24 hours to reduce the swelling. Appropriate analgesics (non-steroidal anti-inflammatory and narcotic) are prescribed and most surgeons continue antibiotic therapy (amoxicillin or clindamycin) for 5–7 days. The patient should use saline rinses after meals. After 48 hours, the patient should use chlorhexidine mouthwash for 2 weeks, in addition to the saline rinses after meals. The diet should be restricted to a clear liquid diet for 24 hours and advanced to a soft mechanical diet for 2 weeks, to minimize the risk of wound dehiscence.

COMPLICATIONS

The complications are generally similar to the symphyseal donor site: haematoma, infection, wound dehiscence and inferior alveolar or lingual nerve injury, although the incidence of sensory deficit following ramus harvest is reported to be lower than symphyseal harvest, at 8 and 16 per cent, respectively. There is also the possibility of fracture during the procedure or in the post-operative healing phase.

Maxillary tuberosity and zygomaticomaxillary buttress

The volume of bone available from these sites is limited but may be mixed with allogenic material and/or supplements such as PRP or BMP (BMP-2 or BMP-7) for added volume. The pre-operative preparation is similar to that used for the mandibular symphyseal and ramus donor sites, and the procedure may be easily performed under local anaesthetic, with or without sedation. Once a standard mucoperiostial flap is elevated, bone shavings can be harvested from these sites using shaving devices such as the MX-grafter, or using ronguers to remove bone from the tuberosity area taking care not to enter the maxillary antrum. There is also the option of removing a small and thin widow of bone from the anterior maxillary wall in the buttress region. This widow is typically only 2–3 mm thick and 1 × 1 cm in dimension.

Calvarial shavings

Calvarial bone has been used to augment and graft the maxillofacial region over many years. Although this usually involves general anaesthesia to obtain corticocancellous blocks, techniques have been described to obtain cortical shavings of up to 14 ml under local anaesthetic and sedation.

PREPARATION

The patient should use a chlorhexidine shampoo before surgery. The hair is not shaved, but instead bunched up using elastic bands to create an area of exposed skin in the midline over the vault of the skull. Peri-operative antibiotic therapy and sterile technique are important.

PROCEDURE

After sterile preparation and draping, a 4-cm saggital skin incision is marked out and local anaesthetic (2 per cent lidocaine with 1:100 000 epinephrine may be mixed with 0.5 per cent bupivicaine) is injected into the scalp. A full thickness incision is made down to bone and the periostium is elevated creating a subperiostial pocket. Once the pocket is created, the bone shaver is introduced and bone is harvested from the outer cortex (Figure 2.7.8). The pocket is then irrigated and the scalp closed in two layers (galea and skin). Bulb suction drains may be needed to prevent haematoma formation.

POST-OPERATIVE MANAGEMENT

Antibiotic ointment is applied to the incision three times a day and the patient may shower after 24 hours, but should avoid submersion of the incision in water. Appropriate analgesics (non-steroidal anti-inflammatory and narcotic) are prescribed, and most surgeons continue antibiotic therapy for 5–7 days.

RECIPIENT SITE TECHNIQUES

Onlay graft

Onlay grafts may be used to augment the width and/or the height of the alveolus, although augmenting vertical height is one of the most challenging augmentation procedures. Once the bone graft has been harvested, it should be stored in saline and kept moist until the time of grafting. The success of onlay grafts relies on recipient bed vascularity,

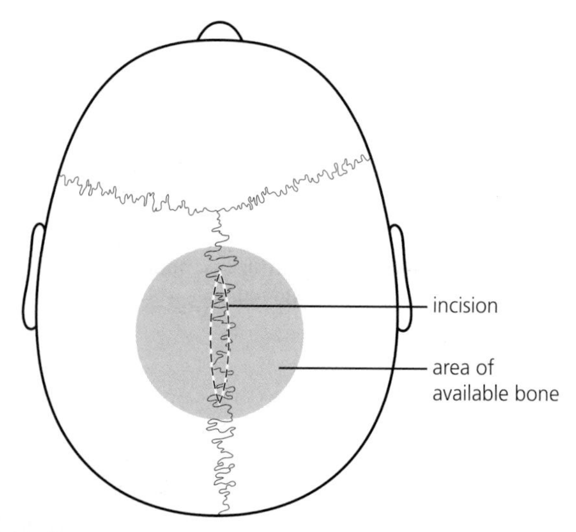

2.7.8 Calvarium donor site.

close approximation and contact between graft and the recipient site, and graft immobilization. In addition, there must be tension-free soft tissue closure over the site to minimize the risk of wound dehiscence which may result in graft failure and loss.

The incision for the recipient site may be made at the crest of the ridge or in the vestibule. Incisions on the crest give easy access, but they are often directly over the graft and are at risk of dehiscence with subsequent graft failure and loss. Incisions placed in the vestibule are away from the graft, but the flap relies on perfusion from the lingual or palatal side and are therefore at risk for breakdown, especially if the crest is composed of dense fibrous tissue.

The recipient bed should be prepared to allow close approximation between the recipient bed and the onlay graft, as well as improve immobilization of the graft. This is often achieved by reducing any significant convexities and mortising the bed to receive the graft. The vascularity of the graft is maximized by perforating the recipient site cortical bone and the graft with a small bur, to encourage early capillary ingrowth and vascularization (Figure 2.7.9). The block is then stabilized using one or two 1.2-mm diameter screws to avoid rotation (Figure 2.7.9). If greater width is desired than the thickness of the graft will allow, the graft may be placed in two layers or secured using positioning screws leaving space under the graft that can be filled with cancellous bone or allogenic bone (Figure 2.7.10). Any sharp edges of the graft are smoothed to reduce the chance of mucosal

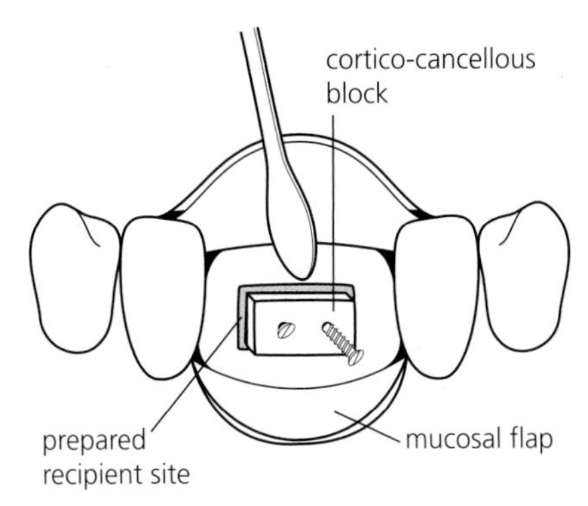

2.7.9 Mortised onlay graft.

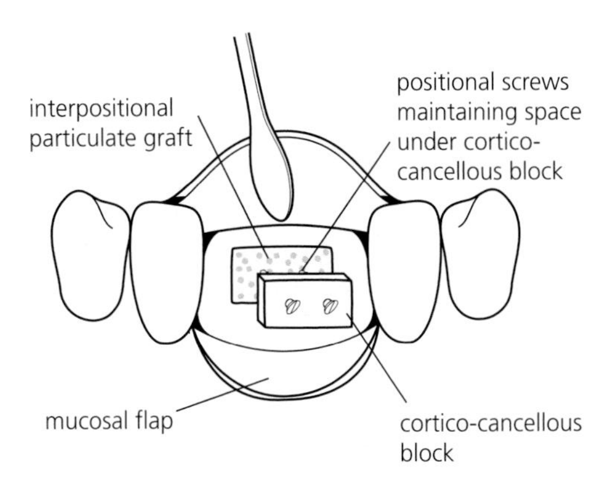

2.7.10 Onlay graft.

breakdown. Cancellous bone or allogenic bone may be placed around the periphery to further augment the site. Membranes may be overlaid onto the graft, although many surgeons feel that this increases the risk of wound dehiscence and infection.

The soft tissue must be closed without tension. Prior to closure, the buccal periostium is incised and undermined to allow advancement of the flap. The incision is closed using non-resorbable sutures.

Appropriate analgesics (non-steroidal anti-inflammatory and narcotic) are prescribed and most surgeons continue antibiotic therapy (amoxicillin or clindamycin) for 5–7 days. The patient should use saline rinses after meals. After 48 hours, the patient should use chlorhexidine mouthwash for 2 weeks, in addition to the saline rinses after meals. The diet should be restricted to a clear liquid diet for 24 hours and advanced to a soft mechanical diet for 2 weeks, to minimize the risk of wound dehiscence. The grafted site should be allowed to heal and consolidate for four to six months prior to implant placement.

Maxillary sinus grafting

Maxillary sinus grafting was first described in the 1970s, but its success has improved since then. The alveolus in the edentulous posterior maxilla is often occupied by a large pneumatized maxillary antrum, resulting in a vertical deficiency in bone. Grafting the floor of the sinus increases the vertical dimension of bone available for successful implant placement. Until recently, this has been performed with simultaneous placement of the implants if there was at least 5 mm of native bone height to provide primary stability for the implant, but if there was less than 5 mm of bone height, implant placement was deferred to a second procedure four to six months following the sinus graft. However, recent literature reports successful implant placement in as little as 1 mm of native bone height, provided there is adequate width (8 mm or more). In these situations, some surgeons will use corticocancellous blocks mortized into the floor of the sinus to provide more stability for the implants.

PRE-OPERATIVE PREPARATION

Panoramic radiographs are adequate to assess the vertical height of bone available at the implant site, but CT scans provide more detailed three-dimensional topographic visualization of the sinus floor and surrounding walls, including the presence of septae within the sinus. In addition, CT scans allow visualization of the sinus mucosa. Patients with sinusitis or sinus disease should be referred for appropriate management before grafting. Local mouth preparation should include chlorhexidine mouth rinse pre-operatively and many surgeons use peri-operative antibiotic that is administered either enterally or parenterally before surgery.

PROCEDURE

Access to the sinus is performed through a Caldwell Luc window in the lateral wall of the sinus. The initial mucosal incision may be placed in the vestibule, although this may increase the likelihood of oroantral fistula formation in the event of wound dehiscence. This may be avoided by utilizing a crestal or sulcular incision away from the bony window. Once a full mucoperiostial flap is elevated and the lateral wall of the maxilla and sinus is exposed, a 1 × 1.5 cm bony window is created anterior to the zygomaticomaxillary buttress (Figure 2.7.11). The superior osteotomy is placed inferior to the infraorbital nerve at the level of the planned graft height, while the inferior osteotomy should lie approximately 3 mm above the floor of the sinus so as to avoid the multiple septations and recesses often encountered along the sinus floor, which make completing the osteotomy and infracturing the bony window problematic. Occasionally, a second window is needed if there is a septum within the sinus. The bony window is created using a diamond bur or a piezosurgery tip to minimize the chance of Schneiderian membrane perforation. Small perforations (less than 3 mm) are inconsequential, but larger perforations should be covered with a resorbable membrane after elevation of the lining and prior to insertion of the graft. Once the bony widow is created and the sinus lining is visible around the periphery, sinus curettes are used to carefully mobilize and elevate the Schneiderian membrane with the oval piece of bone from the window still attached. Once mobilized, the membrane and bony window is turned into the sinus such that the bony segment now becomes the new elevated sinus floor. The space beneath the elevated bony segment and the lining is filled with bone or substitute graft material (Figure 2.7.11). The volume of the graft placed should allow for 20 per cent resorption prior to implant placement. The average volume of graft material required to augment the sinus is 5 ml. Autogenous bone remains the gold standard graft material, but this may be mixed with or even substituted with allogenic bone with good success. Recent literature also report good success with collagen soaked in BMP (BMP-2 or BMP-7).

To close the site, a resorbable membrane is placed over the bony window and the mucoperiostial flap is sutured with non-resorbable sutures which are left in place for 2 weeks.

POST-OPERATIVE MANAGEMENT

In addition to the usual post-operative management of intraoral graft sites as described earlier, the patient should be instructed in sinus precautions. These are especially important if the sinus lining was perforated, and should include no nose blowing, or sucking through straws for at least 3 weeks. Nasal decongestants and saline nasal spray may also be helpful.

COMPLICATIONS

Potential complications include infection, acute maxillary sinusitis, wound breakdown and subsequent failure of the graft, injury to the infraorbital nerve, injury to adjacent tooth roots with devitalization and oroantral fistula.

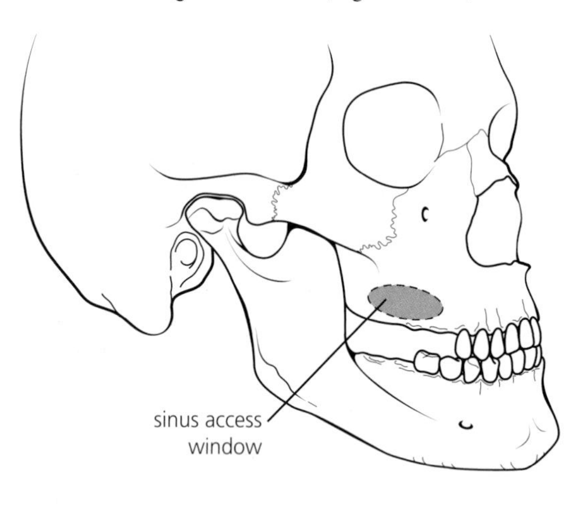

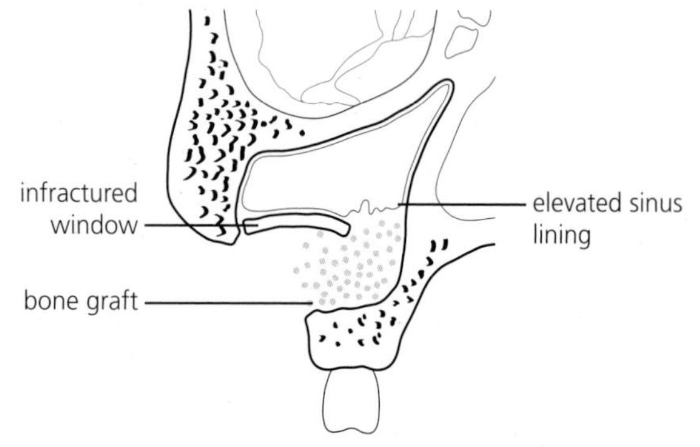

2.7.11 Sinus lift/augmentation.

Alveolar bone splitting/spreading

Osteotomies along the alveolar crest may be performed in the maxilla and the mandible in order to increase the width of the alveolus (Figure 2.7.12). The pre-operative preparation is the same as other grafting procedure outlined above; however, the flap dissection is different. To maintain blood supply to the osteotomized inner and outer segments, the periostium is left attached to the bone. This is achieved by a crestal or vestibular incision as previously described, and a supraperiostial dissection of the labial or buccal mucosal flap. The crestal osteotomy may be made with a saw, a small fissure bur or a piezosurgery tip. The vertical osteotomies may be carried through both inner and outer cortical plates if expansion of both plates is desired. Alternatively, the vertical cut may be through only the buccal/labial cortex if lingual expansion is not required. The vertical osteotomies

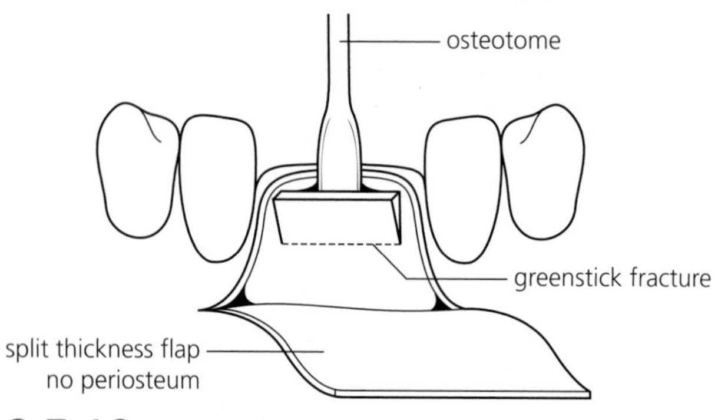

2.7.12 Alveolar ridge splitting.

are usually 1 cm in height. Once the osteotomies are made, osteotomes are driven into the crestal cut and the cortical plate(s) are pedicled on the overlying periostium. The intervening space may then be implanted or grafted with bone or substitute graft materials. The segments and intervening graft may be stabilized using miniplates or screws for immobilization during the healing phase. In addition, many surgeons will cover the site with a resorbable membrane prior to suturing with a non-resorbable suture.

Alveolar distraction osteogenesis

Distraction osteogenesis may have a role where the implant site is deficient in bone height, but has adequate width. It is used most often in the anterior mandible and maxilla. The principle is osteogenesis as the alveolar segment is gradually moved in a coronal direction, thereby generating greater bone height. There are several alveolar distraction devices, but all have common features. Each device has an anchorage and an active component and is operated by a transmucosal element (usually a screw). Patient preparation follows the principles outlined above.

PROCEDURE

A full thickness labial mucoperiostial flap is elevated as described above with the foresight to place the transmucosal element of the distraction device through the incision, and ideally through keratinized mucosa. Once adequate bone has been exposed to allow placement of the distraction device, the device is fixated in position using screws, with careful consideration towards the desired vector of movement, and the osteotomies are marked with the device in place. The device is then removed and the osteotomies are prepared. The osteotomies strive to establish a block of alveolus pedicled on the palatal or lingual mucoperiostium, and is free of mechanical interference that may prevent transposition (Figure 2.7.13). This is achieved by two vertical osteotomies that are connected by a horizontal apical osteotomy. The osteotomy may be made with a saw, a small fissure bur or a piezosurgery tip, and passes through both inner and outer cortical plates. Once the osteotomies are made, they are completed using osteotomes to mobilize the alveolar segment. The distraction device is then reinserted with screws into the pre-existing holes. Once the distraction device is secured it is activated to test the vector of movement and to ensure that there are no bony interferences. It is then returned to its passive position and the flap is sutured closed with non-resorbable sutures.

POST-OPERATIVE MANAGEMENT

The post-operative management is no different than any of the oral grafting procedures described earlier. However, there are specific aspects unique to alveolar distraction. The device is not activated for 7 days to allow a latency period, during which time the osteotomies have vascular ingrowth and early non-bony callous formation. After the latency period, the patient activates the device at a rate of 0.5–1 mm distraction per day, by turning a screw. Therefore, if a 10-mm vertical increase is desired, this can be accomplished in as little as 10 days. The active phase is then followed by a consolidation phase, during which time the distraction is maintained for 12 weeks, allowing the callous to ossify and gain stability.

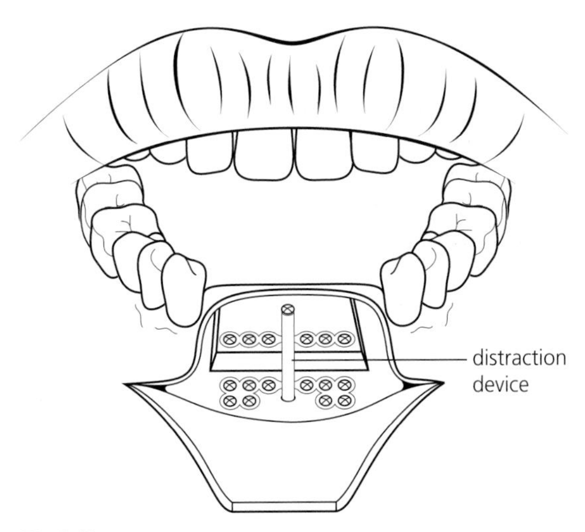

2.7.13 Alveolar distraction.

COMPLICATIONS

In addition to the standard intraoral grafting complications, there may be resorption and loss of the alveolar segment, or movement in an unfavourable direction.

> **Top tips**
>
> - Autogenous bone is considered the gold standard due to its ostoblastic, osteoinductive and osteoconductive properties.
> - Potential bone yields from various donor sites: mandibular symphysis = 5 ml; mandibular ramus = 5–10 ml; proximal tibia = 20–40 ml; anterior iliac crest = 50 ml; and posterior iliac crest = 50–100 ml.
> - Membranous bone grafts show less rapid resorption than endochondral bone grafts.
> - Cancellous grafts vascularize more rapidly the corticocancellous grafts.
> - The mandibular symphysis provides blocks of corticocancellous bone measuring up to 1.5–2 cm in length, 1 cm in height and 4–7 mm in thickness.
> - The mandibular ramus provides corticocancellous blocks of bone measuring up to 3 cm in length, 1 cm in height and 4 mm thick.
> - Implants may be placed simultaneously with sinus floor augmentation if there is 5 mm or more of native bone height, although recent literature shows success in as little as 1 mm of native bone height, if there is adequate width.

FURTHER READING

Block M. *Color atlas of dental implant surgery.* Philadelphia: WB Saunders, 2007.

Esposito M, Grusovin MG, Coulthard P, Worthington HV. The efficacy of various bone augmentation procedures for dental implants: A Cochrane systematic review of randomized controlled clinical trials. *International Journal of Oral and Maxillofacial Implants* 2006; **21**: 696–710.

Garg A. *Bone biology, harvesting, grafting for dental implants: Rationale and clinical applications.* New Maldon: Quintessence, 2004.

Khoury F, Hadi A, Missika P. *Bone augmentation in oral implantology.* New Malden: Quintessence, 2007.

2.8

Basic and advanced implantology: A European perspective

JOHN CAWOOD

INTRODUCTION

The introduction and development of endosteal implants has brought about a revolution in that implant-supported prosthetic devices have become the state of the art.

Nowadays, the establishment and maintenance of osseointegration is very predictable if the relevant factors are taken into consideration, such as favourable anatomical form and environment, biocompatibility and favourable long-term biomechanical conditions. Advances in implant design and surface modification, such as anodic oxidation, encourage direct bone formation on to the implant surface, thus increasing initial implant stability and improving outcome.

At present, the level of evidence indicative of absolute and relative contraindications for implant treatment due to systemic disease is low. Similarly, the evidence base remains weak with regard to pre-existing periodontal disease. Studies at the patient level suggest survival of implants and superstructure are not significantly different from non-periodontally compromised patients. However, at the implant level the incidence of peri-implantitis and marginal bone loss is significantly increased in the periodontally compromised patient. It should be noted that no study has documented that the survival of an implant exceeds that of a tooth properly treated for periodontitis.

The success rate for immediate loading of implants varies between 80 and 100 per cent after one year with higher success rates recorded in the mandible than the maxilla. Survival of conventionally loaded implants is reported as 98 per cent after one year.

In bone graft patients, studies show increased bone contact with implants and increased implant stability when implant placement is delayed for at least three months to allow revascularization of the graft, new bone formation and remodelling of the bone graft.

Advances in both surgical technology and surgical techniques have increased the predictability of pre-implant surgery and have also reduced the morbidity of such surgery. Technological advances include improved imaging techniques, dedicated instrumentation, bone plates and screws and development of biomaterials, such as bone substitutes and membranes for guided tissue regeneration. Computerized tomography allows accurate measurements to be made and provides information on bone density. Interactive planning has refined treatment planning and treatment execution. Computer-generated models (stereolythography) allows for simulated surgery and provision of templates, further increasing the predictability of the treatment outcome (Figure 2.8.1).

PRE-IMPLANT SURGERY

Following tooth loss, there is loss of alveolar bone due to disuse atrophy. At first, bone loss is rapid. After two to three years, the rate diminishes but loss does continue indefinitely (Figure 2.8.2). There is an associated decrease in mucosal coverage of both the keratinized and non-keratinized mucosa which quickly compromises the potential implant site.

Pre-implant surgery is intended not only to improve the implant site *per se*, but also to correct deficiencies in the height and width of the alveolus and to restore or improve the intermaxillary relationship. This is because loss of bone in the edentulous jaw, and to a lesser extent in the partially edentulous jaw, leads to an alteration of the maxillomandibular jaw relationship, encroachment of muscle attachments in relation to the edentulous alveolus and a decrease in the surface area of the overlying mucosa. The effect of these changes combined with ageing, circumoral hypotonia and collapse results in changes of facial form and appearance (Figure 2.8.3).

There must be adequate bone volume both in height and width to allow placement of implants of sufficiently large dimensions to withstand functional loading and permit optimal axial inclination, in order to fulfil the functional and aesthetic requirements without interfering with adjacent anatomical structures, for example the neurovascular bundle, maxillary sinus and adjacent teeth. Vertical transverse and

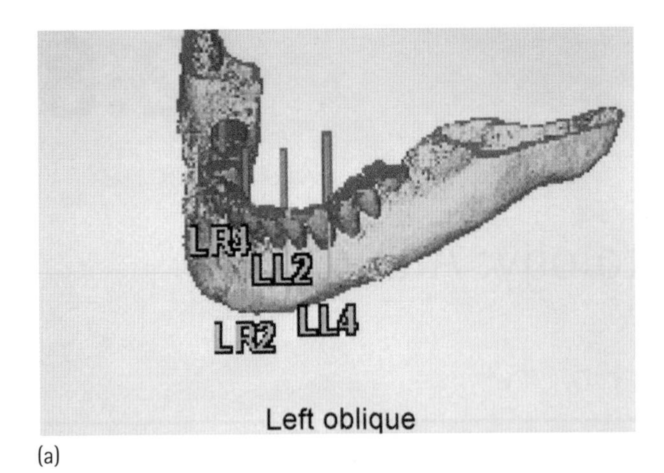

(a)

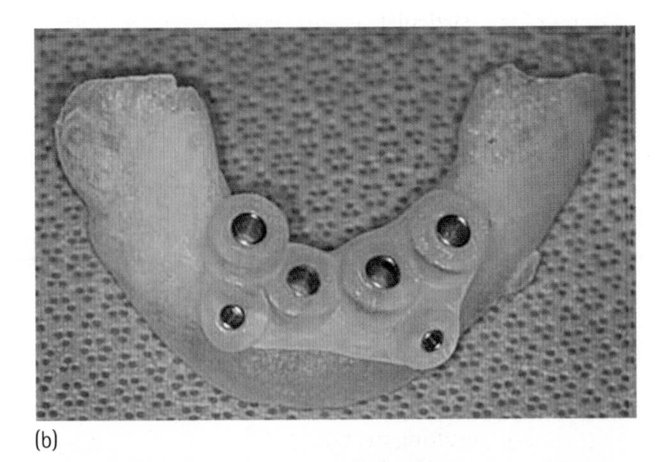

(b)

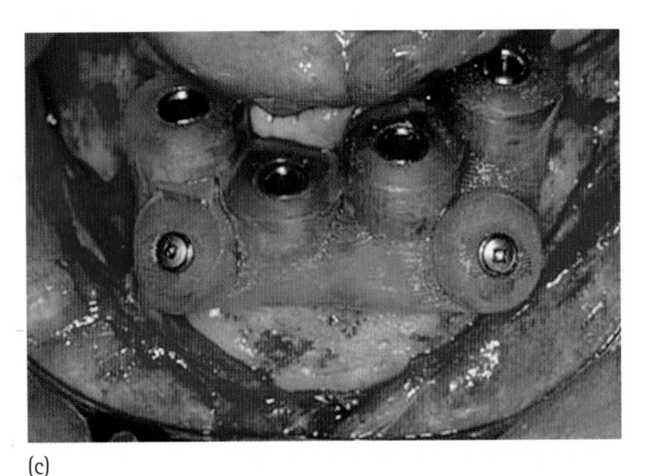

(c)

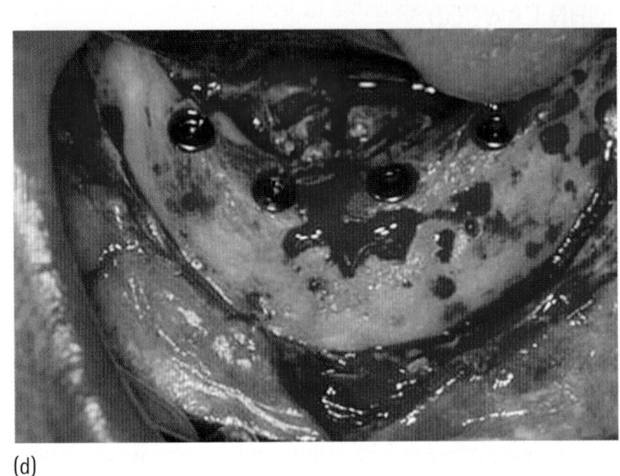

(d)

2.8.1 Computer generated stereolythographic model and surgical guide for control of implant placement. (a) Stereolythographic model of mandible; (b) computer-generated surgical guide for implant placement; (c) surgical guide *in situ* and position secured with screws; (d) radiograph of implants.

anteroposterior intermaxillary relationships should be favourable. If the foregoing conditions do not prevail, pre-implant surgery (including bone augmentation, soft tissue procedures and possibly an osteotomy) may be undertaken.

Based on the Cawood and Howell classification of the edentulous jaws, a scheme for pre-implant surgery has evolved (Figure 2.8.4).

- Class 1, dentate
- Class II, post-extraction
- Class III, adequate height and width
- Class IV, adequate height, inadequate width ('knife-edge ridge')
- Class V, inadequate height, inadequate width ('flat ridge')
- Class VI, loss of basal bone ('submerged ridge').

In a study of 300 edentulous patients by Longman, the type of jaw atrophy was assessed. The most frequently encountered pattern of jaw atrophy is class IV in the maxilla and class V in the mandible (Figure 2.8.4).

In the class IV, V and VI edentulous or partially dentate jaws, implant placement is usually combined with bone augmentation using onlay grafts, inlay grafts and/or interpositional grafts and in addition soft-tissue procedures.

The choice of bone graft is influenced by the type of grafts required, i.e. block graft or particulate graft. The quantity of bone required will determine the donor site, i.e. local (intraoral) or distant (e.g. iliac crest). Corticocancellous block grafts are used to augment areas where there are deficiencies in width and height of the alveolar process. Particulate grafts are used to fill two or three walled defects, e.g. augmentation of the floor of the maxillary sinus or interpositional bone grafts.

There is a fundamental difference in the healing of these grafts, which should be taken into account when using them. Unlike block corticocancellous bone grafts, most of the particulate cancellous bone graft is able to survive with areas of new bone formation occurring throughout the original graft. Even when dehiscence occurs, usually only a small portion of the particulate graft is lost. The primary healing depends on capillary ingrowth, not only from the bone surface of the recipient site, but also from the enveloping soft tissue. Particulate grafts are difficult to use as onlay grafts because containment is a problem. The use of barrier membranes is useful when small alveolar defects have to be filled.

Corticocancellous block grafts provide a scaffold that will be resorbed almost completely to be replaced by new bone by the process of creeping bone substitution. Rigid fixation of corticocancellous grafts to the recipient site is essential for this process to take place unhindered. Any micromovement at the interface between the graft and recipient site will jeopardize capillary ingrowth from the recipient bed, resulting in avascular necrosis and loss of the graft. It is always advisable to use at least two screws to fix the bone to prevent any micromovement. Other important factors are the close adaptation of the graft itself to the recipient bed and tension-free closure of the soft tissue. Depending on the size of the graft, revascularizaton will occur in approximately 2 weeks; subsequently remodelling begins. It is therefore advisable to delay insertions of endosteal implants for at least three months following placement of the bone graft.

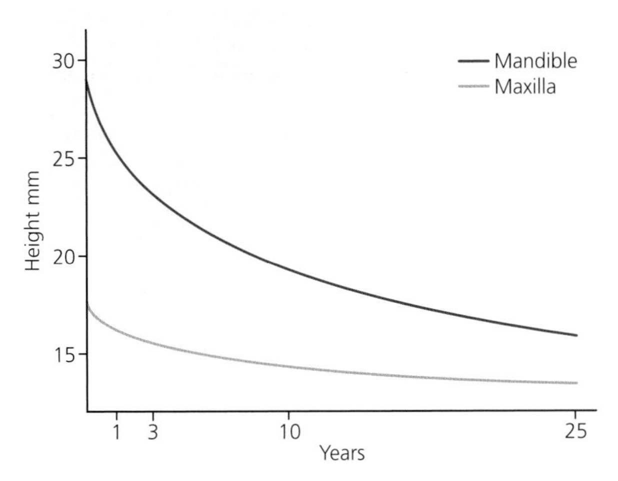

2.8.2 Reduction of ridge height of the edentulous mandible and maxilla over time (after Tallgren 1972).

SOFT TISSUE PROCEDURES

The main objective of soft tissue procedures is to improve the peri-implant environment in order to eliminate mobile mucosa or inflammatory hyperplasia. Ideally, implants should be surrounded by an immobile keratinized mucosa. For this reason, split-thickness mucosal grafts are harvested from the palate in strips, using a mucotome, which are draped around the implants and secured with a dressing plate (Figure 2.8.5 p.98).

Connective tissue grafts are usually harvested from the palate to correct mucogingival defects around implants and also to augment residual small volume soft-tissue defects, mainly in the aesthetic zone (Figure 2.8.6 p.99). Small rotational flaps aid the envelopment of implants with keratinized mucosa and to restore the shape of the interdental papilla. The lip switch technique, first described by Kazanjian, is indicated in those patients who have a shallow buccal vestibule in the mandibular vestibular area or a high attachment of the mentalis muscle to give a deepened sulcus.

CLASS II

Immediate placement of implants in the extraction socket has the advantage of reducing the number of surgical

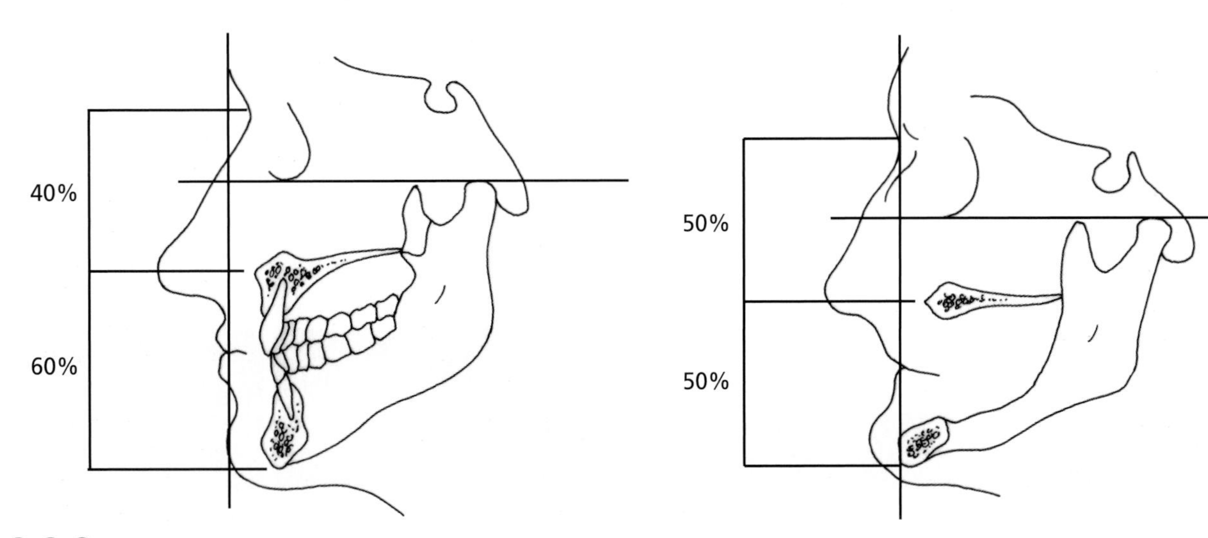

2.8.3 Consequences of jaw atrophy. Decreased lower face height, prognathism and collapse of lower facial soft tissue are shown. Reprinted with permission.

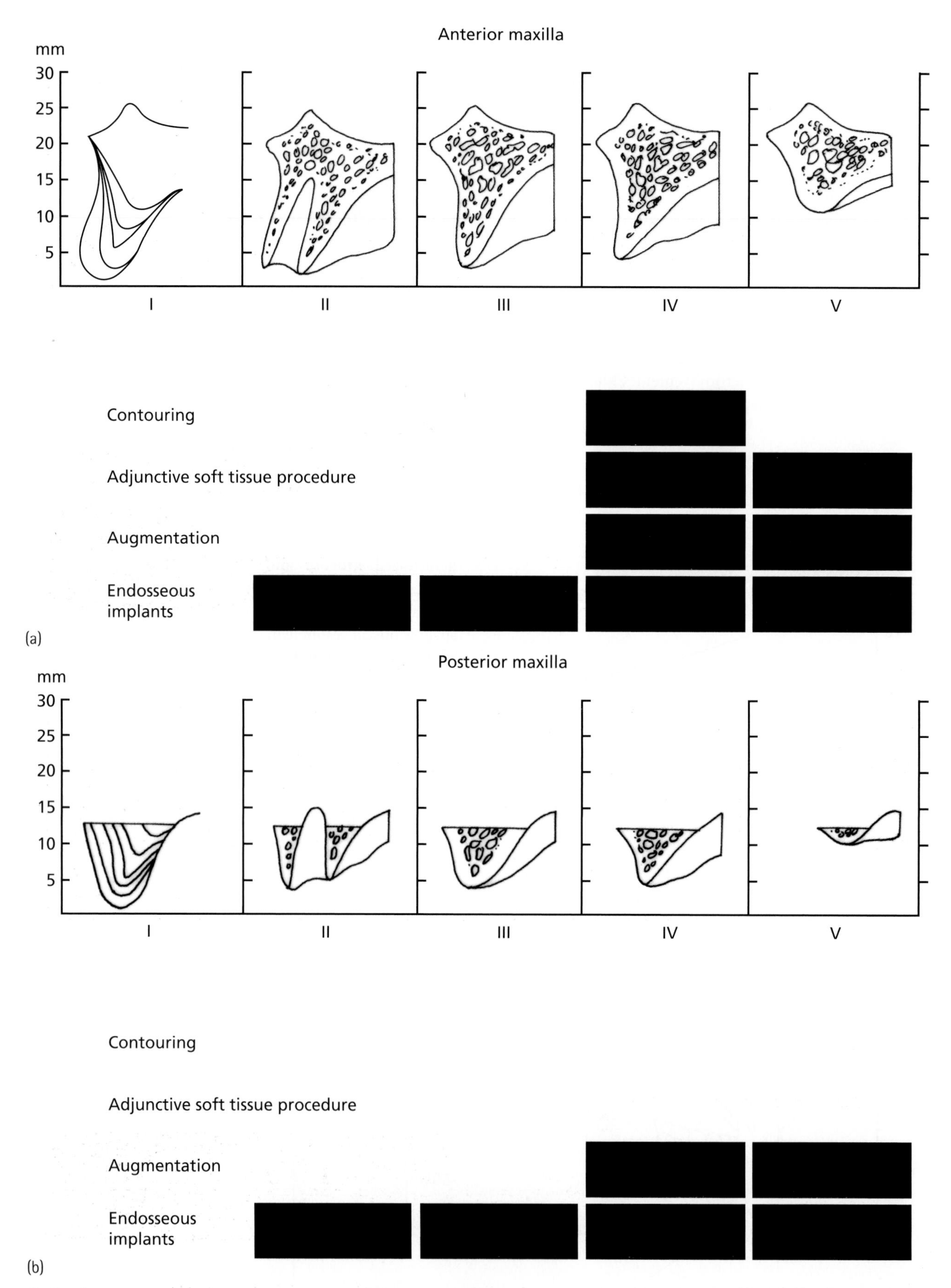

2.8.4 Scheme for pre-implant surgery based on Cawood and Howell classification of the edentulous jaw. (a) Anterior maxilla; (b) posterior maxilla.

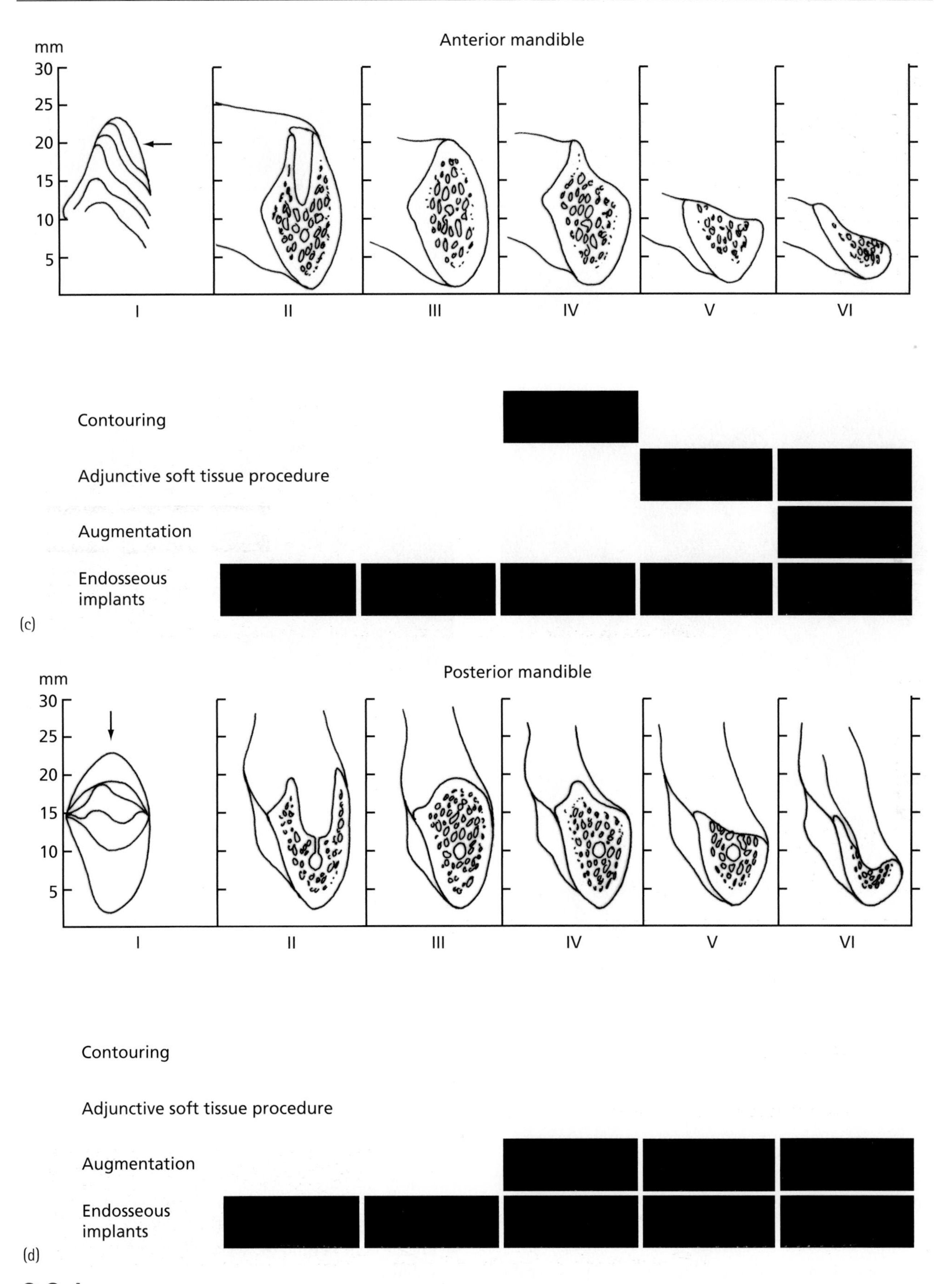

2.8.4 Scheme for pre-implant surgery based on Cawood and Howell classification of the edentulous jaw. (c) anterior mandible; (d) posterior mandible. Reprinted with permission.

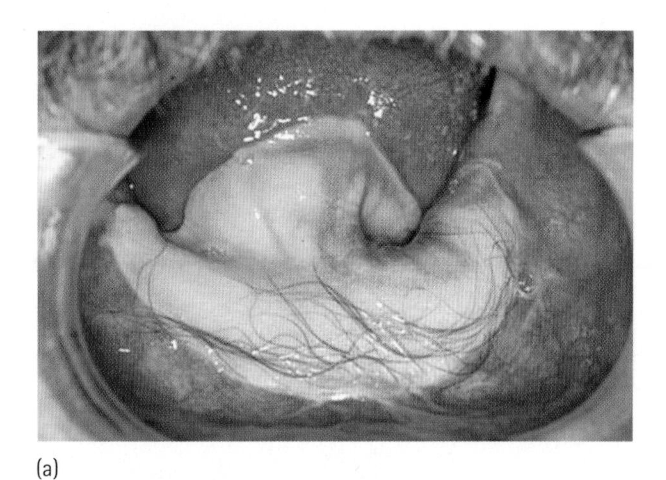

(a)

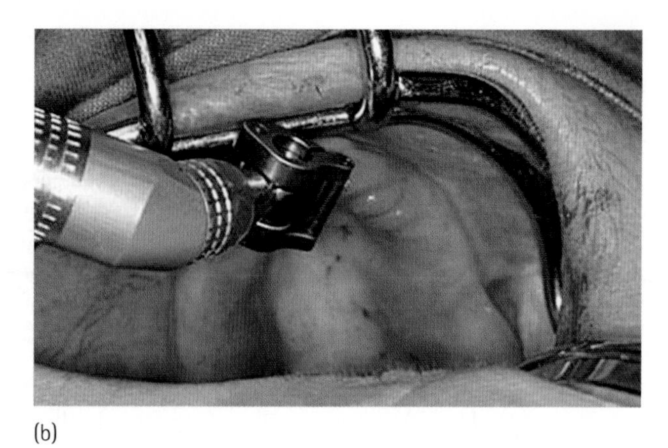

(b)

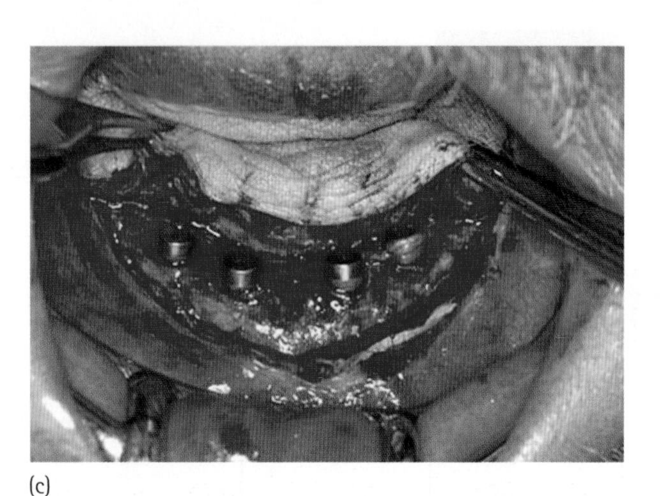

(c)

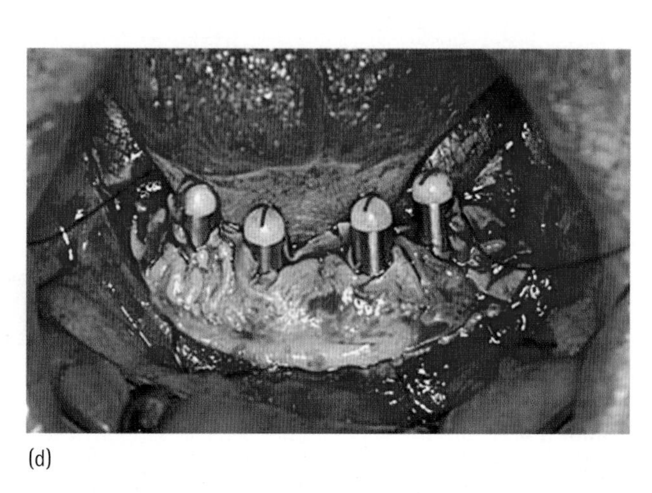

(d)

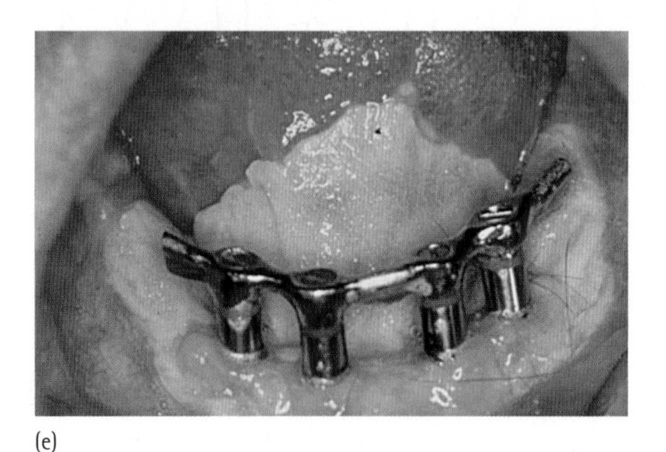

(e)

2.8.5 Split thickness mucosal graft to enhance implant environment, anterior mandible. (a) Fasciocutaneous free flap following anterior floor of mouth and rim resection surgery; (b) harvesting of mucosal graft from palate using a mucotome; (c) alveolar ridge exposed and implants positioned; (d) mucosal graft draped around implants; (e) healed mucosal graft and implant superstructure.

interventions and reducing the time to delivery of the prosthesis.

- Use of periotome and sectioning of roots to preserve the integrity of the alveolar walls.
- Complete removal of the periodontal ligament, any granulation tissue and fibrous connective tissue.
- Acute and subacute peri-apical or periodontal infection is a contraindication to immediate implant placement.
- Engage bone beyond the socket to ensure initial implant stability.
- Coronal aspect of implant should be placed 2 mm apical to the coronal aspect of the socket to allow for bone remodelling and osseous regeneration.

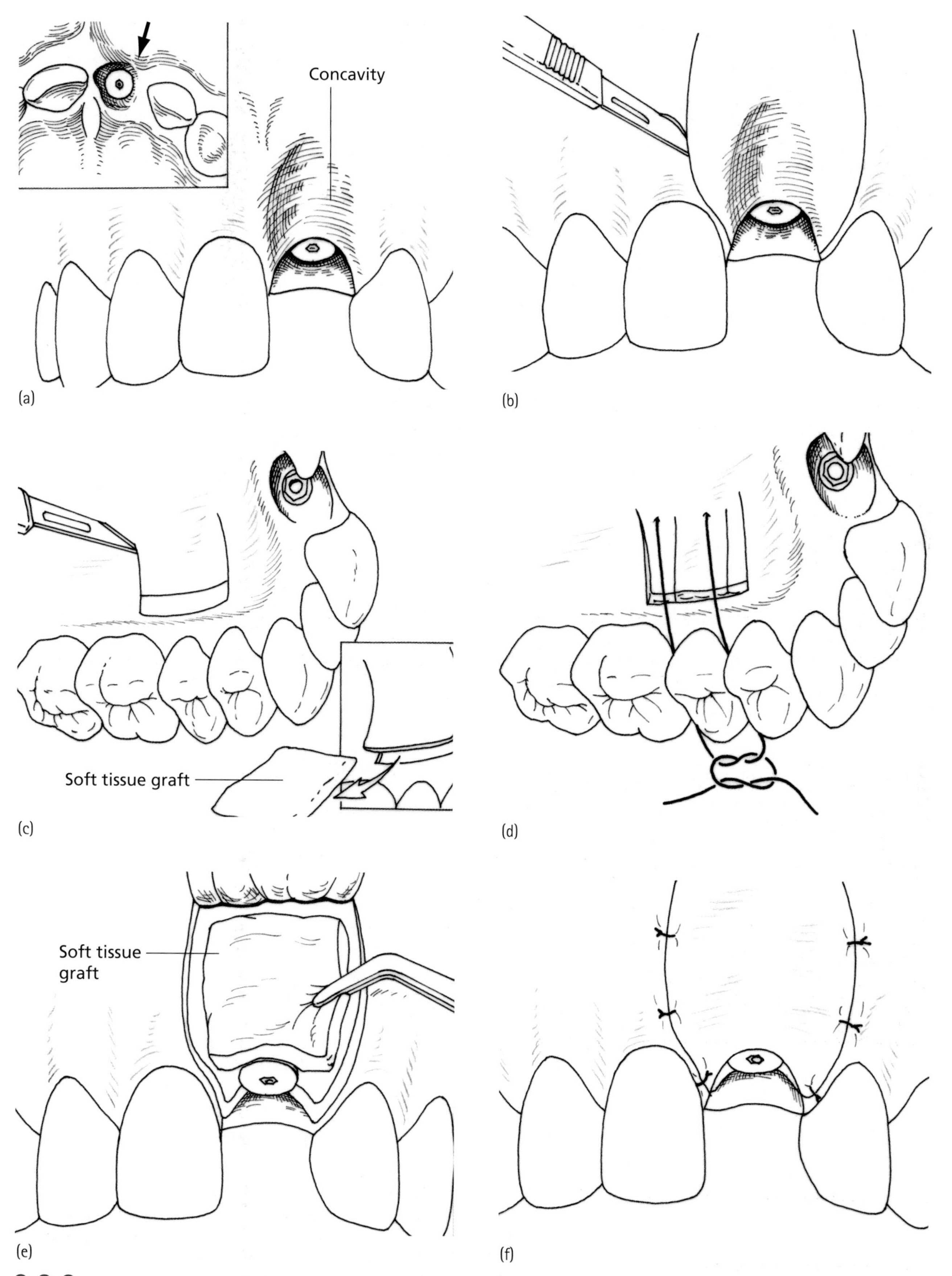

2.8.6 Soft tissue management in implant placement. Connective tissue graft. (a) Concavity over implant site; (b) elliptical incision on labial aspect; (c) connective tissue graft harvested from palate; (d) palatal flap sutured back; (e) connective tissue graft placed over defect; (f) flap replaced over connective tissue graft restoring contour. Reprinted with permission from OMS Knowledge Update, Vol. 1, 1994; IMP/70–71.

- Small alveolar defects may be repaired by placement of a barrier membrane over augmentation material, provided soft-tissue coverage is possible.

Placement of an immediate implant is contraindicated where a defect of the coronal aspect of the socket exists. Instead allow complete healing of the socket. After three months, the residual alveolus can be repaired with an onlay graft (Figure 2.8.7).

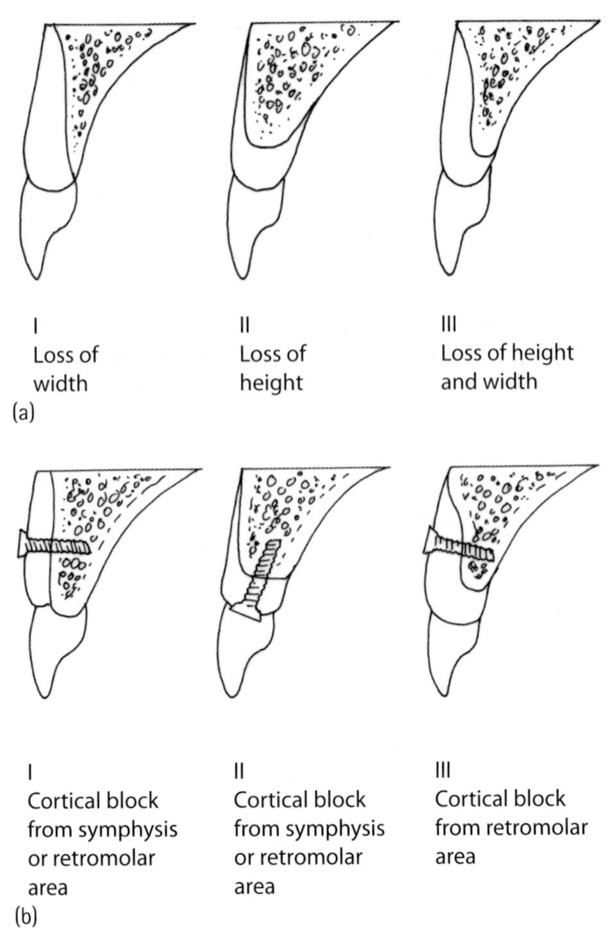

2.8.7 (a) Alveolar local bone deficiencies: I, loss of width; II, loss of height; III, loss of height and width. (b) Correction of local alveolar deficiency with locally harvested block grafts. I, veneer graft; II, onlay graft; III, saddle graft. Reprinted with permission from Sethi A, Kaus T. *Practical Implant Dentistry*. Quintessence, 2005.

CLASS III

Delayed implant placement in mature bone is a safe and predictable procedure. Immediate loading is possible provided there is a minimum height of 12 mm and a minimum width of 6 mm of alveolar bone. However, in the aesthetic zone, the soft-tissue should be level with the papilla of the adjacent teeth, otherwise augmentation is required. For delayed implant loading, a remote incision is preferred to reduce the risk of implant dehiscence. For immediate implant loading, a crestal incision is required. A surgical guide is essential for optimal site selection for implant placement and prosthetic outcome.

The direction of the implant bed is determined by the adjacent teeth and the direction of the cortical plates. Implant positioning should be no less than 2 mm from the adjacent teeth and no less than 3 mm from an adjacent implant. The pilot bur establishes the direction and depth of the implant bed. The diameter of the osteotomy is sequentially enlarged using graduated burs with copious irrigation to avoid thermal trauma to the bone. In low density bone, the use of bone condensers is preferred to enlarge the osteotomy site, which also compacts adjacent bone and aids primary implant stability. In high density bone, the implant's bed must be completely formed using hand reamers and bone taps. The implant bed depth should be 1 mm greater than the implant length.

CLASS IV (BONE EXPANSION)

- Bone expansion is indicated when the residual alveolar height is no less than 12 mm and the nasolabial support is adequate.
- Bone expansion should be carried out in a healed site with mature cortical plate.
- There should be intervening cancellous bone and no fusing of the cortical plates (a computed tomography (CT) scan is helpful for this assessment).
- In the aesthetic zone, the overlying soft tissue should be level with the papillae of the adjacent teeth.
- CT scan should have reference radio-opaque markers, so that the tooth position can be assessed in relation to the future implant position and indicates that the outcome is feasible.
- Surgical guide is required to control implant position.
- Osteotomy is initiated with a scalpel blade.
- Expander is inserted into the cancellous bone between the cortical plates.
- Progressive dilation of implant bed to required dimension.
- Two-stage implant system advised.
- Healing period of six months.

CLASS IV MAXILLA (INADEQUATE NASOLABIAL SUPPORT)

In the anterior maxilla, the direction of bone loss is initially horizontal. This converts the broad class III ridge into a narrow knife-edge ridge which has adequate height, but inadequate width of residual bone to accommodate implants. The anterior maxillary osteotomy is designed to increase the width of the alveolus in order to insert implants and also to provide nasolabial support (Figure 2.8.8).

A CT scan is required to demonstrate that intervening cancellous bone is present and that there is no fusion of the cortical plates.

- A horseshoe-shaped incision is made in the labial mucosa and a mucosal flap dissected to a point approximately 3 mm below the crest of the alveolar crest.
- The periosteum is incised and a full-thickness mucoperiosteal flap reflected on to the palatal aspect.
- A sagittal osteotomy is developed using a scalpel blade to penetrate the cancellous bone. The osteotomy is completed with a fine reciprocating saw. The cortical bone of the nasal floor is cut with a fine osteotome. Vertical bone cuts are made through the buccal cortex in the premolar region.
- The anterior nasal spine is removed and the anterior part of the nasal septum is detached from the anterior segment to be mobilized.
- The labial segment is mobilized anteriorly approximately 6 mm and stabilized with either microplates or position screws.
- An interpositional graft of particulate bone is inserted.
- Tension-free closure of the mucosa is obtained.
- Implants placed after three months.
- The anterior maxillary osteoplasty can be combined with sinus floor augmentation (Figure 2.8.8).

Where there is fusion of the cortical plates, augmentation of the class IV ridge is achieved using a block veneer graft which is stabilized with lag screws (Figure 2.8.9).

For single tooth replacement in the anterior maxilla, augmentation of the alveolus is required for optimal implant placement and soft-tissue support using a veneer graft harvested from the mandible.

- Remote palatal incision extended within the crevicular margin labially to involve one unit either side of the recipient site. Papilla-sparing incisions and bevelled incisions optimize the aesthetic result.
- Bone graft is contoured to fit the recipient site passively.
- Bone graft secured with two microscrews to avoid risk of micromovement.
- Tension-free closure of mucosa is obtained using a periosteal release incision, if necessary.
- Implant placement after three months.

Sufficient bone can be obtained from the mandibular ramus area for placement of up to four implants. An increase in width of 2–6 mm and an increase in height of about 4 mm can be achieved (Figure 2.8.10).

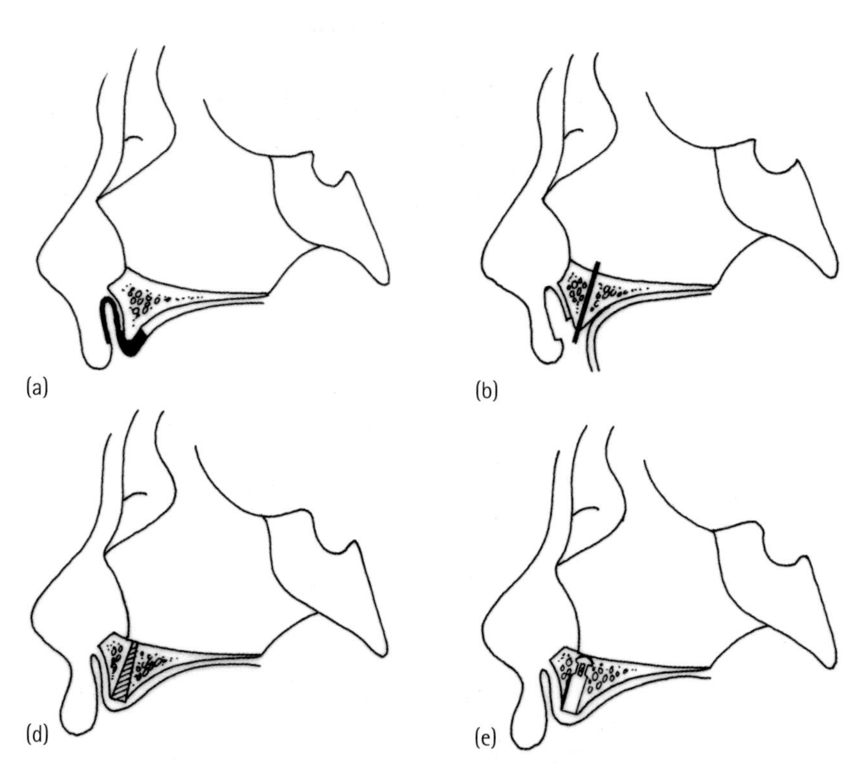

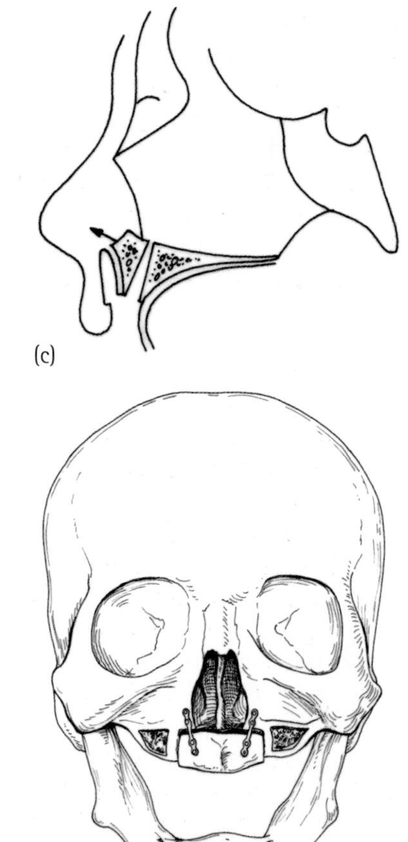

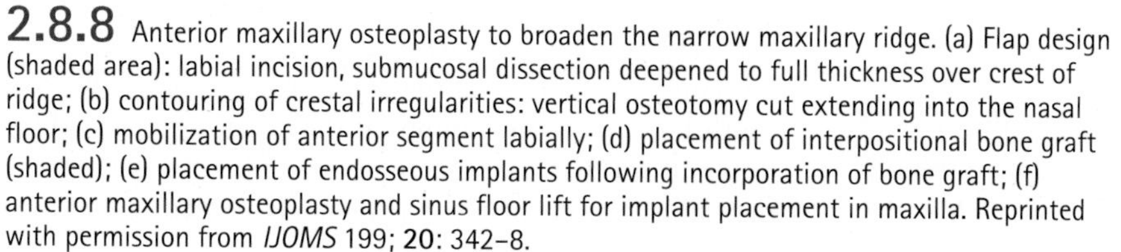

2.8.8 Anterior maxillary osteoplasty to broaden the narrow maxillary ridge. (a) Flap design (shaded area): labial incision, submucosal dissection deepened to full thickness over crest of ridge; (b) contouring of crestal irregularities: vertical osteotomy cut extending into the nasal floor; (c) mobilization of anterior segment labially; (d) placement of interpositional bone graft (shaded); (e) placement of endosseous implants following incorporation of bone graft; (f) anterior maxillary osteoplasty and sinus floor lift for implant placement in maxilla. Reprinted with permission from *IJOMS* 199; **20**: 342–8.

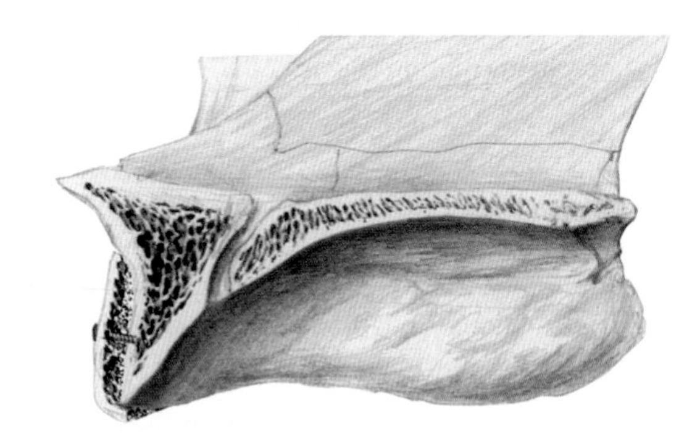

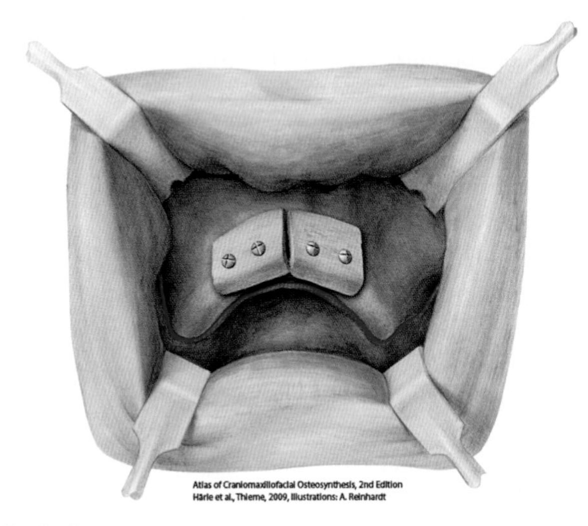

2.8.9 Class IV anterior maxilla augmented with a veneer graft and stabilized lag screws. From *Atlas of Craniomaxillofacial Osteosynthesis*. Reproduced with permission from Thieme.

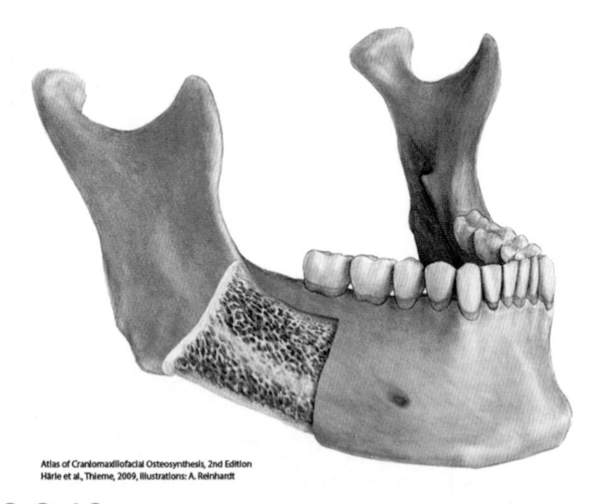

2.8.10 Mandibular ramus veneer graft. From *Atlas of Craniomaxillofacial Osteosynthesis*. Reproduced with permission from Thieme.

CLASS V MAXILLA

The class V maxilla is characterized by loss of the alveolar process resulting in a vertical, transverse and anteroposterior alteration of the interarch relationship. Extensive augmentation with autogenous bone is required to restore the alveolar dimension and provide the necessary facial support. Bone is harvested from the iliac crest.

To determine the quantity of bone to be harvested, the selected tooth position is related to a stone cast of the edentulous ridge by means of a plater matrix. Silicone can be used to form a template to facilitate both the harvesting of bone from the iliac crest area and also to adapt the graft to the recipient site.

The onlay graft is stabilized using position screws. Tension-free closure is obligatory and is facilitated with a periosteal release incision. Implant placement should be delayed for at least three months.

CLASS VI MAXILLA

Resorption of the maxillary alveolar process eventually leads to a relatively posterior and cranial position of the maxilla resulting in a reversed intermaxillary relationship and increased vertical intermaxillary distance. Reconstruction of the class VI maxilla aims at restoration of interarch relationship and augmentation of the alveolar bone to provide support for the collapsed facial musculature and implant placement (Figure 2.8.3).

SURGICAL TECHNIQUE

A horseshoe incision is made high in the vestibule from first molar to first molar. The mucoperiosteum is reflected and the lateral sinus wall and nasal aperture are exposed. A No. 5 round bur is used to make the horizontal osteotomy cut. The thin sinus membrane is elevated (preferably intact). The bone cuts are completed, including the medial sinus wall and nasal septum. The tuberosity is detached from the pterygoid plate using a small osteotome. Due to the fragile nature of the maxilla, the 'down fracture' procedure must be carried out gently. In cases of severe rupture of the sinus membrane, the exposed sinus is sealed with a cortical plate bone stabilized with a microplate. The mobilized maxilla is fixed in the planned position with four microplates. The intervening space is packed with particulate cancellous bone. Tension-free closure of the soft tissues is obligatory and periosteal release incision may be required for this to be achieved. Implants are placed at least three months later in the planned position using a surgical guide (Figure 2.8.11).

ATROPHIC MANDIBLE

Unlike the maxilla, which is composed of trabecular bone predominantly with a thin cortex, the mandible has a thick cortical layer. This provides superior support for endosteal implants, particularly in the anterior mandible. Following tooth loss, the blood supply of the edentulous mandible differs from that of the dentate mandible. In the dentate mandible, blood supply is principally centrifugal arising

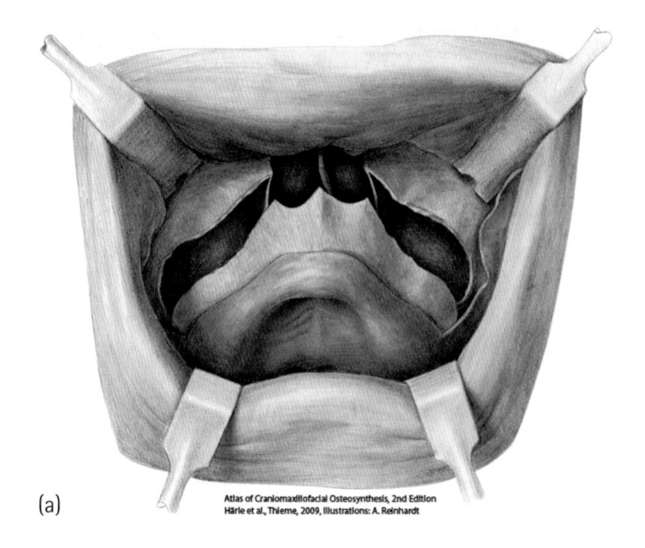

(a)

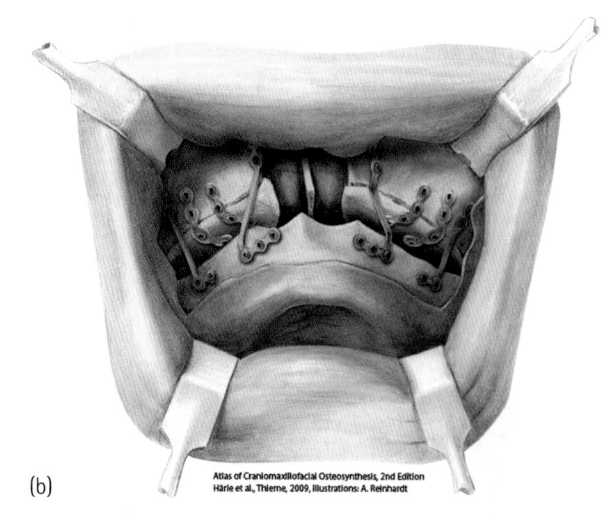

(b)

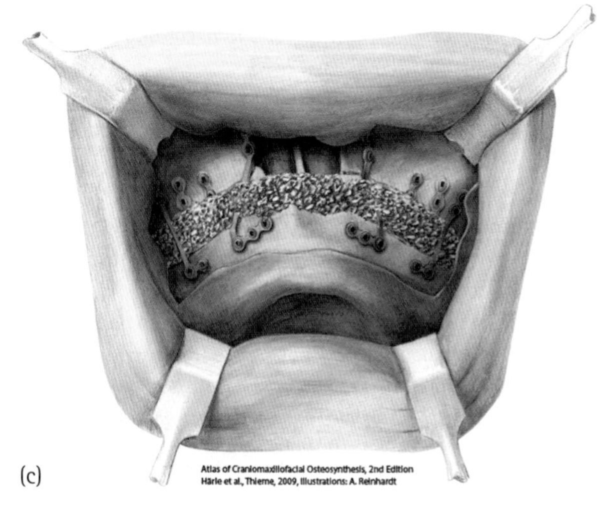

(c)

2.8.11 Surgical technique. (a) Exposure of maxilla via horseshoe incision in sulcus. (b) Repositioning of caudal fragment anteritoly and inferiorly and stabilized with 4 microscrews. Note placement of cortical plate to seal maxillary antrum. (c) Placement of particulate cancellous bone graft (harvested from posterior iliac crest). From *Atlas of Craniomaxillofacial Osteosynthesis*. Reproduced with permission from Thieme.

mainly from the inferior alveolar artery and periodontal arterial arcades. The blood supply of the edentulous mandible is mainly centripetal, being derived via the subperiosteal plexus. Therefore, when carrying out pre-implant surgery of the edentulous mandible, elevation of the mucoperiosteum must be performed carefully to avoid damaging the periosteal layer and subsequent ischaemic necrosis of the underlying bone.

CLASS II AND III MANDIBLE

Similar to the maxilla endosteal implants can be inserted with minimal pre-implant surgery being required. However, it should be noted that any surgical interference with the inferior alveolar nerve may lead to sensory alteration and loss which can be permanent.

CLASS IV AND V MANDIBLE

In the class IV anterior mandible, contouring to remove the narrow ridge or onlay bone grafting will be influenced by the prosthetic requirements. In the class V edentulous mandible anteriorly implants may be inserted without need for bone augmentation. However, the soft tissue environment is unfavourable with reduced keratinized mucosa and a shallow sulcus. A Kazanjian flap is useful to increase the area of attached mucosa and at the same time deepen the labial sulcus.

CLASS VI MANDIBLE

The class VI mandible is characterized by loss of basal bone that can be extensive. Often the inferior alveolar canal is exposed and pain results from compression of the nerve during function. Augmentation of the class VI mandible is indicated when the residual height is less than 10 mm. Augmentation is accomplished either with an interpositional bone graft or an onlay bone graft. The choice between these two techniques is partly operator dependent and partly dependent on the relationship of the soft tissues of the floor of the mouth relative to the residual ridge. If the lax tissues of the floor of the mouth 'spill' over the residual ridge, then an onlay bone graft is more effective in 'damming back' the floor of mouth tissues. Through a subperiosteal tunnel, an onlay graft is placed in the posterior mandible to cover the exposed inferior alveolar canal. Implant placement is delayed for a minimum of three months (Figure 2.8.12).

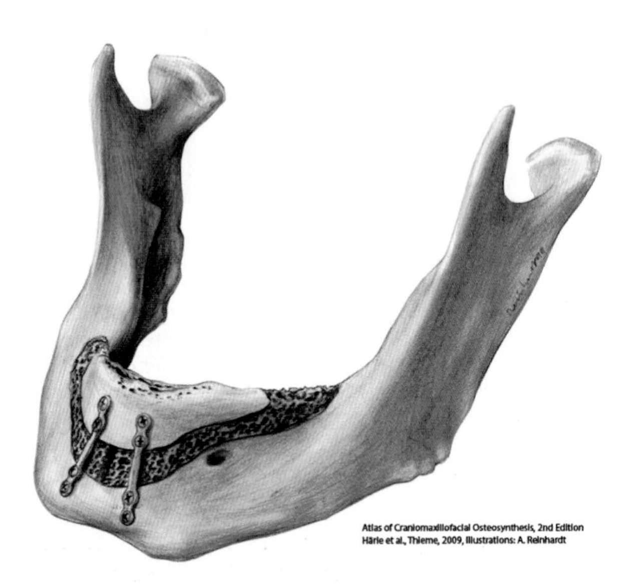

2.8.12 Class VI mandible: augmentation with interpositional particulate bone graft anteriorly and onlay graft posteriorly to protect inferior alveolar nerve. Stabilization with miniplate osteosynthesis. From *Atlas of Craniomaxillofacial Osteosynthesis.* Reproduced with permission from Thieme.

Top tips

- Computerized tomography aids planning and treatment.
- Surgical guide for optimal implant position.
- Bone augmentation for optimal implant size and position.
- Autogenous bone graft remains 'gold standard'.
- Surgical stent aids block graft procurement and adaptation.
- Rigid fixation of block graft using a minimum of two screws.
- Tension free closure of overlying soft tissue after bone augmentation.
- Keratinized mucosa should surround implant.

FURTHER READING

Branemark PI. *The osseointegration book: from calvarium to calcaneous.* Berlin: Quintessenz, 2005.

Cawood JI, Stoelingo PJW, Blackburn TK. The evlolution of preimplant surgery from preprosthetic surgery. *International Journal of Oral and Maxillofacial Surgery* 2007; **36**: 377–85.

Claven J, Lundgren S. Ramus or chin grafts for maxillary sinus inlay and local onlay augmentation: Comparison of donor site morbidity and complications. *Clinical Implant Dentistry and Related Research* 2003; **5**: 154–60.

Sclar AG. *Soft tissue and esthetic considerations in implant therapy.* New Maldon: Quintessence, 2003.

Stoelinga PJW. Chapter 46: Preprosthetic reconstructive surgery. In: Peterson LJ (ed.). *Principles of oral and maxillofacial surgery,* vol 2. Philadelphia: Lippincott Williams and Wilkins, 1992: 1169–207.

2.9

Major preprosthetic surgery, incorporating implants

EUGENE KELLER

MAXILLA (PARTIAL OR TOTAL EDENTULISM) RECONSTRUCTION

Introduction

Implant reconstruction of the severely resorbed edentulous maxilla frequently requires autogenous block bone graft reconstruction. This can be accomplished with iliac, cranial or mandibular corticocancellous block bone grafts. Depending on the degree of bone loss, the patient's functional or esthetic requirements, and the prosthodontic requirements, the bone graft procedures can either be a one- or two-stage reconstruction. The one-stage reconstruction requires simultaneous placement of block bone grafts and endosseous root form dental implants. In the two-stage procedure, bone grafting and implant placement procedures are separated by three to six months to allow for bone graft healing. The bone grafting procedures are classified anatomically as onlay, inlay or interpositional types.

Onlay (one stage) corticocancellous block bone graft (Figure 2.9.1)

INTRODUCTION

For totally edentulous patients with advanced bone loss, there also needs to be adequate bone quality and quantity between the anterior antral walls to accommodate four to six endosseous implants to stabilize the one-stage onlay bone graft. If there is insufficient bone, a two-stage onlay bone graft procedure is performed. In the latter situation, the bone graft is stabilized by miniplates or bone screws. There must also be adequate interarch space to accommodate the onlay bone graft and dental osseoprosthesis. The soft tissue flap used to cover the onlay bone graft must be free of infection and significant scar tissue. A periosteal incision of the labial-buccal flap with mucosal advancement is needed for a critical watertight non-tension everted wound closure.

SURGICAL PROSTHETIC PROCEDURE

1. For full arch reconstruction nasoendotracheal anaesthesia is required.
2. Labial-buccal incision position is critical.
3. Non-traumatic (low heat production) bone graft harvesting is critical to preserve cell viability of the cancellous and cambian layer of osteoblasts. Iliac bone is utilized for large full arch reconstruction and cranial or mandibular ramus or symphysis bone for smaller segmental reconstruction (see under Bone graft harvesting technique).
4. Rigid onlay bone graft stabilization (endosseous implants or miniplates and screws) is important to promote bone graft healing and simultaneous implant osseointegration (one-stage procedure).
5. Non-traumatic bone drilling osteotomy preparation prior to implant placement.
6. Non-tension everted watertight wound closure following periosteal incision.
7. Four to six months of minimal (physiologic) prosthesis loading.
8. Long-term physiologic dental prosthesis loading.

Inlay (antral and nasal) (one stage) corticocancellous block bone graft (Figure 2.9.2)

INDICATIONS

This is indicated for totally edentulous patients with advanced bone resorption but inadequate interarch space to accommodate the onlay bone graft and associated osseoprosthesis. It is also indicated for patients with inadequate soft tissue elasticity for onlay bone graft soft tissue coverage. The surgeon can also elect to perform the inlay versus the onlay bone graft, bearing in mind that the final implant prosthesis will be affected (fixed-removable versus continuous fixed). For partially or totally edentulous patients, a two-stage bone grafting procedure can be

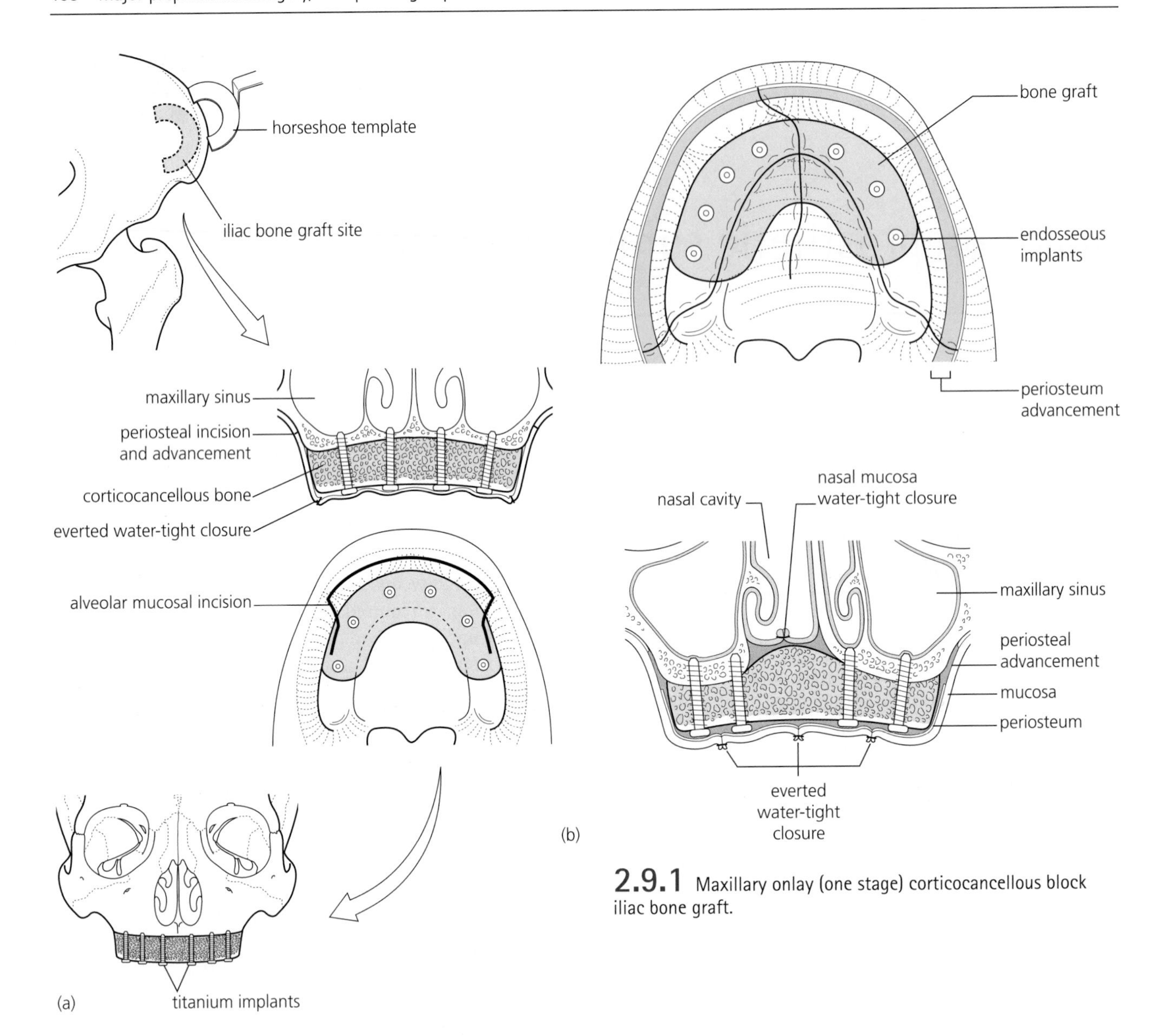

2.9.1 Maxillary onlay (one stage) corticocancellous block iliac bone graft.

performed utilizing either corticocancellous block or particulate bone grafts from the iliac crest, mandible or cranium. Various allogenic and autogenous bone particulate bone grafts can also be mixed to increase the particulate bone graft volume. This is not common in the author's practice as adequate volumes of cancellous bone can be harvested from the anterior and/or posterior iliac crest. If particulate bone grafts are utilized, the sinus membrane or various membranes (collagen preferred) need to be utilized to confine the graft material in the correct position for later secondary implant placement. If there is adequate sinus floor bone (5 mm or more), a one stage procedure can be accomplished. However, in this situation, the author is frequently able to place short-wide diameter implants into the sinus floor without adjunctive bone grafting.

SURGICAL PROCEDURE

1 Nasoendotrachael general anaesthesia is generally required for bilateral antral reconstruction in edentulous patients utilizing autogenous corticocancellous block bone grafts.
2 Crestal incisions are indicated to permit a periosteal releasing incision, limit sulcus scaring and allow periosteum coverage.
3 Rigid block bone graft stabilization (endosseous implant or miniplate and screws) is critical to enhance physiologic bone graft healing (revascularization, remineralization and transfer osteogenesis) to occur.
4 Non-tension watertight everted wound closure.
5 Four to six months of minimal (physiologic) bone graft and implant loading.
6 Long-term physiologic dental prosthesis loading.
7 Documentation of non-infected and properly ventilated antrum prior to antral floor reconstruction (preliminary antral procedures by appropriate surgeon may be indicated).

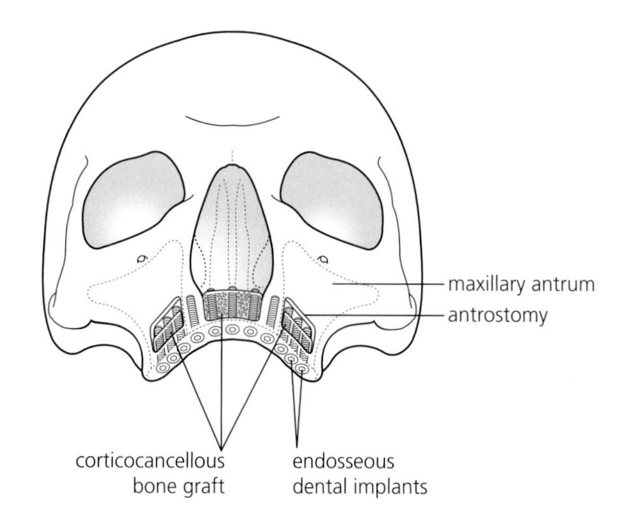

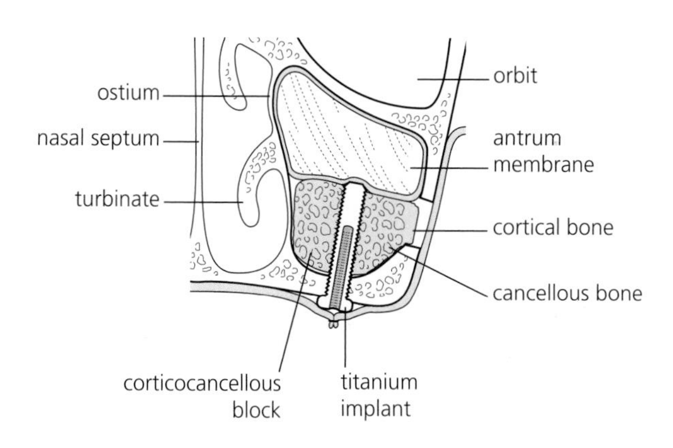

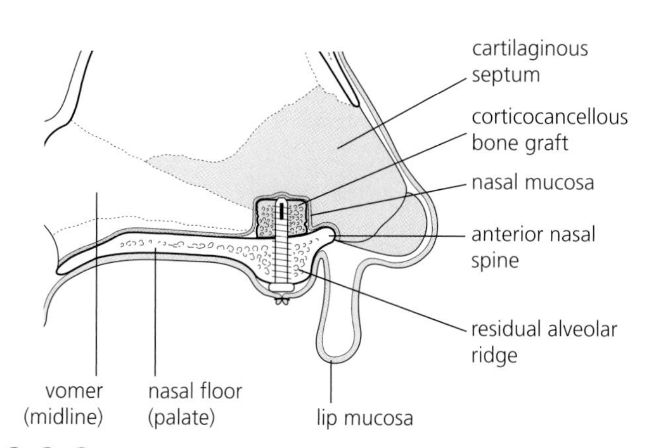

2.9.2 Maxillary nasal/antral inlay (one stage) corticocancellous block iliac bone graft.

Interpositional corticocancellous block bone graft with Le Fort I down-graft osteotomy (Figure 2.9.3)

INDICATIONS

This technique is indicated for partially or totally edentulous patients, who in addition to their edentulism exhibit two complicating factors: (1) horizontal and/or vertical maxillary deficiency with associated facial deformity and skeletal malocclusion, and (2) inadequate bone quality and/or quantity to support endosseous implants in the edentulous area eventually requiring bone-anchored dental prosthesis. These patients are generally younger individuals, who have high functional and aesthetic expectations. They also frequently exhibit high functional disability in mastication, speech, deglutition and nasopharyngeal airflow.

SURGICAL PROCEDURE

1 This reconstructive effort is generally carried out in two stages: (1) the first involves a low Le Fort I osteotomy with correction of the vertical and/or horizontal skeletal deformity and malocclusion, and placement of interpositional block bone grafts to stabilize the repositioned maxilla and (2) provide bone volume and bone density for eventual endosseous implant reconstruction of the edentulous alveolar areas.
2 Adequate miniplate osteosynthesis stabilization of the repositioned maxilla and interpositional bone graft is critical for physiologic bone healing and maintenance of block bone graft volume for adequate numbers and adequate size of endosseous implant.
3 Antral floor membrane removal is important to ensure complete antral floor bone graft incorporation (antral graft for implants).
4 Particulate or block bone grafts across the down-fractured nasal floor is critical in patients missing anterior teeth and alveolar bone. This facilitates eventual endosseous implant reconstruction in this important aesthetic zone.
5 If the Le Fort I interpositional bone grafting is successful, the secondary implant reconstruction four to six months later requires routine implant surgical technique.
6 A one-stage procedure involving simultaneous osteotomy, autogenous bone grafting and endosseous implant reconstruction is technically difficult (requires both sulcus and alveolar ridge incisions) and may result in compromised implant position for final prosthesis fabrication. For these reasons, the one-stage versus two-stage procedure is rarely indicated.

MAXILLARY DISCONTINUITY RECONSTRUCTION (FIGURE 2.9.4)

Indications

Segmental loss of alveolar and basal bone generally is secondary to congenital clefting or postsurgical/post-traumatic aetiology. The surgeon and prosthodontist need to decide whether bone grafting and implant reconstruction of the segmental defect is required, resulting in complete arch reconstruction with fixed or fixed/removable prosthesis, or whether an implant-supported removable obturator

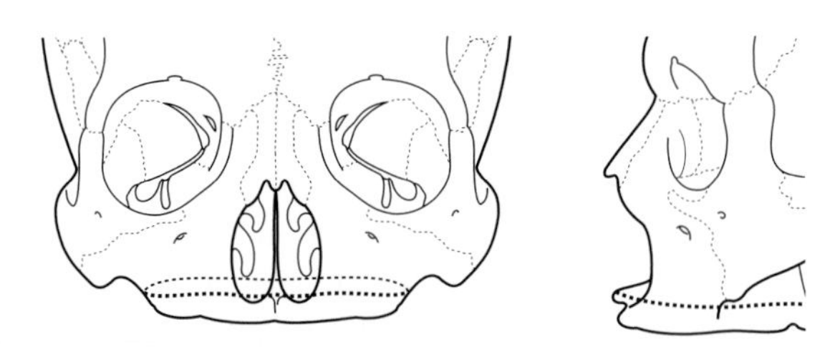

Le Fort I osteotomy

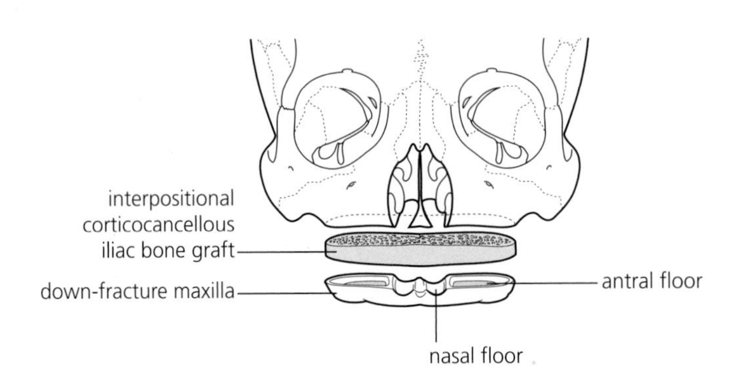

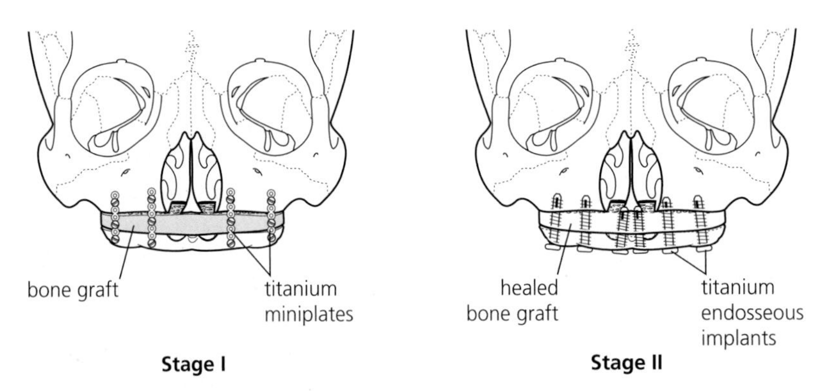

2.9.3 Maxillary interpositional (two stage) corticocancellous block iliac bone graft with LeFort I osteotomy.

prosthesis is required. The size and aetiology of the discontinuity is an important consideration, as well as the patient's functional and aesthetic expectations. In general, the congenital clefts and small defects are bone grafted and secondarily reconstructed with a fixed implant prosthesis, whereas the large (hemi-maxillectomy) defects are reconstructed with implant-supported removable obturator prosthesis. Vasularized composite (bone and soft tissue) are utilized in selected patients to reconstruct the large defects, thus avoiding an obturator removal prosthesis.

SURGICAL TECHNIQUE

1 Alveolar-palatal cleft (and smaller post-oncologic or post-surgical defects) bone grafting needs to be accomplished in a manner where the osseous anatomy of the nasal floor, piriform aperture and anterior portion of the palate are fully reconstructed. In the author's hands, this requires a combination of corticocancellous block and cancellous particulate bone grafts from the iliac crest. In the growing cleft child, these bone grafts are placed between the ages of seven and ten years, when the cuspid roots is one-half to two-thirds formed, and in the adult, four to six months before endosseous implant placement; again, complete reconstruction of the missing anatomy is important, especially in the anterior esthetic zone.
2 In larger post-oncologic or post-traumatic defects (where non-vascularized bone grafts are contraindicated), the endosseous implants and/or onlay or inlay bone grafts are placed in the residual maxillary bone. The surgical techniques are the same as those described earlier (see above under Maxilla (partial or total edentulism) reconstruction). This may be in the form of antral inlay or onlay bone grafts, or pterygoid and zygomatic implants. In this situation, the implant-supported prosthesis is a fixed-removable obturator type. More

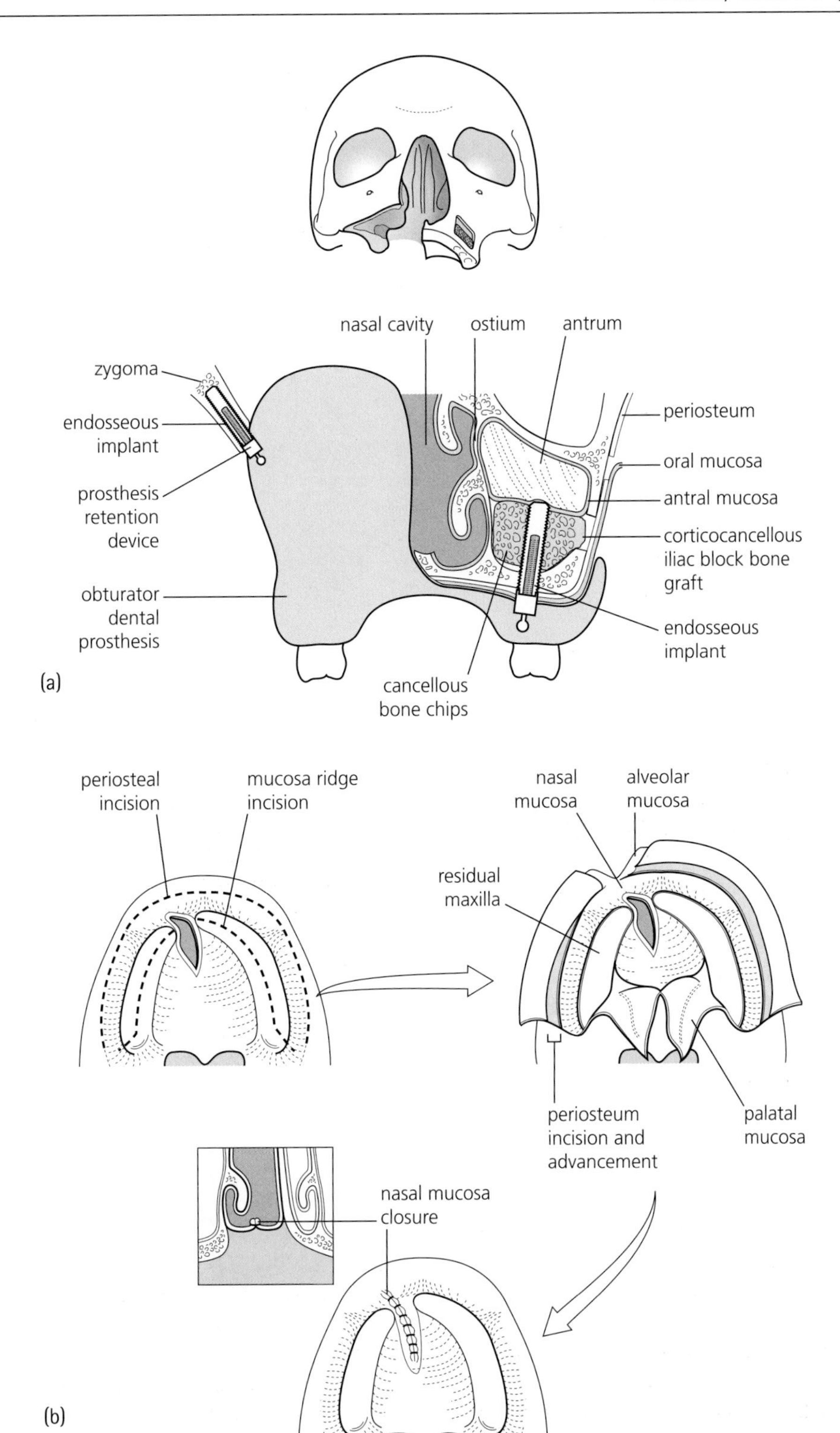

2.9.4 Maxillary discontinuity reconstruction with corticocancellous block iliac bone graft. (a) Hemi-maxillectomy defect; (b) Congenital alveolar/palatal defect.

recently, vascularized composite bone grafts have been utilized for the larger defects. In this situation, it is important to have adequate volume and position of the bone graft; also, the soft tissue portion frequently needs to be debulked to accommodate the dental prosthesis.

MANDIBLE (PARTIAL OR TOTAL EDENTULISM) RECONSTRUCTION

Implant reconstruction of advanced bone resorption without bone grafting (Figure 2.9.5)

INDICATIONS

Patients with bone height equal to or greater than 5 mm and bone width equal to or greater than 6 mm between the mental foramen are candidates for placement of four or five endosseous implants.

SURGICAL TECHNIQUE

Because of the advanced bone resorption, a number of important surgical technique modifications are required: (1) crestal rather than sulcus incisions, to preserve the mentalis integrity; (2) conservative periosteal elevation to preserve a compromised (totally periosteal) blood supply to the residual mandible; (3) isolation of the bilateral mental nerve, which is positioned on the crest of the residual alveolar ridge; (4) low speed-high cooling bone cutting of dense hypovascular bone; (5) bone cutting threading of all osteotomy implant sites through the inferior border; (6) no implant osteotomy site bone bevelling; (7) placement of autogenous osseous coagulum obtained from taping the instrument through the implant preparation site to the inferior border; (8) place the endosseous implant at right angle to the occlusal plane; (9) avoid straight line placement of the anterior implant to avoid unfavourable cantilever prothesis loading (at times, this will require uncovering of the thin bone overlying the inferior alveolar nerve and distalizing of the nerve to allow more posterior positioning of the right and left distal implant); (10) allow implant access holes to exit anterior to the dentition to counteract the dental class III occlusion tendency; (11) accept a high incidence of nonkeratinized peri-implant tissue; (12) understand gradual physiologic increase of bilateral mandibular body height and width following functional prosthetic loading of the anterior mandible (Wolff's law of bone physiology).

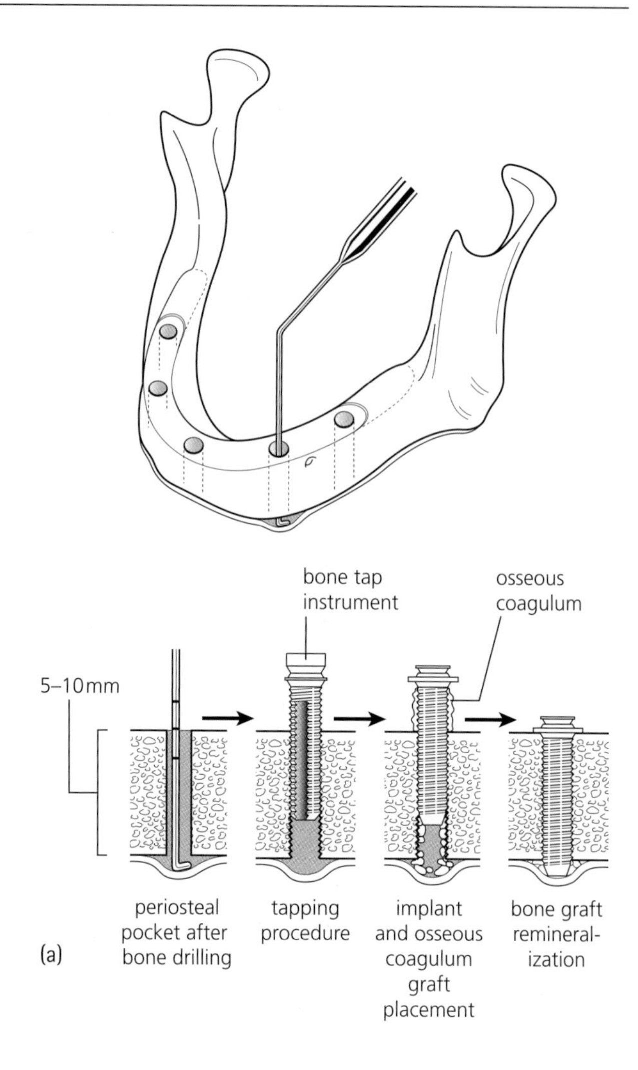

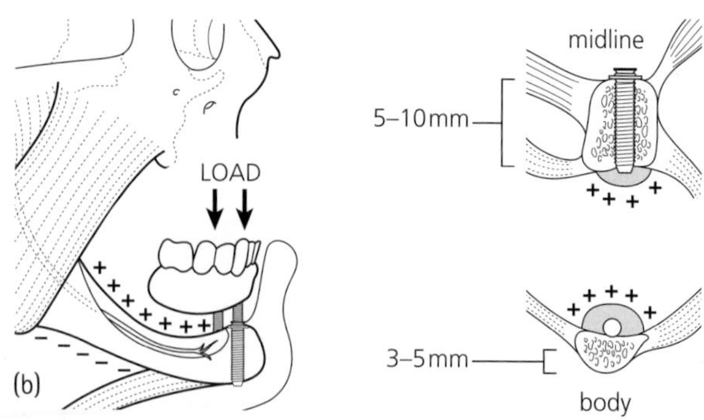

2.9.5 Mandibular endosseous implant reconstruction. (a) Advanced bone resorption; (b) Functional bone remodeling after implant loading (Wolffs law).

Onlay corticocancellous block bone graft reconstruction of advance mandibular resorption (Figure 2.9.6)

INDICATIONS

Adjunctive onlay bone grafting in the advanced bone resorption patient is required when the anterior residual bone is less than 5 mm in height and/or the width is less than 6 mm in the future endosseous implant sites. This group of patients can also avoid the onlay bone grafting procedure if they are willing to function with an over-denture-type prosthesis on two or three midline implants, where there is invariably enough bone (genial tubercle and mentalis muscle attachment area) for implant stability. In this situation, the patient would be willing to accept varying

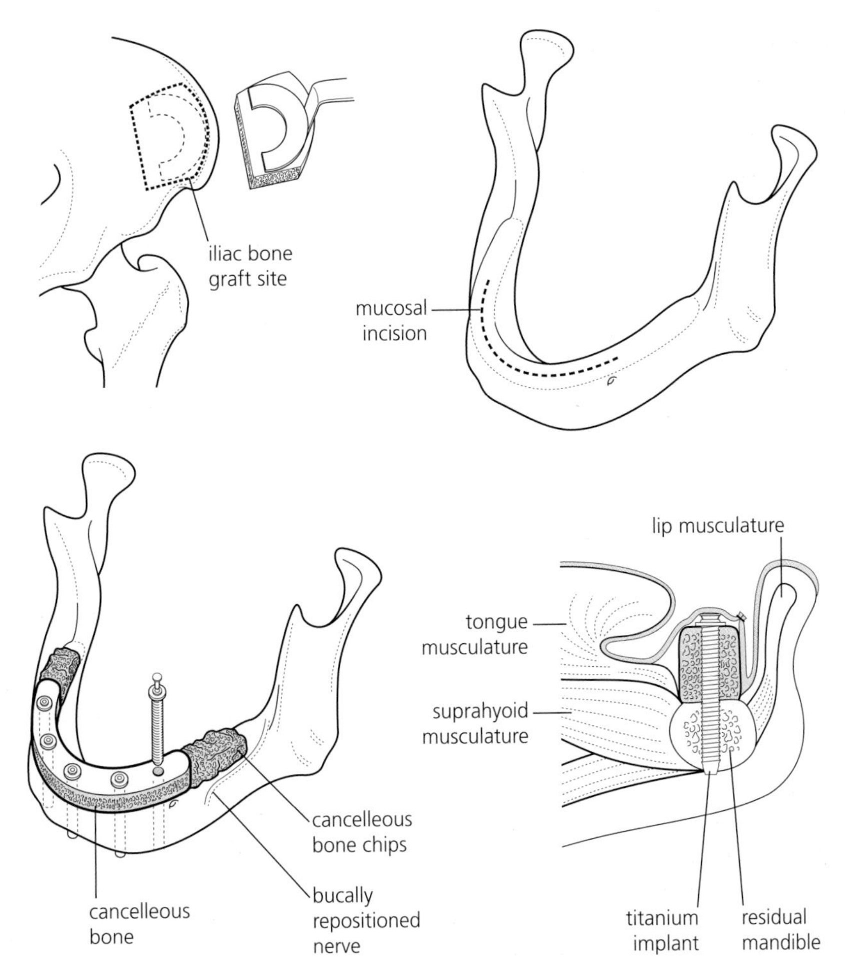

2.9.6 Mandibular onlay (one stage) corticocancellous block iliac bone graft.

degrees of aesthetic and/or functional compromise (lower lip support and tooth position).

SURGICAL TECHNIQUE

In addition to the surgical techniques listed above under Implant reconstruction of advanced bone resorption without bone grafting.

1. Avoid transecting the mentalis muscle and conservative periosteum reflection.
2. Atraumatic bone grafting harvesting and atraumatic recipient site surgery bone healing (bone conduction, bone induction, transfer osteogenesis).
3. Provide watertight, everted tension-free wound closure to ensure early fluid nutrition and revascularization of the bone graft. This requires mobilization of the sublingual mucosa, which is always highly redundant from previous bone loss.
4. Delayed placement (second stage) of the more posterior implant may be necessary due to the narrow width (less than 6 mm) in the mental foramen area. In this situation, the corticocancellous block bone graft may need further stabilization with miniplates or screws. The same situation exists when a unilateral posterior onlay bone graft is placed above the inferior alveolar nerve.
5. Delayed (2–3 weeks) placement of the interim prosthesis to avoid disturbing wound closure and to avoid early bone graft loading.
6. Bone graft placement does not extend more than 1-cm beyond most distal implants as this distal body bone will eventually regenerate in height and width after a period of time (one to three years) of functional loading (Wolff's law of bone repose to physiologic loading tension in the bilateral body portion of the mandible, see Figure 2.9.5b)).

Discontinuity reconstruction with vascularized or non-vascularized block bone grafts and endosseous implants (two-stage procedure) (Figure 2.9.7)

INDICATIONS

When mandibular discontinuity occurs following trauma, infection or oncologic resection, it is generally necessary to establish mandibular continuity prior to implant

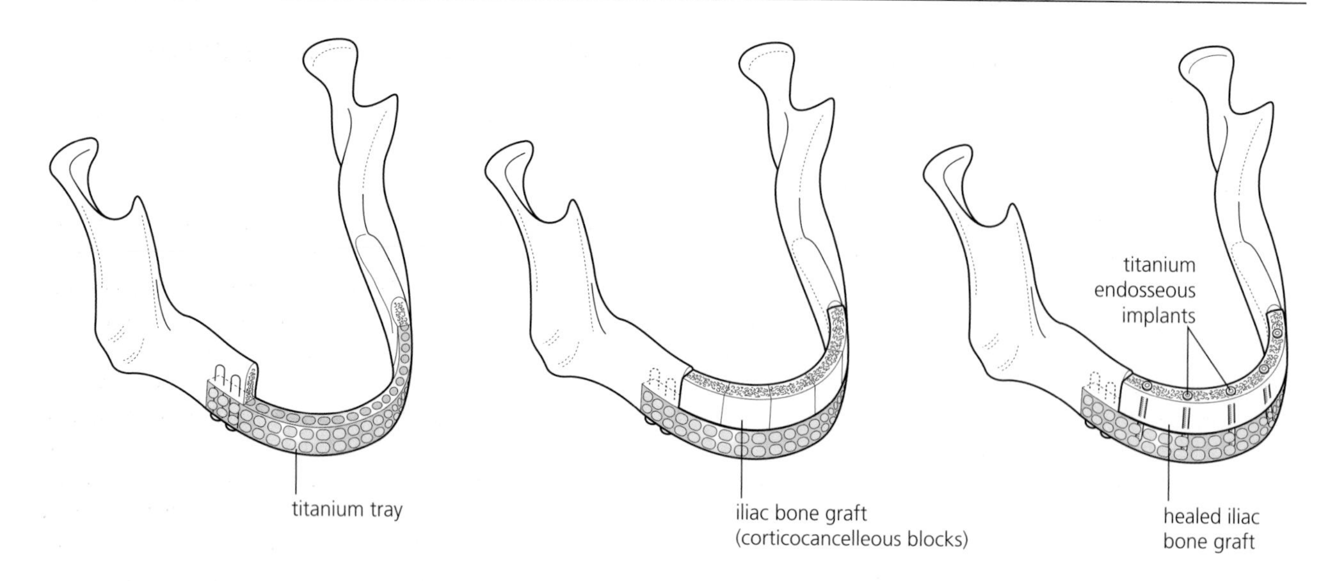

reconstruction. Contraindications to this surgical reconstruction relates to significant patient medical co-morbidity, poor or uncertain oncologic prognosis or severe post-irradiation compromise (decreased vascularity, cellularity and tissue hypoxia).

SURGICAL TECHNIQUE

1 Vascularized or non-vascularized corticocancellous block bone grafts are harvested and skeletally fixed to the osseous defect. Non-vascularized block grafts are primarily obtained from the ilium or calvarium. When severe blood supply compromise is present, when the length of the discontinuity is excessive, or when vascularized soft tissue is required, harvest of vascularized composite bone grafts from various anatomic sites (most common include ilium, fibula or scapula) when bone and/or soft tissue is required, radial, abdominal, lateral thigh or various perforator grafts are indicated when only soft tissue is required. On occasion, various non-vascularized bone grafts are combined with vascular soft tissue grafts (vascularized abdominal with non-vascularized ilium).
2 Endosseous implants are placed four to six months following bone grafts when revascularization and remineralization is nearly complete (two-stage procedure).
3 If bone grafting has been successful from a bone volume and bone position standpoint, endosseous implant reconstruction follows routine implant reconstruction techniques.
4 When placing implant into irradiated bone or into bone graft previously placed into irradiated tissue, special surgical protocol is followed and includes the following: meticulous atraumatic bone drilling with exuberant cooling, conservative periosteal reflection (bone gets all of its blood supply from the periosteum in heavily irradiated patients), meticulous bone tapping and meticulous soft tissue closure in a non-tension everted watertight fashion.

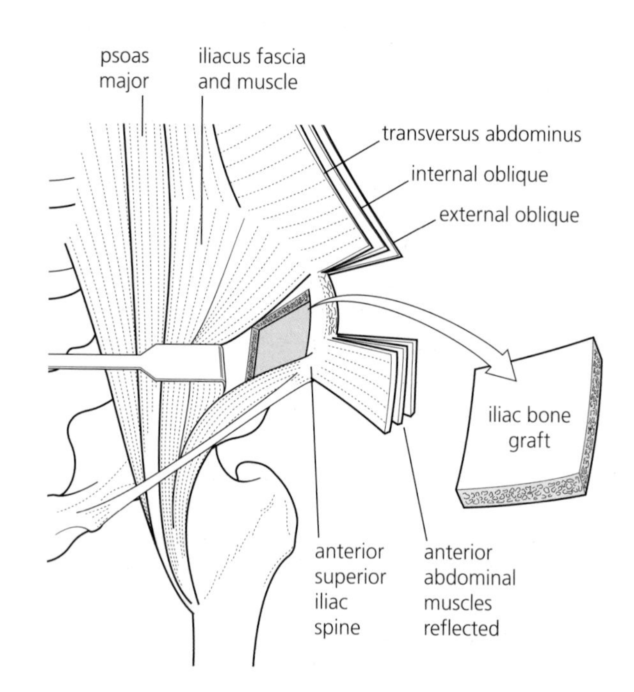

2.9.7 Mandibular oncologic or post-traumatic (two stage) corticocancellous iliac block bone graft with titanium mesh tray (stage I) and titanium endosseous implants (stage II).

5 Prosthetic reconstruction in irradiated patients require fixed continuous prosthesis to avoid compromised soft tissue loading.
6 Endosseous implants placed into the irradiated edentulous mandible are better placed in the interforaminal area where the central irradiation beam creates the least damage to bone and where the cortical/cancellous bone ratio is more favourable than the bone of the mandibular body or ramus of the same patient.

Mental and inferior alveolar nerve management in bone compromised patient (Figure 2.9.8)

INDICATIONS

In the severely resorbed mandible, the mental and inferior alveolar nerve are generally either herniated at the crest of the ridge or are covered by relatively thin bone. The technique of unroofing and repositioning the herniated nerve is relatively straightforward and atraumatic. Once the nerve is uncovered, the incisive branch must be cut at least 2–3 mm anterior to the mental branch. This allows the nerve to be lifted from its canal and repositioned posteriorly away from the implant osteotomy site. If performed correctly, a short period (two to six months) of paraesthesia and/or anaesthesia will follow. If a closed nerve injury (crushing and/or tearing with a rotary drill) is created in a situation where the exact location of the nerve is not appreciated, the long-term potential morbidity is much increased. The author feels a planned minor nerve injury is much preferred over an unplanned closed nerve injury. In addition, implant placement can be greatly enhanced in many situations (such as an atrophic mandible) where improved prosthesis biomechanical loading is achieved. In the mandibular unilateral posterior edentulous patient onlay bone grafting is more difficult, primarily because of the presence of the inferior alveolar nerve. In addition, an onlay block bone graft is technically difficult and more risky to the nerve than the anterior block graft reconstruction described earlier. For these two reasons, the author prefers unroofing and repositioning the nerve prior to onlay bone grafting. In addition, frequently an onlay bone graft is not required once the nerve is out of the operative site. The surgical technique of uncovering and repositioning the mental and inferior alveolar nerve is illustrated in Figure 2.9.8, in the atrophic edentulous mandible and the posterior partially edentulous mandible. Surgical instrumentation is minimal and simple and consists of small round high speed drilling burrs and small No. 2 and a No. 4 molt curette.

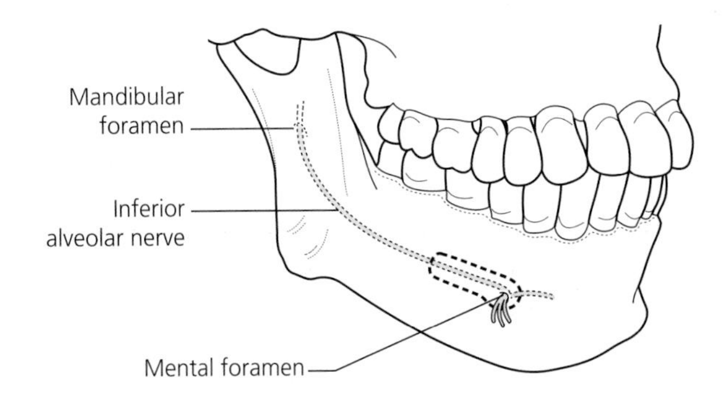

2.9.8 Surgical uncovering of mental/inferior alveolar nerve prior to endosseous implant reconstruction.

MEMBRANES AND BIOLOGIC HEALING ADJUNCTS

Membranes

The author uses very little, if any, alloplastic membranes in bone-grafted patients. Since the periosteum is highly osteogenic and provides significant rigidity and anatomic confinement, its proper use and positioning is preferred. This frequently requires a selective periosteal release (incision) at the height of a flap to allow it to be advanced over a bone-grafted area. The elastic fibres immediately above the periosteum permits up to 12 mm of flap advancement once the periosteum is accurately incised, a significant distance from the surgical defect to be covered. The antrum membrane is also highly osteogenic and can provide adequate confinement of a particulate graft (in addition to its osteogenic potential). If a very thin antral membrane ruptures, an appropriate collagen material is the most physiologic replacement of either the periosteum or antral membrane. An even better solution in the author's opinion is the use of small cortical grafts properly stabilized with endosseous implants (one-stage procedure) or miniplates or screws (two-stage procedure) providing a predictable bone reconstruction of small antral or alveolar defects.

Autogenous biologic healing adjuncts

The hallmark of predictable bone grafting augmentation and endosseous implant reconstruction of various anatomic defects is meticulous and biologically sound surgical planning and surgical technique. Most healing failures follow faulty diagnosis (wrong surgery for a given problem), faulty patient selection (medical or psychologic co-morbidities) or faulty surgical technique. The latter include excessive tissue destruction (cautery, laser, tearing or crushing of tissue), poorly designed or poorly vascularized tissue flaps, inadequate haematosis leading to haematoma, failure to eliminate dead space with drains or suturing, devitalizing bone with excessive heat and failure to achieve watertight non-tension soft tissue (mucosa–periosteum) closure. Extraoral approaches to the mandible where incisions are placed low in the neck potentially eliminate or reduce all the skin arterial perforators and reduce subcutaneous fat. This blood supply compromise combined with excessive cautery and thinning of the skin provides poor soft tissue coverage of the osseous reconstructive efforts. Biologic enhancers will not cover up compromised surgery, but may enhance outcome if all other wound conditions are satisfied. The latter, however, has not been established to date by properly designed prospective studies.

BONE GRAFT HARVESTING TECHNIQUES

Adjunctive bone grafting for all but the most simple osseous defects warrant utilization of fresh autogenous bone, which most agree represents the well-established gold standard of care.

Ideally, the bone graft should provide adequate bulk to repair the anatomic defect, act as a strong bone induction agent and provide viable osteogenic stem cells, which provide transfer osteogenesis when placed in a closed biologic environment. The latter contains cellular nutrition and early revascularized potential. This graft must also be covered with a viable periosteum (osteoblasts) and surrounded with viable bone (cambium layer osteoblasts) to take advantage of the osteoinductive properties of the bone graft. Proper rigid stabilization of the graft is critical to ensure more specialized bone regeneration rather than less specialized collagen production in the osseous defect. The corticocancellous block or cancellous particulate bone from the ilium satisfies most, if not all, of the above-mentioned attributes if properly harvested. Stabilizing the particulate grafts can become a problem, which can lead to a loss of significant graft volume. Cortical grafts from the cranium or mandible, if properly harvested, can provide all but the transfer osteogenic component listed above. Atraumatic harvesting of the bone grafts is just as important as atraumatic preparation of the recipient site. Both are required for predictable bone grafting success. Ideally, the recipient site should be fully prepared before the bone graft is harvested. This allows immediate transfer of the bone graft to the recipient site, which theoretically helps preserve the osteoinductive (protein) and transfer osteogenic (cellular) potential. When proper healing occurs, the bone graft will respond properly to physiologic loading (Wolff's law). The latter will not theoretically occur with allogenic bone grafts, which may take years to be replaced with normal bone. The latter will provide osseous bulk, but not viable bone, which responds appropriately to physiologic loading of an endosseous osseo-integrated implant.

Top tips

- Advanced maxillary bone graft reconstruction requires autogenous corticocancellous block onlay, inlay or interpositional bone grafting. Each type (onlay versus inlay versus interpositional) has specific indications and can be either one or two stage.
- Bone graft reconstruction of small- to medium-sized congenital alveolar–palatal defects requires corticocancellous block bone grafts to completely restore the nasal floor, palate and piriform rim to achieve the most ideal nasal and dental implant aesthetic result.
- The reconstructive surgeon, prosthodontist and patient need to decide whether to replace lost anatomy or obturate lost anatomy in early planning of corrective surgery for large post-surgical or post-traumatic maxillary defects.
- Endosseous implant reconstruction of advanced bone resorption of the edentulous mandible can be achieved with a minimum of 5 mm of bone height and 6 mm of bone width.
- Bone regeneration of severely resorbed mandibular body occurs following functional loading of osseointegrated endosseous dental implants placed in the mandibular symphysis region (Wolff's law of bone physiology).
- Mandibular discontinuity reconstruction with vascularized or non-vascularized block bone grafts requires metal trays or reconstruction plates which are physiologic to avoid bone graft stress shielding during bone graft healing.
- A planned minor nerve injury is preferred to an unplanned major nerve injury when placing endosseous implants close to the inferior alveolar and metal nerve. Therefore, nerve uncovering and removal from the surgical site may be prudent.
- The periosteum provides the most physiologic and effective barrier membrane in all bone grafting situations. This requires selective periosteum incision and repositioning techniques.
- Autogenous bone graft harvesting surgical techniques must be atraumatic to preserve the bone induction (bioactive protein), bone conduction and transfer osteogenic (cellular) potential required for maximum bone graft regeneration.
- Atraumatic management of the covering mucoperiosteum or skin is required to provide a physiologic environment for predictable bone graft regeneration.

FURTHER READING

Keller EE, Desjardins RP, Eckert SE, Tolman DE. Composite bone grafts and titanium implants in mandibular discontinuity reconstruction. *Journal of Oral and Maxillofacial Surgery* 1988; **3**: 261–6.

Keller EE. Mandibular discontinuity reconstruction with composite grafts. Free autogenous iliac bone, titanium mesh trays, and titanium endosseous implants. In: Worthington P, Beirne OR (eds). *Oral and maxillofacial surgery clinics of North America.* Philadelphia: WB Saunders, 1991: 877–91.

Keller EE. The maxillary interpositional composite graft. In: Worthington P, Branemark PI (eds). *Advanced osseointegration surgery: Applications in the maxillofacial region.* Chicago: Quintessence Publishing, 1992: 162–74.

Keller EE, Tolman DE. Mandibular ridge augmentation with simultaneous onlay iliac bone graft and endosseous implants: A preliminary report. *Journal of Oral and Maxillofacial Surgery* 1992; **7**: 176–84.

Keller EE, Gandy SR. Modified mandibular body step osteotomy-ostectomy. *International Journal of Adult Orthodontics and Orthognathic Surgery* 1993; **8**: 37–45.

Keller EE, Eckert SE, Tolman DE. Maxillary antral and nasal one-stage inlay composite bone graft: Preliminary report on 30 recipient sites. *Journal of Oral and Maxillofacial Surgery* 1994; **52**: 438–47; discussion 447–8.

Keller EE. Reconstruction of the severely atrophic edentulous mandible with endosseous implants: A 10-year longitudinal study. *Journal of Oral and Maxillofacial Surgery* 1995; **53**: 305–20.

Keller EE, Tolman DE, Zuck SL, Eckert SE. Mandibular endosseous implants and autogenous bone grafting in irradiated tissue: A 10-year retrospective study. *Journal of Oral and Maxillofacial Surgery* 1997; **12**: 800–13.

Keller EE. Maxillary discontinuity defects: Tissue-integration reconstruction. In: Branemark P, Tolman DE (eds). *Osseointegration in craniofacial reconstruction.* Chicago: Quintessence Publishing, 1998: 187–204.

Keller EE, Tolman D, Eckert S. Endosseous implant and autogenous bone graft reconstruction of mandibular discontinuity: A 12-year longitudinal study of 31 patients. *Journal of Oral and Maxillofacial Surgery* 1998; **13**: 767–80.

Keller EE, Tolman DE, Eckert S. Surgical-prosthodontic reconstruction of advanced maxillary bone compromise with autogenous onlay block bone grafts and osseointegrated endosseous implants: A 12-year study of 32 consecutive patients. *International Journal of Oral and Maxillofacial Implants* 1999; **14**: 197–209.

Keller EE, Tolman DE, Eckert SE. Maxillary antral-nasal inlay autogenous bone graft reconstruction of compromised maxilla: A 12-year retrospective study. *International Journal of Oral and Maxillofacial Implants* 1999; **14**: 707–21.

Tolman DE, Desjardins RP, Keller EE. Surgical-prosthodontic reconstruction of oronasal defects utilizing the tissue-integrated prosthesis. *Journal of Oral and Maxillofacial Surgery* 1988; **3**: 31–40.

Worthington P, Krogh PH, Keller EE. Does the risk of complication make transpositioning the inferior alveolar nerve in conjunction with implant placement a 'last resort' surgical procedure? *Journal of Oral and Maxillofacial Surgery* 1994; **9**: 249–54.

2.10

Craniofacial implantology

GREG BOYES-VARLEY, DALE HOWES

INTRODUCTION AND REVIEW OF THE LITERATURE

Modified reconstruction procedures are applied when the facial skeleton has insufficient bone for conventional implant placement. Extensive bone grafting is recommended to create adequate bone volume for placement of endosseous implants to restore the severely resorbed or resected maxilla with a fixed prosthesis. Bone grafting procedures include onlay grafts, inlay grafts into the floor of the maxillary antrum and Le Fort I maxillary osteotomy with advancement and down-grafting techniques. Newly grafted bone has to remain load-free to allow consolidation and revascularization for four months. Staged bone graft techniques increase treatment time, which is tedious and socially unacceptable for the patient.

ANGULATED IMPLANTOLOGY: ZYGOMATIC IMPLANTS

Maxillary atrophy makes quality of life for denture wearer's unbearable, made worse by continuous physiological bone resorption and maxillary sinus pneumatization. The zygomatic implant has provided the clinician with an alternative to grafting procedures in the reconstruction of the severely resorbed maxilla. Branemark originally designed the technique in 1989 and has a reported success rate of 97 per cent.

This implant traverses the posterior maxillary alveolus and lateral sinus wall into the body of the zygoma. The restorative interface requires angular correction from the long axis to allow for appropriate tooth position. In 2003, Boyes-Varley described the use of a 55° restorative head (Southern Implants, Irene, South Africa) in order to reduce the buccal cantilever by 20 per cent. The use of a modified head angulation of 55° with implant placement as close to the crest of the edentulous ridge as possible allows restorative clinicians to achieve an ideal restorative position in the posterior maxilla.

Diagnostic radiology

Radiological assessment for the zygomatic implant protocol is used to detect the presence of pathology within the maxillary sinuses and to evaluate the volume of bone available in the maxillary alveolus and zygomatic body.

The following radiographic views are recommended:

- Panoramic view to detect bone height within the maxilla and anatomical structures.
- Occipito-mental views to assess the extent of the maxillary sinus and presence of sinus pathology.
- Lateral cephalogram to assess jaw relationship.
- Axial, coronal and reformatted computed tomography (CT) scans give an excellent assessment of the maxilla and maxillary sinus. In oncology and trauma surgery, a three-dimensional spiral reconstruction is useful.

Optimal implant placement is dictated by the position of three distinct anatomical sites:

1. The position of the incisura between the zygomatic arch and the frontal process of the zygomatic bone (Figure 2.10.1, point A).
2. The confines of the lateral wall of the maxillary antrum (Figure 2.10.1, point B).
3. The thickness of the existing alveolar crest (Figure 2.10.1, point C).

For optimal implant placement, the position of the incisura is fixed and provides the superior pivot point of the zygoma implant (Figure 2.10.2). Occasionally, the surgeon can place the exit point of the implant more medially towards the infero-lateral orbital margin and great care should be taken to avoid perforation into the infero-lateral aspect of the orbit. This puts the implant into an upright position and brings the restorative head into the first molar site instead of the second premolar site.

The lateral wall of the sinus is engaged by the implant as far laterally as possible to obtain the most lateral position of the implant in the sinus wall. The head of the implant in the maxillary alveolus is placed as close to the mid-alveolar position of the ridge as possible (Figure 2.10.3).

SURGICAL TECHNIQUE

Placement of zygomatic implants is performed under general anaesthesia. A crestal incision is made extending from 1 cm in front of the maxillary tuberosity to the same position on the contralateral side. Periosteal elevation results in the exposure of the entire maxilla, around the base of the piriform rim, up to the inferior aspect of the infraorbital nerves and finally exposing the inferior aspect of the body of the zygoma bilaterally (Figure 2.10.4).

A round bur is then used to create a lateral window in the superior-lateral aspect of the wall of the maxillary antrum, with sinus mucosa reflection. Using a round burr, the proposed point of entry of the fixture into the zygomatic bone is demarcated through the sinus window (Figure 2.10.5a,b).

The final site preparation follows the graded pilot and twist drills. Care should be taken not to perforate the bony orbit with subsequent disruption of the orbital contents (Figure 2.10.6).

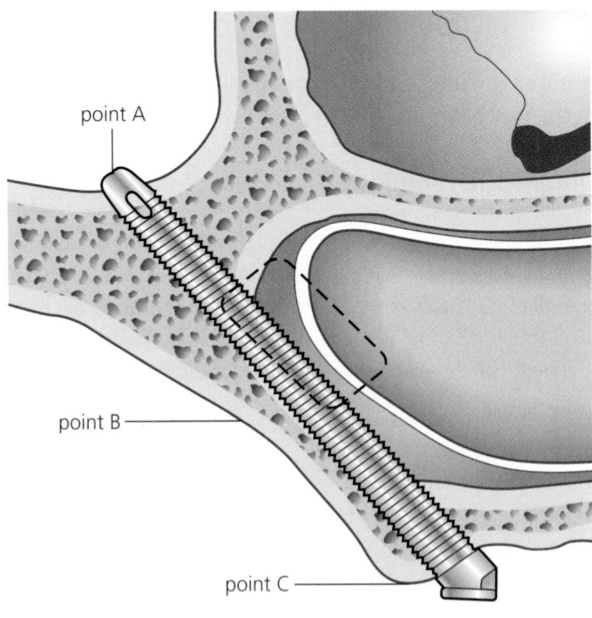

2.10.1 Optimal position of zygomatic implant *in situ*.

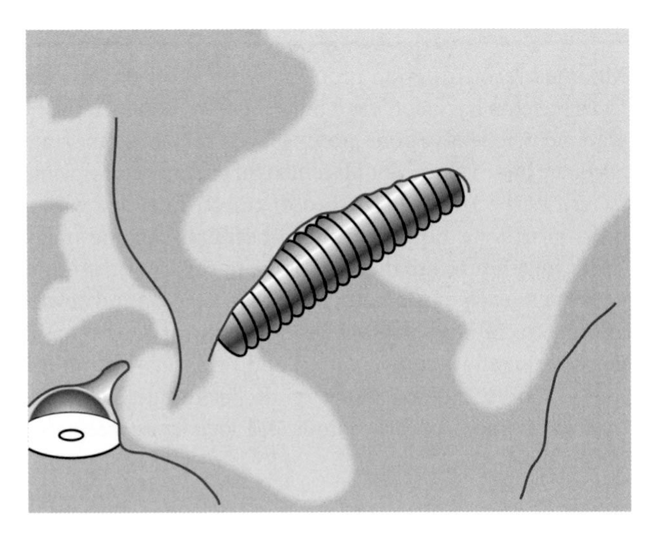

2.10.3 Zygomatic implant body within the lateral wall of the maxillary antrum.

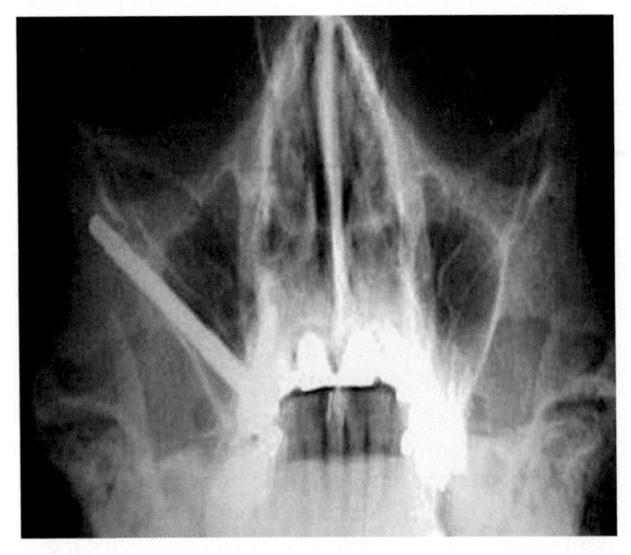

2.10.2 Radiograph of partial zygomatic implant *in situ*.

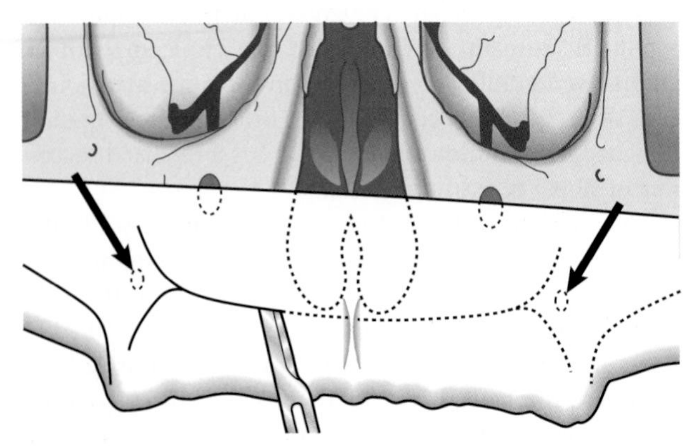

2.10.4 Crestal incision form right to left maxillary tuberosity.

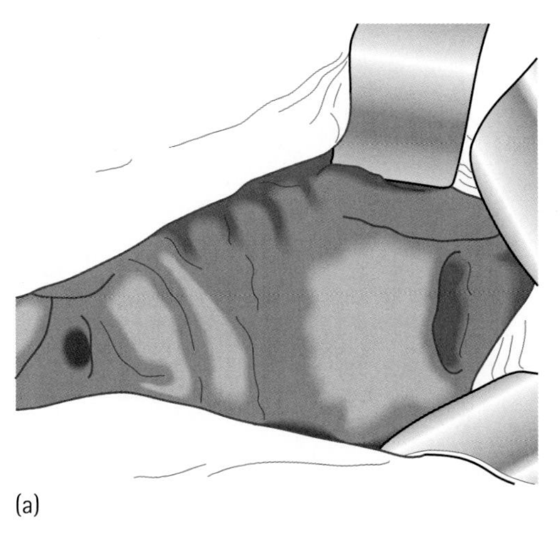

(a)

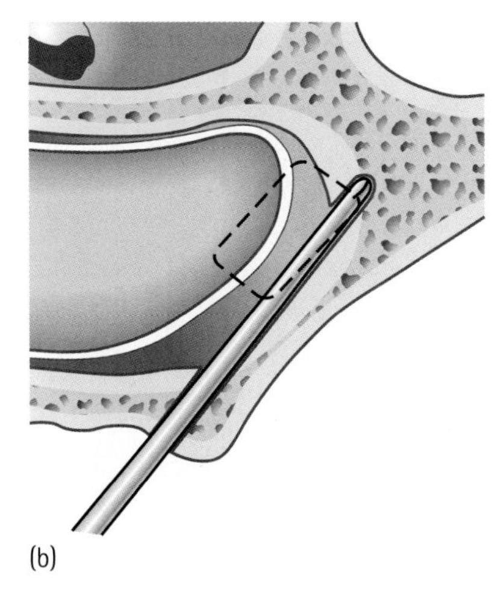

(b)

2.10.5 (a) Bone window in the supero-lateral aspect of the maxillary sinus. (b) Pilot drill into the body of the zygoma.

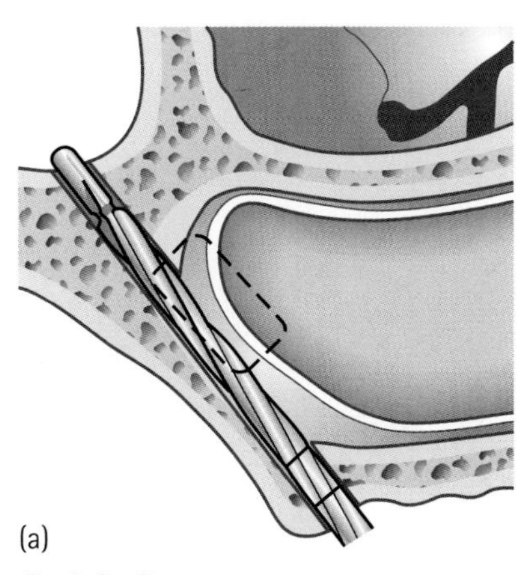

(a)

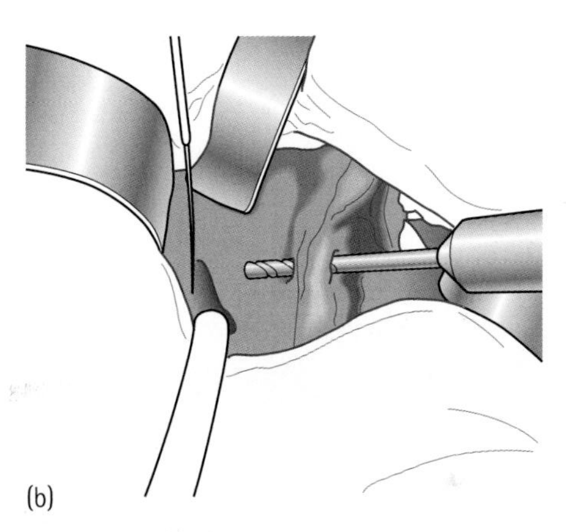

(b)

2.10.6 (a) Intermediate drill into the body of the zygoma. (b) Final drill preparation into the body of the zygoma.

IMPLANT PLACEMENT

A zygomatic implant with a head angulation of 55° (Southern Implants) is the preferred implant as this improves the emergence profile and decreases the buccal cantilever (Figure 2.10.7a). Final placement of the fixture is accomplished by ensuring proper angulation of the implant platform by placement of a guide pin into the implant and the fixture rotation to ensure optimal position (Figure 2.10.7b).

Standard protocol is two zygomatic implants placed posteriorly with four paranasal implants and a fixed porcelain fused to the titanium prosthesis (Figure 2.10.8).

HEMI-ZYGOMATIC IMPLANTS

Reconstruction of hemi-maxillary defects in partially dentate patients where there has been premolar and molar loss often predisposes to sinus pneumatization with minimal bone in this area for conventional implant placement. Treatment options include a unilateral sinus graft or the utilization of a hemi-zygomatic protocol with the placement of one standard endosseous fixture and a zygomatic in the posterior maxillary region (Figure 2.10.9).

QUADRATIC ZYGOMATIC IMPLANTS

Balshi described the use of multiple zygomatic implants in reconstruction of the atrophic maxilla and proposed the use of up to three zygomatic implants per quadrant. The authors' clinical experience has shown that using only two zygomatic fixtures per quadrant has proved adequate for the rehabilitation of the atrophic maxilla with fixed or fixed hybrid prosthesis. An autogenous bone graft can be avoided and is advantageous as the patient is saved the morbidity and possible complications of a bone graft. This allows for an arch of 10–12 teeth even in patients with inadequate anterior width and height of bone (Figure 2.10.10).

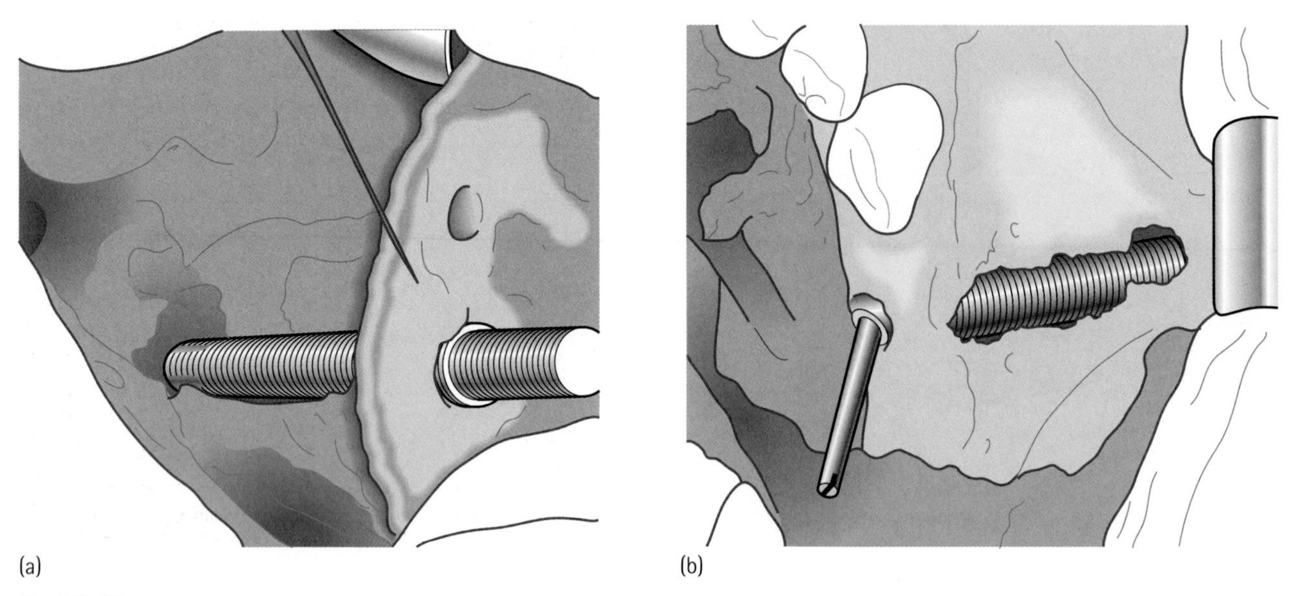

(a) (b)

2.10.7 (a) Placement of 55° zygomatic implant into lateral aspect of the maxilla. (b) Placed 55° zygomatic implant with occlusal projection do the mandibular occlusal plane.

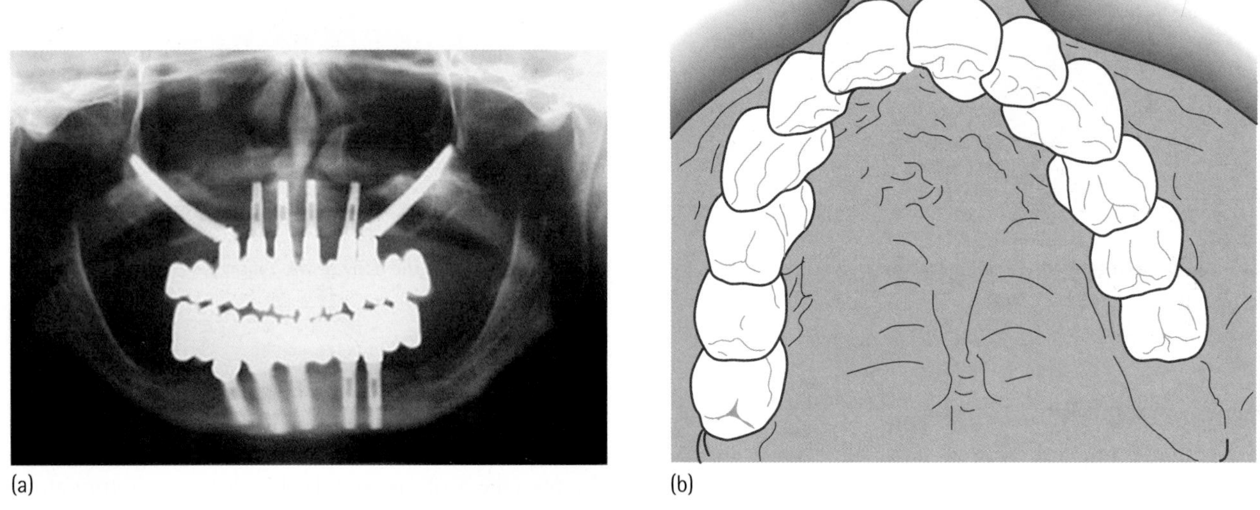

(a) (b)

2.10.8 Standard maxillary zygomatic protocol (a). Restoration of standard zygomatic protocol with full cross arch permanent prosthesis (b).

Surgical technique

Quadratic zygomatic implant placement is usually one fixture placed into the premolar site and the second into the canine or lateral incisor positions. The surgical technique is as for standard zygomatic fixture placement and a more palatal mucosal incision is made to include an adequate band of attached mucosa (Figure 2.10.11).

Care should be taken not to perforate into the inferolateral aspect of the orbit with the more anterior fixture and post-operative radiographs are obligatory. It is possible to immediately load these implants with a fixed hybrid acrylic strengthened prosthesis, which remains in place while healing takes place (Figure 2.10.12, see page 126).

This avoids a second procedure to expose the implants four months after placement. This has cost implications since hospital stay, theatre time and recovery time are all reduced, allowing the patient to be integrated back into society more quickly. After healing has taken place, the temporary prostheses are replaced with fixed porcelain fused to a titanium prosthesis (Figure 2.10.13, see page 126).

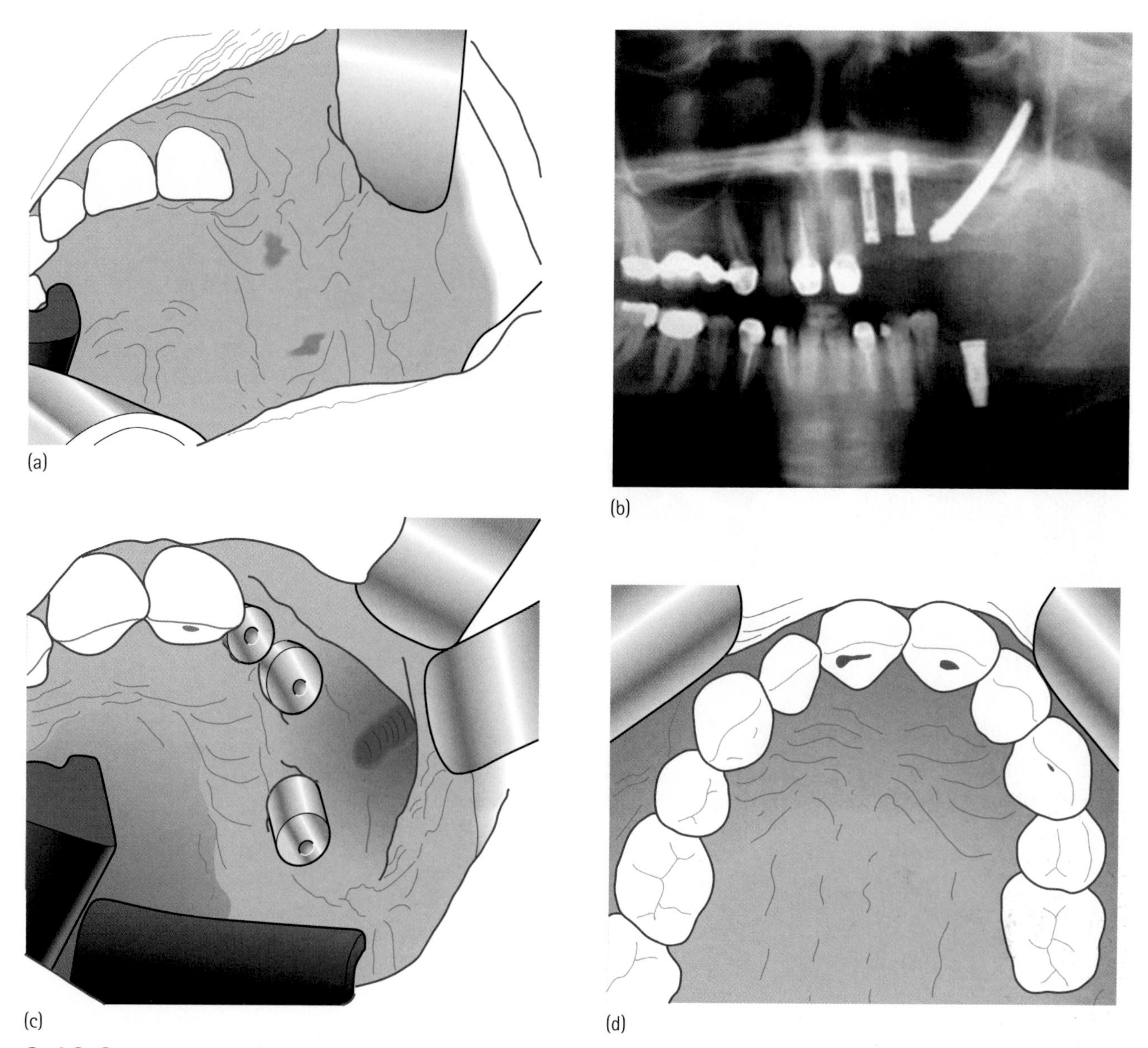

2.10.9 (a) Partial maxillary defect. (b) Post operative radiograph of placed implants. (c) Implants at exposure. (d) Final restored prosthesis in the left maxilla.

ZYGOMA, ZYGOMATIC IMPLANTS AND ONCOLOGY RECONSTRUCTION

Tumour ablative surgery and trauma to the mid-facial complex involves structures integral to phonetics, deglutition and mastication, and makes reconstruction both difficult and controversial. The surgery is complex and involves sealing of the oral cavity from the nasal cavity, re-establishment of the paranasal sinuses and restoration of the facial contour. Dental rehabilitation is also a massive functional and aesthetic consideration that should be considered when planning the proposed reconstruction.

Several methods have been proposed for post-surgical reconstruction. Reconstruction depends on the extent of the resultant bony and soft tissue defect and obturation requires a working relationship between the surgical and prosthetic teams. The prosthetic design has evolved over decades and osseointegration has revolutionized facial reconstruction in these cases. This technology can mostly circumvent the need for vascularized osseomyocutaneous grafts or these grafts in combination with non-vascularized free bone grafts. The advantage of endosseous implant rehabilitation over vascularized free flaps is the ability of the surgeon to inspect the resection cavity for recurrent disease. Visual inspection for recurrences in today's world is trumped by interval radiographic assessment, with the use of computed tomography (CT), magnetic resonance imaging (MRI) and positron emission tomography (PET) scans. These investigations are costly, are often unavailable to patients with recurrent disease and make maxillary rehabilitation

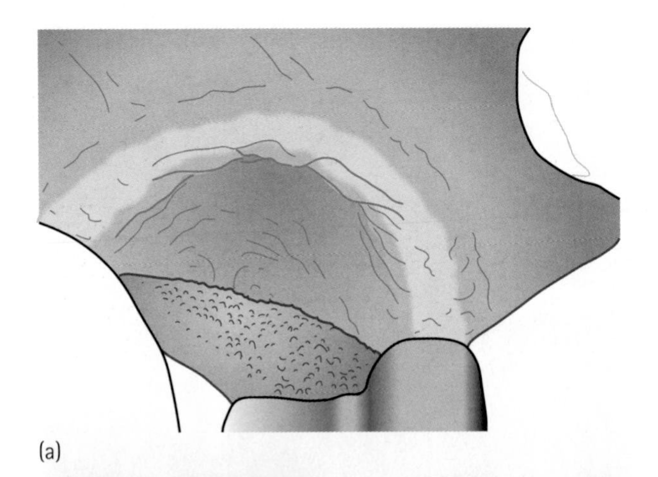
(a)

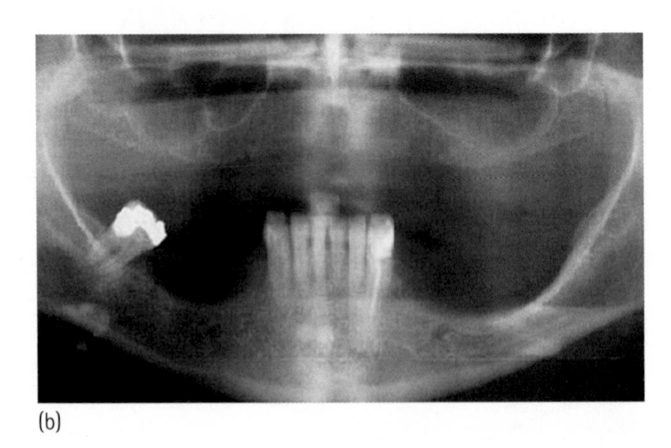
(b)

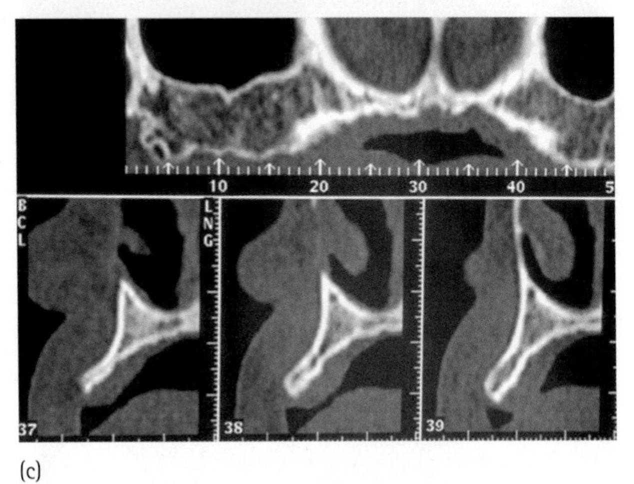

(c)

2.10.10 (a) Cawood Class IV maxillary ridge. (b) Panoramic radiograph of Cawood Class IV maxilla. (c) Reformatted CAT scan of anterior maxillary ridge in Cawood Class IV.

with endosseous implants a more viable and inexpensive treatment modality. The placement of endosseous implants facilitates prosthodontic rehabilitation, which allows for secure, aesthetic and functional replacement of ablated hard and soft tissues and minimizes the disadvantages of silicone bulbs, obturators and dentures.

ONCOLOGY RECONSTRUCTIVE PROTOCOL

Diagnosis

Patients requiring resection for oncology are subjected to a standardized pre-operative radiological survey. This includes routine orthopantomogram, occipito-mental views, lateral cephalogram taken in occlusion and CT scan of the affected area and neck. Incisional biopsy of the tumour is performed to obtain a definitive histological diagnosis and tumour grading and helps to establish the surgical and post-operative chemotherapeutic or radiotherapy protocols (Figure 2.10.14, see page 127).

PROSTHODONTIC PREPARATION AND STEREOLITHOGRAPHIC SIMULATED SURGERY

Where possible, a stereolithographic acrylic model is grown from the Dicom Format CT scanning data. Resection surgery is simulated on this model and allows for optimal implant positions and conformation of prosthetic design. Diagnostic casts are modified according to the expected resection and a surgical obturator prepared and a temporary obturator made (Figures 2.10.15–2.10.17, see page 127).

Tumour resection, immediate implant placement and obturation

Airway management is achieved most often by tracheostomy. Extraoral access to the tumour is achieved in most cases by a modified Weber–Ferguson flap with a wide soft tissue resection margin and hemi-maxillectomy. After tumour resection, frozen sections of the resection margin are done to ensure complete tumour excision (Figure 2.10.18a,b, see page 128).

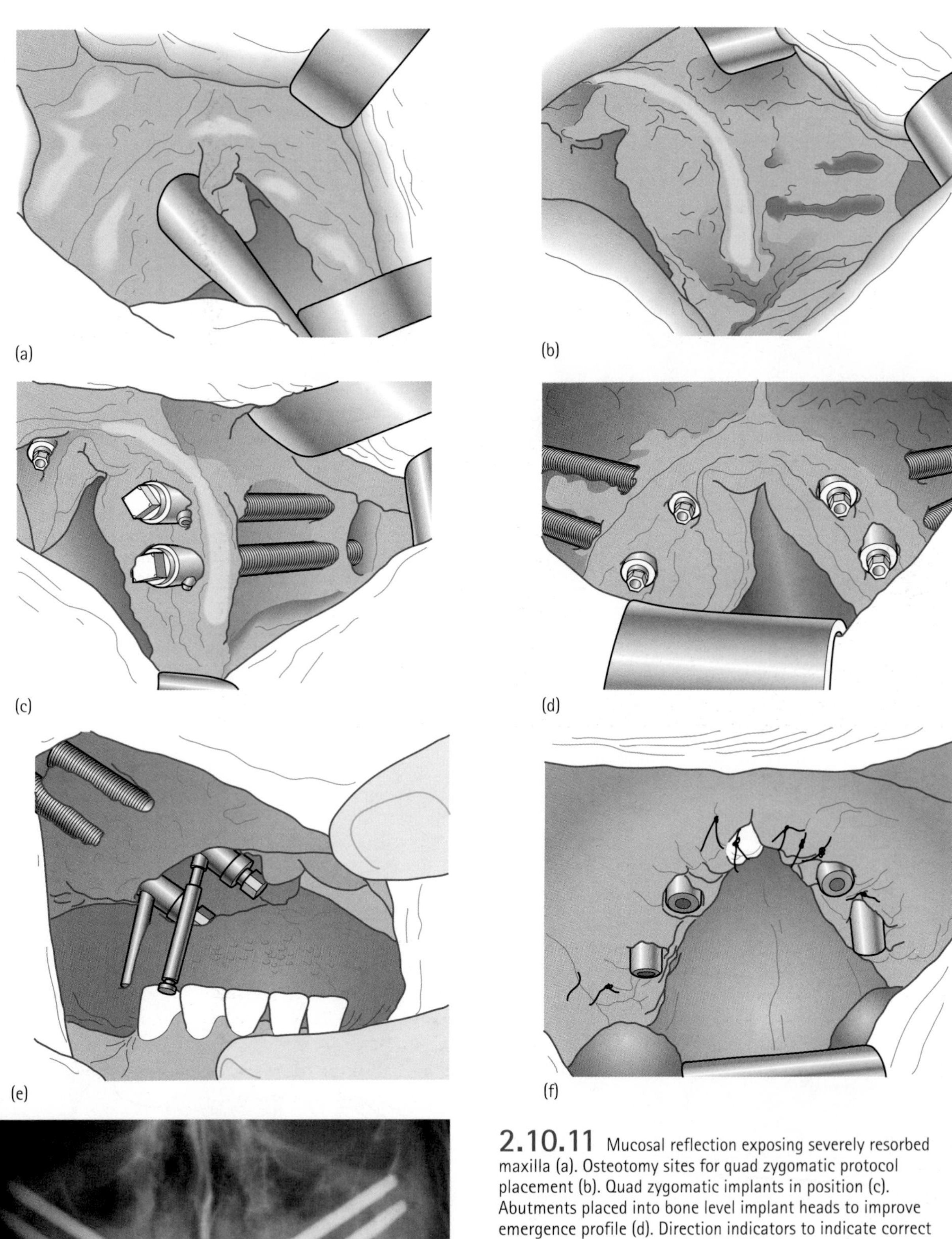

2.10.11 Mucosal reflection exposing severely resorbed maxilla (a). Osteotomy sites for quad zygomatic protocol placement (b). Quad zygomatic implants in position (c). Abutments placed into bone level implant heads to improve emergence profile (d). Direction indicators to indicate correct implant head position in the arch (e). Healing abutments placed and suturing of mucosa (f). Post operative Occipito mental radiograph of implants in the maxilla (g).

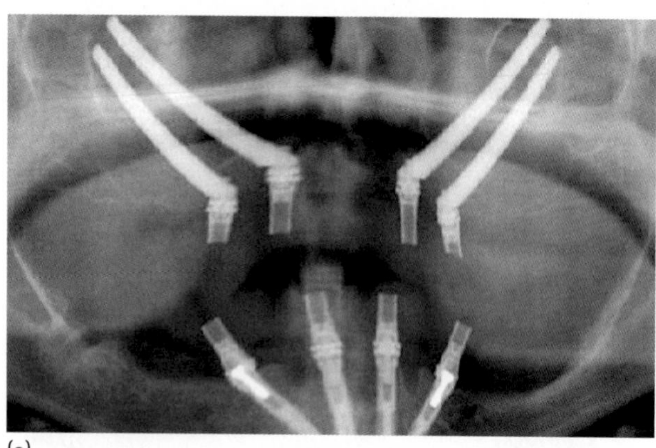

(a)

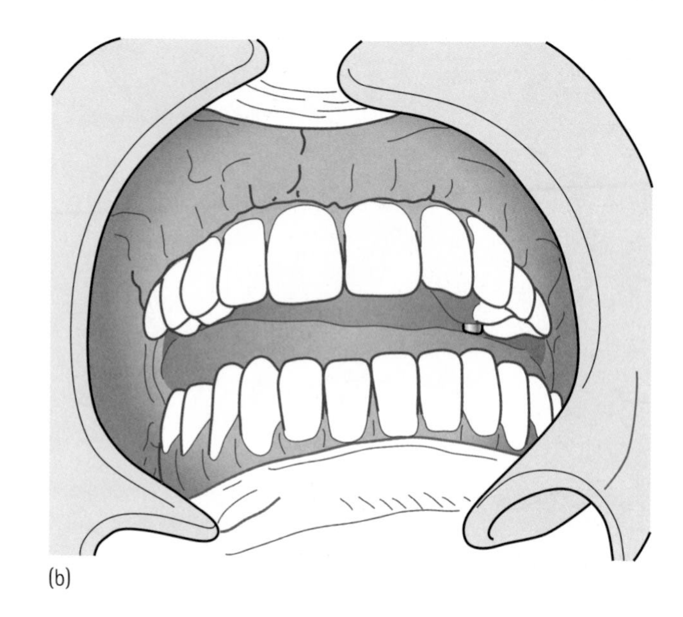

(b)

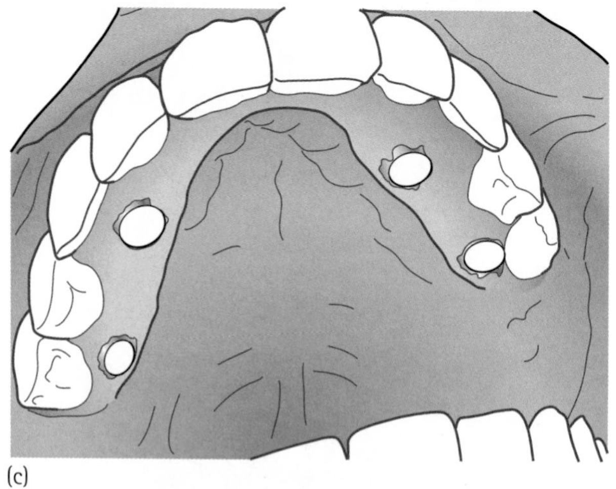

(c)

2.10.12 Radiograph of temporary restorative titanium cylinders for temporary prosthesis (a). Temporary acrylic prosthesis placed 5 hours after surgery (b). Occlusal view of temporary acrylic prosthesis placed 5 hours after surgery (c).

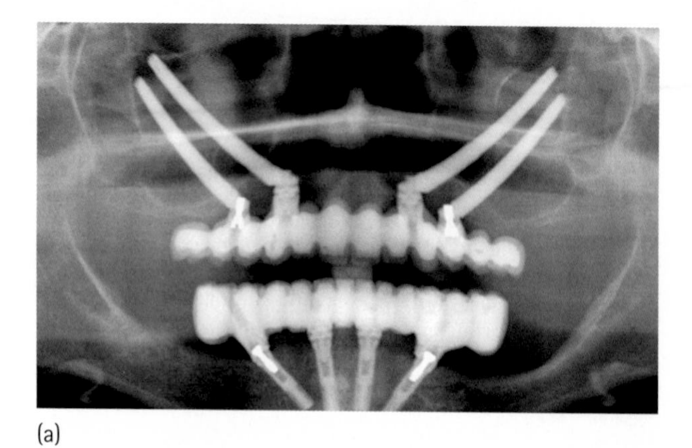

(a)

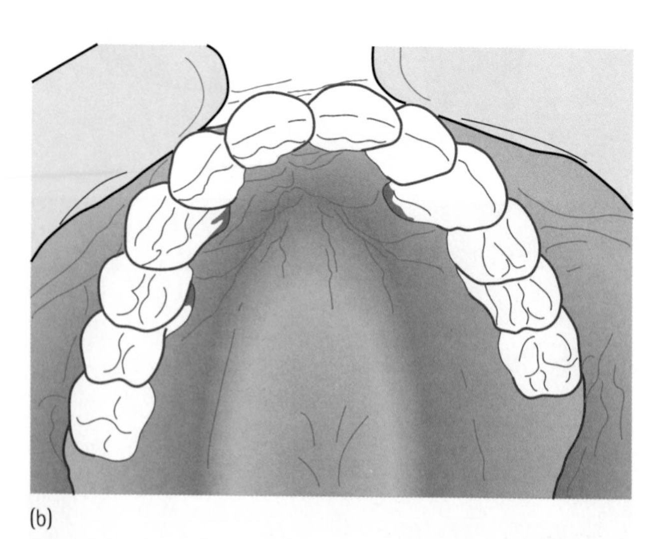

(b)

2.10.13 Radiograph of final fixed prosthesis 3 months post placement (a). Occlusal view of final fixed prosthesis 3 months after implant placement (b).

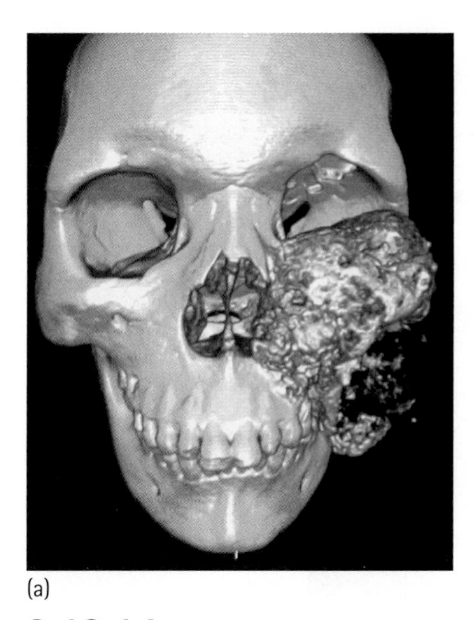

(a)

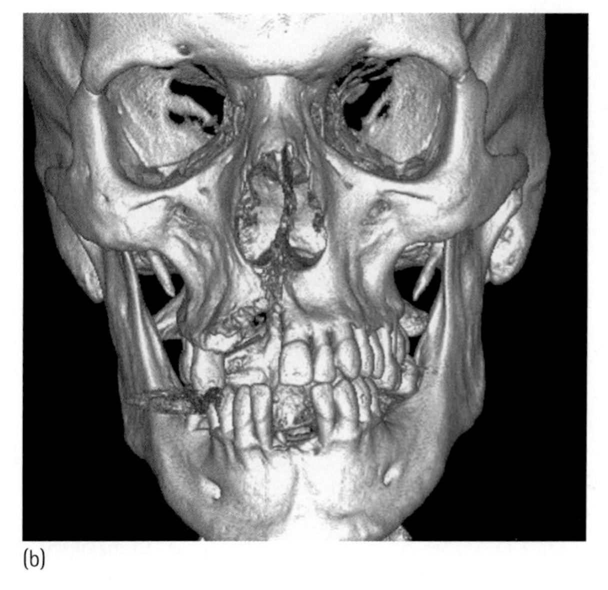

(b)

2.10.14 3-D Spiral CAT scan pre-oncology resection of maxillary chondrosarcoma (a). 3-D Spiral CAT scan pre resection of right maxillary squamous cell carcinoma (b).

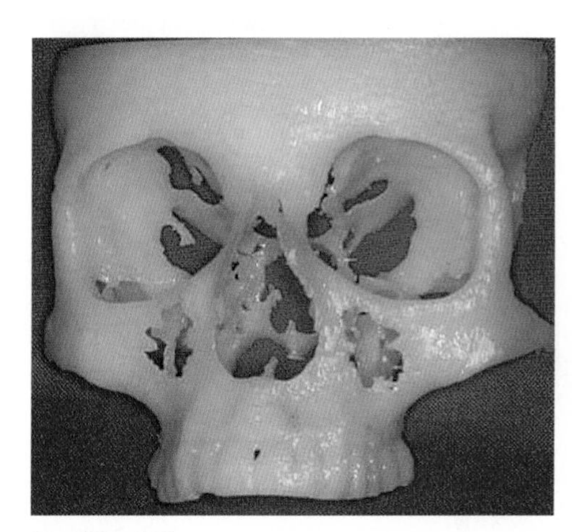

2.10.15 Stereolithographic model.

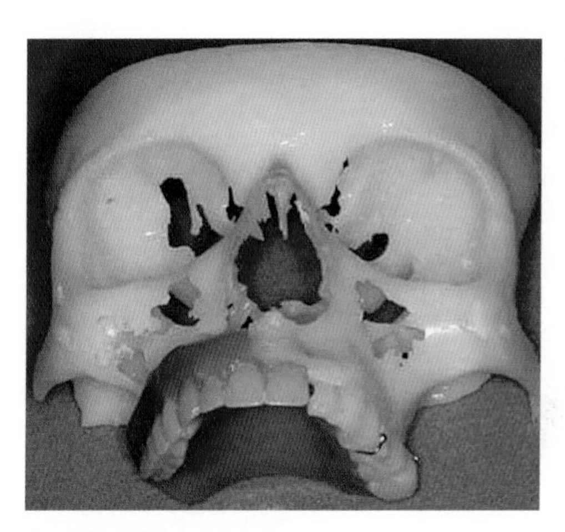

2.10.17 Temporary obturator fitted on to stereolithographic model and confirmation of obturator design.

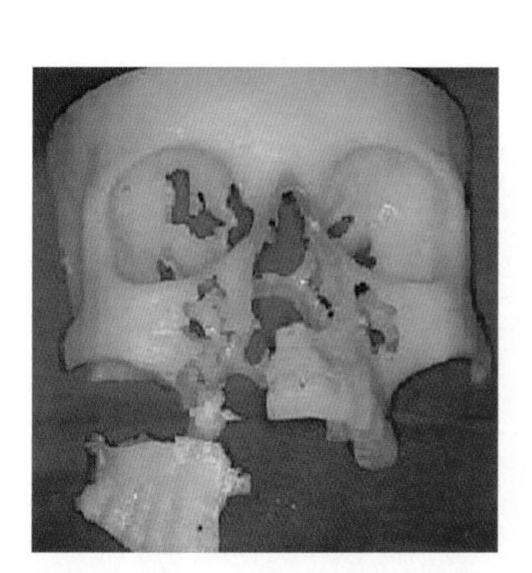

2.10.16 Simulated hemi maxillectomy on stereolithographic model.

IMPLANT PLACEMENT

The objective of implant placement is to 'recreate' the buttresses and processes of the maxilla, allowing for appropriate force distribution of the prosthetic rehabilitation with the remaining facial skeleton. Both standard and zygomatic implants are used and the use of the zygomatic implant allows for the lowering of the restorative platform to the level of the palate (Figure 2.10.19a,b).

A modified zygomatic implant was placed into the maxillary resection stump. This implant has been termed an oncology implant, with the soft tissue portion of the implant being a smooth machined surface (Southern Implants) (Figures 2.10.20 and 2.10.21).

A low nasal antrostomy is performed at the floor of the intact sinus allowing for drainage of the maxillary sinus inferiorly, as well as through the osteum.

(a)

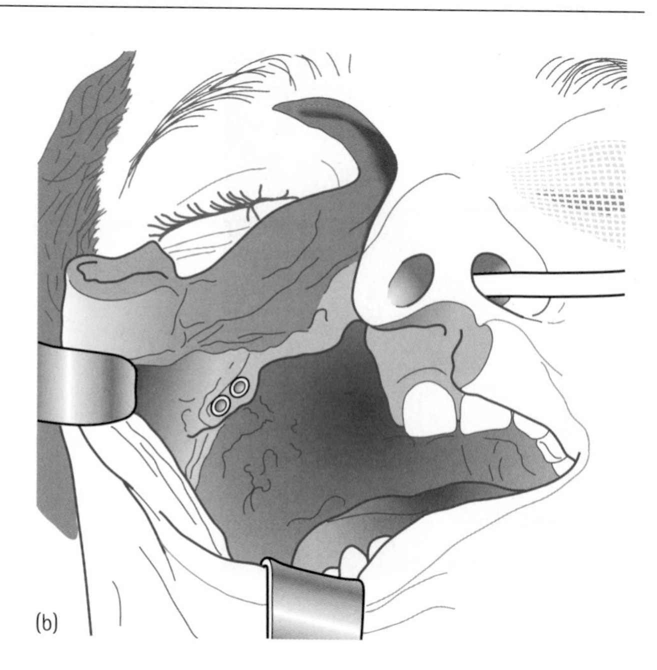

(b)

2.10.18 Weber-Ferguson incision to expose left maxillary tumour (a). Hemi maxillectomy with implants placed into zygomatic boby stump (b).

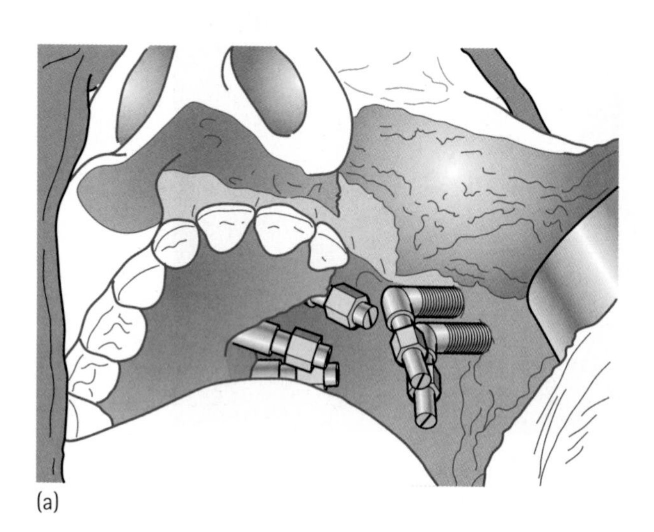

(a)

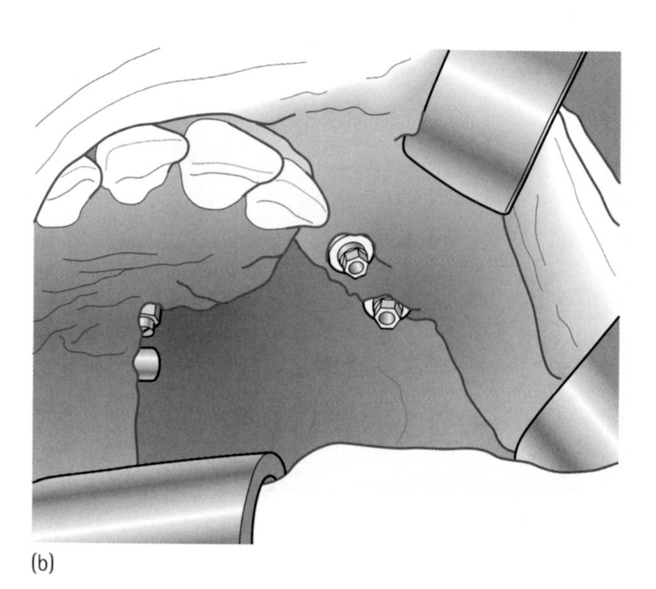

(b)

2.10.19 Position and angulation of zygomatic fixtures within the zygomatic stump projected toward the occlusal plane using the palatal height as a guide (a). Position and angulation of zygomatic fixtures within the healed tissue 3 months after resection and implant placement (a,b).

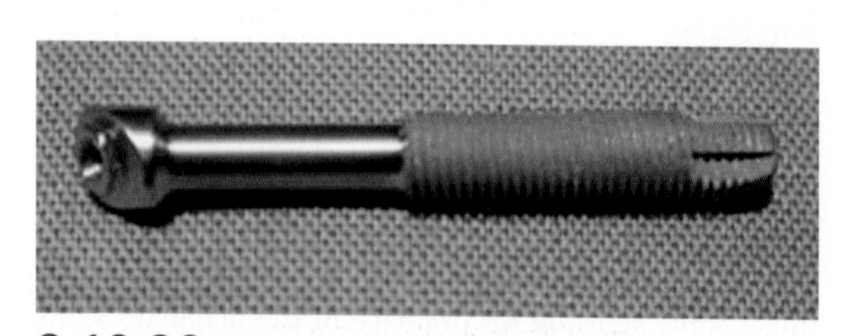

2.10.20 Oncology zygomatic implant.

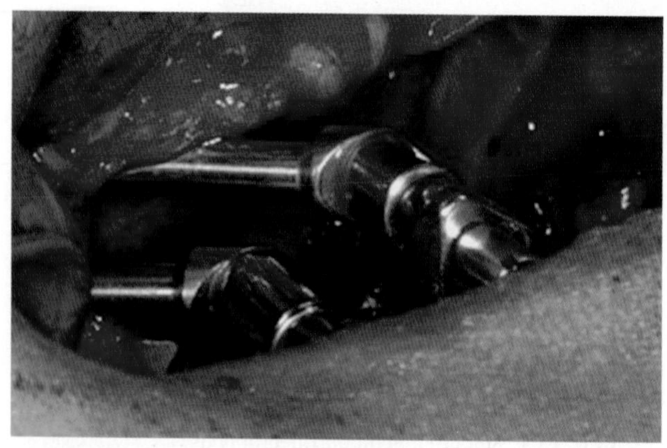

2.10.21 Oncology zygomatic implant *in situ*.

SURGICAL OBTURATION AND SKIN CLOSURE

The surgical obturator is modified intra-operatively after implant placement to restore normal soft tissue facial contour over the resection site and guide soft tissue healing. This obturator is secured by two 15-mm transosseous titanium screws in the remaining palate and supported by the zygomatic implants on the affected side. The Weber–Ferguson flap is closed with a two-layered technique and a nasogastric feeding tube placed in the contralateral nostril (Figure 2.10.22).

Laboratory fabrication of definitive superstructure and interim obturator

Master casts are poured and mounted on an articulator using the jaw relation from the modified duplicate surgical obturator. The superstructure and the interim obturator are then fabricated (Figure 2.10.23).

Prosthodontic rehabilitation can be achieved with an over denture protocol (Figure 2.10.24a,b) or with fixed dento-alveolar elements and a separate removable implant supported (Figure 2.10.25a,b).

Post-operative radiographs are taken to confirm the position of the implants within the bone and to ensure that the prosthesis is firmly secured to the implants (Figure 2.10.26).

Maintenance

The surgical site is monitored closely by both the oncologist and reconstructive teams for adequate post-operative healing and long-term recurrence. Prosthetic maintenance is ongoing, particularly in the first year, where soft tissue changes can be extensive. The obturators may require

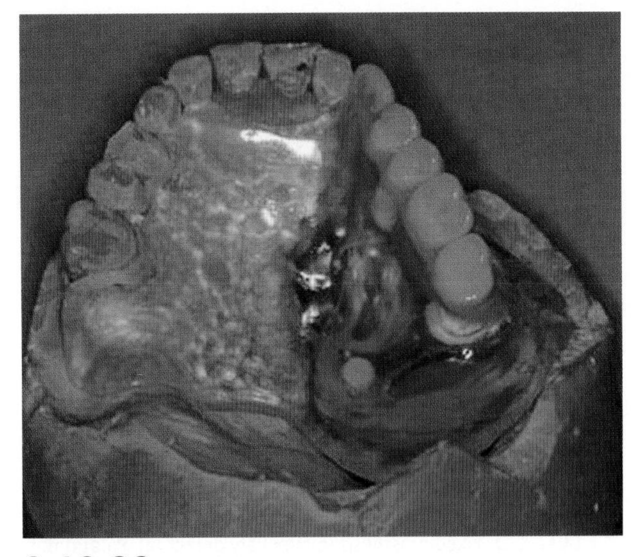

2.10.23 Interim obturator fitted onto model.

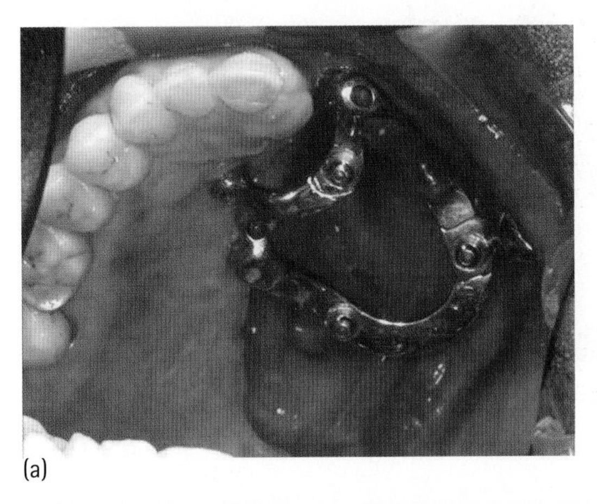

(a)

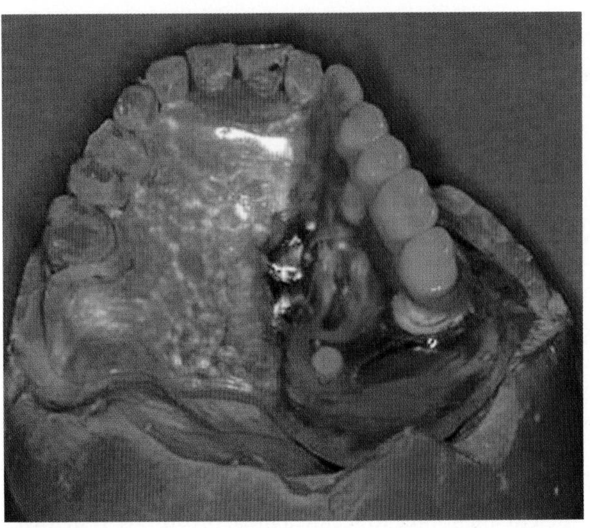

(b)

2.10.24 Definitive splinted superstructure with interim obturator on model (a). Interim obturator fitted onto model (b).

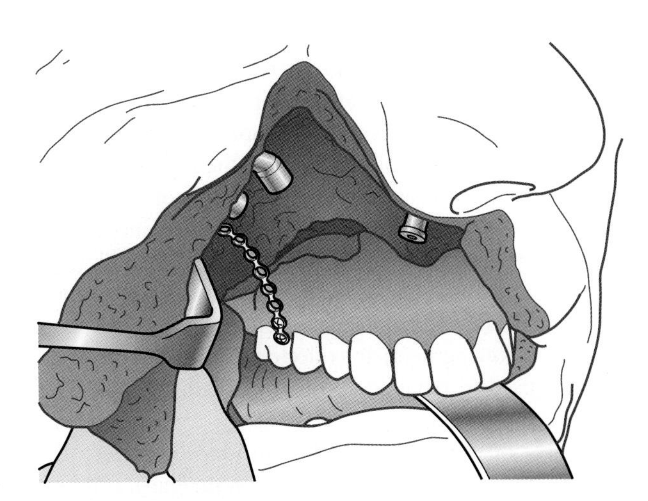

2.10.22 Placement of temporary obturator into hemi-maxillary defect.

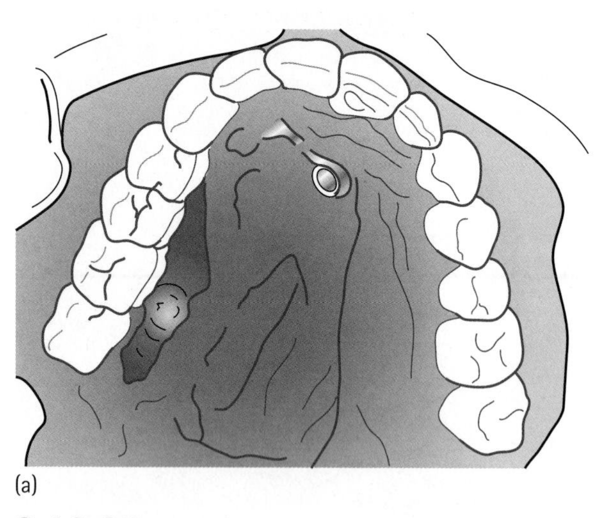
(a)

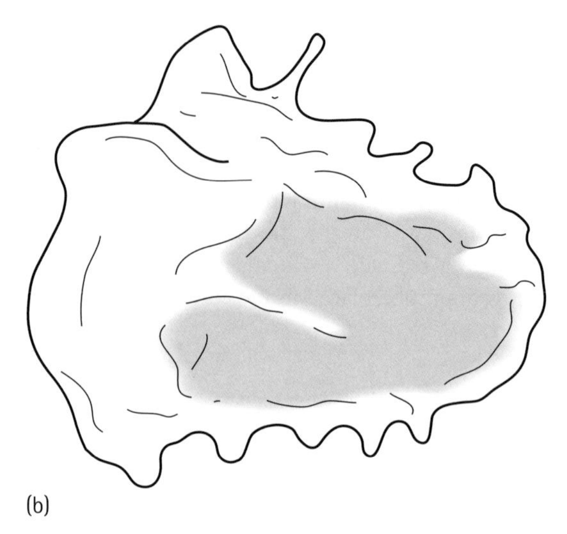
(b)

2.10.25 Fixed prosthesis in maxillary defect (a). Palatal obturators (b).

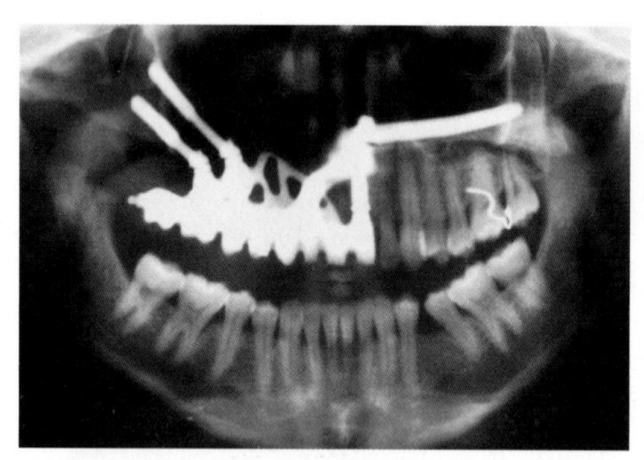
(a)

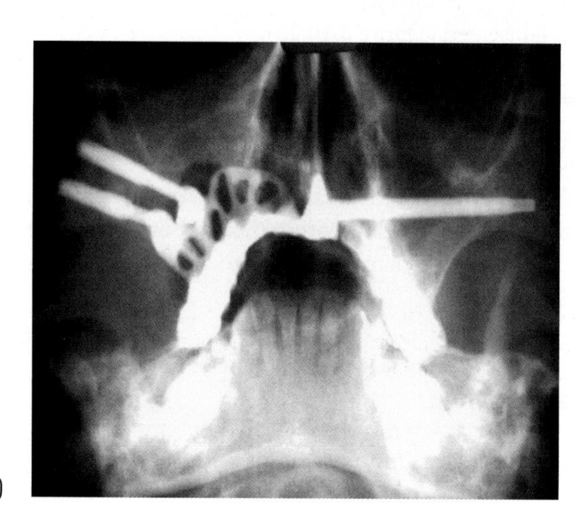
(b)

2.10.26 Implant radiographs.

continual peripheral adjustment and oral hygiene training is undertaken using brushing techniques and pulsating irrigation.

ZYGOMATIC IMPLANTS AND NASAL AND NASOMAXILLARY RECONSTRUCTION

Oncology cases which present in the anterior maxilla often require anterior maxillary and nasal resection in order to resect the tumour. Rehabilitation in these cases often requires the provision of a combination of an intraoral and extraoral prosthesis (Figure 2.10.27a–f).

Nasal prostheses are generally implant retained and a modified placement technique can be done to achieve sufficient anchorage to secure a nasal prosthesis. It involves the placement of two standard zygomatic fixtures almost horizontally in combination with standard implantology into the anterior maxillary floor (Figure 2.10.28a–c).

ZYGOMATIC IMPLANTS AND GUNSHOT RECONSTRUCTION

The rehabilitation of the midface after a gunshot wound to the face ablates structures which are in the path of the missile. The resultant facial deformities after gunshot wounds to the face can create serious psychological and aesthetic complications for the patients. Facial trauma from gunshot wounds is common in many countries, especially when sustained in war. Little has been published about reconstruction following gunshot wounds and other trauma to the face after anatomical disruption of the maxillofacial complex akin to oncology resection following hemi-maxillectomy, and the treatment protocols used to rehabilitate these patients are similar to oncology reconstructions.

The area of cavitation which is produced between the entrance and exit wounds produces both hard and soft tissue defects. There is a secondary missile effect of the bone and fractured tooth fragments, and soft tissue is destroyed in

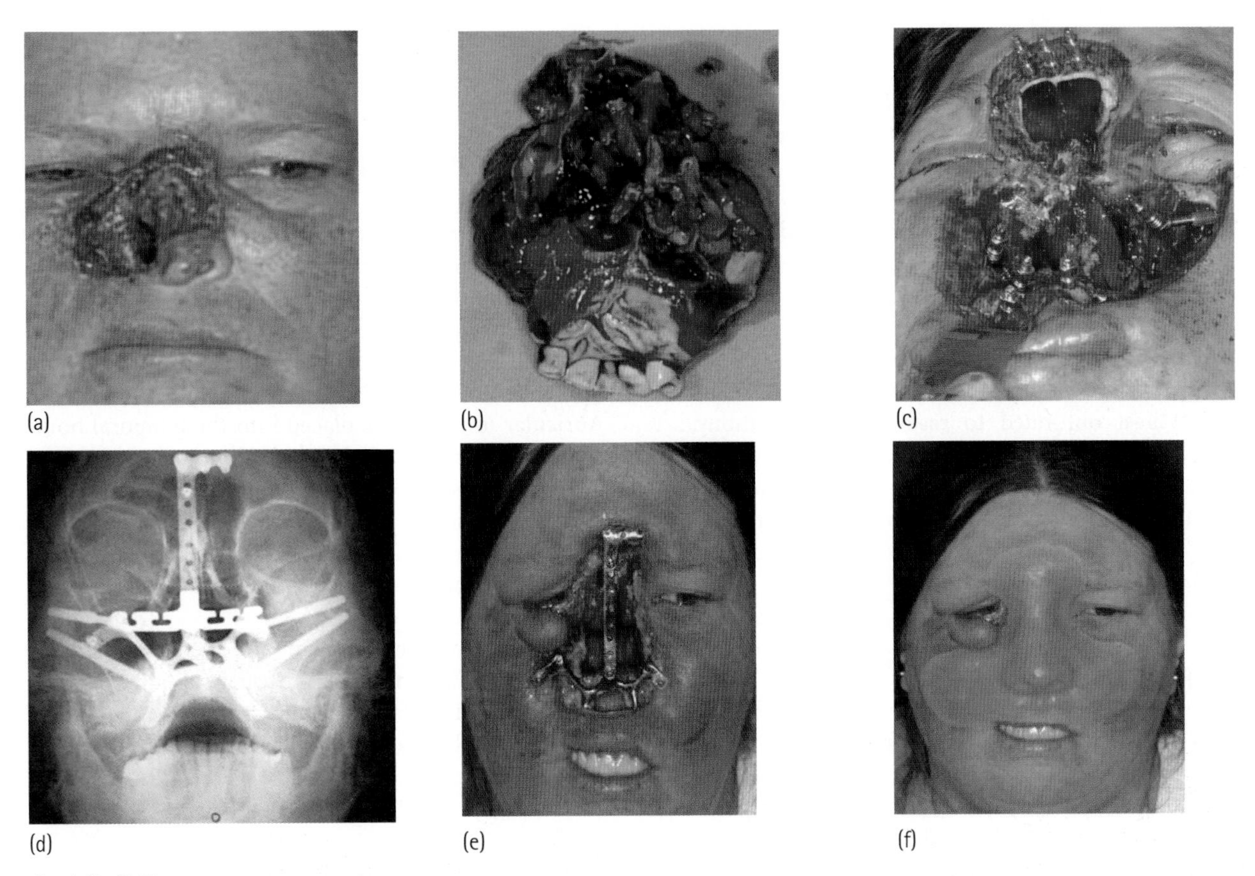

2.10.27 (a) Squamous cell carcinoma of the naso-maxillary complex. (b) Resection specimen. (c) Facial defect with implants placed at time of resection surgery. (d) Radiograph of titanium prosthesis attached to the facial implants. (e) Titanium prosthesis *in situ*. (f) Temporary facial obturator.

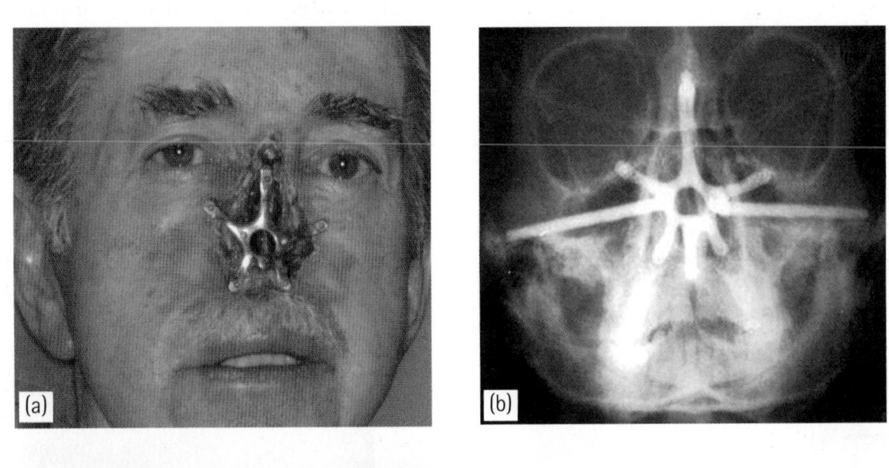

(c)

2.10.28 (a) Titanium framework *in situ* for nasal prosthesis. (b) Radiograph of titanium prosthesis attached to the facial implants. (c) Nasal prosthesis *in situ*.

the process. The initial treatment is aimed at resuscitation of the patient with debridement of the avulsed area and attempts to obtain soft tissue closure and repositioning and reduction of facial bone fractures with titanium miniplates (Figure 2.10.29).

Rehabilitation takes place roughly three months after initial repair of the hard and soft tissue. A full radiological examination is undertaken and this gives the restorative team the necessary information required to plan rehabilitation. Three-dimensional spiral CT scan imaging is the most useful in this regard. Facial gunshot wounds usually traverse the midline and the soft and hard tissue defects are best obturated to restore facial harmony. Occasionally, bone grafts are performed into the area and sort tissue defects are closed prior to bone grafting. Implant placement is done using a combination of standard and zygomatic implants and an immediate loading technique is employed (Figure 2.10.30).

FIXED PROSTHESIS

Almost all maxillary defects resulting from anatomical disruption of the maxillofacial complex can be particularly well rehabilitated functionally and aesthetically using this protocol in conjunction with standard implantology and fixed/fixed-removable prosthodontic principles (Figure 2.10.31, see page 134).

PTERYGOID IMPLANT

The posterior maxilla has limitations in the extent of the maxillary sinus and the tuberosity and pterygoid plate region is an alternative to sinus lifting procedures. The placement of a tapered implant into this region requires the correct angulation and is placed into the maxillary tuberosity and angulated up the posterior wall of the maxillary antrum. This is technically demanding, has limited access and has an 85 per cent success rate (Figure 2.10.32, see page 134).

EXTRAORAL IMPLANTS: CRANIAL, AURICULAR AND ORBITAL

The placement of extraoral implants to replace missing ears, eyes and cranium are accomplished with the placement of small length implants, which are placed into very dense regions of the frontal bone, supraorbital margin and temporal bone (Figure 2.10.33).

Auricular implants are placed into the temporal bone, roughly 20–22 mm behind the external auditory meatus and orbital implants into the supraorbital margin. These implants are usually about 4–5 mm in length and are splinted by a titanium dolder bar, on to which the auricular or orbital prosthesis is attached (Figure 2.10.34, see page 135).

Orbital implants are placed into the lateral and superior orbital margin. These implants are usually about 4–5 mm in length and are splinted by a titanium dolder bar, on to which the orbital prosthesis is attached (Figure 2.10.35, see page 135).

BONE-ANCHORED HEARING AID

Hearing problems are one of the most common handicaps found in children and affects 15 out of every 1000 children under the age of 18 years. The most common hearing losses are sensorineural (found in the cochlea, and can include vestibulocochlear neural damage, conductive hearing loss due to damage or infection of the middle ear and auditory ossicles and noise-induced hearing loss. Medicine offers little for those patients with cochlear impairment and cochlear implants and hearing aids are most commonly prescribed. Hearing aids are commonly attached around the affected ear, with the air-conductive appliance inside the

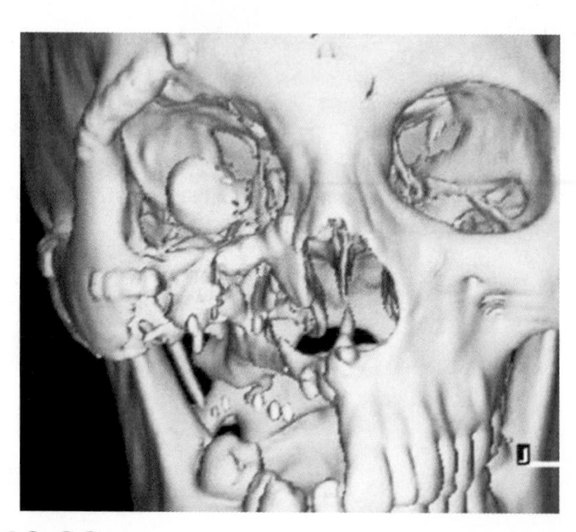

(a)

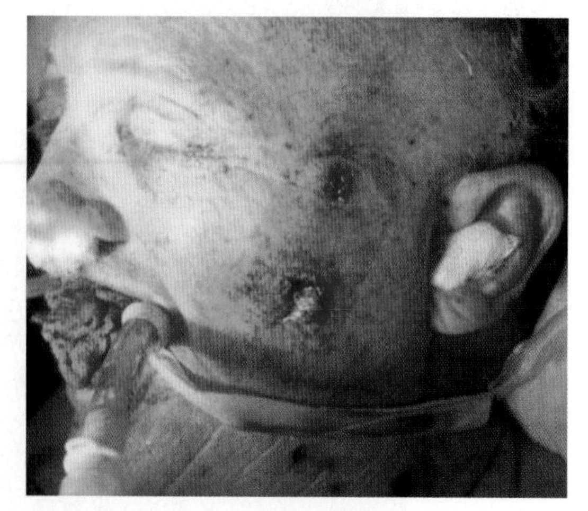

(b)

2.10.29 (a) CAT scan of initial facial bone repair. (b) Facial gunshot wound in the trauma unit prior to initial repair.

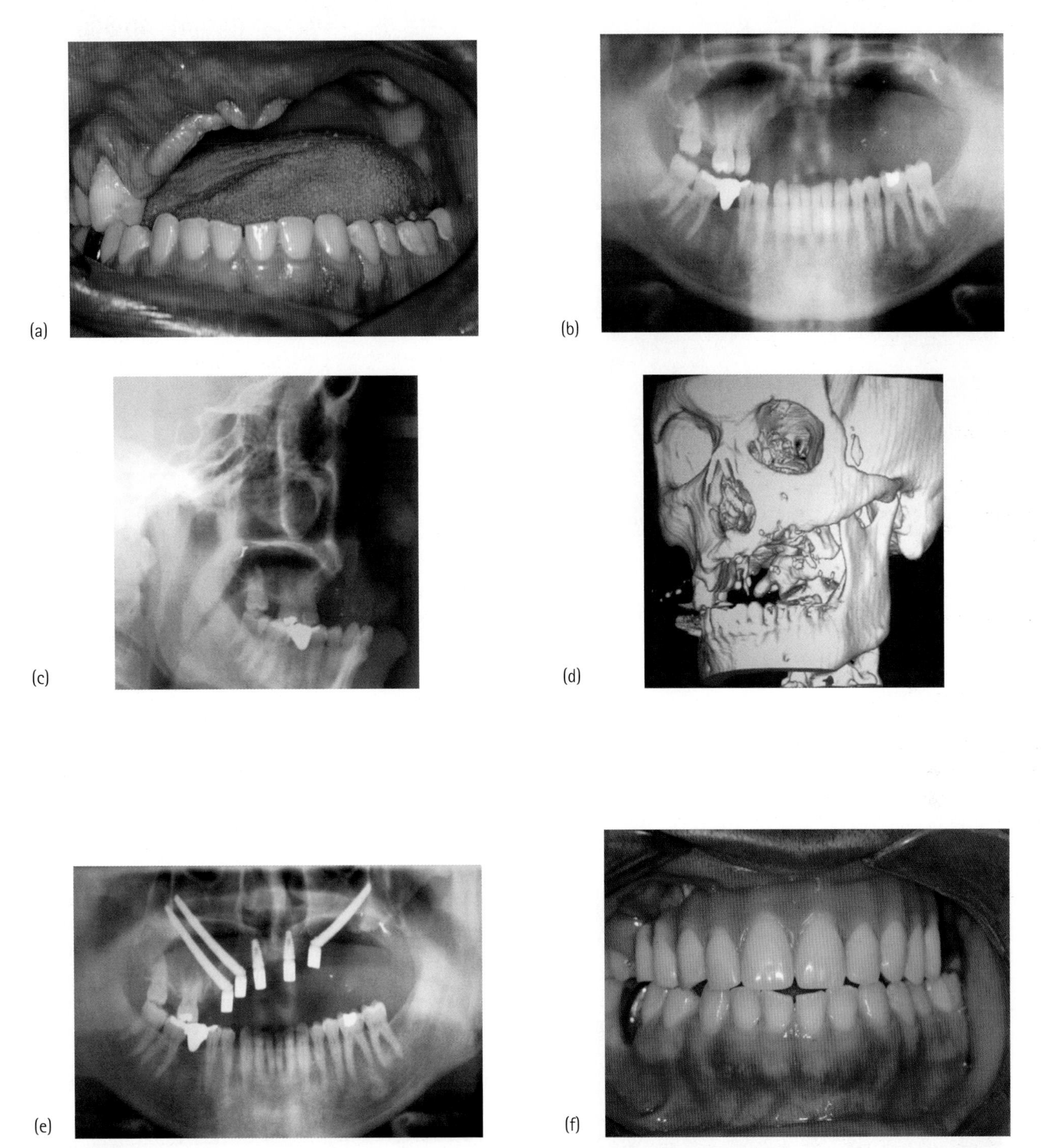

2.10.30 (a) Healed defect after initial gunshot repair. (b) Panoramic radiograph of the resultant defect. (c) Lateral cephalogram of defect. (d) CAT scan of facial bone defect after facial gunshot wound. (e) Panoramic radiograph of inplants *in situ*. (f) Obturator fixed onto implants.

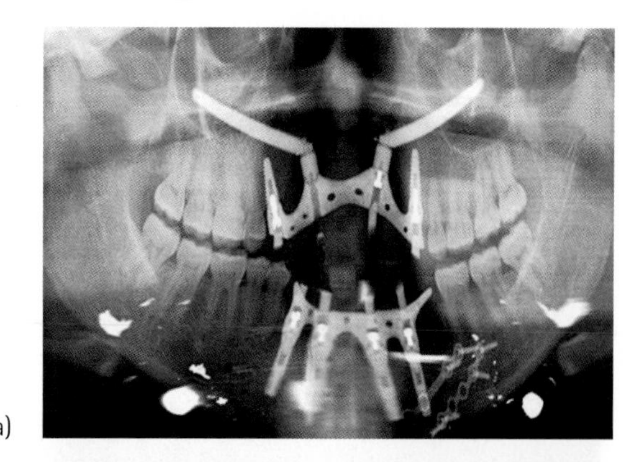

(a)

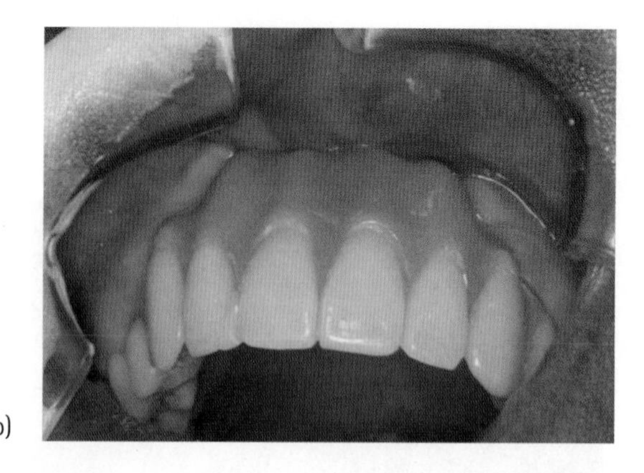

(b)

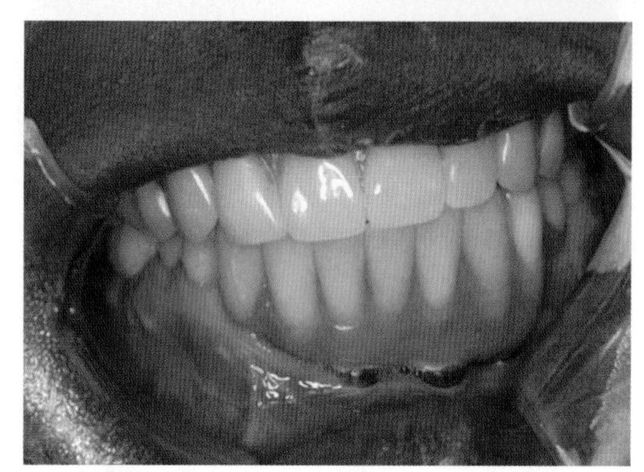

(c)

2.10.31 (a) Panoramic radiograph of implants and framework *in situ*. (b) Maxillary fitted temporary obturator. (c) Maxillary and mandibular temporary prostheses.

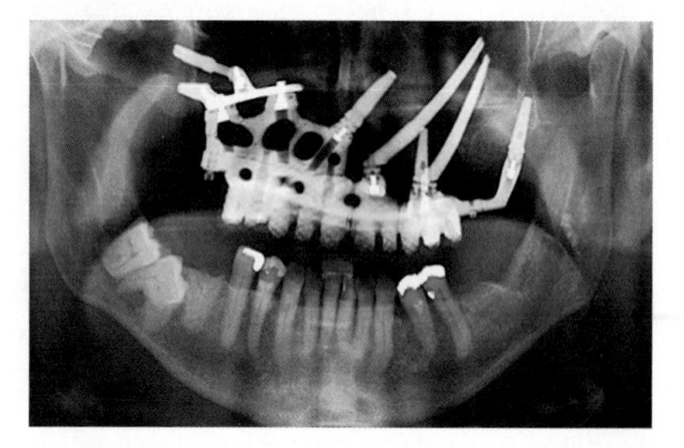

2.10.32 Pterygoid implant in combination with standard and zygomatic implants.

external auditory meatus. An alternative to the conventional hearing aid is a bone-anchored hearing aid (BAHA), which is used for amplification of sound and improving conductive hearing loss through bone conduction of the sound waves. Cochlear function is imperative for the success of bone-conducted hearing aids placed into the mastoid region of the affected ear.

Surgical technique for placement of the titanium fixture into the lateral aspect of the skull is the same as the placement of the superior implant placed for ear loss and the implant is placed in a two-stage procedure and the hearing aid attached to the implant about 8–12 weeks later (Figure 2.10.36, see page 136).

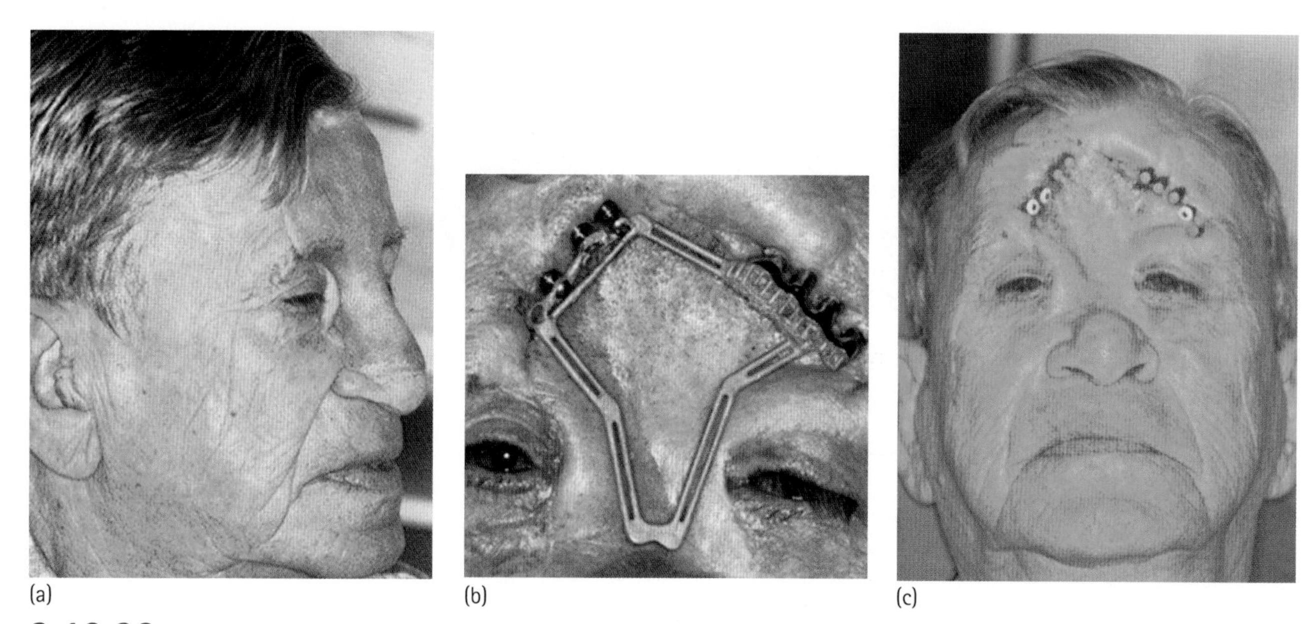

2.10.33 (a) Frontal bone defect after frontonasal resection. (b) Frontal implants and fixed rigid titanium bar *in situ*. (c) Implants and healing abutments prior to doder bar placement.

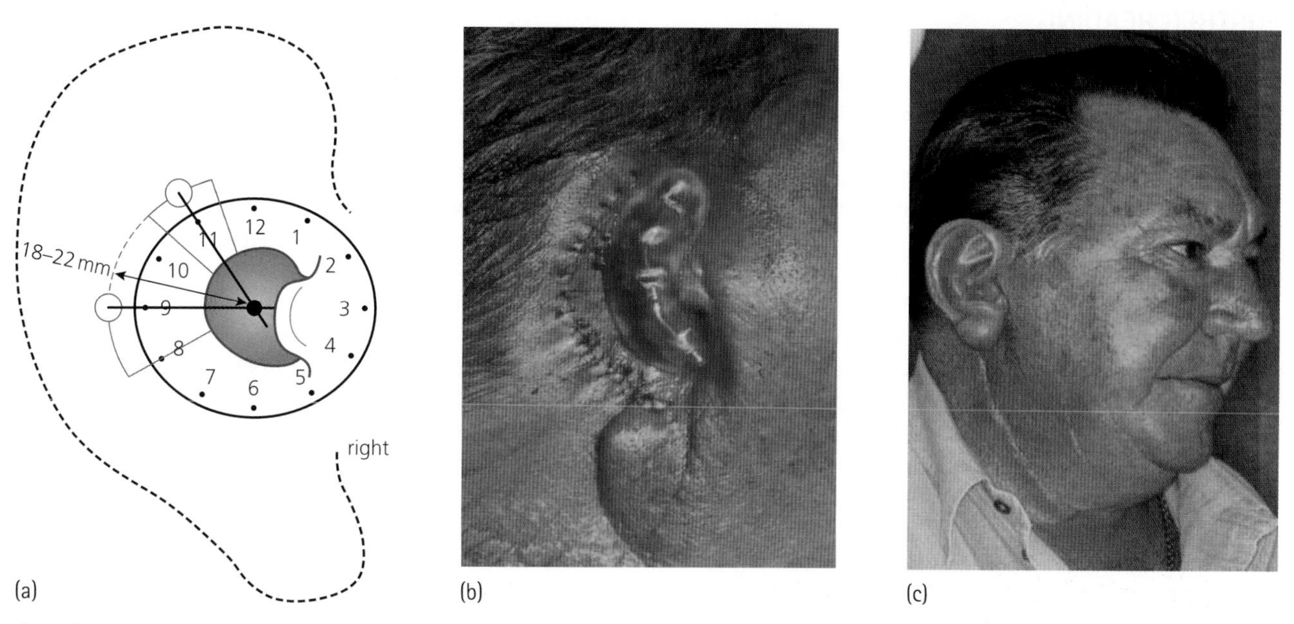

2.10.34 (a) Schematic diagram of cranial implant sites for ear replacement. (b) Post placement sutured incision with healing plate. (c) Final attached ear prosthesis.

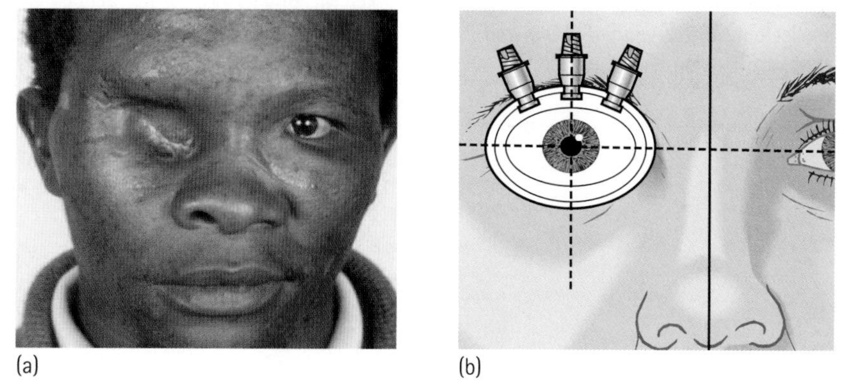

2.10.35 (a) Orbital defect prior to implant insertion for orbital prosthesis. (b) Schematic diagram of orbital implant sites.

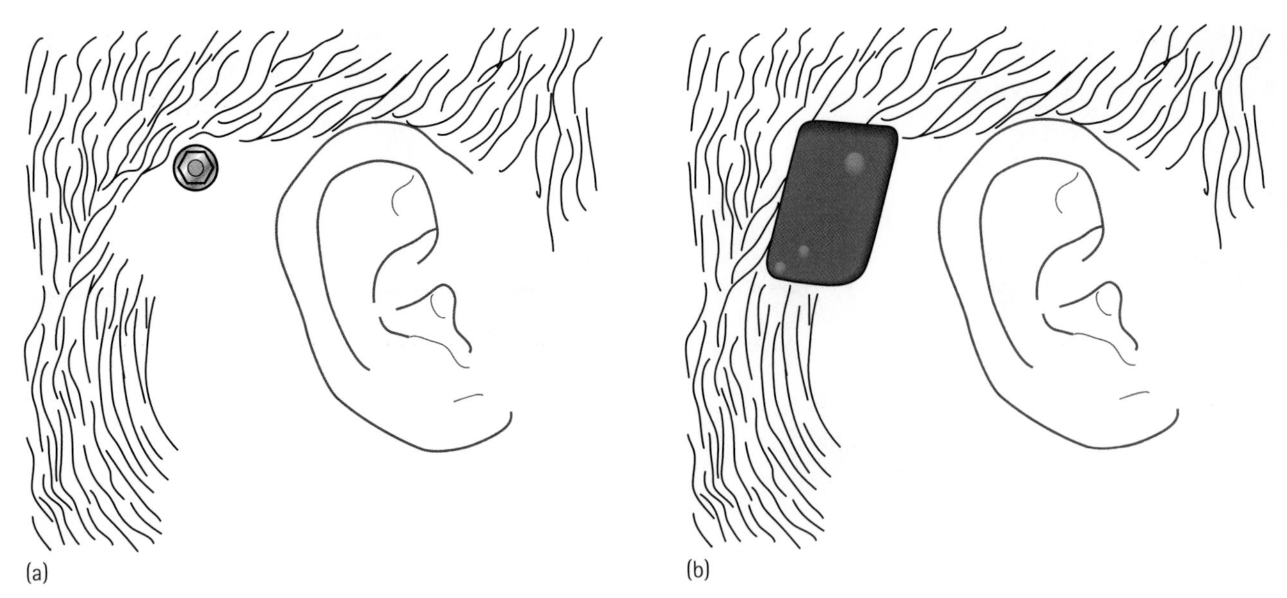

2.10.36 (a) Temporal implant placement for BAHA. (b) BAHA fitted onto implant.

FURTHER READING

Balshi TJ, Wolfinger GJ, Petropoulos VC. Quadruple zygomatic implant support for retreatment of resorbed iliac crest bone graft transplant. *Implant Dentistry* 2003; **12**: 47–53.

Bothur S, Jonsson G, Sandahl L. Modified technique using multiple zygomatic implants in reconstruction of the atrophic maxilla: A technical note. *International Journal of Oral Maxillofacial Implants* 2003; **18**: 902–904.

Boyes-Varley JG, Howes DG, Lownie JF, Blackbeard GA. Surgical modifications to the branemark zygomaticus protocol in the treatment of the severely resorbed maxilla: A clinical report. *Journal of Oral and Maxillofacial Implants* 2003; **18**: 232–7.

Boyes-Varley JG, Howes DG, Davidge-Pitts KD *et al.* A protocol for maxillary reconstructions following oncology resection using zygomatic implants. *International Journal of Prosthodontology* 2007; **20**: 151–61.

Branemark P-I, Svensson S, Van Steenberghe D. Ten year survival rates of fixed prostheses on four or six implants ad modum Branemark in full edentulism. *Clinical and Oral Implants Research* 1995; **6**: 227–31.

Brown JS, Jones DC, Summerwill A *et al.* Vascularized iliac crest graft with internal oblique muscle for immediate reconstruction after maxillectomy. *British Journal of Oral and Maxillofacial Surgery* 2002; **40**: 183–90.

Lekholm U, Wannfors K, Isaksson S, Adielsson B. Oral implants in combination with implants. A 3 year retrospective multicenter study using the branemark implant system. *International Journal of Oral Maxillofacial Surgery* 1999; **28**: 181–7.

Malevez C, Daelemans P, Adriaenssens P, Durdu F. Use of zygomatic implants to deal with resorbed posterior maxillae. *Periodontology* 2000; **33**: 82–9.

Mustafa AR, Adams Jr WP, Hartog JM *et al.* Maxillary reconstruction: Functional and aesthetic considerations. *Plastic and Reconstructive Surgery* 1999; **104**: 2172–83.

Okay DJ, Genden E, Buchbinder D, Urken M. Prosthodontic guidelines for surgical reconstruction of the maxilla. A classification system of defects. *Journal of Prosthetic Dentistry* 2001; **86**: 352–63.

Smolka W, Iizuka T. Surgical reconstruction of maxilla and midface: Clinical outcome and factors relating to postoperative complications. *Journal of Craniomaxillofacial Surgery* 2005; **33**: 1–7.

Ten Bruggenkate CM, Johan P, van den Bergh A. Maxillary sinus floor elevation: A valuable preprosthetic procedure. *Journal of Periodontology* 2000; **1998**: 176–82.

Urken ML, Bridger AG, Zur KB, Genden EM. The scapular osteofasciocutaneous flap: A 12-year experience. *Archives of Otolaryngology, Head and Neck Surgery* 2001; **127**: 862–9.

2.11

Tissue engineering

MILLER H SMITH, KENJI IZUMI, STEPHEN E FEINBERG

INTRODUCTION

In order for oral and maxillofacial surgery to advance as a specialty, we must continuously investigate new treatment options. Over the past 20 years, the scope of tissue engineering has exploded in an attempt to provide solutions to improve hard and soft tissue healing. Restoring three-dimensional form and function is of utmost importance through reconstruction of tissue defects, and tissue-engineered products can minimize morbidity associated with the harvest of autogenous soft and hard tissue grafts. Materials and techniques continue to evolve and many are being investigated to be able to provide unique alternatives to the oral and maxillofacial surgeon in the near future. Soft tissue constructs attempt to decrease scar tissue formation and maximize our innate healing potential. Regeneration of osseous and cartilaginous tissues requires the use of engineered scaffold constructs fabricated from various materials with a combination of numerous biological factors. In addition, investigation into regeneration of craniomaxillofacial structures is on the rise and some have even evaluated prefabricated free vascularized hard tissue grafts for use in maxillofacial reconstruction.

INDICATIONS

Tissue engineering is indicated in the following:

- preprosthetic surgery
- following pathological resection
- following trauma
- developmental deformities.

SOFT TISSUE RECONSTRUCTION

Principles and justification

Oral mucosa and skin are the most common autogenous soft tissue grafts used for preprosthetic surgery and resurfacing of oral mucosa defects. Both require a second surgical donor site, resulting in significant patient morbidity. Oral mucosa is limited in supply, while the functional and aesthetic outcomes of skin grafts are often unfavourable. Skin and oral mucosa substitutes prevent donor site morbidity, provide more therapeutic options and accomplish better outcomes than conventional therapies in reconstructive surgery. One method of creating a tissue-engineered soft tissue substitute is through the manufacture of an *ex vivo* produced oral mucosa equivalent (EVPOME) in which an epithelial layer of autogeneous oral keratinocytes is developed and grown on top of AlloDerm® (LifeCell, Branchburg, NJ, USA), an acellular, non-immunogenic, human cadaver dermis (Figures 2.11.1 and 2.11.2). AlloDerm confers excellent

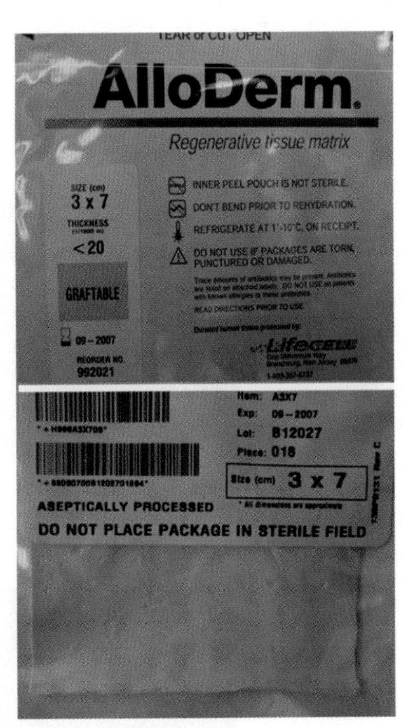

2.11.1 Package of AlloDerm, 3 × 7 cm in size (top); inner pouch (bottom). The author prefers the thinnest piece (0.009–0.013 inches, 0.22–0.33 mm).

handling characteristics, resulting in a supple nature to the grafts, and is a tissue product well established in the field of oral and maxillofacial surgery. The EVPOME graft is then used for reconstruction of the desired soft tissue defect by suturing it in place over a recipient bed with adequate blood perfusion to allow rapid vascularization of the graft to occur. EVPOME is utilized as a full-thickness oral mucosa substitute and has characteristics of keratinization identical to that of native oral mucosa (Figure 2.11.3).

Ideally, a number of principles must be adhered to for proper success of a soft tissue graft:

1. The recipient bed must be vascularized.
2. The graft must not be placed on bare cortical bone.
3. Stabilization and immobilization allows for vessel inosculation from the underlying capillary network.
4. Close adaptation to the recipient bed is essential.
5. Bolsters or surgical stents acting as a pressure dressing must be used to ensure haematoma formation is avoided under the graft.

Procedure

The patient is usually scheduled 4 weeks prior to the desired reconstructive surgery in order to harvest a biopsy of the oral mucosa. A tissue punch provides an adequate number of compatible keratinocytes to manufacture EVPOME grafts prior to transplantation, while causing minimal morbidity. Palatal tissue provides a keratinized mucosa equivalent, while the retromolar pad or buccal mucosa provides non-keratinized mucosa equivalent. The patient is anaesthetized using local infiltration techniques. A small 4–6-mm punch biopsy is performed to the level of the dermis (Figure 2.11.4). At the palate, local haemostasis is obtained with pressure and the wound is dressed with a haemostatic collagen material stabilized with a figure-of-eight suture. At the retromolar area or buccal mucosa, the wound is closed primarily. The harvested tissue is transferred into a culture medium and transported into the laboratory.

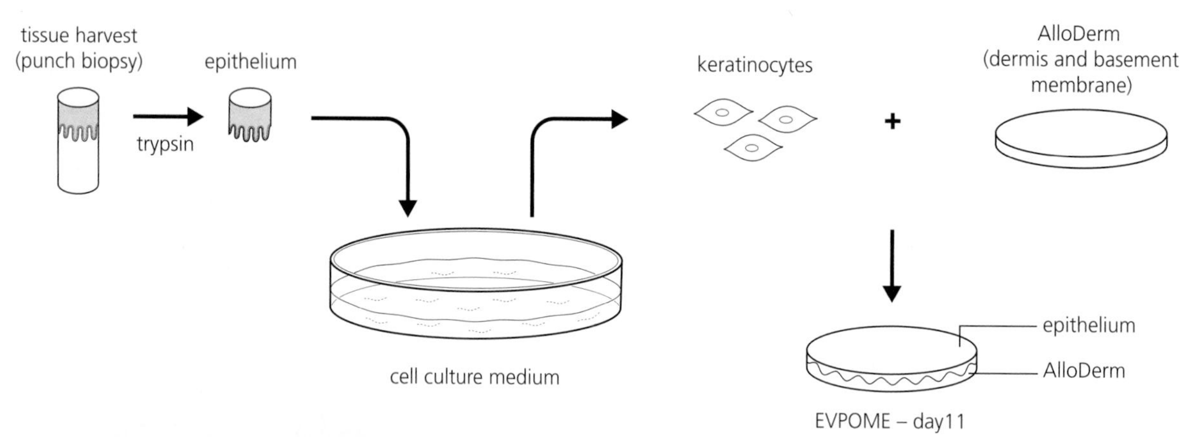

2.11.2 Tissue punch is used to isolate keratinocytes which are then cultured and seeded onto a basement membrane of AlloDerm.

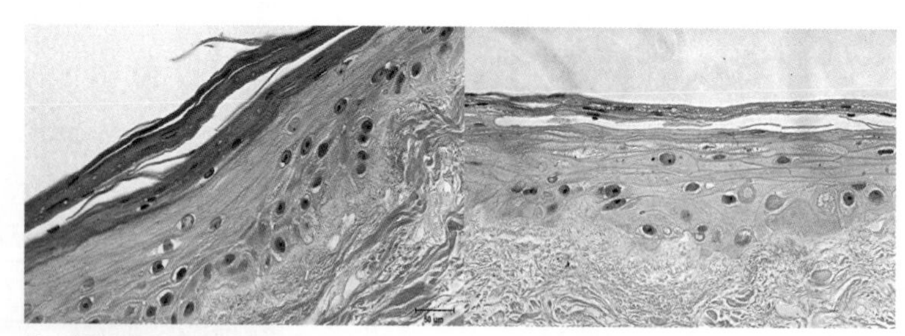

2.11.3 Haematoxylin and eosin stains of EVPOME graft at days 11 and 18, demonstrating integration of keratinized layer overlying AlloDerm.

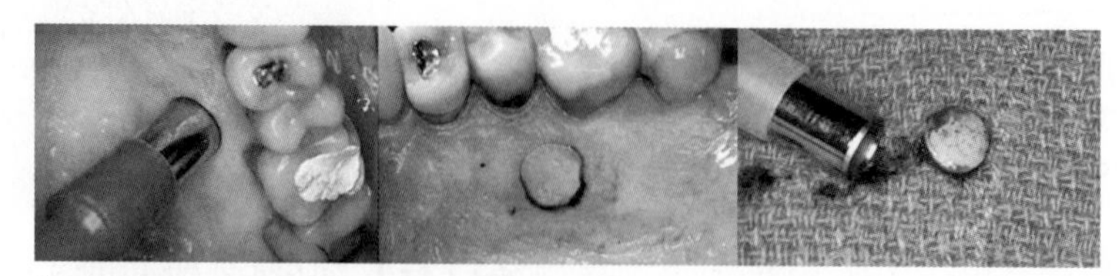

2.11.4 Tissue punch for tissue harvest from hard palate for isolation and growth of keratinocytes.

The manufacturing and culturing procedures of the EVPOME have been described in detail elsewhere. Briefly, oral keratinocytes are dissociated by soaking the harvested biopsy tissue in 0.04 per cent trypsin solution (Figure 2.11.2). The cells are grown in a culture medium free of bovine serum, mouse feeder cells and pituitary extracts. The lack of foreign xenogenic cells avoids any cross-contamination or immunization. Following growth of a sufficient number of keratinocytes over 2 weeks (Figure 2.11.5), cells are seeded on to pieces of type IV collagen-presoaked AlloDerm (cells are seeded on the roughened basement membrane side). For the first 4 days, a composite of keratinocytes and AlloDerm is incubated in a submerged culture. For the next 7 days, the composite is raised at an air–liquid interface culture. Upon reaching day 11 after seeding, the dermis with keratinocytes, the EVPOME grafts are ready to transplant (Figure 2.11.6).

Preparation of the recipient bed is created through conventional surgical procedures, such as vestibuloplasty and tumour excision. These basic procedures are found in Chapters 2.7 and 4.5, respectively. Vestibuloplasty is often used to create an appropriate environment for the placement of implants or denture support in case of insufficient vestibular depth and/or complete loss of a keratinized (attached, immobile) gingiva (Figure 2.11.7). A supraperiosteal split thickness dissection is made with a scalpel or metzenbaum scissors. The tissue is then pushed apically to the desired height of the vestibule and then sutured to the underlying periosteum (Figure 2.11.8).

For cases of tumour excision, such as the lateral border of the tongue, it is common to place a soft tissue graft for suitable healing. Appropriate margins surrounding the tumor are inked (Figure 2.11.9) and tissue is incised using electrocautery. Haemostasis is achieved most commonly using electrocoagulation and rarely with ligation to maximize preservation of the vascularity of the recipient site (Figure 2.11.10).

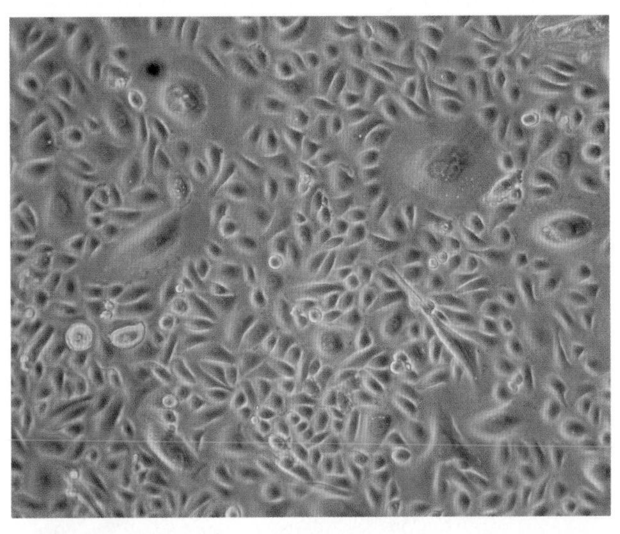

2.11.5 Oral mucosa keratinocytes in culture are poised to be seeded on to AlloDerm.

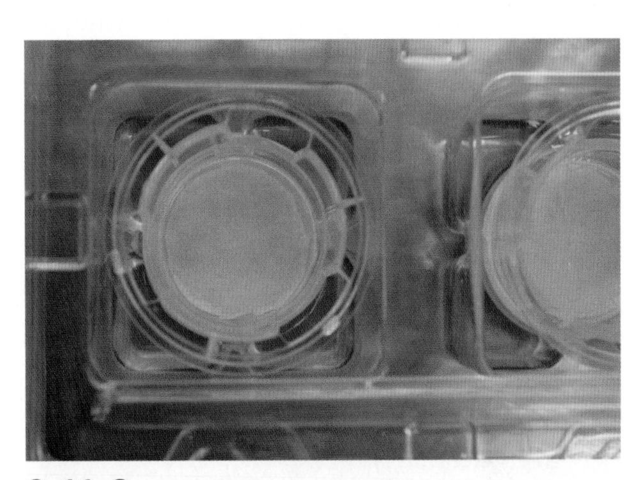

2.11.6 Rehydrated AlloDerm is soaked in human type IV collagen ensuring that the epidermal side (retained intact basement membrane) is positioned uppermost. A composite of oral keratinocytes and AlloDerm is then submerged in culture and transferred to an air–liquid interface.

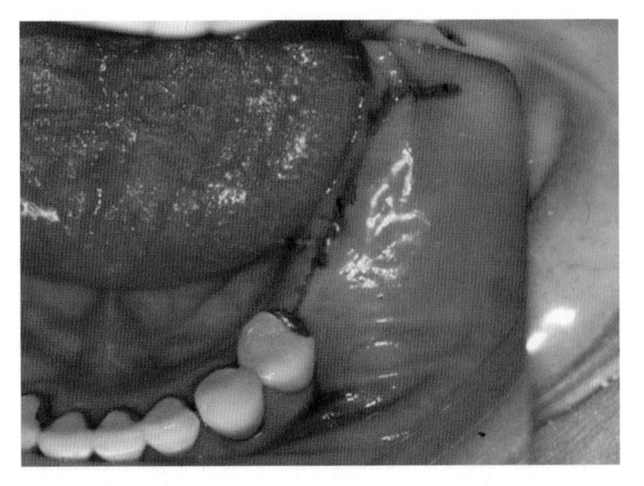

2.11.7 Thick unattached oral mucosa overlying posterior alveolar ridge is an impediment for dental implant success and must be corrected prior to endosseous implant placement.

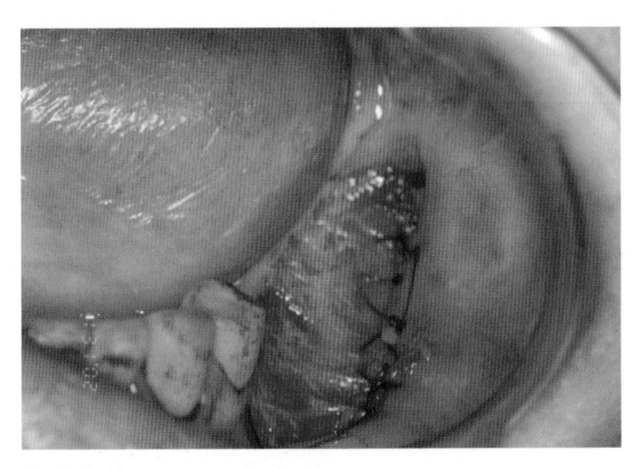

2.11.8 Split thickness supraperiosteal dissection to the desired vestibular depth with the leading margin tacked to the underlying periosteum with sutures.

The EVPOME is then trimmed to the desired size and shape using a sharp No. 10 blade scalpel rotating over the belly of the blade without pulling or dragging the blade, to avoid disruption of the keratinocyte cell layer. In the process of handling the grafts for reshaping and suturing, one should be careful to avoid touching and rubbing the EVPOME surface (Figure 2.11.11). The graft should be blot-dried only with sterile cotton gauze being as atraumatic as possible, avoiding any wiping motion. EVPOME grafts are placed with the AlloDerm side down over the recipient bed and fixed in place to the surrounding mucosa with 4/0 silk on a cutting needle. The graft is secured within the defect using interrupted sutures cut short to the knot. Long uncut marginal sutures opposing one another are tied over a bolster of antibiotic-soaked gauze to apply pressure to the defect to minimize dead space and haematoma formation (Figures 2.11.12 and 2.11.13 (tumour excision), Figures 2.11.14 and 2.11.15 (vestibuloplasty)). The gauze bolster and sutures are removed at post-operative day 7 after grafting. The underlying EVPOME grafts possess a characteristic red hue indicative of early revascularization (Figure 2.11.16). For vestibuloplasties, a rigid surgical stent can be created pre-operatively and secured in place intraorally with miniscrews or circumosseous wires (Figure 2.11.17). After a period of four months, the graft will have integrated and will possess adequate keratinization to allow for implant placement (Figure 2.11.18).

HARD TISSUE RECONSTRUCTION

Principles and justification

The underlying hard tissues offer the framework for overlying facial aesthetics, as defects in osseous and cartilaginous tissues are visibly portrayed through the soft tissues. Classically, significant morbidity and deformity is traded in a distant area for reconstruction of craniofacial structures. Allogeneic grafts are available; however, in order to achieve minimal immunologic response, all cellular tissues are removed reducing the potential for reliable integration. Lastly, alloplastic materials are at risk for foreign body reaction, with significant inflammation and increased risk of infection. Tissue-engineered scaffolds have been created to capitalize on a patient's innate healing response, while adding specific factors at the local site to attempt to

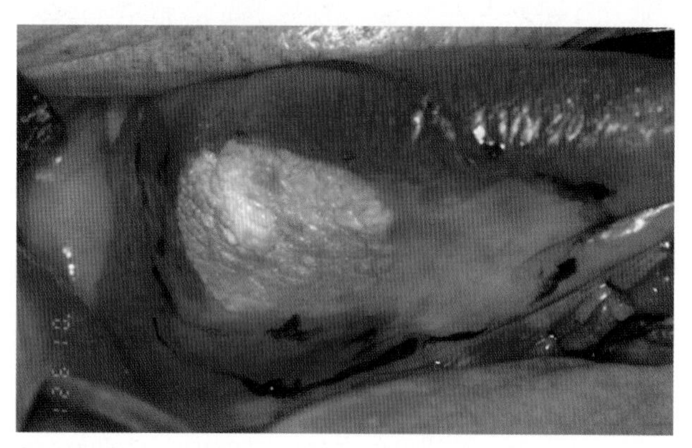

2.11.9 Tumour to the right lateral border of the tongue (squamous cell carcinoma T2N0M0) with inked margins. Reproduced with permission from Wakita M *et al. Oral histology and embryology*. Tokyo: Ishiyaku Publishers, 2006.

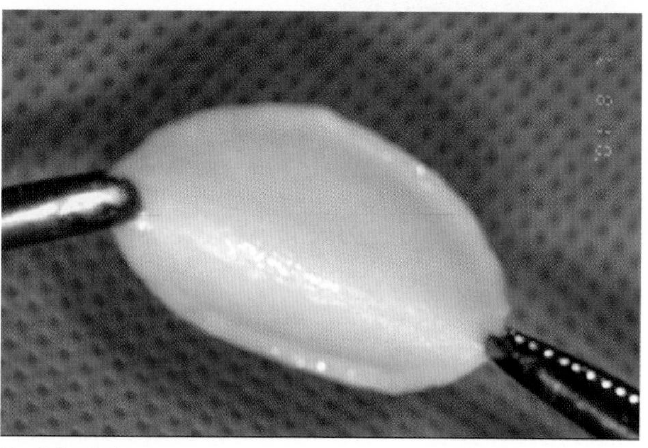

2.11.11 EVPOME graft prior to transplantation.

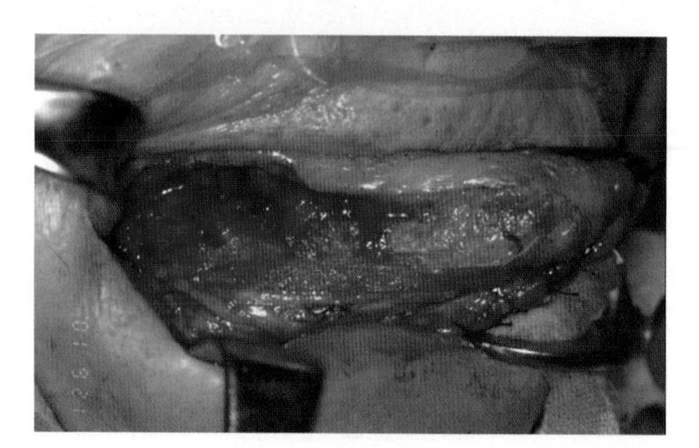

2.11.10 Wide local excision using electrocautery. Reproduced with permission from Wakita M *et al. Oral histology and embryology*. Tokyo: Ishiyaku Publishers, 2006.

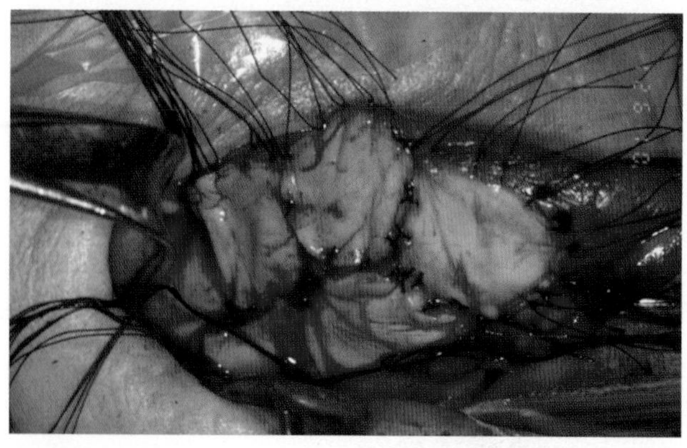

2.11.12 Six pieces of EVPOME are sutured over the wound bed in place. Reproduced with permission from Wakita M *et al. Oral histology and embryology*. Tokyo: Ishiyaku Publishers, 2006.

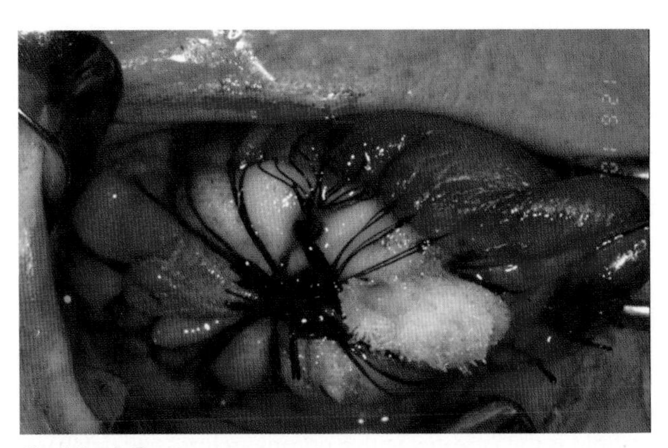

2.11.13 A bolster of antibiotics-soaked gauze is used to apply pressure to the EVPOME grafts for prevention of haematoma formation. Reproduced with permission from Wakita M *et al. Oral histology and embryology*. Tokyo: Ishiyaku Publishers, 2006.

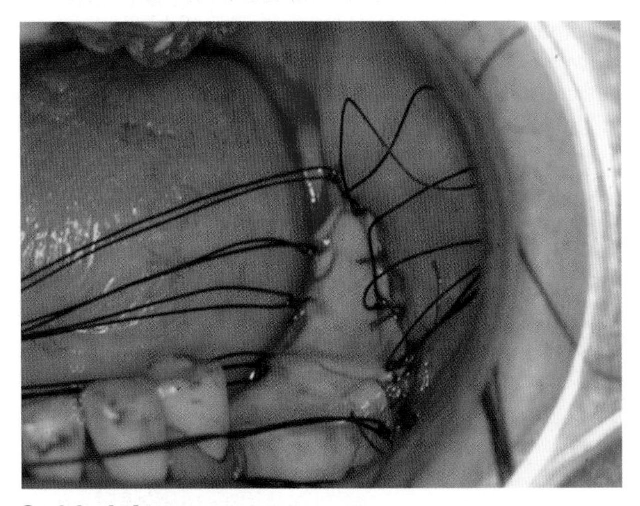

2.11.14 Two pieces of EVPOME configurated and sutured in place to the left posterior alveolar ridge.

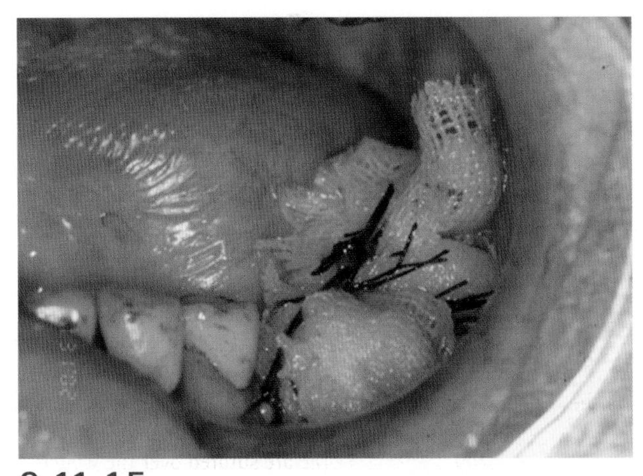

2.11.15 Bolster secured using opposing sutures used to stabilize the graft.

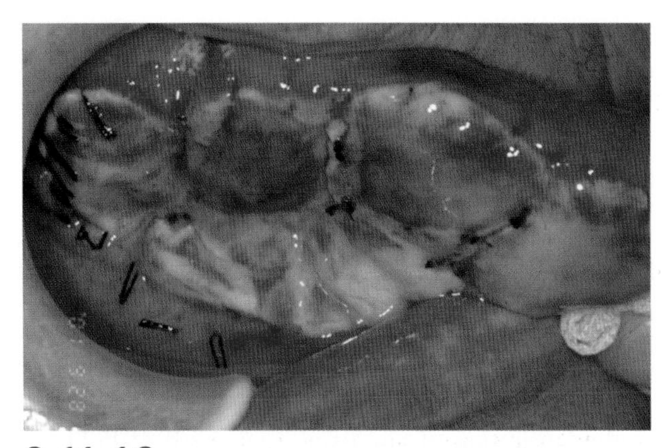

2.11.16 Healing EVPOME grafts seven days following placement demonstrating early vascularization from the underlying tissue.

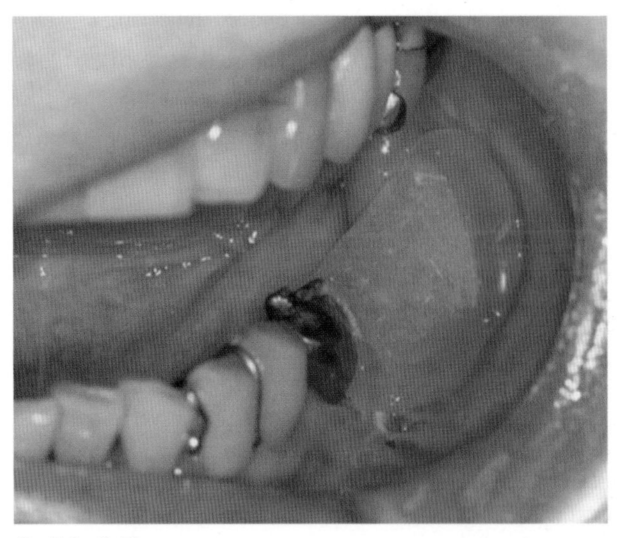

2.11.17 Conversely, grafts can be secured with a surgical resin stent lined with tissue conditioner to avoid pressure areas.

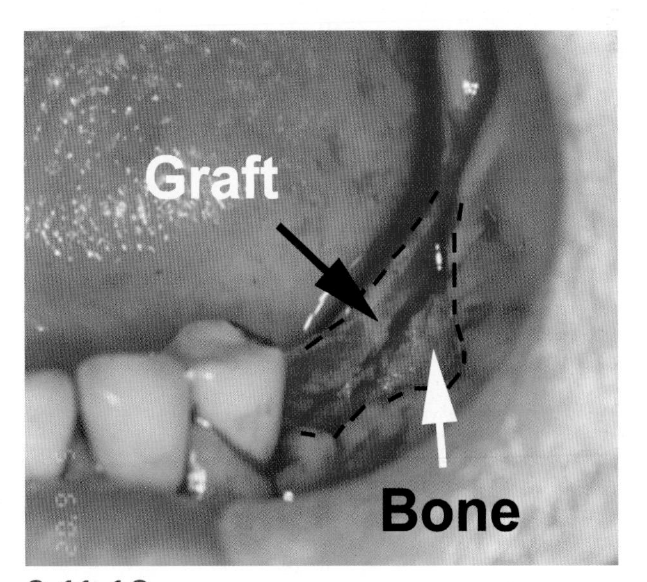

2.11.18 Incision made four months post-operatively revealing healthy attached gingiva acceptable for implant placement.

improve hard tissue regeneration. Tissue engineering has explored a number of materials for the creation of scaffolds including polymers, ceramics and composites. Polymers (polylactic acid, polyglycolic acid, polycaprolactone, polypropylene fumarate) have variable properties and offer reliable biodegradation. More permanent ceramics (hydroxyapetite, tricalcium phosphate) can be used alone, but are frequently combined with polymers in composite grafts. Composites can also include biofactors, such as purified concentrated growth factors, transduced cells with various viral vectors, and autogenous bone marrow cells.

Ideally, a number of principles must be adhered to prior to the fabrication of any tissue-engineered scaffold for replacement into osseous defects:

- replace complex three-dimensional defects
- biocompatible with minimal inflammatory response
- offer functionality and immediate load bearing
- bioresorbable, allowing native structures to assume load bearing as they degrade
- mechanical properties similar to native tissues
- prevent ingrowth of harmful fibrous tissues
- delivery of biofactors:
  - inserted at time of fabrication
  - inserted at time of surgery
  - from adjacent native bone.

Procedure

The surgeon will often obtain pre-operative imaging to determine the extent of the current or surgically created defect. Computed tomography, both conventional and cone-beam, as well as magnetic resonance imaging can be used for this purpose depending on the structures being evaluated (Figure 2.11.19). The patient's dataset is captured on file and a three-dimensional image is rendered for treatment planning using a variety of image processing software (Figure 2.11.20). Depending on the location, shape and size of the defect, an ideal scaffold template contour can be created *de novo* electronically by virtual design, or by inversing the data from the patient's normal contralateral side (Figures 2.11.21 and 2.11.22). Image software includes ANALYZE (www.analyzedirect.com), PV-WAVE (www.ittvis.com) and MATLAB (www.mathworks.com). Once the template is created through a mapping dataset, the microstructure of the scaffold is then created with a porous architecture database. Various microstructures can be applied based on the material used and mechanical properties desired to attempt to promote growth of either cartilaginous or osseous tissues. Mathematically designed interconnecting porous cylinders and interconnecting porous spheres are two examples (Figure 2.11.23) where effective modulus (strength) and porosity are inversely proportional (Figure 2.11.24). Additionally, shells without internal microstructure can offer delivery of well-contained bone marrow directly to the defect, while minimizing load-bearing capabilities. Portions of the scaffold are extended beyond the defect and dilated over adjacent native bone for securing the scaffold once implanted. A scaffold is then fabricated using solid free-form fabrication techniques, such as fused deposition modelling, stereolithography or selective laser sintering (SLS) (Figure 2.11.25). SLS is a rapid prototyping method that offers layer-by-layer fusion of particles to create complex geometric shapes, as well as intricate microstuctures with porous spaces that can be smaller than 1 mm. Virus-transfected cells and biofactors can be directly linked to the scaffold structure

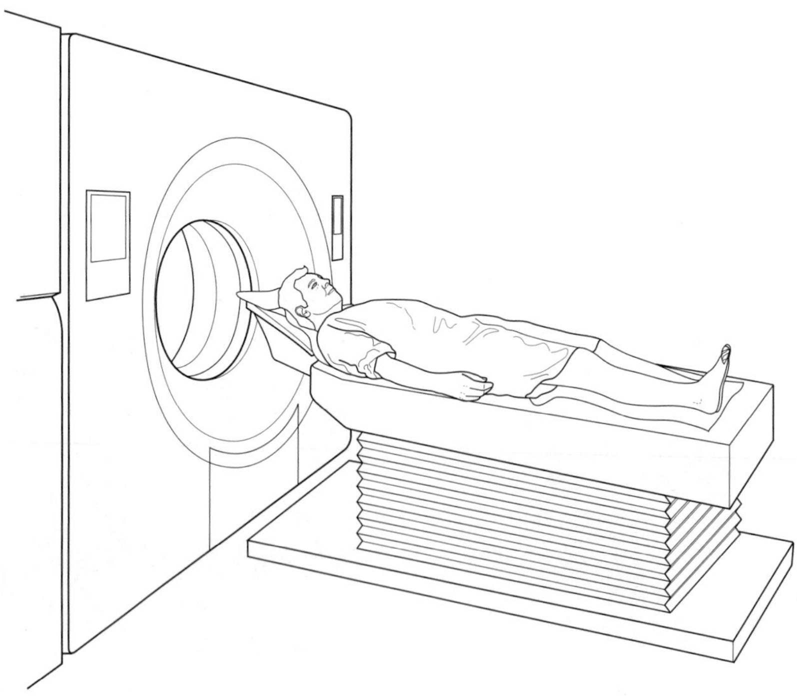

2.11.19 Patient is imaged using computed tomography or magnetic resonance imaging.

using various culture media and techniques described elsewhere (Figure 2.11.26). Conversely, at the time of surgery, bone marrow stromal cells can be harvested and isolated from aspirates and inserted directly into the scaffold immediately prior to implantation (Figure 2.11.27).

Specific structures that have been attempted for regeneration include mandibular condyles, orbital rims and segmental defects in the mandible (Figure 2.11.28). The scaffolds themselves are of varying size and shape to fill the defect as precisely as possible. Based on the area of interest, standard surgical techniques are used as discussed in previous chapters. Wide exposure of the bone and cartilaginous tissues is performed through elevation and

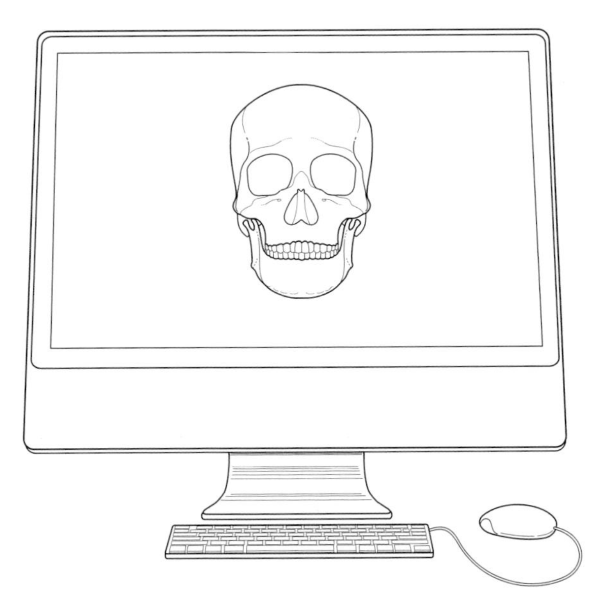

2.11.20 Using image processing software, dataset reconstructed into three-dimensional image for treatment planning.

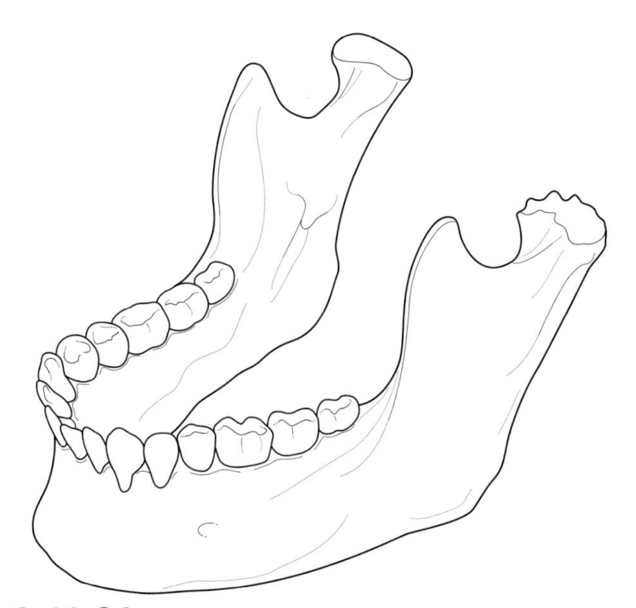

2.11.21 Degenerative joint disease of the left mandibular condyle.

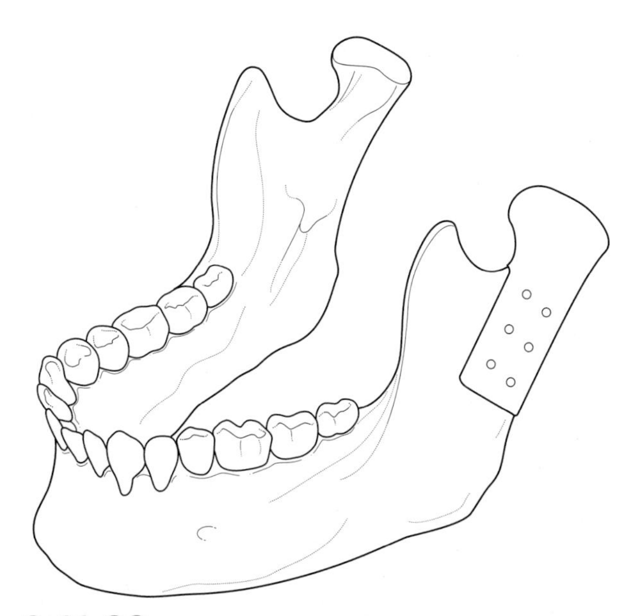

2.11.22 Using image-based design, mandibular condyle can be created to specific dimensions based on the treatment plan or replicated from the normal contralateral condyle. The remainder of the scaffold developed with well-adapted overlying sleeve to secure the condyle in place.

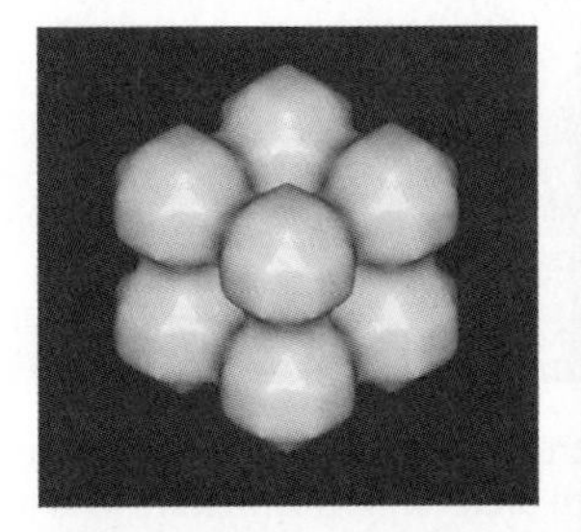

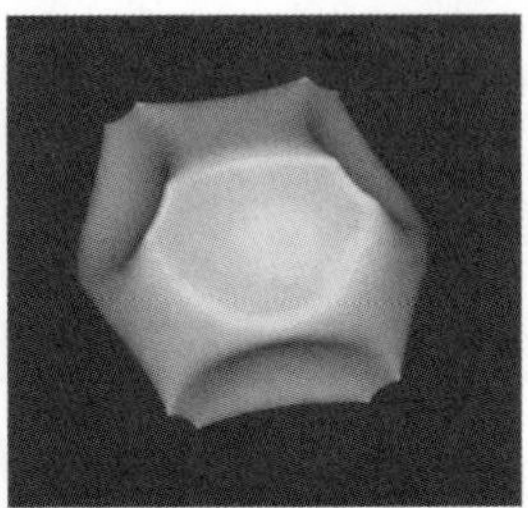

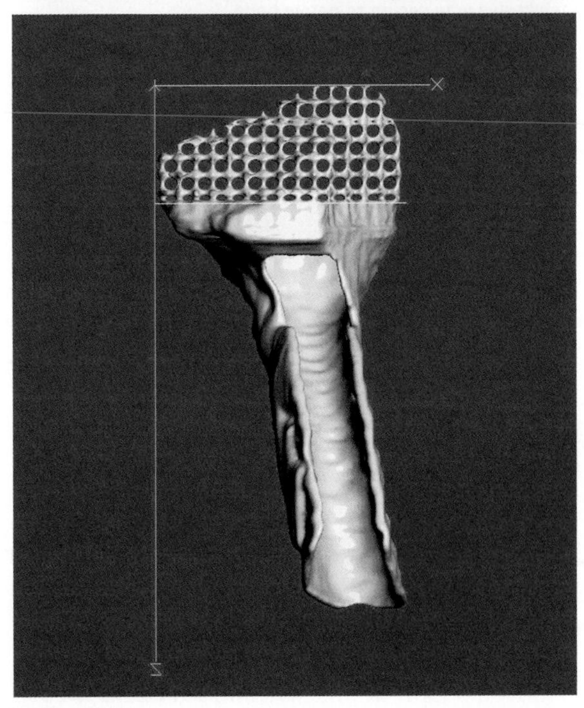

2.11.23 Sphere (upper left) and cylinder (upper right) unit cells can be used to create microstructure to portions of the scaffold.

retraction of subperiosteal tissues, being careful to avoid excessive trauma to the overlying mucosa and periosteum. In cases of trauma or developmental deformity, the defect is isolated, and an acceptable tissue bed for placement of the scaffold is created in order to ensure appropriate primary closure of the tissues. Conversely, in cases of pathological resection, presurgical evaluation determines approximate margins, which may change at the time of surgery depending on the specimen resected. The scaffold may need to be trimmed partially in order to fit into the defect precisely. Bone marrow can be harvested from the hip either by conventional exposure as described in Chapters 3.5 and 9.5, or using a micro-aspiration device. Bone marrow stromal cells can be isolated using a microfluidic device, or cancellous marrow spicules can be crushed with mortar and pestle, and cells or small cancellous fragments can be injected within the

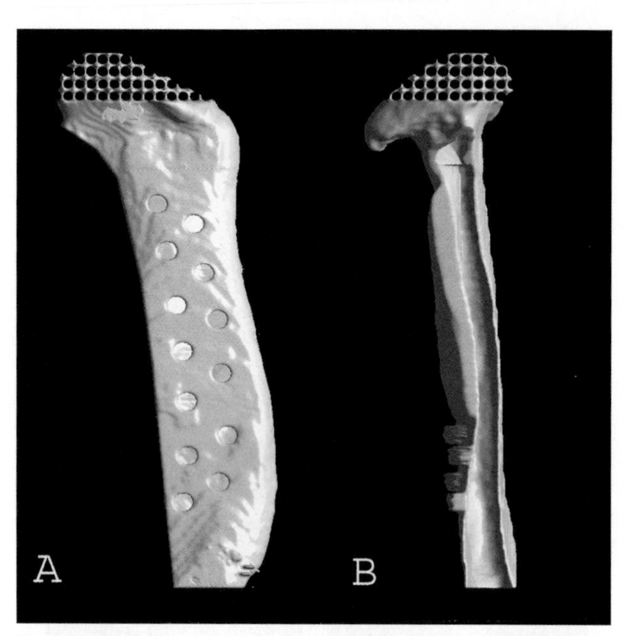

2.11.24 Scaffolds can be created to replace complex three-dimensional shapes, with localized areas of microstructure, and an attached sleeve to secure to native bone.

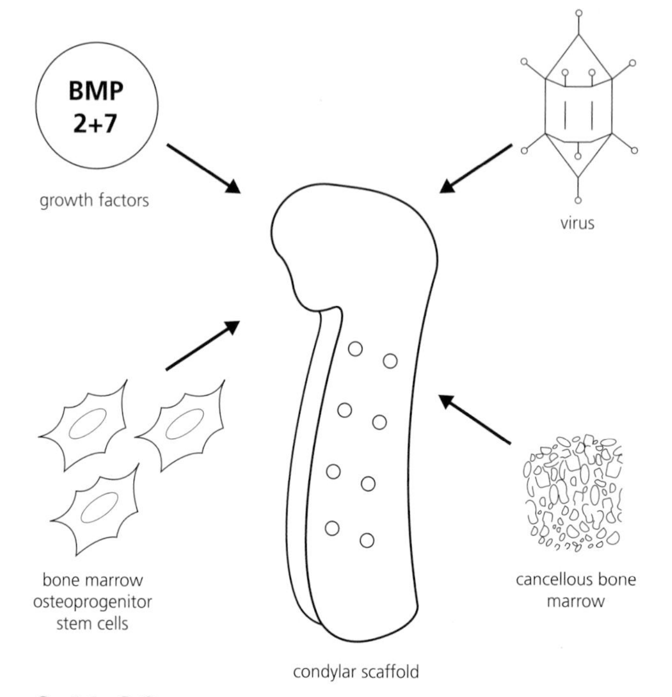

2.11.26 Various biologics can be used for creation of composite scaffolds. Concentrated recombinant bone morphogenetic proteins, viral transfected cells, bone marrow osteoprogenitor stem cells and harvested cancellous bone marrow are some examples.

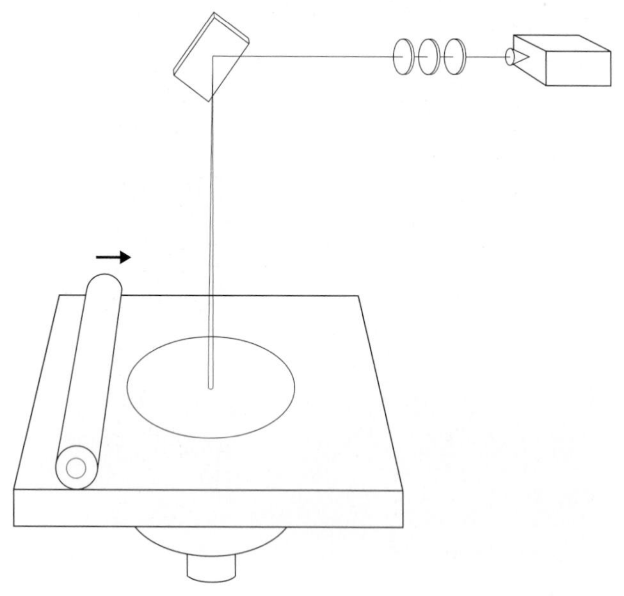

2.11.25 Selective laser sintering.

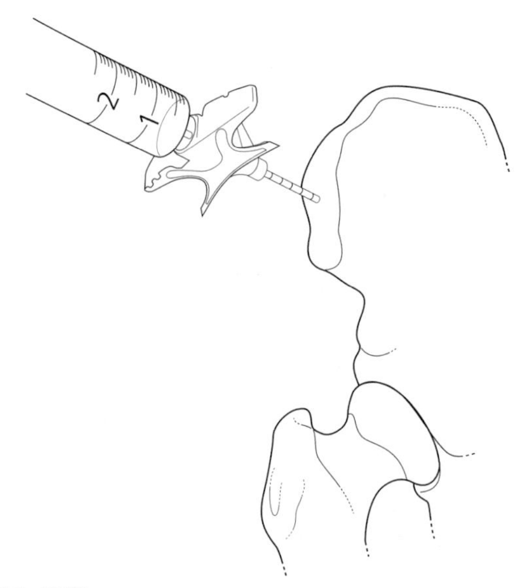

2.11.27 Bone marrow is aspirated from the anterior iliac crest to harvest osteoprogenitor stem cells.

scaffold porosities (Figure 2.11.29). Miniplates and screws are used to secure the scaffold to the native bone to ensure four-point stabilization. In order to advance the tissues over the scaffold to obtain primary closure, the periosteum is cross-hatched using a scalpel (Figure 2.11.30). Metzenbaum scissors can also be used to dissect the tissues for larger advancements. The overlying tissues are closed primarily in layers using interrupted sutures. Horizontal mattress sutures may be used to release tension if tissues are tight to close.

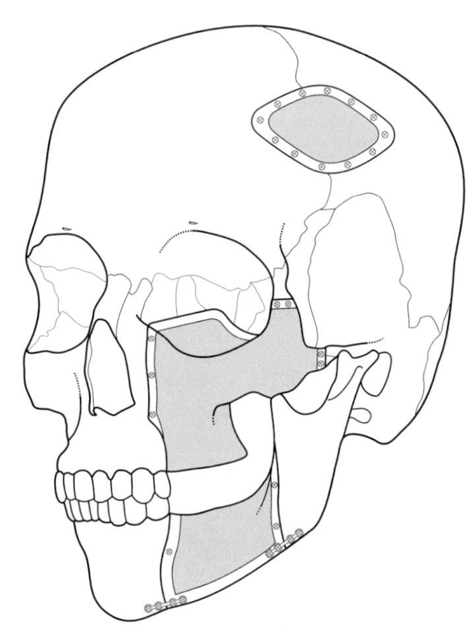

2.11.28 Scaffolds can be created to correct complex geometric shapes of the craniomaxillofacial complex.

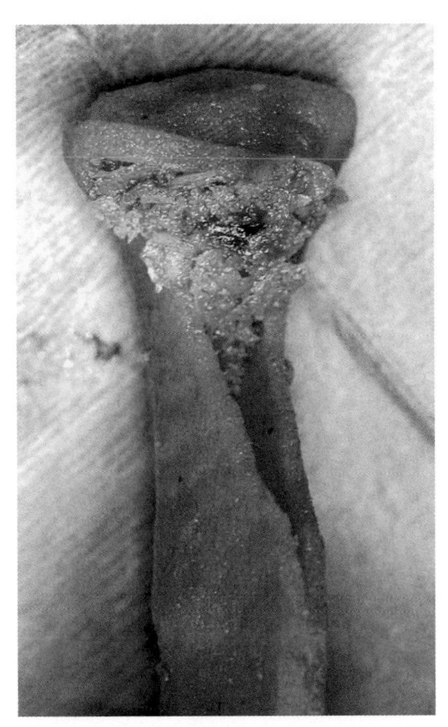

2.11.29 Cancellous bone marrow, harvested via a conventional surgical approach, is packed into the hollow shell of a mandibular condylar–ramus scaffold.

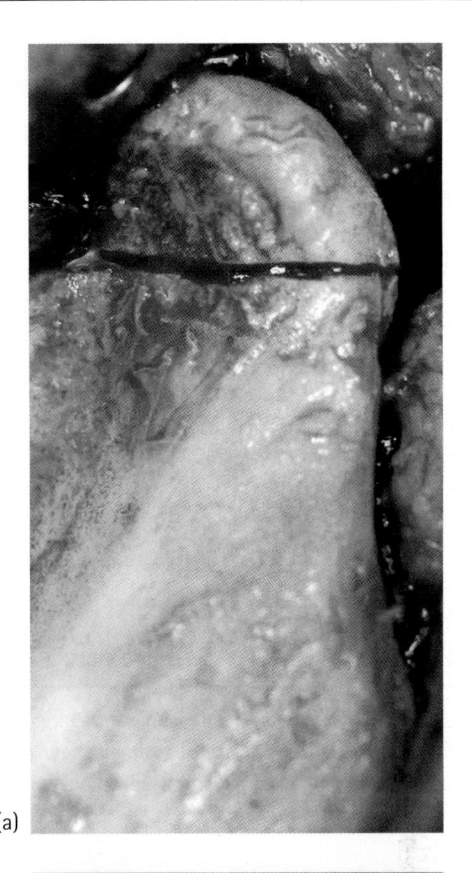

(a)

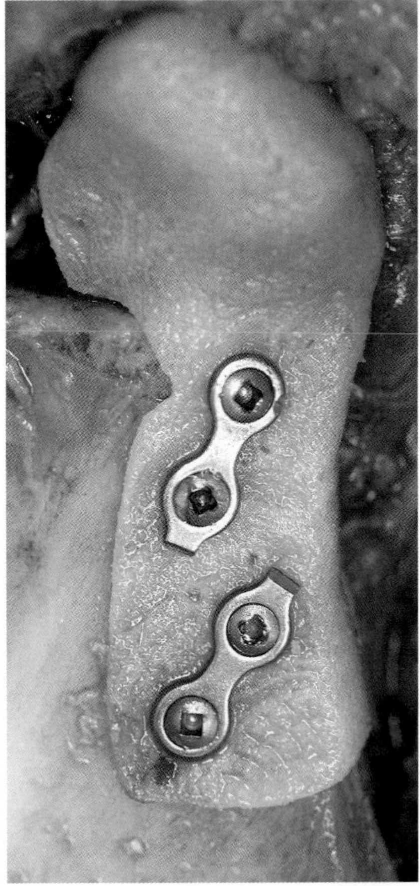

(b)

2.11.30 In animal models, following condylectomy, a well-adapted condylar–ramus scaffold is secured in place using miniplates and screws, allowing for immediate function.

Top tips

- A multidisciplinary team approach utilizing the services of oral and maxillofacial surgeons, biomedical and mechanical engineers, radiologists and adjunct scientists is necessary for proper investigation and fabrication of tissue-engineered materials
- Soft tissue defects have the potential to be reconstructed with minimal morbidity with the use of combination grafts.
- Computer-engineered scaffolds have the ability to be combined with various biological components to attempt to improve regeneration of osseous and cartilaginous tissues.
- Further research is imperative for continued advancement.

FURTHER READING

Hokugo A, Sawada Y, Sugimoto K *et al.* Preparation of prefabricated vascularized bone graft with neoangiogenesis by combination of autologous tissue and biodegradable materials. *International Journal of Oral and Maxillofacial Surgery* 2006; **35**: 1034–40.

Hollister SJ, Lin CY, Saito E *et al.* Engineering craniofacial scaffolds. *Orthodontics and Craniofacial Research* 2005; **8**: 162–73.

Hollister SJ, Maddox RD, Taboas JM. Optimal design and fabrication of scaffolds to mimic tissue properties and satisfy biological constraints. *Biomaterials* 2002; **23**: 4095–103.

Hutmacher DW. Scaffold design and fabrication technologies for engineering tissues – state of the art and future perspectives. *Journal of Biomaterials Science. Polymer Edition.* 2001; **12**: 107–24.

Izumi K, Song J, Feinberg SE. Development of a tissue-engineered human oral mucosa: From the bench to the bed side. *Cells, Tissues, Organs* 2004; **176**: 134–152.

Izumi K, Feinberg SE, Iida A, Yoshizawa M. Intraoral grafting of an *ex vivo* produced oral mucosa equivalent: a preliminary report. *International Journal of Oral and Maxillofacial Surgery* 2003; **32**: 188–97.

Mikos AG, Herring SW, Ochareon P *et al.* Engineering complex tissues. *Tissue Engineering* 2006; **12**: 3307–39.

Rohner D, Hutmacher DW, Cheng TK *et al.* 2003. *In vivo* efficacy of bone-marrow-coated polycaprolactone scaffolds for the reconstruction of orbital defects in the pig. *Journal of Biomedical Materials Research. Part B, Applied Biomaterials* 2003; **66**: 574–80.

Schek RM, Wilke EN, Hollister SJ, Krebsbach PH. Combined use of designed scaffolds and adenoviral gene therapy for skeletal tissue engineering. *Biomaterials* 2006; **27**: 1160–66.

Smith MH, Flanagan CL, Kemppainen JM *et al.* Computed tomography-based tissue-engineered scaffolds in craniomaxillofacial surgery. *International Journal of Medical Robotics* 2007; **3**: 207–16.

PART 3

SURGICAL TECHNIQUES

3.1

Emergency procedures

DAVID W MACPHERSON, CLIVE A PRATT

INTRODUCTION

There are relatively few 'life- or limb-threatening' emergencies in oral and maxillofacial surgery and as a result wide experience of dealing with them is relatively sparse. This chapter is aimed at giving a 'hands-on' text of how to assess and perform these procedures. Because oral and maxillofacial surgery (OMFS) is a very specialized field, physicians from other specialties are likely to have even less experience in dealing with these problems and it is therefore essential that OMFS surgeons should be trained and competent to deal with these emergencies should they occur.

SURGICAL AIRWAY

Emergency surgical airway

INDICATIONS

The indications for an emergency surgical airway are failure to provide a definitive airway by either an oro- or naso-tracheal approach. A disrupted airway would indicate maxillofacial trauma, while an obstructed airway would indicate the presence of a foreign body.

This may be either as a result of the airway being disrupted or obstructed. Severe maxillofacial trauma, with significant disruption of the midface anatomy and associated profuse haemorrhage occasionally may make standard endotracheal intubation impossible, even by an experienced anaesthetist. If it is impossible to oxygenate the patient and protect the airway by other means, then an emergency surgical airway must be performed. All procedures described should be performed using universal precautions.

There are only two emergency surgical airways:

1 needle cricothyroidotomy
2 surgical cricothyroidotomy.

In children, the same procedures must be carried out, using the same techniques. Emergency tracheostomy is fraught with the same dangers and difficulties in children as in adults and needle and surgical cricothyroidotomy are quicker, more straightforward and therefore less risky procedures.

NEEDLE CRICOTHYROIDOTOMY

Needle cricothyroidotomy is performed as an absolute emergency on a patient dying from hypoxia and is carried out when oxygenation and protection of the airway is failing by conventional means.

If the patient is in the resuscitation room, with cervical collar, sandbags and tapes to immobilize the cervical spine, it is easier to carry out this procedure if these are removed and an assistant performs in-line cervical immobilization supporting the head (Figure 3.1.1).

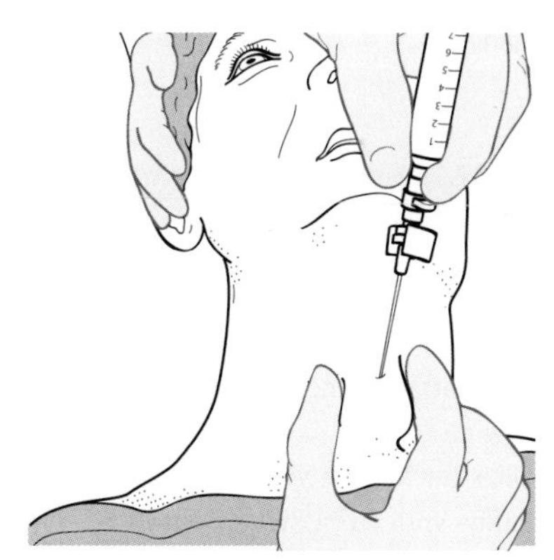

3.1.1 Needle cricothyroidotomy. Insertion of large-bore venflon at 45° caudally, in the midline, into the trachea. Inline immobilization of cervical spine by assistant.

Equipment needed

Alcohol wipe.
12–14G Venflon (+ spare).
10 mL syringe.
Connecting tube with Y-connector.
Oxygen source, 12–15 L/min.

The cricothyroid membrane is identified by finding the superior end of the thyroid cartilage (Adam's apple) and sliding down the thyroid cartilage in the midline. The finger drops in to the cricothyroid membrane. Confirmation that this is the cricothyroid membrane is made by carrying on down to the hard cricoid cartilage.

Unfortunately, if there is any risk of cervical spine injury the neck must not be extended.

Wipe the skin with an alcohol wipe; attach a 10 mL syringe, with 1 mL of air in it, to the large-bore (12–14G) venflon and pass it through the cricothyroid membrane, aiming 45° inferiorly (Figure 3.1.2). There is a 'give' as the needle goes through the membrane, which is quite superficial. Eject the air and skin-plug from the syringe and aspirate on the syringe. Getting air back shows the needle must be in the trachea. Slide the venflon in, sliding out the trocar – just like putting a venflon into a vein.

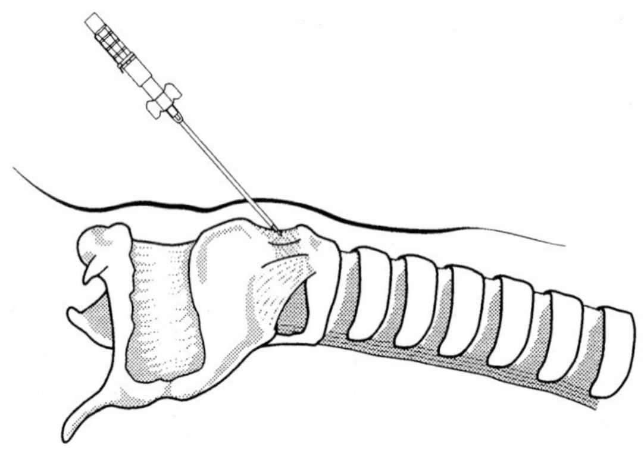

3.1.2 Jet insufflation of oxygen via a needle cricothyroidotomy.

Technique

1 In-line immobilization of head by assistant.
2 Universal precautions.
3 Identify cricothyroid membrane.
4 Alcohol wipe.
5 Immobilize trachea between finger and thumb.
6 12G venflon with 10 mL syringe with 1 mL of air in it.
7 Insert the needle in midline aiming 45° down the trachea.
8 Eject air (+plug of skin) from syringe and aspirate.
9 Remove trocar, connect to oxygen supply at 15 mL/min.
10 Y-connector (or hole in tube) 1 second on, 4 seconds off.
11 Monitor oxygen saturations.
12 Prepare for surgical cricothyroidotomy.

The connecting tube must have a Luer-type lock to attach to the venflon at one end, have a Y-connector (or just cut a hole in the tubing) in the middle and a connector at the other end to attach to the oxygen cylinder or wall oxygen supply. The oxygen should be running at 12–15 L per minute. Put a finger over the hole in the tubing in a ratio of 1 second on and 4 seconds off.

Jet insufflation via needle cricothyroidotomy can provide adequate oxygenation but unfortunately does not enable sufficient ventilation and there will therefore be a gradual rise in the pCO_2. It also does not protect the airway. Although theoretically a needle cricothyroidotomy with jet insufflation may give 30–40 minutes before the pCO_2 rises to a critical level, it should only be looked upon as a very temporary (life-saving) measure before conversion to a surgical cricothyroidotomy.

This may enable time for a more experienced surgeon to arrive, but the time should anyway be spent preparing the necessary equipment.

A needle cricothyroidotomy should only be considered as an immediate life-saving manoeuvre and should be converted into a formal surgical cricothyroidotomy as soon as possible.

In the case of a patient with severe maxillofacial trauma and a head (brain) injury, management must be aimed at:

1 preventing any rise in pCO_2 which would exacerbate the brain injury;
2 protecting the airway from the associated haemorrhage.

Surgical cricothyroidotomy

As soon as the oxygen saturations start to rise following the needle cricothyroidotomy, confirming that oxygen is reaching the lungs, equipment must be collected to convert this to a surgical cricothyroidotomy, with an inflated cuffed tube protecting the airway.

Local anaesthetic with vasoconstrictor (lidocaine 2 per cent with adrenaline 1:100 000) should be infiltrated around the area so that this can be working while the necessary equipment is gathered (Figure 3.1.3) and an experienced surgeon is called.

Equipment needed

1 Local anaesthetic – lidocaine 2 per cent + adrenaline 1.100 000.
2 Scalpel with No. 11 blade.
3 Tracheal dilator – or curved artery clip.
4 Suction with Yankaeurs-type sucker.
5 Size 6 or 6.5 cuffed tracheostomy tube + spare.
6 Syringe to inflate cuff.
7 Connector with Ambu-bag attached.
8 Oxygen supply.
9 Stethoscope to check air-entry to lungs.
10 Spare 12G venflon + 10 mL syringe.

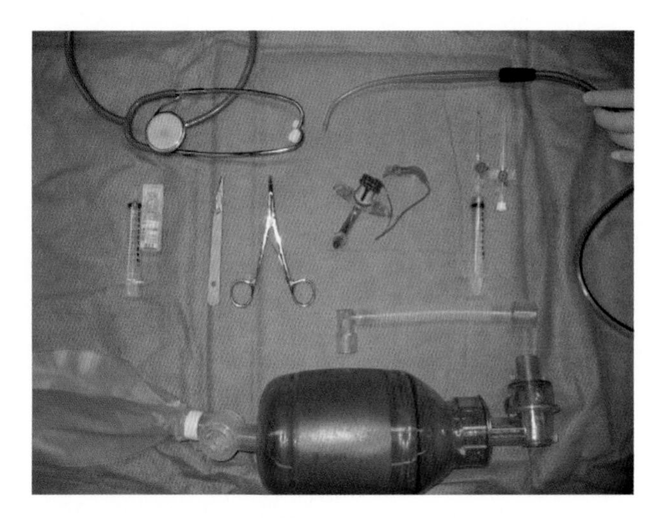

3.1.3 Equipment needed for surgical cricothyroidotomy.

Surgical cricothyroidotomy is a more controlled procedure and the skin should be properly prepared with antiseptic and local anaesthetic with vasoconstrictor given to make the procedure easier. It also protects against the risk that the patients conscious level may rise as a result of the improved oxygenation and the pain associated with a procedure not carried out with local anaesthetic. An experienced surgeon may elect to go straight to surgical cricothyroidotomy, bypassing the needle and jet insufflation. It is important to familiarize yourself with the equipment and to check the cuff on the tube before proceeding.

If a needle cricothyroidotomy has been performed, once the area has been cleaned with antiseptic, local anaesthetic given and the necessary equipment is to hand, then conversion to surgical cricothyroidotomy should be made. Ideally, this should be within 5–10 minutes of the needle cricothyroidotomy.

Remove the venflon – it is in the way, making the procedure more difficult and runs the risk of cutting the venflon with the scalpel if it is left *in situ*. Hold the skin under tension and make a 3 cm horizontal incision so that the skin edges part, revealing the membrane. Stab vertically down with the blade through the membrane and draw the blade towards you, making a hole ~1 cm long. Do not twist the blade in your hand or turn the scalpel round in your hand to use the handle to open up the membrane. These risk either snapping the blade (the thyroid and cricoid cartilages can become calcified) or sustaining a sharps injury.

Put the scalpel down, pick up the tracheal dilator and insert it into the cut membrane horizontally (so that it engages against the inferior surface of the thyroid cartilage and the superior surface of the cricoid) and open it so that the cut edges of the membrane are separated, exposing the trachea.

Technique

1. In-line immobilization of head by assistant.
2. Universal precautions.
3. Prepare the skin with antiseptic and local anaesthetic + vasoconstrictor.
4. Tense the skin with finger and thumb.
5. Remove the cricothyroidotomy venflon.
6. 3 cm horizontal incision through the skin so that skin edges part.
7. Stab vertically down through membrane and make 1 cm incision.
8. Insert tracheal dilator (or curved haemostat) horizontally and open it so that it separates the thyroid and cricoid cartilages.
9. Keep dilator in place. Insert Yankaeurs sucker to clear trachea.
10. Insert tracheostomy tube, remove introducer, inflate cuff.
11. Connect to Ambu-bag and oxygen supply.
12. Assess oxygen saturation, end-tidal CO_2 and air-entry to lungs.
13. Fix tracheostomy tube with tapes or sutures.

Suction out the trachea with the Yankaeurs sucker and assess the trachea. Insert the tracheostomy tube into the trachea. After removing the central introducer, inflating the cuff and connecting to an Ambu-bag and oxygen supply, assess air entry to both sides of the chest and start to monitor oxygen saturations and end-tidal CO_2.

Potential complications

1. Failure to insert tracheostomy tube into trachea.
2. Haemorrhage.
3. Damage to trachea, oesophagus and neighbouring structures.
4. Aspiration of blood and asphyxia.
5. Damage to vocal cords.
6. Creation of false passage.
7. Surgical emphysema.

If all is well, then secure the tracheostomy tube with either the tapes provided or sutures. If insertion fails then either open up the trachea again with the dilator, apply oxygen, suction and reassess or even go back to reinserting a venflon and further jet insufflation.

OTHER SURGICAL AIRWAYS

1. Percutaneous tracheostomy
2. Surgical tracheostomy.

As the trachea passes caudally below the cricoid cartilage, it becomes progressively posterior (deeper) and access to the trachea becomes more difficult and hazardous both because of poorer visibility and also the rich vasculature of the area and the thyroid gland.

Neither of these techniques should therefore be considered as an emergency procedure. Ideally, they are performed on an already endotracheally anaesthetized patient, as an elective operation. This may be as a prelude to major head and neck cancer surgery or before definitive treatment of severe maxillofacial trauma, enabling the airway to bypass the planned operative field. Alternatively, they may be required for a patient on long-term ventilation to enable bronchial toilet. Both techniques provide a definitive airway – a cuffed tube in the trachea.

Occasionally, an awake tracheostomy must be carried out under local anaesthetic on a patient maintaining his own airway (but in danger of losing it) where oro- or naso-tracheal intubation cannot be performed. Severe fascial-space infections, such as Ludwig's angina, with tense swelling of the tissues of the neck and around the upper airway, often with associated trismus, make either endotracheal intubation or awake tracheostomy a difficult and hazardous procedure. Frequently, an experienced anaesthetist may be able to perform an awake nasotracheal intubation with an intubating fibreoptic bronchoscope, thereby avoiding the need for the tracheostomy. However, it is wise to have the potential incision marked out and the local anaesthetic already injected in case the attempted intubation fails.

Percutaneous tracheostomy

Percutaneous tracheostomy is an elective procedure that enables a definitive airway to be placed using an essentially blind (closed) technique. It is not suitable for children as the airway is small and the trachea is mobile and soft, making the procedure technically much more difficult. It is therefore a procedure that can be carried out, on adults, in the intensive care unit, particularly for an already orotracheally intubated patient requiring a tracheostomy for longer term airway support.

This is a sterile 'surgical' procedure and the field should be properly cleaned and draped. The tracheal rings should be palpated below the cricoid cartilage and local anaesthetic with vasoconstrictor injected both subcutaneously and also more deeply down to the trachea. Assuming there is no risk of cervical spine injury, the neck can be fully extended, facilitating the procedure.

The operation is based on the Seldinger technique, whereby a guidewire is slid down through a large-bore venflon inserted into the trachea, usually between tracheal rings two and three. As soon as the guidewire is in the trachea, its position can be checked by viewing down the orotracheal tube with an intubating bronchoscope. The guidewire is left *in situ* while the venflon is removed and then progressively larger dilators are introduced over the guidewire. When the tract is adequately dilated, the tracheostomy tube can be slid into place. Usually it is sensible to let the orotracheal cuff down (to reduce the risk of puncture by the venflon or guidewire) at the beginning of the procedure and to withdraw the tube slightly to facilitate insertion of the dilators and tracheostomy tube. The orotracheal tube must still remain through the vocal cords until satisfactory position and function of the tracheostomy tube is confirmed. Percutaneous tracheostomy is a time-consuming procedure that should be carried out when the airway is already protected with a definitive tube in place.

Surgical tracheostomy

Surgical tracheostomy is an elective 'open' technique which again is ideally performed on an already intubated patient. Before fibreoptic intubation and the wider acceptance of surgical cricothyroidotomy, emergency tracheostomy was more frequently attempted. Under such circumstances, it is an extremely hazardous procedure and was associated with significant mortality due to distorted anatomy, poor access and visibility and associated haemorrhage.

Indications

1. Elective procedure for airway to bypass planned operative field.
2. Long-term respiratory support.
3. Protection of airway from obstruction by tumour.
4. Congenital anomalies, e.g. subglottic stenosis.
5. Retention of secretions.

If the patient is anaesthetized and assuming there is no risk of cervical spine injury, the neck should be fully extended. If tracheostomy under local anaesthetic is being performed, the patient may well not tolerate lying back and a compromise position may be needed with the patient partially sitting up.

Whether under general or local anaesthetic, local anaesthetic should be liberally injected throughout the whole operative field, both into the skin and also down through the deeper tissues to the trachea. A 5 cm transverse incision should be made halfway between the cricoid cartilage and the suprasternal notch (Figure 3.1.4). Subcutaneous fat and platysma are divided and retracted and fastidious haemostasis must be maintained throughout the procedure. Blunt scissor-dissection absolutely in the midline will show the strap muscles on either side which should be retracted. Keep palpating the tracheal rings through the incision to ensure that dissection continues in the midline.

The thyroid isthmus will be seen. Although it may be possible to retract this, it is safer to divide it (Figure 3.1.5). The pretracheal fascia should be divided at the superior end and the thyroid isthmus gradually lifted off the trachea from above downwards before clamping, dividing and tying the ends off and retracting them to the sides (Figure 3.1.6). There is still some pretracheal fascia that must be carefully dissected to come down on to the tracheal rings. Identify the second and third rings.

The anaesthetist should be warned that the trachea is about to be incised, so that the endotracheal tube cuff can be let down and the tube retracted a couple of centimetres to avoid risk of cutting into the cuff. The tube must remain between the vocal cords until safe and satisfactory placement of the tracheostomy tube has been confirmed by checking the end-tidal CO_2 and O_2 saturation.

Using a No. 11 scalpel incise transversely through the membrane between the second and third tracheal rings. Cut down through the third ring and excise a window about 1 cm in diameter (Figure 3.1.7). In children, a vertical incision in the midline through the third and fourth tracheal rings should be made. Stay sutures should be inserted either side of the incision and retracted, opening up the incision into the trachea (Figure 3.1.8). Having sized (the same as the orotracheal tube *in situ*) and checked the tracheostomy tube cuff, insert it into the trachea, inflate the cuff, connect up to the anaesthetic tubing and assess the end-tidal CO_2. If all is satisfactory, then the skin incision can be closed around the tracheotomy tube and the tube secured either with the tapes provided or by suturing the flanges with heavy duty sutures. Once airway entry has been identified in both lung fields, the orotracheal tube can now be removed.

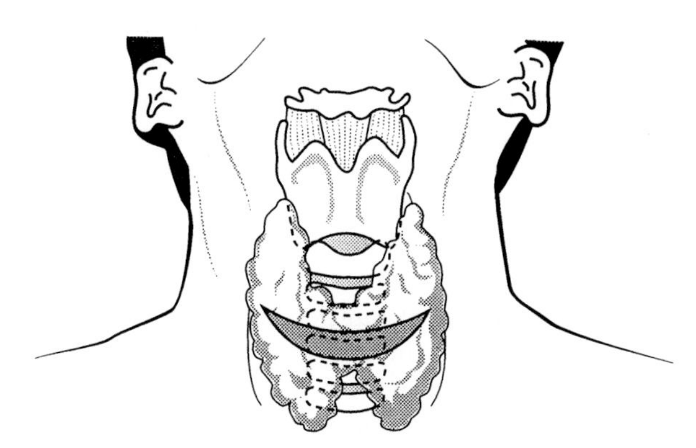

3.1.4 Skin incision for elective tracheostomy.

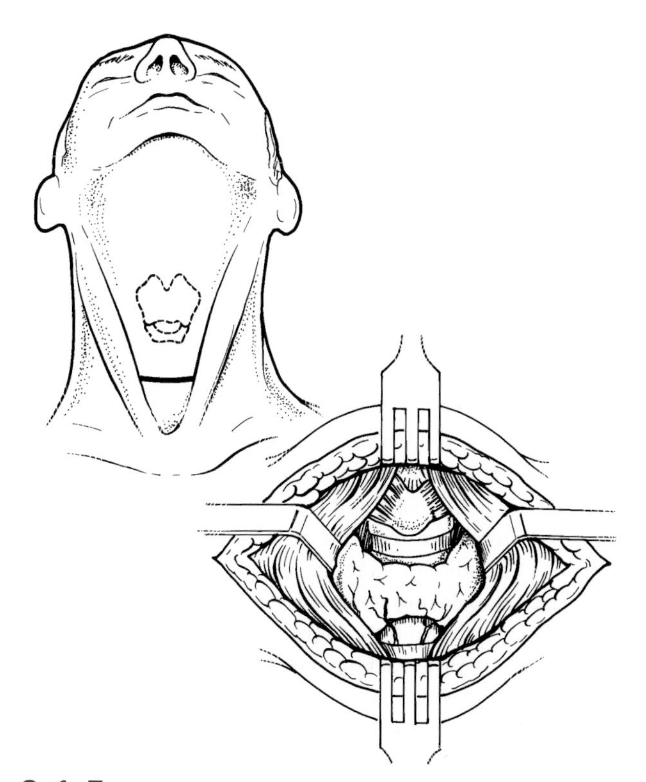

3.1.5 Tracheostomy dissection showing the thyroid isthmus overlying the trachea.

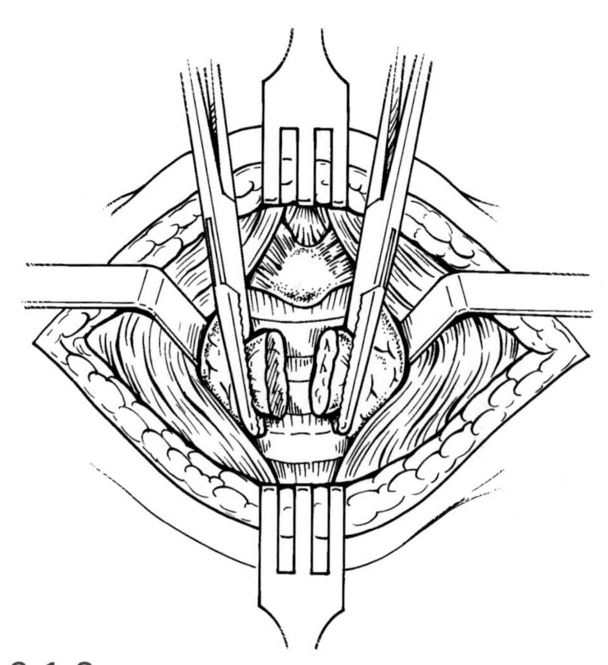

3.1.6 The thyroid isthmus is clamped and divided.

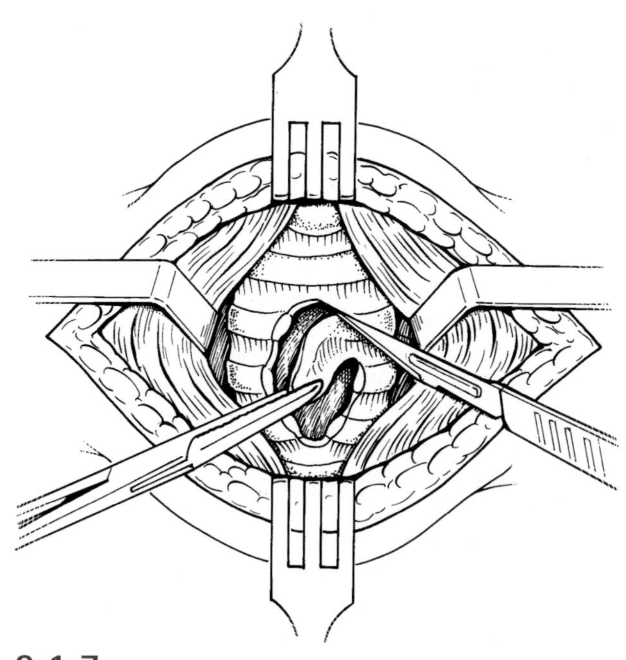

3.1.7 A circular window is created using a scalpel with a No. 11 blade.

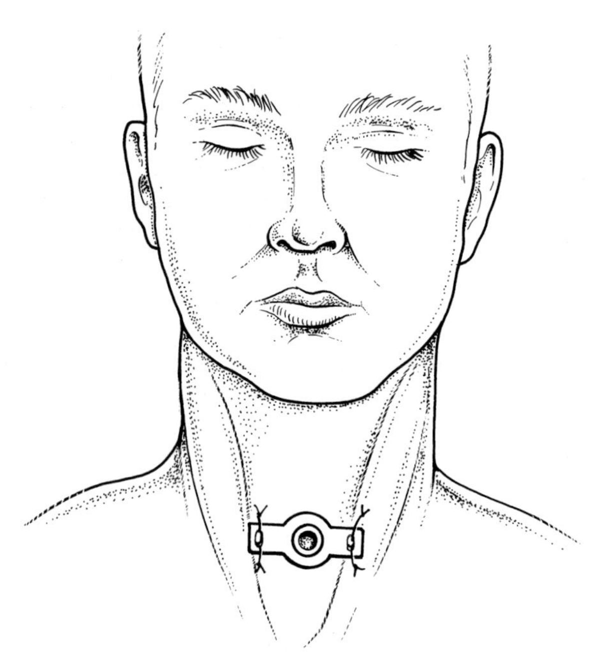

3.1.8 The tracheostomy tube flanges are sutured to the skin.

Technique

1. Neck fully extended, patient anaesthetized and intubated.
2. Universal precautions and site prepared and draped.
3. Local anaesthetic with vasoconstrictor both to skin and deeper tissues.
4. 5 cm slightly curved (smiling) incision in skin crease, halfway between cricoid cartilage and suprasternal notch.
5. Careful haemostasis with bipolar diathermy throughout.
6. Dissection down through fat and platysma in midline, exposing the strap muscles of the neck.
7. Blunt scissor-dissection in midline separating strap muscles and retracting them laterally.
8. Thyroid isthmus should be identified, clamped, divided and tied off.
9. Continue careful dissection down to tracheal rings – identify second to third tracheal rings.
10. Inform anaesthetist to let down cuff and slightly withdraw tube.
11. Check tracheostomy tube size (same as orotracheal tube being used) and cuff.
12. Cut with No. 11 scalpel blade horizontally through membrane between rings two and three; continue this to excise a window, including the anterior surface of the third tracheal ring.
13. Suck out trachea, insert tracheostomy tube.
14. Inflate cuff, connect to anaesthetic tube, check end-tidal pCO_2 and oxygen saturations.
15. Close skin incision around tube with 3o sutures.
16. Secure tracheotomy tube with tapes or 1o sutures.

It is important to ensure adequate humidification of the air or oxygen to prevent crusting within the lumen and potential obstruction. If the tracheostomy is being performed for longer term use, then a double lumen tube can be inserted. This enables the inner tube to be removed and cleaned without affecting the position of the tube itself.

UNCONTROLLED MAXILLOFACIAL HAEMORRHAGE

It is important to be familiar with measures which can be employed to arrest maxillofacial haemorrhage.

Intraoral haemorrhage following exodontia usually can be addressed with the use of local anaesthesia with vasoconstrictor, packing and suture. Elsewhere in the maxillofacial region, haemorrhage needs to be dealt with promptly and effectively as large volume blood loss can occur quickly if not adequately controlled. As always, airway and breathing must be addressed first and a secure definitive airway placed and supplemental oxygen supplied before addressing the circulation. While the patient continues to haemorrhage, fluid resuscitation alone will be unsuccessful; blood loss must also be controlled.

Haemorrhage may be arrested by direct pressure on a wound when a bony structure lies deep to the laceration, as in the scalp. In the face, lip, peri-orbital area and neck, such compression seldom controls blood loss and in these circumstances, clamping and ligation of transacted vessels will be required. Where the soft tissues are extensively disrupted as in high energy injuries such as gunshot wounds, haemorrhage control may only be achievable with ligation of the external carotid (see below).

Where severe mid-facial bony trauma has occurred (with Le Fort II or III fractures) and torrential nasal haemorrhage has resulted, and where anterior and posterior nasal packs have been unsuccessful, forward manipulation of the maxillary segment may stop maxillary artery haemorrhage. If this fails, external carotid artery ligation is indicated.

Insertion of Foley catheter to nasal cavity

SEVERE NASAL HAEMORRHAGE

This commonly follows maxillofacial trauma, but may also occur in uncontrolled hypertension or indeed spontaneously. When there is no history of trauma, sitting the patient up and applying pressure to the area may result in sufficient control to be able to examine the nose and, if necessary, cauterize the bleeding point using local anaestheic, bipolar diathermy or silver nitrate sticks.

An anterior nasal packing with ribbon gauze soaked in a fluid such as Sofradex® should control anterior bleeds. Expansile cellulose devices such as Merocel® are a simple method of haemorrhage control.

Post nasal packing will be required if bleeding is from the post nasal space or if severe trauma has resulted in severe bleeding requiring both anterior and post nasal packing. Either Epistats (a preformed device with inflatable balloons for both posterior and anterior packing) can be used or, alternatively, Foley catheters are introduced into both nasal cavities and advanced along the nasal floor until they reach the soft palate (Figure 3.1.9). The balloons are inflated with sterile saline and then gentle traction is applied to both catheters until the balloons lodge at the posterior nasal choanae. The catheters can be held in position by tying them together around the anterior nasal spine. The catheters are deflated at 24 hours and, if no epistaxis ensues, can be removed.

In patients with Le Fort II or Le Fort III fractures and disruption of the cribriform plate, care must be taken to ensure that the Foley catheters and packing are not aimed cranially, with risk of forcing them into the cranial cavity.

Nasal packing is only effective by tamponading the bleeding vessels against a solid base provided by the rigid floor of nose. Occasionally, with severe midface trauma and Le Fort I level fracture, such packing just acts to displace the maxillary fracture rather than compressing the bleeding vessels. Placing bilateral mouth props to support the maxilla against an intact mandible may help. In the additional presence of displaced or comminuted mandibular fractures, then cranial (barrel) bandaging may help until such time as definitive intervention can be provided.

Rarely, severe nasal haemorrhage is not controlled by the above approach. Ethmoidal artery ligation can be considered and is usually achieved endoscopically. Where these skills are not available, the anterior ethmoid artery can be ligated via a medial orbital approach (Figure 3.1.10).

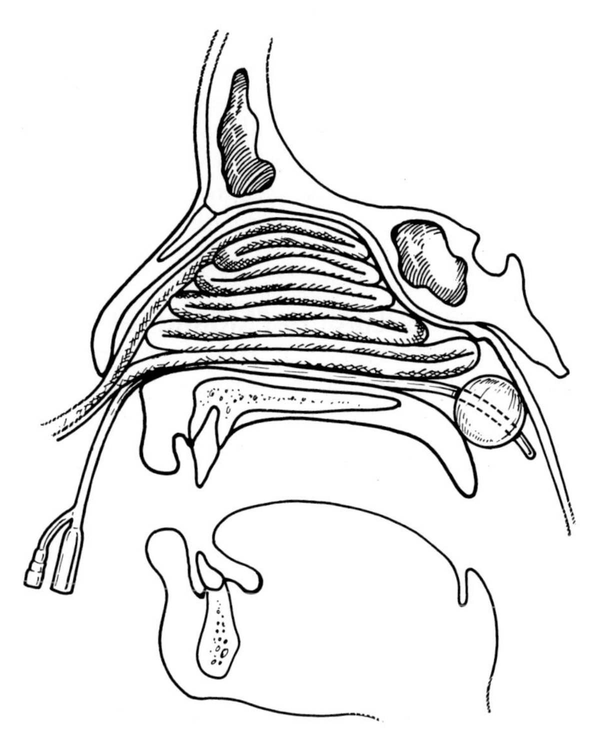

3.1.9 Nasal packing showing Foley catheter in postnasal space and anterior nasal packing with ribbon gauze.

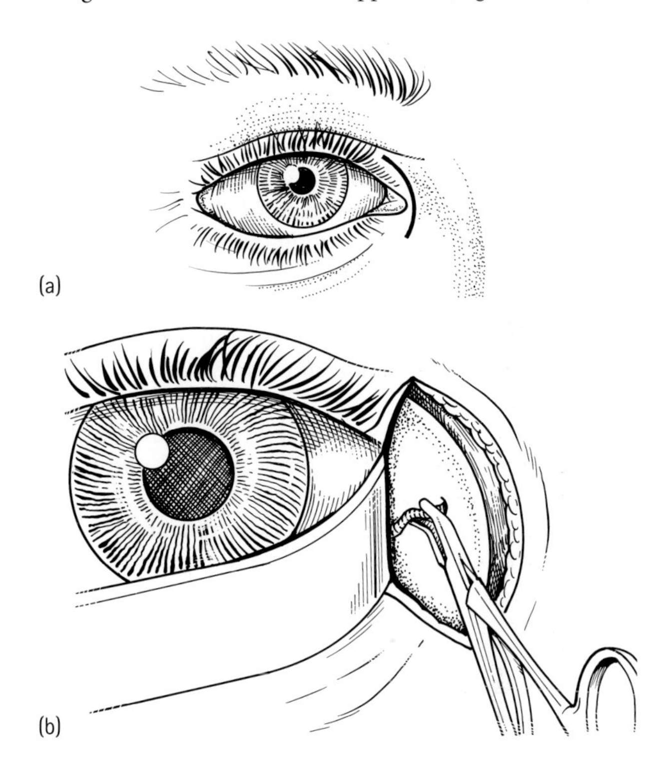

3.1.10 (a) Inner canthal incision; (b) the anterior ethmoidal artery is clamped with a ligaclip.

Post nasal packing

1 Push Foley catheter with 20 mL balloon along floor of nose until it is visible behind the soft palate; repeat for the second side.
2 Inflate the balloons.
3 Pull the catheters forward until the inflated balloons occlude the postnasal choanae.

Anterior nasal packing

Pack the nasal floor and cavity with 5 cm ribbon gauze, soaked with Sofradex® or BIPP (bismuth iodoform paraform paste).

Technique for ligation of the anterior ethmoidal artery

1 General anaesthesia.
2 Also give local anaesthetic and vasoconstrictor.
3 2.5 cm curved incision at inner canthus – see Figure 3.1.10.
4 Deepen down to bone.
5 Elevate periosteum, aiming posteriorly subperiosteally.
6 Anterior ethmoidal artery is identified at its foramen, 2.5 cm from the orbital rim and just above the medial canthal ligament.
7 Ligate either with ligaclips or bipolar diathermy.

EXTERNAL CAROTID ARTERY LIGATION

This procedure is indicated where torrential haemorrhage in the area supplied by that artery has not been controlled by other means. This may arise as a result of maxillofacial trauma but is very occasionally warranted during ablative oncological surgery of the tongue or maxilla. In general terms, if significant haemorrhage is anticipated during an oncological procedure, a neck dissection, if appropriate, with vessel exposure should be performed prior to the ablation. Very rarely, it is required during orthognathic procedures.

The patient is prepared, anaesthetized and positioned with the neck extended and rotated to the contralateral side. Where the neck has already been accessed for another procedure, such as a neck dissection, this approach is used. In non-oncology cases, rapid access is best achieved with a 5 cm incision along the anterior border of sternomastoid. Dissection through the subcutaneous fat and platysma exposes the muscle. The deep cervical fascia investing sternomastoid is divided, the muscle retracted posteriorly and the internal jugular vein is exposed. The jugular vein is mobilized by dissecting the carotid sheath and freeing the vein superiorly and inferiorly. The common carotid artery will be seen medially (see Figure 3.1.11). At this point the anaesthetist should be warned as manipulation of the carotid bulb at the bifurcation may cause cardiac dysrhythmias.

The artery is followed superiorly to the bifurcation and the (anterior, multiple branching) external carotid is identified. The hypoglossal nerve is an adjacent structure and should not be damaged. Prior to ligation of the vessel, the external carotid should be clamped with a non-crushing vascular clamp to confirm that haemorrhage can be controlled by this procedure. Very occasionally, especially in midface trauma, exposure of the contralateral external carotid may be required to achieve haemorrhage control. In very difficult situations, the assistance of an interventional radiologist may be required to identify the disrupted vessel or consider translumenal methods of haemorrhage control.

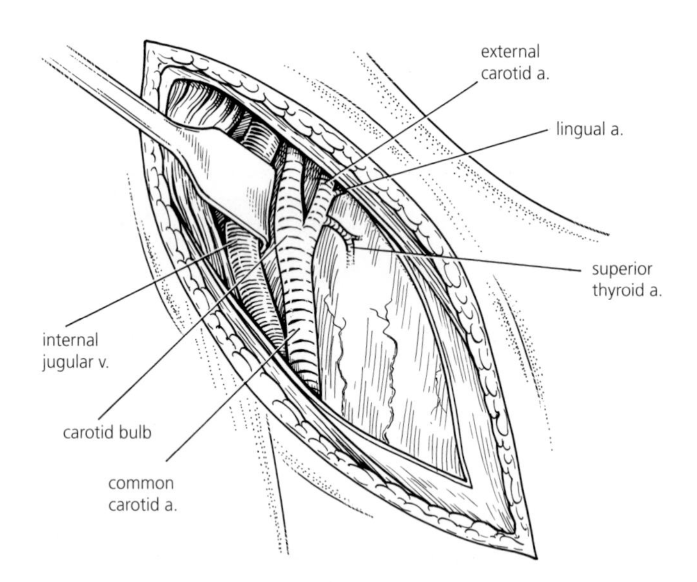

3.1.11 The carotid sheath is opened to expose the internal jugular vein and carotid artery.

Technique

1. G.A., patient's head up, neck extended and rotated contralaterally.
2. 5 cm incision along anterior border of sternomastoid.
3. Dissect down through fat, platysma and deep cervical fascia.
4. Retract sternomastoid posteriorly.
5. Open up carotid sheath exposing internal jugular vein.
6. Free up vein inferiorly and superiorly, exposing common carotid artery deep to the vein.
7. Follow artery superiorly to bifurcation.
8. Clamp external (more anterior + with branches) carotid.

ACUTE RETROBULBAR HAEMORRHAGE

This condition is one of the few true emergencies in maxillofacial surgery. The presence of orbital pain, reducing visual acuity, proptosis and ophthalmoplegia in the acute presentation of midface trauma or following surgical management should be assumed to be a retrobulbar haemorrhage. Fundoscopy to note a pale optic disc is the only investigation required – computed tomography (CT) imaging wastes time and rarely assists the diagnosis.

Symptoms and signs

Acuity – reducing.
Pain – increasing.
Proptosis.
Paralysis of ocular muscles – ophthalmoplegia.
Pupils – dilating.
Pale optic disc.

Management

On diagnosis, several simple preliminary steps are of value in preserving or restoring vision.

1 Basic steps:
- sit the patient up if their condition permits;
- remove all dressings around the eye;

- remove the skin and deep sutures immediately if periorbital lacerations (or surgical incisions) have been sutured. This may allow decompression of the orbit;
- site two venous cannulae.

2 Medical management which includes:
- 1 g of methylprednisolone i.v. stat;
- 200 mL of 20 per cent mannitol infused over 15–20 minutes;
- Acetazolamide 500 mg i.v. if available.

3 Perform a lateral canthotomy:
- Two mL of 2 per cent lignocaine and adrenaline are injected into the lateral canthal region. Sharp dissecting scissors are used to divide the lateral canthus through the lateral fornix down to periosteum – this will release some pressure and will buy time before formal intra-conal decompression.

Following this intervention, book theatres and an anaesthetist, explaining the urgency of sight preserving surgery. Surgical decompression is almost always required and should never be delayed. However, some clinicians advocate megadose steroid therapy alone, with surgical intervention only if no clinical improvement is seen within 30 minutes. The surgical aim is to decompress the intraconal space and a surgeon who performs this procedure for the first time should not expect to encounter a copious bleed.

Surgical decompression

There are several approaches which are possible:

1 through an existing laceration or surgical incision;
2 via a lateral eyebrow incision (Figure 3.1.12);
3 via an infra-orbital approach.

It is important to avoid an incision in eyelid skin, such as a blepharoplasty approach, since this technique also confers a risk of a retrobulbar bleed.

The peri-orbita is incised and the intraconal space entered by blunt dissection between the lateral and inferior rectus muscles (Figure 3.1.13). Any surgical implants should be removed.

A small drain (or the finger of a surgical glove) is sutured in place and left for at least 24 hours.

No attempt should be made to treat any bony injuries at this stage. A retrobulbar haemorrhage is commonly associated with comminution of the orbital floor and therefore required detailed CT evaluation. Additionally, there is an increased risk of a further bleed when definitive treatment is undertaken. Surgical treatment would therefore be contraindicated where the contralateral eye is visually impaired because of pre-existing pathology.

Following medical and surgical management, close eye observations are mandatory. Any increasing pain or visual deterioration may indicate re-exploration. Further doses (250 mg) of methylprednisolone are warranted at 8-hourly intervals for 24 hours, but the blood glucose should be monitored, especially in diabetics.

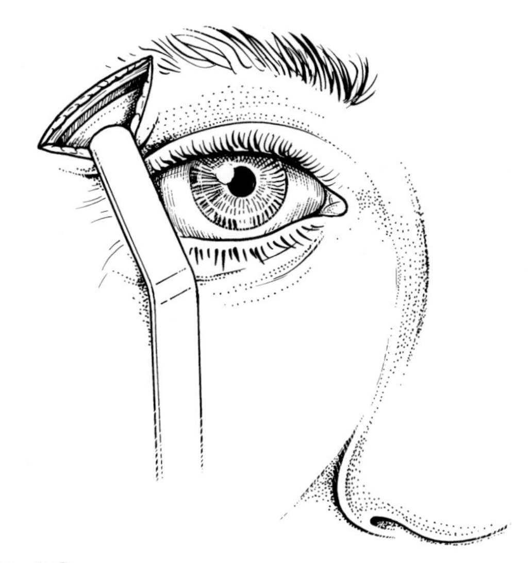

3.1.12 A lateral brow incision is performed and the peri-orbita incised.

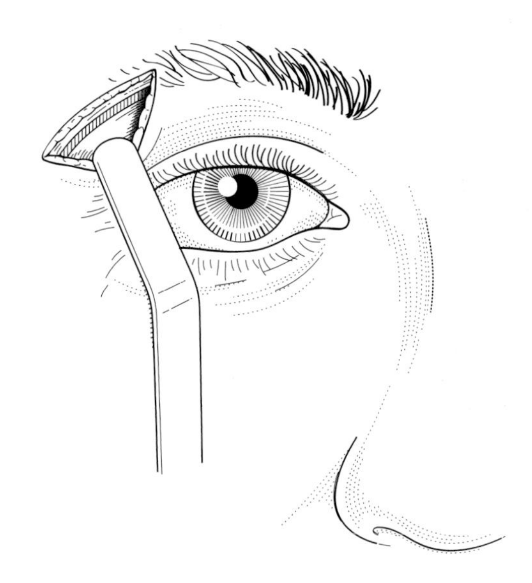

3.1.13 The intraconal space is opened by blunt dissection.

Top tips

- Airway and haemorrhage are two of the most significant emergencies to be dealt with in maxillofacial surgery.
- Surgical tracheostomy is always an elective procedure once initial airway control has been achieved.
- The technique of needle cricothyroidotomy is a life-saving procedure with which all trainees need to be conversant.
- Arrest of haemorrhage is critical – i.v. resuscitation alone cannot be effective with an open circulation.
- Retrobulbar haemorrhage is a medical and surgical emergency. Always consider this diagnosis as it can be missed or recognized too late to save vision.

3.2

Reconstructive surgery – orofacial flaps and skin grafting

JOHN LB CARTER

Z PLASTY FOR FRAENECTOMY

Principles and justification

Fraenectomy may be indicated for release of tight bands in the upper or lower labial vestibules, beneath the tongue tip or in the buccal sulci. Simple division across the bands results in loss of tissue and sulcus depth and may result in delayed healing with prolonged discomfort and scarring.

Anaesthesia

Local anaesthetic is infiltrated beneath the whole length of the fraenular band and encouraged to spread in the tissue planes by gentle massage.

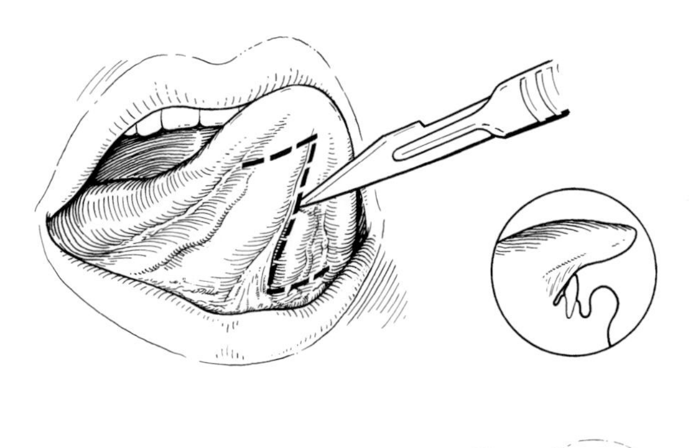

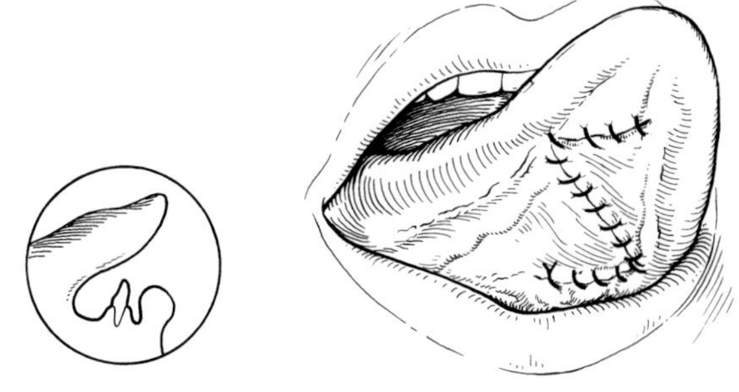

3.2.1 Z-plasty for release of lingual fraenum.

Incision

The length of the fraenum is incised with a scalpel and at each end limbs are incised, at between 60 and 90°, of equal length to the length of the band. Using fine-toothed forceps with care not to damage the apices of the flaps, dissect the submucosal tissues beyond the base of each flap, into loose non-attached tissue planes.

Flap repositioning

The flaps thus created are mobilized and transposed through 90°. If accurate repositioning is not possible without tension, further release by undermining the bases of the flaps may be indicated. Simple sutures using 3/0 resorbable suture on a 5/8 circle cutting needle are placed, first through the apices of the flaps to ascertain the adequacy of flap repositioning then evenly spaced along the edges of the flaps to close the wounds. Gentle pressure over the repair for a few minutes will aid haemostasis.

Outcome

No tissue need be lost when this technique is used. The gain in length along the centre limb of the 'Z', which increases in proportion to the increase in angulation of the limb incisions, should be 75–100 per cent with consequent benefit to sulcus depth and reduction in tension at the ends of the fraenum.

ADVANCEMENT AND ROTATIONAL FLAPS

Principles and justification

Wherever small amounts of tissue, sufficient to preclude primary closure without tension, are excised or lost, local flaps may be mobilized and either advanced into the defect or rotated around a pivot point into the defect to be closed. In random pattern flaps (submucous plexus vasculature), the pivot point can vary around the arc of the flap. In axial flaps (substantial submucous vessels), the pivot point must be contiguous with the base of the vascular pedicle; this limits their application, though the latter are capable of survival to a 50 per cent greater length.

The base of such flaps may fold under the tension of the pull of the flap and this occasionally warrants a small relieving backcut to relieve excessive tension, although this carries the risk of reducing the blood supply to the flap and should be avoided with careful flap planning or by the use of excision of a Burow's triangle to minimize the problem.

Advancement flaps

Good examples of the use of advancement flaps in the mouth are seen in the closure of bone defects resulting from the removal of erupted wisdom teeth, for the closure of oroantral fistulae and for resurfacing the vermillion surface of the lip.

INCISION

Commencing at the margins of the defect, two diverging incisions are made, spaced as wide apart as the anticipated length of the pedicle. For coverage of a bone defect, the incision passes down onto bone through the attached mucosa and laterally, submucosally, into the buccal tissues. Incision of a clean cut edge around the defect defines the margin to be repaired and must extend beyond the rim of the bony defect.

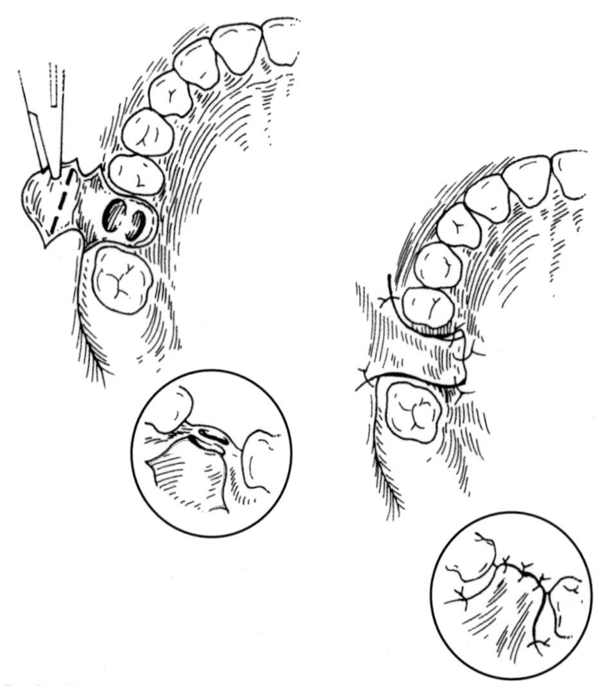

3.2.2 Division of submucosal periosteum underneath the pedicle to facilitate flap advancement.

FLAP DESIGN

Periosteal elevation of the flap allows its elevation and the reflected flap is carefully incised parallel to the base, through periosteum only, with a fine scalpel blade. This releases the elasticity inherent in the mucous membrane and, together with the laxity of the buccal mucosa at the base of the flap, allows its advancement into the defect. When an oroantral fistula has been long-standing or it is likely that maxillary sinus is contaminated, the success of this procedure will be enhanced by the use of 4/0 monofilament non-resorbable sutures for flap closure.

POST-OPERATIVE CARE

In this situation, where bone has been exposed, the use of prophylactic antibiotics is recommended. Consideration should be given to performing an intranasal antrostomy, to allow sinus irrigation for 24–48 hours post-operatively, for antral toilet.

Rotation flaps

PRINCIPLES

Rotational flaps have applications despite the relatively restricted surface areas of the mouth and are primarily used in closing palatal defects. It is often impossible to achieve complete defect coverage from the tissue available. Fortunately, the excellent regenerative capability of oral tissues ensures that good healing at the donor site will occur without the need for grafting if the donor area is covered by a simple splint or dressing and protected from direct trauma. Variants of pivotal movements of flap pedicles include simple single lobe and bilobed flaps, transposition flaps of the Limberg (rhomboid) type and island interpolation flaps.

INCISION

Design of the incision of a rotation flap is greatly influenced by the necessity for the end of the flap adjacent to the defect to extend beyond the defect so that the shortening effect along the radius of the arc of rotation accommodates the required length at the tip of the flap. This will accommodate adequate repair without undue tension.

Bilobed flaps are effective by displacing the tension secondarily away from the primary donor site towards areas of greater tissue laxity. Island flaps and rhomboid flaps similarly rely on the facility of more distant tissue laxity to provide importable donor material.

OPERATION

Careful planning, as outlined above, is the secret of success in rotating flaps. The surgical techniques differ little from Z-plasty or advancement.

The primary flap of tissue to be transposed demands a clean incision to create right-angled cuts and the thickness of the flap should closely match the thickness of the mucosal margin of the defect. Tip necrosis is less likely if the tip of the flap is rounded. If a bone defect is to be covered then

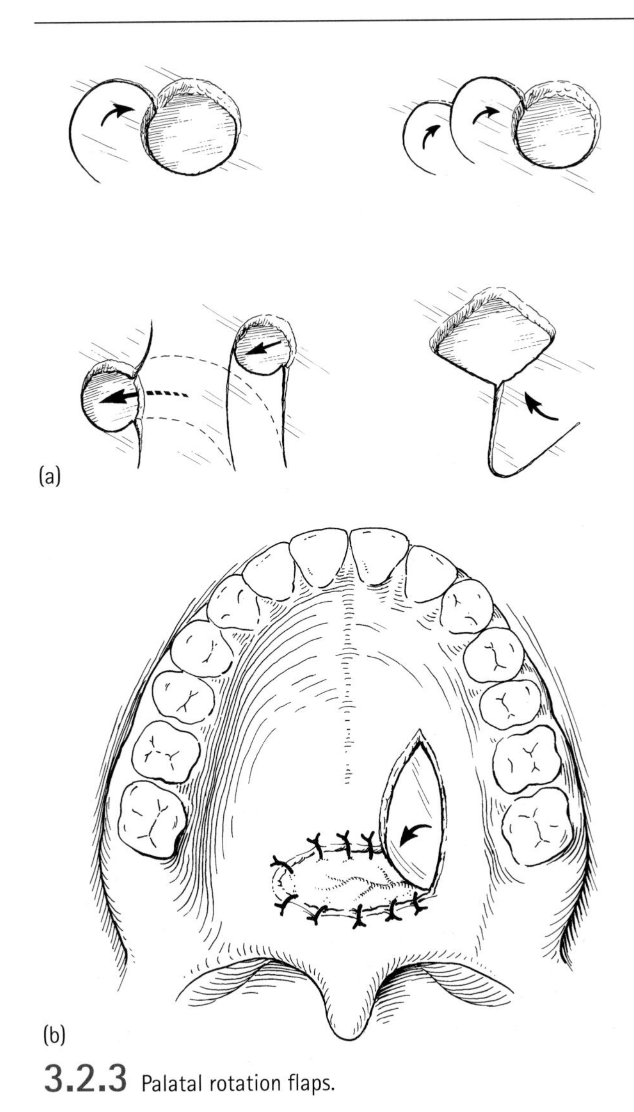

3.2.3 Palatal rotation flaps.

periosteum should be included with the flap, but if this is not required, a supraperiosteal dissection will retain cover over the donor defect and accelerate healing. The presence of an identifiable functioning axial vascular pedicle, such as the greater palatine vessels, within a flap, increases the likelihood of its success and the length to base-width ratio which can be successfully transposed. The avoidance of undue pressure from overlay splints is essential and relief of acrylic over the flap must be ensured. Meticulous attention must be paid to haemostasis to avoid the accumulation of haematoma on the flap bed.

TEMPORALIS FLAP

Principles and justification

The use of the majority of large pedicled flaps for orofacial reconstructions is reliant on the principle of transposition of tissue with a functioning axial blood supply. The four main arteries concerned in reconstruction in this area are the facial, transverse facial, superficial and deep temporal arteries. The position and relative size of the vessels show significant variation between individuals and between sides in the same individual. Tortuosity of these arteries increases with advancing age and may contribute to increased liability to atherosclerosis.

The temporalis muscle takes its blood supply from the anterior and posterior branches of the deep temporal artery, supplemented by the middle temporal branch of the superficial temporal artery.

Two of the five motor branches of the facial nerve, its temporal branches to the frontalis muscle and zygomatic branches, which mainly supply orbicularis oculi, traverse the undersurface of the temporoparietal fascia running across the zygomatic arch and are surgically significant. Sensation to the hair-bearing area of skin over the temple and lower third of the auricle is supplied via the auriculotemporal nerve which passes over the posterior root of the zygoma, behind the superficial temporal vessels on the surface of the temporoparietal fascia.

Uses

This flap has extensive application in the orofacial region. Within the mouth, it is useful for repairing defects on the oropharynx, the hard and soft palate and buccal mucosa, and its use has been reported for repairs to the floor of mouth and tongue. Together with calvarial bone it has been used for mandibular reconstruction. On the face, malar reconstruction and the repair of orbital defects are described and other uses include the obliteration of mastoid cavities, facial reanimation, eyelid reconstruction and skull base surgery. A purely fascial variant may be raised when only a thin vascularized covering is required.

Operation

INCISION

Infiltration along the proposed incision line with 10–20 mL adrenaline solution (1:5000) is carried out 5 min prior to incision to enhance haemostasis.

The skin incision commences, subcutaneously only, at the upper junction of the auricle with the face (Figure 3.2.4b). A gentle arc defines the outer limit of the temporoparietal fascia and should remain within the hair-bearing area. It is customary to shave the operative area completely, however; this defines the incision area as a fine, shaved line and reduces post-operative embarrassment and does not seem to increase the risk of wound infection.

If care is taken, the posterior branch of the superficial temporal artery can be identified and exposed to permit its preservation, if this is anatomically compatible with the desired flap extent. More commonly, the vessel runs obliquely posterosuperiorly and will need to be ligated and divided. Good haemostasis at the skin wound edges can be

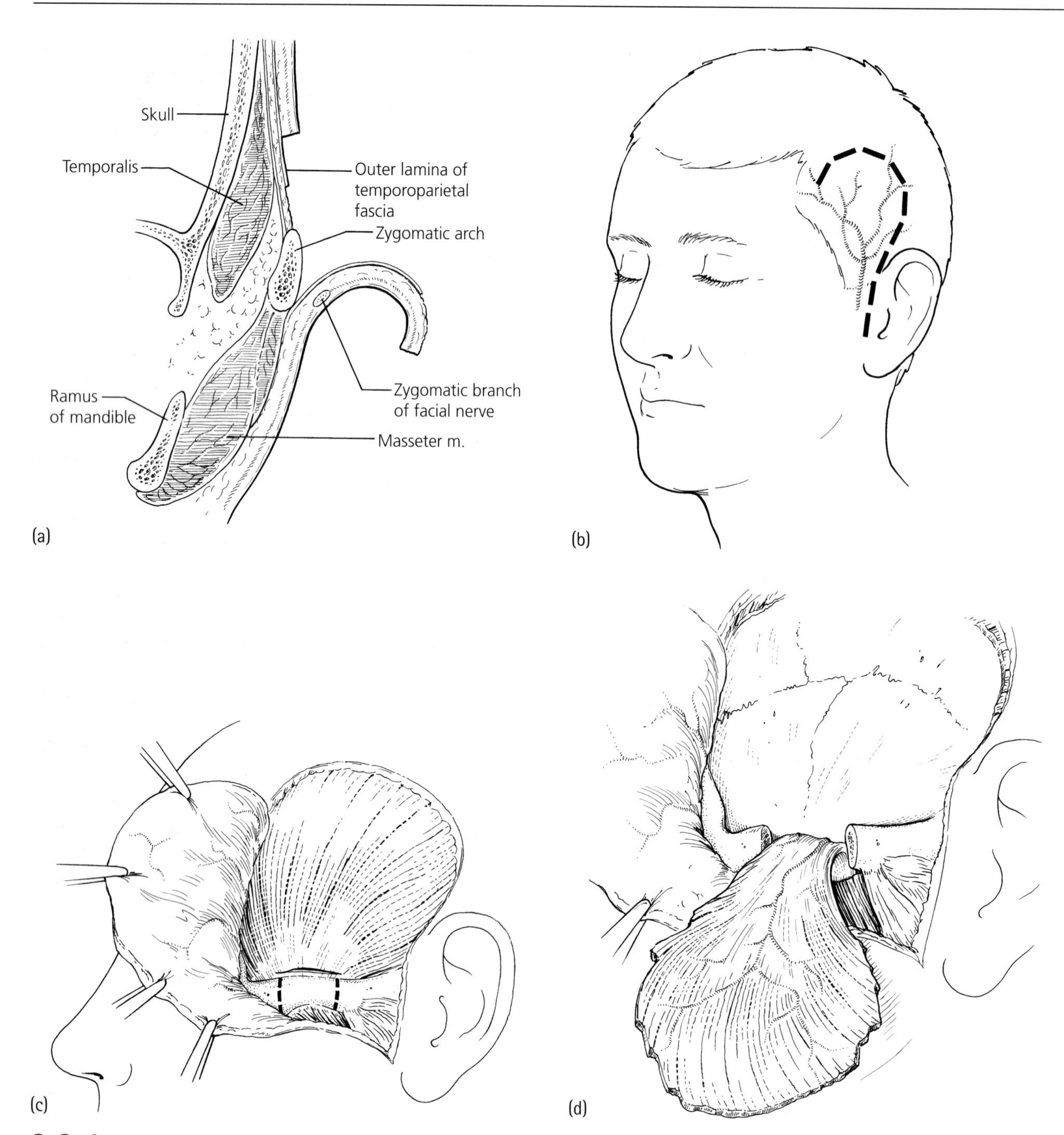

3.2.4 Temporalis flap: (a) anatomy; (b) skin incision; (c) sectioning of the zygomatic arch; (d) mobilization of the temporalis muscle.

achieved using haemostatic clamps at approximately 2 cm intervals, on both sides of the incision.

Meticulous dissection is required to expose the fascial plane with minimal damage to fine surface veins, just deep to the hair follicles. As the belly of the flap is exposed, it should be protected from drying by overlay with saline-dampened swabs.

The temporalis fascia splits into two laminae some 2 cm above the zygomatic arch and yellow fatty tissue between them is seen. Incising only through the outer lamina allows vertical dissection through the fat plane to the upper border of the zygomatic arch, from which the outer lamina and the periosteum of the arch can be elevated and reflected laterally, including the upper two branches of the facial nerve.

The exposed zygomatic arch is now sectioned from above using a fine saw with adequate irrigation and the 3–4 cm osteotomized segment can either be removed or pedicled inferiorly for later realignment. The exposed narrowing portion of the muscle is tendinous in this area as it descends to take origin from the coronoid process and the medial ramus of the mandible; its deep surface forms the pivotal zone of vascular supply about which the flap will rotate.

FLAP DESIGN

Before raising the flap, attention is now directed to its transfer route to the recipient defect area. Careful dissection intraorally may be required to allow development of a tunnel to allow transposition of the flap to the donor site. If access is tight or if coronoid bone is to be included on the pedicle, a coronoidotomy must be performed.

The belly of the flap is now exposed and the area required for repair is assessed. All muscle contracts on sectioning and allowance must be made for this to reduce the useful flap area available for transfer by some 30 per cent.

If less than the whole muscle bulk is needed it is suggested that the tissue anteriorly is left undisturbed to minimize the cosmetic defect post-operatively. When the vascular pattern causes concern about sectioning the flap, or the whole muscle bulk is needed, the insertion of an acrylic prosthesis may be considered.

Subperiosteal elevation now enables the body of the flap to be lifted, rotated carefully on its pedicle, advanced to the defect and inset with 3/0 Vicryl sutures using a round bodied needle.

The skin flap is inspected carefully and haemostasis assured. A vacuum drainage cannula is placed, exiting through a small incision in the scalp and secured with a silk suture before removal of the haemostatic clamps from the wound edges. Final wound closure is effected using 4/0 subcutaneous sutures and 5/0 cutaneous monofilament nylon or Prolene sutures.

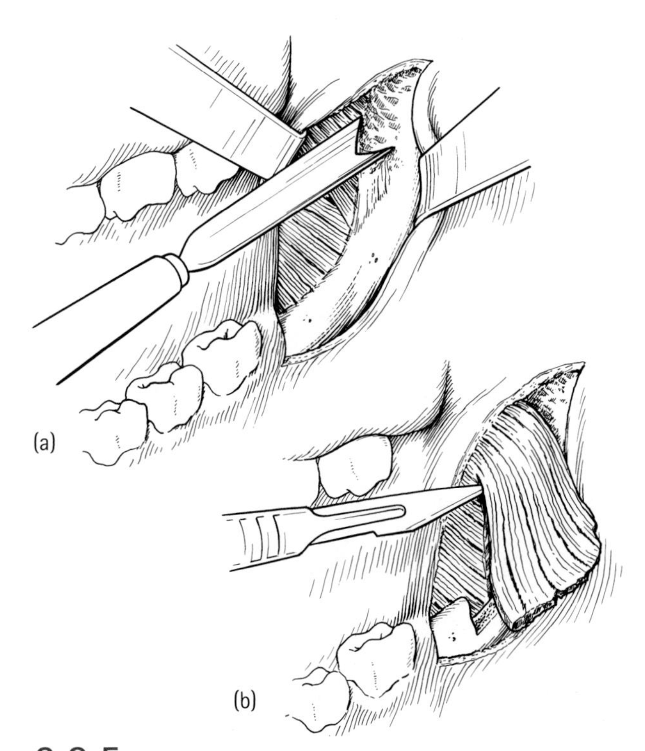

3.2.5 Masseter flap: (a) stripping the temporalis tendon; (b) freeing the periosteal attachment of the masseter muscle.

Provided effective vacuum seal is obtained, pressure dressing should be avoided. The author prefers the use of 1 per cent hydrocortisone ointment along the sutured wound edge, applied 8-hourly for 5 days, to other dressings because of potential benefit from the drug and because the oily nature of the preparation discourages clot adherence.

MASSETER FLAP

Principles and justification

The masseter muscle is a single fused structure anteriorly where, from its origin at the anterior border of the zygomatic arch, it passes obliquely down at 45° to its insertion at the lower border of the mandible. Posteriorly, like the pages of a three-page book, potential spaces allow the passage of the masseteric nerve between the inner two pages and the masseteric artery between the outermost two pages. The outermost page is the bulkiest arising from the anterior two-thirds of the inferior border of the zygomatic arch and inserting onto a wide area of the lateral aspect of the lower ramus, across the angle of the mandible and along the lower border overlapping the second molar tooth position. The middle and inner pages arise from the middle and inner portions of the mid third of the zygomatic arch, respectively, and insert only onto the lateral aspect of the ramus. The muscle takes its blood supply from the superficial temporal artery via the masseteric branch of the transverse facial artery which arises within the upper portion of the parotid gland. It is supplemented by one or two branches of the maxillary artery which pass across the ramus of the mandible through the sigmoid notch. Damage to the latter vessels during surgery should not prejudice flap vitality but may result in troublesome haematoma if not recognized.

Uses

This flap is most useful for providing cover within the oral cavity for resection defects close to its medial aspect yet protected from tumour contiguity by the intervening bone of the ramus of the mandible. Its use has been described for simple closure of the intraoral defect following retromolar bone or mandibular ramus resection where prolonged procedure is contraindicated, and for repair to the palatal mucosa.

Operation

INCISION

When this flap is used in the repair of a palatal defect, standard exposure requires a mucosal incision along the anterior edge of the ascending ramus. This exposes the tendinous attachment of the temporalis muscle which must be stripped from the ramus; this is best achieved by using the concave forward edge of a nasal septal chisel. With a clean bone edge thus exposed, a scalpel is used to incise the anterior periosteal attachment of the masseter muscle.

Dissect close to bone to elevate the masseteric periosteum entirely, laterally from its attachment to the ramus. For closure of a buccal mucosal defect lying completely anterior to the forward edge of the ramus, it is theoretically possible to incise through periosteum at the posterior vertical edge of the masseter; then by dint of forward horizontal incisions through periosteum and muscle close to the zygomatic arch origin and the lower border insertion, the inner muscle leaves can be reflected forward to cover the defect. In practice, the need for coronoid or ramus resection is most likely to have influenced the decision to use this flap and access for raising the flap is expedited.

Relief incisions must be used judiciously to achieve spreading and lengthening of the flap. After insetting into the recipient defect, the option of split skin grafting onto the muscle is straightforward, but this may not be necessary as the exposed vital muscle, in the oral environment, will epithelialize spontaneously within 2–3 weeks to produce oral epithelium.

Use of buccal fat pad

Buccal fat transposed into the mouth can be used without skin graft to cover small mucosal defects and to close oroantral communications. It epithelializes readily within 2–3 weeks. The procedure is easily achieved with the use of local anaesthesia and is particularly indicated when loss or tearing of the mucosal tissue, which might otherwise be used for a local advancement flap, has occurred.

Access to the pad of buccal fat is achieved either via a mucosal incision directly creating wound continuity with the defect to be covered, or by raising a submucosal tunnel between the fat pad and the defect. In either case, the release of a fatty pedicle must occur by controlled herniation into the oral cavity and extreme delicacy must be exercised in teasing out a pedicle and during inset suturing. Incision of the fine capsule enclosing the fat pad should be only 5 mm long or may be achieved through a tunnel by careful dissection using the tips of fine mosquito forceps.

Herniation of the fat can be encouraged by gentle pressure over the fat pad site on the cheek just anterior to the anterior border of the masseter muscle towards the first molar tooth. Inset is achieved using 4/0 resorbable sutures on a round-bodied needle.

Use of abdominal dermofat

The principle of using abdominal dermofat as a graft for bulk replacement in contour deficiency, such as that seen in first arch syndrome, relies upon harvesting a segment of abdominal skin with attached adipose tissue after

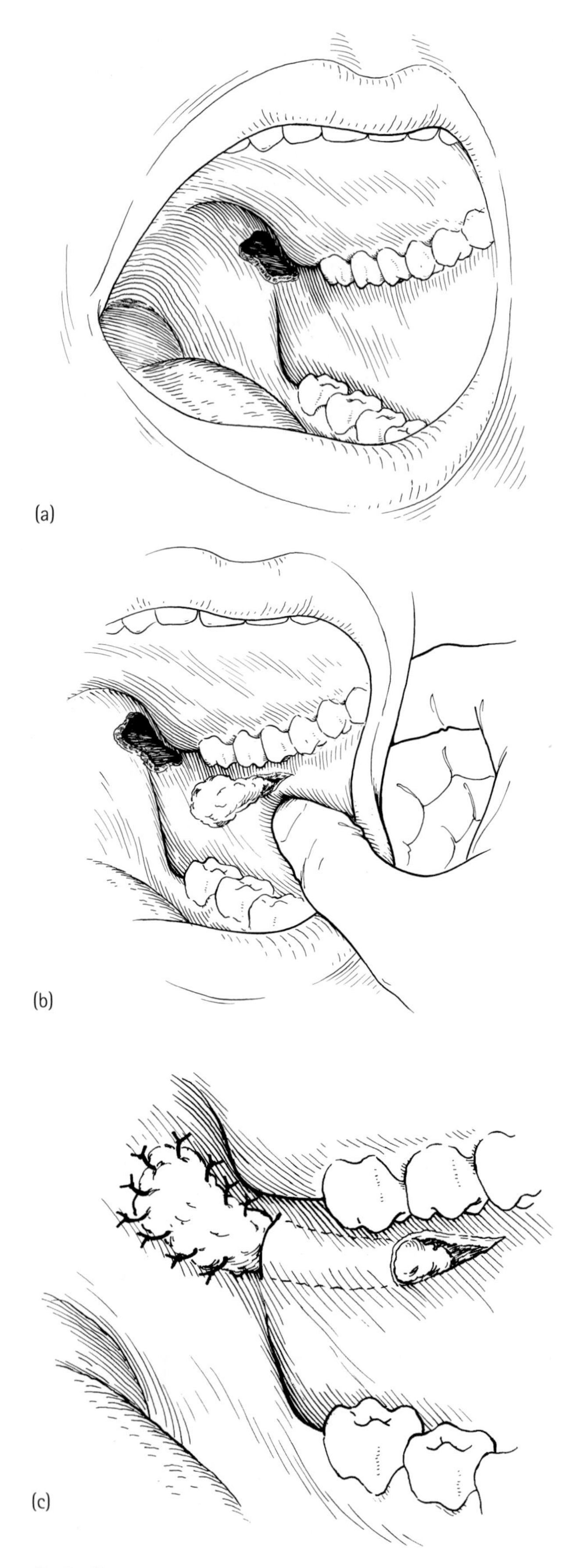

3.2.6 Buccal fat flap: (a) defect; (b) mobilization; (c) insertion of flap.

de-epithelialization, and implanting the graft into a subdermal or submucosal pocket. It is not appropriate for open surface defects. The fat provides the bulk for defect filling whilst the dermis provides a raw surface for vascular budding during healing. Tissue survival is unpredictable; at least 20 per cent of the fat bulk is lost and this loss is often represented by the fluid degeneration of the fat which may require aspiration.

The techniques of microvascular transfer of tissue have rendered this procedure obsolete in most situations.

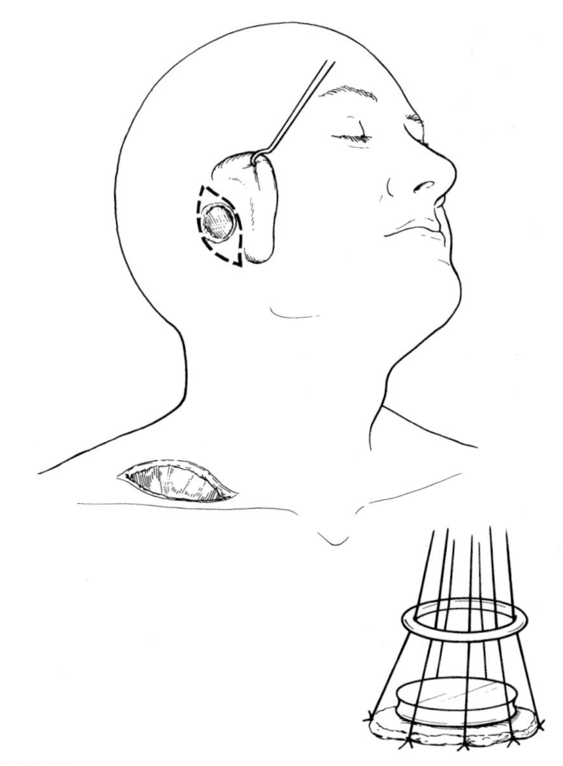

3.2.7 Full-thickness skin graft.

FREE SKIN GRAFTS

Principles and justification

The use of free skin grafts demands that the bed of the recipient site is biologically clean and adequately perfused to permit rapid vascularization of the graft, and substantial enough to provide stability during the healing phase. Infected soft tissues, dense bare cortical bone and cartilage are unsuitable for this treatment although grafting can be delayed with storage of the graft wrapped in saline-moistened gauze at 4°C for several days whilst wounds are cleaned, and bare bone can be decorticated. Bone within the mouth in the maxillary and palatal regions can be sufficiently vascular to accept direct grafting.

Tissues where vasculitis is present due to systemic disease or radiotherapy may also give poor support to free skin grafts.

In order to encourage good graft take, close adaptation of the graft to the recipient bed is essential for capillary budding, and haematoma interference must be avoided. Split skin grafts are generally more applicable for resurfacing large superficial defects exceeding 5 cm in diameter and can be further expanded by meshing. Successful full thickness skin grafts undergo little shrinkage.

On the skin surface the most common needs of maxillofacial surgeons for split skin grafts are the donor site defects after the transposition of trunk or limb pedicled and free flaps for microvascular procedures. In these situations, the supple nature of full thickness abdominal skin grafts, for example on the radial aspect of the forearm, are proving advantageous over split skin where primary closure is difficult.

Operations

FULL THICKNESS SKIN GRAFT

Classically, the use of defatted postauricular, supraclavicular and abdominal skin donor sites is most common in descending order of frequency for full thickness skin grafts. Which is chosen depends largely on aesthetic considerations of donor/recipient compatibility, area of deficit and anaesthetic technique. Grafts exceeding 2 cm in diameter usually exclude the postauricular crease as a potential donor site.

The chosen site is infiltrated with local anaesthetic to enhance tissue plane definition. A template of the defect size is used to outline the graft, but incision of extra tissue is usually required to allow cosmetically attractive donor site tissue closure. Incision depth includes the dermis and an excision plane is defined through the underlying adipose layer. The graft is lifted and stored in saline-moistened gauze, while the donor defect is closed primarily

The undersurface of the graft is now exposed and all fat attached to the dermis is planed off using curved scissors. The defatted graft surface is laid onto the recipient bed and any overlap excised. The margins of the graft are exactly in apposition to the defect margins by inserting interrupted 4/0 resorbable sutures around the circumference of the graft, with one end of the suture left longer than the graft diameter and the other cut short to the knot. Before suturing is completed, suction is gently applied beneath the graft to remove residual haematoma.

Either a bolus of flavine-soaked wool or a proprietary flanged button of appropriate size to the graft is placed over the graft and the long ends of the sutures are used to secure this and exert equal gentle tamponade over the entire graft surface.

The graft should be left undisturbed for 10 days when the pressure dressing is removed. Antibiotic prophylaxis with metronidazole is appropriate to discourage anaerobic infection. It is salient to point out that full thickness skin grafts taken from hirsute donor areas will continue to support hair growth at the recipient site.

SPLIT SKIN GRAFT

Any graft which contains less than the complete dermal layer is included in this definition. The thickness of the graft may be tailored for different recipient site requirements by choice of dermatome blade setting and by selection of the donor site skin quality. In principle, the thinner the graft the more likely its survival until vascularization is complete, but the greater the shrinkage occurring as the graft matures. Adaptation of split thickness skin must be ensured on similar principles to full thickness grafts.

Meshing of split skin grafts helps the exclusion of haematoma, but further increases shrinkage.

In lining maxillectomy defects, shrinkage is of little consequence but the avoidance of haematoma under the graft is a major benefit. The close approximation of graft to the recipient bed in this situation is best achieved by carriage on a closely adapted obturator or, for sulcus deepening procedures, a denture flange. This is usually adapted preoperatively to achieve perfect contouring by the use of a thermoplastic lining of stent or gutta percha. The split skin graft is draped over the mould and inserted into the recipient space. Unlike full thickness grafts, a marginal overlap of graft is acceptable and residual excess can be trimmed away at the first obturator change between 10 days and 3 weeks post-operatively.

For surface coverage of soft tissues such as the cheek, when large areas of leukoplakia are excised, the technique of quilting by the use of multiple resorbable sutures through the surface of the graft, in addition to marginal sutures, is designed to ensure continuing intimate graft to bed approximation.

Outside the mouth, the use of thin split skin grafts can be disappointing with maturation causing fibrotic bunching of tissue at the radial forearm site in particular. Pressure bandaging has long been used by surgeons to reduce the tendency of grafts to contract in this manner. The application of a tight Tubigrip bandage over the graft, with a tailored sheet of Silastic interposed between graft and bandage, has been found to greatly improve this problem.

KERATINOCYTE GRAFTING

The technique of tissue culture of skin grafts has only recently become possible because of developments in tissue culture technique. A 2 cm diameter biopsy specimen can be grown from the patient's mucosa to 50 cm^2 over 2 weeks with increasing reliability. However, the resulting graft is only a few cells thick and is extremely fragile because it lacks intercellular adhesion. Grafts have been applied by the author, but stability is problematic and successful outcome may have resulted from healing by natural epithelialization as well as by graft-influenced cellular growth. The potential of this technique is enormous (see also Chapter 2.11, p. 135).

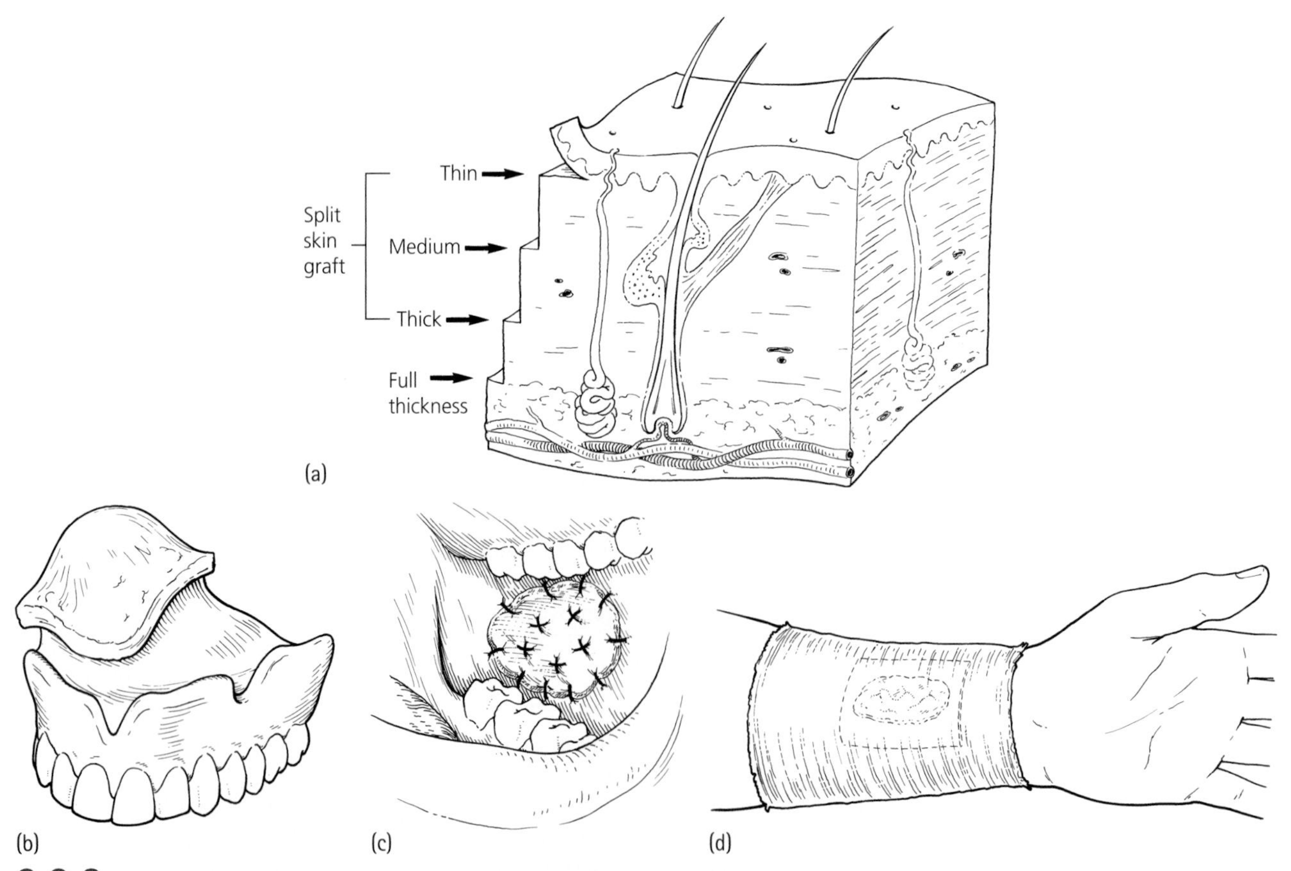

3.2.8 Split skin grafting: (a) depths; (b) split skin graft for maxillectomy defect; (c) graft for buccal defect; (d) graft to cover radial flap defect.

Top tips

- When performing lingual fraenectomies do not sacrifice tissue as this will increase the tethering.
- Advancement and rotational flaps must lie passively in their desired position. Periosteal release may be needed.
- Handle soft tissues with care and avoid crushing the edge of flaps with forceps.
- Ensure that the tunnel for the temporalis flap does not constrict the blood supply.
- Free grafts must be immobilized and closely applied to the underlying recipient bed – use either quilting stitches or a tie-over bolster.

FURTHER READING

Cheung LK, Samman N, Tideman H. The use of mouldable acrylic for restoration of the temporalis flap donor site. *Journal of Cranio-Maxillofacial Surgery* 1994; **22**: 335–42.

Falconer DT. Reconstruction of the defect at the donor site of the temporalis muscle flap. *British Journal of Oral and Maxillofacial Surgery* 1991; **29**: 16–19.

Langdon JD The masseter muscle cross-over flap. *British Journal of Oral and Maxillofacial Surgery*, 1989; **27**: 124–31.

Langdon JD, Patel MF (eds). *Operative maxillofacial surgery.* London: Chapman and Hall, 1988.

Sleeman D, Carton ATM, Stassen AFL. Closure of radial forearm free flap defect using full-thickness skin from the anterior abdominal wall. *British Journal of Oral and Maxillofacial Surgery* 1994; **32**: 54–6.

3.3

Pectoralis major

ANDREW LYONS

PRINCIPLES AND JUSTIFICATION

First described by Ayrian in 1979, the pectoralis major rapidly became the workhorse in head and neck reconstruction. Raised as either a myocutaneous or muscle flap, only the flap developed a reputation for a reliable easy-to-use reconstruction. It is based on vessels of the thoracromial artery. The muscle exists as two portions: a clavicular head, from its sternal half, and a sternocostal head, from the sternum to the level of the seventh costal cartilage, and from the upper sixth ribs. The muscle is attached by a flat tendon into the lateral lip of the intertubercular sulcus of the humerus.

Its blood supply is based on vessels of the thoracromial artery. This artery, on entering the deep 'clavipectoral fascia' of the muscle, splits into a deltoid branch to supply the humeral head and a pectoral branch to supply the remainder of the muscle. The pectoral potion of the muscle also gets its blood supply from the lateral thoracic artery and perforators from the internal mammary artery. Both of these vessels are almost always sacrificed to enable mobilization of the flap, as the pectoral branch is almost always the dominant vessel. However, this axial patterned flap is not without limitations and problems. The first is bulk; although the muscle bulk disappears with time, this deformity is never lost. As the muscle traverses the neck much needed cover of exposed vessels may be desirable.

Pedicle length may be a problem particularly where a myocutaneous flap is desired for a cutaneous defect. Although it is adequate for most intraoral defects, except those where maxillary obturation is required, where external skin coverage is required pedicle length is lost as the skin flap is effectively doubled over to achieve the correct skin orientation.

The biggest problem is skin reliability although a total necrosis rate of between 3 and 7 per cent was found, a partial necrosis rate of 29 per cent was noted of the skin paddle. Other operators have published better results. The paddle is usually taken at the extreme end of the flap. In the female, it is not possible to harvest skin more superiorly as the breast tissue will make the flap bulky and awkward. The viability of skin is dependent on perforators in the area that come predominantly from the pectoral branch. In the author's experience, skin will be lost in 1:10 male flaps and 1:3.5 female flaps. Fortunately, this is not usually a problem as the underlying muscle will usually obturate the defect to prevent a fistula, but this cannot be guaranteed.

For greater safety therefore, a muscle only flap can be raised. This may cause some loss of mobility in oral reconstructions and diminish the bulk where it may required.

INDICATIONS

Many surgeons justify the use of this flap over a free flap to reduce operating time and by conjecture operative morbidity. In the author's experience, this is a fallacy. It is difficult to raise this flap synchronously unlike most free flaps, and the time taken in raising this flap is not that much less than the time taken for an experienced microvascular surgeon to complete an arterial and venous anastomosis.

It is certainly an option where previous surgery and or radiotherapy have made access to reliable vessels for microvascular anastomosis difficult, particularly when this affects both sides of the neck. It is certainly useful to obturate defects where a free tissue transfer has failed.

It provides a useful myocutaneous flap for larger rather than small defects as this increases the number of perforators to the skin. It can be used for large tongue and floor of mouth defects, particularly total glossectomy defects. It is useful for lateral mandibular defects where a reconstruction plate is not to be used. By conjecture this is not a useful reconstruction for defects involving an anterior segment of the mandible where some form of spacer such as a reconstruction plate would be required. Dehiscence for plates use in conjunction with pectoralis major flaps has been recently put at 30 per cent for lateral defects and 50 per cent for anterior defects. It can be used as a tubed flap in laryngeal reconstruction, but leakage and dehiscence is high.

If used for cutaneous defects in the neck, the reliability of the flap can be enhanced by using a myocutaneous flap and overlying this with a split skin graft. Within three to six months, a surprisingly good aesthetic result can be achieved.

OPERATION

Position of the patient

The patient is supine with the arm on a board and abducted to 90°. A line should be drawn from the medial tip of the coracoid process to the tip of the xiphisternum (Figure 3.3.1). This approximates to the surface markings of the pedicle; the thoracoacromial vessels. The muscle extends inferiorly to the costal margin of the fifth, sixth and seventh ribs. It is not recommended to mark or develop the skin paddle beyond the costal margin, it is surprisingly easy to incorporate parts of the rectus abdominis muscle into the flap in an effort to increase pedicle length, but this should be avoided if possible to achieve maximum skin reliability.

The skin paddle (if required) should therefore be situated on the line of the pedicle with the costal margin as its lower margin. In males, ellipsoid paddles should be orientated lengthways along the pedicle marking. In females, for cosmesis, the pedicle can be orientated horizontally in a submammary position.

Incision

The skin paddle should be incised through subcutaneous fat to the underlying muscle (Figure 3.3.2). To increase the number of perforators, a layer of subcutaneous fat can be raised along the length of the muscle pedicle (Figure 3.3.3), this will mean at the superolateral aspect of the skin paddle the incision passes only down to the subcutaneous fat. However, this still does not guarantee success of the skin layer and, as the pedicle passes directly below the breast, at least some subcutaneous fat should be left in females.

Raising the flap

The skin paddle having been defined, the muscle should be dissected off the underlying chest wall. Although it is less well defined inferiorly, a plane can be developed on the surface of the rib periosteum and the fascia over the intercostal muscles. Proceeding first in a superolateral and then lateral direction, dissection and elevation of the flap can begin. Laterally, it should be easy to palpate and see the lateral border of the muscle. During the dissection, perforators will be encountered running into the muscle from the chest wall. They can usually be left on the muscle but those on the chest wall should be diathermised.

Exposure of pectoralis minor

As the muscle is dissected off the chest wall midway, the pectoralis minor will be encountered (Figure 3.3.4). This muscle should be spared and is separated from the pectoralis major by its fascia. At this stage, the pedicle should be visible through a thin layer of fat below the pectoralis major muscle. At the lateral part of the dissection, the antechostal brachial nerve will be encountered and should be divided. Just above

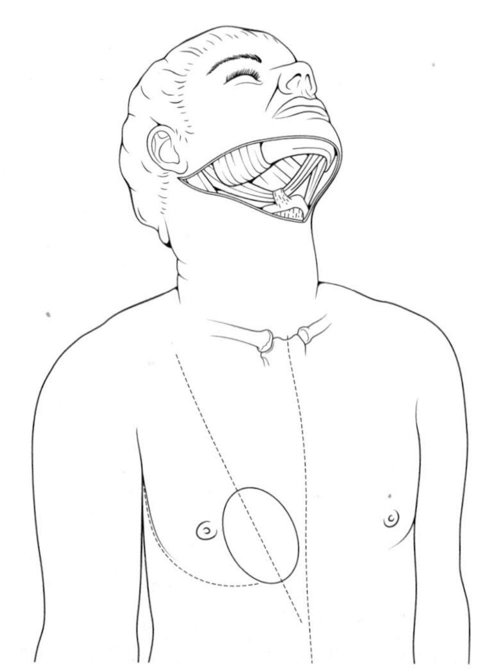

3.3.1 Skin markings in male. Note the straight dotted line indicating the position of the pedicle.

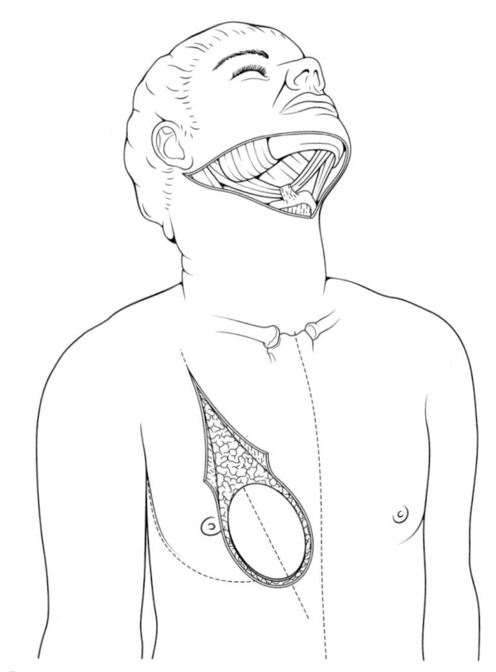

3.3.2 Incision around skin paddle and superiorly to allow layer of subcutaneous tissue to be raised along the pedicle.

this are the lateral pectoral vessels. Unless the flap is required for the lower neck, providing the thoracoacromial vessels have been identified, these should be divided as its integrity will restrict the vertical movement of the flap.

If the thoracoacromial vessels have not been visualized at this stage the dissection should proceed no further, as the thoracoacromial vessels are laterally disposed beneath the muscle and can conceivably be confused with the lateral pectoral vessels. Having divided the vessels, it will probably be necessary to diathermy muscles in the axillary fat. At this stage with the pedicle visualized, the humeral head should be divided in the axilla and this will add considerable length to the flap.

Elevation of the flap is almost complete and should proceed upwards to just below the clavicle if necessary, which in most cases it will be to ensure adequate pedicle length.

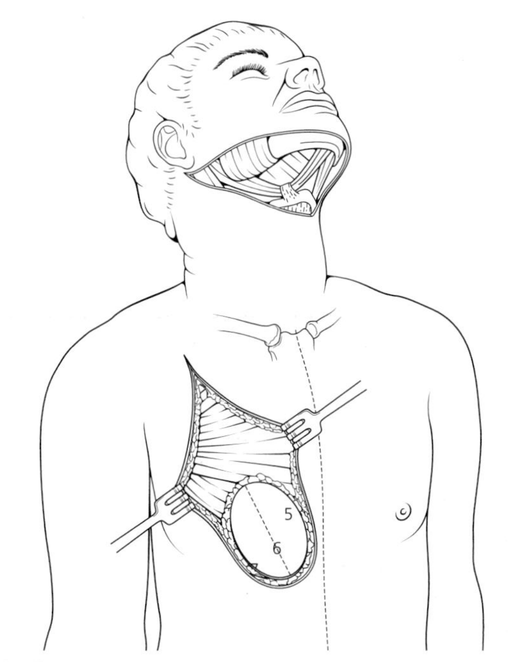

3.3.3 Subcutaneous fat along pedicle and skin flap prior to raising pectoralis major muscle.

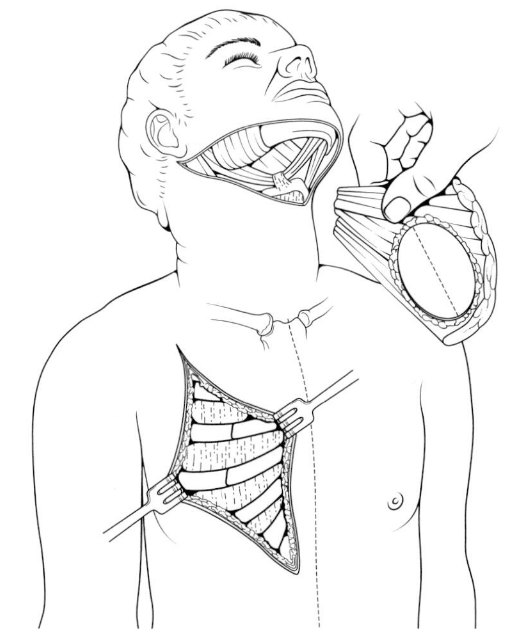

3.3.4 Exposure of pectoralis minor, pectoralis major muscle is out of view as it has been placed in the neck.

Making the tunnel

A tunnel should be made above the clavicle and below the skin and subcutaneous tissue into the neck (Figure 3.3.5). This is usually achieved by dissecting downwards from the neck and upwards from the donor site wound. The space within this tunnel can be assessed by inserting the four fingers of a hand.

The upper border of the skin paddle or lower border of the muscle should be grasped from above by a large clip after its insertion through the tunnel and then pulled gently upwards. If resistance is encountered, the tunnel and pedicle should be reassessed to see where there is snagging. Some surgeons suture the edges of the skin paddle to the muscle below to prevent shearing of the skin paddle. In the author's opinion, this is unnecessary providing the flap is handled with care and respect.

Insetting the flap

When the flap has been placed *in situ* it must not be under any tension. Not only might this affect the flow within the pedicle, but over the next 2 weeks as the muscle scars and contracts it will pull the healing wound edges away inferiorly leading to wound dehiscence. The flap can reach further if muscle only is used, but again lack of tension is vital. The flap should be secured with muscle, subcutaneous and skin layers.

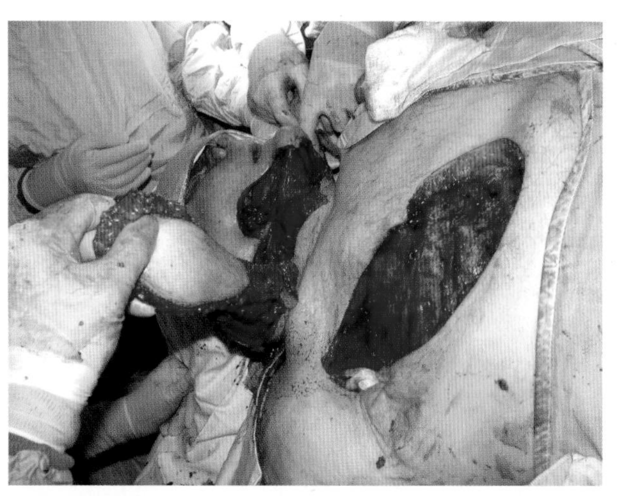

3.3.5 Flap just after tunnelling and pulling through from donor site.

The donor site can usually be closed primarily (Figures 3.3.6 and 3.3.7) and the cosmetic result is particularly good after a submammary incision in females. Suction drainage is recommended, particularly in the axilla.

POST-OPERATIVE CARE

Monitoring is less crucial than free tissue transfer. Twice a day should suffice as little can be done to correct any apparent arterial or venous problem, and certainly in the immediate post-operative phase, pallor and the colour and quantity of blood on pinpricking are unreliable.

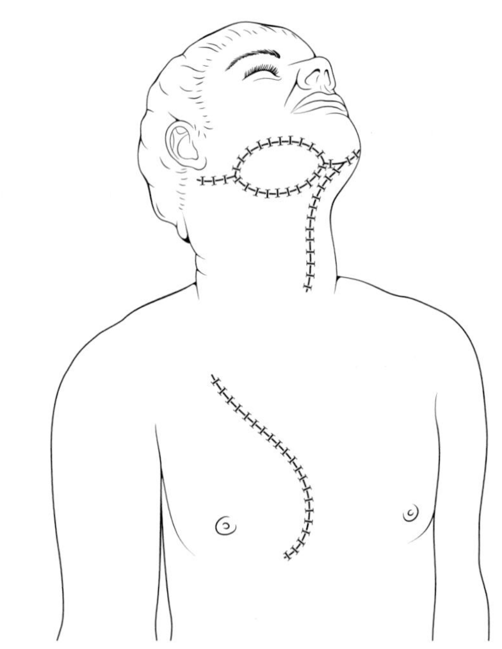

3.3.6 Closure of incision on male patient.

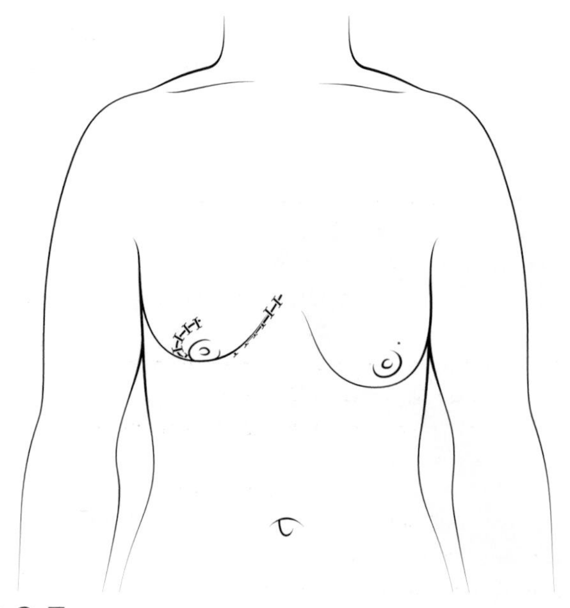

3.3.7 Closure of incision on male patient.

COMPLICATIONS

Intra-operative

The pedicle may be damaged during flap elevation.

Post-operative

- Flap necroses. It is extremely unusual, though not impossible, for the entire flap to become ischaemic and necrose.
- Partial necroses. More commonly, this applies to the skin and subcutaneous fat. If this occurs intraorally, a leak into the neck and fistula formation are not inevitable in the presence of viable muscle. The dead tissue should be debrided and, if carried out in an operating room, local anaesthetic may be an option in patients who are not ASA 1.

Top tips

- Leave the subcutaneous fat along the line of the pedicle to increase the number of perforators supplying the flap.
- In women, always use a submammary incision and avoid taking too much fat with the flap.
- If replacing external skin in the neck, using split skin over a muscle only flap will increase flap length and reliability. In time, a very acceptable aesthetic result will result from the skin graft with less donor site morbidity

FURTHER READING

Baek SM, Lawson W, Biller HF. An analysis of 133 pectoralis major myocutaneous flaps. *Plastic and Reconstructive Surgery* 1982; **69**: 460–67.

Mariani PB, Kowalski LP, Magrin J. Reconstruction of large defects postmandibulectomy for oral cancer using plates and myocutaneous flaps: a longterm follow-up. *International Journal of Oral and Maxillofacial Surgery* 2006; **35**: 427–32.

Ord RA. The pectoralis major myocutaneous flap in oral and maxillofacial reconstruction: a retrospective analysis of 50 cases. *Journal of Oral and Maxillofacial Surgery* 1996; **54**: 1292–5.

Shah J, Haibhakti V, Loree TR, Sutaria P. Complications of the pectoralis myocutaeous flap in head and neck reconstruction. *American Journal of Surgery* 1990; **160**: 352–5.

Vartanian JG, Carvalho AL, Carvalho SM *et al.* Pectoralis major and other myofascial/myocutaneous flaps in head and neck cancer reconstruction: Experience with 437 cases at a single institution. *Head and Neck* 2004; **26**: 1018–23.

Zbar RI, Funk GF, McCulloch TM *et al.* Pectoralis major myofascial flap: a valuable tool in contemporary head and neck reconstruction. *Head and Neck* 1997; **19**: 412–18.

3.4

Reconstructive surgery – harvesting, skin mucosa and cartilage

PETER WARD BOOTH

SKIN

Indications

The most common requirement for cutaneous tissue in the head and neck is after removal of skin lesions such as skin cancers. Mucosal replacement is another indication, but nowadays free skin grafts are rarely used for this purpose. Some free tissue free flap harvest sites may require skin cover, but this is outside the head and neck, for example to cover a radial forearm flap harvest.

Surgical options

There are a variety of options for closure of cutaneous defects, each having advantages and disadvantages (see Table 3.4.1).

Surgical technique

See Figures 3.4.1–3.4.5.

Table 3.4.1 Surgical options.

Procedure	Advantages	Disadvantages
Direct closure	Incision lines can be kept along the lines of natural tension, improving aesthetic outcome Using local skin from the same aesthetic zone	Limited defects only, as closure will create excessive tension leading to wound breakdown and infection
Local flap harvest – advancement	Allows much larger lesions to be closed	Unlikely that all the skin incisions will run along natural tension lines
Rotation procedures	Usually can be raised from the same aesthetic zone	
Skin graft – full thickness	Large area of skin can be covered Better aesthetics, in terms of thickness of the graft and aesthetic skin match than split skin but not as good as local flap	Problems of a donor site, produces a second area of scarring Poor skin colour and thickness match Takes 10–14 days to heal
Skin graft – split skin	Almost limitless amount of skin in terms of the head and neck	Very poor skin, texture and thickness match Painful donor site Both sites take 10–14 days to heal Significant wound contraction, about 20 per cent
Skin – free tissue transfer	Large area No delay in healing Usually possible to get the correct thickness	Long surgical procedure Poor colour and texture match

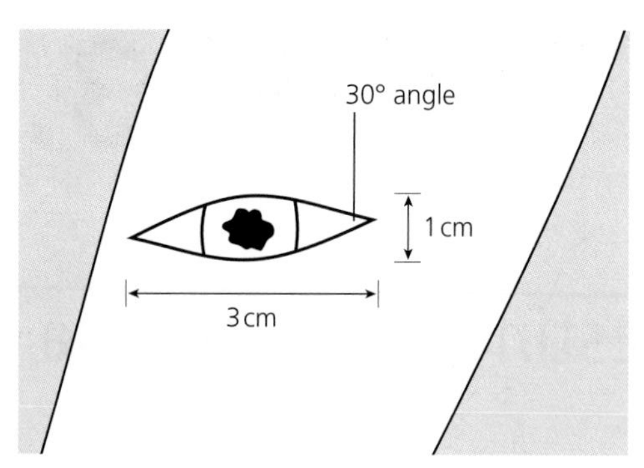

3.4.1 Direct closure; the ratio of length to width should be 3:1 and create 30° angles.

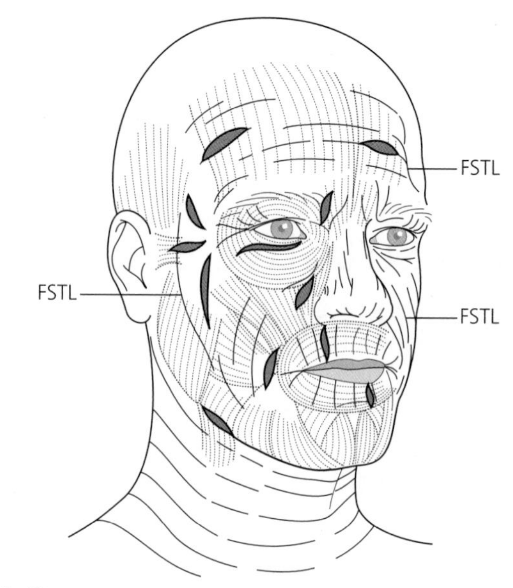

3.4.3 These tension lines are even more important in the facial region. FSTL, favourable skin tension lines.

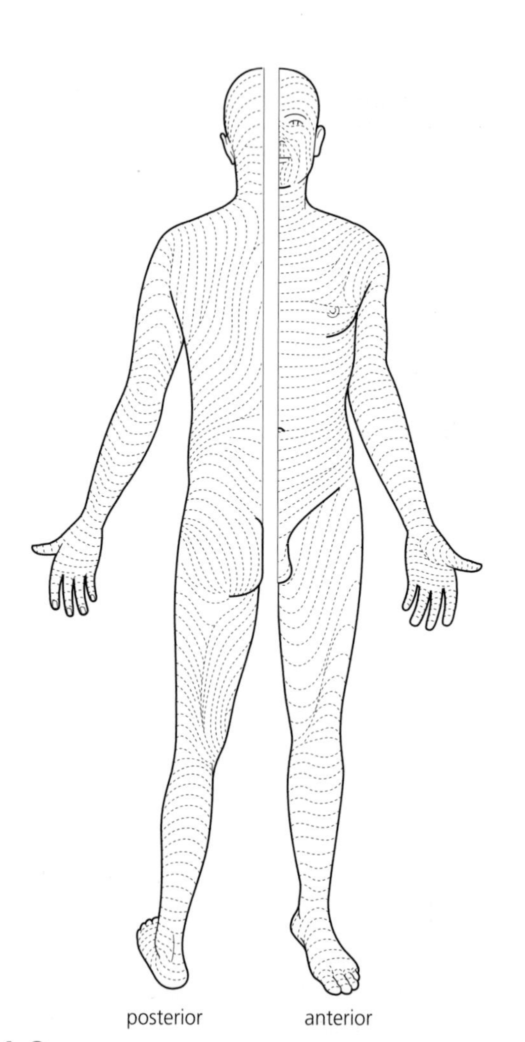

3.4.2 Incisions along the lines of tension, as shown, create narrow scars. Crossing these lines produces a broad ugly scar

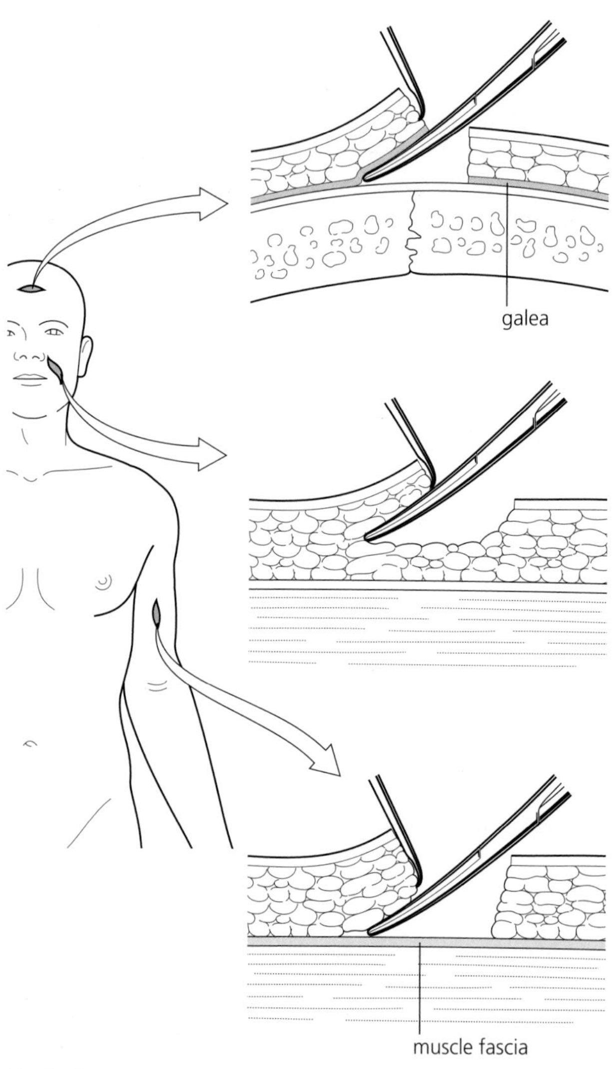

3.4.4 Undermining of the tissues should be in the subcutaneous level and only about 1 cm distance. Sharp dissection is better but may induce more bleeding than blunt dissection.

Direct closure

Best done as an elliptical incision parallel to the lines of tension. Certain basic principles should be followed:

- incision made at right angles to the skin;
- should follow the line of tension;
- aim to have a length of the excision which gives:
  - 30° angles at the end of the excision;
  - a 3:1 length to width ratio;
- local undermining of tissue to allow a passive closure.

Local flap closure

Again, there are certain surgical principles as outlined below (see Figures 3.4.6–3.4.9).

- The local flap can be either 'advanced' or 'rotated' into the defect. Some also consider the transposition flap as a separate category, but this is normally a variation of rotation and/or advancement.
- The flap should be brought from within the same aesthetic zone.
- The final scar should, as much as possible, lie along lines of tension, but this is rarely possible with all the incisions.
- The choice of flap is dictated by seeking tissue from an area of lax tissues. Thus the decision as whether to rotate or advice is based on the site of the lesion and the site of available tissue.

3.4.5 Careful suture and creating skin eversion is essential.

- On the face, the flap length to width ratio should be no more than 4:1 and the flap should be about 10 per cent larger than the defect.

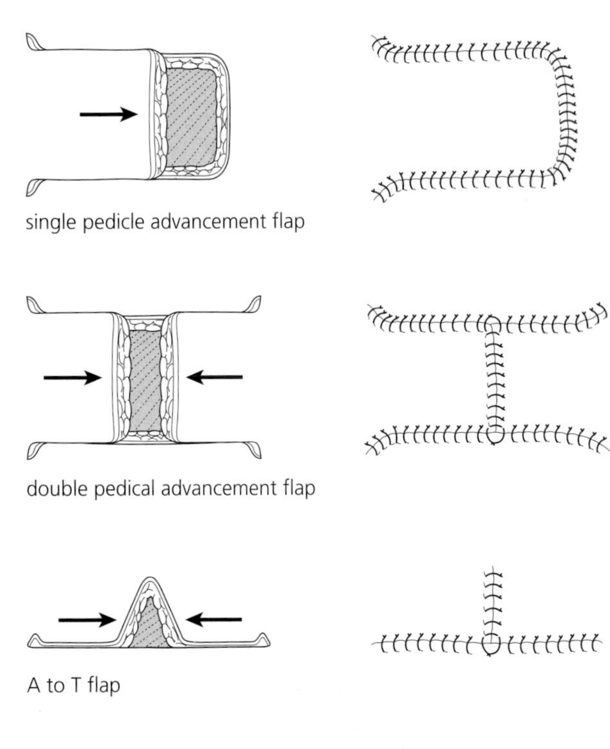

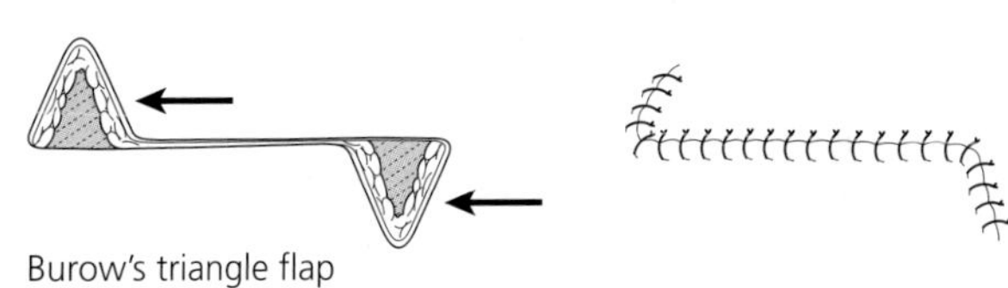

3.4.6 The principles of an advancement procedure.

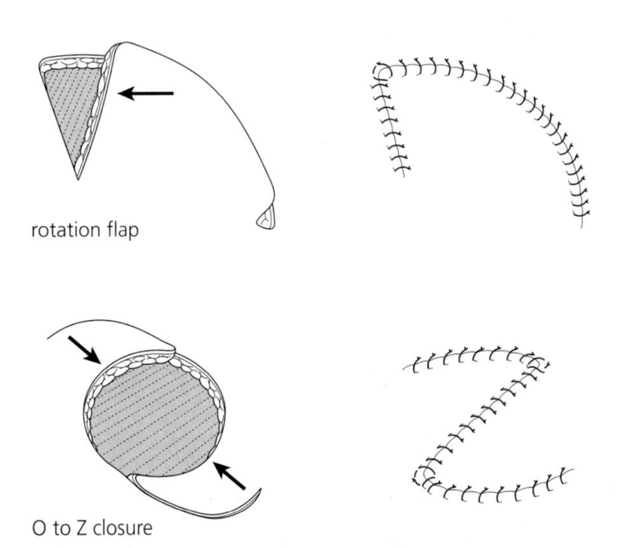

3.4.7 The principles of a rotation procedure.

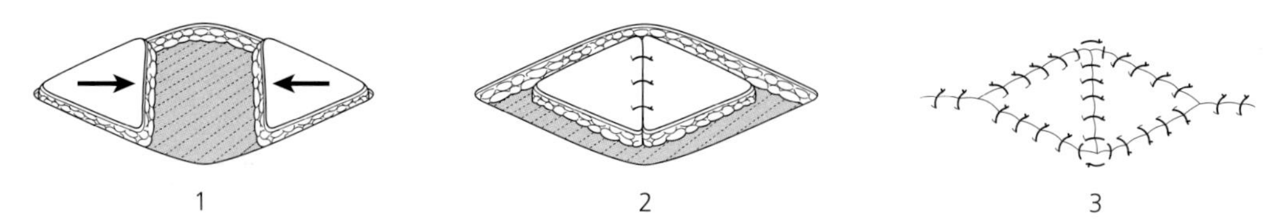

3.4.8 Island flaps rely on the subcutaneous tissues for their blood supply, so the rotation or advancement is over a short distance, lest the tension will impair the blood supply.

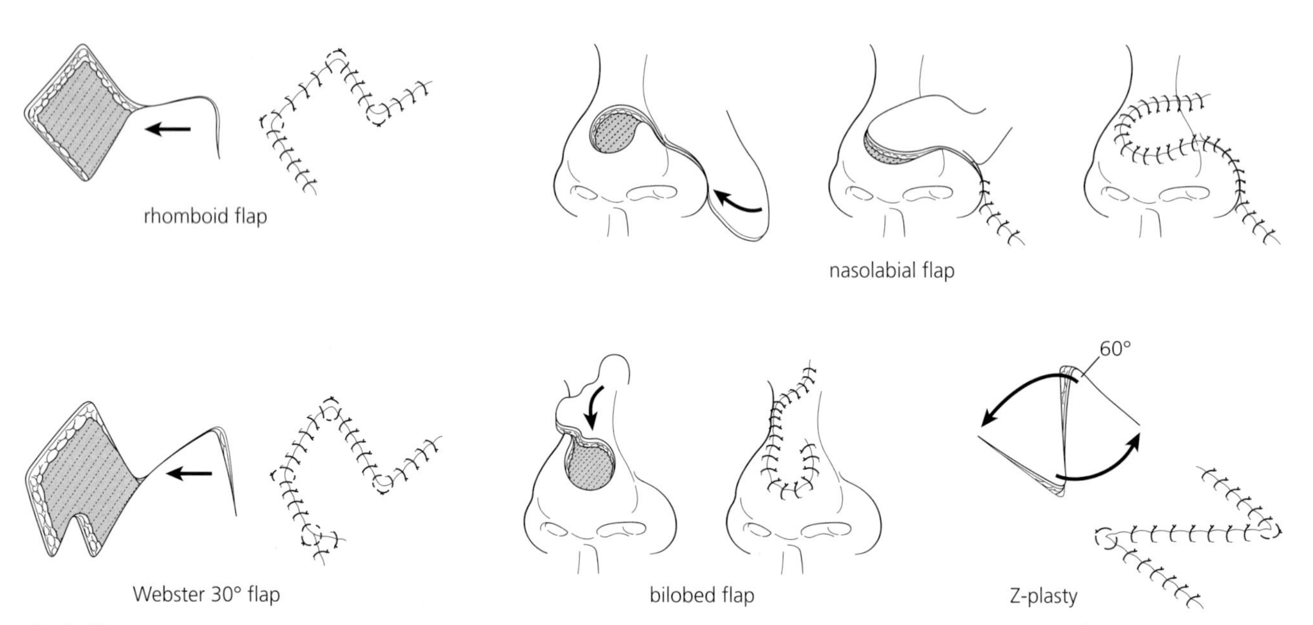

3.4.9 Different examples of rotation procedures.

SKIN GRAFTING

Full thickness

Again, certain surgical principles pertain (see Figures 3.4.10 and 3.4.11).

The donor site should be selected for:

- availability of skin;
- provide good colour and thickness match;
- not in an obvious visible site.

In practical terms, the following donor sites are frequently used.

- Root of the neck:
  - usually able to provide 4–6 cm grafts;
  - not readily visible;
  - pale but thin skin.
- Post-auricular:
  - limited size, 2–3 cm;
  - not easily seen;
  - thin skin with good colour match.
- Pre-auricular:
  - good colour and texture match;
  - limited size, 3 cm length but not much more than 1 cm in width.

With both split and full thickness grafts, it is important to have meticulous haemostasis of the excised site to allow intimate contact between graft and wound bed – small stab perforations in the graft are ideal for this. The harvested graft should be de-fatted using scissors. Dressings should be firmly placed on the wound bed. Silicone mesh covered by flavin wool dressing or foam dressing all secured by tie over sutures are ideal.

The donor site should be normally directly closed in layers. It may be helpful to place a small suction drain for the first 24 hours. Pain is not a feature of the donor site (compared with split graft harvest).

The wound at the surgical site should ideally be left undisturbed for 10 days, although it should be regularly inspected to check for haematoma and wound infection.

Split skin grafts

Clearly, anywhere in the body is a potential donor site, but in reality the need to find a flat surface which is not too visible and has adequate dimensions means that the inside of the thigh or upper arm are usually used. For facial reconstruction the inside of the upper non-dominant arm is ideal. It does not immobilize the patient, normally has enough skin, is easily kept clean and can be readily observed (see Figures 3.4.12 and 3.4.13).

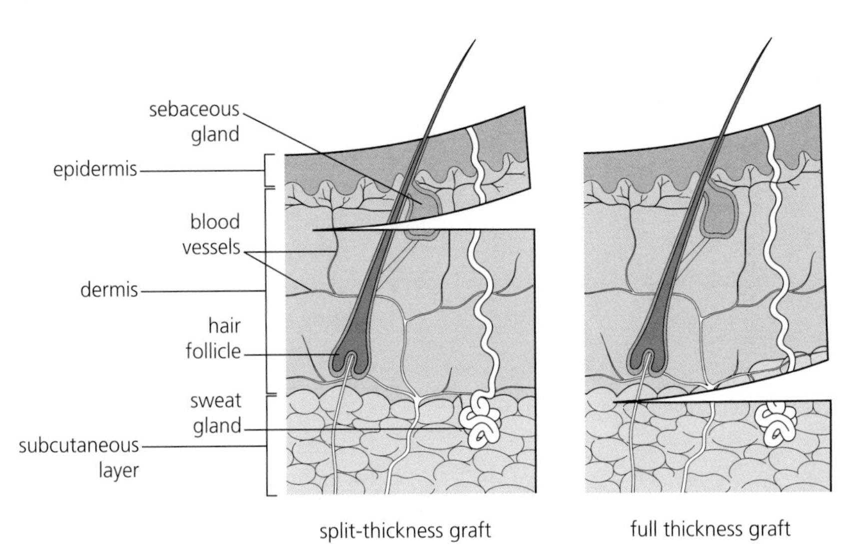

3.4.10 The differences between spilt and full thickness grafts.

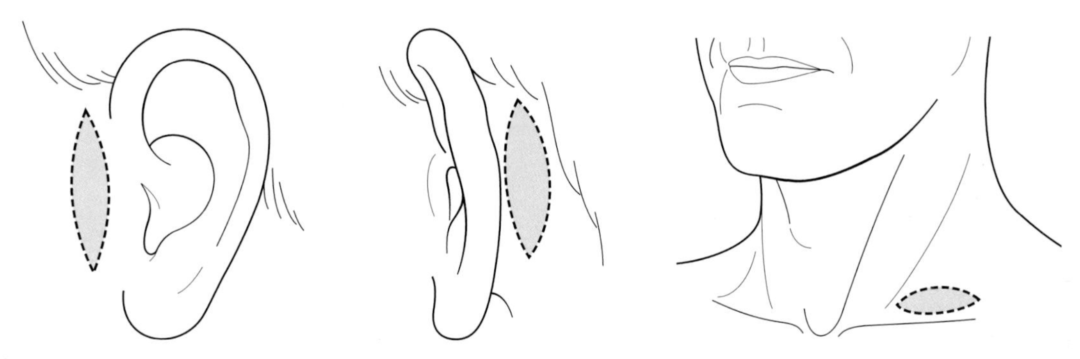

3.4.11 Good sites for full thickness grafts.

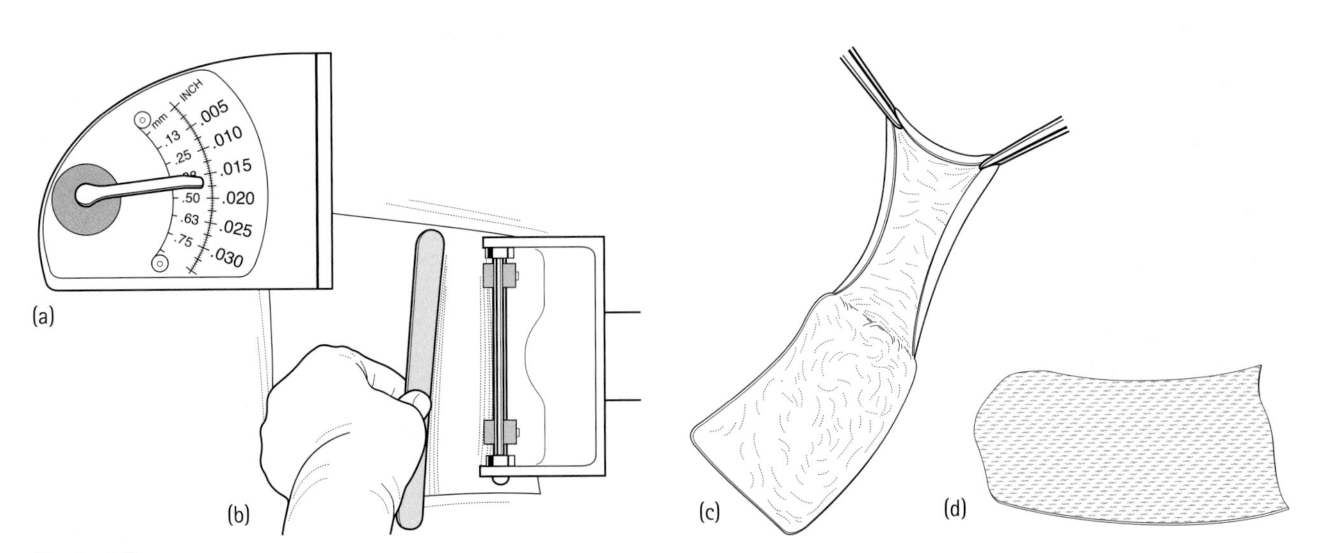

3.4.12 The stages of split skin grafting: (a) setting the correct thickness, the width of a No 1 blade is a good guide: (b) the area must be well lubricated and the piece of wood just ahead of the dermatome ensures an even thickness across the whole width of the cut: (c) typical appearance: (d) the graft should have small perforations to prevent haematoma formation.

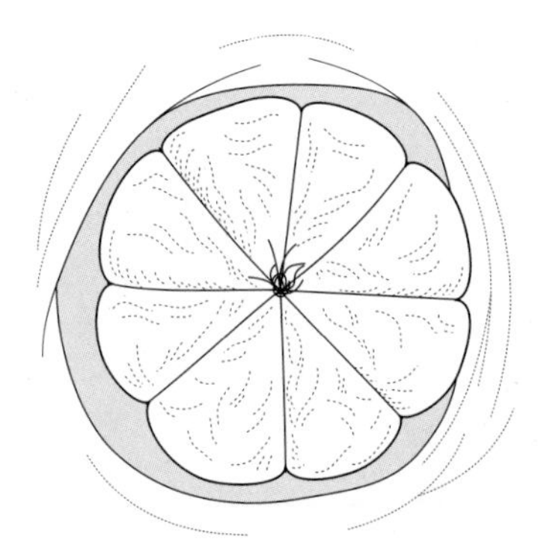

3.4.13 Tie over sutures maintain stability and prevent haematoma under the graft.

The principles of applying the skin graft are similar to full thickness.

- Topical cleaning prior to and after surgery may be helpful, but the routine use of antibiotics is not indicated.
- Meticulous haemostasis is needed to ensure good contact between the graft and the nutritional wound bed.
- Firm pressure to stabilize the graft and prevent a haematoma forming beneath the graft. A similar dressing technique as used with a full thickness graft is ideal.
- Again, stab perforations or meshing of the graft helps to prevent haematoma formation.
- Ideally the wound should be left untouched for 7–10 days.

The thinner the graft the better the 'take' but the greater contraction. Normally, the graft should be about 0.3 mm, which is about the thickness of a No. 15 blade.

The skin can be harvested with a conventional hand held blade, but it is very difficult to get an even thickness. The standard traditional skin grafting knife has more or less been replaced by a powered dermatome. This produces a very even thickness graft, but more importantly the width of the graft can be more easily predicted. The success of the technique is very much related to acquiring the experience to get a good 'feel' for the depth of the cut. However, certain techniques can make it more predictable.

- All the skin and cutting surfaces should be well lubricated with mineral oil.
- A flat board should be advanced just in front of the dermatome to ensure a flat surface is presented to the blade.
- A slow even progression of the dermatome prevents folding of the skin ahead of the blade producing a more even cut.
- Meshing of the graft can increase the size of the graft by about 30 per cent but in most cases the meshing is merely to create small perforations to prevent haematoma formation.

The donor site can be extremely painful and this must be anticipated and prevented. A commonly used technique is to apply an alginate dressing impregnated with long acting local anaesthetic, such as buvicaine, or the non-steroidal volterol in an i.v. preparation. The alginate dressing is then, and importantly, stabilized with an adhesive dressing such as Tegaderm™. The wound should be left untouched for 14 days. It is essential to keep the wound under observation to check for haematoma formation or infection as the wound may need to be exposed and cleaned up.

Free tissue transfer is covered elsewhere in the textbook.

CHOICE OF SUTURE MATERIAL

Resorbable materials are in theory highly desirable, since it avoids another procedure for the patient. Unfortunately, these materials have a number of problems:

- The resorption process is equivalent to a foreign body reaction, producing significant inflammation.
- The process is too slow for facial wounds, here the material should have disappeared within 5–7 days.
- The use of subcutaneous resorbable sutures may mask these problems somewhat (see Figures 3.4.14–3.4.16).

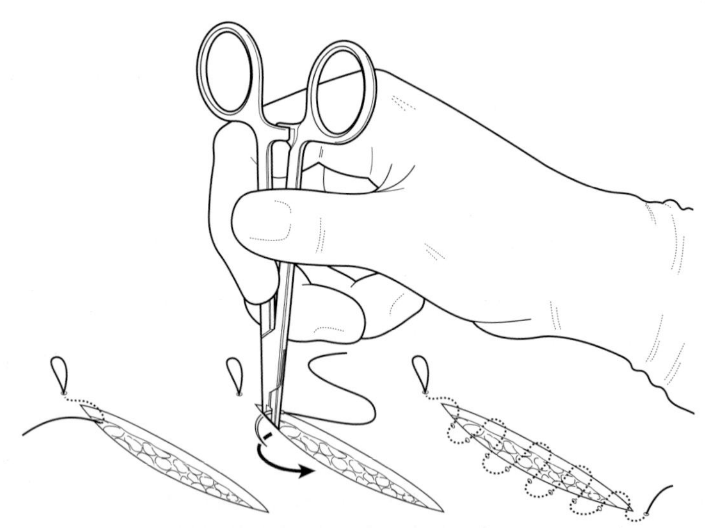

3.4.14 Subcuticular sutures are easy to remove than interrupted sutures, and may help to prevent 'stitch' marks if a resorbable suture is used.

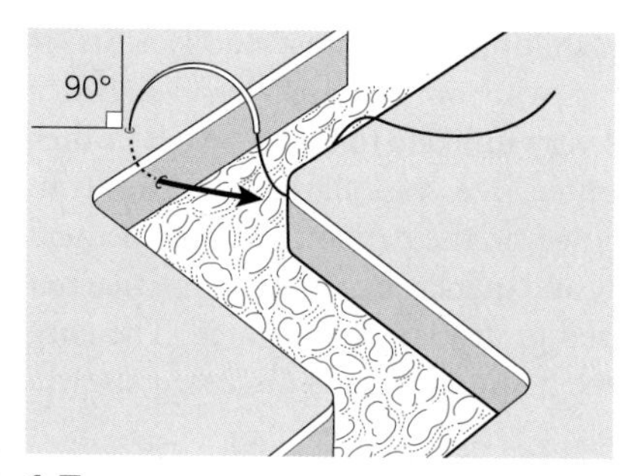

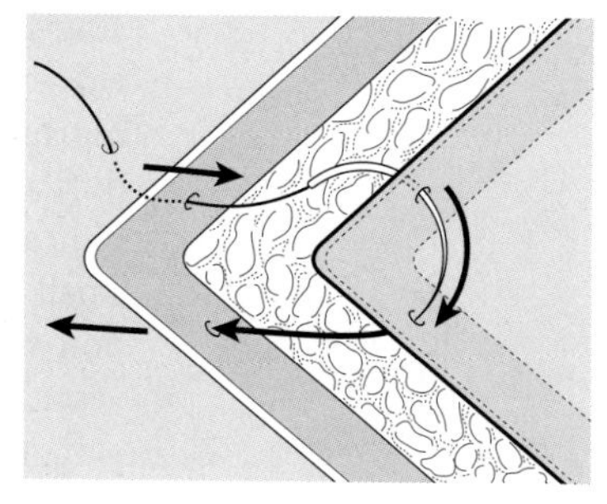
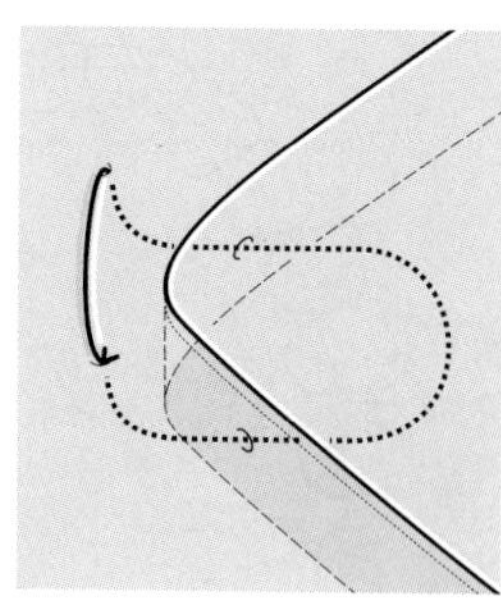

3.4.15 This avoids the pressure of the suture causing necrosis of the tip of such a sharp angle incision.

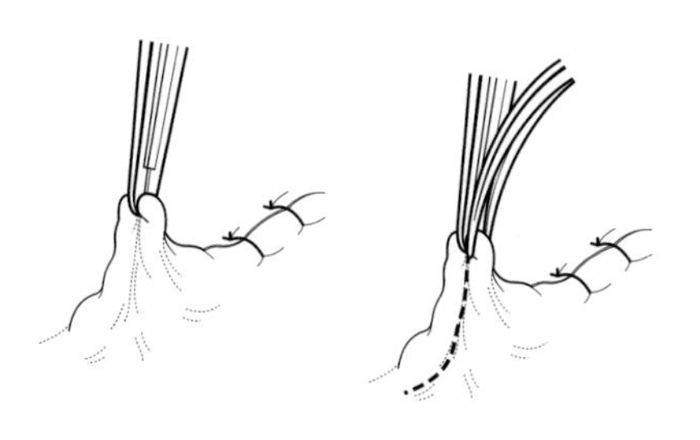
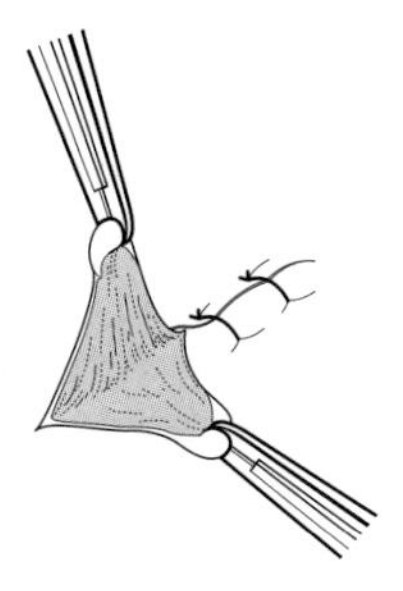
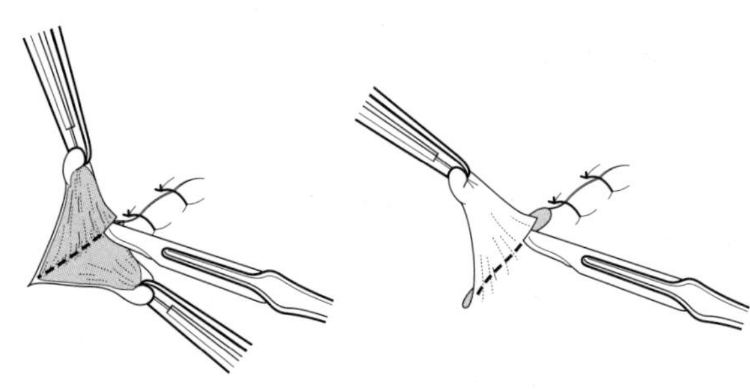

3.4.16 Removal of a 'dog ear'.

The ideal material is a polypropylene material (e.g. prolene), which has minimal tissue reaction and can be removed at 5–7 days. The use of a resorbable material, such as vicryl rapide, has the shortest resorption time of around 14 days but is a textured material leading to more tissue reaction.

MUCOSAL FLAPS

As with the skin, these flaps can be direct closures, local rotational and advancement flaps.

For a successful outcome:

- Excessive tension will reduce blood supply and lead to dehiscence and infection.
- The flap length/width ratio is about 4:1.
- The only non-muscle flap with a true vascular pedicle is based on the greater palatine vessels, the rest are random pattern flaps.
- Unlike skin, the local anatomical variations of the mucosa do demand special attention. It is most important that attached mucosa is attached to the gingiva of the teeth. This means flaps must be designed to ensure that relationship. In some cases this is not possible and free full thickness attached mucosa, normally harvested from the palate, may have to be used. A micro dermatome is an excellent way of achieving such a harvest (see Figures 3.4.17 and 3.4.18).

NON-VASCULARIZED BONE HARVESTING

Non-vascularized bone grafts do not survive once transplanted, but provide growth factors and a hard tissue skeleton. The latter prevents the in-growth of soft tissue and

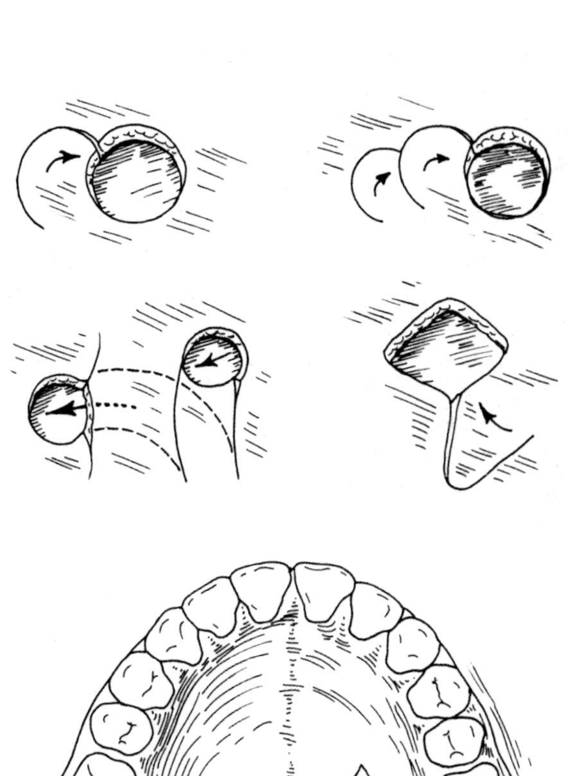

3.4.17 Posterior view of the right shoulder showing the blood supply to the trapezius muscle and spine of the scapula.

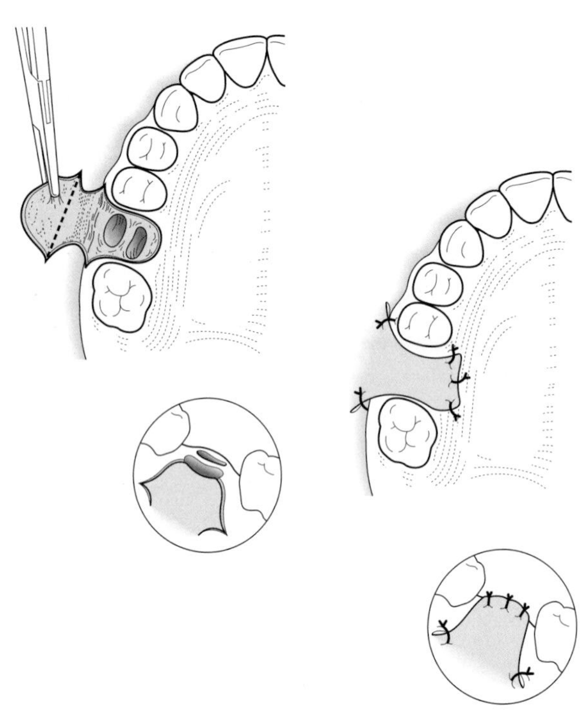

3.4.18 Incisions for harvest of the right trapezius/scapular myo-osseous flap. Dotted line denotes incision when no radical neck dissection is necessary and dashed line denotes incision if radical neck dissection if performed.

the former stimulates angiogenesis and ultimately new bone formation. This process takes time and it is essential that the graft is placed in a highly vascularized environment free from any infection. In practical terms, the graft in the mouth needs to be a sealed vascularized environment with good vascularized mucosa covering the graft. Clearly, in young growing children this is most readily achieved but in elderly patients who smoke and have significant co-morbidity it is very unlikely to be achieved. In these more difficult patients, free vascularized tissue transfer is indicated. If, however, the patient is young or the defect is small and easily and quickly becomes re-vascularized, a free non-vascularized graft may be indicated. The surgery for vascularized free tissue transfer is discussed elsewhere.

Indications

As mentioned above, these grafts have only limited use, yet sadly the literature continues to expound their use, primarily in surgical centres which do not have access to microvascular techniques; this, however, is not a proper 'indication'. By the criteria above the indications are:

- alveolar defects in children with cleft lip and palate defects;
- small 'three surface' defects in the jaws, whereby the bone defect is surrounded by bone walls except at the surface (e.g. after removal of a benign tumour from the alveolus);
- small bone defects in which an implant is to be placed;
- post-traumatic grafting in young patients. This is replacing acutely, prior to contracture of the soft tissue envelop. This may be to an orbital floor or nasal graft;
- secondary jaw reconstruction of small continuity defects, in which the fragments have been stabilized by bone plates. Again only small defects in patients with well-healed soft tissues with excessive scarring will be successful;
- it has very little value because of the predictable poor outcome in reconstruction after oral cancer ablation.

Table 3.4.2 Common donor sites.

Site	Indications and disadvantages
Cranium, outer cortical plate	Hard stable bone, scar normally hidden in the hair. Difficult to carve and manipulate. Reported risk of precipitating intracranial bleeding. Small volume
Rib with or without costal cartilage	Small volume, very soft but pliable bone. With the cartilage in 30 per cent of cases harvested in young children it will continue to grow. Small risk of chest complications especially in the elderly, pneumothorax and chest infection. Can be painful In young females, the harvesting may, if too high, damage breast development
Ilium anterior approach	One of the commonest sites yields large volumes of bone (especially with the posterior approach), it has an unobtrusive scar. While it is very painful, unless a trephine is used, it has few significant side effects. Damage to the lateral cutaneous nerve of the thigh should be easy to avoid, but it does happen and is a significant problem. Fractures of the iliac crest can occur. The posterior approach is much less frequently used as it is necessary to rotate the patient prevent synchronous surgery to the mouth and bone harvest
Tibia	This is a trephine approach which yields small volumes but ideal for alveolar defects. Few complications and little pain, but unrewarding in elderly patients as the bone is replaced by fat and blood
Intraoral – used predominately in implantology where small volumes of particulate bone are required	Chin: easily accessed, small volume, quite vascular, but leaves anterior teeth numb for some time Lateral posterior mandible: better volume, deal for alveolar augmentation for implants. Little visible bone defect, haematoma may produce swelling Cortical bone scarification. This involves paring off the cortical surface of the lateral mandible. It produces a good volume of particulate bone, ideal in implantology, but no value for continuity defects, unless very small

Common donor sites

Clearly any part of the bony skeleton can be used, but in reality only a few are regularly used (see Table 3.4.2).

SURGICAL TECHNIQUE

Cranium

The incision is an angular one over the prominence of the parietal bone, care being taken to avoid damaging hair follicles (see Figure 3.4.19). It may of course be accessed as part of a coronal flap. The incisions are down to bone, and the periosteum elevated. The outline of the bone graft is cut in the outer palate and, either with a very thin flexible oscillating saw or small curved chisels, the outer plate is raised. In children it may be helpful to do a pre-operative computed tomography (CT) scan to ensure adequate bone thickness to remove the outer plate.

In some circumstances, if working with neurosurgeons, the full thickness can be removed and the inner plate plated into the outer plate position to prevent any hollowing over the calvarium.

As the bone is very rigid and hard, it has to be fashioned with cuts and bending forceps to the desired shape. It may be necessary to grind the bone to produce small fragments to pack around the main graft and produce a smooth contour at the recipient site.

Closure usually requires a small vacuum drain and should be in layers.

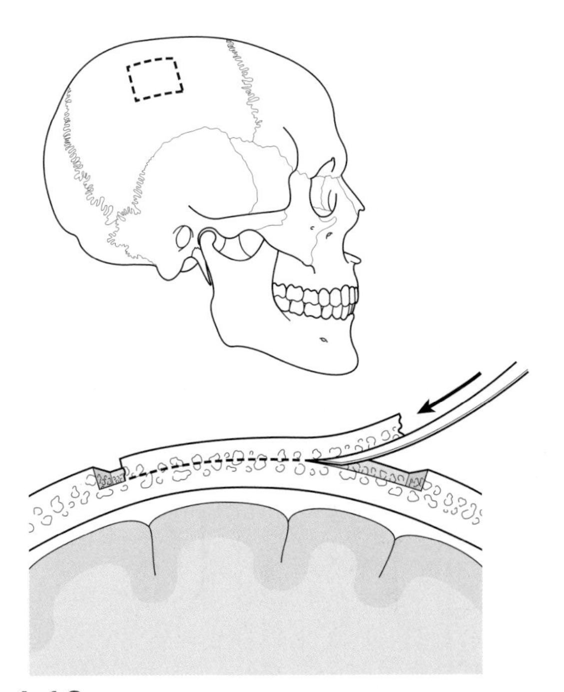

3.4.19 A groove is scored through the outer table and the outer table is removed with fine chisels.

Rib

The incision is in the submammary area, usually 5–7 rib, but no more than two consecutive ribs, to prevent a flay segment. The incision is usually made in the mid-clavicular line unless a costochrondral graft is needed, then it is more medial. The incision is down to bone and a careful circumferential subperiosteal dissection is carried out using a curved stripper. If the cartilage is to be harvested, then a sliver of periosteum is left to hold the cartilage to the bone. Care is needed to stay subperiosteal to prevent pleural damage. The rib is then cut again with care to avoid damaging the pleural lining. Once removed, the cavity should be filled with saline and the chest expanded to look for any air leaks. Closure is in layers with a vacuum drain in place for 24 hours. It may be helpful to perfuse or inject long-acting local anaesthetic solution into the overlying muscle after deep closure for pain relief (see Figures 3.4.20–3.4.23).

Ilium

The anterior approaches are the most common graft site (see Figures 3.4.24–3.4.27). The incision for an open approach should be made on the lateral side of the crest to avoid a painful scar being traumatized by clothes. The approach is straight down to bone through muscle and periosteum. The incision should not be too medial or too low to avoid damaging the lateral nerve of the thigh. Once down to bone, either the lateral or medial tissues should be elevated depending on which surface is to be harvested. On most occasions it will be the medial side, since less muscle stripping is needed and it is said to be less painful. The bone cuts should be made so that most of the crest remains intact. This is done by elevating the crest and hinging lateral, so

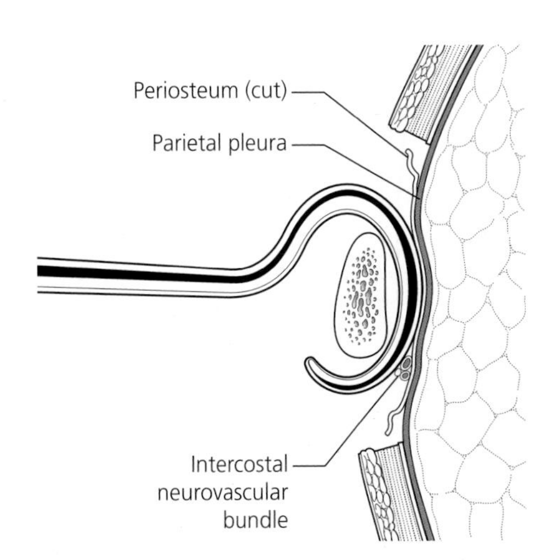

3.4.20 Skin incision for harvesting right scapular blade or lateral border.

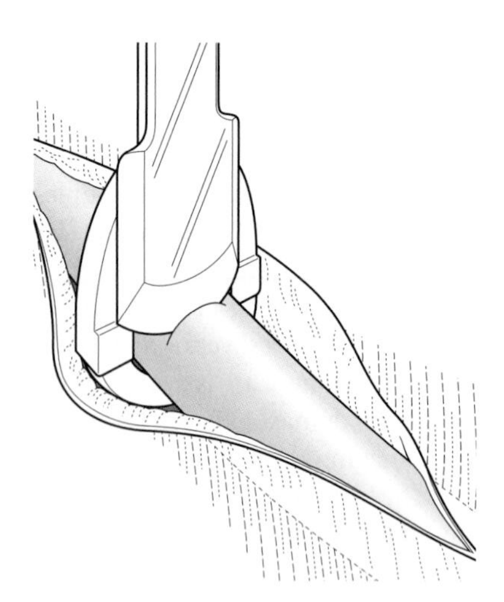

3.4.21 (a) Posterior view of the muscles overlying the right scapula and the triangular space with the circumflex scapular vessels. (b) Exposure of the lateral scapular border after retraction of infraspinatus medially and detachment of the teres major muscle from the inferior angle of the scapula.

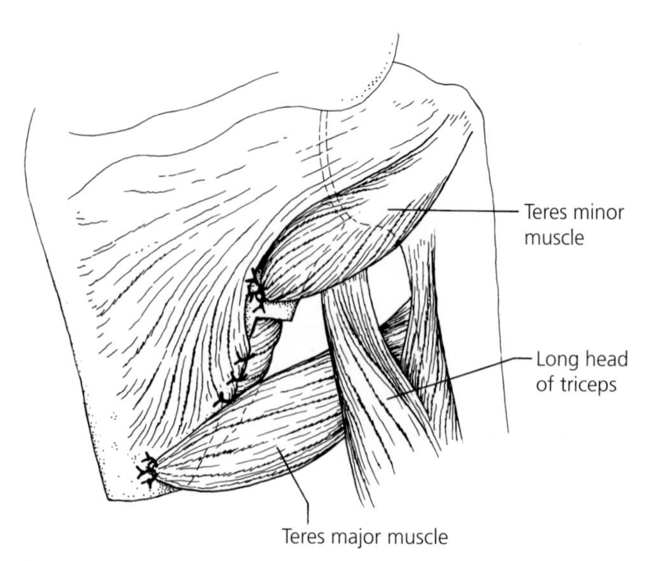

3.4.22 Muscle repair suturing subscapularis muscle to infraspinatus over the bare bone of the lateral scapular border and re-attachment of teres major and minor muscles.

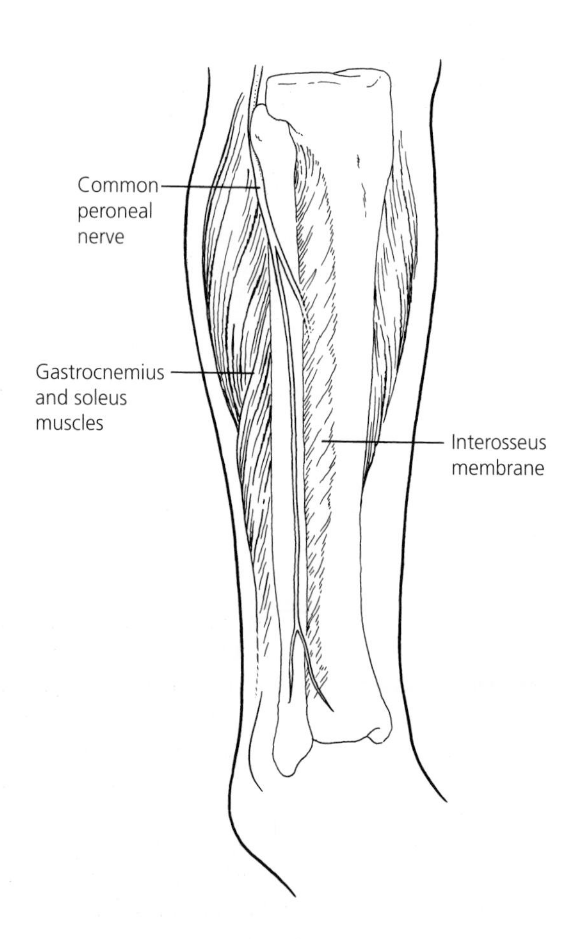

3.4.23 Anterolateral view of right fibula and tibia showing common peroneal nerve coursing lateral to the neck of the fibula.

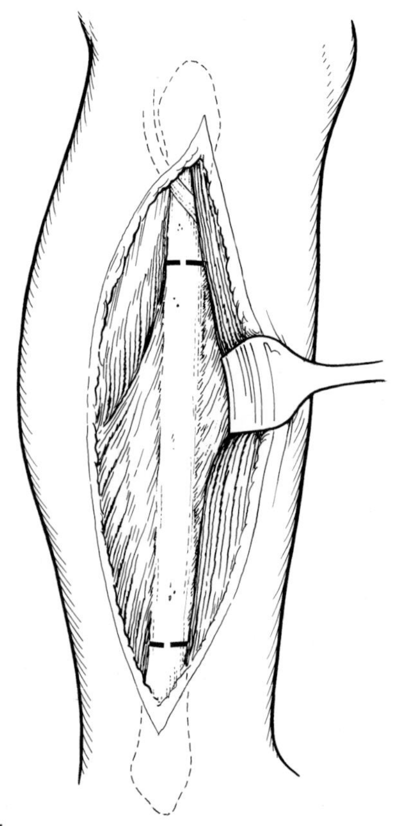

3.4.24 Lateral view of right fibula after retraction of the peroneal muscles anteriorly and soleus muscles posteriorly with proposed sites of bone section.

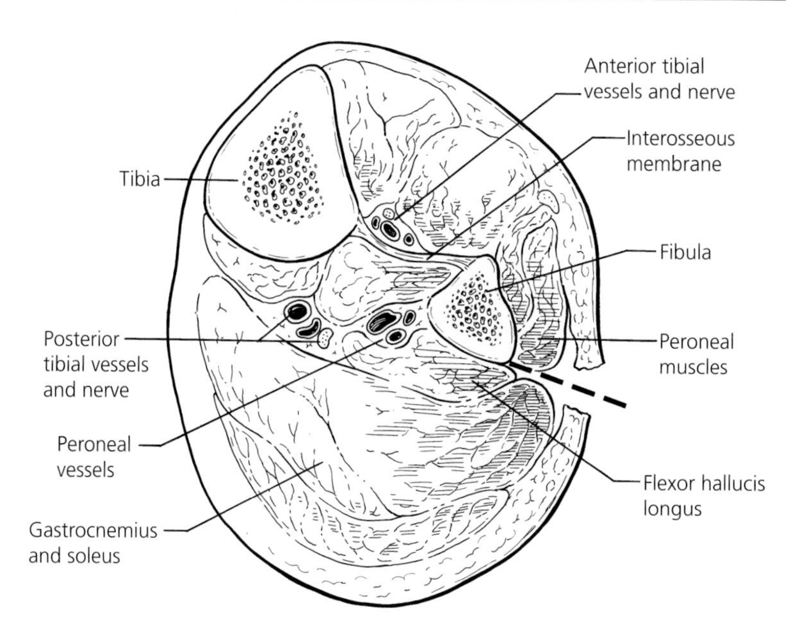

3.4.25 Transverse section of right tibia and fibula from above.

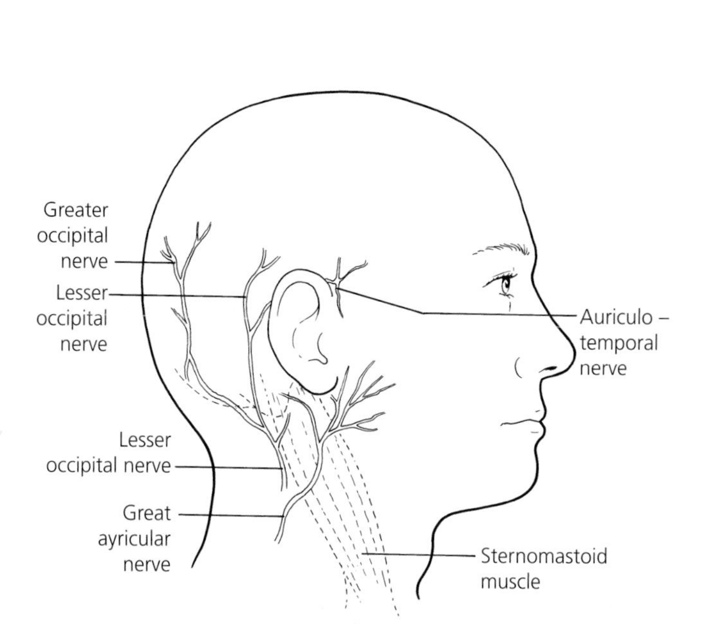

3.4.26 Nerve supply to the right external ear.

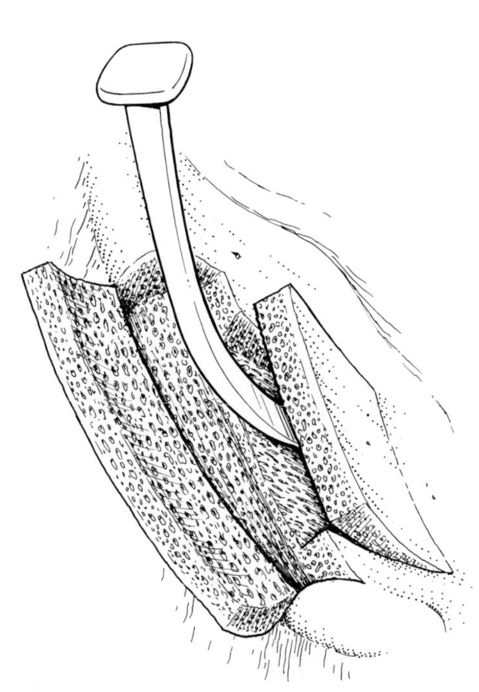

3.4.27 View of left auricle to show potential sites of cartilage harvest

allowing access to the bone for harvesting, and then returned once the harvest is complete. In some circumstances, if only a thin piece of bone is needed, two-thirds of the crest can be preserved and a thin sliver of medial bone removed, if say an orbital floor is being grafted. The iliac crest if temporarily hinged laterally, should be kept attached to periosteum to preserve the blood supply and stability to the replaced crest. Supplementary fixation is not normally needed.

Prior to closure, an epidural catheter should be placed beneath the muscle so a perfusion of long-acting local anaesthetic can be established for the first 24 hours for pain relief. The use of suction drains is controversial. If the drain is placed on the cut bone surface it seems to keep draining blood for days. If the periosteum and muscle are tightly approximated, this seems to reduce the haematoma by tamponade action. Bone wax should be avoided as this produces a foreign body reaction often requiring further exploration of the wound. It may be helpful to place the suction drain just subcutaneously to avoid a more superficial haematoma.

The process can be made less painful by a trephining technique. A small 1 cm stab incision is made on to the anterior crest and a trephine is directed posteriorly/inferiorly. This produces a core of cortical cancellous bone and a much smaller volume than an open procedure. It is closed in two layers.

Tibia

Normally a trephined procedure so cores of cortico-cancellous bone are harvested (see Figure 3.4.28). The bone is taken from the pyramidal shaped plateau, above the shaft and away from the joint, and in children away from the epiphyseal growth centre.

The landmark to make the 5 mm stab incision down to bone is on the medial aspect just above the patella protuberance. The head of the fibula provides a useful guide to the position of the growth centre at the epiphysis, which is above this imaginary horizontal line. Multiple cores are harvested into the pyramidal area. Closure is normally a single layer.

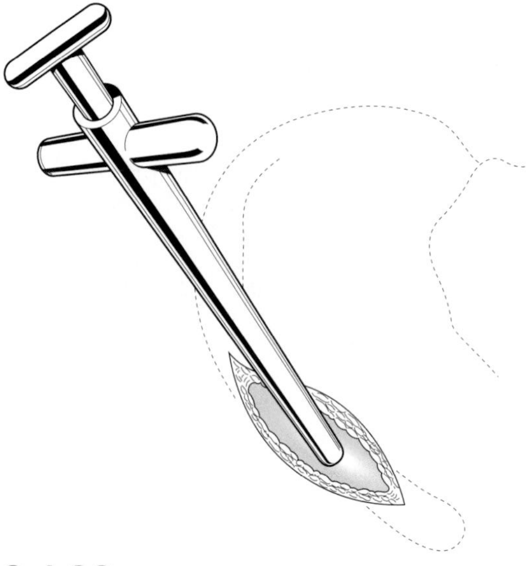

3.4.28 The outer sleeve of the trephine stabilises the trephine on the iliac crest, so a core can be extracted. Normally only a small 'stab' incision is needed.

Intraoral sites

SURGICAL TECHNIQUE

After infiltration with a long-acting local anaesthetic solution, wide exposure via a mucoperiosteal flap is performed to identify and preserve important structures (such as the mental nerve). It is advisable to use a suction device with a bone trap to supplement the harvest.

If the bone is to be removed from the anterior mandible, a small strut of bone is preserved in the midline to maintain the contour of the chin. Two small box-shaped cuts are made in the cortical plate and lifted free. The bone is then curetted from the cavity, which is usually very vascular. It is not necessary to have any suction drainage, but closure of the mucosa should be in two layers, the deeper sutures should pick up the mentalis muscle and ensure its re-insertion high up the alveolus. An elastic adhesive dressing is then applied in the mental groove further pulling up and supporting the muscle insertion to prevent ptosis. Patients will be aware of a feeling of numbness to their anterior teeth, which may persist for a considerable time.

Posterior lateral harvest from the mandible follows the same principle, removing the lateral cortical plate from behind the last molar to the lateral ramus. Closure has less tension as it is supported by the masseter and a drain is not needed.

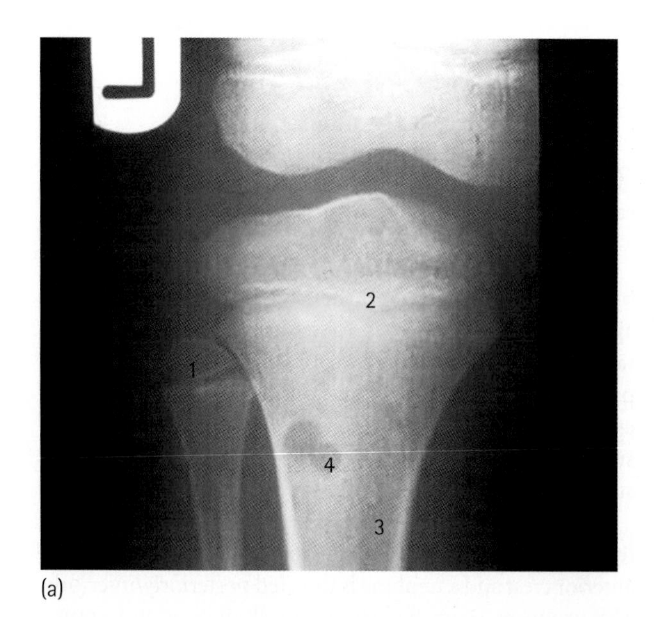

(a)

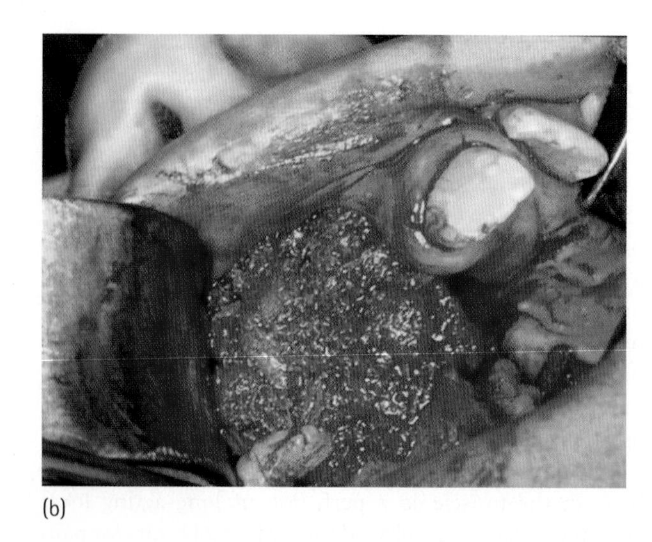

(b)

3.4.29 (a) 1 Head of fibula, which can be easily palpated, below the epiphysis; 2 epiphysis; 3 the trephine should not enter the shaft; 4 entry site. (b) The tibial graft easily fills this cleft alveolar defect.

Table 3.4.3 Frequently used sites for cartilage grafts,

Site	Advantages and disadvantages
Rib	Can be harvested with bone
	Good bulk, but limited length
	May 'grow' in children
	Painful
Ear	Small area, and thin
	Not 'flat'
	Painful
Nasal septum	Invisible scar
	Flat
	Good size, but thin
	Few complications

As with all intrabone harvesting, the yield is small and it is necessary to grind up the cortical plate as well as use the bone trapped from the suction.

Vascularized bone grafts are discussed elsewhere.

Cartilage grafts

There are a number of frequently used sites as outlined in Table 3.4.3.

SURGICAL TECHNIQUE

See Figures 3.4.30–3.4.32.

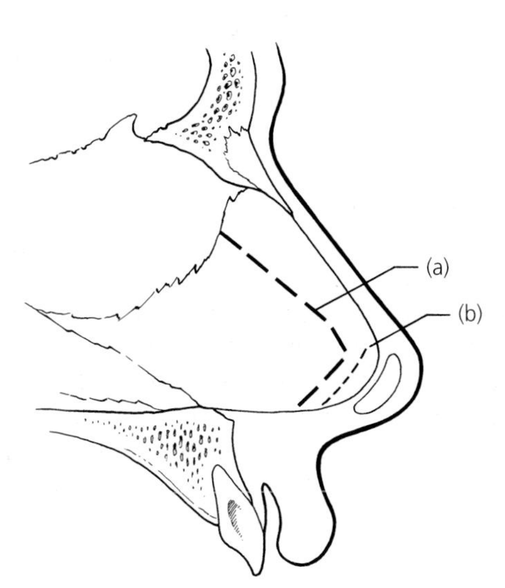

3.4.30 Right lateral view of nasal septum to show (a) mucosal cut anteriorly and (b) septal cut a few millimetres posterior to this.

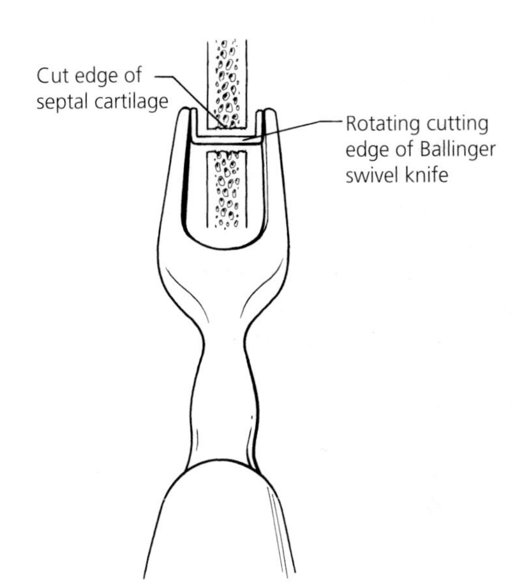

3.4.31 Ballinger swivel knife cutting the septal cartilage.

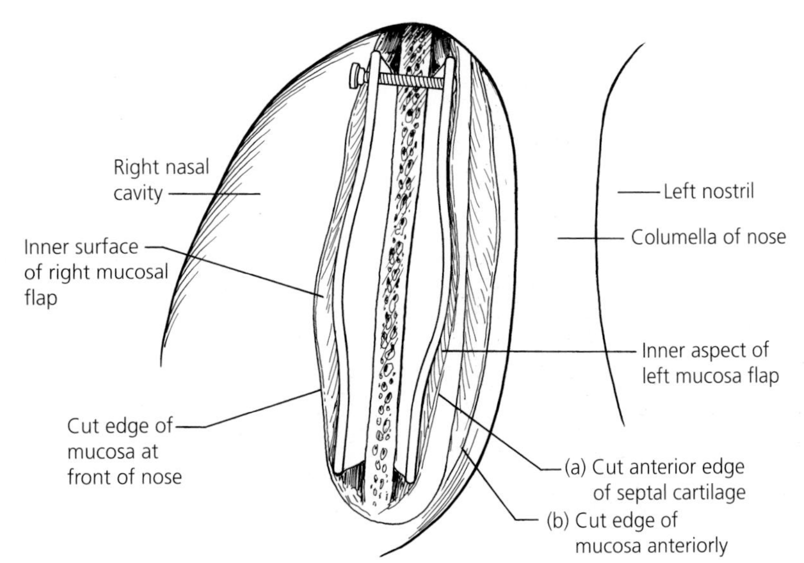

3.4.32 View of the cut surface of the septal cartilage from the front through the right nostril after retraction of the mucoperichondrial flaps with a Killian's speculum.

RIB

This has been described above.

EAR

There are two sites, the small concave conchal bowl area and the longer curved area between the helix and antihelix. The site is infiltrated with long-acting anaesthetic for pain relief and to help the dissection. The flap is raised and the clean cartilage surface exposed. Both sites are approached anteriorly, although they can be harvested from behind if prevention of a visible scar is essential.

The skin flaps are sutured in one layer and a compression dressing with tie over sutures placed to prevent haematoma formation.

NASAL SEPTUM

After infiltration with long-acting local anaesthetic, two approaches can be used. Traditionally, a small curved anterior incision is made on one side of the septum. An alternative is to make a high anterior intraoral incision around the nasal spine. This has the advantage of picking up the septal cartilage low down on the palatal shelf and the stripping of the mucoperiosteum is significantly simpler and easier than the traditional approach.

Stripping of the mucoperiosteum is the difficult part of the procedure and a sharp dissector is essential, to ensure no perforations of the mucosa occur. If perforations occur in both surfaces, a permanent fistula is likely to create an irritating whistling on breathing. Once the mucoperiosteum has been raised on the operative side an incision is made through the cartilage and stripping commenced on the contralateral side. The septum can then be excised and harvested. If the nose is not to 'collapse' a horizontal and anterior vertical strut of cartilage about 5 mm in width must be preserved.

Closure is in a single layer and supplemented by through and through mattress sutures to prevent haematoma formation. Sometimes bilateral packs are placed to prevent haematoma formation but, while a traditional approach, its value in producing compression in the right place is doubtful.

Top tips

- Skin: direct closure is the ideal option.
- Local flaps should be from the same aesthetic zone.
- Grafts rarely have the same colour, texture or thickness and are the worst option.
- Vascularized free tissue transfer is ideal for large defects.
- Bone: non-vascularized bone works well in children, but poorly in older patients.
- Vascularized bone grafts are ideally in the older cancer reconstructions, non-vascularized have a very limited role in these circumstances.
- The bone graft donor sites can have significant morbidity.

FURTHER READING

Fewkes JL, Cheney ML, Pollack SV. *Illustrated atlas of cutaneous surgery.* Philadelphia: JP Lippincott, 1992.

Fonseca RJ, Davis WH. *Reconstructive preprosthetic oral and maxillofacial surgery.* Philadelphia: WB Saunders, 1986.

Jackson IT. *Local flaps in head and neck reconstruction.* St Louis: QMP, 2002.

Miloro M, Larsen P, Ghali GE, Waite P. *Peterson's principles of oral and maxillofacial surgery,* 2nd edn. Philadelphia: BC Decker Inc., 2004.

Ward Booth P, Schendel S, Hausamen J. *Maxillofacial surgery,* 2nd edn. Oxford: Churchill Livingstone, 2006.

3.5

Microvascular surgery – principles

CYRUS J KERAWALA

INTRODUCTION

Within the head and neck, microsurgical reconstruction is employed when other options such as local and distant flap transfers are deemed inappropriate. Although microsurgery is not the first choice in the reconstructive ladder, and may not be the best solution for all defects, it offers the surgeon a wide range of possibilities for complex reconstruction.

INDICATIONS

These include:

- replacement of vital structures, e.g. glossectomy defect;
- obliteration of cavities, e.g. maxillectomy defect;
- bone reconstruction, e.g. following mandibular resection;
- replacement of muscle and nerve function, e.g. facial reanimation;
- alimentary tract reconstruction, e.g. after laryngo-pharyngectomy.

CONTRAINDICATIONS

Microsurgical transfers are commonly long and technically demanding operations. In addition, emergency re-intervention may be necessary. Contraindications for this type of procedure therefore include medical illnesses that preclude the ability of a patient to tolerate prolonged anaesthesia. Advanced age is not necessarily a contraindication, nor is a potentially severe medical problem as long as it is well controlled.

PRE-OPERATIVE WORK-UP

A comprehensive history and physical examination is mandatory, as is close liaison with involved anaesthetic staff. Pre-optimization of patients may be advantageous in selected cases. Many patients undergoing microsurgery will have already undergone imaging dependent on their primary disease but additional investigations specific to the reconstruction may also be appropriate, for example angiography.

SELECTION OF DONOR SITE

Decision-making is critical to the success of microsurgery. The choice of optimal flap is based on a combination of factors that include the type of tissue required, pedicle length and flap reliability. In addition, consideration should be given to donor site morbidity.

Within the head and neck, a large number of options exist. The microsurgeon should be familiar with the majority although some will be used more than others. There should be avoidance of flap 'favourites' since ultimately each defect should be reconstructed on its merits.

Within the head and neck, most forms of reconstruction can be comfortably undertaken with ten flaps:

- radial forearm free flap (RFFF);
- anterolateral thigh flap (ALT);
- lateral arm flap;
- rectus abdominus;
- latisimus dorsi;
- fibular;
- vascularized iliac crest (DCIA);
- scapular/parascapular;
- jejunum;
- gracilus.

In broad terms, the above can be divided into three groups, namely soft tissue flaps, hard tissue flaps and combinations. The choice of soft tissue flap very much depends upon the volume of the defect. The body habitus of the patient in part determines bulk although variation in operating technique may overcome this (e.g. intraoperative thinning of ALT). In bony reconstruction, the operating surgeon has a lesser degree of control (e.g. double-barrelled fibular).

MICROSURGICAL PRINCIPLES

Attention to detail is mandatory. Having planned the flap based on the size and type of tissue needed, an alternative reconstruction should always be considered as a 'lifeboat'. Recipient vessel location should be planned outwith potential zones of injury (e.g. previous radiotherapy fields). Two-team operating should be employed wherever possible to ensure that a well-rested surgeon is available for the more technically challenging aspects of the operation.

The overall plan should be discussed with the anaesthetist, including details of the length of procedure and required positioning of the patient. Potential donor sites should be devoid of vascular access. During the operation and in the immediate post-operative period, vasoconstrictors should be avoided. The patient should be adequately hydrated with a good central venous pressure. Likewise, the patient's core temperature should be maintained to avoid vasospasm. If hypotensive anaesthesia is adopted at any stage (e.g. during ablation) then this should be reversed prior to microsurgery.

The main enemy of the microvascular surgeon is fatigue. Physical exertion, alcohol and caffeine should be avoided for at least 24 hours in individuals prone to a tremor. The operator should take short breaks to minimize waning performance that can accompany long periods of concentration. Above all, both the microsurgeon and assistant should feel physically comfortable throughout with appropriate seating.

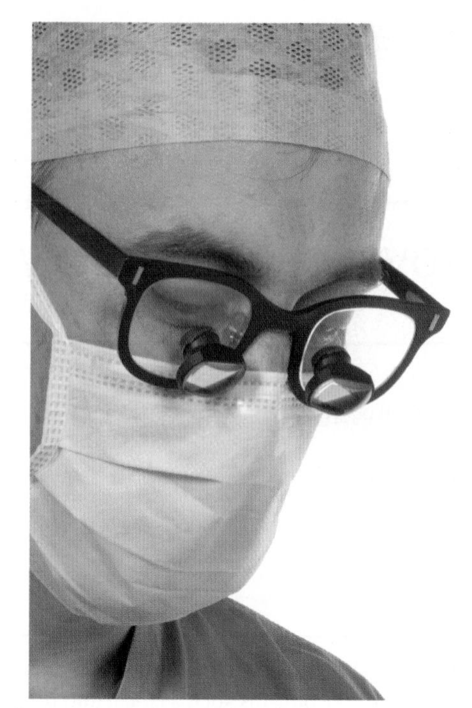

3.5.1 Binocular loupes.

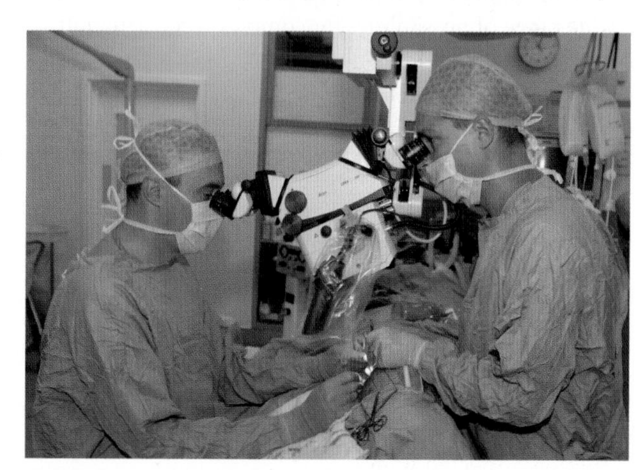

3.5.2 Double-headed operating microscope.

Optical systems

- **Magnifying ocular loupes**. Loupes are often more convenient than the microscope for preliminary dissection and can be used for anastamosis of vessels greater than 3 mm in diameter. Simple models with elasticated headbands magnify up to 1.8×, while more sophisticated binocular loupes fitted to spectacles can provide up to 4× magnification (Figure 3.5.1). Loupes with higher magnifications tend to have small fields of vision and depth of focus.
- **Operating microscope.** Although the operating microscope has many advantages in providing magnification and illumination, it brings with it additional problems of cost, set-up time and intraoperative positioning. A double-headed operating microscope with the surgeon and assistant at opposite sides is essential for head and neck reconstruction (Figure 3.5.2). Most commonly, this set up is achieved through the use of beam splitters so that the surgeon and assistant have the same view. Coaxial illumination is also important to avoid shadows. Due to the frequent need for changing magnification, zoom systems operated by either a foot or finger should be incorporated. Through-the-microscope photographic or DVD capabilities enhance teaching and documentation.

Instrumentation

Most microsurgical procedures can be performed with a simple, well-maintained basic set of instruments (Figure 3.5.3).

- **Jeweller's or watchmaker's forceps** (hereafter called microsurgical forceps). The tips of these must meet evenly over a length of at least 2 mm.

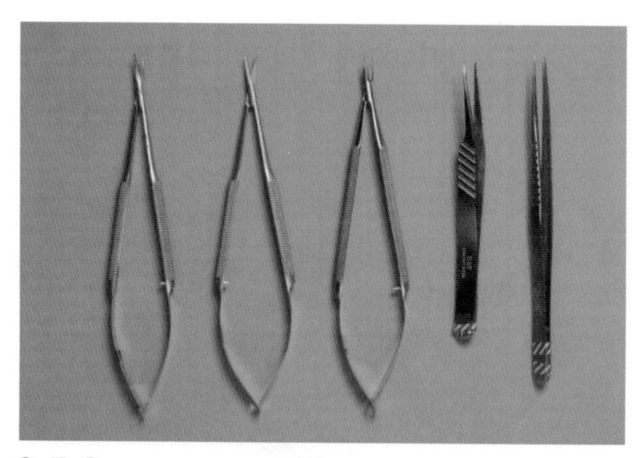

3.5.3 Microvascular instruments.

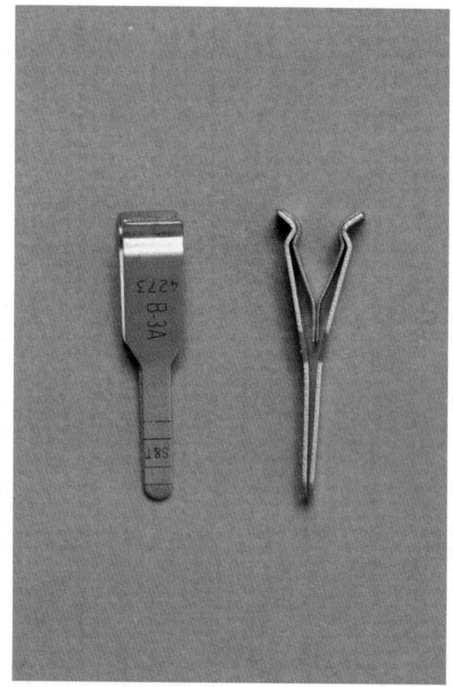

3.5.4 Vessel clamps

- **Vessel dilators.** These are microsurgical forceps rounded and polished at the tip. Closed tips can be inserted into the end of a divided vessel with minimal trauma.
- **Needle holders.** Purpose-designed models have spring-loaded handles that have a round or flat grip and are curved, angled or straight depending on operator preference.
- **Dissecting scissors.** These should be spring-handled. The curved blades can be short or long.
- **Adventitia scissors.** These are identical to dissecting scissors but have straight blades.
- **Vessel clamps** (Figure 3.5.4). Spring-loaded varieties are available for arteries and veins. Some surgeons also use double-approximater clamps to aid anastamosis.
- **Instrument case.** A metal-lined case with rubber spigots provides insurance against instrument damage.

At least two sets of microvascular instruments should be available in case emergency re-operation is necessary. Whenever instruments are not in immediate use the tips should be protected with rubber tubing. Regular demagnetization is necessary.

BASIC ANASTAMOTIC TECHNIQUE

Essentials for a patent anastamosis

There are several essential requirements to ensure an adequate anastamosis with long-term patency.

- There should be meticulous, atraumatic dissection of involved vessels with ligation or coagulation of branches.
- The vessel wall and the intima at the site of the intended anastamosis must be resected to apparently normal tissue.
- Adequate blood flow should be demonstrated from the recipient artery prior to anastamosis. If flow is impaired, dilation can be attempted or pharmacological agents applied (e.g. papaverin).
- Anastamoses should be completed without tension, employing vessel immobilization or vein grafts as necessary.
- Overhanging adventitia should be removed and sutures placed without trauma to the intima. All traces of contaminants should be irrigated with heparinized solutions (100 U/mL) prior to completion of the anastamosis.

End-to-end anastamosis techniques

Personal preference means that some surgeons use interrupted sutures and some prefer a continuous pattern. The technique most commonly taught is the joining of vessels end-to-end using a triangulation method whereby two stay sutures are inserted 120° apart so that when they are placed under tension the front wall of the anastamosis is stretched laterally (Figure 3.5.5). As a result, the back wall tends to fall away and is less likely to be picked up inadvertently. In the clinical situation this is not always possible and many prefer two sutures at 180°.

After vessels have been prepared, the two stay sutures should be placed and the ends left long, such that they can be anchored to the cleats of a double clamp or held by an assistant. The front wall is then sutured using square or reef knots that must lie flat against the anastamosis line so that the threads do not project into the vessel lumen (Figure 3.5.6). Two or more co-optation sutures are then placed between the stay sutures before the vessel is rotated through

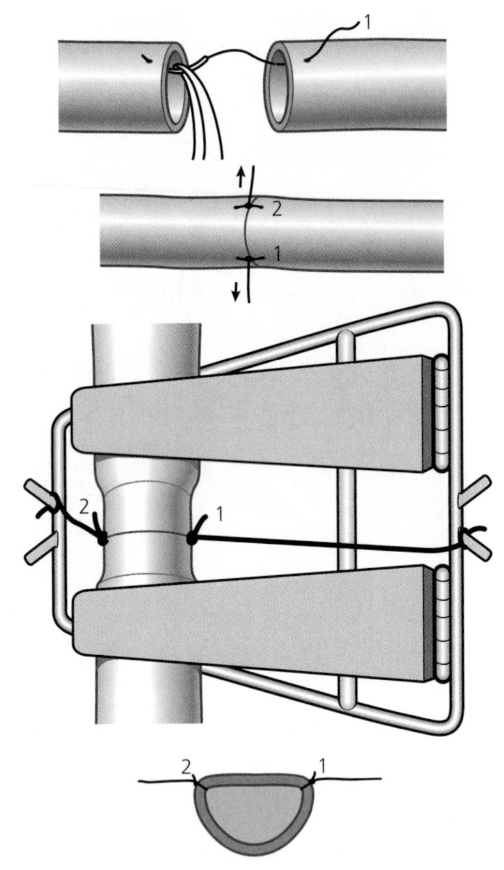

3.5.5 Triangulation method of vessel approximation.

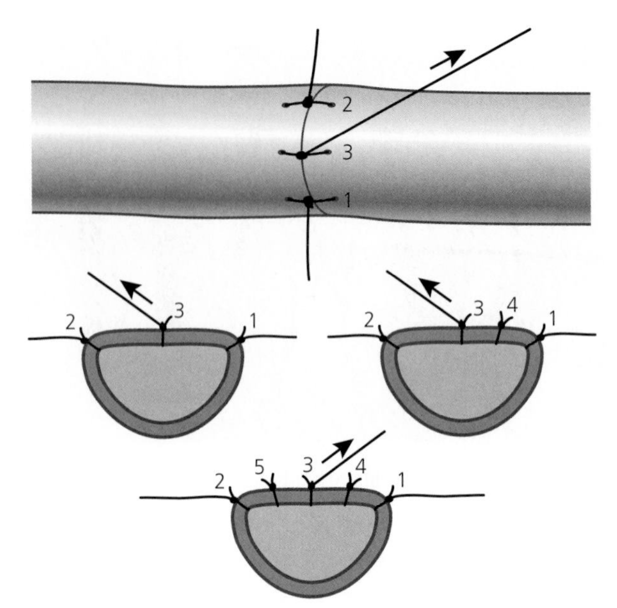

3.5.6 Completion of front wall co-optation.

180°. The anastamosis should be critically appraised before the back wall is closed (Figure 3.5.7).

The venous anastamoses is performed in an identical manner to the artery but it can be technically more demanding because the absence of a substantial muscularis means the vein wall collapses easily. Minimal adventitial stripping is therefore recommended.

Once the anastamosis is complete, the necessary clamps are released and blood flow observed under magnification. An initial small ooze commonly occurs, but generally stops within a few minutes. Pulsatile bleeding requires placement of further sutures.

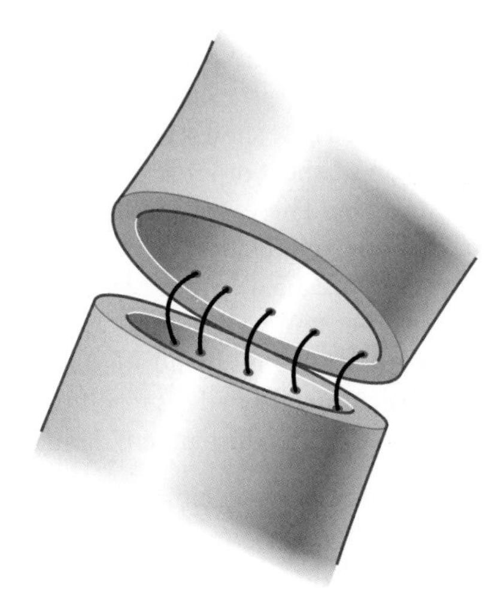

3.5.7 Critically appraise rotated vessel before back wall closure.

End-to-side anastamosis technique

The arteriotomy or venotomy in the recipient vessel is the most critical step in this procedure since it must match the size of the vessel to be anastamosed. The adventitia around the intended site should be carefully removed so that it does not protrude into the newly formed lumen. Stay sutures are initially placed at the proximal and distal ends of the arteriotomy or venotomy (Figure 3.5.8). Secondary co-aptation sutures are then inserted along the anastamosis line with either the front or back wall being closed first depending on operator preference (Figure 3.5.9).

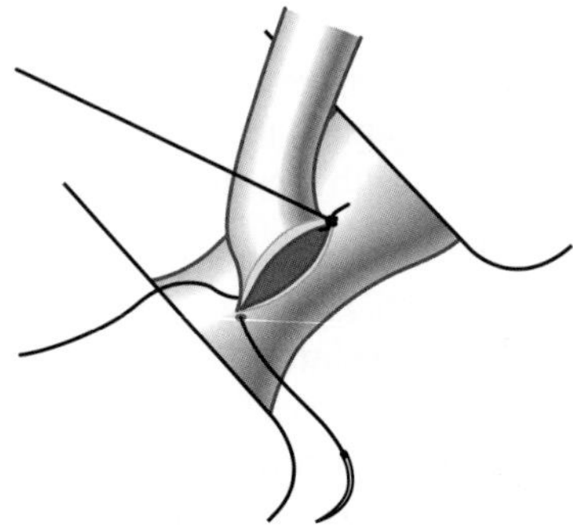

3.5.8 Stay sutures in end-to-side anastamosis.

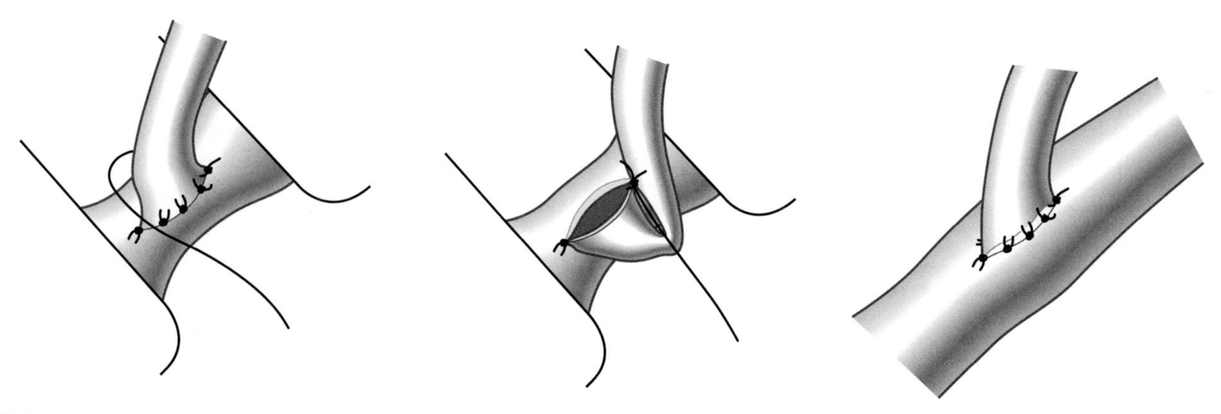

3.5.9 Completion of end-to-side anastamosis.

Size discrepancy

Discrepancy in vessel size can be solved by performing an end-to-side anastamosis. Alternatively the smaller vessel can be dilated, transecting on a 45° diagonal (Figure 3.5.10) or incised to create a fishtail (Figure 3.5.11).

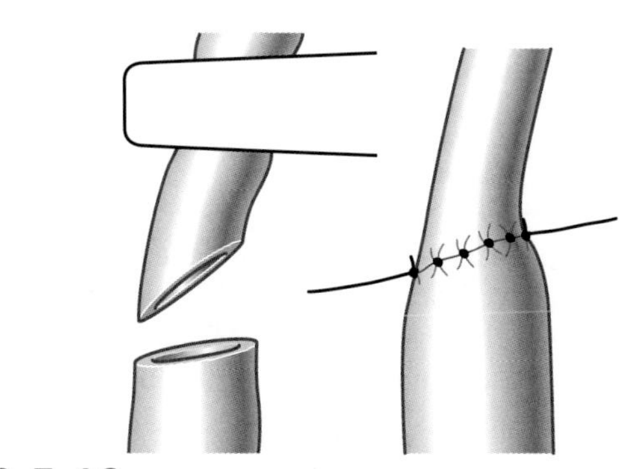

3.5.10 Diagonal transaction of vessel.

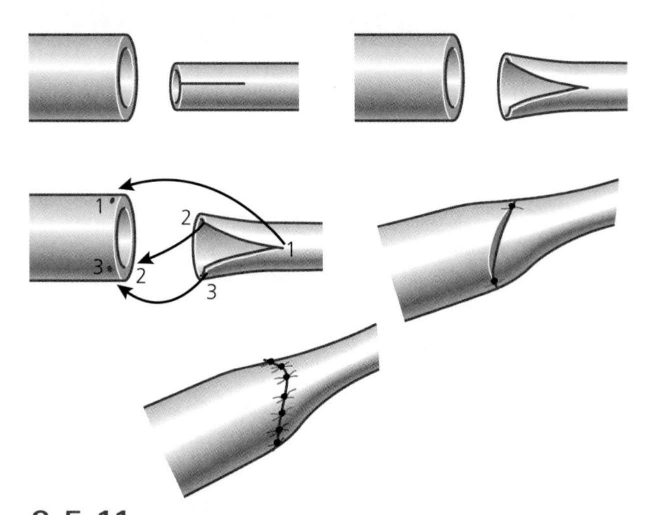

3.5.11 Fishtail technique.

Assessment of suture lines

A critical assessment should be made prior to accepting the anastamosis. The most common errors in technique include:

- stitches too tight;
- stitches too loose so that a loop of material intrudes into the lumen;
- too many or too few sutures;
- suture holes not equidistant from the edge;
- uneven spacing between sutures;
- inversion or eversion of tissue edges.

Patency test

Anastamotic patency can be assessed in a variety of ways. Arterial patency is indicated by well-dilated vessels demonstrating either pulsatile elongation or expansile pulsation. The empty and refilled patency test ('milking' an anastamosis) is traumatic and should be performed as gently and infrequently as possible. Ultimately, anastamotic patency can be assessed by a return of colour and capillary refill to the revascularized tissue.

POST-OPERATIVE CARE

Post-operative staff must be familiar with free flap monitoring and the general care of the microsurgery patient. A hyperdynamic circulation with adequate hydration, filling pressures, urine output and body temperature should be the aim. Pain should be controlled to prevent anxiety that in turn leads to vasoconstriction. Anti-coagulation may be used depending on the surgeon's preference (e.g. Dextran 40, heparin, aspirin).

Free flap monitoring is also dependent on preference. The criterion standard remains careful and regular clinical examination of the flap (colour, skin turgor, refill etc.). Some surgeons prefer a needle test which should result in the oozing of bright red blood up to a minute after the needle is withdrawn. Other monitoring techniques include:

- surface/implantable Doppler ultrasound;
- temperature monitoring;
- pulse oximetry;
- intravenous fluorescein;
- near infrared spectroscopy.

If vascular compromise is suspected within a free flap, immediate measures should be taken:

- general assessment of the patient (e.g. exclusion of hypotension);
- repositioning of the patient to relieve possible pedicle compromise;
- exclusion of haematoma;
- in the absence of haematoma release of the vacuum on any relevant drain in case the pedicle is in contact with the drain holes;
- removal of compressive dressings or tight sutures.

If such simple manoeuvres are not successful, immediate re-exploration is critical as long as the patient's general condition allows it.

COMPLICATIONS

Microsurgical operations are by their very nature physiologically traumatic for the patient. Potential major complications may occur including myocardial infarction, stroke and death. Informed consent is mandatory and should include detailed discussions with appropriate warnings to include:

- intra- and post-operative bleeding, with possible transfusion;
- donor and recipient site infection;
- morbidity specific to the free flap used;
- the need for emergency re-operation;
- partial or total flap loss;
- possible revisionary operations (e.g. flap thinning).

RECIPIENT VESSEL SELECTION

The delivery of blood into and out of the flap depends on meticulous harvesting of the nutrient pedicle, careful preparation of the recipient vasculature and a technically perfect anastamosis. Care must also be given to the geometry of the pedicle to prevent tension and kinking caused by head mobility.

General considerations

Recipient vessel selection is one of the most critical steps in ensuring a successful outcome. Careful intraoperative selection greatly facilitates the process of revascularization and as a result vessels should be selected and isolated prior to flap division to minimize the ischaemic period. The majority of the flap insetting should be completed prior to the anastamosis since this is not only facilitated by working on an ischaemic flap but the position of the donor vessels becomes fixed after insetting which allows tension on the vascular pedicle to be predicted.

Apart from availability, a number of other factors must be considered when selecting recipient vessels. The choice of vessel is in part limited by the site of the defect and particular flap employed (e.g. in the DCIA, the venae commitantes can be unsuitable for anastamosis until they join to produce a vein of sufficient calibre). The presence of a previous ipsilateral radical neck dissection may limit the availability of recipient vessels. Advanced age and previous irradiation may also lead to athrosclerosis.

Recipient artery selection

The two major sources of arteries are branches of the external carotid artery and the thyrocervical trunk. Due to their proximity to defects, the lower branches of the former are the most commonly employed. However, the thyrocervical trunk and in particular its transverse cervical artery (TCA) are almost always preserved following neck dissections and provide a useful alternative. The TCA can be traced for a significant distance underneath the trapezius muscle and comfortably transposed into the mid portion of the neck. This vessel is far less prone to athrosclerosis than the external carotid artery and usually lies outside the area of most intense radiation therapy.

Recipient vein selection

There are three primary recipient veins in the neck. While the internal jugular vein or its immediate branches serve an excellent outflow, the external jugular and transverse cervical veins are alternatives. The anterior jugular veins should be avoided since its caudal portion is at risk during tracheostomy. The cephalic vein may be used as a source of vein grafts or can be used as a recipient vein if traced distally into the arm and then transposed over the clavicle.

Top tips

- For the novice microvascular surgeon repeated *in vitro* practice is essential.
- The microsurgeon should be well rested prior to the operation and comfortable throughout it.
- Flaps used should reflect anatomical and functional considerations rather than the surgeon's favourite.
- The surgeon should be critical about every suture placed. If he or she is not satisfied then that suture should be replaced.
- The surgeon should be critical about the completed anastamosis. It is far better to repeat an anastamosis during the time of primary surgery than return to it once vascular compromise is apparent hours later.
- Recipient artery and vein selection is imperative with vessels being chosen outside any potentially compromised field.

FURTHER READING

Brown JS, Devin JC, Magennis P *et al.* Factors that influence the outcome of salvage in free tissue transfer. *British Journal of Oral and Maxillofacial Surgery* 2003; **41**: 16–20.

Bui DT, Cordeiro PG, Hu QY *et al.* Free flap reexploration: indications, treatment, and outcomes in 1193 free flaps. *Plastic and Reconstructive Surgery* 2007; **119**: 2092–100.

Chalian AA, Anderson TD, Weinstein GS, Weber RS. Internal jugular vein versus external jugular vein anastamosis: implications for successful free tissue transfer. *Head and Neck* 2001; **23**: 475–8.

Chen KT, Mardini S, Chuang DC *et al.* Timing of presentation of the first sings of vascular compromise dictates the salvage outcome of free flap transfers. *Plastic and Reconstructive Surgery* 2007; **120**: 187–95.

Urken M, Cheney M, Sullivan M, Biller H. *Atlas of regional free flaps for head and neck reconstruction.* New York: Raven Press, 1995.

3.6

Radial forearm flap

ANDREW E BROWN, CHRISTOPHER M AVERY

PRINCIPLES AND JUSTIFICATION

The radial forearm flap may be harvested as a fasciocutaneous, septocutaneous, fascial or osteocutaneous flap, including a sensory nerve or the palmaris longus tendon if required. The flap is an accepted 'workhorse' for oral reconstruction, providing a large area of relatively hairless and thin pliable skin. It is straightforward to raise with a long vascular pedicle. Any criticism is levelled at the morbidity of the donor site; in particular the cosmetic defect, poor or delayed skin graft healing, and tendon exposure. Over 70 per cent of the strength of the original radius is lost after harvest of an osteocutaneous flap. The mean incidence of reported fracture of the remaining radius is 25 per cent. Fracture results in significant morbidity and often requires secondary surgery. Steps that can be taken to minimize these complications include a suprafascial dissection technique to improve donor site healing and use of prophylactic internal fixation to reduce the fracture risk.

INDICATIONS

- Reconstructing mobile areas of the oral cavity and oropharynx.
- Not an ideal cosmetic replacement for facial skin but useful for reconstruction of lip and circumoral defects when the palmaris longus tendon improves lip competence.
- Fascial flaps are less dimensionally stable and heal by secondary 'mucosalization'. They can be used for small palatal defects or over areas of exposed bone.
- Indications for the osteocutaneous flap have declined as other donor sites offer greater volume of medullary bone or better quality cortical bone. It retains a 'niche' role for small volume bone defects, such as the anterior maxillary alveolus and orbital rim. It may still be useful for reconstructing the thin edentulous mandible, particularly if associated with a significant soft tissue defect or when implant placement is unlikely, and where the general medical or vascular status precludes the use of alternative flaps.
- The role of sensate flaps remains controversial with no proven functional or quality of life benefit.
- A fascial flap may be prelaminated with a mucosal graft as a delayed procedure for elective reconstruction of intraoral defects.

SURGICAL ANATOMY

In the distal forearm, the radial artery lies in the superficial subcutaneous tissues between the brachioradialis and flexor carpi radialis tendons (see Figure 3.6.1). It is enveloped by the conjoining of two layers of deep fascia and gives off multiple small vessels (septocutaneous perforators) to form a subdermal plexus supplying the overlying skin. Similar branches pass to the underlying musculature and periosteum of the radius. Drainage of the flap is via the radial venae comitantes and/or the superficial subcutaneous veins, often the cephalic vein. A single vena comitans or confluent vein provides satisfactory venous drainage.

Although conventionally raised as a fasciocutaneous flap, the deep fascia is not essential for skin perfusion (see Figure 3.6.2). The enveloping fascia around the pedicle may be opened and a septocutaneous flap elevated in the suprafascial plane. If the fascial covering of the flexor tendons is retained, the problems associated with skin graft healing are minimized when compared with the subfascial donor defect.

A branch of the lateral or medial cutaneous nerve of the forearm is incorporated if a sensate flap is required.

PRE-OPERATIVE

The non-dominant forearm is preferred (see Figure 3.6.3). The sufficiency of the residual ulnar supply to the hand is confirmed by an Allen test, supplemented by Doppler studies if required. The entire skin of the forearm may be safely transferred but most intraoral defects are reconstructed with flaps of 7 cm × 5 cm or smaller. The flap is designed with the artery towards the lateral aspect to avoid the more hirsute skin and an unsightly extension over the radial aspect of the forearm. Small defects may be closed with an ulnar rotation flap or a V to Y closure technique, although this may cause additional oedema and numbness.

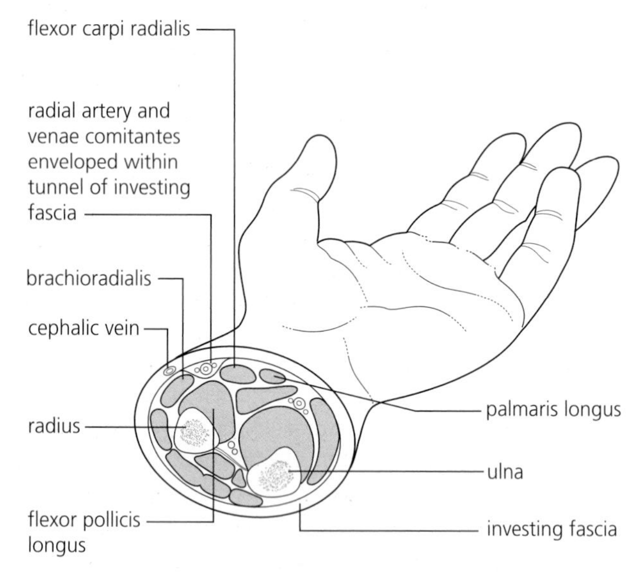

3.6.1 Transverse section through left forearm.

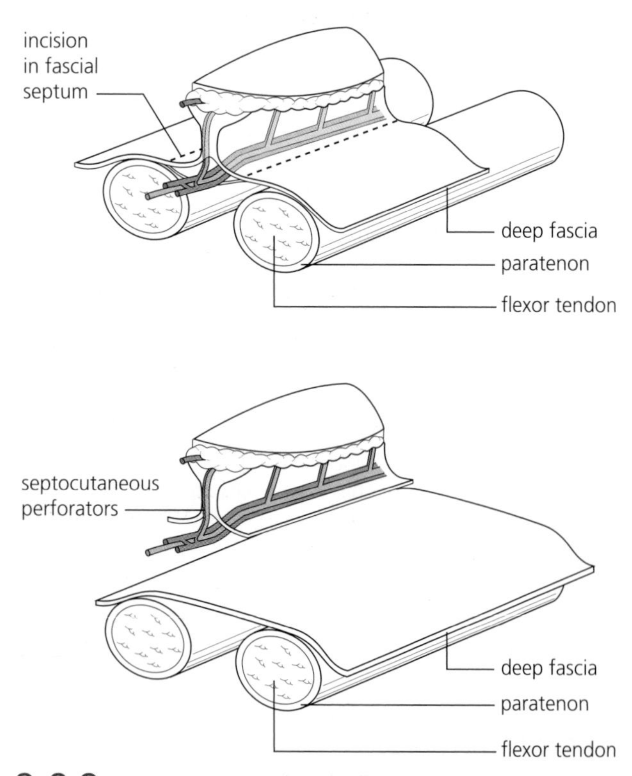

3.6.2 Relationship of investing fascia to vascular pedicle and underlying tendons (septocutaneous perforators illustrated longer than *in vivo* for clarity).

OPERATION

Fasciocutaneous flap

INCISION AND INITIAL DISSECTION

The flap is raised under tourniquet control (200 mmHg pressure) following partial exsanguination by elevation. Binocular loupes are useful to identify small feeding vessels that should be carefully managed with bipolar diathermy or ligation clips. Starting at the medial (ulnar) border of the skin paddle, the incision is made through skin, subcutaneous fat and fascia to expose the underlying muscle. The incision is extended around the proximal and distal aspects. The assistant applies gentle traction to facilitate sharp dissection beneath the fascia from medial to lateral. If required, a superficial vein or sensory nerve is preserved at the proximal aspect. Remain in the subfascial plane and take care to avoid damaging the paratenon as palmaris longus and the medial edge of the flexor carpi radialis are exposed (see Figure 3.6.4).

IDENTIFICATION OF THE PEDICLE

As the lateral (radial) border of flexor carpi radialis is approached, take care to continue in the subfascial plane and identify flexor pollicis longus lying at a deeper level. This avoids inadvertent detachment of the vascular pedicle now seen on the undersurface of the flap. Identify, clamp and divide the radial artery at the distal edge of the flap (see Figure 3.6.5).

FLAP MOBILIZATION

The circumferential incision is completed on the lateral (radial) aspect ensuring that the pedicle lies within the

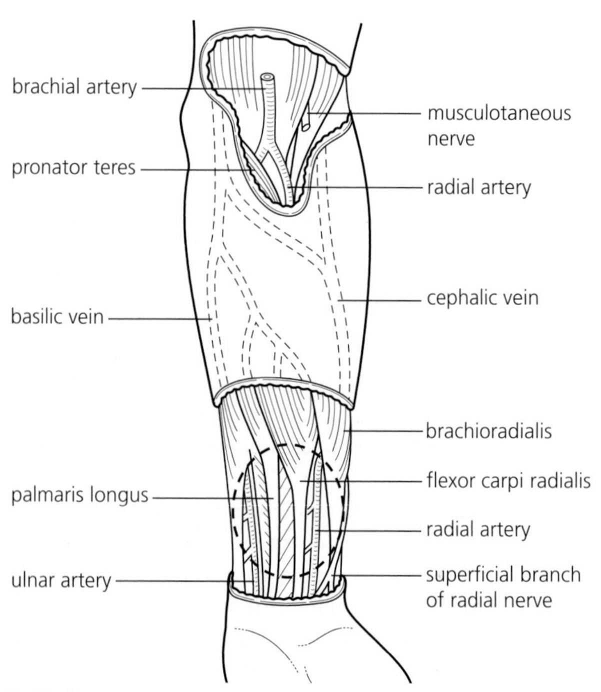

3.6.3 Anterior aspect of left forearm showing relevant anatomical structures.

margins of the flap. The brachioradialis tendon is exposed and retracted laterally to identify and protect the superficial sensory branch of the radial nerve. The skin paddle is now elevated taking care to cauterize any small vessels passing from the radial artery to the underlying muscle and bone. Elevation is facilitated by opening the distal part of the forearm incision. Proximal subcutaneous dissection of a superficial vein or sensory nerve will be required if these are to be included. The cephalic vein, with the lateral cutaneous nerve, usually lies at the lateral edge of the positioned flap (see Figure 3.6.6).

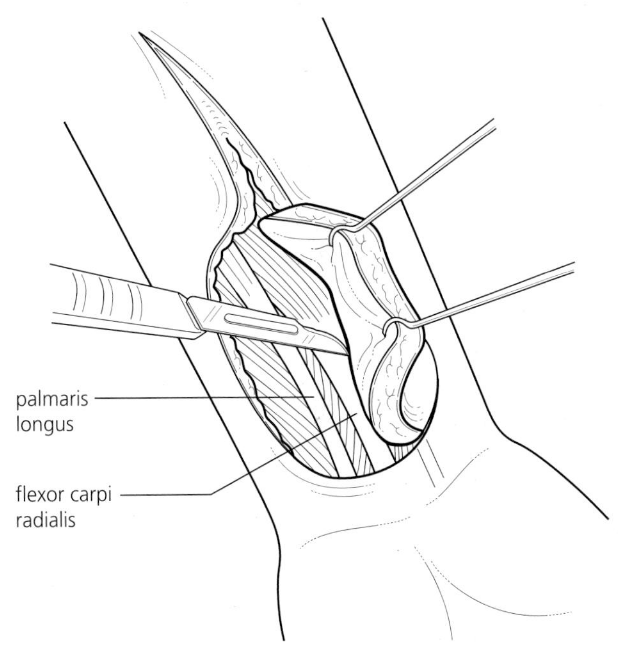

3.6.4 Fasciocutaneous flap – medial (ulnar) elevation in subfascial plane.

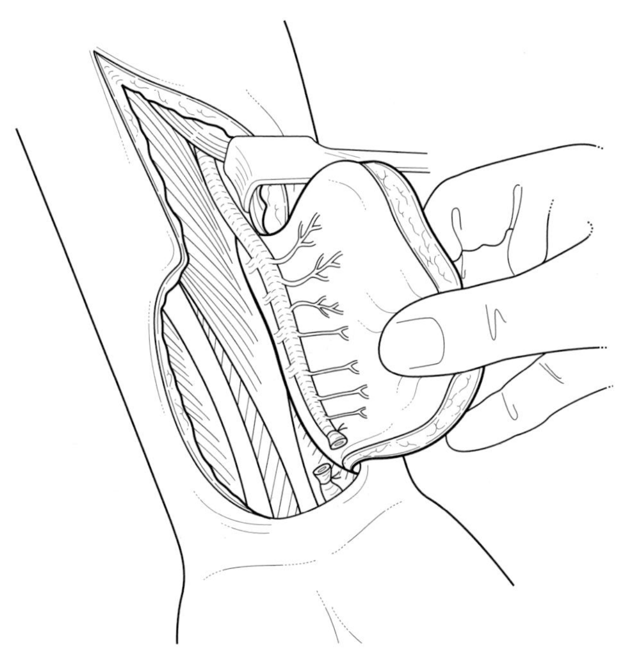

3.6.5 Fasciocutaneous flap – identification of radial vascular pedicle on deep surface with ligation distally.

COMPLETION OF ELEVATION

The forearm incision is opened fully, incorporating a z-plasty in the cubital fossa if extended into this area. The fascial septum between brachioradialis and flexor carpi radialis is opened to expose the whole arterial pedicle. The skin flap is held in a damp swab and gently lifted as dissection along the pedicle proceeds. Small side branches are carefully ligated or cauterized. The limit of the arterial pedicle is the bifurcation of the brachial artery but such length is rarely needed and the radial recurrent artery, just distal to the bifurcation, can often be spared. The deep and superficial venous systems usually unite at the cubital fossa and the superficial vein can be dissected beyond this confluence to provide additional venous pedicle length if required.

DETACHMENT OF THE FLAP AND DONOR SITE CLOSURE

The tourniquet is released and perfusion of the flap and hand is checked. Complete hemostasis is obtained along the pedicle and on the undersurface of the flap. Allow time for relaxation of small vessel spasm and apply topical papaverine if necessary. Closure of the distal forearm incision may be performed at this stage. The flexor tendons are oversewn with muscle if possible and the donor defect repaired with a full thickness skin graft from the inguinal crease or inner arm. A partial thickness graft from the upper outer arm or thigh is used for large defects. The veins may be divided first to assess the venous outflow before clamping and dividing the arterial pedicle. A suction drain is inserted and the proximal forearm wound closed. Alternatively, a negative pressure wound dressing is applied which has the advantage of helping the skin graft to adhere to the donor site.

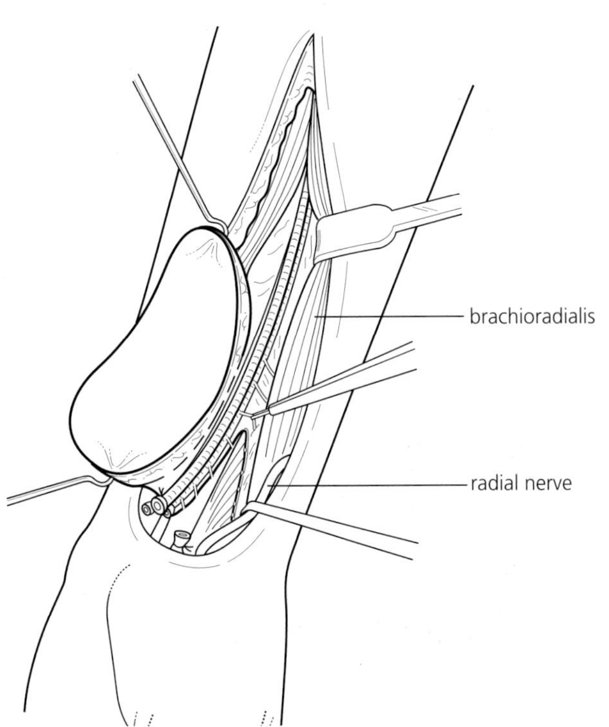

3.6.6 Fasciocutaneous flap – completion of elevation from lateral (radial) aspect with diathermy of communicating vessels passing to deeper structures.

Septocutaneous flap

PLANE OF THE SUPRAFASCIAL DISSECTION

The skin is incised to expose the deep fascia. Sharp dissection is carried out in the immediate suprafascial plane. The technique is slightly more demanding and binocular loupes are advised. Elevation begins at the ulnar (medial) border as usual and progresses laterally over flexor carpi radialis, stopping short of the radial artery. A few small perforating vessels to the inferior surface of the flap are cauterized (see Figure 3.6.7).

DISSECTION ALONG THE DISTAL PEDICLE

The distal end of the arterial pedicle is ligated and divided. Lifting the pedicle exposes the floor of the fascial envelope between the flexor tendons. The medial and lateral aspects of this envelope are incised parallel and close to the pedicle. The floor of the fascial envelope becomes progressively thinner as the flap is elevated and larger perforating vessels from the undersurface of the pedicle are ligated. Dissection on the radial aspect is in the plane of the superficial radial nerve, taking care not to disrupt the overlying subcutaneous plexus. The forearm skin and fascia overlying the brachioradialis and flexor carpi radialis is incised to retract these muscles and the proximal dissection of the pedicle is completed as described above. Once the proximal edge of the flap has been reached the forearm, skin and fascia overlying the brachioradialis and flexor carpi radialis is incised to retract these muscles. The proximal dissection of the pedicle is completed as described above. The donor site remains largely covered with investing deep fascia and often some deep subcutaneous tissue on the radial aspect. It is usually repaired with a full thickness skin graft together with a negative pressure wound dressing (see Figure 3.6.8).

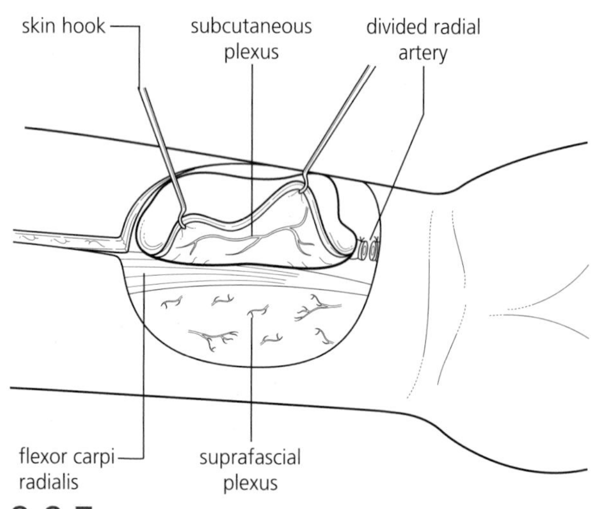

3.6.7 Suprafascial flap – dissection deep to subcutaneous plexus and immediately superficial to investing fascia.

Composite osteocutaneous flap

SURFACE MARKINGS

The skin paddle and bone graft are marked out. A maximum of 11–13 cm can be harvested. The limiting factor is the attachment of pronator teres. Allow at least 2 cm from the distal osteotomy to the radial styloid to allow placement of a bone plate prior to closure (see Figure 3.6.9).

SKIN FLAP ELEVATION

Dissection of the skin flap is easiest in the subfascial plane. Starting on the ulnar aspect, proceed as far as the lateral (radial) border of the flexor carpi radialis. The distal pedicle is ligated and divided. If the initial dissection is in the suprafascial plane, the fascia must be incised along the lateral border of the flexor carpi radialis (see Figure 3.6.10).

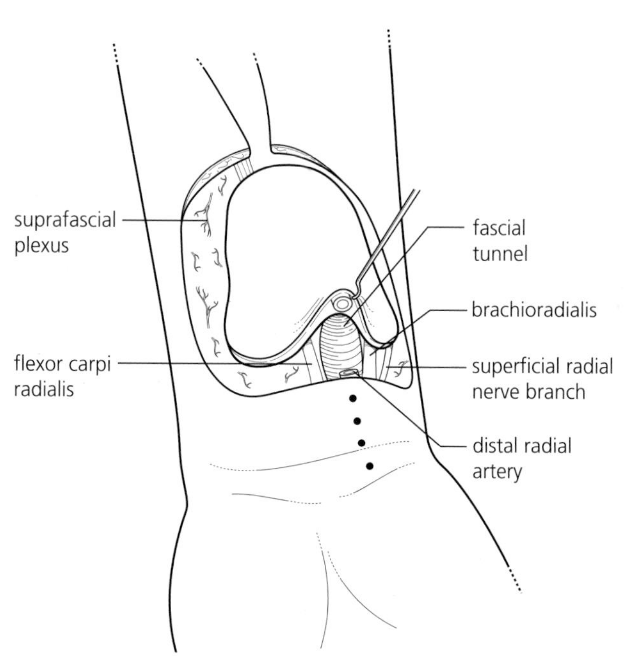

3.6.8 Suprafascial flap – vascular pedicle elevated from floor of enveloping fascial tunnel (see also Figure 3.6.2).

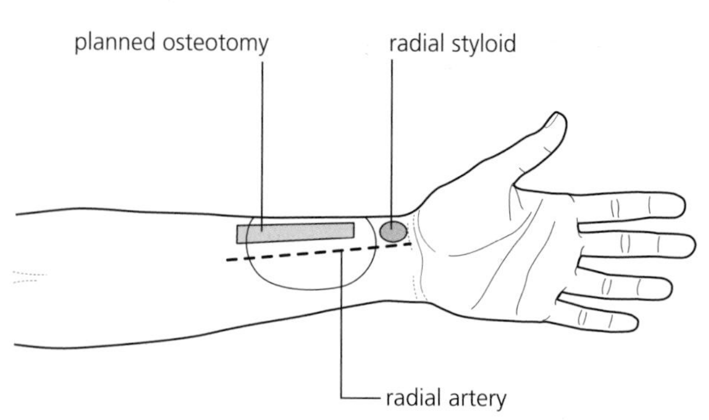

3.6.9 Osteocutaneous flap – surface markings.

PRESERVATION OF MUSCLE CUFF ATTACHMENT TO BONE

The proximal investing fascia is divided to retract the flexor carpi radialis. Avoid damaging the median nerve which lies medial to the distal aspect of the tendon. Retraction exposes the flexor pollicis longus and pronator quadratus, which are incised along the length of the bone graft to reach the ulnar (anteromedial) aspect of the radius. Preserve sufficient muscle cuff to protect periosteal perforating vessels passing through the muscles from the inferior surface of the radial pedicle. Most perforators run close to or in the lateral intermuscular septum which remains attached to the lateral aspect of the bone graft.

BONE EXPOSURE AND OSTEOTOMY PLANNING

The periosteum is incised and the cuff of flexor pollicis longus sparingly elevated to mark out the osteotomy site. The interosseous membrane and lower border of the radius are identified to avoid excessive bone removal, particularly in the mid-section where it curves upward in a convex manner. Plan to remove one-third to one-half of the radial circumference (see Figure 3.6.11).

OSTEOTOMY TECHNIQUE

The end osteotomies are bevelled to avoid over-cutting and stress concentration. The horizontal anteromedial osteotomy is performed from the ulnar aspect with a fine fissure burr using the 'postage stamp' method. Take care to protect the attached cuff of flexor pollicis longus. Complete the cortical cut with a fine oscillating saw, then angle this towards the radial (lateral) border ensuring that no more than half the radius is harvested. The graft is gently mobilized with a fine curved osteotome (see Figure 3.6.12).

DISSECTION ON THE RADIAL ASPECT AND MOBILIZATION OF FLAP

Retract the brachioradialis and dissect on the deep surface of the muscle to identify the osteotomy site, taking care to preserve the attachment of the intermuscular septum to the lateral aspect of the bone. The flap is lifted superiorly by incising the periosteum along the line of the osteotomy and dividing any other retaining soft tissues, taking due care to avoid damaging the pedicle. The proximal dissection is completed as normal (see Figure 3.6.13).

BONE PLATING THE RADIUS

The distal osteotomy must be at least 2 cm proximal to the radial styloid to allow space for a minimum of two screws and to avoid the wrist joint. The proximal and distal muscle attachments are stripped and repositioned later. A 3.5 mm dynamic compression plate is adapted to bridge the defect

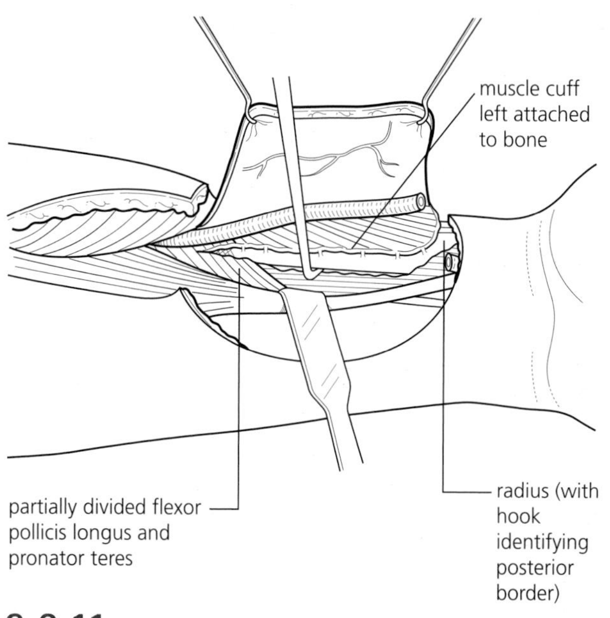

3.6.11 Osteocutaneous flap – preservation of muscle cuff and dissection to posterior border of radius.

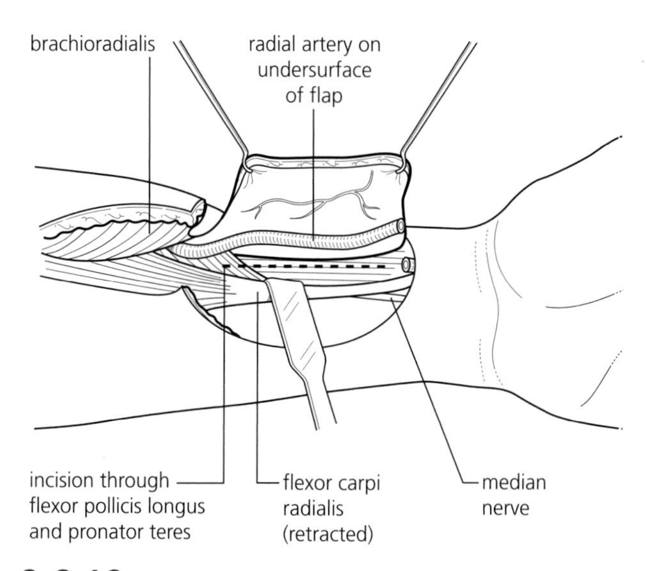

3.6.10 Osteocutaneous flap – dissection through muscle to gain access to anteromedial aspect of radius.

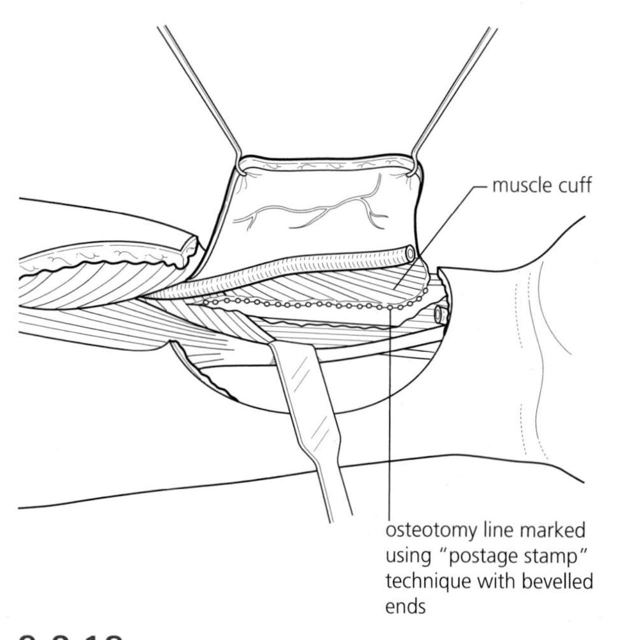

3.6.12 Osteocutaneous flap – osteotomy design (typically 40–50% of the circumference of the radius can be harvested).

on the anteromedial surface of the radius. At least two bicortical screws are inserted at each end in a neutral (non-compressive) position ensuring that both medial and lateral cortices are engaged. A weaker but more malleable 3.5 mm pelvic reconstruction plate may be placed over longer defects. A T-shaped plate is helpful if distal space is limited (see Figure 3.6.14). Anatomically contoured low contact radial plates with a T-shaped end and a unilocking screw system are quick to apply and provide excellent fixation.

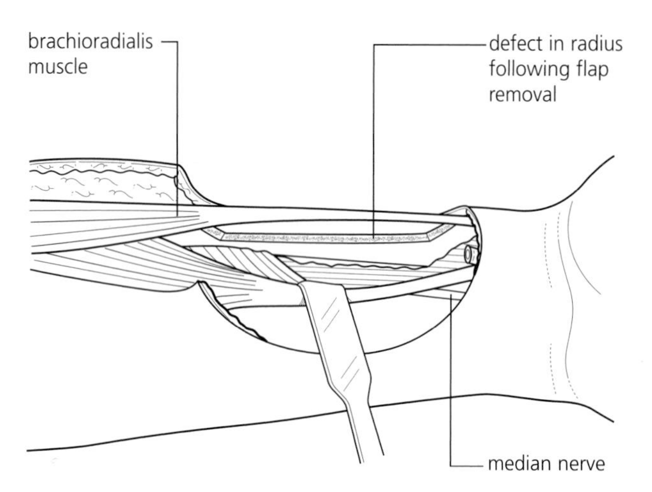

3.6.13 Osteocutaneous flap – typical donor site defect.

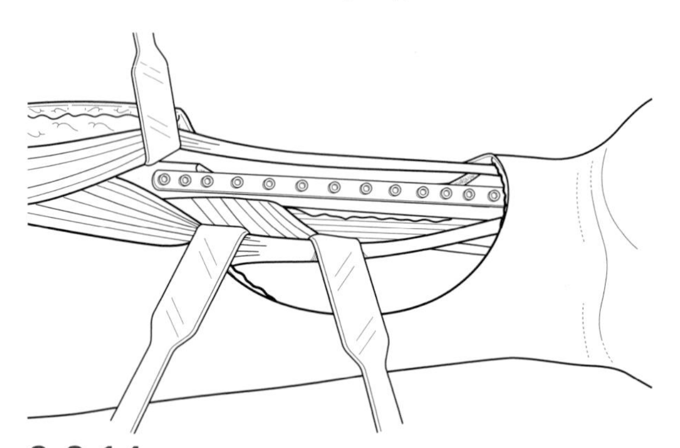

3.6.14 Osteocutaneous flap – prophylactic bone plate on anteromedial aspect fixed with minimum of two screws at each end but none within the defect.

Top tips

- Plan flap with artery at the lateral edge for better donor site aesthetics and to avoid hair.
- Simplify and achieve faster elevation of flap by using deep venous system drainage only (venae comitantes).
- Let flap rest at donor site to allow small vessel spasm to relax. Meticulous haemostasis should be achieved to avoid later haematoma and flap compromise.
- Skin graft healing is improved with minimal risk of tendon exposure if a suprafascial dissection technique and negative pressure wound dressing are used.
- Take between 30 and 50 per cent of the radial circumference with a composite flap.
- Prophylactic plating substantially reduces the risk of fracture allowing up to 50 per cent of the radial circumference to be removed.

DONOR SITE MANAGEMENT

The flexor pollicis longus and brachioradialis are approximated to cover the plate and the soft tissue donor site repaired as usual. A complete above-elbow cast, which may be prefabricated, is applied and the arm supported in a sling. A below-elbow cast is placed when the skin graft is inspected. The supporting cast is applied for 6 weeks. The plate rarely requires removal.

FURTHER READING

Avery CM. A Review of the Radial Free Flap: Still Evolving or Facing Extinction? Part One. *Br J Oral Maxillofac Surg* 2010; **48**: 245–252.

Avery CM. A Review of the Radial Free Flap: Still Evolving or Facing Extinction? Part Two. *Br J Oral Maxillofac Surg* 2010; **48**: 253–260.

Avery CM, Iqbal M, Orr R, Hayter JP. Repair of radial free flap donor site by full-thickness skin graft from inner arm. *British Journal of Oral and Maxillofacial Surgery* 2005; **43**: 161–5.

Avery CM, Danford M, Johnson PA. Prophylactic internal fixation of the radial osteocutaneous donor site. *British Journal of Oral and Maxillofacial Surgery* 2007; **45**: 576–8.

Avery CM, Best A, Patterson P *et al.* Biomechanical study of prophylactic internal fixation of the radial osteocutaneous donor site using the sheep tibia model. *British Journal of Oral and Maxillofacial Surgery* 2007; 45: **441–6.**

Avery CM. Prospective study of the septocutaneous radial free flap and suprafascial donor site. *British Journal of Oral and Maxillofacial Surgery* 2007; **45**: 611–6.

Bowers KW, Edmonds JL, Girod DA *et al.* Osteocutaneous radial forearm free flaps. The necessity of internal fixation of the donor-site defect to prevent pathological fracture. *Journal of Bone and Joint Surgery* 2000; **82**: 694–704.

Lutz BS, Wei FC, Chang SC *et al.* Donor site morbidity after suprafascial elevation of the radial forearm flap: a prospective study in 95 consecutive cases. *Plastic and Reconstructive Surgery* 1999; **103**: 132–7.

Martin IC, Brown AE. Free vascularized fascial flap in oral cavity reconstruction. *Head and Neck* 1994; **16**: 45–50.

Richardson D, Fisher SE, Vaughan ED, Brown JS. Radial forearm flap donor-site complications and morbidity: a prospective study. *Plastic and Reconstructive Surgery* 1997; **99**: 109–15.

Thoma A, Khadaroo R, Grigenas O *et al.* Oromandibular reconstruction with the radial-forearm osteocutaneous flap: experience with 60 consecutive cases. *Plastic and Reconstructive Surgery* 1999; **104**: 368–78; discussion 379–80.

Villaret DB, Futran NA. The indications and outcomes in the use of osteocutaneous radial forearm free flap. *Head and Neck* 2003; **25**: 475–81.

Werle AH, Tsue TT, Toby EB, Girod DA. Osteocutaneous radial forearm free flap: its use without significant donor site morbidity. *Otolaryngology–Head and Neck Surgery* 2000; **123**: 711–17.

3.7

Scapular and parascapular flap (with or without bone)

XIN PENG, CHI MAO, GUANG-YAN YU

PRINCIPLES AND JUSTIFICATION

Scapular and parascapular flaps with or without bone is a unique system of flaps available for free tissue transfer based on the subscapular artery and its branches. A wide variety of tissue combinations have been used extensively for head and neck reconstruction of both the mandible and maxilla. The ease of harvest, reliability and limited morbidity associated with the use of this flap make it a desirable donor site in select patients. The disadvantages are few, including the need for repositioning the patient, lack of sensation in the flap and limited bone stock for osseointegration, particularly in females.

INDICATIONS

Mandibular reconstruction

Osseous defects of the mandible of up to 14 cm, in conjunction with large cutaneous or intraoral mucosal defects, are well suited for this application. Great freedom in spatial orientation of skin and bone is allowed.

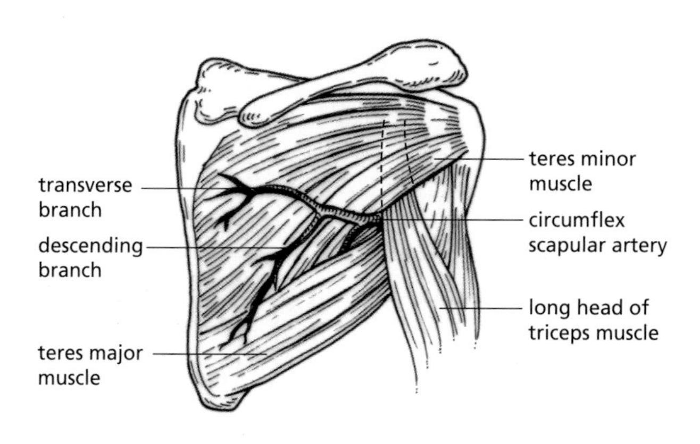

3.7.1 Muscle and vascular anatomy of scapular site.

Through-and-through oromandibular defects

Through-and-through defects of the cheek, combined with sagittal mandibular defects, can be reconstructed with this flap, as can anterior mandible defects.

COMPLEX MIDFACE DEFECTS

The scapular bone can be used for the maxilla and the infraorbital rim in maxillectomy defects. A great amount and variety of soft tissues are available for restoring complex defects involved in the skull base, orbit and midface.

ANATOMY

The scapular flap is supplied by the circumflex scapular branch of the subscapular artery and may be harvested as either a fasciocutaneous flap or osteofasciocutaneous flap with the lateral border of the scapular bone. The circumflex scapular artery (CSA) runs through the muscular triangular space and branches into transverse and descending cutaneous branches, which form the basis of the scapular and parascapular fasciocutaneous flaps (Figure 3.7.1).

The lateral aspect of the scapula bone is available for harvest based on the periosteal branches of the circumflex scapular artery (CSA). Approximately 10 cm of bone is available for harvest in females, and 14 cm of bone is available in males. The distal third of the scapula is supplied additionally by the terminal branches of the thoracodorsal artery.

The vascular pedicle is derived from the subscapular artery, derives a length about 4–5 cm to the lateral border of the scapular. A longer pedicle of 6–9 cm is possible for fasciocutaneous flap. The diameter of the subscapular artery is 2.0–2.5 mm. Paired venae comitantes accompany the circumflex artery, then join into a single large vein near the axillary vein.

One beneficial feature of the scapular flap is that the bone and skin paddle have a large degree of mobility relative to one another that facilitates flap insetting in complex composite reconstruction.

ANAESTHESIA

The operation is performed under general anaesthesia.

OPERATION

Position of patient

Flap harvest is performed with the patient in a prone or lateral decubitus position. Shoulder, back, lateral thorax and upper arm are circularly prepared to allow for movement of the extremity and exposure of the subscapular system from an axillary approach. In the lateral decubitus position, vacuum beanbags are used to stabilize the patient and to protect the dependent shoulder. An axillary roll is required to reduce traction on the opposite brachial plexus. Simultaneous oral–maxillofacial operation and flap harvest is tenuous at best and usually cannot be achieved.

Flap design

Scapular and parascapular flaps can be harvested along the axis of the transverse or descending branch of the CSA. The harvest is begun by first identifying the muscular triangular space. Draw the outline of the scapula and locate the upper margin of the latissimus insertion along the posterior axillary line. Approximately 2 cm superior to this, a depression between teres major and teres minor can usually be palpated alongside the lateral border of the scapula, representing the triangular space, where the CSA runs along the fascial septum between the teres major and minor muscles to enter the posterior thoracic fascia and the skin. The handheld Doppler device can be used to confirm the presence of the vascular pedicle. The width of the flap may not exceed 8–10 cm to make direct closure possible. The bone segment is harvested from the lateral scapular border, inferior to the glenohumeral joint and mostly including the inferior angle (Figure 3.7.2).

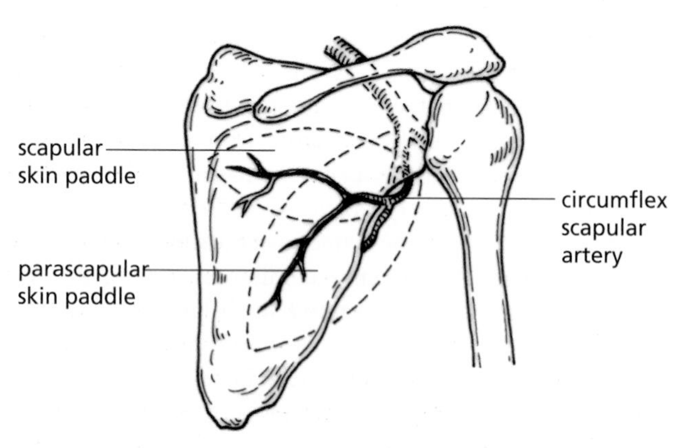

3.7.2 Design of scapular and parascapular skin paddle.

Operative technique

Starting medially, the skin and subcutaneous fatty tissue are incised to the deep fascia overlying the infraspinatus muscle. Elevate the fasciocutaneous skin paddle from medial to lateral just above the deep muscular fascia and below the dorsal thoracic fascia. The pulsation of the cutaneous branch, which is enveloped in the fascia, can now be seen and palpated easily. After the cutaneous branch has been exposed, the skin paddle is circumcised at its lateral portion and completely elevated (Figure 3.7.3).

Identify the teres major muscle. The circumflex artery will be identified within the omotricipital triangle just superior to the teres major muscle. The CSA is traced proximally, and the fascia space between the teres minor and major muscles is opened. Follow the circumflex vascular pedicle to the subscapular and axillary artery, several branches to the teres major and subscapular muscles are ligated to accomplish the vascular preparation.

The lateral margin of the scapula is identified by retracting the teres minor medially to expose the perforators to the bone, branching off from the deep segment of the CSA. To gain access to the scapular bone, the infraspinatus and teres minor muscles are incised 3 cm parallel to the

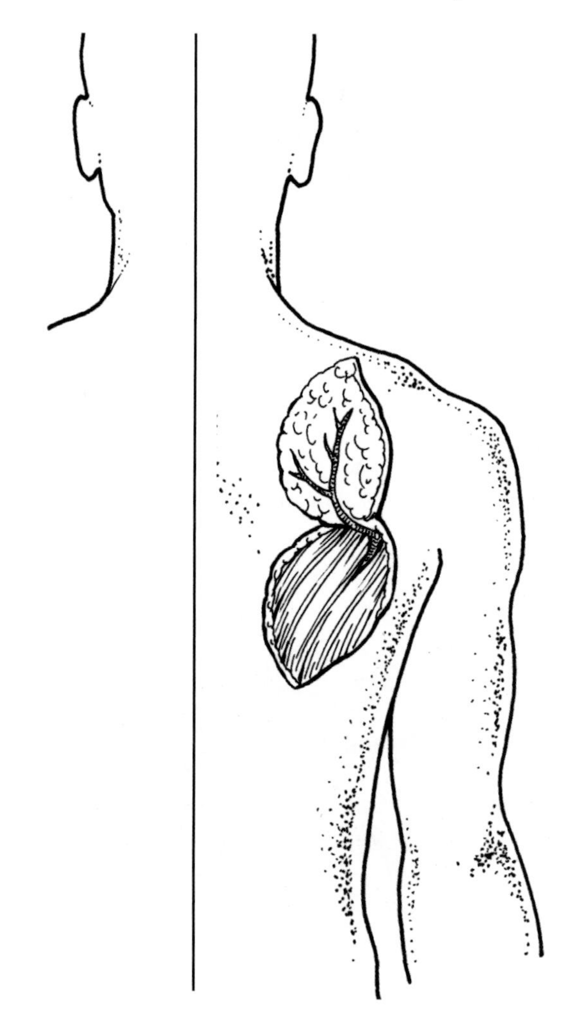

3.7.3 Elevation of parascapular skin paddle.

lateral border of scapula, leaving a muscle cuff attached to the bone. Cranially to the branches of the CSA to the bone, the teres minor and infraspinatus muscles are transected perpendicular to the muscle fibres to prepare for the osteotomy. Doing this, the vascular branches of the CSA to the bone must carefully be protected (Figure 3.7.4).

The osteotomy is performed, beginning 1–2 cm inferior of the glenohumeral joint. Here, care must be taken not to injure the vascular pedicle. The osteotomy is normally carried out 2–3 cm parallel to the lateral border of scapula and can include the whole inferior angle. The scapular angle may be harvested independently if the angular vessels are identified and preserved. After completion of the osteotomy, retracting the scapular bone segment laterally, the remaining fibres of the subscapular muscle are divided (Figure 3.7.5).

The osteocutaneous scapular flap is now completely elevated and ready for microvascular transfer. To lengthen the vascular pedicle, the CSA can be traced to the subscapular artery. To prevent winging of the scapula, the teres major muscle is reattached by drill holes in the lateral border of the residual scapula. A deep drain is inserted, and wound closure is accomplished after wide undermining (Figure 3.7.6).

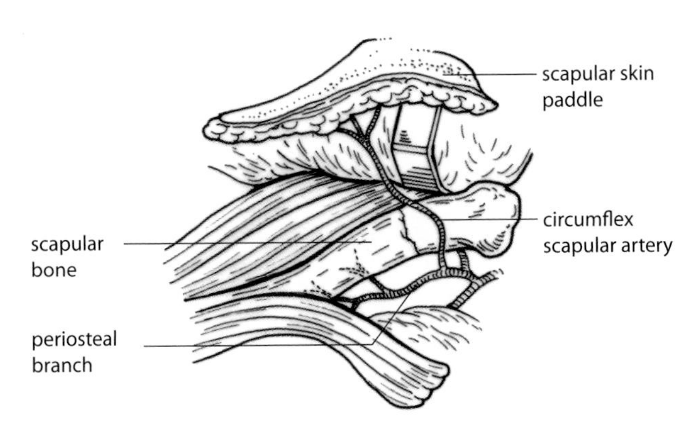

3.7.4 Osteocutaneous scapular flap.

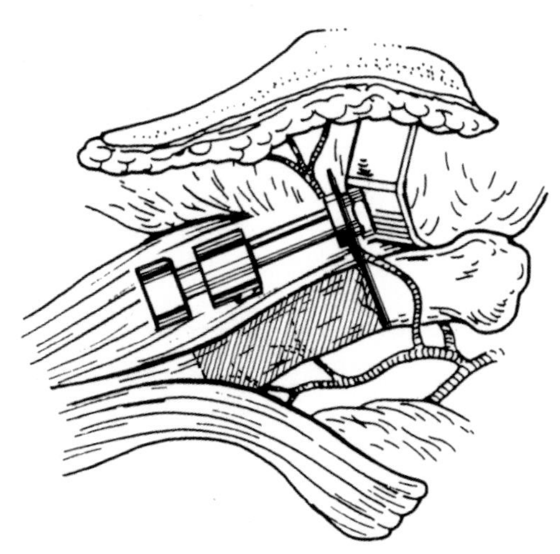

3.7.5 Osteotomy of lateral scapular rim.

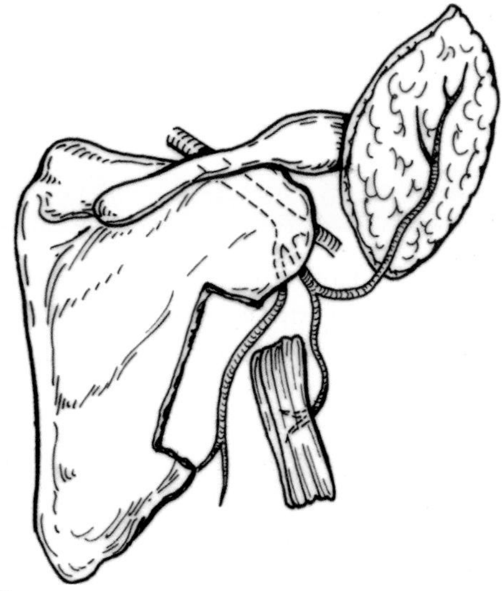

3.7.6 Raised osteocutaneous scapular flap.

POST-OPERATIVE CARE

Post-operatively, the donor arm should be kept immobilized for 1 week. Physical therapy can then be instituted to improve passive and active range of motion. Intensive home physical therapy to improve shoulder strength can begin within 3 weeks after surgery. This greatly limits post-operative morbidity.

Post-operative monitoring of flap vascular flow with serial examination, external Doppler, pinprick or an implantable Doppler device is at the discretion of the reconstructive surgeon. Use of anticlotting agents, such as heparin, aspirin and dextran, are also used at the judgement of the surgeon.

COMPLICATIONS

- **Haematoma formation.** This may result from inadequate haemostasis or coagulopathy.
- **Seroma formation.** It can develop given the amount of dead space present after harvest. Maintaining large suction drains for several days post-operatively helps to alleviate this problem.
- **Wound dehiscence and skin breakdown.** These complications can also develop at the donor site. This is particularly problematic with large defects that are closed under tension. Significant undermining of adjacent tissue may be required to obtain primary closure. Skin grafting in this dependent mobile area should be avoided.
- **Wound infection.** It is a rare complication. Use separate instruments and clean gloves and gowns at the donor site to avoid contamination and subsequent wound infection. The donor site is closed prior to working on the recipient site. Antibiotic prophylaxis should be used.
- **Injury of the long thoracic nerve.** Take care to avoid injury to the long thoracic nerve, which supplies the serratus anterior, because this can result in a winged

scapula. The injury can be observed with scapular flap harvest because of patient positioning. Take care to avoid extreme elevation of the arm, and support for the head should be provided during harvest.

Top tips

- It is important for flap design to identify the triangular space between the teres minor, major and long head of triceps muscles. A Doppler device can be used to confirm the vascular pedicle.
- The lateral pole of the skin paddle should not be defined until the circumflex scapular artery is identified.
- Make sure that no branch to the bone is transected during dissection of the deep segment of the circumflex scapular artery.
- When preparing the scapula for the osteotomy, care must be taken not to injury the circumflex scapular artery and its branches to the bone.
- Direct closure of the donor site under excessive tension should be avoided.

FURTHER READING

Funk GF. Scapular and parascapular free flaps. *Facial Plastic Surgery* 1996; **12**:57–63.

Langstein HN. Scapular osseous flap. In: Evans GRD (ed.). *Operative plastic surgery.* New York: McGraw-Hill, 2000: 399–406.

Nassif TM, Vidal L, Bovet JL, Baudet J. The parascapular flap: a new cutaneous microsurgical free flap. *Plastic and Reconstructive Surgery* 1982; **69**: 591–600.

Swartz WM. Scapular osteocutaneous flap. In: Strauch B, Vasconez LO, Hall-Findlay EJ (eds). *Grabb's encylopedia of flaps,* 2nd edn. Lippincott-Raven, Philadelphia. 1998: 714–18.

Urken ML, Bridger AG, Zur KB, Genden EM. The scapular osteofasciocutaneous flap: a 12-year experience. *Archives of Otolaryngology–Head and Neck Surgery* 2001: **127**: 862–9.

Wolff K-D, Hölzle F. Scapular flap. In: Wolff K-D, Hölzle F. (eds). *Raising of microvascular flaps: A systematic approach.* Heidelberg: Springer-Verlag, 2005: 83–106.

3.8

Rectus abdominis

XIN PENG, CHI MAO, GUANG-YAN YU

PRINCIPLES AND JUSTIFICATION

The rectus abdominis flap has been used extensively for breast reconstruction because of its ease of harvest and reliability. The advent of microsurgical techniques has allowed this versatile flap to be transposed to repair soft tissue defects of the head and neck for decades. It can be harvested as a muscle-only flap or as a myocutaneous flap, which can be used to replace soft tissue bulk. The pedicle is of adequate length for anastomosis in the neck or temporal region. Vascularized skin and fat resist atrophy, but denervated muscle shrinks with time. Although not optimal for small or shallow defects, the rectus flap provides the reconstructive surgeon with an excellent option to reconstruct large defects. This flap is most commonly used for orbital-maxillary defects, skull base reconstruction and glossectomy defects.

INDICATIONS

Orbital-maxillary reconstruction

Reconstruction following orbital exenteration and maxillectomy is facilitated with a rectus flap. The muscle bulk adequately fills the defect. The rectus abdominis myocutaneous flap is very suitable for the extensive defects resulting from radical maxillectomy with zagoma because of its large soft tissue volume.

Skull base reconstruction

The rectus abdominis flap is also commonly applied for the reconstruction of skull base defects in which a large volume of conformable, vascularized muscle is required to obliterate a skull base defect and bolster a dural closure. In these cases, the flap is harvested without a cutaneous paddle unless skin closure of a palatal defect is required.

Glossectomy defects reconstruction

As a myocutaneous flap, it is particularly suitable for reconstructing total glossectomy defects. Fat volume is well preserved in a denervated free myocutaneous flap, but it loses muscular bulk with time. Preservation of bulk can be of functional benefit in the glossectomy patient.

ANATOMY

The rectus abdominis is a long, broad strap muscle, broader above and extending the full length of the anterior abdominal wall. This muscle has a dual dominant blood supply. The upper vessel is the superior epigastric artery, one of the two terminal branches of the internal mammary artery. The lower vessel is the inferior epigastric artery that arises from the external iliac artery above the level of the inguinal ligament (Figure 3.8.1).

The rectus abdominis muscle is enclosed in the rectus sheath, which consists of an anterior and posterior lamina. The anterior sheath should never be harvested below the arcuate line where there is no posterior sheath. This is particularly important in the restoration of abdominal wall integrity after raising the rectus abdominis muscle or musculocutaneous flap.

The commonly used inferior rectus abdominis flap is a musculocutaneous flap based on the deep inferior epigastric artery and vein and terminal musculocutaneous perforators. These vessels arise from the external iliac artery and vein and course superomedially to run along the deep lateral aspect of the muscle. Within 1–2 cm of the arcuate line, the vessels enter the muscle. The deep inferior epigastric vein is frequently found to be a system of paired venae comitantes running with the artery. Just proximal to the external iliac vein, this system often forms one dominant vein.

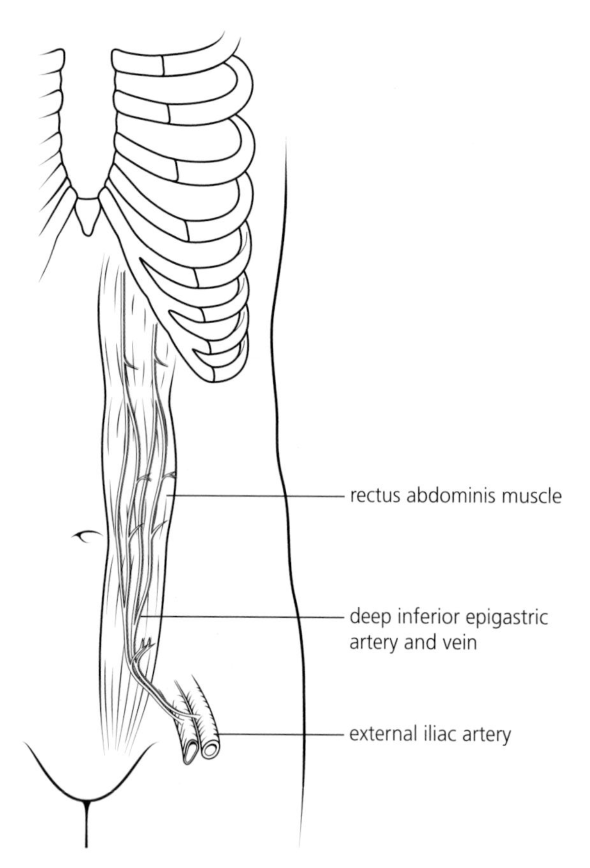

3.8.1 Muscle and vascular anatomy of rectus abdominis site.

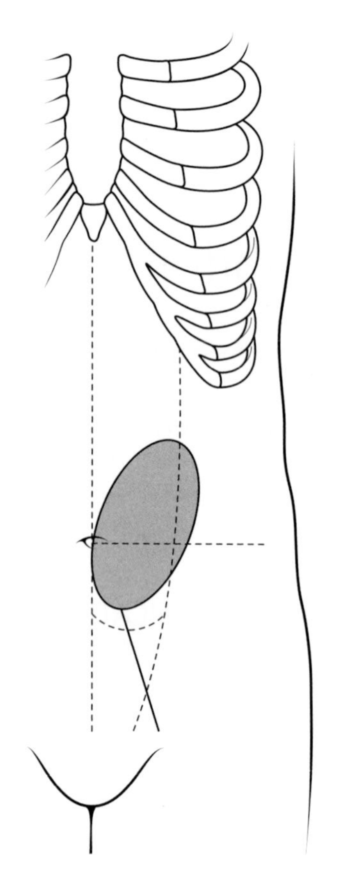

3.8.2 Design of rectus abdominis flap.

ANAESTHESIA

The operation is performed under general anaesthesia.

OPERATION

Position of patient

The patient is placed in a supine position. The operating field is prepped between lower rib arch, posterior axillary line and upper thigh. The flap can be harvested simultaneously by two teams.

Flap design

Draw linea alba, linea semilunaris, inguinal ligament, symphysis, costal margin and approximate position of arcuate line at level of anterior iliac spine. Landmarks are palpated, which include the ribcage, pubis and anterior superior iliac spine. The dissection does not extend beyond these landmarks. The defect size is measured or estimated, and a flap that is slightly larger than the defect is designed. A unilateral flap that includes a periumbilical portion is created. This ensures capture of the perforators (Figure 3.8.2).

Depending on tissue requirements, the skin paddle can be designed vertically, totally overlying the rectus muscle, or obliquely, along an axis between the umbilicus and the tip of the scapula with much of the skin paddle lateral to the linea semilunaris. This latter orientation is possible because of an axial blood flow pattern from the portion of skin overlying the muscle in the periumbilical area parallel along this axis. When designed in this manner, the lateral aspect of the flap is much thinner than the portion overlying the muscle and can be useful when the defect requires soft tissue of varying thickness.

Operative technique

The skin is incised, and cautery is used to dissect through the fat. Use caution when working with the rectus muscle because musculocutaneous perforators may be violated. Placing tacking sutures from the skin to the anterior sheath can preserve the viability of the perforators. The anterior rectus sheath is identified. The sheath is transected superiorly and inferiorly beneath the skin incision. The inferior incision is placed above the arcuate line in order to facilitate closure without the use of mesh. Laterally, the linea semilunaris is used as a landmark for the lateral sheath incision (Figure 3.8.3).

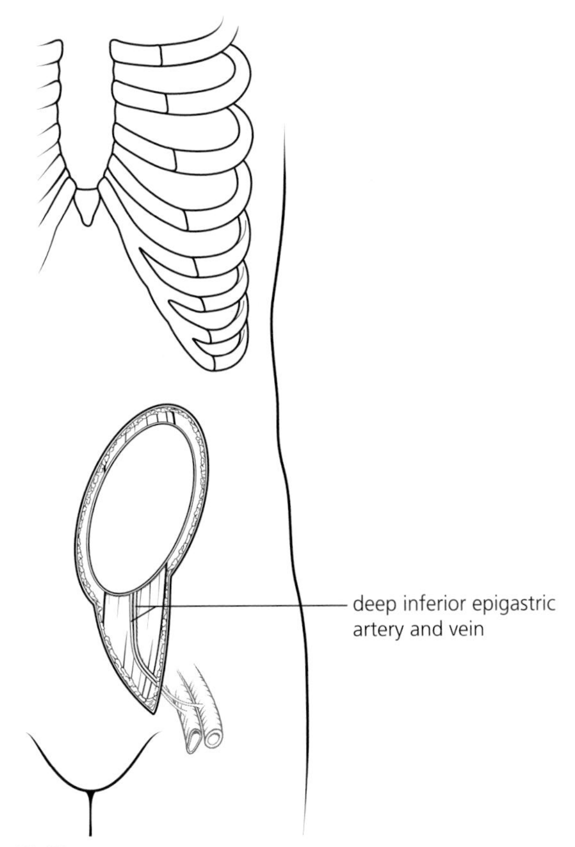

3.8.3 Elevation of rectus abdominis flap.

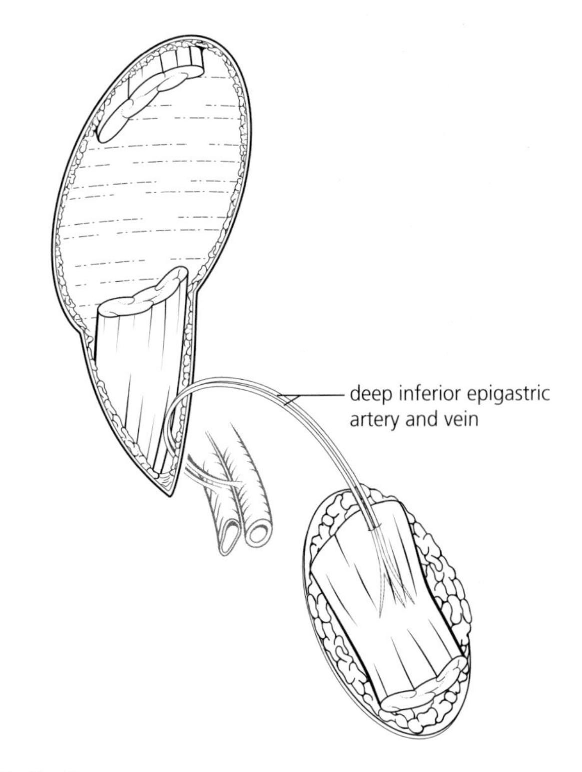

3.8.4 Raised rectus abdominis flap.

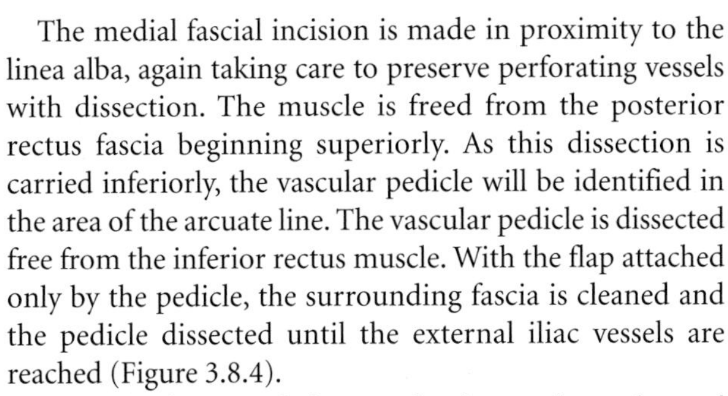

The medial fascial incision is made in proximity to the linea alba, again taking care to preserve perforating vessels with dissection. The muscle is freed from the posterior rectus fascia beginning superiorly. As this dissection is carried inferiorly, the vascular pedicle will be identified in the area of the arcuate line. The vascular pedicle is dissected free from the inferior rectus muscle. With the flap attached only by the pedicle, the surrounding fascia is cleaned and the pedicle dissected until the external iliac vessels are reached (Figure 3.8.4).

When the flap is ready for transfer, the vessels are clamped and the pedicle is divided. The abdomen is closed in a primary fashion. Proper and careful closure of the anterior sheath is important to prevent a hernia. Mesh is also routinely applied to reinforce the closure, this is particularly important if the sheath has been violated inferior to the arcuate line. A suction drain is placed and wound closure is completed (Figure 3.8.5).

POST-OPERATIVE CARE

Post-operatively, the patient wears the abdominal binder for 2 weeks and is instructed against any heavy lifting for 6 weeks. A pillow is placed on the abdomen to assist with coughing. Stool softeners are also useful to minimize abdominal strain.

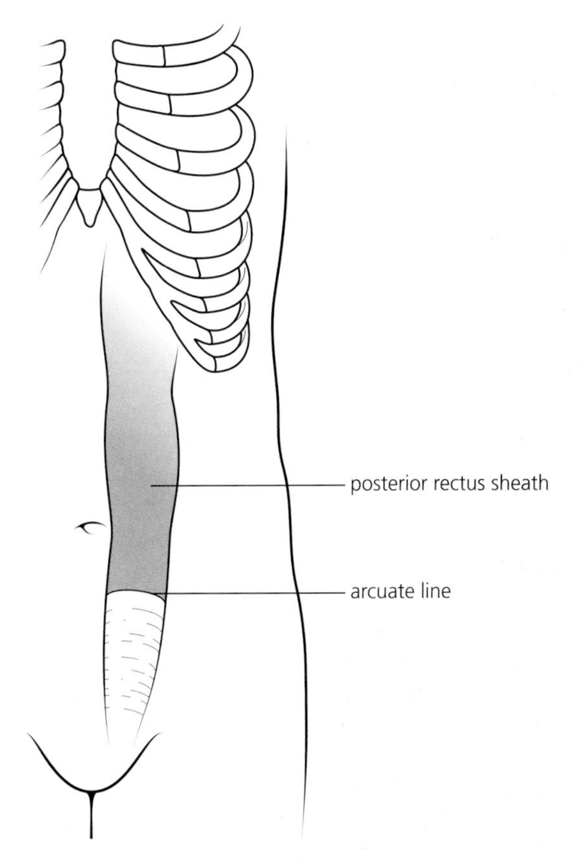

3.8.5 Posterior rectus sheath and arcuate line.

Post-operative ileus is common for a short time following surgery and generally resolves spontaneously. Ambulation is helpful for hastening the resolution of ileus, heralded by the return of bowel sounds.

Patients are monitored closely in the hospital. The skin paddle is monitored frequently for signs of vascular compromise. Post-operative monitoring of flap vascular flow with serial examination, external Doppler, pinprick or an implantable Doppler device is at the discretion of the reconstructive surgeon. Use of anti-clotting agents, such as heparin, aspirin and dextran, are also used at the judgement of the surgeon.

Intensive physical therapy from speech pathologist, physical therapist or other specialists can begin within 3 weeks after surgery.

COMPLICATIONS

Donor site complications are uncommon but possible.

- **Hernias.** It may occur when the rectus sheath has not been properly closed or is insufficient for adequate closure.
- **Wound infections.** This may also occur. A general surgeon may be of assistance in wound closure in patients at risk.
- **Haematomas.** It may occur as a result of inadequate haemostasis and anticoagulation. Drains should be placed carefully in the operating room and not removed until the heparin has been discontinued.

Top tips

- The rectus abdominis flap is not very suitable for head and neck reconstruction in obese patients.
- The inferior incision of the flap should be placed above the arcuate line in order to facilitate closure without the use of mesh.
- When the dissection is carried inferiorly in the area of the arcuate line, care must be taken not to injury the deep inferior epigastric artery and vein.
- Proper and careful closure of the anterior sheath is important to prevent hernia. Mesh may be applied to reinforce the closure.

FURTHER READING

Dinner MI, Labandter H, Dowden RV. Rectus abdominis musculocutaneous flap. In: Strauch B, Vasconez LO, Hall-Findlay EJ (eds). *Grabb's encylopedia of flaps*, 2nd edn. Philadelphia: Lippincott-Raven, 1998: 1309–13.

Ebihara H, Maruyama Y. Free abdominal flaps: variations in design and application to soft tissue defects of the head. *Journal of Reconstructive Microsurgery* 1989; **5**:193–201.

Pryor SG, Moore EJ, Kasperbauer JL. Orbital exenteration reconstruction with rectus abdominis microvascular free flap. *Laryngoscope* 2005; **115**: 1912–16.

Urken ML, Turk JB, Weinberg H *et al.* The rectus abdominis free flap in head and neck reconstruction. *Archives of Otolaryngology–Head and Neck Surgery* 1991; **117**: 857–66.

West CA, Towns G, Bachelor AG *et al.* Reconstruction of skull base and dura using rectus abdominis muscle combined with a vascularised fascial perforator flap. *Journal of Plastic, Reconstructive and Aesthetic Surgery* 2006; **59**: 631–5.

3.9

Latissimus dorsi flap

ANDREW W BAKER

DEVELOPMENT

- The first musculocutaneous flap was described in the medical text by Tansini in 1896.
- It was used initially for the primary reconstruction of the post mastectomy defect.
- The first use of a pedicled latissimus dorsi flap for reconstruction in the head and neck area was described by Quillen in 1978.
- Watson reported the first successful microvascular transfer of a free latissimus flap in 1979, and exploited a wide variety of applications for head and neck reconstruction.

FEATURES

This is a popular donor site for the transfer of tissue to the head and neck region due to:

- the ease of dissection;
- the length and diameter of the vascular pedicle, rarely compromised by arteriosclerosis;
- it can be raised as a pedicled or free flap;
- the large surface area of muscle only or musculocutaneous flap available;
- minimal donor site morbidity;
- access to the dissection requires turning and usually prohibits simultaneous harvest.

The latissimus dorsi is a large broad flat muscle that covers the posterior inferior portion of the trunk (Figure 3.9.1).

It has a broad and crescentic origin from the lower four ribs; the spinous processes of the lower six thoracic vertebrae; the thoracolumbar fascia and laterally it also arises from the fascia that is attached to the iliac crest.

The muscle curves around the lower border of the teres major, and is twisted upon itself, so that the superior fibres become at first posterior and then inferior, and the vertical fibres at first anterior and then superior. It ends in a quadrilateral tendon, about 7 cm long, which passes in front of the tendon of the teres major, and is inserted into the bottom of the intertubercular groove of the humerus; its insertion extends higher on the humerus than that of the tendon of the pectoralis major.

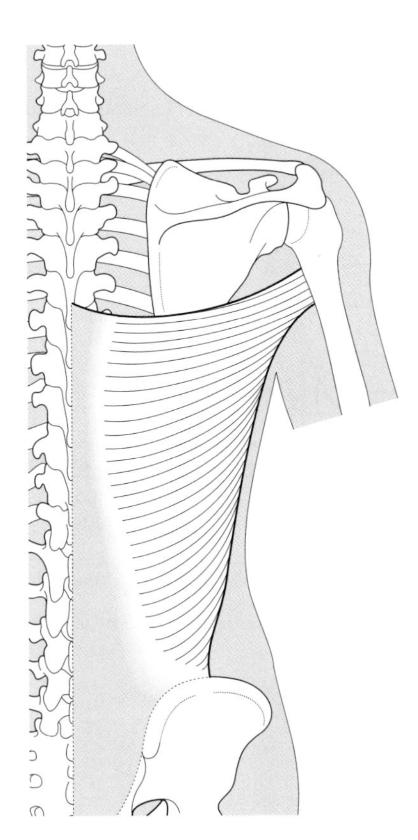

3.9.1 Anatomy of the latissimus dorsi muscle.

The lower border of its tendon is united with that of the teres major, the surfaces of the two being separated near their insertions by a bursa; another bursa is sometimes interposed between the muscle and the inferior angle of the scapula.

NEUROVASCULAR ANATOMY

The main superior pedicle of the muscle is the thoracodorsal artery and vein, which eventually supplies a rich network of musculocutaneous perforators, particularly over the anterior border of the muscle. It should be noted that as a type 5 muscle, there are a further two minor vascular supplies and therefore angiosomes are supplied by the posterior intercostal segmental perforators in the mid portion and the lumber artery segmental perforators in the distal paraspinal area (Figure 3.9.2).

The thoracodorsal vessels are terminal branches of the subscapular artery and vein which arise from the third part of the axillary vessels. These vessels initially run inferiorly through the axilla, and then for a short distance below the lat dorsi muscle before penetrating the muscle at the vascular hilum. At this point, the vein can be identified laterally with the artery medial, the thoracodorsal nerve being sandwiched between the two. In its extramuscular course, there are branches to subscapularis, teres major and serratus anterior and the important angular branch to the tip of the scapula. Just within the muscle the vessels typically bifurcate into transverse and longitudinal branches. The transverse branch runs an average of 3.5 cm below the upper border of the muscle and the longitudinal branch usually 2.0 cm from the lateral edge. This feature allows the potential development of two separate skin paddles.

- The average diameter of the thoracodorsal artery is 2.5 mm, the diameter of the vein is 3.5 mm.
- The length of the pedicle is between 6 and 16 cm.
- By extending the dissection proximally to the origin of the subscapular vessels at the axillary artery, the subscapular artery pedicle can provide a diameter of 6 mm on average. The pedicle length is also extended by at least 4 cm.

The thoracodorsal nerve supplies the motor innervation to the latissimus dorsi. It arises from the posterior segment of the brachial plexus. It enters the axilla from behind the axillary vessels and then descends with the thoracodorsal artery and vein to the neurovascular hilum. The thoracodorsal nerve usually crosses the axillary vessels approximately 3 cm proximal to the subscapular artery and vein.

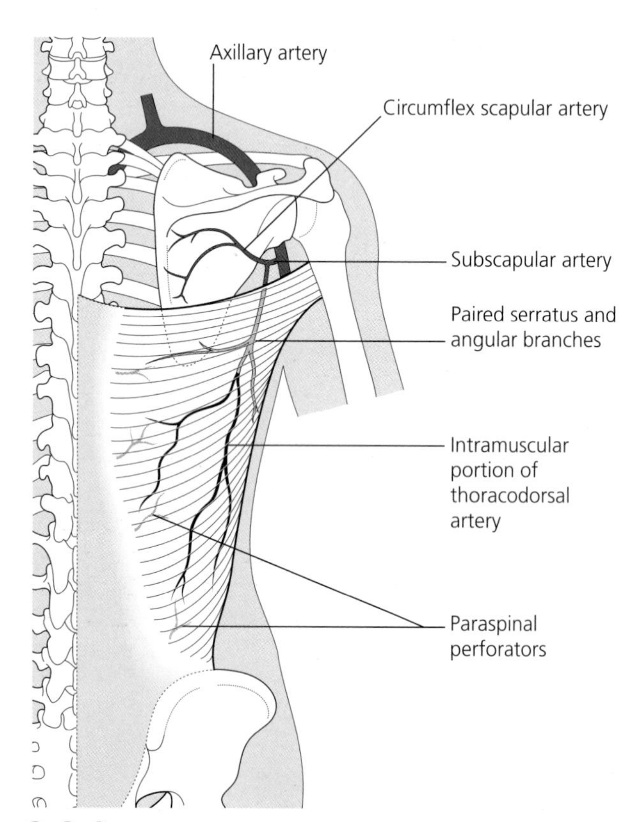

3.9.2 The key branches of the vascular supply to the latissimus dorsi muscle.

FLAP DESIGN AND UTILIZATION

The length of the pedicle is generous and even as a pedicled flap, most defects of the head and neck area can be reached after the flap is passed through the axilla and then between the pectoralis minor and major muscles of the chest wall. By exteriorizing the pedicle, even posterior scalp defects may be reconstructed.

Division of the arterial branches to the serratus anterior prevents inferior tethering of the thoracodorsal pedicle.

Complete isolation of the pedicle by division of the circumflex scapular branch can be achieved. However, once this is performed then there is no mechanical method to stop rotation and kinking of the pedicle as it arises from the axillary artery. Complete transaction of the tendon of the latissimus dorsi at the superior insertion provides an ultimate freedom of rotation.

Fashioning the skin paddle over the distal portion of the muscle can extend the flap's reach, but here it should be noted that unlike the number of perforators at the anterior edge of the muscle in the distal territories, the density of musculocutaneous perforators is much reduced and thus viability of the skin is potentially reduced. Additionally, one should also consider that the blood supply to the skin in this area will have had to cross at least one angiosome via choke vessels, further compromising the viability of the distal skin (Figure 3.9.3).

The total area covered by the latissimus dorsi muscle is approximately 25×40 cm. The maximum size of the skin paddle that can be transferred is naturally determined by

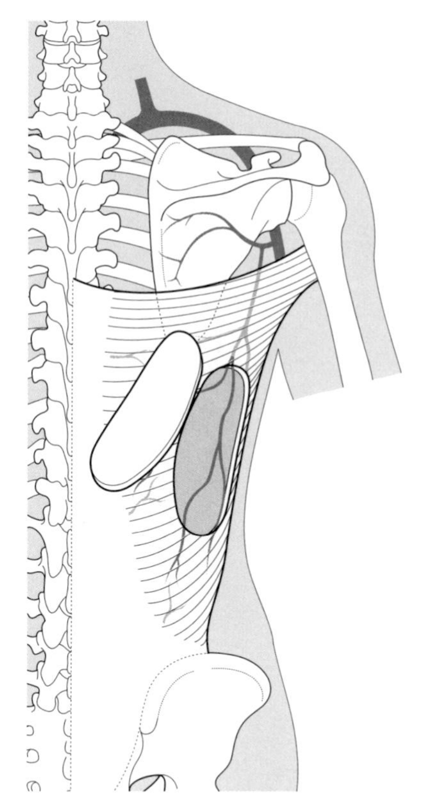

3.9.3 The skin paddle can be based on the transverse or vertical limbs of the thoracodorsal artery. However, the highest density of perforators favours the anterior edge of the muscle, as indicated.

the size of the particular patient. Although the defect can be skin grafted, rarely is this advised or required.

Through and through defects of the head and neck involving skin and mucosa can be reconstructed by folding and de-epithelializing a portion of a single large latissimus dorsi musculocutaneous paddle or by using two separate musculocutaneous paddles based on the transverse and descending branches as described by Tobin in 1981.

The early 1980s saw much interest in the potential development of the vascularized bone transfer with the latissimus dorsi flap and rib, this was based on lab based radio-opaque injection studies of the subscapular vessels in dogs which suggested retrograde filling of the posterior intercostal perforators and therefore potential blood supply to dorsal aspects of the fifth to tenth ribs. Very few examples exist in the literature of this demanding technique.

The important clarification of the angular branch of the thoracodorsal artery by Coleman and Taylor in 1991 defined a separate vascular supply to the caudal tip of the scapular. This finding not only provides a separate vascular section of the scapular for the scapular flap system, but importantly provides a dependable segment of bone for use in a thoracodorsal flap setting.

Harii advocated the use of the innervated latissimus dorsi flap in facial reanimation. The advantages of the latissimus dorsi for this procedure are the length and calibre of the neurovascular pedicle and its division into two segments, which allows the transfer of two separate muscle units. One unit being used for reanimation of the mouth and the other, for the lower eyelid. The latissimus dorsi musculocutaneous flap has also been used for dynamic reconstruction of composite cheek defects that include the loss of the mimetic muscles of the midface. In this case, the musculocutaneous unit is transferred and revascularized and the thoracodorsal nerve is anastomosed to the ipsilateral facial nerve.

The use of innervated latissimus dorsi flap for the dynamic reconstruction of the tongue, following glossectomy has been proposed. However, it is accepted that duplication of the complexity of the tongue's musculature in both form and function by a simple muscle flap consisting of fibres running in one direction is limited. Haughey and Frederickson described the use of the reinnervated latissimus dorsi musculocutaneous flap for total tongue reconstruction. The thoracodorsal nerve was anastomosed to the cut end of the hypoglossal nerve. In this and subsequent studies, useful tone without purposeful movement could be demonstrated in the neo-tongue.

Watson and Lendrum reported a one-stage tubed latissimus dorsi flap for circumferential pharyngoesophageal reconstruction. Watson described several technical considerations in using the latissimus dorsi flap for pharyngeal defects. The authors advised transferring a large segment of muscle around the circumference of the skin paddle that is to be tubed. The muscle was sutured to the surrounding tissues to provide a second-layer seal (Figure 3.9.4).

Recently, Kim proposed the latissimus dorsi perforator flap. The concept allows harvest of vast areas of trunk skin, without the necessity of simultaneous muscle harvest. The musculocutaneous perforators are dissected free of the muscle, on their course to the skin. Indeed, it has been suggested that a large skin paddle may be sustained by the inclusion of a singular perforating vessel group. This recent discovery may well prove invaluable for head and neck reconstruction as it can provide plentiful thin pliable tissue.

PRE-OPERATIVE ASSESSMENT

It is useful to asses the patient pre-operatively, and the muscle can be easily visualized by pushing with the outstretched arm against a wall. Note should be made of previous axillary surgery, as this may have already compromised the thoracodorsal vessels. The anterior border of the latissimus dorsi can be readily palpated in the thin patient as it descends out of the posterior axillary fold, laterally on the trunk. Localization with Doppler probes is not necessary.

FLAP HARVESTING TECHNIQUE

Typically, the patient is usually turned into the lateral decubitus position. The ipsilateral arm is prepared and

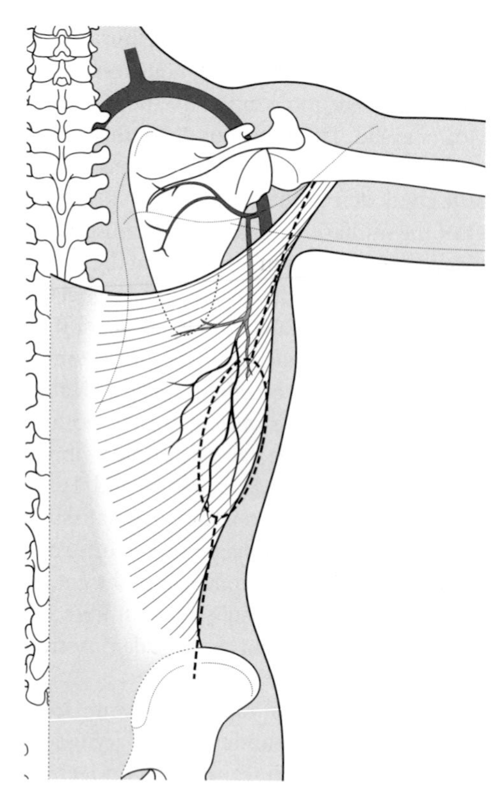

3.9.4 The anterior border of the latissimus dorsi is marked on the patient as a line between the posterior axillary fold and a point halfway between the anterior superior iliac spine and the posterior superior iliac spine.

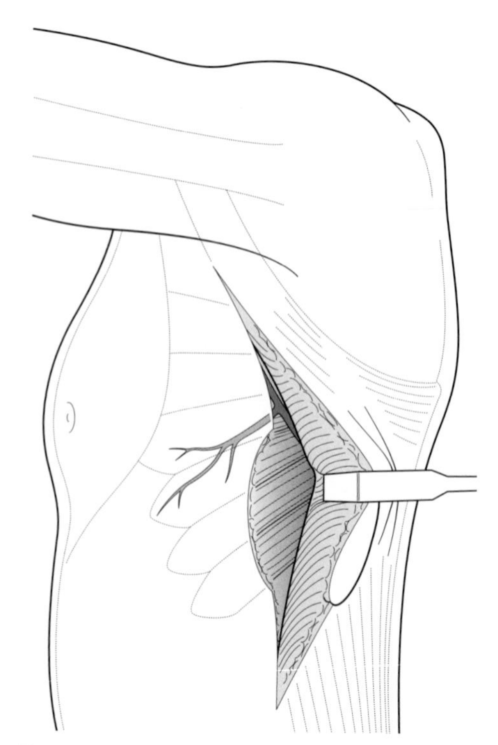

3.9.5 By retracting the free edge of latissimus dorsi, the extramuscular pedicle can be identified by tracing the last extramuscular branch to serratus anterior back to the main vessel.

draped together with the lateral thorax, shoulder, axilla and back. The anterior border of the latissimus dorsi is marked on the patient as a line between the posterior axillary fold and a point halfway between the anterior superior iliac spine and the posterior superior iliac spine. On this line, approx 2 cm below the level of the tip of the scapula is where the vessels penetrate the muscle and divide into the horizontal branch, which runs a few centimetres below the scapula tip, and a more vertically directed branch, which runs 3–4 cm posterior to the anterior edge of the muscle. A skin paddle should be centred over one of these main branches, preferably over the vertical limb which bears the highest density of skin perforators (Figure 3.9.5).

The initial incision is from the axilla along the marked line or cutaneous paddle. Then identify the anterior leading edge of the latissimus.

Superiorly, the pedicle can be found within the adipose tissue of the axilla, then descending to provide branches to the muscles and the angular branch to the scapula before entering the hilum of the latissimus dorsi. By retracting the free edge of latissimus dorsi, the extramuscular pedicle can be identified by tracing the last extramuscular branch to serratus anterior back to the main vessel. It is important to note that typically the branch to the angle of the scapula arises also at this same level (Figure 3.9.6). After careful recognition of the pedicle, these opposing branches are ligated and secured so that significant cranial mobilization of the flap can continue. Depending on the requirements of the flap, the whole or part of the muscle is harvested by dissection from the chest wall and surrounding muscles. If it is required to maximize the amount of muscle harvested, the author uses the GIA linear stapling device to both cut and cauterize the muscle edge. The staples also make a suitable edge to suture to the recipient site (Figure 3.9.7).

Complete mobilization of the latissimus dorsi requires transection of the tendinous insertion to the humerus. This manoeuvre should be performed with caution while protecting the vascular pedicle and keeping it under direct vision.

Passage of the pedicled flap requires preparation of a tunnel between the pectoralis major and minor. The lateral edge of these muscles is identified in the deep part anterior axilla through the superior aspect of the incision.

A carefully placed neck dissection incision can facilitate delivery of the pedicle in the neck or an incision parallel and inferior to the clavicle may be required to access of the pedicle through the tunnel. Natural passage through

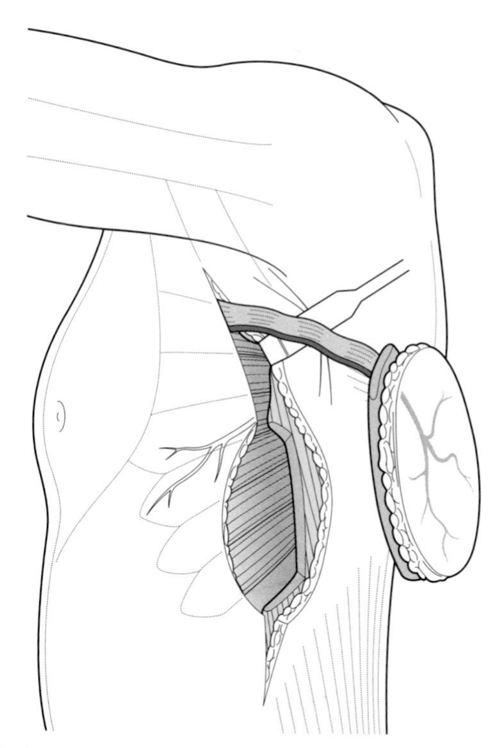

3.9.6 With the pedicle isolated and the muscle and skin flap elevated, the flap is ready for delivery to the neck.

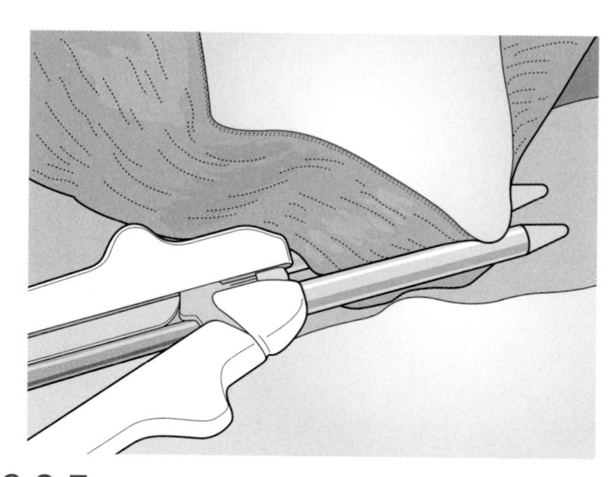

3.9.7 GIA linear stapling device to cut and control bleeding from the muscle.

pectoralis major attachments at the clavicle is required and room for the vascular pedicle should be generous.

Carefully, the latissimus dorsi flap is passed through the tunnel while maintaining the pedicle's orientation and being certain not to twist or kink the pedicle.

Primary closure of the donor site can usually be accomplished by wide undermining to produce a linear scar. A number of deep tension sutures may be required to stabilize the wound closure.

FURTHER READING

Haughey B, Fredrickson J. The latissimus dorsi donor site. Current use in head and neck reconstruction. *Archives of Otolaryngology–Head and Neck Surgery* 1991; **117**: 1129–34.

Haughey B. Tongue reconstruction: concepts and practice. *Laryngoscope* 1993; **103**: 1132–41.

Mathes S, Nahai F. *Reconstructive surgery, principles, anatomy, and technique.* New York: Churchill Livingstone, 1997.

Quillen C. Latissimus dorsi myocutaneous flaps in head and neck reconstruction. *Plastic and Reconstructive Surgery* 1979; **63**: 664–70.

Tansini I. Spora il mio nuovo processo di amputazione della mammaella per cancre. *Riforma Med (Palermo, Napoli)* 1896; **12**: 3.

Tobin G, Moberg A, DuBou R, Weiner L, Bland K. The split latissimus dorsi myocutaneous flap. *Annals of Plastic Surgery* 1981; **7**: 272–280.

Urken ML, Cheney ML, Sullivan MJ *et al. Atlas of regional and free flaps for head and neck reconstruction.* New York: Raven Press Ltd, 1995.

Watson JS, Craig R, Orton C. The free latissimus dorsi myocutaneous flap. *Plastic and Reconstructive Surgery* 1979; **64**: 299.

Watson JS, Lendrum J. One stage pharyngeal reconstruction using a compound latissimus dorsi island flap. *British Journal of Plastic Surgery* 1981; **34**: 87–90.

Wolff K-D, Hölze F. *Raising of microvascular flaps: a systematic approach.* Berlin: Springer-Verlag, 2005.

3.10

Anterolateral thigh flap

ANDREW LYONS

PRINCIPLES AND JUSTIFICATION

The anterolateral thigh flap is a perforator flap (Figure 3.10.1). A perforator flap is a flap of skin or subcutaneous tissue that is based on the dissection of a perforating vessel. A perforating vessel or, in short, a perforator, is a vessel that has its origin in one of the axial vessels of the body. It passes through certain structural elements of the body besides interstitial connective tissue and fat before reaching the subcutaneous fat layer. As a perforator flap, the anterolateral thigh flap is relatively simple to raise and in most hands has been reported as an extremely reliable flap for a variety of defects. If the flap pedicle is harvested at its junction with the profunda vessels, the artery is typically 4 mm in diameter and the vein 6 mm in diameter, and it is extremely long. The lateral cutaneous nerve can be incorporated for either motor or sensory nerve reconstruction. Like most perforator flaps it has the advantage of not removing a bulk of muscle and of the skin being closed primarily. It can be raised as a free myocutaneous flap and, provided a large enough flap is raised, the distribution of perforators can be ignored. However, in a Western population, the added bulk is seldom necessary and there are better alternatives if this is desired.

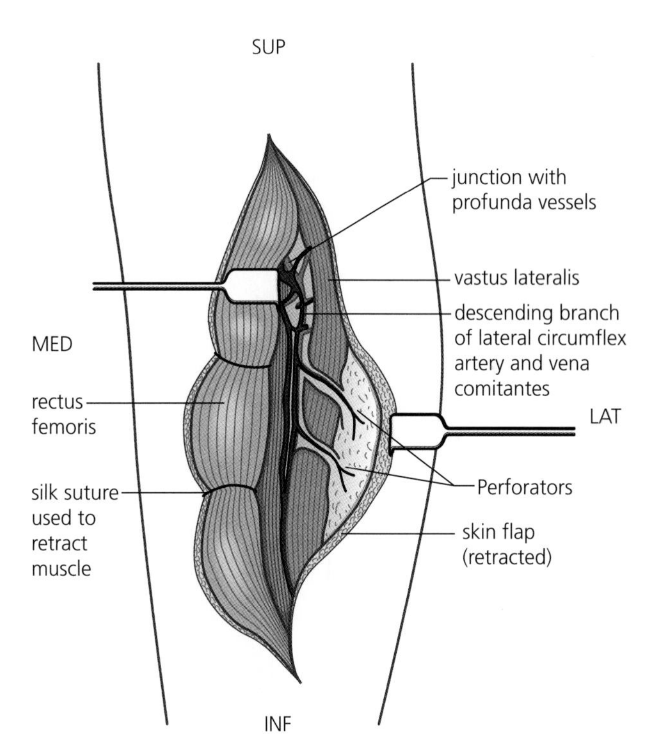

3.10.1 Anatomy of anterolateral thigh flap based on descending branch of lateral circumflex femoral artery.

INDICATIONS

The anterolateral thigh flap is indicated for the coverage of any soft tissue defect of the head and neck including tubed flaps for laryngeal reconstruction and as an obturator flap for maxillary defects. Although popularized in the Far East as the first choice or default flap for intraoral reconstruction, the apparent increase in flap thickness exhibited in Caucasian Western populations, particularly females, can make this flap less than ideal for many defects, and its use should be avoided for patients with a BMI higher than 30. Despite the possibility of a flap that may be 5 cm thick, this is a very useful flap for larger intraoral defects. The flap thickness may be an advantage in replacing a composite parotid resection, total glossectomy where loss of bulk due to muscle atrophy is not a problem, and in maxillary obturation. According to some authors, fairly radical flap thinning can be undertaken, circumventing the thickness problem, perhaps aided by the use of the operating microscope. However, although some flap thinning can be easily undertaken at the margins of the flap, reduction of the entire flap to say 50 per cent would not be recommended, particularly to surgeons new to this technique.

PRE-OPERATIVE

The size and thickness of the proposed defect should be estimated and will indicate whether this flap should be used. The thickness of the flap can be assessed by simply squeezing the skin and subcutaneous tissue in the area of the thigh to be harvested between the thumb and forefingers. If another flap such as the radial forearm flap could be used, to some extent the patient should be offered the choice between the alternative flaps. Even though closed primarily, the donor site scar and thigh dimpling that occurs after healing is not ideal and the patient may prefer the defect in the forearm caused by the radial forearm flap. A line is drawn between the anterior superior iliac spine and the lateral border of the patella (Figure 3.10.2). At a point midway along this line a 4 cm circle is drawn. Perforating vessels are searched for using a 10 MHz hand-held Doppler probe, the most common site to find a perforator is in the inferolateral section (Figure 3.10.3).

Nearly all patients have usable perforators (96%) and hand-held Doppler only has a positive predictive value of 65 per cent, so this is a guide only and should not be a reason for abandoning the flap. Either leg can be used for any defect so the leg that has the loudest perforators should be used. However, all patients should be warned that an alternative flap might have to be utilized.

OPERATION

Position of the patient

The patient should be supine without the aid of any sandbags or splinting of the leg. This permits synchronous harvesting of the flap with the head and neck resection. Though not essential, ideally all monitoring lines should be placed in the other leg.

Incision

The incision is placed along a line drawn between anterior superior iliac spine and the lateral border of the patella (Figure 3.10.2) unless it crosses where a perforator can be heard on the Doppler (in which case the line should be moved to give at least 1 cm clear skin between the signal and the flap margin). If a sensate flap is required, the lateral femoral cutaneous nerve can be harvested. Conveniently this runs along the line joining the anterior superior iliac spine to the lateral border of the patella and is found to lie in the deep subcutaneous tissue just above the fascia. No further flap marking is carried out to permit relocation when the perforator(s) are visualized much later. The incision should be angled at 45° laterally to protect any nearby perforator(s) and is deepened to incise the deep fascia to expose the underlying rectus femoris or vastus lateralis muscle.

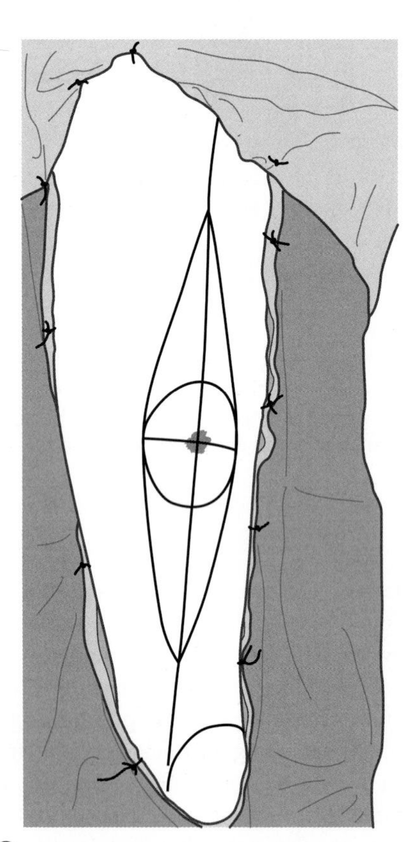

3.10.2 Anterolateral thigh flap marked out. Note inferolateral segment of 4 cm radius circle is most likely to contain perforator(s).

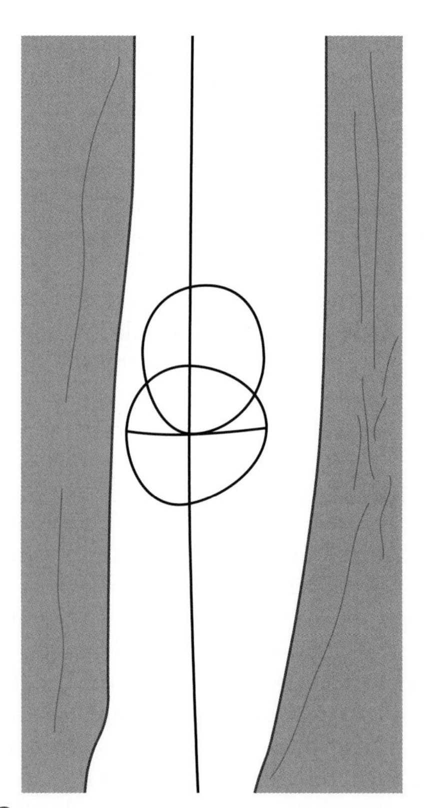

3.10.3 After Doppler mapping, this circle that will be included in the flap has been moved 4 cm away from the anterior superior iliac spine, at top left of picture.

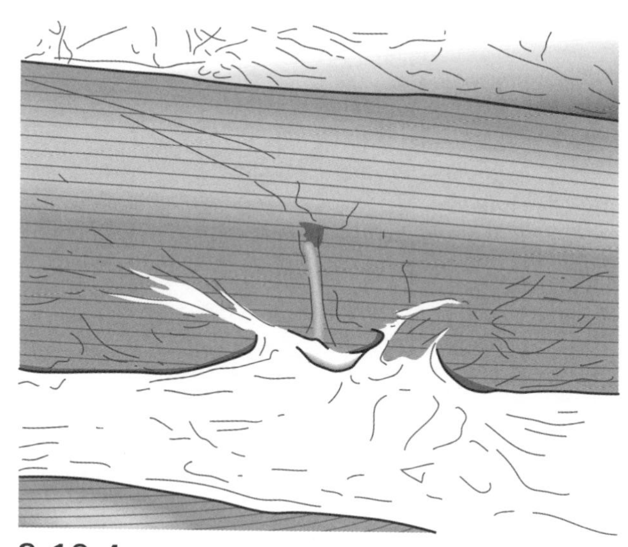

3.10.4 Dissection of perforator.

Perforator location

Dissection under the fascia is undertaken with a pair of small blunt ended scissors in a lateral to medial direction to permit identification of the perforator(s) (Figures 3.10.4 and 3.10.5). Nearly all perforators (>85 per cent) will run through the vastus lateralis muscle. Perforators with a combined diameter of the artery and vena comitantes of 1 mm or less should not be used as the sole perforator that can be used as a supplementary perforator. These myocutaneous perforators will require a more difficult tracing and dissecting out than any septocutaneous perforators found.

In the rare event that no perforators are found within or lateral to the septum between vastus lateralis and rectus femoris, perforators can be searched for medial to this septum. Perforators here are also likely followed into the descending branch. This resultant 'anteromedial thigh flap' is likely to produce a very fat bulky flap with a relatively short pedicle but it may still be useful. The transverse branch of the lateral circumflex femoral artery gives rise to perforators to form the tensor fascia lata flap. The pedicle is situated at the superior end of the line joining the anterior superior iliac spine to the lateral border of the patella and lies between the tensor fascia lata and rectus femoris muscle. Perforators may be located in a similar fashion by dissecting below the fascia in a medial to lateral direction. Again this flap will tend to offer a bulky flap with a shorter pedicle than the anterolateral thigh flap.

It is recommended to first trace out the perforators by careful dissection to the main pedicle rather than dissect them out completely as the latter manoeuvre is more easily performed once the entire pedicle can be visualized. Side branches from the perforators should be coagulated with a bipolar diathermy or ligated with small metal clips, particularly if close to the perforator. Perforators are followed through muscle and or fascia until the main pedicle (descending branch of the lateral circumflex femoral artery) is reached within the groove between rectus femoris and vastus lateralis muscles.

It is not recommended to locate the descending branch of the lateral circumflex femoral artery by dissecting down into the groove between the rectus femoris and vastus lateralis then follow branching lateral perforators in a lateral direction towards the skin, as most of this perforators will end in muscle.

Musculocutaneous non-perforator flap

Alternatively, providing the skin flap is no less than 100 cm^2 and no less than 10 cm in length along the artery, a 1.5 cm sheet of vastus lateralis muscle can be raised with a myocutaneous flap by dissecting below this layer of muscle in a lateral direction. However, if such a bulky flap is desired there may well be better alternatives.

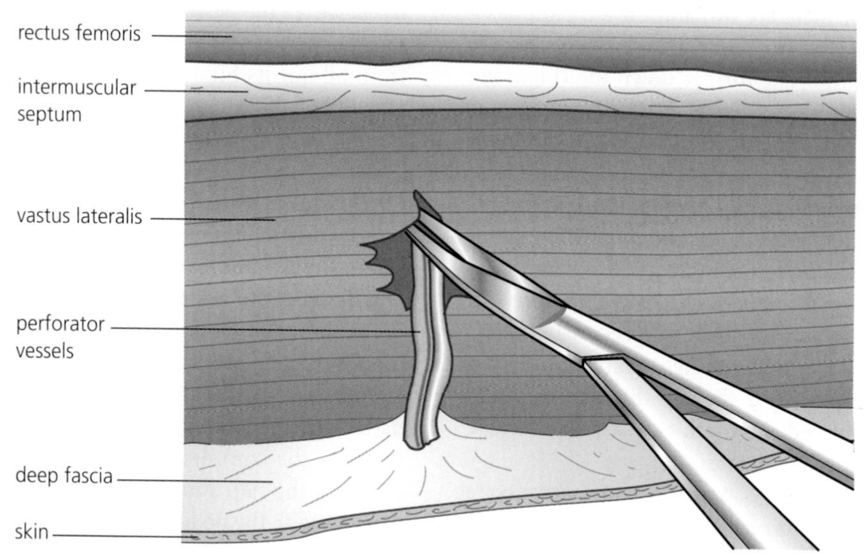

3.10.5 Dissection of perforator.

Pedicle dissection

The artery and its venae comitantes are followed from the junction with the perforator(s) to the junction with the profunda femoris artery and vein if the entire length of the pedicle is required (Figure 3.10.6). During this dissection, it is helpful to self retain the muscle by placing large sutures from its underbelly to the lateral skin. Once the juncton has been identified, full dissecting out of the pedicle and perforators can take place in a proximal to distal direction. If the entire length is not required then it is not necessary to dissect out the entire descending lateral circumflex vessel, however, the artery and venae comitantes may be much smaller (at around 2 mm) before both transverse and ascending vessels join so it may be preferable to accommodate a lengthy pedicle in the neck rather than have an ideal length with small vessels. During this dissection many branching arteries and veins will be encountered and will require ligation. This may include the ascending and transverse lateral circumflex vessels (Figure 3.10.7). Branches of the femoral nerve run underneath the pedicle and will have to be dissected out carefully. This becomes more problematic as the diameter of both the pedicle and nerves become smaller, and it may be preferable to sacrifice a small nerve branch which will have little, if any, impact on motor function rather than damage the pedicle or perforator(s). During the dissection of the musculocutaneous perforators, by leaving a 5 mm cuff of muscle around these perforators the dissection is made less hazardous and the perforators are made more robust.

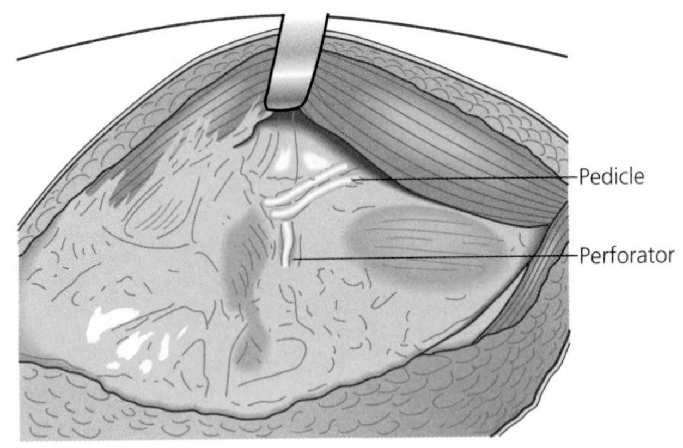

3.10.6 Exposure of the pedicle: descending superficial circumflex femoral artery and vena comitantes with perforator in foreground.

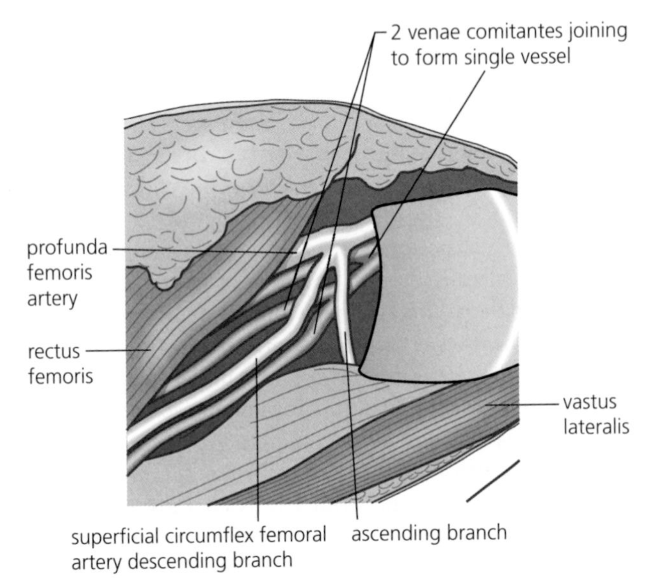

3.10.7 Junction of pedicle and profunda vessels.

Flap design and skin paddle elevation

Once the main pedicle and perforator(s) have been fully dissected out, the skin flap can now be designed. If two perforators are present then, unless the flap is very large, it will encompass both at either ends of its length. If there is just one perforator, or there are two and the surgeon has a specific requirement, the position of the paddle can be varied according to need. The further down the thigh, the thinner the tissue becomes (Figure 3.10.8), but if it is planned to anastomose at the large termination part of the pedicle this will produce a very long pedicle.

According to some authors, flap thickness in Caucasians is 4 cm in the upper thigh, 3 cm in the mid thigh and 2 cm in the lower thigh. The tissue is much thicker as a result of fat deposition in the superior thigh, but the pedicle is often an ideal or manageable length for most oral reconstructions and the increased bulk may be desirable. A compromise may be reached to end up with a slightly thicker flap than necessary, with a slight pedicle length excess but with very large vessels to use in an anastomosis.

To ensure that the 'backcut' flap incision does not violate the perforator(s) it is recommended to pass a small needle from the fascia towards and out of the skin at a point situated a minimum of 1 cm from the pedicle below the fascia where the perforators can be visualized. The flap can then be marked around this, and the flap raised and isolated from all but its blood supply to permit evaluation of the viability of the flap.

Observing the undivided flap

There should be clear evidence of bleeding subcutaneous flap tissue at this time. If two perforators have been raised, the viability of either perforator can be assessed using a microvascular clamp on the pedicles (Figure 3.10.9).

This manoeuvre is essential if the flap is to be divided and used as two separate or chimeric flaps. During the interval between the completed elevation of the flap and pedicle division, the flap should be sutured to one of the wound margins with the pedicle under no tension. This will prevent the flap accidentally falling off the leg downwards, which might produce a force sufficient to tear the pedicle.

Dividing the flap

This is straightforward and the same as for any other flap, the vessels in the thigh should be transfixed if harvesting at the profunda junction. The flap should be irrigated with heparinized saline. If clotted blood becomes dry in the perforators, it will be difficult to get them running again. If there is only one perforator before the pedicle is divided, a stitch should be run from part of the perforator (preferably the muscle) cuff to a flap margin to prevent torsion or kinking of the perforator.

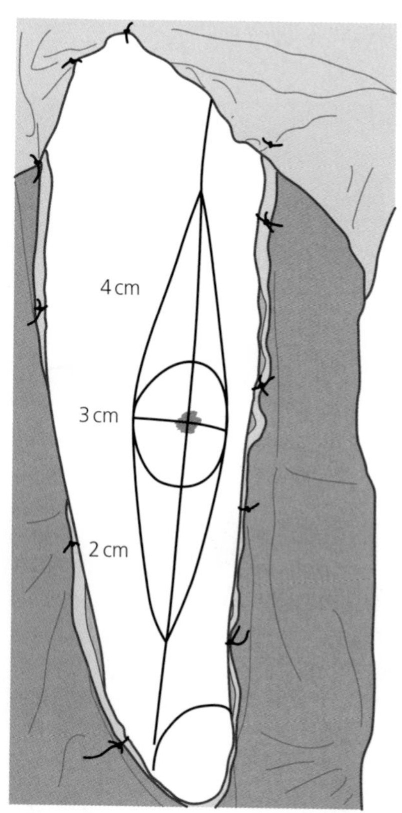

3.10.8 Flap thickness at different thigh levels.

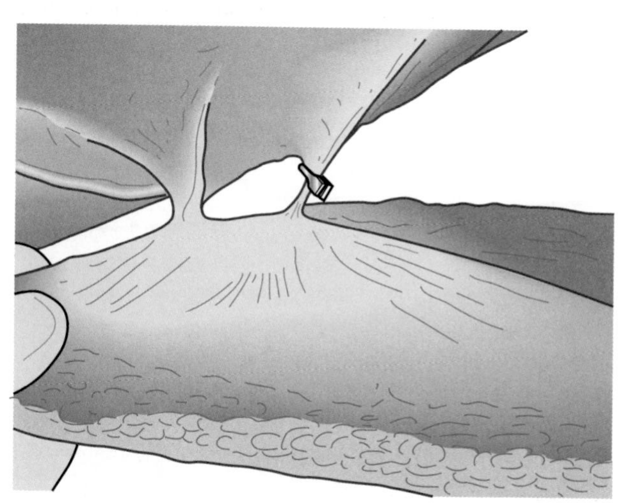

3.10.9 Flap with microvascular clamp to assess flow of unclamped perforator.

Closure of the donor site

This can be commenced as soon as the flap has been completely raised and a large part of the closure can be carried out prior to pedicle division. If closure is not to be carried out immediately, three sutures (2/0 or larger) should be used to close the donor site temporarily, as swelling will otherwise make closure very difficult.

After diathermising any bleeding points, closure should commence with repair of any muscle that has been divided to permit perforator dissection. A resorbable 3/0 stitch is recommended. Closure of the fascia and subcutaneous tissue should then be carried out using a 2/0 resorbable suture. If the pedicle has not been divided, the superior part of the wound can be left open, to be closed after pedicle division. The skin can be closed with either non-resorbable sutures or clips. It is not recommended to insert a drain in the leg, although a tight crepe bandage is desirable. Flaps of up to 10 cm width can be closed primarily but nylon tension sutures will probably have to be used to achieve this.

Insetting the flap

Flap insetting may be made difficult if it is too bulky for the defect (Figure 3.10.10). Certainly trimming the fat, particularly at the margins of the flap, is helpful in this scenario. If the flap is tight as it is inset, it is recommended to orientate it with a minimum number of sutures (say four) and then proceed to anastomosis (Figure 3.10.11). The flap is then allowed to run before insetting. If the flap is to be tubed, the deep fascia can be closed around the skin layer as a double closure.

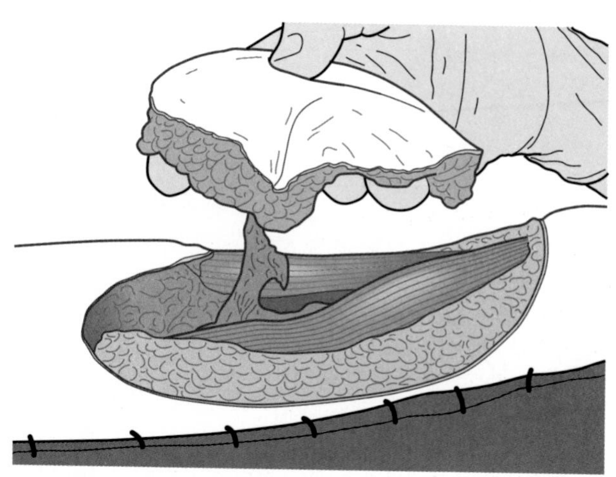

3.10.10 Bulky anterolateral thigh flap.

POST-OPERATIVE CARE

Monitoring the flap

The skin is easily monitored and a Doppler probe can be placed on the site of the perforator in the flap as before it was raised; this is easily achieved for flaps used for skin replacement but more problematic for intraoral flaps, although this is easier with a detachable internal monitoring probe. Otherwise, monitoring the pedicle in the neck is usually adequate. If the blood flow is to be evaluated using a needle prick, blood flow may be slower than that seen in other flaps. After radiotherapy or at least one month, the flap can be safely thinned if it is too bulky.

COMPLICATIONS

Intraoperative

Damage to the fine perforators is the obvious and catastrophic complication. Fortunately, this is most likely to

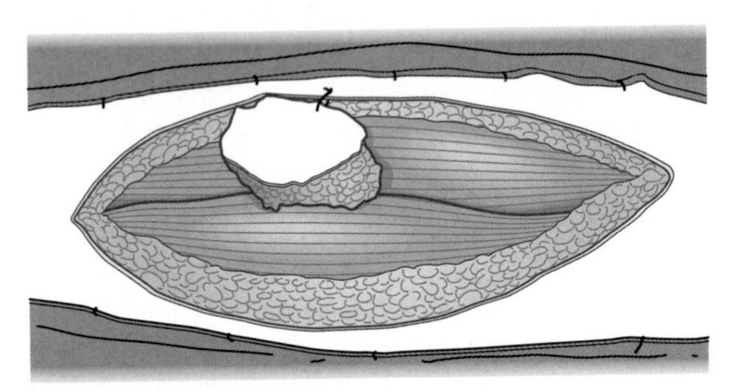

3.10.11 Flap temporarily attached to skin.

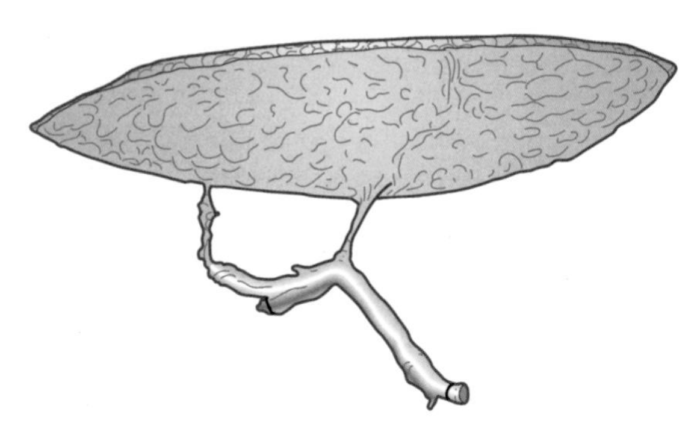

3.10.12 Detached flap.

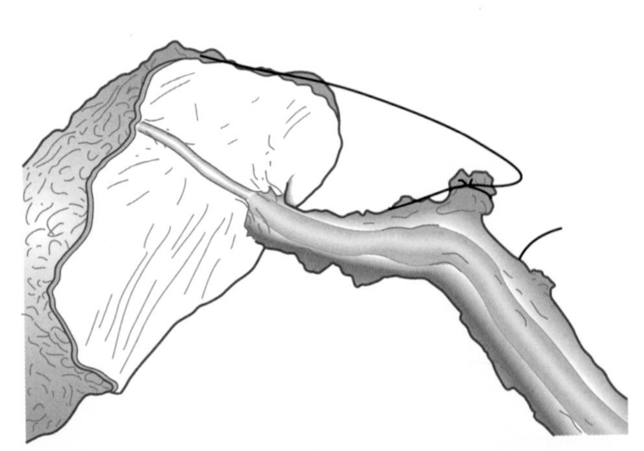

3.10.13 Detached with single perforator and anti-twisting stitch.

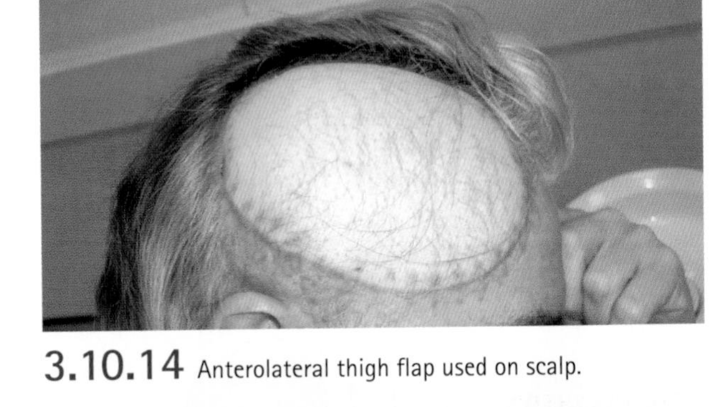

3.10.14 Anterolateral thigh flap used on scalp.

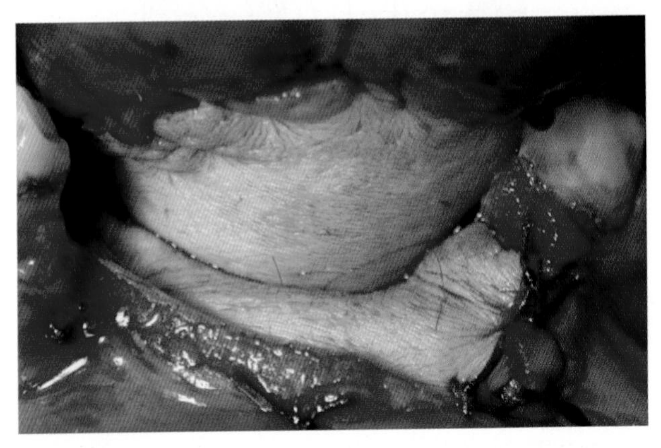

3.10.15 Anterolateral thigh flap used for floor of mouth reconstruction.

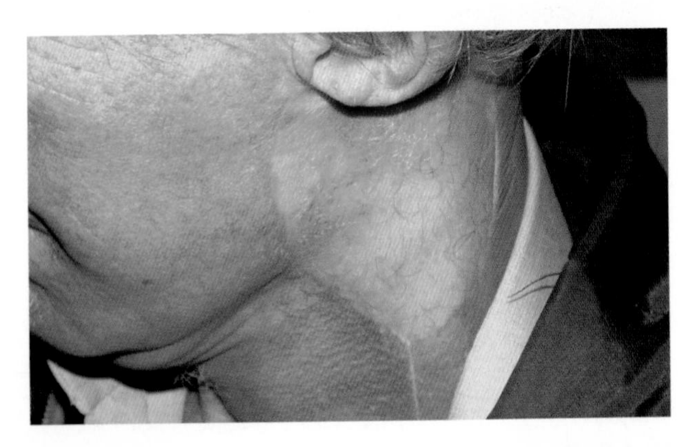

3.10.16 Anterolateral thigh flap used for parotid area reconstruction.

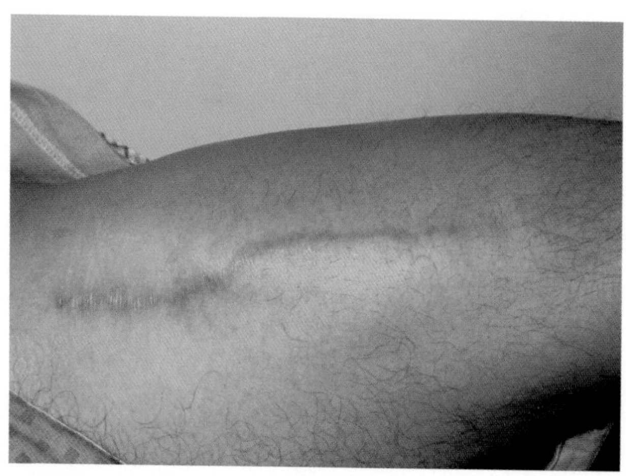

3.10.17 Donor site after six months.

Top tips

- Always get consent from the patient for another flap, particularly if you are inexperienced as you may not be able to find a perforator, and can at least use what was going to be an anterolateral thigh flap as a Wolfe Graft!
- Do not underestimate the bulk of fat that you might be obliged to inset with this flap and, if it is going to be 'tight', tack the flap in to orientate it, then do the anastomoses to get it running. Insetting a tight 'running flap' will not stop the blood flow.
- Always be vigilant against twisting the pedicle, particularly if there is only one perforator; use a suture to safeguard this as described in the text.

occur in the very early stages of the flap, when it can be abandoned for an alternative. Twisting a single perforator is a hazard that should be avoidable by placing the safety stitch as described earlier.

Post-operative

In the author's experience, this is an extremely reliable flap, but vigilance for arterial and venous failure is clearly essential. Even partial flap necrosis is rare. Gait problems may require months to resolve if a large number of femoral nerve branches have been sacrificed. Thigh numbness may result, but is likely to be of little significance to the patient.

FURTHER READING

Burd A, Pang P. The antero-lateral thigh (ALT) flap: a pragmatic approach. *British Journal of Plastic Surgery* 2003; **56**: 837–9.

Celik N, Wei FC, Lin CH *et al.* Technique and strategy in anterolateral thigh perforator flap surgery. An analysis based on 15 complete and partial failures in 439 cases. *Plastic and Reconstructive Surgery* 2002; **109**: 2211–16.

Coskunferat OK, Ozkan O. Free tensor fascia lata perforator flap as a backup procedure for head and neck reconstruction. *Annals of Plastic Surgery* 2006; **57**: 159–63.

Demirkan F, Chen HC, Wei FC *et al.* The versatile anterolateral thigh flap: a musculocutaneous flap in disguise in head and neck reconstruction. *British Journal of Plastic Surgery* 2000; **53**: 30–36.

Kimura N, Satoh K. Consideration of a thin flap as an entity and clinical applications of the thin anterolateral thigh flap. *Plastic and Reconstructive Surgery* 1996; **97**: 985–92.

Mardini S, Tsai FC, Wei FC. The thigh as a model for free style flaps. *Clinics in Plastic Surgery* 2003; **30**: 473–80.

Ross GL, Dunn R, Kirkpatrick J *et al.* To thin or not to thin: the use of the anterolateral thigh flap in the reconstruction of intraoral defect. *British Journal of Plastic Surgery* 2003; **6**: 409–13.

Song YG, Chen GZ, Song Y. The free thigh flap: a new free flap concept based on the septocutaneous artery. *British Journal of Plastic Surgery* 1984; **37**: 149–59.

Yu PU. Characteristics of the anterolateral thigh flap in a western population and its application in head and neck reconstruction. *Head and Neck* 2004; **26**: 759–69.

Yu P, Youssef A. Efficacy of the handheld Doppler in preoperative identification of the cutaneous perforators in the anterolateral thigh flap. *Plastic and Reconstructive Surgery* 2006; **118**: 928–33.

3.11

Gracilis flap

HENNING SCHLIEPHAKE

RECONSTRUCTIVE USE

The gracilis flap is most frequently used in free neuromuscular tissue transfer for facial reanimation after long-standing facial paralysis. The low profile of the muscle and the organization in small innervated segments make this flap particularly suitable for the reconstruction of mimic muscles. Gracilis muscle free flaps are, however, also used as innervated muscle segments for tongue reconstruction and for skull base repair as muscle only flaps. The skin overlying the muscle has been reported to be unreliable, but myocutaneous gracilis free flaps have been successfully transferred as transverse gracilis (TUG) flaps for breast reconstruction. Moreover, the muscle is extensively used as pedicled flap for reconstructive procedures in the perineal area.

ANATOMY

The gracilis muscle is a flat and thin adductor muscle of the thigh. It originates from the ramus of the pubic bone and inserts at the medial tibial tuberosity below the knee. The gracilis muscle is a type II muscle with its dominant vascular supply arising from the adductor artery and vein, which themselves branch off the profunda femoris artery and vein. The vascular pedicle commonly has two comitans veins and enters the gracilis muscle 8–10 cm distal to the pubic tubercle. Minor vascular pedicles arise from the superficial femoral artery (distal) and from the medial circumflex artery (proximal). The motor nerve supply comes through the anterior branch of the obturator nerve and enters the muscle approximately 2 cm proximal to the vascular pedicle.

OPERATION

Position of the patient

The patient is positioned supine with the hip of his donor leg flexed, abducted and rotated outward and the knee moderately flexed so that the foot rests on the operation table at the height of the opposite lower leg (Figure 3.11.1). This position is secured by support against the calf and the thigh preventing the knee from stretching and the thigh from rotating back inward. Care must be taken to provide adequate padding for the calf in order to prevent pressure ulcers on the skin overlying the tibia. The leg and the pubic hair should be shaved pre-operatively and the site draped in a way that the inner half of the thigh and the landmarks (medial tibial tuberosity and the pubic tubercle) are exposed and can be clearly palpated. The surgeon is positioned on the side of the operation table opposite to the donor leg.

Skin incision

A straight line is drawn between the pubic tubercle and the tibial tuberosity. In an upright position, this would delineate the anterior margin of the gracilis muscle. In a horizontal position in relaxation, the muscle drops down and the anterior margin is located approximately 15 mm posterior

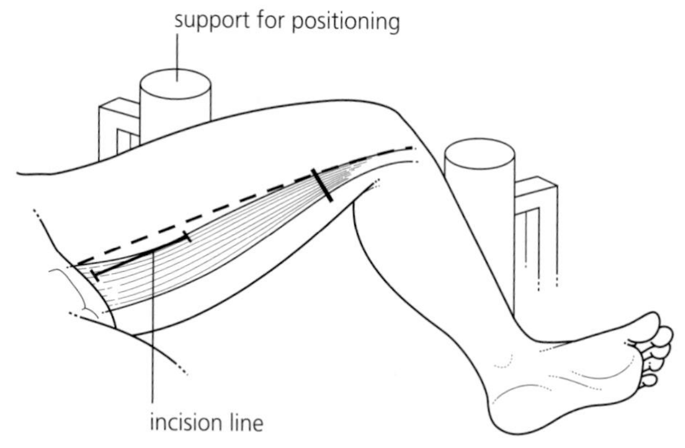

3.11.1 Positioning of the donor leg.

to the straight line, where it should be marked with an additional line (Figure 3.11.1). The incision through the skin and subcutaneous fat tissue is carried out along this line approximately 20 cm in length starting below the pubic tubercle. The incision goes through the superficial fascia down to the fascia lata.

Exposure of the gracilis muscle

The gracilis midbelly is identified after incision of the overlying fascia and clearly distinguished from the sartorius muscle, which is located anterior to the gracilis in the surgical position of the leg in the mid thigh and from the adductor longus muscle that is located immediately anterior to the gracilis muscle in the proximal thigh (Figure 3.11.2). Separation of the skin and the subcutaneous fat tissue from the lateral aspect of the muscle can help to identify the gracilis from the small anterior–posterior dimension. The intermuscular septum between the adductor longus and the gracilis muscle is carefully divided superficially and small vessels that may enter the anterior margin of the muscle can be coagulated and divided.

Identification of the vascular pedicle and the motor nerve supply

The vascular pedicle runs in the intermuscular septum between the adductor longus and the adductor magnus before entering the gracilis muscle (Figure 3.11.3). It is first envisioned when carefully dividing the adductor longus from the gracilis muscle at the anterior margin of the gracilis by blunt dissection while reflecting the gracilis muscle. In this position, the vessels are running across the surface of the adductor magnus muscle that becomes visible between the adductor longus and the gracilis muscle (Figure 3.11.4). After identification of the artery and the two comitans veins, the motor nerve supply is dissected and exposed by continuing the dissection slightly more proximal, where the anterior obturator nerve can be identified from its oblique course across the surface of the adductor magnus muscle. The nerve enters the gracilis muscle approximately 20 mm proximal to the entry of the vascular pedicle.

Dissection of the vascular pedicle

Before entering the gracilis muscle, the vascular pedicle gives off small branches to the adductor longus muscle (Figure 3.11.4). These branches have to be ligated to get access to the full pedicle length. During this procedure it is helpful to pull up the adductor longus muscle with two small retractors placed proximally and distally to the vascular pedicle. Fine scissors and forceps are necessary to accomplish blunt release of the tiny branches from the adductor longus muscle surface. After elevation of the branches, haemostat clips are used for ligation. Electrocautery of the small vessels is not recommended in order to avoid thermal damage to the main pedicle. After separation of the branches, the adductor longus muscle can be pulled fully upwards giving way to the dissection along

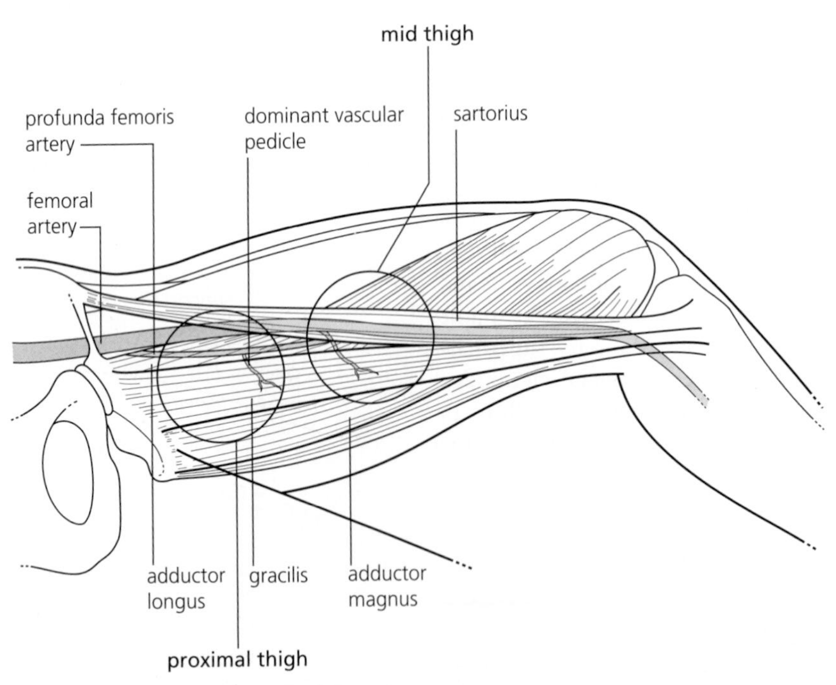

3.11.2 Spatial relationship of the gracilis muscle at mid thigh and proximal thigh. Adapted from Manktelov [3].

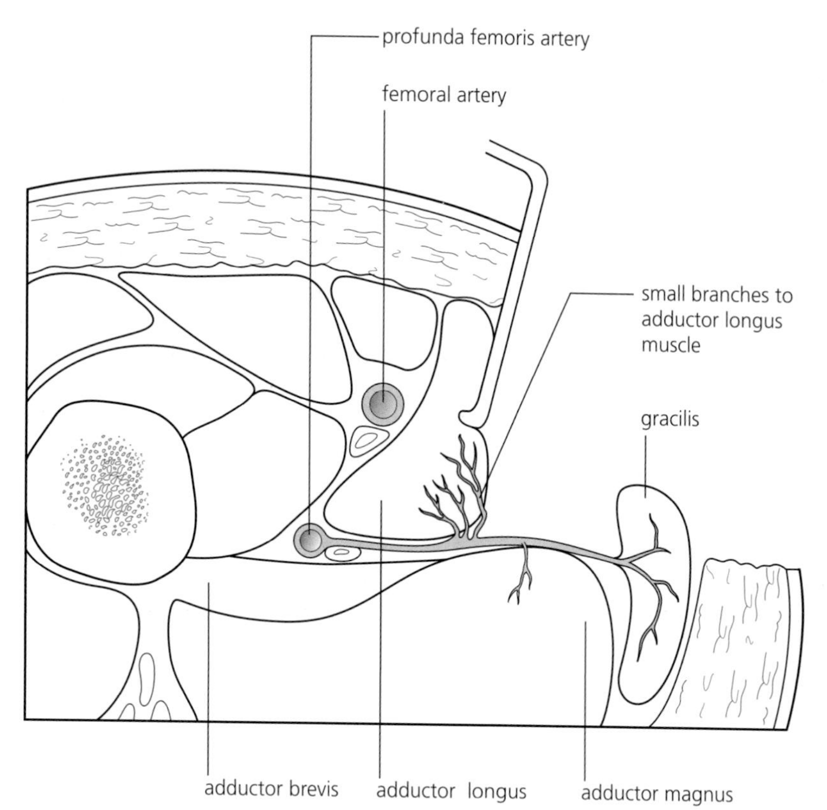

3.11.3 Anatomy of the course of the vascular pedicle. Adapted from Manktelov [3].

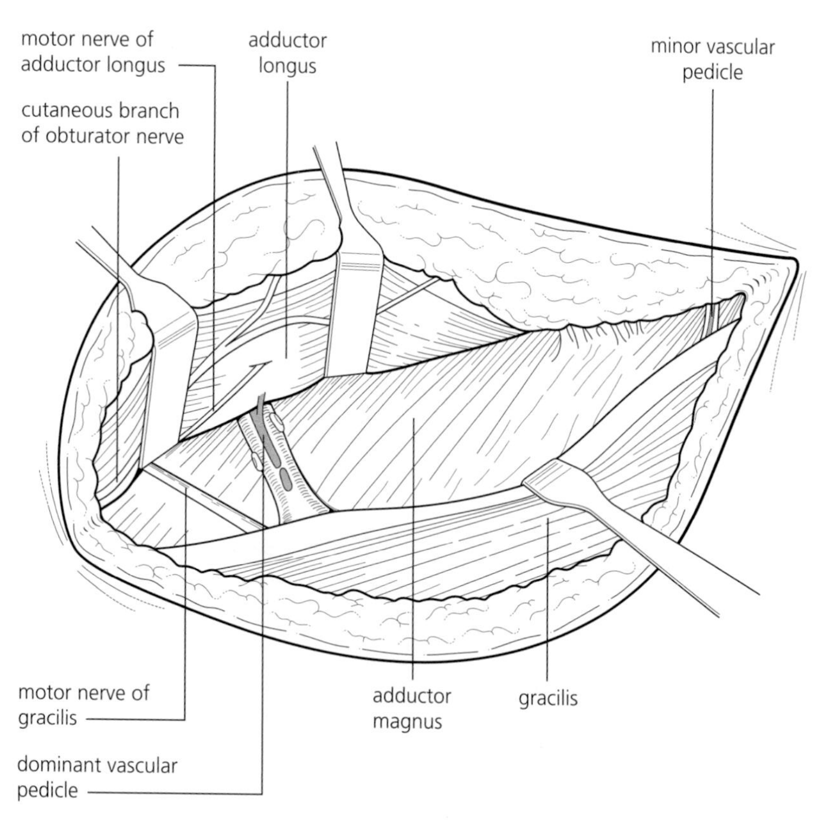

3.11.4 Identification of the vascular pedicle between adductor longus and gracilis, lying on the adductor magnus. Adapted from Manktelov [3].

the pedicle to the profunda femoris vessels. There may well be branches that run off into the underlying adductor magnus muscle, these have to be identified and ligated by carefully elevating the vascular pedicle from the muscle surface before the pedicle is separated from the profunda femoris vessels. During ligation of the pedicle, care must be taken not to compromise blood flow in the profunda femoris vessels. Therefore, a minimum distance of 5 mm from the junction between the pedicle and the profunda femoris artery and vein should be observed when the pedicle is cut. After completion of the dissection of the adductor artery and veins, a pedicle length of approximately 6 cm should be available. The diameter of the vessels can be expected to be between 2 and 2.5 mm on average.

Dissection of the obturator nerve and definition of the graft size

The obturator nerve that has been previously identified is easily followed along its course proximally by blunt dissection until a length of approximately 8 cm is achieved. A nerve stimulator is used to define neuromuscular units. If very small muscle segments are planned, dissection of the nerve under the microscope can be carried out and individual neuromuscular units identified after stimulation of individual fascicles (Figure 3.11.5). The nerve usually contains three fascicles, although there may be up to seven present. The anterior half of the muscle belly is commonly innervated by one fascicle; the posterior half is supplied by the remaining ones with some overlap in the mid line. The width of the muscle segment that is used for facial reanimation commonly occupies half of the width of the muscle belly, so that the anterior half of the muscle is divided for harvesting. In the proximal half, the muscle fibres run parallel which makes division in longitudinal direction easy. The length of the muscle required has to be identified beforehand during pre-operative planning and the dissection of the recipient site in the cheek (see Chapter 3.14). Usually, a length of approximately 8 cm is needed. To avoid inadvertent damage to the neurovascular pedicle during release and circumcision of the deeper muscle portions, a small retractor is inserted underneath the pedicle close to its entry into the muscle and gently pulled upwards (Figure 3.11.6). During final separation and mobilization, the epimysium is preserved on the surface of the muscle to provide a sliding layer for easier movement of the muscle during contraction after transfer. Before the pedicle is divided, adequate perfusion of the muscle segment is checked.

After complete separation, the function of the obturator nerve segment included in the graft should also be checked with the nerve tester after placing the graft on a moist

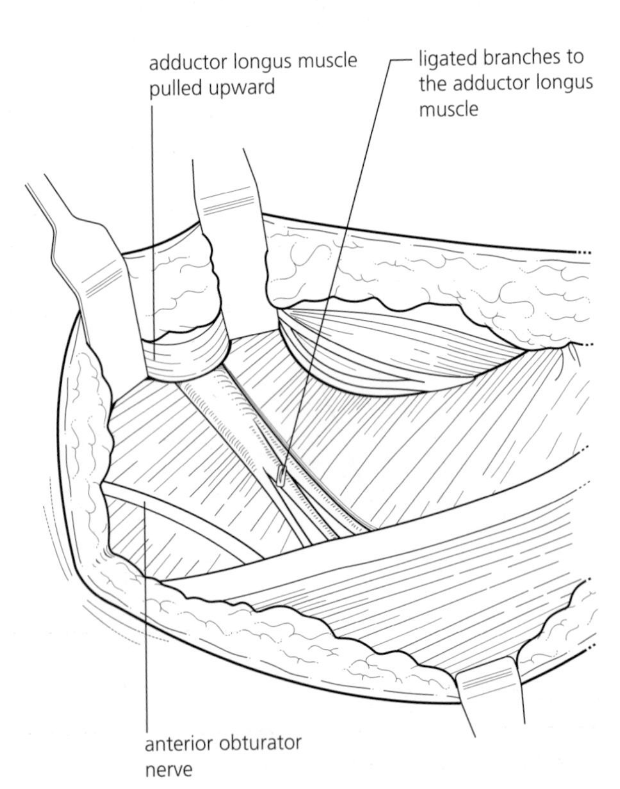

3.11.5 Complete exposure of the vascular pedicle and the nerve supply.

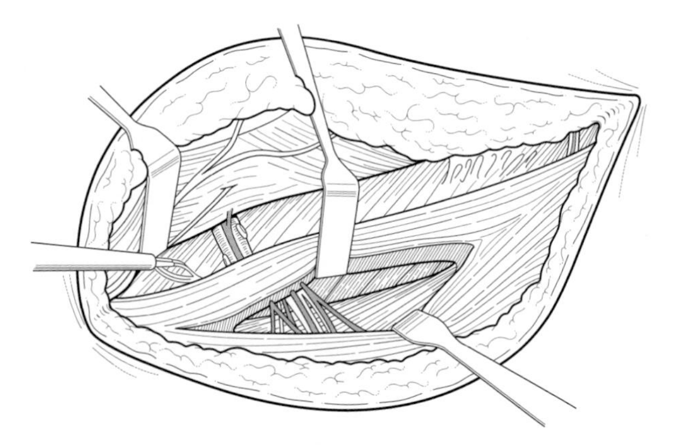

3.11.6 Dissection of the muscle to identify individual muscular units. Adapted from Manktelov [3].

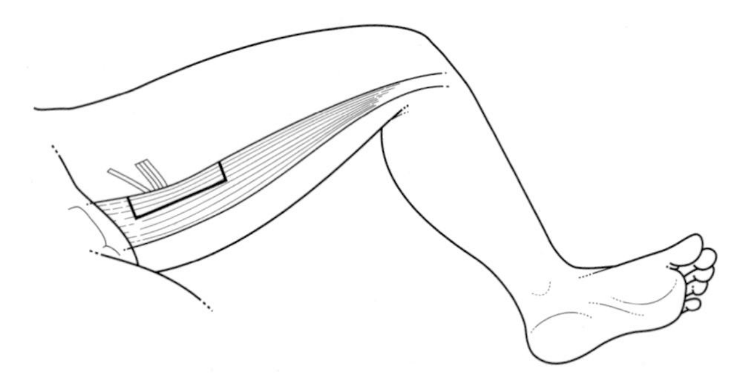

3.11.7 Location and size of the graft removed from the muscle.

surgical towel on the patient's skin (Figure 3.11.7). The graft is then stored in moist surgical towels until definite graft fixation and microvascular anastomosis are performed.

Wound closure and post-operative care

Meticulous control of bleeding from the transectioned muscle tissue is performed by electrocautery. The anterior margin of the remaining parts of the gracilis muscle is attached to the fascia of the adductor longus muscle to stabilize the gracilis muscle and restore easy function of the adductor muscles. A 10 gauge suction drainage is placed on the reconstructed fascia and the wound is closed in layers. The leg is bandaged with decreasing pressure from distal to proximal or a pressure stocking is applied to avoid post-operative thrombosis.

Routine post-operative prevention of thrombosis is applied by administration of fractionated heparin (e.g. enoxaparin). The operated leg should be positioned in a slightly elevated position for a couple of days until complete mobilization of the patient is achieved. Post-operative mobilization with the help of a physical therapist can be performed from the first post-operative day on as the muscle function of the adductor group remains grossly unaffected by the removal of the small gracilis segment and its nerve supply. If no substantial bleeding occurs, the suction drainage can be removed on the second post-operative day.

COMPLICATIONS

In general, harvesting of the gracilis muscle has very low morbidity and complications are rarely encountered associated with this procedure.

Intraoperative complications

- Damage to the pedicle may occur during release of the branches to the adductor longus and adductor magnus muscle. The use of the microscope during dissection and the use of clips rather than electrocautry during ligation are helpful in avoiding this problem.
- Damage to the profunda femoris vessels may occur during separation and ligation of the pedicle. In particular, the profunda femoris veins are prone to compromised blood flow and subsequent thrombosis. This can be avoided by observing an adequate distance of 5 mm pedicle length during ligation and separation of the pedicle from the profunda femoris vessels and by using clips rather than sutures for ligation.
- Nerve damage is unlikely to occur as the dissected segment of the obturator nerve is only short and interference with other nerves is not encountered.

Post-operative complications

- **Haemorrhage.** Post-operative bleeding is unlikely to occur as the site of harvest does not contain high volume flow vessels and the dissection is carried out only along intermuscular septa without dividing or cutting vessels with relevant blood flow that could be violated inadvertently and overlooked during wound closure. Nevertheless, improperly seated ligation clips after separation of the pedicle from the profunda femoris vessels can become detached and cause substantial haemorrhage. Thus, great care is required during this part of the dissection to make sure that ligations of the adductor vessels are reliable. Secondary bleeding from the transected muscle may occur if haemostasis has been inadequate. The careful use of electrocautery after identification of individual intramuscular branches under the microscope before wound closure minimizes this risk.
- **Thrombosis.** Thrombosis is also unlikely to occur if routine heparin prophylaxis is administered and early mobilization is accomplished. The saphenous vein that drains the superficial venous system is located above the site of harvest. This vein is commonly not encountered during dissection and thus can be easily preserved. Deep venous thrombosis may occur if ligation clips or sutures compromise the blood flow in the profunda femoris veins, which can be avoided by observing an adequate distance to the vein during ligation as described above.

Top tips

The dissection of the flap is very straightforward, with little chance for it to go grossly wrong. Nevertheless, a few things can ease the surgical work and improve the results.

- During flap dissection, the division of the branches that go off into the adductor longus is a crucial point. Use magnification to make sure that this is done carefully and take your time. Use clips or microcautery.
- As the pedicle is rather short, use as much length as you can get, however, keep in mind to preserve a 5 mm cuff for ligation to avoid thrombosis of the profunda femoris vein.
- When defining the muscle volume, take care not to obtain too much tissue. Careful nerve testing and definition of functional muscle units will improve the result in terms of cosmetics, as unsightly bulging of the grafted muscle during contraction is avoided. Trimming of the muscle after transfer is always more difficult and carries the risk of removing the wrong muscle units.

FURTHER READING

Arnez ZM, Pogorolec D, Planinsek F, Ahcan U. Breast reconstruction by the free gracilis (TUG) flap. *British Journal of Plastic Surgery* 2004; **57**: 20–26.

Hari K, Ohmori K, Torii S, Free gracilis muscle transplantation with micorvascular anastomosis for the treatment of facial paralysis. *Plastic and Reconstructive Surgery* 1976; **57**:133–5.

Manktelow RT. *Microvascular reconstruction.* New York: Springer, 1986, 37.

Mathes SJ, Nahai F, Classification of the vascular territory of muscles: experimental and clinical correlation. *Plastic and Reconstructive Surgery* 1981; **76**: 177.

Sullivan MJ, Urken ML. Gracilis. In: Urken ML, Cheney ML, Sullivan MJ, Biller HF (eds). *Atlas of regional and free flaps for head and neck reconstruction.* New York: Raven Press, 1995, 139–48.

Yousif N, Matloub H, Kabachalam R *et al.* The transverse gracilis musculocutaneous flap. *Annals of Plastic Surgery* 1992; **29**: 482–90.

3.12

Fibular flap

PETER A BRENNAN, ANDRÉ ECKARDT

INTRODUCTION

The fibula is a long slender triangular-shaped bone that is said to have two functions – ankle joint stability and microvascular reconstruction of bony defects! It is mainly composed of cortical bone, giving it great stability. The advantages of the fibula are that it offers an abundant supply of tubed bi-cortical bone, which is useful for reconstruction of long segmental defects across the midline – 25 cm or more of bone can be harvested. There is usually little morbidity at the donor site, and it is highly reliable with a 95 per cent success rate (when used, the skin paddle component is reported to be less reliable). It is also possible to harvest the fibula simultaneously with the tumour resection as no change in the patient's position is required. Bone height is the main potential disadvantage, especially when reconstructing the dentate mandible. To overcome this problem, the osteotomized fibula can be folded back onto itself while maintaining intact soft tissue and periosteum on one side ('double barrelling'). Distraction osteogenesis, followed by implant placement, can also give a very good result (Figure 3.12.1). It is usual to leave the flap for several months before distraction to allow bony union with the recipient bed and enable the fixation plates to be removed.

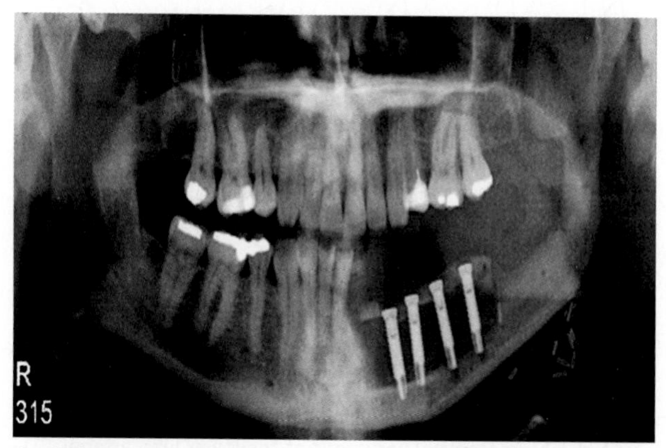

3.12.1 Implants placed in a recently distracted fibula.

HISTORICAL DEVELOPMENT

The first vascularized fibula flap transfer was used for ulnar reconstruction in 1974 (series of cases published in 1983). Free fibula transfer for two tibial defects were subsequently reported in 1975. As the flap was increasingly used, modifications were made, such as including large parts of the soleus muscle, and skin paddles. Whereas these first fibula transfers were performed without a skin paddle, an osteocutaneous fibula flap was first reported in 1983. The use of the vascularized fibula in mandibular reconstruction was reported in 1989 and this opened a new field in maxillofacial reconstructive surgery.

The fibula is the longest bone flap available and it can be transferred as a bone flap or in combination with a skin island for soft tissue coverage if required. Therefore, it has a broad spectrum of indications ranging from bony reconstruction of the extremities to partial or total mandibular reconstruction including closure of perforating defects of the oral cavity. The disadvantage of the skin paddle is that it cannot be rotated separately from the bone (as compared to a scapula flap).

SURGICAL ANATOMY

An understanding of the relevant anatomy of the fibula itself and the arrangement of muscles, compartments and vascular supply of the lower limb below the knee is vital (Figure 3.12.2).

The lateral compartment of the lower leg (lateral to the fibula itself) is formed by peroneus longus and brevis muscles (the latter muscle arising from the fibula more distally). In the anterior compartment, extensor hallucis longus (EHL) and extensor digitorum longus are attached to

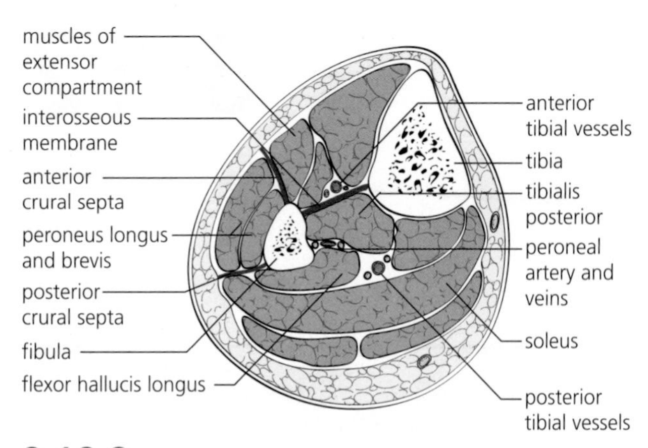

3.12.2 Cross-section of the mid calf. The inter-osseous membrane and anterior/posterior crural septae have been highlighted in bold (nerves have not been shown).

the anterior surface of the fibula. The large tibialis anterior muscle is found nearer the tibia. Separating the anterior and posterior compartments is the anterior inter-osseus membrane – a white fibrous band that is attached to both fibula and tibia. The anterior tibial artery and deep tibial nerve can be found running close to this membrane. In the posterior compartment, lying between tibialis posterior and flexor hallucis longus (FHL) muscles (and close to the deep surface of the fibula) are the peroneal vessels. The soleus and gastrocnemius form the muscle bulk of the posterior compartment. Finally, the anterior crural septum runs between peroneus longus and brevis and EHL, while the posterior crural septum runs between the peroneus longus and FHL – the latter septum is usually used to reach the fibula itself during the dissection.

VASCULAR ANATOMY

- The fibula is supplied by periosteal branches of the peroneal artery, and by an endosteal vessel which directly enters the bone at the middle third/distal third junction. The peroneal artery arises from the posterior tibial artery, and runs between the chevron-shaped fibres of tibialis posterior and FHL, running close to the fibula itself, along its deep surface. The vascular pedicle is relatively short (approximately 6 cm), but it can be made longer by harvesting the fibula more proximally than that required for the reconstruction – following detachment of the flap the pedicle is dissected free from this excess bone, which is subsequently discarded.
- Between two and six cutaneous perforator vessels emerge from the peroneal artery, and run behind the fibula to perforate FHL and soleus before supplying a longitudinally oriented area of calf skin. A paddle of skin can be harvested with the main bone flap. There is anatomical variation in location, course, size and number of these cutaneous perforators according to anatomical studies and various clinical reports. Different survival rates of the skin island have been reported and various proposals have been made to improve its reliability. In an anatomical study, an average of 4.2 cutaneous perforators were found and most of them had a myocutaneous passage through the FHL and soleus muscles. The most reliable region for harvesting the skin paddle was found to be 8–12 cm above the ankle, an area corresponding to the junction between the middle and distal thirds of the fibula. To facilitate identification of the cutaneous perforators, pre-operative mapping using a handheld Doppler probe is advisable. The perforators can also be seen on pre-operative imaging (see below).
- There are a number of important anatomical variations of the lower limb arterial supply which need to be known (Figure 3.12.3). The normal arterial supply is found in 88 per cent. Although some information can be obtained by a standard vascular examination and duplex assessment, accurate assessment of the patient's lower limb vasculature can only be provided by conventional angiography or magnetic resonance angiography (MRA). The latter is becoming widely used, especially as it avoids arterial puncture and its associated complications. In the authors' opinion, such vascular assessment is mandatory before harvesting a fibula flap to exclude congenital peroneal artery anomalies. These include a dominant peroneal artery (0.2 per cent of patients) or congenital absence of the peroneal vessels (less than 0.1 per cent). Because many of these congenital and acquired peroneal artery anomalies are unilateral, it is advisable to obtain bilateral leg imaging before harvesting a fibula flap. One of the authors (PAB) has encountered a variation of the abnormally long tibio-peroneal trunk, where the peroneal artery joined the fibula some 26 cm from the fibula head (Figure 3.12.4). However, not all surgeons routinely request these tests, with some relying instead on duplex scanning alone.

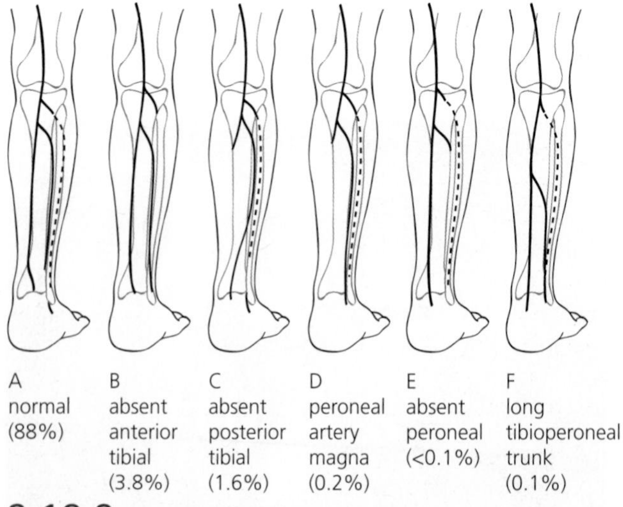

3.12.3 Anatomical variations of the lower limb arterial supply.

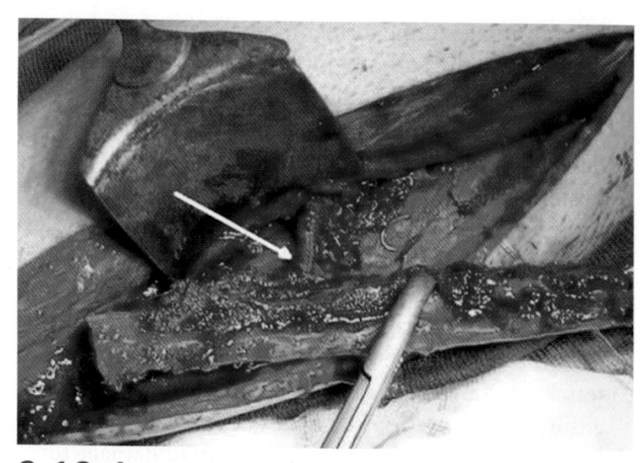

3.12.4 Anatomical variant with peroneal artery joining fibula some 26 cm below the fibula head.

- Peripheral vascular disease occurs quite frequently in head and neck cancer patients, and the peroneal artery typically serves as an important collateral blood supply to the foot. Clearly, if there is significant atheroma in the lower limb vessels, and/or an anatomical variant with one or more vessels missing, it is better not to carry out a fibula free flap. Foot loss following this procedure has been reported in the literature!

CLINICAL USE OF FIBULA FLAP IN MAXILLOFACIAL SURGERY

In maxillofacial surgery, the fibula flap is mainly used for primary or secondary reconstruction of extensive mandibular bone defects. When greater depth of bone is required in large mandibular defects, it may be possible to fold the bone back on itself (double barrelling), or perform interval distraction osteogenesis. The flap can also be used for congenital malformations, and some have recommended its use in pre-prosthetic surgery. It has many other uses outside the head and neck region.

SURGICAL TECHNIQUE

The fully anaesthetized patient is placed on their back and the leg is flexed at both the hip and knee joint and brought into a prone position for better access to the lateral and posterior aspect of the calf. We have described a simple triangular shaped padded device that, when placed under the knee, greatly facilitates this position. It can be easily constructed by a competent dental technician.

1 The entire lower extremity is prepared with antiseptic solution, and the foot is enclosed in a sterile drape. Both authors do not routinely use a tourniquet for flap harvest. If a tourniquet is preferred, this should be inflated to over 300 mmHg, and should be released after a maximum of 2 hours to prevent re-perfusion injury. The fibula head and lateral malleolus (as constant anatomical landmarks) are identified and marked. Drawn between the two is the surface marking of the posterior inter-crural septum (one of the approaches to the lateral fibula, the other being via the anterior crural septum).
2 For a bone-only fibula graft, a skin incision is made along this line, in the middle to distal one-third of the palpable bone. Superiorly, the incision should not pass too close to the fibula head for risk of subsequent damage to the common peroneal nerve. Inferiorly, at least 6–7 cm of bone should be left to maintain ankle joint stability. When a skin paddle is required, the initial linear incision can be modified and placed more anteriorly than the line marked as above. Once the skin flaps have been raised and the perforator(s) identified emerging from the posterior surface of the fibula (Figure 3.12.5), the skin paddle itself can be marked and raised centred on these perforators. As previously mentioned, a Doppler probe can also be used to mark the perforator sites.
3 The skin and subcutaneous fat is raised from the underlying muscle fascia by sharp dissection. The posterior crural septum will come into view, appearing as a white line directly over the lateral aspect of the fibula. Posteriorly soleus is identified and peroneus longus and brevis with their longitudinally running muscle fibers are retracted anteriorly. The septum can then be followed onto the bone itself.
4 Peroneus longus and brevis are detached from the lateral surface of the fibula using sharp dissection. The dissection passes anteriorly, along the whole length of the incision in a broad front, with detachment of the anterior crural septum, extensor digitorum longus and extensor hallucis longus. The safest way to do this is with sharp dissection, staying close to the bone but leaving a small cuff of muscle attached to it.

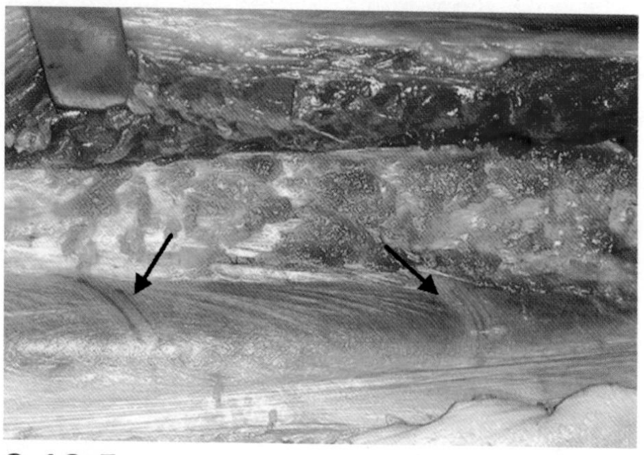

3.12.5 Two perforators can be seen emerging posterior to the fibula (arrowed).

5 A thick white membrane (the inter-osseus membrane) will be encountered next (Figure 3.12.6). The anterior tibial artery and vein and the deep peroneal nerve are sometimes visible lying between this membrane and the underside of the tibialis anterior muscle. This vascular pedicle is retracted and the membrane is incised along its length using a pair of sharp scissors which are opened and slid along the membrane from proximal to distal (or vice versa) at a distance of about 1 cm from the fibula.
6 Attention should now be paid to the fibula bone cuts. The periosteum at the proposed bone cuts is incised. An instrument (such as a Macdonalds or Howarths retractor) is gently passed around the deep surface of the fibula in a subperiosteal plane to protect the underlying pedicle. The bone cuts (both proximal and distal) are performed with an oscillating saw. Some surgeons complete the cuts with an osteotome. The fibula is now carefully retracted laterally using bone clamps. This procedure gives greater access to the peroneal vessels. When a longer pedicle is required, the amount of bone harvested can be increased by making a more proximal bone cut. The pedicle can be dissected free from this bone (and the latter discarded by making a further bone cut at the required length) once the flap is detached.
7 Gentle lateral traction of the fibula reveals the chevron shaped fibres of tibialis posterior (Figure 3.12.7). The next stage depends on operator preference. Most surgeons will dissect through tibialis posterior at the distal bone cut site, using sharp and blunt dissection and staying close to the fibula itself (it is usual to leave 1 cm or so of tibialis posterior attached to the fibula). The peroneal vessels (artery and two accompanying veins) will readily come into view (Figure 3.12.8) and can be ligated and divided, thereby allowing the bone to be further retracted laterally. Others prefer to expose the length of the pedicle by dissecting along the length of tibialis posterior using sharp and blunt dissection. The advantage of the former method (and that preferred by the authors) is that the peroneal artery can be identified early and followed up the fibula, in a manner not dissimilar to following the facial nerve during a parotidectomy – the overlying tibialis posterior can be lifted off the pedicle and safely cut.
8 If skin is required, the skin incision around the paddle is now completed (see step 2 above). It is sensible to include a cuff of both FHL and soleus when completing this part of the dissection to include as many perforating muscular branches as possible. The laterally retracted fibula flap can be moved from side to side to ensure that this is done from both sides (laterally and medially), thereby reducing any chance of damage to either the main pedicle (Figure 3.12.9) or these perforators. As the skin and muscle paddle are released,

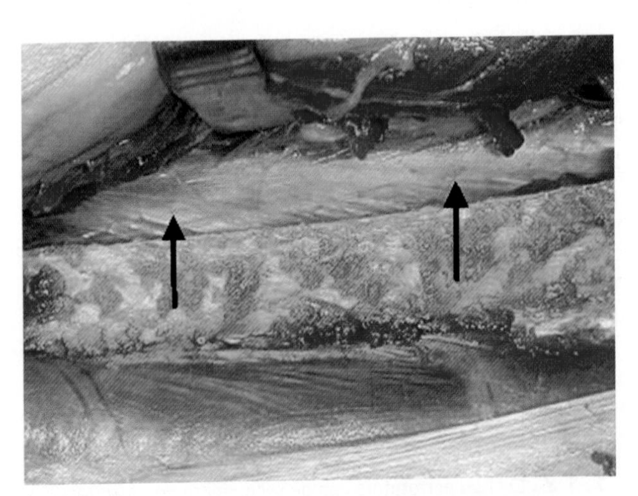

3.12.6 The white inter-osseous membrane (arrowed).

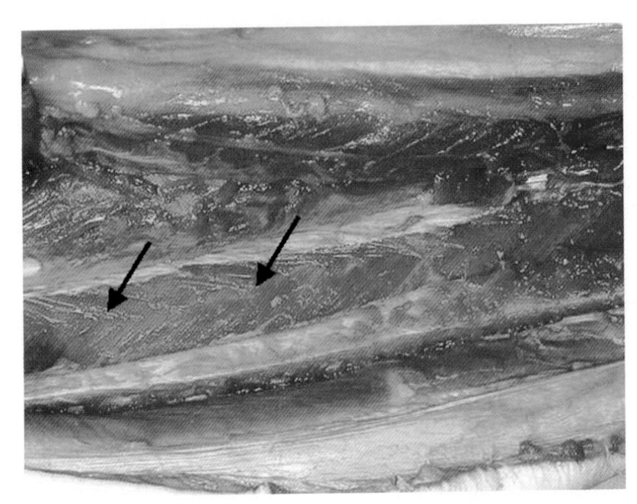

3.12.7 The chevron arrangement of the tibialis posterior muscle fibres.

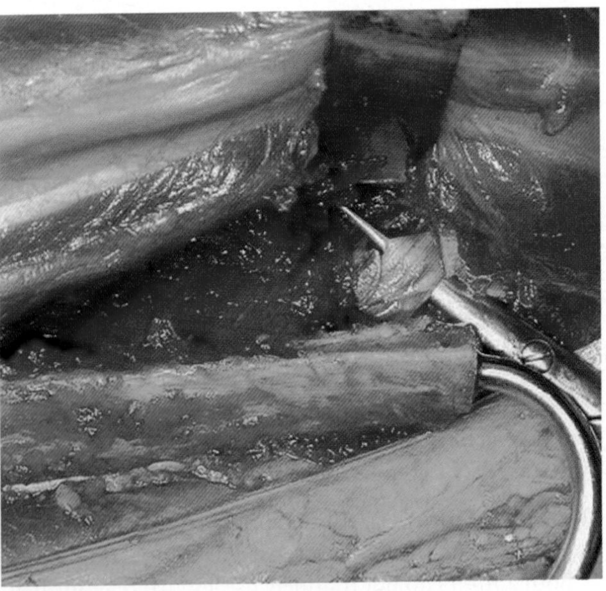

3.12.8 Identification of the distal pedicle.

it is wise to temporarily suture the paddle to the muscle cuff attached to the fibula to reduce the chance of shearing.

9 As more of the tibialis posterior is released, the flap can be retracted further laterally (Figure 3.12.10) revealing the FHL and the posterior inter-muscular septum. The FHL is released from the fibula itself, taking care to ensure that the pedicle is not damaged during this procedure. Several perforating vessels arise from the peroneal artery and enter the FHL, and if care is used, these can be identified and dealt with before they are cut! The posterior tibial vessels are found more medially and should be left undisturbed.

10 Finally, any remaining muscle attachments are released from the fibula. Once the flap has been raised, it can be 'rested' in a heparinized saline-soaked gauze swap and temporarily placed back in the wound with the pedicle still running until it is needed for the reconstruction. When finally tying off the artery, a transfixation suture as well as conventional ligation ensures that the divided vessel will not inadvertently start bleeding post-operatively!

11 If osteotomies are needed to allow the fibula to satisfactorily fit the defect, these can be done from the lateral aspect of the bone after the pedicle has been divided. Before these osteotomy cuts are made, the soft tissues and periosteum at the proposed bone cuts are carefully stripped off using sharp dissection and subsequently protected using a periosteal retractor. The cuts can be made with an oscillating saw on a sterile table, and completed with an osteotome. With the advent of modern imaging and software, it is possible to accurately plan the osteotomy cuts in three dimensions, and to perform these cuts while the flap is still attached on the peroneal pedicle. The flap is secured at the recipient site using the surgeon's choice of fixation (either a reconstruction plate or multiple 2 mm mini-plates). As mentioned above, the pedicle is sharply dissected off any excess bone to increase its length.

12 The wound is closed in layers by carefully suturing muscle groups together. A suction drain is also placed. When a skin paddle has been harvested, the defect is closed with either a full thickness or split thickness skin graft. The latter can be taken from the thigh of the same leg, preferably using a powered dermatome.

13 Patients should mobilize early, initially with partial weight-bearing. Ankle and foot movements are encouraged. Skin grafts should be managed in the conventional way. When patients are slow to mobilize, low molecular weight heparin prophylaxis should be considered.

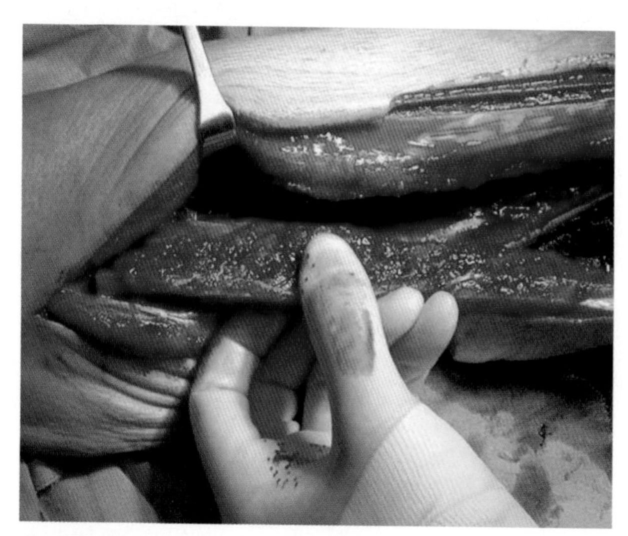

3.12.9 The flap is retracted laterally to aid dissection proximally.

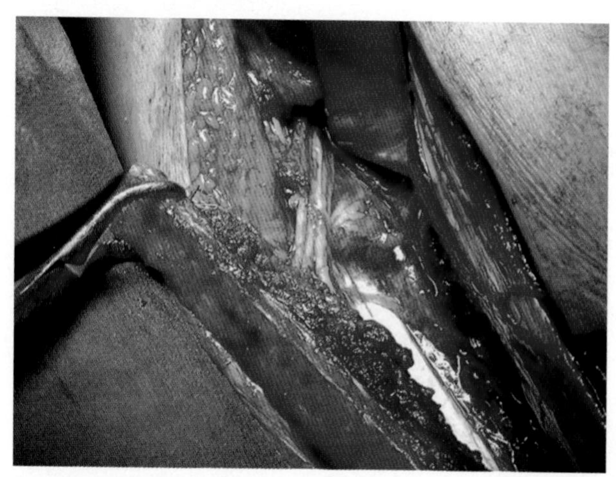

3.12.10 The proximal vascular pedicle.

Top tips

- Careful pre-operative assessment with imaging is recommended (either angiography or MRA).
- Correct leg positioning with adequate stabilization facilitates access.
- Surgical landmarks: mark the fibula head and lateral malleolus and draw a line between them. Leave at least 7 cm of bone proximally and distally to prevent damage to the common peroneal nerve and maintain ankle joint stability.
- Always dissect on a broad front, and leave a small cuff of muscle attached to the bone.
- Identify cutaneous perforators early if a skin paddle is to be used (they emerge posterior to the fibula).
- Place a retractor subperiosteally during proximal and distal bone cuts to prevent pedicle damage.
- Include a generous muscle cuff (FHL and soleus) when a skin paddle is raised.

FURTHER READING

Anand R, Brennan PA, Panchbhavi V, Ilankovan V. Stabilising the leg to harvest a fibular flap: a new device. *British Journal of Oral and Maxillofacial Surgery* 2002; **40**: 438–9.

Anand R, Mourouzis C, Wilbourn M *et al.* An unreported variation of the course of peroneal artery during fibula flap harvest. *British Journal of Oral and Maxillofacial Surgery* 2007; **45**: 588–9.

Baker NJ. Modification of the skin incision to allow versatility in placement of the skin paddle when raising a fibular osteocutaneous flap. *British Journal of Oral and Maxillofacial Surgery* 2005; **43**: 535–6.

Beppu M, Hanel DP, Johnston GH *et al.* The osteocutaneous fibula flap: an anatomic study. *Journal of Reconstructive Microsurgery* 1992; **8**: 215–23.

Chen ZW, Yan W. The study and clinical application of the osteocutaneous flap of fibula. *Microsurgery* 1983; **4**: 11–16.

Eckardt A, Swennen G. Virtual planning of composite mandibular reconstruction with free fibula bone graft. *Journal of Craniofacial Surgery* 2005; **16**: 1137–40.

Hidalgo, DA. Fibula free flap: a new method of mandible reconstruction. *Plastic and Reconstructive Surgery* 1989; **84**: 71–79.

Kelly AM, Cronin P, Hussain HK *et al.* Preoperative MR angiography in free fibula flap transfer for head and neck cancer: clinical application and influence on surgical decision making. *AJR. American Journal of Roentgenology* 2007; **188**: 268–74.

Taylor, GI, Miller GDH, Ham FJ. The free vascularized bone graft. *Plastic and Reconstructive Surgery* 1975; **55**: 533–44.

Ueba Y, Fujikawa S. Nine year follow-up of a vascularised fibula graft in neurofibromatosis: A case report and literature review. *Orthopaedic and Trauma Surgery* 1983; **26**: 595–600.

Whitley SP, Sandhu S, Cardozo A. Preoperative vascular assessment of the lower limb for harvest of a fibular flap: the views of vascular surgeons in the United Kingdom. *British Journal of Oral and Maxillofacial Surgery* 2004; **42**: 307–10.

Wolff, KD, Ervens J, Herzog K, Hoffmeister B. Experience with the ostecutaneous fibula flap: an analysis of 24 consecutive reconstructions of composite mandibular defects. *Journal of Cranio-Maxillofacial Surgery* 1996; **24**: 330–38.

3.13

Vascularized iliac crest grafts

ANDREW LYONS

PRINCIPLES AND JUSTIFICATION

Of all the free vascularized bone containing flaps, the vascularized iliac crest graft undoubtedly provides the best bone stock for orofacial reconstruction, supplying tissue to reconstruct the facial skeleton accurately, with ample bone for the placement of dental implants. Most flaps are probably raised to include some or all of the internal oblique muscle without skin. Although it is usually rather bulky, skin can be included and even raised with the exclusion of muscle as a perforator flap.

The blood supply is from the deep circumflex iliac artery (DCIA) and venous drainage is from its vena comitantes. The pedicle is fairly short and fragile but the artery, and particularly the vein, are of adequate diameters of 2–4 and 2–7 mm, respectively. In most cases, there is a single artery and vein coming off the external iliac artery which usually divides within 1 cm into a deep branch supplying the ilium and lower transversalis, and an ascending branch supplying the muscles of the abdominal wall. Three approaches to the deep circumflex vessels may be utilized. The first approach is subinguinal. The femoral vessels are isolated below the inguinal ligament and the deep circumflex iliac vessels are identified by upward retraction of the inguinal ligament. The transinguinal approach involves identification and retraction of either the spermatic cord or round ligament and dissection through the transversus abdominus to expose the external iliac vessels. However, Taylor, who first described this flap in 1979, noted the variability in the location of the large ascending muscular branch and warned that because of its size it was a potential point of confusion when trying to locate the DCIA. It is mainly for this reason that the superior approach using location of the distal pedicle on the undersurface of the internal oblique muscle is the one preferred by the author.

The donor site can almost always be closed primarily and if careful attention is paid to closure of the deeper tissues there should be little long-term morbidity.

INDICATIONS

Vascularized iliac crest grafts are indicated for reconstruction of segmental mandibular defects in dentate patients, particularly anterior defects, and for reconstruction of maxillary defects that extend outside the maxillary alveolus. Where a cutaneous defect exists, the flap can be used to cover skin defects resulting from both maxillary and mandibular pathology. Additionally, where a large partial glossectomy has been carried out *en bloc* with an anterior mandible defect, the skin paddle can be used as a tongue resting on the internal oblique used as the floor of the mouth. In either mandibular or maxillary reconstruction the ipsilateral hip should be used. In the mandible, this can provide an ideal lower border angle or symphysis. In the case of midline defects, the flap should be raised ipsilaterally to the side where the pedicle is to be anastomosed.

Using the ipsilateral side in the maxilla gives optimal pedicle orientation and bone to bone apposition. The flap is contraindicated where there has been a previous iliac crest graft, an inguinal hernia repair or abdominal incision for an operation such as appendicectomy. Patients with gait problems are not good candidates for this procedure in either limb. Obesity is only a consideration where a skin paddle is to be taken. In most cases of mandibular reconstruction, the contralateral side can be harvested instead, though some contouring may be lost at the lower border of the mandible.

PRE-OPERATIVE

The area around the iliac crest should be checked for visible scars in case this was missed in the history. There is a large thickness of subcutaneous fat in this area and in many patients this will render the skin unsuitable for reconstruction. If a skin paddle is to be harvested, the use of a handheld Doppler is advocated to locate the perforators. There is a fairly consistent perforator 5 cm lateral and 2.5 cm above the anterior superior iliac spine and other perforators may be found laterally at a similar distance above the iliac crest. A template can be used to aid in bone harvest, and this should ensure accurate fast bone harvest. This should be constructed pre-operatively, with the aid of a 3D CT of the jaw which can be converted into a model and template. The patient should be warned of post-operative pain and discomfort, numbness at the front of the thigh and that gait is likely to be abnormal for at least three months.

OPERATION

Positioning the patient

With the patient supine, a large sandbag is placed beneath the hip, and skin preparation should be across the midline medially, at a lower level than the greater trochanter inferiorly, laterally past the post axillary line and superiorly just above the costal margin. A sigmoidal line is drawn from the pubic symphysis along the superior border of the iliac crest, which should be palpated, to the posterior axillary line. If a skin paddle is to be harvested, it should be marked out following perforator location with a Doppler probe (Figure 3.13.1).

Incision

Along the length of the incision, the skin and fat is incised through Scarpa's and Campa's fasciae to the external oblique muscle whose fibres run in a downwards and forwards direction, this should obviously run around the skin paddle if one is to be raised. The muscle should be incised in the direction of its fibres to the underlying internal oblique muscle which has a very distinctive downwards and slightly backwards orientation (Figure 3.13.2). If a skin paddle is to be raised, the perforators should be identified and a cuff of external oblique muscle left around the perforators.

The only exception to this is if it is planned to raise an osseocutaneuos flap devoid of muscle where the muscle layers are opened to permit tracing the pedicle to the ascending or main branch of the DCIA (Figures 3.13.3 and 3.13.4). This technique will not be discussed further; only surgeons with extensive experience of vascularized iliac crest grafts should carry out this procedure, which has been well described by Kimata.

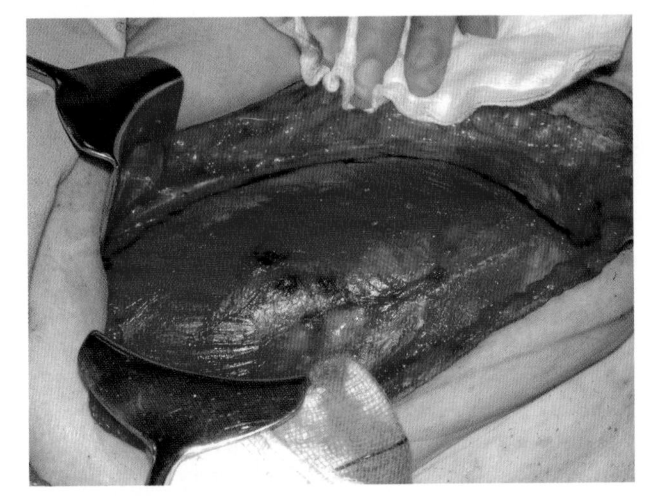

3.13.2 Exposure of internal oblique muscle, left-sided flap.

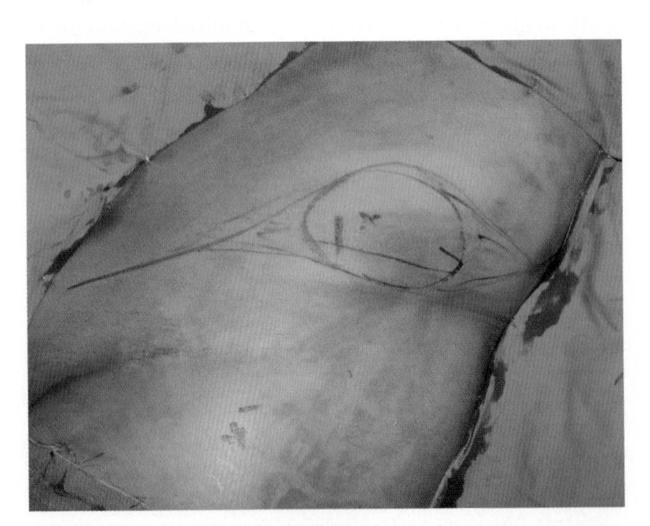

3.13.1 Skin markings or flap with skin paddle, the X marks the Doppler signal point. The lower line would be appropriate for a myo-osseus flap (left side).

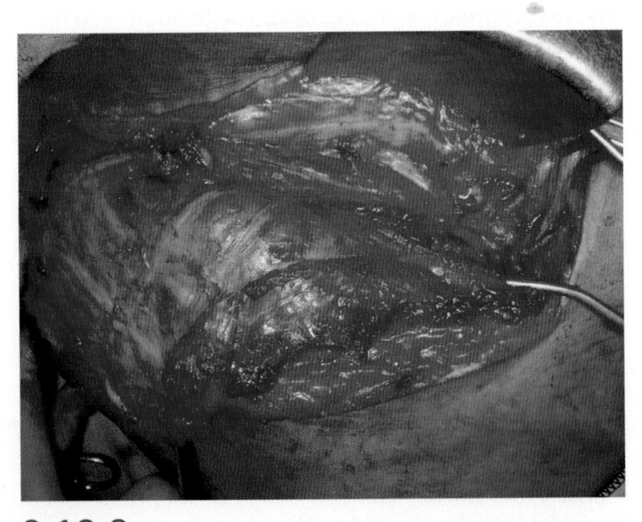

3.13.3 Undersurface of internal oblique showing ascending branches and DCIA in a right-sided flap.

Exposure of the internal oblique

The external oblique muscle should be incised along the whole length of the crest and this incision should be extended medially along its lower border to the inguinal ligament. The muscle should then be elevated superiorly detaching it from the underlying internal oblique muscle.

Raising the muscle flap

Once the internal oblique muscle has been exposed, commensurate with the amount to be harvested, the portion required should be marked out with ink. In mandibular reconstruction, the iliac crest is best utilized as the lower border and the estimate for the amount of muscle to be harvested should include that required to run from 'the lower border' into the buccal sulcus. It is recommended to harvest at least 4 cm of muscle from the upper border of the iliac crest. In the rare event that there is only an ascending branch of the DCIA, the flap will have to rely on this vessel.

The incision through the internal oblique muscle should commence at the superolateral aspect of the muscle and should extend below the transversalis fascia onto this muscle. The internal oblique and transversalis fascia should be raised by sharp dissection. Meticulous haemostasis to the many perforating vessels which run through the two muscles is required using bipolar diathermy. Dissection should proceed in an infero-lateral direction as this will release the assistant from the tiresome job of pulling a large bulk of skin fat and external oblique muscle upwards.

Dissection of the pedicle

The ascending branch will soon be visualized and as dissection proceeds this will become larger. At this stage, dissection should proceed inferiorly to expose a possible 'lower ascending branch', as there is frequently branching of the ascending branch. As the dissection proceeds inferiorly the DCIA itself will be encountered. This may be above or below the iliacus muscle as it inserts into the ilium but a small, 1 cm or less, cuff of muscle should be left around the vessel to safeguard it. The author realizes that other descriptions involve not locating the DCIA alongside the ilium but harvesting 2 cm of iliacus to preserve it. In the author's experience, this is the minimum muscle required for a safe 'blind approach'.

Dissection should now proceed medially and the internal oblique muscle incised supero-medially laterally to aid this. There should at least be a small length of muscle left above the ascending branch but more muscle may be required and the only limitation is the extent of the muscle at the costal margin superiorly and rectus sheath medially, although a cuff of muscle should always be left to aid in repair. It is tempting to harvest as little internal oblique muscle as possible, but it should be remembered that in reconstructing high dentate mandibles 4 cm of muscle may be lost just to bring the muscle into the mouth!

As the dissection proceeds medially to the ilium the overlying internal and external oblique muscles will need to be incised to the medial end of the ilio-inguinal ligament.

Attention must be paid to vessels branching off the pedicle which, if violated, will bleed causing a loss of pedicle visualization (Figure 3.13.5). These are best ligated with metal clips rather than diathermied to protect the pedicle. About 2 cm from the external iliac vessels, the ascending branches will join the pedicle and at about this point the vein, which is 2–3mm in diameter, will start to dilate as it curves upwards and medially to course over the DCIA and external iliac artery before joining with the external iliac vein at a diameter of 4–8 mm. This requires meticulous dissection as the veins can be quite thin walled and the wide vein with the 1.5–2 cm length over the artery that can be achieved may be crucial. As the defect may not be ready for the flap, it is recommended to delay this dissection until the time has been reached for pedicle division and delivery of the flap.

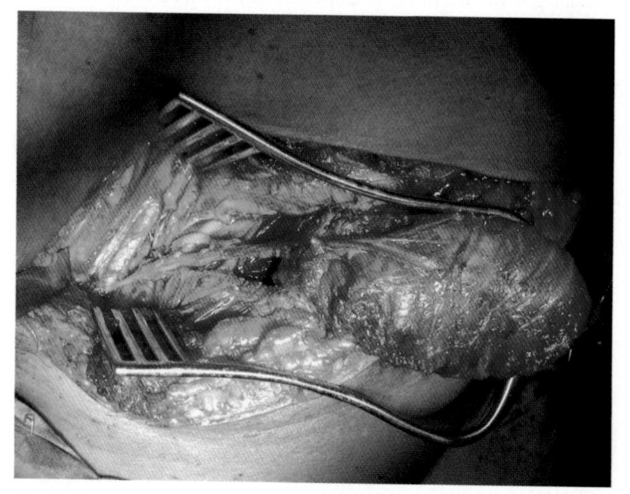

3.13.4 Complete flap with pedicle (left side).

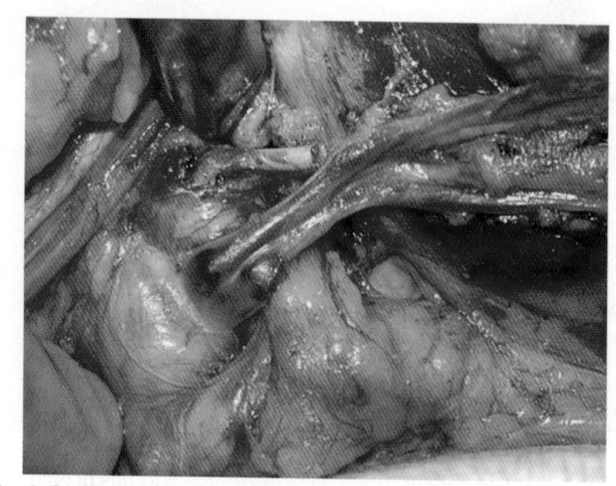

3.13.5 Junction of pedicle and external iliac vessels (right side).

Although the anatomy of the pedicle is fairly constant, there is some variability. The ascending and main deep circumflex vessels may join the iliac vessels separately, giving duplicate pedicles. Although it may be possible to run the flap on one set of vessels, ideally all these vessels, which are usually less than 2 mm in diameter, should be anastomosed. Occasionally, only the ascending branch will originate from the external iliac artery with the main DCIA originating from the internal iliac artery. The pedicle should now be traced backwards towards the ilium, separating the pedicle from the underlying psoas muscle. At a point 2–3 cm medial to the ASIS, the lateral cutaneous nerve of the thigh will be identified and the pedicle should be dissected off this structure. It is, however, advocated that those with early or little experience of this flap should sacrifice this nerve if they are in any doubt about the pedicle being at risk.

Bone harvesting

The point at which bone harvest should commence along the length of the ilium is dependent on three factors:

1 The quantity of bone required: this flap will reach the contralateral ramus with total mandibular reconstruction, but the entire length of the ilium that can be harvested with the muscle and pedicle will be required.
2 The part of the mandible to be reconstructed: the anterior crest is an ideal shape for mandibular angle reconstruction. The anterior mandible does not require the anterior crest and by taking the bone 3 cm lateral to the ASIS, this will be 3 cm extra pedicle length.
3 If the maxilla is to be reconstructed, the requirement for bone length is not usually great, but the requirement for pedicle length may be critical. Therefore, the bone harvest should commence as far away laterally from the ASIS as possible.

If the anterior crest is to be harvested after detaching the inguinal ligament, the gluteus medius muscle should be stripped from the outer aspect of the ilium to match the template. If the anterior crest is not to be harvested, the periosteum should be stripped from the inner aspect of the ilium to where the medial bone cut is to be made. It is important to leave the gluteus medius attached to the outer aspect, otherwise the anterior crest can become avascular and may dehisce through the wound! The bone is cut with a saw and the medial and lateral beginning and end cuts should be made with a small copper retractor or periosteal elevator protecting the underlying periosteum and pedicle. The template, even if just constructed intraoperatively, should give an idea of where any 'intra-flap' osteotomy cuts are located and it is the author's preference to make theses cuts *in situ* as the bone is held rigid here. These osteotomy cuts should not perforate the inner cortex, this can be greenstick fractured later to preserve the periosteum (Figure 3.13.6). The horizontal cut can now be made with a retractor situated medially to protect the peritoneum. Once the osteotomy cuts have been made, an osteotone should be used gently to mobilize the bony flap, which should be carefully handled out of the pelvis (Figure 3.13.7).

Closure of the donor site and pedicle division

Any obvious bleeding should be attended to, bipolar diathermy only can now be used on the flap. Bone wax should be placed over the trabecular bone of the donor site.

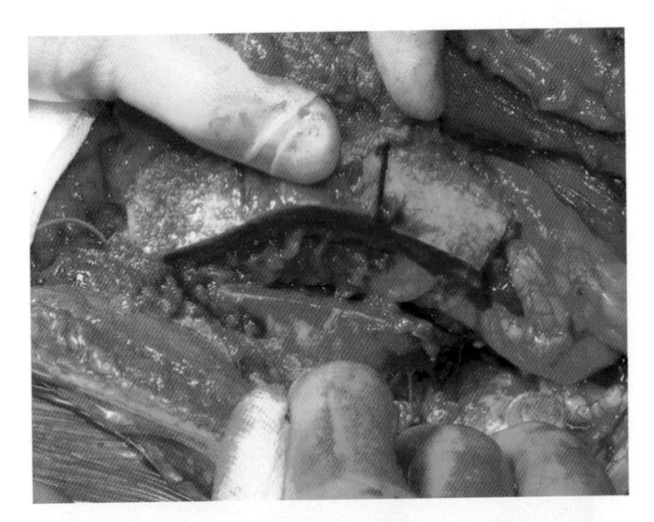

3.13.6 Osteotomy cuts in left-sided flap. This has been made to preserve the ASIS and inguinal ligament. Note that the two incomplete osteotomy cuts that will be greenstick fractured later.

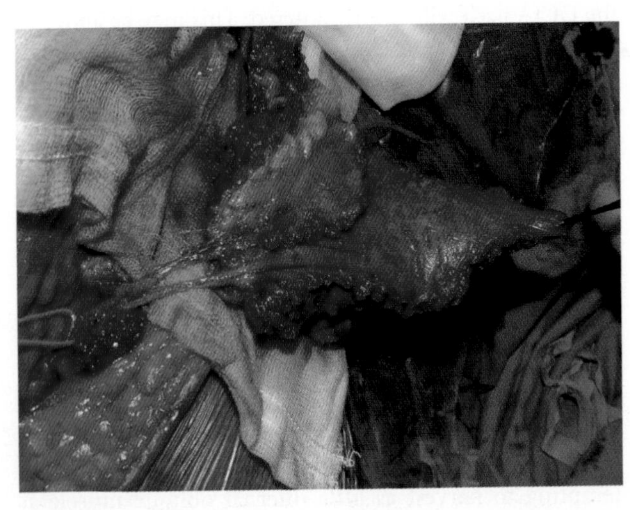

3.13.7 Left-sided flap and pedicle.

Once it has been ascertained that the flap including the bone is bleeding, attention should be drawn to the donor site, most of which can be closed before detaching the pedicle. Bone wax should be placed over the trabecular bone. The abdomen should then be closed in layers. To aid this, a series of holes are made approximately 1 cm apart along the inner and outer cortex of the bony defect in the ilium.

It is recommended to use 1 or 1/0 nylon sutures and temporarily hold them with artery clips until all the sutures have been placed before tying the knots. A piece of non-resorbable mesh should be trimmed to the size of the internal oblique defect. This is sutured to the outer cortex of the ilium and the internal oblique muscle with a round-bodied needle, 1 or 1/0 nylon suture with the knots being tied immediately (Figures 3.13.8 and 3.13.9). A suction drain with a minimum intraluminal diameter of 3 mm should be placed over this layer and an epidural catheter teased through one of the sutured muscle layers. Both of these devices should be secured to the skin with a suture immediately after introduction. Closure of the muscle layers medial to the ilium has to be delayed until pedicle division.

Division of the pedicle

Final dissection of the proximal pedicle should be undertaken and the artery and vein divided and ligated. The flap should be carefully handled to avoid twisting the pedicle. The lumen of the artery is identified and a small nylon cannula is introduced into it to permit flushing of the flap with 20–50 mL of heparinized saline.

The muscle medial to the donor site is closed in layers. If detached, the inguinal ligament is sutured to the ilium and the external oblique muscle is closed to itself medially and to the gluteus medius muscle laterally. Even if a large skin flap has been harvested, direct skin and subcutaneous tissue closure is assured.

Insetting and anastomosis

The bony component of the flap should be adjusted with a saw if required, rotary instruments are not recommended in case the pedicle is snagged and torn. The bone should be fixed with the appropriate screws and plates. In contrast to the fibula, the iliac bone is contoured using opening osteotomies with simple splitting of the bone prior to spreading the bone around the cut. This will increase the bone length. Cancellous bone chips can be used to fill the resultant bone gaps. The muscle and skin should just be tacked in place to orientate the pedicle, and the anastomosis prepared and carried out at this stage.

In the author's personal experience, the vein is best anastomosed first. This allows no interruption of flow through the artery once this anastomosis is complete. At 5 minutes before the artery is allowed to run, 5000 units of heparin are administered intravenously, this is not the author's usual practice for any other flap. The DCIA is a relatively small vessel and before it was the author's practice to use heparin, many flaps would start to run before stopping after 10–20 minutes. It may be that the heparin prevents fibrin degradation products in the previously ischaemic tissue, setting off the clotting cascade

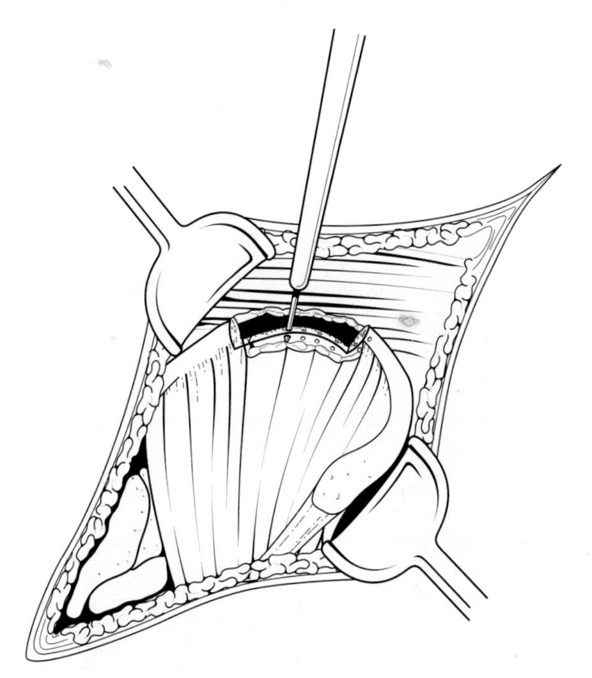

3.13.8 The transversalis and parts of the iliacus are sutured into these holes with a round body needled 1 or 1/0 nylon suture. It is recommended to temporarily hold the sutures with an artery clip until all the sutures have been placed before tying the knots.

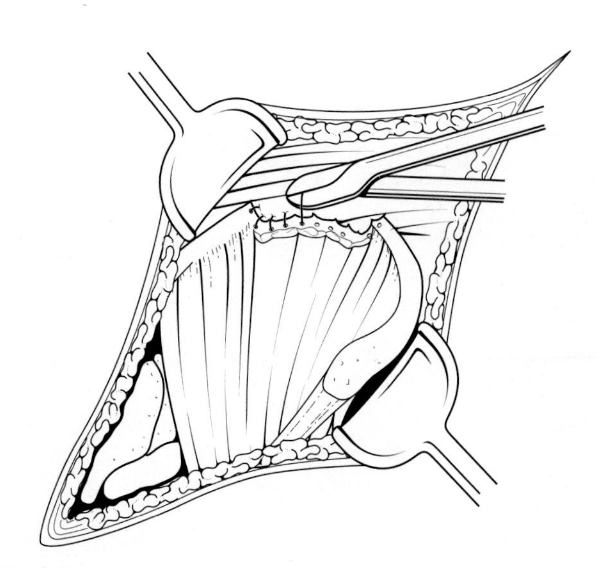

3.13.9 A piece of prolene mesh or similar material is trimmed to the size of the defect in internal oblique.

when fresh blood enters the vessels, and to date this technique has allowed 40 consecutive DCIA based flaps to run perfectly following clamp removal.

After the flap is running, the internal oblique muscle is sutured into the intraoral defect. Some muscle trimming may be required but, although the flap may appear very bulky at this stage, it is likely to shrink back in a matter of weeks and certainly after radiotherapy. If there is a skin flap, this can now be inset.

POST-OPERATIVE

If there is a skin paddle the artery can be easily monitored with a handheld Doppler probe and assessed for pallor, although it is possible that the state of this flap based on a small perforator may appear less perfused and less drained than the muscle and bone. A handheld Doppler can assess arterial flow to the pedicle within the neck. For venous monitoring, the colour of the flap, which will obviously appear dark if engorged, is useful. Stabbing the muscle may be useful, bright red blood should flow rapidly and if individual muscle fibres can be seen it probably signifies the flap is not working. The muscle should ideally have a 'glazed toffee apple appearance'. A Doppler probe sutured around the flap side of the venous anastomosis may also be helpful. None of these methods is 100 per cent reliable, and it is fair to say this is a difficult flap to monitor. The muscle component of this flap should be epithelized by 72 hours. Local anaesthetic can be infused through the epidural catheter to aid in analgesia. A very good aesthetic result can be achieved with this method of reconstruction (Figures 3.13.12 and 3.13.13).

COMPLICATIONS

Intraoperative

- Damage to the small delicate pedicle is always possible. This is most likely to occur to the main DCI vein behind the medial portion of the ilium where it can be buried in the iliacus muscle.
- Violation of the thin transversalis muscle to produce herniation of pre-peritoneal fat is always a possibility but can be closed.
- Snagging of the pedicle with a rotary instrument is possible and potentially disastrous; use of these instruments should be minimized in this operation!

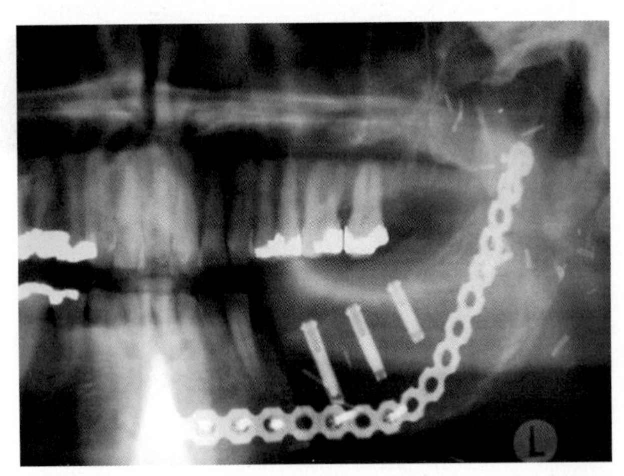

3.13.10 Mandibular reconstruction showing excellent bone bulk for dental implants.

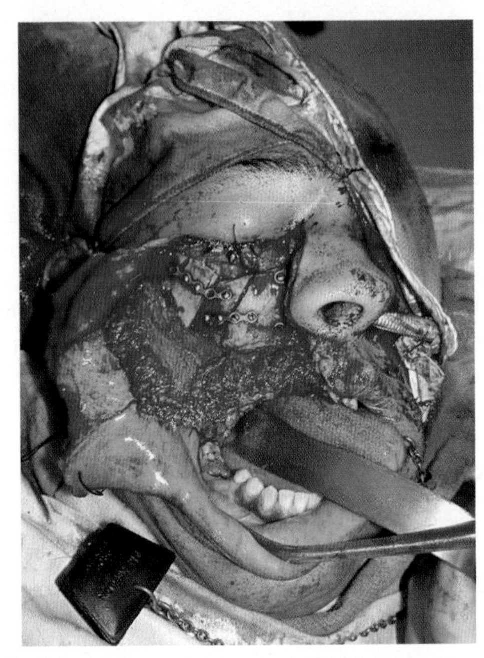

3.13.11 Maxillary reconstruction. Note multiple osteotomies and internal oblique muscle prior to suturing into position.

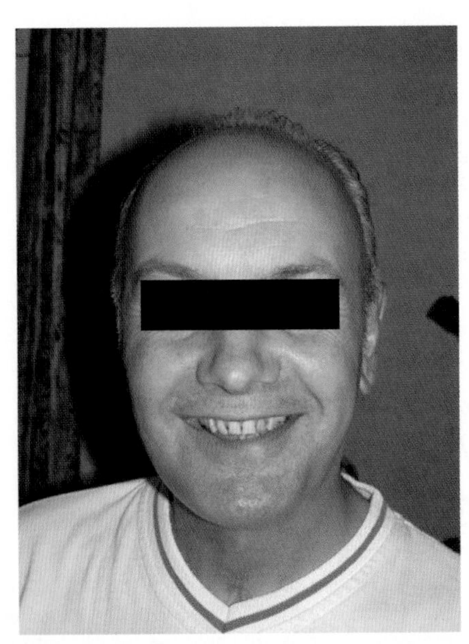

3.13.12 Mandibular reconstruction on right (pre-implants).

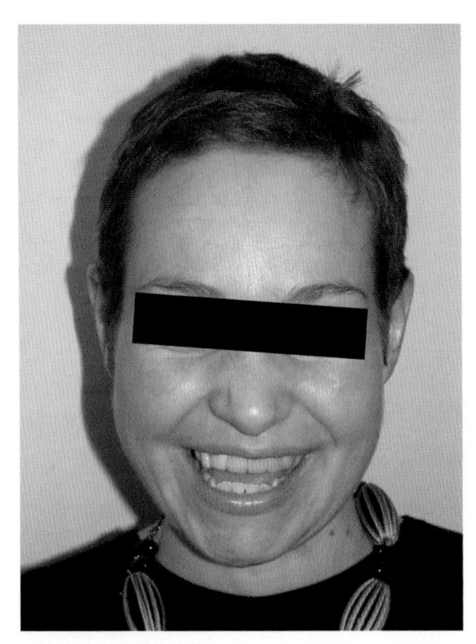

3.13.13 Maxillary reconstruction. Note reconstruction crosses midline.

Post-operative

- Loss of flap perfusion and venous drainage are particular problems in maxillary reconstruction.
- Partial necrosis of the internal oblique muscle may occur, but is not usually a problem as granulation over vital bone will resolve this.
- Partial bone necrosis can be more of a problem and is of course more likely to occur with small distal segments of osteotomized bone.
- Seromas may occur, probably as a result of damage to the external iliac lymphatics.
- Post-operative infection, particularly associated with the internal oblique mesh, can be very troublesome and may even require removal of the mesh. It is advisable to handle this material carefully and apply topical antiseptics to the mesh bed and mesh itself to reduce this.
- Incisional hernia is always possible if the layers of the donor site are not closed with care.
- Numbness to the anterior thigh due to damage to the lateral cutaneous nerve may be troublesome to some patients.
- Gait problems may last six months or even longer, especially in the elderly.

Top tips

- Always ensure enough muscle is harvested in mandibular defects. Distal bone fragments can sometimes have a precarious blood supply. A thick covering of richly supplied muscle will hence sometimes be invaluable.
- Where pedicle length is likely to be an issue (usually maxillary cases) use the smallest amount of bone harvested as far back along the iliac crest as possible, to lengthen the pedicle.
- Do not underestimate the time, complex nature and importance of carefully closing the donor site defect. In some quarters, this flap has acquired a reputation for medium- and long-term morbidity, both of which can nearly always be avoided by attention to detail!

FURTHER READING

Brown JS. Deep circumflex iliac artery free flap with internal oblique muscle as a new method of immediate reconstruction of maxillectomy defect. *Head and Neck* 1996; **18**: 412–21.

Forrest C, Boyd B, Manktelow R *et al.* The free vascularised iliac crest tissue transfer: donor site complications associated with 82 cases. *British Journal of Plastic Surgery* 1992; 45: 89–93.

Kimata Y, Uchiyama K, Sakuraba M *et al.* Deep Circumflex iliac perforator flap with iliac crest for mandibular reconstruction. *British Journal of Plastic Surgery* 2001; **54**: 487–90.

Kimata Y. Deep circumflex iliac perforator flap. *Clinics in Plastic Surgery* 2003; **30**: 433–8.

Lyons AJ, James R, Collyer J. Free vascularised iliac crest graft: an audit of 26 consecutive cases. *British Journal of Oral and Maxillofacial Surgery* 2005; **43**: 210–14.

Shpitzer T, Neligan PC, Gullane PJ *et al.* The free iliac crest and fibula flaps in vascularized oromandibular reconstruction: comparison and long term evaluation. *Head and Neck* 1999; **21**: 639–47.

Urken ML, Vickery C, Weinberg A *et al.* The internal oblique-iliac crest osseomyocutaneous microvascular free flap in head and neck reconstruction. *Journal of Reconstructive Microsurgery* 1989; **5**: 203–14.

3.14

Facial reanimation

HENNING SCHLIEPHAKE

INDICATIONS

Facial reanimation is indicated in cases of acquired long standing facial paralysis or in congenital disorders associated with a decrease in facial muscle activity such as the Möbius Syndrome, congenital unilateral lower lip palsy (CULLP syndrome) or even haemifacial microsomia. Acquired long standing facial paralysis most frequently results from neurosurgical or otolaryngological interventions for intracranial tumours as central palsy, but may as well occur after ablation of malignant parotid tumours as peripheral palsy.

Facial reanimation encompasses surgical measures that support or restore facial movement in cases of facial nerve palsies. In contrast to static reconstructions, such as suspension plasties to raise the oral commissure or lateral canthopexy to alleviate the sequelae of orbicularis oculi muscle palsy, these procedures allow for active movement of facial muscles either by supporting existing muscular activity or by transferring neuromuscular units from adjacent or distant sites to the deficient area. As voluntary and involuntary facial movement is accomplished by 18 separate muscles that are unique in the way they produce individual facial expression, even dynamic functional reconstruction using revascularized transfer of neuromuscular units cannot fully restore symmetry in unilateral facial palsy. However, functionally and aesthetically most disturbing deficits, such as the inability to raise the oral commissure to achieve oral continence or to close the eyelids to protect the globe, can be repaired.

PRE-OPERATIVE PLANNING

Timing

Symmetric innervation of the transferred muscle segment is crucial for a successful reconstruction. This does not only relate to voluntary movement but even more to spontaneous emotional expression. As the facial nerve is the only cranial nerve that spontaneously produces impulses during facial expression, it is considered as the source of choice for neurotization. The hypoglossal nerve and the motor nerve supply to the masseter muscle have also been used as a source of innervation to a muscle graft, but could not achieve the degree of symmetry that the facial nerve provides.

In cases of peripheral nerve palsy, the ipsilateral facial nerve stump could be used. However, as the individual fascicles of the nerve are assigned to different facial regions, appropriate selective neurotization through one of these fascicles is difficult without the possibility to check for their original assignment and avoid synkinetic movement of 'wrong' contralateral muscles. Therefore, in peripheral and even more in central facial nerve palsy, the contralateral facial nerve is the preferred source of innervation. Nerve impulses from the contralateral side are conducted to the paretic side through a cross-face nerve graft. Thus, free neuromuscular tissue transfer for facial reanimation is a two step procedure with the first step being the cross-face nerve graft from the opposite side and the second step performing the muscle transfer 9–12 months after nerve grafting.

OPERATION

Cross-face nerve graft

GRAFT PROCUREMENT

The sural nerve is commonly used as the donor nerve for the cross-face nerve graft as it provides adequate length to cross over to the opposite side of the face. The nerve runs down the leg on the posterolateral aspect of the calf where it passes to the lateral side of the foot approximately 2 cm posterior to the ankle. Here it is easily exposed from a small horizontal incision of 1–2 cm length. After identification of the nerve trunk, a second transverse incision some 4–5 cm proximal is placed on the calf, slightly more posterior than the first one. The nerve is identified and connection with the exposed nerve segment further distal is established by subcutaneous dissection. The same is carried out again 4–5 cm more proximally. The nerve is then divided below the most distal incision and removed in a proximal direction. Care must be taken to avoid tearing of the branches, which have to be identified by subcutaneous dissection and separated from the main trunk. In this way a nerve segment of 10–12 cm length can be obtained. The small incisions are closed and moderate compression dressing with decreasing pressure from distal to proximal is applied.

FACIAL NERVE PREPARATION

The sural nerve graft is connected to one or two branches of the facial nerve on the opposite site that provide impulses to the area that is supposed to be reconstructed on the paralyzed side. In this way, symmetric innervation and facial expression are intended. Commonly, the muscles that elevate the oral commissure receive motor nerve supply from the buccal branches of the facial nerve. This part of the nerve contains multiple branches that are connected to each other, so that division of one or two small branches does not compromise facial nerve function on the non-paralyzed side of the face. In order to allow for identification and selective dissection of these branches using electrotesting, general anaesthesia has to be carried out without muscle relaxation.

The patient should have his endotracheal ventilation tube inserted through the nose. His head has to be positioned and draped in a way that allows turning of the head and provides access to both parotid areas, as well as visual control of perioral and periorbital muscles.

Exposure of the facial nerve branches starts from a preauricular incision after elevation of the facial skin superficially to the parotid fascia (Figure 3.14.1). Good visualization is mandatory for safe exposure and reliable identification of the individual nerve branches, as well as microsurgical coaptation between the branches and the sural nerve graft later on. Thus, if required, the incision is extended superiorly across the hair line and inferiorly around the mandibular angle into the submandibular area. Despite a rather long incision line, the resulting scar is less conspicious than the vertical cheek incisions that are otherwise recommended for direct access to the nerve branches.

When the anterior edge of the parotid gland is reached, dissection is continued along the fascia into the fat tissue where the branches leave the gland. As the branches are below 1 mm in diameter, this part of the operation requires careful dissection with repeated use of the nerve stimulator to identify the precise function of the individual branches (Figure 3.14.2). Redundance of innervation is mandatory for those functions that are provided by the branches selected for coaptation with the cross-face nerve graft to avoid loss of function on the non-paretic side. Thin rubber ropes are used to mark these branches and the dissection is carried on in the subcutaneous plane anteriorly to the naso-labial crease.

The pathway for the nerve graft to the opposite side of the face runs through a subcutaneous tunnel in the upper lip. This tunnel is dissected from bilateral curved incisions at the alar base and a contralateral preauricular incision. The former ones are used for subcutaneous dissection from midline to the nasolabial fold (Figure 3.14.3). The latter incision is placed in a facelift-like fashion and the parotid area is exposed by extracapsular dissection after elevation of a facial skin flap. When the subcutaneous tunnel is finished, a thin and curved long forceps is inserted from the paretic to the non-paretic side. The proximal end of the nerve graft is grasped and guided through the tunnel to the paralyzed side. In this way, coaptation of the facial nerve branches is not inadvertently done to fascicles that run into side branches that have been divided or torn during harvest. The nerve is placed high in the upper lip immediately underneath the collumella and the alar base in order to avoid interference with the dissection during muscle transfer lateron.

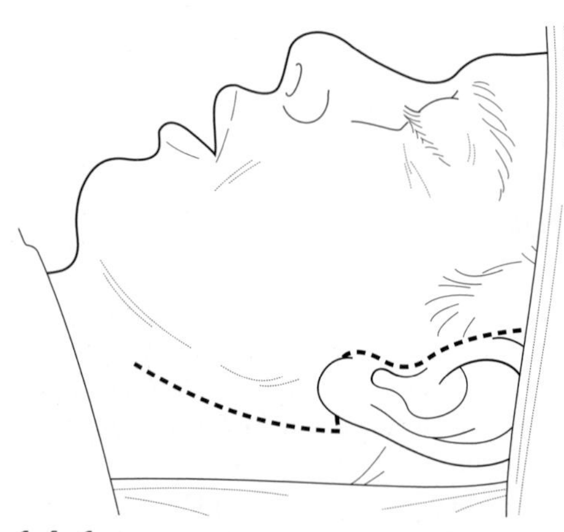

3.14.1 Preauricular incision line that is extended submandibular.

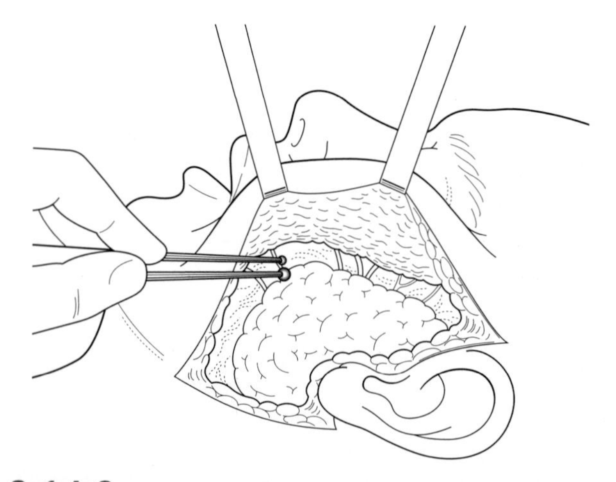

3.14.2 Dissection of small branches of the facial nerve exiting the gland at the anterior margin. Nerve testing to prove redundance of nerve supply in the buccal and zygomatic region.

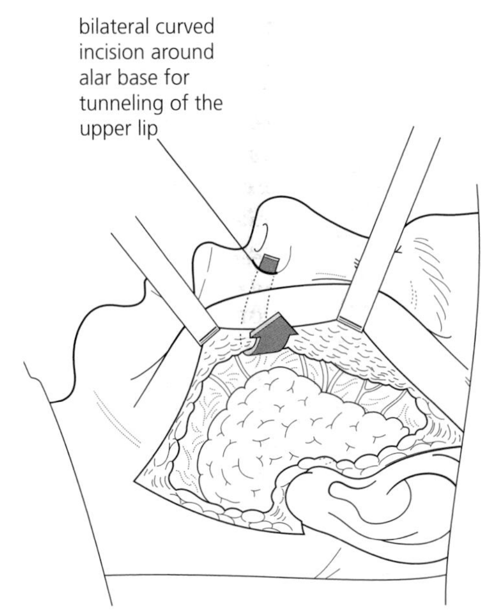

3.14.3 Preauricular incision and subcutaneous dissection to the upper lip, continued to the contralateral side by bilateral bow-shaped incisions at the nasal alar base.

Interfascicular nerve coaptation between the selected facial nerve branches and the sural nerve graft is done under the microscope using 11/0 sutures. It will not be possible to connect all fascicles of the nerve graft to the small facial nerve branches, but it is important to make sure that the fascicles of the facial nerve branches are securely connected to individual fascicles of the sural nerve graft. The end of the nerve graft on the paralyzed side is fixed to the parotid fascia by a non-resorbable 3/0 suture that can be easily identified and dissected 9–12 months later during muscle transfer. Suction drainage with one 10 gauge drain on either side and skin closure in layers end the operation. It is important to make sure that the drain is not located in the vicinity of the coapted nerve branches, to avoid inadvertent damage during drain removal.

Muscle transfer

PLANNING

After a minimum waiting period of nine months, the muscle transfer can be planned for restoration of oral commissure movement and/or eye closure. In order to achieve a symmetric smile it is important pre-operatively to:

- define the desired position of the modiolus at rest with the patient sitting in an upright position;
- identify the vector and the extent of movement of the commissure during smiling.

The commissure and the nasolabial crease are marked on both sides with a waterproof pen on the immediate pre-operative day. The difference between the actual and the planned position of the commissure at rest is registered on the paralyzed side with a ruler. The extent of movement of the commissure during smile on the non-paralyzed side is also measured directly using the ruler and the direction of movement is marked on the skin with an arrow. These marks will have to be renewed after facial skin disinfection and draping immediately before the operation starts. The required length of the muscle graft can be estimated from the distance between the zygomatic bone prominence and the position of the modiolus at rest.

PREPARATION OF THE RECIPIENT SITE

The facial skin on the paralyzed side is elevated from the perauricular incision, which is extended to the submandibular area. Subcutaenous dissection is carried on to the lower border of the mandible where the facial vessels are identified and exposed to be used as recipient vessels for the muscle graft. The end of the cross-face nerve graft that had been fixed to the parotid fascia is released and adequate regeneration is approved clinically by a positive Tinel's sign and histologically after removal of a small portion of the nerve for frozen section analysis. Elevation of the skin is continued medially until the oral commissure and the malar prominence are reached. This exposes the paralyzed zygomaticus muscles, the action of which is supposed to be replaced by the muscle graft (Figure 3.14.4a).

The tissue underlying the commissure is grasped with a forceps and pulled gently in a cranial direction towards the zygoma, while the formation of creases and the change in the shape of the commissure is observed (Figure 3.14.4b). The traction points will have to be modified slightly and the procedure repeated until a satisfactory smile shape results. This traction point is secured with a permanent suture that is left open. Commonly, one or two more traction points are needed to produce a movement and shape that mimics that of the normal side. These are explored while the central point in the commissure is 'activated' by pulling the suture. In this way, additional points are identified and secured with sutures. The additional points are commonly found slightly more medial to the commissure in the upper lip and below the central point in the lateral portion of the lower lip.

INSERTION OF THE MUSCLE GRAFT

The muscle is harvested according to the procedure described in Chapter 3.11. The graft is placed on the recipient site with the point of entry of the vascular pedicle and the nerve on the undersurface of the muscle. The muscle length should be roughly adapted according to the distance between the commissure in a simulated position at rest and the malar prominence. This is advisable to avoid asymmetric positioning of the neurovascular pedicle that may occur if the muscle is shortened after one end has already been fixed. Usually, a length of 6–7 cm is used in this position.

The graft end that faces the commissure is divided into two or three portions depending on the number of traction points identified (Figure 3.14.5). The muscle ends are

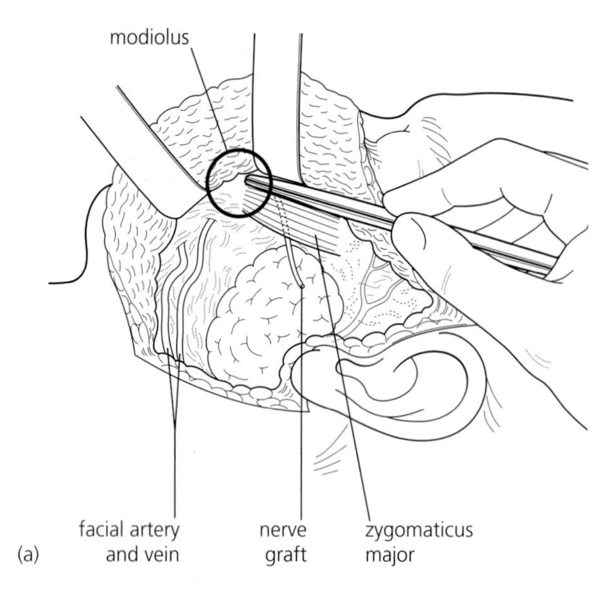

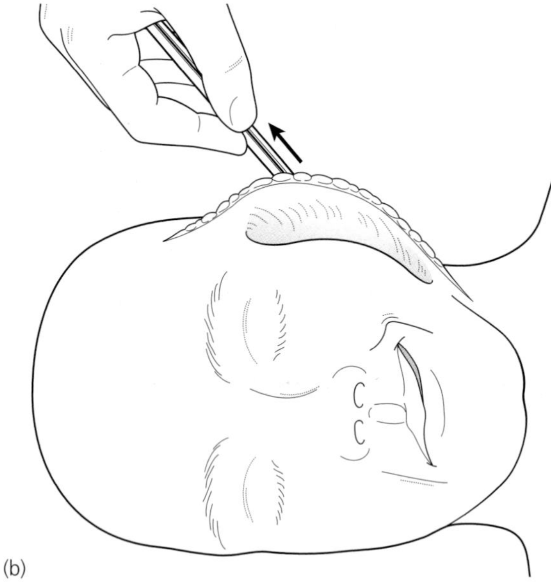

3.14.4 (a) Exposure of the zygomaticus muscle and identification of the modiolus. (b) Traction to the commissure to define the 'smile pattern'.

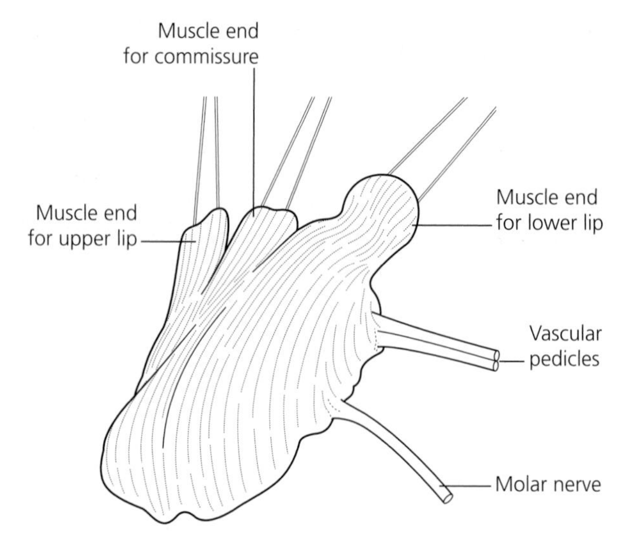

3.14.5 The graft end is divided into three parts before it is fixed to the oral commissure.

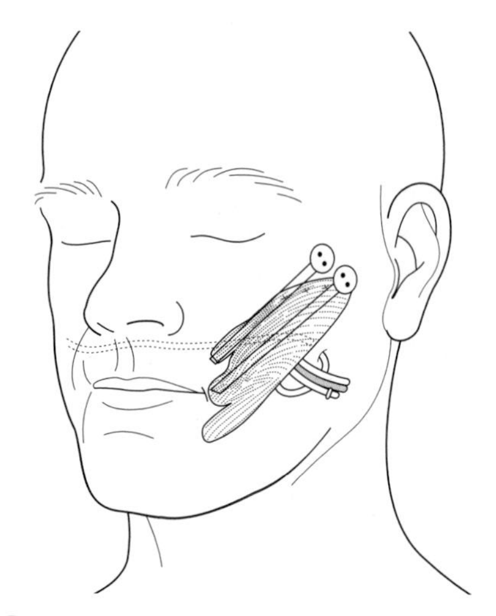

3.14.6 Positioning of the graft and the stay sutures.

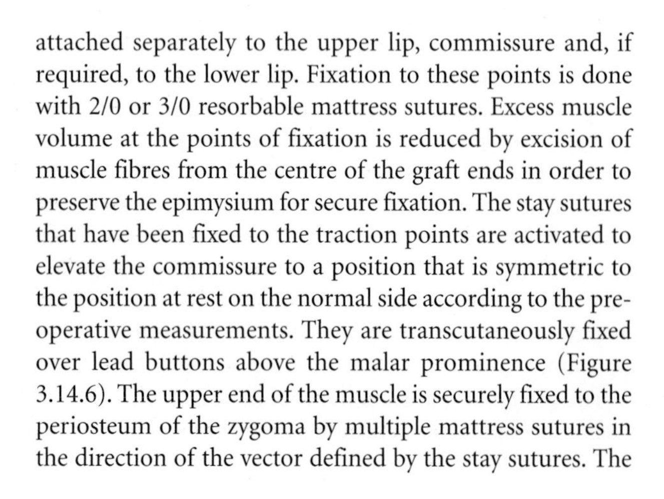

attached separately to the upper lip, commissure and, if required, to the lower lip. Fixation to these points is done with 2/0 or 3/0 resorbable mattress sutures. Excess muscle volume at the points of fixation is reduced by excision of muscle fibres from the centre of the graft ends in order to preserve the epimysium for secure fixation. The stay sutures that have been fixed to the traction points are activated to elevate the commissure to a position that is symmetric to the position at rest on the normal side according to the preoperative measurements. They are transcutaneously fixed over lead buttons above the malar prominence (Figure 3.14.6). The upper end of the muscle is securely fixed to the periosteum of the zygoma by multiple mattress sutures in the direction of the vector defined by the stay sutures. The muscle length should be adapted in a way that there is slight tension on the muscle.

Vascular anastomoses of the graft vessels with the facial vessels are done under the microscope using 9/0 or 10/0 sutures, depending on the diameter of the graft vessels. Occasionally, spasm of the facial artery occurs, which can be released by carefully applying papaverine to the end of the facial artery. Interfascicular coaptation of fascicles of the muscle's motor nerve to the cross-face nerve graft is done using 11/0 sutures. Coaptation should be close to the muscle as possible to allow early reinnervation by regenerating axons from the cross-face nerve graft.

Before wound closure, the stay sutures should be checked to make sure that the new position of the commissure is held

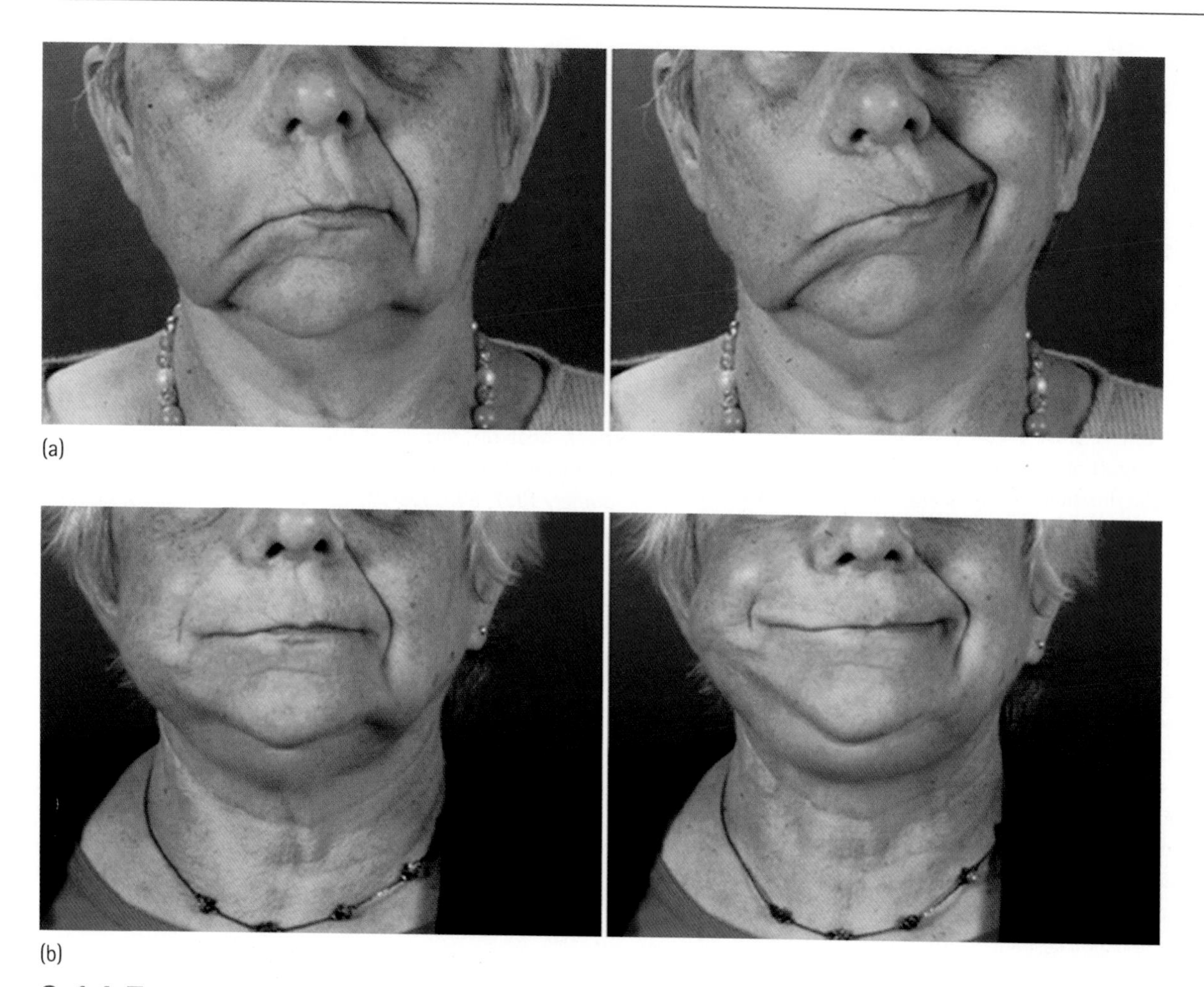

3.14.7 (a) Long-standing facial paralysis at rest (left) and during activation (right). (b) Three months after repair (gracilis graft) at rest (left) and during activation (right).

by the sutures and not by the muscle. A 10 gauge suction drain is placed in the submandibular area and the tip of the drain is kept away from the facial vessels to avoid damage during removal.

POST-OPERATIVE CARE

Post-operative care of the donor leg is described in Chapter 13.2. The suction drainage is routinely removed on the second post-operative day. Patients are asked not to activate their facial muscles on the normal side of the face to avoid tension and dislocation on the reconstructed side. The stay sutures are left for 3–4 weeks to allow for consolidation of the connection between the grafted muscle tissue in the points of fixation. Four weeks after the operation, transcutaneous electrical stimulation of the grafted muscle is started to avoid muscle atrophy during nerve regeneration (Figure 3.14.7a and b).

COMPLICATIONS

Complications are rare with respect to bleeding or wound break down. A major complication is the inability of the muscle graft to take on action. This only becomes evident some 25–30 weeks after the muscle transfer. Electromyography at this time can prove existing or missing voluntarily muscle contractions. Failure to show signs of activity may be due to insufficient vascularization or missing reinnervation. Insufficient vascularization has to be excluded by a meticulous technique of microvascular anastomosis as monitoring of the graft after wound closure is impossible. Reliable graft perfusion through patent anastomoses has to be proven by a positive Accland test and clear signs of muscle perfusion before wound closure. Failure to reinnervate the muscle may occur if the cross-face nerve graft has too few actively regenerating axons. This has to be excluded during muscle transfer by a positive Tinel's sign and histologically by frozen sections.

Top tips

Success in facial reanimation by neuromuscular tissue transfer is very much based on symmetry of facial expression. In order to achieve this, a few things should be kept in mind during the surgical procedures.

- A crucial point is a functioning nerve supply. Thus, coaptation of the cross-face nerve graft to the facial nerve on the non-paretic side must be done with the greatest possible care in that the fascicles of the selected branches are reliably connected to fascicles at the distal end of the nerve graft.
- The nerve graft should be long enough to reach the preauricular incision line to allow for a tensionless coaptation with the graft nerve, which in turn should be as short as possible to shorten neurotization time.
- The muscle graft should be positioned in an almost vertical fashion from the modiolus to the malar prominence to ensure vertical movement of the commissure during activation.
- The position of the commissure at rest must be safely secured by the stay sutures and the lead buttons and the grafted muscle should be under moderate tension in this position. A slight overcorrection will compensate for the tendency of sagging of the soft tissues after removal. Correction of the position of the commissure lateron by activation of the stay sutures is barely tolerated by the patients.

FURTHER READING

Hari K, Ohmori K, Torii S. Free gracilis muscle transplantation with microvascular anastomosis for the treatment of facial paralysis. *Plastic and Reconstructive Surgery* 1976; **57**: 133–5.

Kempe LG. Topical organization of the distal potion of the facial nerve. *Journal of Neurosurgery* 1980; **52**: 671.

Manktelow, R.T. *Microvascular reconstruction.* New York: Springer, 1986: 128.

O'Brien B, Franlin JD, Morrison WA. Cross-facial nerve grafts and microneurovascular free muscle transfer for long established facial palsy. *British Journal of Plastic Surgery* 1980; **33**: 202–12.

Terzis JK, Noah ME. Analysis of 100 cases of free-muscle transplantation for facial paralysis. *Plastic and Reconstructive Surgery* 1997; **99**: 1905–21.

Ueda K, Harii K, Yamada A. Free neurovascular muscle transplantation for the treatment of facial paralysis using the hypoglossal nerve as a recipient motor source. *Plastic and Reconstructive Surgery* 1994; **94**: 808–17.

3.15

The use of lasers – general principles

MADANAGOPALAN ETHUNANDAN

INTRODUCTION

LASER is an acronym for Light Amplification by Stimulated Emission of Radiation. The laser light is a type of electromagnetic (EM) radiation and is derived from the optical part of the EM spectrum. Radiation is considered energy in transit and its propagation can be influenced by changes in the energizing source. The laser light travels in waves, which have characteristic wavelengths and frequency.

PHYSICS AND DEVICES

The physics of laser is a complex topic. In brief, atoms consist of a positively charged nucleus and negatively charged electrons, which orbit in precise energy levels. At rest, these electrons remain at the lowest energy level (ground state) and when energy is added, are elevated to an excited state. The excited state is unstable and the atoms return to the ground state by emission of a photon (spontaneous emission), which can be in any direction.

A laser beam on the other hand, which is generated by a device, consists of photons which are of the same wavelength (monochromatic), coherent (all components of the waveform are in phase) and collimated (very little beam divergence). The basic laser generator consists of three components: (1) an active or lasing medium; (2) an optical chamber or resonator; and (3) an energizing source (Figure 3.15.1).

When energy is pumped into the lasing medium it is absorbed by the individual atoms in the medium, which are elevated to an excited state (stimulated absorption). The photons released as these atoms try to revert to a ground state collide with other excited atoms which are forced to emit an identical photon (stimulated emission), which are of the same wavelength, direction and phase. The stimulated photons produced are reflected back and forth by parallel mirrors in the optical chamber and the number of photons amplified by each reflection (amplification). The front of the output mirror is designed to be partially reflective and allows a small percentage of the energy to be emitted as a laser beam. This beam is further passed through a series of focusing lens to reduce its diameter and increase its intensity and energy to make it suitable for clinical applications.

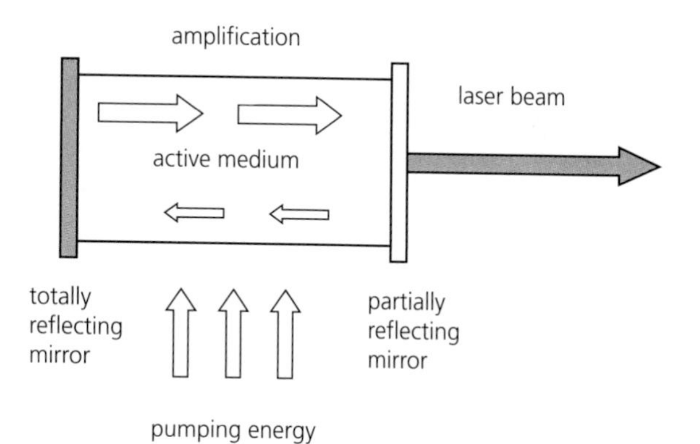

3.15.1 Laser generator.

The differing types of laser now available is determined by the active (lasing) medium producing the beam (Table 3.15.1). The lasers used in maxillofacial surgery are often delivered to the tissues via optical cables or through mirrors in an articulated arm and are dependent on the wavelength and power of the laser beam. Carbon dioxide (CO_2) laser is traditionally delivered with an articulated arm and others such as neodymium: yttrium-aluminium-garnet (Nd: YAG) and potassium-titanyl-phosphate (KTP) are delivered by fibreoptic cables.

LASER–TISSUE INTERACTIONS

The effect of laser on the tissue is principally dependent on its wavelength, power and delivery sequence in addition to the particular characteristics of the tissues. The outcome of these interactions are due to thermal (coagulation, vaporization, carbonization and ignition) and non-thermal (photomechanical, photochemical and photoablative)

Table 3.15.1 Types of laser.

Laser type
Gas lasers
Carbon dioxide (CO_2)
Argon (Ar)
Helium-neon (He-Ne)
Solid/Crystal lasers
Neodymium: yttrium-aluminum-garnet (Nd: YAG)
Ruby
Alexandrite
Pottasium-titanyl-phosphate (KTP)
Excimer laser
(Mix of rare gas and active elements)
Argon fluoride (ArFl)
Dye lasers
Organic dye in solvent

events. Photothermal effects are due to the production of heat from the absorption of laser energy; photochemical effects are due to changes in the chemical composition of the tissue resulting from the absorption of laser light and photomechanical effects results from the target area being mechanically destroyed by laser absorption.

Selective photothermolysis is the ability to achieve temperature-mediated localized injury to the target tissue through a specific chromophore, while minimizing damage to the surrounding tissue, and is dependent on the use of a laser with an appropriate wavelength, energy fluence and pulse duration. Thermal relaxation time is defined as the time required for a given heated tissue to lose 50 per cent of its heat through diffusion and therefore significant thermal diffusion (thermal damage) can be minimized if the duration of the laser pulse is shorter than the thermal relaxation time of the target tissue. The laser beam can be delivered as a continuous wave, pulsed wave (nanoseconds to seconds) or Q-switched (very fast pulses 10^{-9} seconds).

Therefore, for proper selective thermolysis to occur, the target tissue (through its chromophores) must possess greater optical absorption than the non-targeted surrounding tissue and the laser of choice must have a pulse duration shorter than the thermal relaxation time of the target tissue. Further, the power, focus and duration that the beam dwells in a particular spot also influences the tissue effects (focused beam, incision; defocused beam, vaporize at high power, coagulate at low power). The wavelengths, target chromophores and principle uses of the commonly used lasers in maxillofacial surgery are highlighted in Table 3.15.2.

In general, there is very little inflammation associated with laser wounds with a resultant decrease in pain and scarring. This is thought to be due to the denaturation of proteins, including the inflammatory mediators, with subsequent underestimation by the body of the damage caused by the laser. The denatured collagen is also partly responsible for the haemostasis obtained following CO_2 laser wounds, though this is restricted to vessels less than 0.5 mm in diameter.

PRACTICAL LASER SAFETY

Operational and environmental safety

Lasers are safe if used appropriately, though the risks to patient and staff can be significant if used improperly. The clinician using the laser is responsible for the safety of the patient and the staff. Local policies should, however, be in place to allow use of lasers by only trained clinicians, in a safe laser environment staffed by a trained support team. These operational aspects are often overseen by laser protection supervisors and laser protection advisors in the hospital.

The clinician should demonstrate appropriate training, understanding and experience with lasers in addition to being aware of the local safety guidelines. The supporting team, which usually includes a senior nurse, prepares the theatre, checks and starts up the laser and assists with the setting during its use. The key to the laser machine is often

Table 3.15.2 Laser characteristics and common clinical uses.

Laser type	Wave length	Target chromophore	Clinical uses
Carbon dioxide (CO_2)	10600 nm	Water	Cutting, vapourization, skin resurfacing, scar revision
Erbium: yttrium-aluminum-garnet (Er:YAG)	2940 nm	Water	Skin resurfacing, scar revision
Neodymium: yttrium-aluminum-garnet (Nd:YAG)	1064 nm	Oxyhaemoglobin, melanin, black, yellow, red, orange pigment	Vascular lesions (venous malformations), tattoos, pigmented lesions, hair removal
Alexandrite	755 nm	Melanin, black, blue, green pigment	Tattoos, hair removal, pigmented lesions
Ruby	694 nm	Melanin, black, blue, green pigment	Tattoos, hair removal, pigmented lesions
Pulsed dye laser (PDL)	577–595 nm	Oxyhaemoglobin, melanin, yellow, red, orange pigment	Vascular lesions (capillary, venous malformations), pigmented lesions, tattoos, scar revision
Pottasium-titanyl-phosphate (KTP)	532 nm	Oxyhaemoglobin	Vascular lesions (venous malformations)

kept by this person, who keeps it with their house key to ensure that it is not left near the laser machine. The number of keys in circulation is also strictly controlled.

A safe environment involves the creation of a laser light-tight envelope to the theatre in addition to provision of a regularly serviced and inspected laser machine. The access should be limited to essential personnel instructed in laser safety and doors should be locked and all windows and ventilation pathways covered with shutters. Clear warning with illuminated signs should highlight that a laser procedure is in progress and local safety rules apply. These signs are usually interlocked with the electrical supply of the laser machine and illuminate automatically when the power is switched on. Some hospitals have interlocks on the doors, which inhibit laser emission if the door is opened and interrupts clinical procedures. In these instances, it would be sensible to have additional door locks to prevent interlocks cutting the laser emission.

Clinical staff and patient protection

All the staff in the theatre, including the surgeon, should wear eye protection designed for the particular laser in use. These are designed to provide protection from accidental exposure and are not intended to allow direct viewing of the laser beam!

It is essential that the hand piece is not waved around carelessly when the laser is switched on. When active, it should only be aimed at the operation site and at all other times should be switched to the safe standby mode. The support staff in charge of the machine should always keep an eye on the clinician and should switch to standby mode if the laser is being pointed away from the operative site. Mirrors and highly polished surfaces should be excluded from the operative site.

The key areas of patient safety in maxillofacial surgery relates to the airway, eyes and sites adjacent to the target. Though it is rare for explosive gases to be used in anaesthesia nowadays, it is good practice to discuss this with the anaesthetist. There are, however, inflammable combinations of agents, such as nitrous oxide and oxygen, used regularly and it is vitally important that the laser beam does not penetrate the lumen of the airway or endotracheal tube with a significant risk of a catastrophic airway fire. There are specially designed armoured laser resistant endotacheal tubes available, which are often placed per orally. This can restrict access for treatment in the mouth and in these instances a nasal tube can be used, with the additional protection of a metal foil and saline-soaked gauze throat and post nasal pack, to protect the tube in this area. It is important to be particularly aware of the possibility of perforating the palate and entering the nasal airway and causing damage to the nasal tube in this region. In the same way, a cleft palate is a potential risk and an armoured oral tube would be a better option.

Eye protection is vitally important and depends on the particular procedure being undertaken. Lead corneal protectors are used for procedures involving the eyelids and periorbital areas, whereas special laser safety glasses are used for other procedures. The areas surrounding the operative site are protected by a thick layer of saline-soaked gamgee, in which a small hole can be cut to allow access to the target site.

Laser plumes contain dust, hazardous chemicals and biological agents (bacteria, viral DNA), which can cause potential harm. A laser grade smoke evacuation system (high flow; two stage filtration; filtration efficiency >99.99 per cent; down to a particle size of 0.05 μm) is therefore essential for scavenging, in addition to the wearing of surgical masks and gloves.

CLINICAL APPLICATIONS

The common clinical uses of laser are highlighted in Table 3.15.2 and specific applications are described in detail in other chapters in this book. When a CO_2 laser is used it is important to check on each occasion that the He-Ne visible light indicator laser and the invisible CO_2 beam coincide. This is done by aiming the He-Ne laser at a target spot on a wooden spatula and firing the CO_2 laser and comparing the target spot with the burn spot. Do not rest your spatula on your lap when you do this!

The CO_2 and erbium laser is often used for cutaneous resurfacing and the recent advent of computerized pattern generator and scanning capabilities have allowed for large areas to be treated rapidly and safely. CO_2 laser resurfacing has been associated with the reactivation of herpes simplex virus (HSV) causing delayed re-epithelialization and scarring. Antiviral prophylaxis (famciclovir, valacyclovir) should be instituted in this group of patients.

NEWER TECHNOLOGIES

Fractional photothermolysis (Fraxel) works by producing thermal damage to microscopic zones of the epidermis and dermis and therefore it is postulated that following fraxel skin resurfacing, the surrounding normal skin will help in faster healing and less 'down time' between treatments.

Intense pulsed light (IPL) is not a laser, but a non-coherent, multi-wavelength light source, in which appropriate filters are placed to produce light with wavelengths ranging from 590–1200 nm. It is primarily used for hair removal, pigmentary disorders and non-ablative skin tightening.

FURTHER READING

Anderson RR, Parrish JA. Selective photothermolysis: precise microsurgery by selective absorption of pulsed radiation. *Science* 1983; **220**: 524–7.

3.16

The use of lasers – photodynamic therapy

COLIN HOPPER

INTRODUCTION

Photodynamic therapy (PDT) is a process that describes an oxygen-dependent reaction between drug and light within tissue. This results in the generation of oxygen species that cause apoptotic cell killing and vascular shutdown. The end result of this is tissue destruction but in a non-thermal way so that connective tissue elements, such as collagen and elastic, are preserved undamaged. There are a number of drugs available for the treatment of head and neck cancer and these are shown in Table 3.16.1.

Table 3.16.1 Photosensitizers in current head and neck clinical use.

Treatment parameters	Photofrin	ALA	Foscan
Drug dose	2 mg/kg	60 mg/kg	0.15 mg/kg
Light dose	100 J/cm^2	100 J/cm^2	20 J/cm^2
DLI	48 h	5 h	96 h
Wavelength	630 nm	635 nm	652 nm

MECHANISM OF PHOTODYNAMIC THERAPY

Initially, a drug is applied either topically or systemically. This is selectively retained by tumour target tissue. After a period of time when the differential of drug accumulation between the tumour and normal surrounding tissue is maximal, the target area is illuminated. Treatment of early basal cell carcinomas and actinic keratosis can be effected by using aminolaevulinic acid (ALA). This is usually applied as a cream over the area then covered with an occlusive dressing. After 4 or 5 hours, the normal surrounding tissue is masked and the target area is illuminated using light of 635 nm, either from a laser or from a light emitting diode source. Following this treatment the area blisters and crusts and heals over time, leaving little or no scarring. The treatment itself is usually carried out under a local anaesthetic as the period of illumination can be quite uncomfortable, although cooling of the area with a simple fan is often sufficient. The limitations of this therapy are really the depth of effect as tissue necrosis only extends down to a depth of 1–2 mm limiting the application of this technique in larger or nodular skin tumours (Figure 3.16.1).

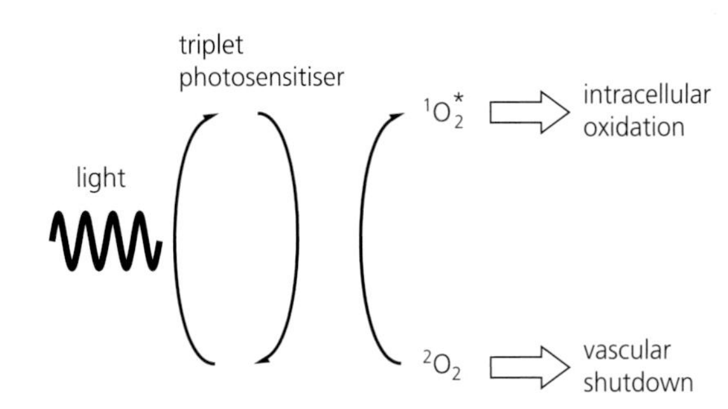

3.16.1 Mechanism of photodynamic therapy.

SYSTEMIC PHOTOSENSITIZERS

There are a number of these available for clinical use, although the only drug to be licensed for the treatment of head and neck cancer is foscan. There have been previous studies using a blood-derived product, photofrin, which is licensed in the United States for a number of applications. With both of these therapies the drug is administered intravenously. In the case of photofrin, it is given in a drug dose of 2 mg/kg with a drug–light interval of 2 days. With foscan, the drug dose is 0.15 mg/kg with a drug–light interval of 4 days. The major drawback of both of these drugs is systemic photosensitization, i.e. the patients remains very sensitive to sunlight. With photofrin, this can be quite prolonged, up to 8–10 weeks and with foscan the period of photosensitivity usually persists for a period of 2–3 weeks.

DRUG ADMINISTRATION

Both drugs are administered intravenously. Foscan, in particular, is quite an irritant solution and has to be given into a large vein. Any leakage of the drug into the surrounding tissue results in marked sensitivity of the tissue which can persist for two to three months. It is often prudent to give a little lignocaine into the vein before administering the foscan itself. From the time of drug administration, the patient is markedly photosensitive and has to take significant light precautions. In the early phase following administration of the drug, the patient has to be fully protected from sunlight. There then follows a period of gradual re-exposure to sunlight. In the case of foscan, this is over the next 14 days, at which point the patient can gradually be exposed to sunlight. Failure to comply with these recommendations may result in the patient sustaining sunburn and there have been cases where this has required hospitalization.

SURFACE ILLUMINATION TECHNIQUE

At the time of illumination, it is important that normal tissues are shielded by whatever technique is available (Figures 3.16.2 and 3.16.3). The use of black wax is often a convenient way to shield normal tissues and identify a target area. It is also important that the light is administered at a right angle to the surface to ensure equal dose symmetry of the light across the treatment field. This may be difficult in the oral cavity and sometimes multiple smaller spots are required to treat a large surface area of tumour.

Surface illumination PDT is a very good treatment for field change disease. The surgical and radiotherapeutic options are quite morbid for these patients who have synchronous dysplastic areas in their oral cavity which may extend over large areas. The treatment of early oral cancer has been described and it is clear that this is a suitable treatment for extensive thin disease. Just because early oral cancer could be treated with PDT does not necessarily mean it should be treated in this fashion. With thin T1 tumours it is quicker and simpler just to excise the lesion with a conventional technique. Where PDT has a clear advantage is where an early tumour is associated with a large area of dysplasia, often termed 'field cancerization'. Foscan is actually licensed for the treatment of advanced head and neck cancer where the patient has failed or is not suitable for conventional chemo-radiotherapy or surgery. In this group of patients, tumour down to a depth of over 1 cm can be destroyed. Complete response rates in this group of patients are in the order of 13 per cent, but subgroup analysis shows that if the total surface area of the tumour can be illuminated and the tumour is less than 5 mm in thickness, then complete response rates up to 50 per cent have been recorded.

INTERSTITIAL ILLUMINATION TECHNIQUE

An alternative to the surface illumination technique is to deliver the light interstitially (Figures 3.16.4 and 3.16.5). This can be done in one of two ways. Either using bare fibres which act as a point source for light distribution within the tissues or using diffuse fibres which can deliver light in a similar way to the techniques used in brachytherapy.

Thicker tumours need to be treated with interstitial techniques and this is an area where a great deal of research is being carried out at the current time. As with any tumour treatment, the aim is to accurately map the full extent of the malignant tissue and then ensure that all of this area is encompassed within a treatment field. The technique for fibre placement may require the adjunctive use of imaging techniques, either ultrasound, CT or MR scans (Figure 3.16.6). Using these techniques, needles can be placed within the tumour and, using a pull back technique, a volume of tumour tissue can be treated. The alternative is to use plastic after-loaders through which diffuser fibres can be passed and light delivery is calculated so that sufficient light reaches all aspects of the tumour and hence is able to treat the volume.

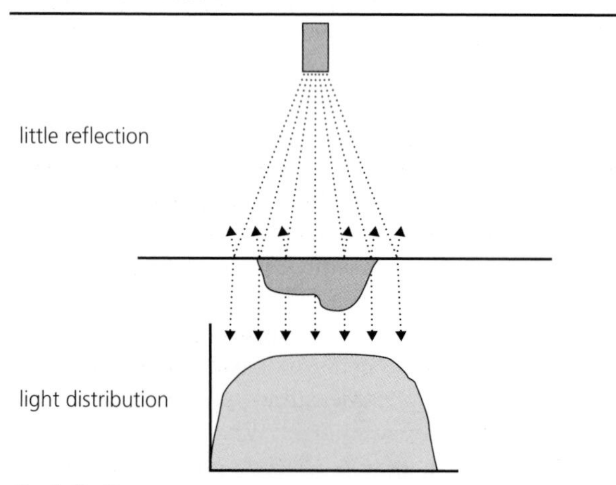

3.16.2 Illumination technique – at right angles to surface.

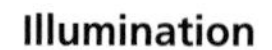
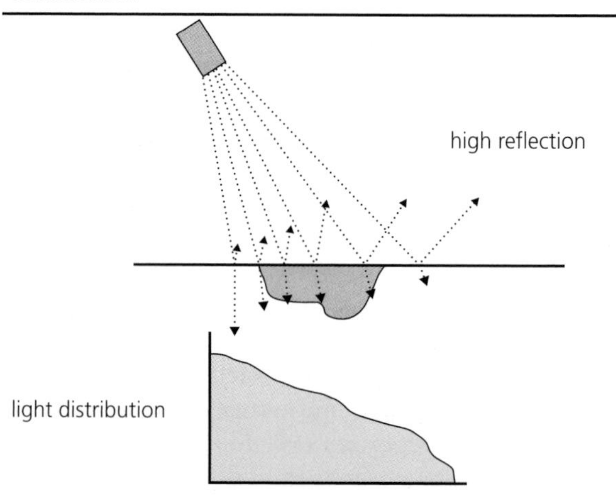

3.16.3 If illumination is not at right angles, then homogeneous illumination is not achieved.

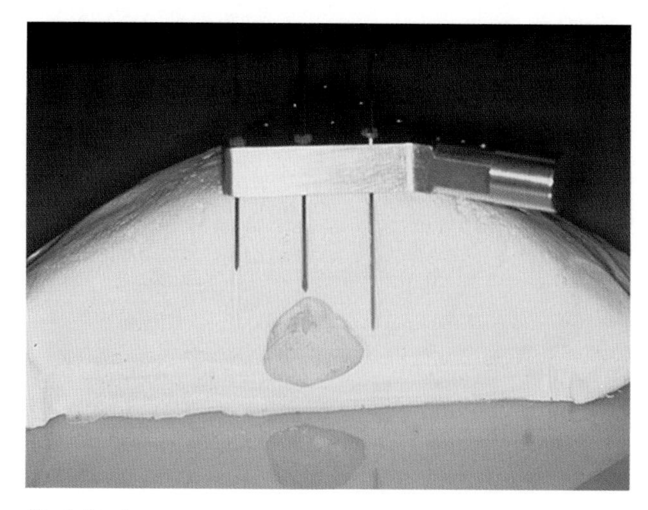

3.16.4 Interstitial technique laser fibres placed through needles and a step back technique is used.

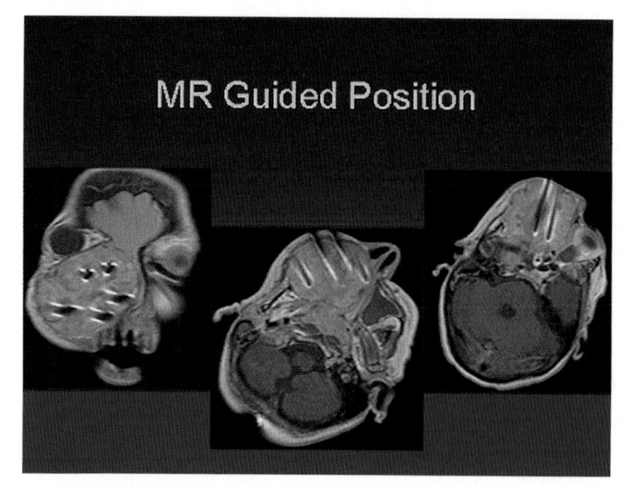

3.16.6 MR positioning of titanium needles avoids damage to sensitive structures.

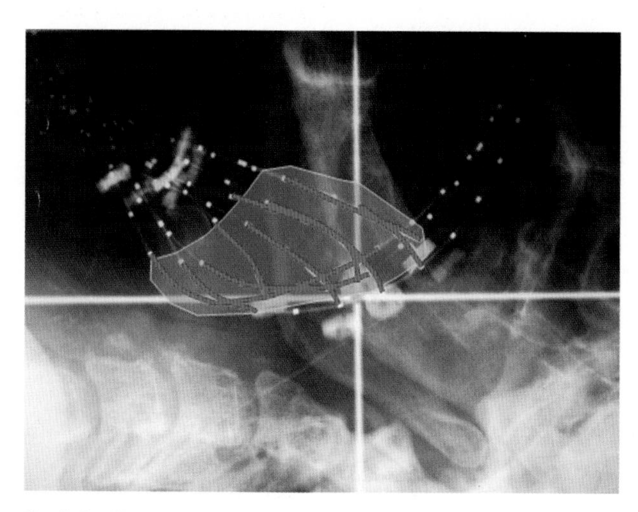

3.16.5 Interstitial approach using afterloading technique to treat tumour volume (in yellow). Diffuser fibres (in red) placed through clear plastic conduits (dotted lines).

POST-OPERATIVE CARE

After these extensive treatments, the patient may experience swelling that may be covered with systemic corticosteroids for a few days or, if treatment compromises the airway, a prophylactic tracheostomy should be performed. It should be remembered that if this is carried out after administration of the photosensitizer, then the patient will be at risk of photochemical burning and low light settings or a headlamp should be used.

The patient also commonly has a flu-like condition for a week or so following treatment and this is associated with a moderate leukocytosis. The treatment itself may be relatively painless, but certainly post-treatment pain does start to be a problem after 2 or 3 days. If surface illumination is used, then there are large areas of necrotic tissue that are sloughed off. These can become offensive and require treatment with topical antibiotics such as metrotop. Analgesia should not be withheld from the patient and the full extent of an analgesic ladder from minor analgesics up to fentanyl patches and opiates may be required for a couple of weeks after treatment. The important advantages of PDT in this group of patients are that the treatment can debulk tumours. It reduces bleeding from a fungating tumour by its direct vascular effect and also of great importance is the fact that nerves and blood vessels are immune to the PDT effect. This should be interpreted with some caution if there is any suggestion that tumour is actually eroding through blood vessel walls. Under these circumstances, caution should be exercised as a carotid blow-out could be precipitated if tumour is eroding through a great vessel. It is interesting to note that, as nerves seem to be spared by the PDT effect, this therapy can be used for the treatment of difficult benign disease, such as lymphangiomas, haemangiomas and neurofibromas. At the current time, this therapy is still in its infancy but shows great promise, especially in the treatment of cystic hygroma which brilliantly transilluminates, making it an ideal target for PDT.

FURTHER READING

Betz CS, Jager HR, Brookes JA *et al.* Interstitial photodynamic therapy for a symptom-targeted treatment of complex vascular malformations in the head and neck region. *Lasers in Surgery and Medicine* 2007; **39**: 571–82.

D'Cruz AK, Robinson MH, Biel MA. mTHPC-mediated photodynamic therapy in patients with advanced, incurable head and neck cancer: a multicenter study of 128 patients. *Head and Neck* 2004; **26**: 232–40.

Hopper C, Kubler A, Lewis H *et al.* mTHPC-mediated photodynamic therapy for early oral squamous cell carcinoma. *International Journal of Cancer* 2004; **111**: 138–46.

Jager HR, Taylor MN, Theodossy T, Hopper C. MR imaging-guided interstitial photodynamic laser therapy for advanced head and neck tumors. *American Journal of Neuroradiology* 2005; **26**: 1193–200.

Lou PJ, Jager HR, Jones L *et al.* Interstitial photodynamic therapy as salvage treatment for recurrent head and neck cancer. *British Journal of Cancer* 2004; **91**: 441–6.

PART 4

MALIGNANT DISEASE OF THE MOUTH AND JAW

4.1

Assessment and principles of management of head and neck cancer

PETER A BRENNAN

INTRODUCTION

Despite many advances in the diagnosis and treatment, the crude overall five-year survival of patients with head and neck mucosal cancer is still around 50 per cent. Modern treatments have resulted in much better local control and improvements in quality of life. With the arrival of new chemotherapy agents and targeted monoclonal antibodies (such as the epidermal growth factor receptor antagonist, cetuximab), used in conjunction with standard modalities of treatment, overall survival will hopefully improve. The incidence of head and neck cancer in younger patients who are both non-smokers and have minimal alcohol intake is cause for concern. Recently, the human papilloma virus, HPV16, has been strongly implicated in the development of oropharyngeal cancer.

The management of mucosal head and neck cancers is complicated by the involvement of and close proximity to many anatomical structures, which are vital for normal function. Speech, swallowing, eating and speaking are all potentially affected by both the disease process itself and the resulting treatment. It is therefore essential that these patients are carefully assessed by a multidisciplinary team (MDT) before any treatment is given. In addition to surgeons, oncologists, radiologists, nurses, speech therapists, dieticians and pharmacists, it is often helpful to have a clinical psychologist and palliative care consultant available as well. We have found that taping the consultation is valuable as the patient is then able to listen with relatives outside the hospital setting.

INVESTIGATIONS PRIOR TO APPOINTMENT IN THE HEAD AND NECK CLINIC

The main routine investigations for a patient with suspected head and neck cancer are summarized in Table 4.1.1. Some specific investigations are discussed.

General examination

Examination of the patient for evidence of other disease (which might influence the choice of treatment) is important. Isolated suspicious neck lumps (in the absence of an obvious primary tumour) warrant examination of the other lymph node sites and abdomen. Suspicious lumps in the supraclavicular fossa should alert the clinician for primary pathology in the lung, gastrointestinal (particularly on the left side) and in women, breast primary pathology, and appropriate investigations should be arranged as necessary. Nutritional status should be assessed, especially if major surgery is planned – the biochemical changes of the catabolic state following treatment lower serum albumin and may impair wound healing and recovery if the patient is already cachetic. It should be noted that up to 10% of head and neck tumours may be associated with a metachronus tumour.

Examination under anaesthetic

Examination under anaesthetic is recommended for all complex tumours, those involving the posterior structures of the oropharynx and those of the tongue base. It also enables the specialist anaesthetist to see the patient at an early stage and assess airway and medical issues that may affect any future major surgery. It is worthwhile using prefabricated drawings of the oral cavity, oropharynx and laryngeal inlet to record the dimensions and extension of the tumour. Nasendoscopy can be used in the outpatient setting to examine inaccessible sites both before and after treatment.

Biopsy

When performing a biopsy, either under local anaesthesia or during an examination under anaesthetic (EUA), it is important to take a sufficiently large piece of tumour and ideally include some normal looking mucosa. Tumour

Table 4.1.1 Summary of investigations.

Basic investigations	
Nasendoscopy	
Examination under anaesthesia (may not be necessary for small and/or anterior tumours)	
Biopsy/fine needle aspiration cytology	
OPG	
Chest x-ray	
Full blood count	
Urea and electrolytes	
Liver function tests including clotting (INR)	
Staging CT or MRI of oro-pharynx and neck	
Chest imaging (see text)	
Special investigations (as required)	**Reason**
Doppler studies of radial and ulnar artery	Radial forearm free flap
Doppler studies of other areas	Perforator flaps
Arteriogram of lower limb, duplex scan	Fibula free flap
Fine needle aspiration cytology	Suspected neck metastasis
Ultrasound	Neck nodes of uncertain character on CT/MRI
PET/CT	Unknown primary, chest evaluation

CT, computed tomography; INR, international normalized ratio; MRI, magnetic resonance imaging; OPG, orthopantomogram; PET, positron emission tomography.

depth is sometimes difficult to assess on a small incisional biopsy, but a generous biopsy may provide some idea of deep invasion (and therefore help plan definitive treatment in the likelihood of neck metastasis), as well as providing information about possible dysplasia at the tumour margins. Tumours greater than 4-mm thickness have a much higher propensity to metastasize to the neck. It is often worthwhile taking biopsies of apparently normal looking mucosa close to the tumour itself, as these may show dysplastic changes which might influence management. Blind biopsies are also useful (for example of the tongue base and posterior nasal space), particularly in patients with an unknown primary tumour.

Fine needle aspiration cytology

Fine needle aspiration cytology (FNAC) is useful in the assessment of enlarged neck nodes. Even small suspicious nodes of 5–6 mm can be biopsied using ultrasound-guided FNAC. Bear in mind that FNAC can lead to false-negative results (when tumour cells are not included in the aspirate) and therefore it is only one method for assessing nodal status. A recent study found that a 23-G (blue in the UK) needle is as diagnostically accurate and results in less patient discomfort than a 21-G (green) needle and the author recommends this smaller needle for head and neck FNAC.

Orthopantomogram and chest x-ray

An orthopantomogram (OPG) provides information about the state of the teeth, as well as gross bone destruction (Figure 4.1.1) and it is also helpful in osteotomy planning when an access procedure is required. It is always sensible to obtain a dental opinion before any treatment is commenced and especially prior to radiotherapy, as early extraction of teeth with poor prognosis minimizes the later risk of osteoradionecrosis. Extractions can usually be performed at the time of EUA. A routine chest x-ray will reveal lung pathology (such as emphysema) and may even show pulmonary metastasis.

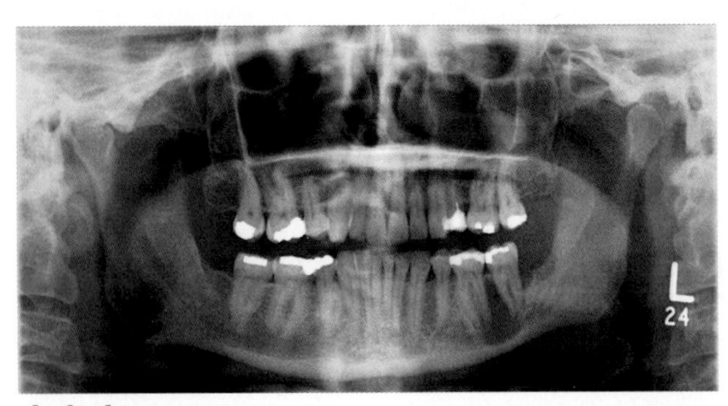

4.1.1 Orthopantomogram showing bone destruction in the lower left quadrant.

Routine blood investigations

Full blood count, urea and electrolytes and liver function tests are routine baseline tests that should be performed in any newly diagnosed head and neck patient. With the increased use of chemotherapy, renal function needs to be known before these toxic drugs are administered. Head and neck patients may have liver disease as a result of chronic alcohol ingestion. If major surgery is planned, chronic alcoholic patients should ideally be detoxified for a week or so before their operation to minimize the complications of acute alcohol withdrawal. One should remember that liver disease may result in changed clotting factors, and indeed an international normalized ratio (INR) is one of the most sensitive tests of liver function.

Cross-sectional imaging

Both computed tomography (CT) and magnetic resonance imaging (MRI) have advantages and disadvantages. Both can be used to image the neck for possible lymph node metastasis, but neither is sufficiently sensitive to detect micro-metastases. However, both CT and MRI will show necrosis within lymph nodes, a finding which is usually indicative of squamous cell carcinoma, rather than lymphoma (Figure 4.1.2). MRI cannot be used to assess the lungs and some claustrophobic patients find the examination intolerable. In future, open magnet machines may make the examination easier for these patients. While cortical bone is poorly imaged on MRI (due to the lack of water molecules), bone marrow provides high signal, and loss of this signal can be a sign of bone invasion (Figure 4.1.3). MRI is also useful in complex anatomical areas, such as the infra-temporal fossa and tongue base. MRI may overestimate the size of tumours due to associated inflammation, but with all imaging, tumour size can be underestimated. An example is the superficially invasive tongue cancer, which might not even be evident on a cross-sectional scan.

CT is a much quicker procedure, but a considerable amount of ionizing radiation is used (8 mSV, equivalent to 400 chest x-rays) and there is a greater risk of an adverse reaction to the intravenous contrast. There is still controversy about whether to use CT for scanning the chest in patients with head and neck cancer. The incidence of lung metastasis in patients with small T-stage tumours is low and higher in patients with multiple or large neck metastasis, particularly if in the low neck levels (III–V).

Ultrasound

Ultrasound (US) is ideal for assessing lymph nodes both prior to and following treatment. Its ability to assess the size, shape, consistency (presence or absence of normal node hilum) and vascularity (with colour flow Doppler) of a node is invaluable. Ultrasound is more sensitive than CT in assessing small metastatic nodes (less than 6 mm), particularly when used with FNAC. It is also helpful in guiding fine needle biopsies in deep or impalpable nodes. The use of US in following up patients after treatment is to be encouraged. With appropriate training, surgeons can perform US in the clinic and they have the advantage of knowing the underlying anatomy in great detail. Liver ultrasound may be indicated with deranged liver function

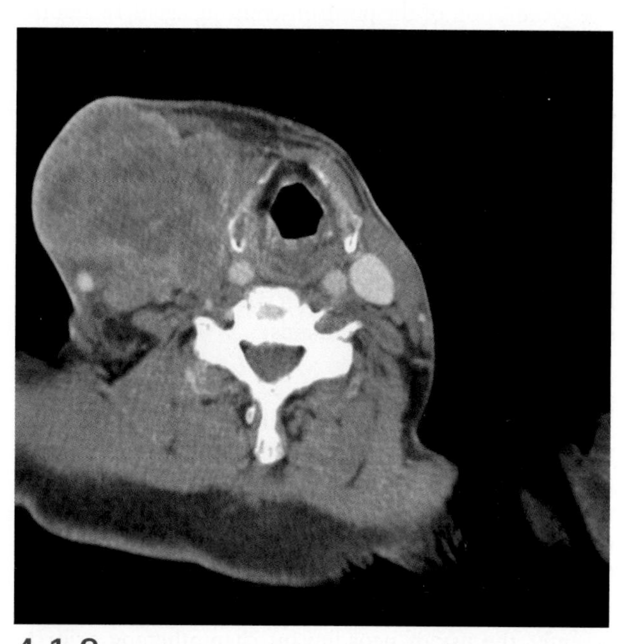

4.1.2 Computed tomography scan showing necrosis within lymph nodes indicative of squamous cell carcinoma.

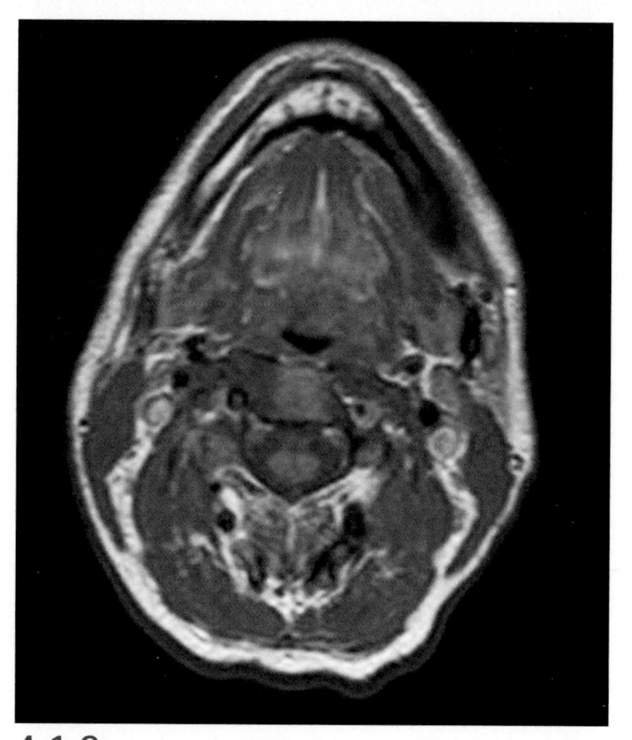

4.1.3 T_1-weighted magnetic resonance image from the same patient as in Figure 4.1.1, showing extensive loss of bone marrow signal indicating tumour spread.

tests, or when a liver is palpated during routine examination. Some advocate the use of intra-operative US with small, high resolution probes to guide primary tumour resection, although this technique is not in widespread use.

Positron emission tomography–computed tomography

The localization of the positron-emitting agent 18-fluoro-deoxyglucose (FDG) with CT has enabled even small tumours to be localized. Positron emission tomography–computed tomography (PET-CT) may have a role to play in the assessment of the unknown primary tumour and to evaluate suspicious chest nodules. However, FDG is also taken up following biopsy (even several weeks later) and therefore may give rise to false-positive results. In time, there may be specific monoclonal antibodies developed that will bind to cancer cells enabling their detection (for example to specific cellular adhesion proteins).

PRINCIPLES OF MANAGEMENT

As mentioned previously, all patients need to be seen in a multidisciplinary combined head and neck clinic so as to ensure that the appropriate treatment is given. Historically, patients would have been treated initially either by surgery or radiotherapy, or with a combination of both. More recently, the use of neoadjuvant chemotherapy prior to definitive treatment is gaining popularity, particularly with large volume disease, and tumours involving structures such as the soft palate. The concept of 'organ-preserving treatment' should be considered. Although resection and reconstruction of, for example, the soft palate may produce a good surgical result, it will never function in the same way as before treatment. Neoadjuvant chemotherapy often shrinks the primary tumour considerably, but whether resection of the primary tumour should be to the same margins as before chemotherapy is controversial, since there is no randomized clinical trial comparing this in head and neck cancer. Treatment will either have curative or palliative intent and it is important to establish at an early stage whether there is a realistic chance of cure.

FACTORS INFLUENCING THE CHOICE OF TREATMENT

All of the following factors need to be considered when planning treatment.

General parameters

General parameters, such as age, medical co-morbidity (such as ischaemic heart disease, peripheral vascular disease, obstructive airway disease, nutritional status, liver and renal compromise), as well as social implications, including smoking and alcohol consumption all need to be considered. For example, an elderly patient with a life-long smoking history who drinks 70 units of alcohol per week may require 'medical optimization' and a high calorie and protein diet (possibly by nasogastic or gastrostomy feeding) to reduce the likelihood of significant post-operative complications if major surgery is planned. For posterior oropharyngeal tumours, it is sensible to place a percutaneous endoscopic gastrotomy (PEG) placement at an early stage to enable feeding post-operatively. This is also important when radiotherapy fields may result in a severe pharyngitis, making eating difficult or impossible.

Tumour site

Both surgery and radiotherapy can be used for the treatment of lip cancers, although radiotherapy is arguably better in advanced disease. Primary surgery or radiotherapy can be used for definitive curative treatment of intraoral tumours, but only surgery is likely to be curative when bone is involved. Neoadjuvant chemotherapy (given before surgery or radiotherapy) may also be indicated, particularly with large tumours and/or those involving such sites as the tongue base or soft palate. Concurrent chemotherapy (given at the same time as radiotherapy) is also used in some centres. Radiotherapy can be used for palliation, but may result in osteoradionecrosis and its associated complications. Radiotherapy can also be used for palliation but even this can result in osteoradionecrosis and its associated complications if the patient survives longer than expected.

Tumour size

Surgery is ideal for small T1 and early T2 tumours, as long as function is not severely compromised. With larger tumours, each case will be discussed at an MDT and an appropriate treatment decision will be made. In many cases, ablative surgery with microvascular reconstruction is followed by radiotherapy if this is indicated following pathological analysis of the resection specimen. Neoadjuvant chemotherapy (using a combination of drugs such as 5-fluorouracil, cisplatin and docetaxel) is particularly useful in large tongue base and soft palate/pharyngeal wall tumours prior to surgery or radiotherapy. To date, there have been no clinical trials comparing neoadjuvant chemotherapy versus surgery or radiotherapy alone on patient survival.

Histology

The likelihood for neck metastasis is increased with poorly differentiated primary tumours. However, many surgeons would consider a tumour depth of 4 mm or more to be a greater predictor of neck metastasis. Peri-neural and vascular invasion are also bad prognostic indicators, as is an infiltrating tumour front (as compared to a cohesive pattern). Field change at the tumour margin, which may be present clinically or be apparent from dysplastic changes in biopsies, is a worrying feature. Radiotherapy can change these dysplastic areas into invasive carcinoma, so it is not surprising that surgery is usually used in these cases.

Neck status

Neck status should be considered with the primary tumour when deciding treatment. Even with small T1 tongue cancers, with a depth greater than 4 mm, the risk of nodal micro-metastasis can be above 20 per cent. In this situation, most clinicians would advocate an ipsilateral selective I–IV neck dissection both to stage the disease pathologically and to remove possible micro-metastatic disease that may not be evident on the pre-operative imaging. The management of the node-positive neck is less controversial and may be treated either by surgery or chemoradiotherapy, depending on the MDT decision. A modified radical neck dissection (ideally with preservation of the accessory nerve) is the usual surgical treatment, but recently the value of dissecting level V has been questioned in certain circumstances, and some would advocate a more limited procedure.

Previous radiotherapy

It is not usually possible to re-irradiate the same target volume twice and recurrent disease in these situations is best treated surgically. For recurrent neck disease, it is sometimes useful to bring new vascularized tissue (including skin) into the area which will enable further radiotherapy to be given if needed. The use of intensity-modulated radiotherapy (IMRT) enables radiotherapy to be delivered to a tumour volume with greater precision than conventional techniques, thereby reducing its side effects (for example, parotid gland sparing).

BASIC PRINCIPLES OF CURATIVE SURGERY

Primary tumour

The surgeon should have a three-dimensional impression of the tumour in their mind. The resection should be marked to include a clinical margin of at least 10 mm. The author routinely uses a Colorado monopolar diathermy needle both to mark and perform the resection. Meticulous haemostasis is paramount, for example, the lingual artery can be tied off posteriorly early on during a lateral tongue resection. Access osteotomies are useful for posterior tongue, some soft palate and pharyngeal/parapharyngeal tumours, as well as for those in the infra-temporal fossa. There is controversy about the use of frozen sections at the time of resection. Inevitably, there will be some shrinkage both after resection and placing the specimen in formalin and the definitive pathological margin may be less than that obtained clinically. Close and involved margins are associated with poor prognosis.

Neck dissection

Once again, meticulous technique is essential. Depending on the disease process, as many anatomical structures as possible should be preserved (particularly the accessory and marginal mandibular nerves). It is debatable whether the primary resection needs to be included en bloc with the neck dissection for floor of the mouth and tongue tumours. In tumours close to the midline, a bilateral neck dissection should be considered.

Reconstruction

The details of the different reconstructive techniques are provided elsewhere in this book. The reconstructive options depend on size of the defect, patient co-morbidity and operator preference. Small defects can be closed primarily or by using a small local flap, such as the buccal fat pad. Alternatively, they can sometimes be left to granulate. For larger defects, microvascular free tissue transfer has revolutionized reconstructive options. It is always sensible to have a plan B so that in the event of problems with the first choice of reconstruction, another option is available (whether that is a different microvascular flap or pedicled flap). In these long cases, it is important to ensure that the surgeon protects his own health: take regular breaks and consider using an operating chair or risk back problems in later life!

Temporary tracheostomy

This should be discussed at the MDT and is dependent on tumour size, site and co-morbidity. Patients can often be decannulated at an early stage.

PALLIATIVE SURGERY

Surgery has a role in the palliative patient. Debulking of tumours, including fungating neck metastases often improves quality of life even if only briefly. It is wise to consult the palliative care team at an early stage for their input. Potentially mutilating surgery when there is no chance of cure is to be deprecated, especially if this leaves the patient in a worse state. In this respect, functional outcome needs to be considered before embarking on major palliative surgery. Palliative neck surgery is sometimes useful (Figures 4.1.4–4.1.6), but skin incisions need to be planned carefully to minimize great vessel compromise and possible blow out at a later stage. Occasionally, palliative surgery gives unexpectedly good long-term results (Figure 4.1.7).

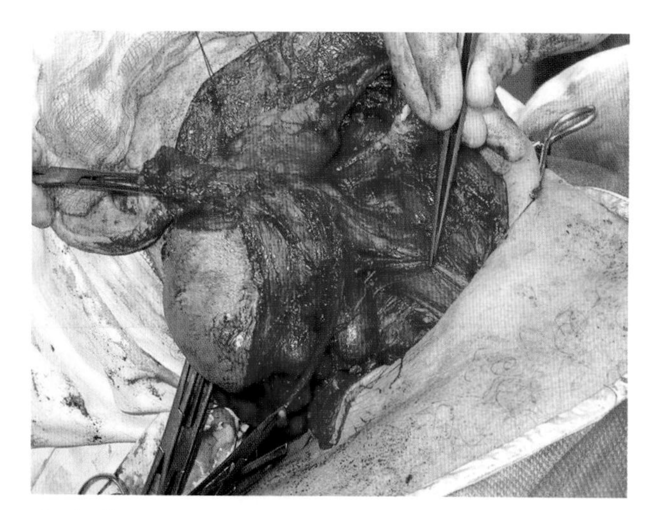

4.1.4 Same patient as in Figure 4.1.2, showing modified radical neck dissection type I, with preservation of the accessory nerve.

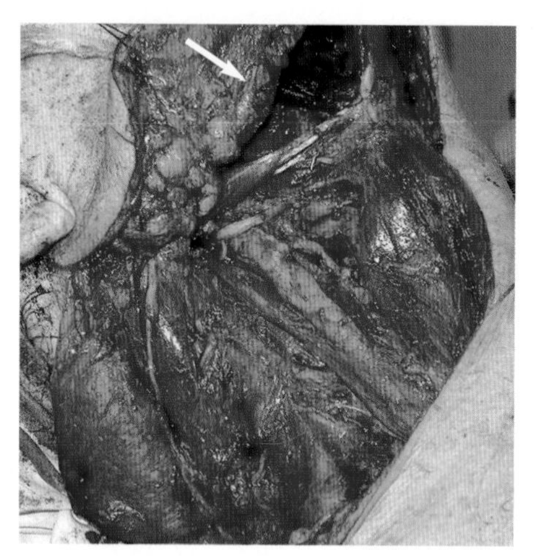

4.1.5 Same patient as in Figures 4.1.2 and 4.1.4 showing completed neck dissection. Marginal mandibular nerve is arrowed and accessory can be clearly seen.

Top tips

- Think of the whole patient – consider medical history and co-morbidity when making treatment decisions.
- For large and/or posterior tumours, consider placing a percutaneous endoscopic gastrotomy at an early stage.
- Concept of organ preservation and function after treatment.
- Open treatment discussions taking into account the views of the patient and all members of the multidisciplinary team.
- Advanced disease at initial presentation might be best managed palliatively – just because you can operate, doesn't mean you should!
- Think about your own health – take regular breaks and consider using an operating chair.

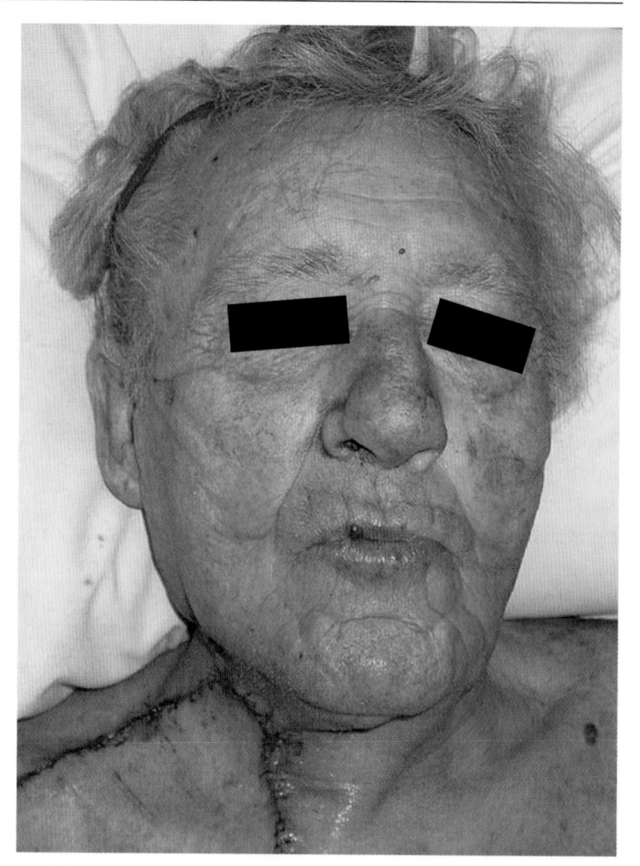

4.1.6 Good nerve function immediately post-surgery.

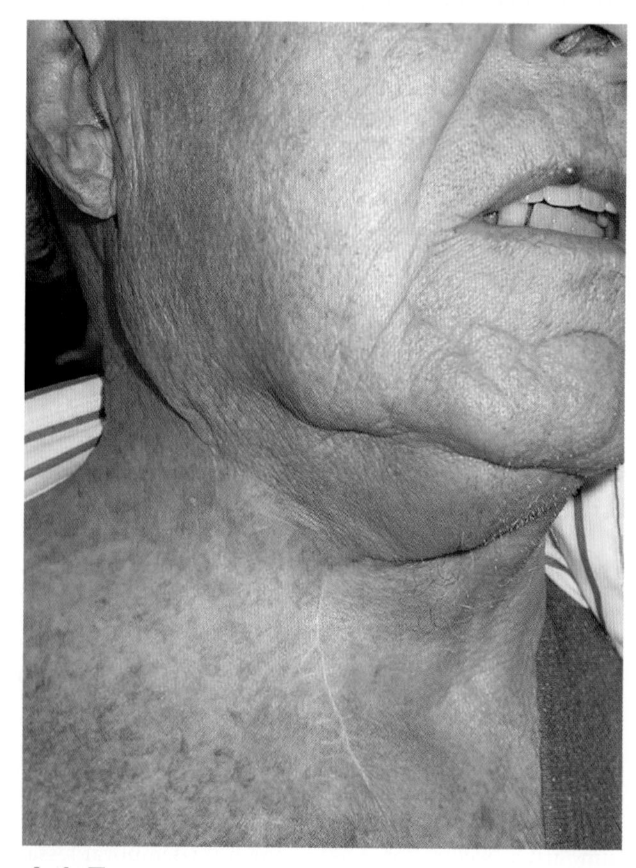

4.1.7 Patient still alive with no evidence of disease two years post-palliative surgery.

FURTHER READING

Bonner JA, Harari PM, Giralt J *et al.* Radiotherapy plus cetuximab for squamous-cell carcinoma of the head and neck. *New England Journal of Medicine* 2006; **354**: 567–78.

Bowden JR, Brennan PA, Butler-Keating R, Zaki GA. Use of audiotaped patient consultations in a head and neck oncology clinic and survey of patient attitudes to this facility. *Journal of Laryngology and Otology* 2003; **117**: 879–82.

Brennan PA, Mackenzie N, Oeppen RS *et al.* Prospective randomized clinical trial of the effect of needle size on pain, sample adequacy and accuracy in head and neck fine-needle aspiration cytology. *Head and Neck* 2007; **29**: 919–22.

Brouwer J, Senft A, de Bree R *et al.* Screening for distant metastases in patients with head and neck cancer: Is there a role for (18)FDG-PET? *Oral Oncology* 2006; **42**: 275–80.

D'Souza G, Kreimer AR, Viscidi R *et al.* Case-control study of human papillomavirus and oropharyngeal cancer. New England Journal of Medicine 2007; **356**: 1944–56.

Ferlito A, Rinaldo A, Silver CE *et al.* Elective and therapeutic selective neck dissection. *Oral Oncology* 2006; **42**: 14–25.

Guerrero Urbano MT, Nutting CM. Clinical use of intensity-modulated radiotherapy: Part I. *British Journal of Radiology* 2004; **77**: 88–96.

King AD, Tse GM, Ahuja AT *et al.* Necrosis in metastatic neck nodes: Diagnostic accuracy of CT, MR imaging, and US. *Radiology* 2004; 230: 720–726.

McMahon J, O'Brien CJ, Pathak I *et al.* Influence of condition of surgical margins on local recurrence and disease-specific survival in oral and oropharyngeal cancer. *British Journal of Oral and Maxillofacial Surgery* 2003; **41**: 224–31.

Pentenero M, Gandolfo S, Carrozzo M. Importance of tumor thickness and depth of invasion in nodal involvement and prognosis of oral squamous cell carcinoma: A review of the literature. *Head and Neck* 2005; **27**: 1080–91.

van den Brekel MW, Castelijns JA, Stel HV *et al.* Modern imaging techniques and ultrasound-guided aspiration cytology for the assessment of neck node metastases: A prospective comparative study. *European Archives of Otorhinolaryngology* 1993; **250**: 11–17.

4.2

Percutaneous endoscopic gastrostomy

SUSANNAH GREEN, PRADEEP BHANDARI

INTRODUCTION

Many patients with maxillofacial disorders, and especially neoplasias, will at some point require nutrition or medication to bypass the oral cavity. As the remainder of the gastrointestinal (GI) tract remains functional, the enteral route remains the favoured option. Oro-enteral or naso-enteral tubes may be impossible to insert and are not ideal for long-term use as they can be inconvenient, unstable and carry additional risks in chronic use. A gastrostomy tube is often a more suitable alternative in these patients. The insertion procedure is necessarily invasive and the associated early morbidity and rare mortality (Table 4.2.1) preclude their use for short-term support. Once in place though complications are infrequent (Table 4.2.1), they can be used in either the inpatient or community setting and they can be easily removed when no longer needed. They are therefore often an excellent option in the medium to long term. Many would suggest if the tube is predicted to be required for over a month then the benefits of a stable permanent access are likely to outweigh the early risks.

There are no absolute contraindications to placement of a feeding gastrostomy, but many situations in which the careful consideration must be given to whether it is the most appropriate option (see Box 4.2.1).

METHOD OF INSERTION

Gastrostomies can be inserted endoscopically, surgically or radiologically. Surgical placement is usually reserved for those requiring abdominal surgery and radiological for those in whom it is not possible to reach the stomach with an endoscope, although some would argue that this method is underused.

Endoscopic placement is usually possible. In patients with oropharyngeal tumours, it does carry the rare added risk of seeding the tumour cells to the gastrostomy site, but provides the careful endoscopist an invaluable opportunity to detect the synchronous oesophageal cancers present in almost 10 per cent of these patients. If early oesophageal cancer or high-grade dysplasia is detected prior to treatment for a known head and neck cancer then the treatment can often be adapted to take both tumours into account, for example radiotherapy fields can be expanded or larger resections taken at surgery. If an advanced, incurable oesophageal cancer is found then a patient may choose to avoid unpleasant but potentially curative treatment for the head and neck cancer.

The most commonly used technique for endoscopic gastrostomy insertion is known as the 'pull method', first described by Gauderer and Ponsky in 1980. It requires two skilled practitioners, who work as a team to pull a cord through the abdominal wall to the stomach and then out through the mouth endoscopically and then use that cord to pull the percutaneous endoscopic gastrotomy (PEG) apparatus back through the mouth into position. It is described in detail below.

PREPARATION

Many institutions will have a clinical nutrition team who will routinely spend time with patients and their carers prior to PEG placement to ensure there is a clear understanding of the procedure and a plan for both aftercare and use of the PEG. The patient must provide informed consent and be fasted. It is sensible to use an oral antiseptic prior to the procedure, particularly in those with malignancy who are likely to have oral bacterial or fungal infections. Most patients will require intravenous sedation for the procedure and a single dose of 2.2 g intravenous co-amoxiclav 30 minutes before the procedure has been shown to be useful in reducing wound infections.

Table 4.2.1 Important complications of percutaneous endoscopic gastrotomies

	Complication	Comments
Procedure related	Drug reaction	To local anaesthetic or sedative used for procedure
	Hypoxia	Oxygen saturations should be measured throughout the procedure
	Aspiration pneumonia	More likely than in standard upper gastrointestinal endoscopy as the patient is required to lie supine for the procedure
	Perforation of abdominal viscous	Particularly the transverse colon (see Transillumination). Air under the diaphragm is normal after the procedure and should not cause concern if seen on x-ray
Early complications	Local discomfort	May be due to gastric necrosis, can improve with loosening of the traction
	Peristomal leakage	Likely to reflect poor wound healing, may respond to loosening the traction
	Bleeding from wound tract	May respond to tightening of the traction
	Wound infection	Rates reduced with use of pre-procedure prophylactic antibiotics
	Ileus	Usually resolves spontaneously
	Accidental removal	Particularly in confused patients
	Peritonitis	Particularly if the tube is removed within a few days, before the tract has had time to epithelialize
Later complications	Tube blockage	Avoid by flushing with water before and after feeds. Many blocks can be reversed by flushing with dilute vinegar or pancreatic enzyme supplements
	Peristomal leakage	When occurs late may respond to tube removal for 24 hours to allow partial closure of tract before re-insertion
	Buried bumper syndrome	Excessive traction between the inner and outer bumper can cause ulceration and necrosis, allowing the inner bumper to migrate through the stomach wall towards the anterior abdominal wall
	Hypergranulation	May be prevented by turning the external part daily or weekly in accordance with the manufacturer's recommendations. Can be treated with silver nitrate
	Accidental removal	Even after the tract has epithelialized, it can close within hours if the tube is removed. The tract can be maintained by inserting a urinary catheter and blowing up the balloon inside the stomach until replacement can be organized
	Necrotising fasciitis	Risk increased by poor patient immunity, absence of prophylactic antibiotics, small abdominal incision, high traction
	Gastrocolic fistula	Probably form during the procedure but often present as diarrhoea after a tube change as the new tube follows the tract into the colon. It should be noted though that diarrhoea is more likely to be feed-related
	Seeding of oropharyngeal tumours to gastrostomy site	More than just a theoretical risk. There are at least 16 case reports in the literature. Can be avoided by surgical or radiological placement

Box 4.2.1 Relative contraindications to feeding gastrostomy.

- Gastro-oesophageal reflux
- Gastroparesis
- Gastric ulceration
- Infiltrating gastric or disseminated intra-abdominal disease
- Gastric varices
- Portal hypertension
- Previous upper gastrointestinal surgery
- Intestinal obstruction
- Functional bowel disease
- Small bowel motility problems
- Crohn's disease, although recent studies show few complications
- Concurrent infection
- Diabetes/severe malnutrition/poor wound healing
- Uncorrectable coagulopathy (international normalized ratio above 1.5, platelets below 50)
- Ascites
- Peritoneal dialysis
- Hepatomegaly
- Late pregnancy
- Recent myocardial infarction
- Obesity.

EQUIPMENT

Commercially available standard PEG kits will include:

- a gastrostomy tube with one end tapered and an internal bumper or balloon at the other
- an external bolster and feeding line attachment
- a long insertion thread
- a wide (e.g. 14-G) needle/cannula

Also needed for the procedure are:

- an upper GI endoscope with a port of adequate diameter to allow passage of a snare
- either fibreoptic or video endoscopes can be used. Fibreoptic endoscopes have a brighter light for more effective transillumination, but a video monitor enables all (in particular, the assistant) to see the procedure from within the stomach, which can be helpful with insertion and angling of the needle.
- a snare
- a mouthguard
- in those with restricted mouth opening, a paediatric mouthguard and small diameter endoscope can be used
- a sterile scalpel
- two small (e.g. 21- and 25-G) needle for local anaesthetic infiltration
- a sterile syringe
- sterile gloves
- antiseptic fluid
- sterile gauze swabs
- sterile drape
- scissors.

Some thought should be given to the type of PEG catheter selected. There are many different types available with a variety of characteristics. When choosing an appropriate type for an individual patient, particular consideration should be given to the following:

- How easy it is to accidentally displace/remove the tube (particularly for confused patients).
- The normal life span of the tube and hence frequency of necessary replacement (which could be of great importance for an otherwise fit patient requiring long-term nutritional support, but will be less relevant for temporary feeding or when the prognosis is poor).
- The procedure required for replacement (some require repeat endoscopy, whereas others can be replaced percutaneously in the community).
- The internal diameter of the tube.
- How many external ports are likely to be needed.
- The cosmetic appearance of the external portion ('button'-type devices are available, which lie flat on the skin and are easy to hide underneath clothing. They can be placed either as a primary procedure or to replace a previously established tube).

INTUBATION

Standard upper gastrointestinal endoscopy is performed with the patient lying on their left side, but for PEG insertion the patient must lie supine. Risk of aspiration is therefore higher and careful oropharyngeal suction is essential. Most practitioners will perform a full upper GI endoscopy to the duodenum at the beginning of all PEG placements for completeness.

SITING THE GASTROSTOMY

Digital indentation

The endoscope is passed into the stomach and then air is insufflated to ensure good gastric distension and apposition with the anterior abdominal wall. The endoscopist then directs the camera anteriorly, while the assistant uses a finger to firmly push on the abdominal wall in a series of short prodding motions. When the area of abdominal wall being pressed upon overlies the stomach then the gastric mucosa can be seen on the camera to indent. As the assistant presses in various places around the anterior abdominal wall, a good estimate can be made of where the stomach lies most closely abutted to the anterior abdominal wall, the optimal site for the PEG, and of the angle at which it should be inserted. Placement sites vary remarkably between individuals, but most will be somewhere slightly caudal and left of the xiphisternum.

Transillumination

It is important to confirm the position and ensure that the stomach is in direct contact with the abdominal wall without any intervening tissue. This is done by transillumination of the anterior abdominal wall with the light from the endoscope. Some video endoscopes have a bright light facility specifically for this purpose. Using this, sometimes with gentle pressure from the assistant's hand over the skin and lowering of the room lights, it should always be possible to see the light from the endoscope illuminating the overlying skin, even through a large amount of adipose tissue.

INSERTION

Placing the insertion thread

Once the best site has been selected, the assistant puts on sterile gloves, cleanses the site and surrounding area and infiltrates local anaesthetic to the skin and subcutaneous tissue. Pushing the small diameter needle used to infiltrate the local anaesthetic through to the stomach until it is visible on the camera allows a final safe confirmation of the site and angle of insertion of the trocar/cannula apparatus.

A skin incision of about 1 cm is then made and the trocar/cannula pushed through until a tall tented impression is seen endoscopically on the anterior gastric wall. With a jab from the wrist, the tip will pass through the wall into the stomach, which is being kept distended by the endoscopist with continuous air insufflation in order to avoid trauma to the opposing wall.

The endoscopist then passes the snare down the biopsy channel of the endoscope and over the trocar/cannula closing it gently. The trocar can then be removed leaving the cannula in place and the insertion thread (or wire) passed through the cannula until about 10 cm lies within the gastric lumen. The snare is then loosened from the cannula and slipped off, to be tightened securely on to the insertion thread. The endoscope and snare are then removed together, trailing the thread all the way back out of the mouth. The snare can then be opened to leave the thread lying between the endoscopist's hand outside the mouth, through the oesophagus and stomach and anterior abdominal wall, to the assistant's hand.

Pulling the gastrostomy into position

The endoscopist ties the tapered end of the gastrostomy tube to the insertion thread at the mouth and the assistant then pulls the abdominal end of the thread until the attached tube abuts the cannula (which can be felt as the thread stops running freely). The cannula and gastrostomy tube are then pulled through together to prevent the thread 'cheese-wiring' the abdominal wall. The remaining length of the tube is then pulled through until the internal bumper is felt to come into contact with the stomach wall. The tube can then be cut to a sensible length and the external bolster and feeding line attachment threaded on. It is vital that the external bolster pulls the tube tightly enough for the stomach to appose the abdominal wall in order for a fistulous tract to form, but not tightly enough to cause ulceration or tissue necrosis (see Table 4.2.1). Opinion is split as to whether it is necessary to repass the endoscope to check the bumper position internally.

POST-PROCEDURE

Institutions will have local guidelines, but a normal regime would be to hold the patient nil by mouth or PEG for 12 hours after the procedure and then infuse only sterile water for a further 12 hours. Bowel sounds should be audible before feed is commenced. Patients should receive hourly temperature, pulse and blood pressure observations for 6 hours post-procedure and the site should be inspected the following day for any signs of infection. Patients and their carers will require significant post-operative support and guidance in the use and care of their PEG.

When no longer required, PEGs are easy to remove. Those with internal balloons can be pulled out with firm traction after the balloon is deflated. Some types can be removed simply by cutting off the external portion and pushing through the internal portion, allowing it to pass naturally. There is a small risk of impaction or perforation when using this technique though and endoscopic removal may be preferable.

ALTERNATIVE PEG INSERTION TECHNIQUES

Some clinicians prefer to use the 'push method' or 'peel-away sheath method' of insertion. In the push method, a strong guidewire is used in place of the insertion thread, but is placed in the same way. The gastrostomy tube is long enough to allow it to be railroaded on the wire from the patient's mouth to the abdominal wall and has a firm tapered end that can be pushed through. In the peel-away sheath method, the optimal site is assessed endoscopically and the stomach inflated. A needle is then inserted into the stomach and a short guidewire passed through it. The needle is removed and a dilating introducer with an outer peel-away sheath is inserted. The introducer is removed, leaving the sheath through which a Foley-type balloon catheter is passed. The balloon is then inflated and the sheath peeled away.

ALTERNATIVE FEEDING TUBES

If it is not possible to feed into the stomach (e.g. functional gastroparesis in diabetics or obstructive pathology at or near the gastric outlet), a post-pyloric option may still be viable. It is fairly simple to add a jejunal extension to a PEG (PEG-J), but these are prone to falling back into the stomach, or to becoming detached and getting lost in the bowel. A more stable alternative is a percutaneous endoscopic jejunostomy (PEJ) which is similar to a PEG but inserted directly into the jejunum. Placement of PEJ tubes is more technically demanding, but in good hands the complication rate should be little different from that seen in PEG insertions.

CONCLUSION

Insertion of a PEG is a relatively quick, simple and safe method of maintaining vital medications and adequate nutrition to patients with swallowing difficulties and oropharyngeal neoplasms requiring extensive surgery or radiotherapy. Variations in body habitus, hiatus herniae and abdominal viscera can make the insertion procedure challenging and both endoscopist and assistant require skill and training. The ideal opportunity for insertion in maxillofacial patients will often be while they are under general anaesthetic either for assessment or for definitive surgery. It may be that the delay and discomfort associated with a visit to the endoscopy unit could be avoided if appropriately trained maxillofacial surgeons were able to perform the procedure at this time.

Top tips

- Use the opportunity of inserting the PEG to survey the upper gastrointestinal tract. This is of particular importance if the indication is for a head and neck cancer – 10 per cent of these patients will have a synchronous oesophageal cancer.
- The assistant performs a skilled part of the procedure – appropriate training and experience are essential.
- A lack of transillumination (visualization of the endoscopic light through the skin) may be due to liver or colon lying between the stomach and the anterior abdominal wall. Have a low threshold for abandoning the procedure and seeking radiological guidance.
- The external bumper should be fitted with only gentle pressure. Excessive traction will lead to tissue necrosis.
- For those in whom gastric feeding is problematic (e.g. gastroparesis, peri-pyloric obstruction), a tube similar to a PEG can be placed into the jejunum (a PEJ).
- If the tube is pulled out inadvertently at a time when a replacement cannot be immediately organized, then insert a urinary catheter and inflate the balloon in the stomach. This will maintain the epithelialized tract to allow easy and safe permanent replacement.

FURTHER READING

Gauderer ML, Ponsky JL, Izant RJ. Gastrostomy without laparotomy: A percutaneous endoscopic technique. *Journal of Paediatric Surgery* 1980; **15**: 872–5.

Green SR, Duncan HD. Selecting the most appropriate route of feeding. *European Journal of Gastroenterology and Hepatology* 2007; **19**: 359–64.

Hussain A, Woolfrey S, Massey J *et al.* Percutaneous endoscopic gastrostomy. *Postgraduate Medical Journal* 1996; **72**: 581–5.

Larson DE, Burton DD, Schroeder KW, DiMagno EP. Percutaneous endoscopic gastrostomy. Indications, success, complications, and mortality in 314 consecutive patients. *Gastroenterology* 1987; **93**: 48–52.

Nightingale J. Gastrostomy placement in patients with Crohn's disease. *European Journal of Gastroenterology and Hepatology* 2000; **12**: 1073–5.

Preclik G, Grune S, Leser HG *et al.* Prospective, randomised, double blind trial of prophylaxis with single dose of co-amoxiclav before percutaneous endoscopic gastrostomy. *British Medical Journal* 1999; **319**: 881–4.

Shike M, Latkany L, Gerdes H, Bloch AS. Direct percutaneous endoscopic jejunostomies for enteral feeding. *Gastrointestinal Endoscopy* 1996; **44**: 536–40.

Wollman B, D'Agostino HB, Walus-Wigle JR *et al.* Radiologic, endoscopic, and surgical gastrostomy: An institutional evaluation and meta-analysis of the literature. *Radiology* 1995; **197**: 699–704.

4.3

Oral and oropharyngeal squamous cell carcinoma: Pathological assessment of resection specimens and neck dissections

JULIA A WOOLGAR

INTRODUCTION

PRESENTATION OF THE SPECIMEN AND TRANSPORT TO THE LABORATORY

- Lay the specimen on a tile or block (heavy card, foam or polystyrene) in the correct anatomical position (Figure 4.3.1).
- Secure with pins or sutures. Avoid critical areas of the surgical margins. Avoid overtight sutures (risk of poor fixation and tearing of tissues).
- For modified and selective neck dissections, label the centre of each anatomical nodal level with a tag or suture (Figure 4.3.1). Submit any additional nodal groups (parapharyngeal, facial, etc.) in separate labelled containers.
- Immerse the specimen fully in fixative. 'Routine' is a formaldehyde-based solution. The volume of fixative should be at least ten times the volume of tissue.
- Alternatively, divide the neck dissection into separate anatomical levels, mark the superior aspect and submit each level in a separate labelled container. Take care not to disrupt the integrity of the primary tumour when dividing level I from primary tumour in en bloc resection specimens.

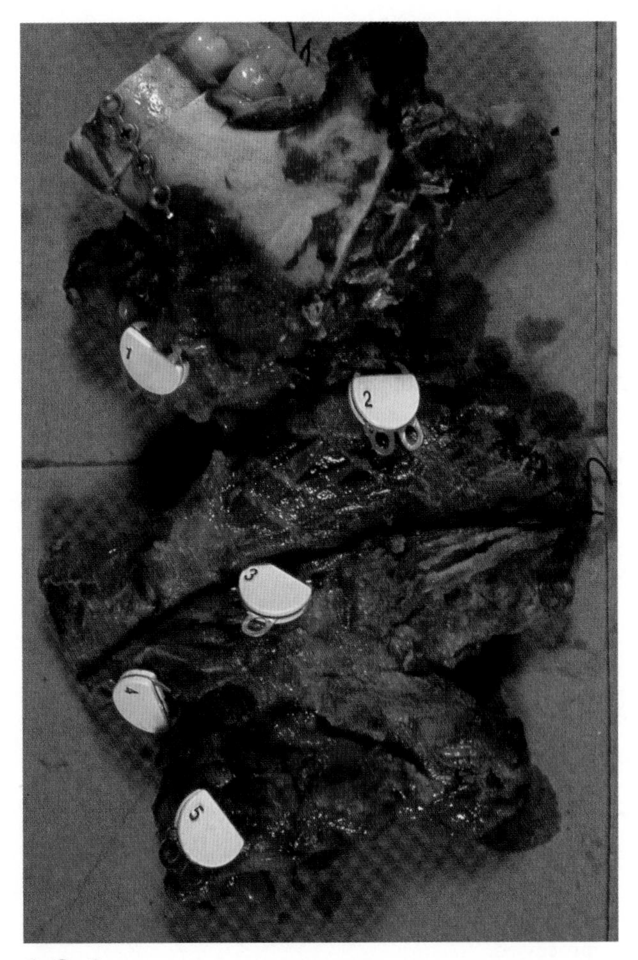

4.3.1 The specimen is laid out in the correct anatomical position with tags indicating the centre of each anatomical nodal level.

THE PATHOLOGY REQUEST FORM

- Give complete, accurate details of the name, address (essential for Cancer Registry), gender and date of birth of the patient.
- State the requesting surgeon and hospital, and contact details.
- State the clinical TNM (tumour, nodes and metastases) stage, details of previous histology including the

laboratory reference number and details of previous radiotherapy, chemotherapy or surgery.

- State the type of surgery: curative intent/palliative.
- Describe the clinical features and extent of the lesion, and the extent of the resection, ideally supplemented by annotated photographs or line diagrams (either free hand or preprinted).
- Give the key to the markers (sutures or tags) used to indicate critical margins, other features of particular interest and the anatomical cervical node levels. In neck dissections, deal with the left and right sides of the neck separately by reference to the anatomical levels included (I–III, I–IV, etc.) plus brief details of other structures.
- Label each pot with the patient's identification and the site/nature of specimen. Use waterproof ink. Check the clarity of preprinted patient identity labels.
- Give contact details of a designated member of the surgical team if an urgent report is requested or in case of a query.

OVERSIGHT OF LABORATORY PROCEDURES FOR 'ROUTINE' HISTOPATHOLOGICAL STAGING ASSESSMENT

- Macroscopic examination and description of the extent of the surgical resection/dissection specimen and the lesion, including measurements, ideally supplement by photography and when appropriate, radiography.
- Surgical margins are painted with Indian ink or a dye to facilitate histological assessment of the proximity of carcinoma to the resection margins.

The primary tumour

- Generally, the specimen is cut into 3–5-mm slices using a coronal plane for specimens from the central and lateral regions of the mouth and a sagittal plane for anterior specimens. If the tumour is close to/involving bone, preliminary assessment of amenable soft tissue margins is often possible prior to decalcification of the bone and remaining closely bound soft tissues.
- The tissue slices showing the maximum extent of the tumour (diameter and depth) and the closest resection margins are selected for processing (Figure 4.3.2). Generally, at least one tissue slice per 10 mm of tissue is processed.
- Routine histological assessment is based on one haematoxylin and eosin (HE)-stained section from each tissue block. Step-serial sectioning and immunohistochemistry may be used in difficult cases.
- The maximum dimension (diameter) and depth (reconstructed tumour thickness) is measured to the nearest millimetre using an optical micrometer to supplement the macroscopic measurements (Figure 4.3.3). No compensation is made for the tissue shrinkage that occurs during fixation and processing.
- Detailed histological assessment of the body and in particular the invasive front of the tumour is made.
- The width of the surgical resection margins (mucosal, deep and later on demineralized, bone) is measured to the nearest millimetre using an optical micrometer.

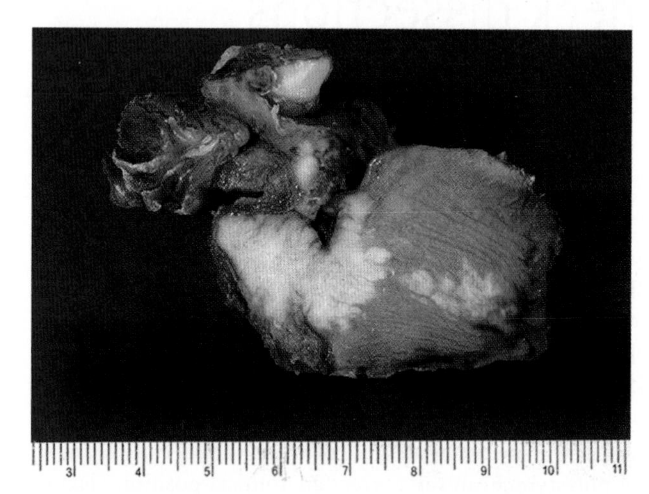

4.3.2 The tongue is sliced in a coronal plane. A streak of tumour well ahead of the main front has resulted in a close deep resection margin. Such streaks may only be present in a single tissue slice and can be missed if the specimen is not sampled thoroughly.

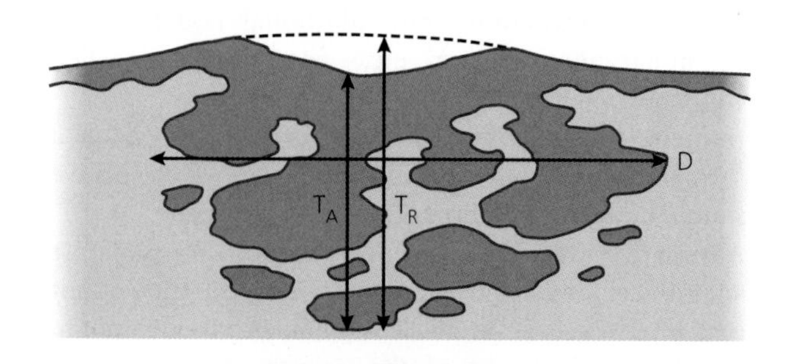

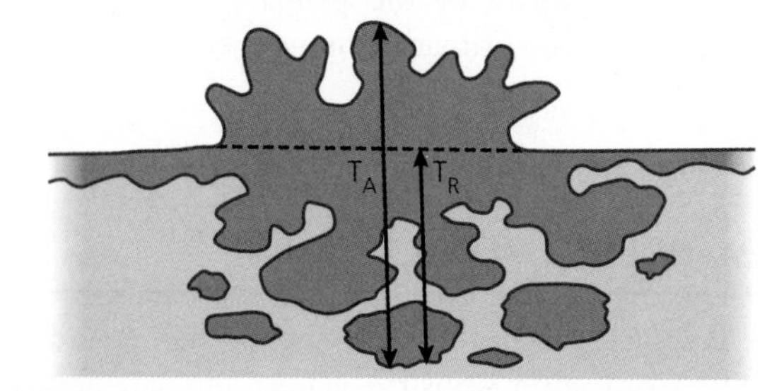

4.3.3 T_A represents the actual tumour thickness. The more important measurement is T_R – the reconstructed tumour thickness which compensates for surface ulceration or an exophytic component. D represents tumour diameter. It is important to include all satellite tumour islands ahead of the main invasive front in the T and D measurements.

Neck dissections

- The adipose tissue of the fixed specimen is searched by observation and palpation in order to identify all lymph nodes >3–4 mm in size.
- Within each anatomical nodal level, each lymph node is harvested (surrounded by its immediate perinodal fibroadipose tissue).
- Lymph nodes are placed in labelled cassettes, slicing larger nodes as shown in Figure 4.3.4.
- Ideally, the position of each node is indicated on a line diagram or photograph.
- The 'tissue bocks' are processed by standard means.
- Histological assessment is based on assessment of a single HE-stained section from each tissue block. Step-serial sections are cut in selected cases (such as further assessment of potential micrometastases or early extracapsular spread).

Sentinel node biopsy

- Sentinel nodes that appear negative macroscopically are subject to a more meticulous assessment.
- The node is bisected or sliced into 2.5-mm slices and each slice is processed.
- If the node is negative on initial routine HE-stained section, then:
  - Step-serial sections at 150-micron intervals are prepared.
  - One HE-stained section from each step-serial level is assessed.
  - If the HE-stained sections are negative, one slide from each level is stained immunohistochemically for cytokeratin using an antibody, such as AE1/3.

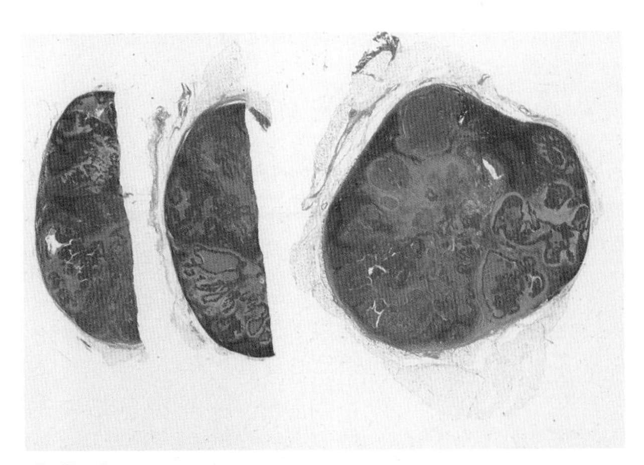

4.3.4 Larger lymph nodes are bisected and then one-half is sliced in a perpendicular plane to give several additional nodal profiles which permit a more thorough sampling.

HISTOPATHOLOGICAL STAGING: CORE DATASET

Certain features of mucosal carcinomas have been shown to be related to clinical outcome in terms of local recurrence, regional and distant metastases and survival, and hence, provide information that can help in management and prognosis prediction. Core data sets include only evidence-based features, and to be of value, it is essential that the pathological assessment is made according to standard protocols that include definitions and guidance on practical aspects. The UK Royal College of Pathologists introduced a core dataset (outlined below) in 1998 with a second edition in 2005.

Pathological data: Primary tumour

Site and subsite.
Maximum diameter (mm) (see Figure 4.3.3).
Maximum depth of invasion/reconstructed tumour thickness (mm) (see Figure 4.3.3).
Histological type: squamous cell carcinoma (SCC), conventional or subtype.
For conventional SCC: degree of differentiation (well/moderate/poor).
Subtypes: State subtype
Invasive front cohesive/non-cohesive (see Chapter 1.3, Figure 1.3.2).
Lymphovascular invasion: detected/not detected.
Invasive front neural/perineural invasion: detected/not detected.
Bone/cartilage invasion (detected/not detected) and type (erosive/infiltrative).
Distance of invasive tumour to mucosal resection margin (mm) and status.
Distance of invasive tumour to deep resection margin (mm) and status.
Distance of invasive tumour to bone resection margin (mm) and status.
Overall status of resection margins: clear, close, involved.
Severe epithelial dysplasia: present/not detected.
Severe epithelial dysplasia at resection margin: present/not detected.

Notes:

- In SCC with a multifocal origin, the maximum diameter is based on the overall area of involvement by SCC. Any simultaneous tumour(s) (separated by non-dysplastic mucosa) should be described separately after details of the index tumour.
- The histological degree of differentiation (tumour grade) is based on the degree of keratinization, cellular and nuclear pleomorphism, mitotic activity.
- Histological subtypes include verrucous carcinoma, carcinoma cuniculatum, papillary SCC, adenoid (acantholyic) SCC, adenosquamous carcinoma, basaloid

SCC, spindle cell carcinoma, giant cell (pleomorphic SCC), undifferentiated carcinoma.
- Prognosis of verrucous carcinoma and carcinoma cuniculatum is generally good since nodal metastases do not occur. Adenocarcinoma and basaloid SCC have a poor prognosis due to early regional and distant metastases.
- Lymphovascular invasion is defined as aggregates of tumour cells within endothelial-lined channels or invasion of the full-thickness vessel wall with ulceration of the intima and fibrin deposition/thrombosis.
- Only nerve/perineural invasion at the advancing front is included.
- Optional additional features that may be mentioned include the presence of sialoadenotropism (extension of dysplasia down orifices of minor salivary glands) and ductal invasion.
- Status of resection margins: clear is >5 mm, close is 1–5 mm, involved is <1 mm. Involved with histological cut-through is 0 mm.
- Further details, such as the precise site of involvement, apparent explanation (single streak, lymphovascular or neural/perineural invasion ahead of main tumour front, etc.) are optional.

Pathological data: Left neck dissection

Yes/no
Type: Standard radical/modified comprehensive/selective
Information on nodal yield, number and size of metastases, and extracapsular spread (see grid below for example).

Table 4.3.1 shows an example of a selective levels I–III dissection.

Notes:

- 'Size' refers to the total profile diameter of the metastatic deposit not the size of node.
- Matted nodes are described by an estimate of the number of nodes involved and the overall maximum size of the largest matted mass.
- ITC denotes isolated tumour cells. These may be detected by detailed histological examination of routinely stained sections or immunohistochemistry or molecular methods. Assessment for ITC is not routine, but may be used for examination of sentinel nodes.
- Extracapsular spread (ECS) ranges from gross invasion of anatomical structures such as muscle (Figure 4.3.5a) to invasion of perinodal adipose tissue down to pericapsular stromal reaction only detectable on histology (Figure 4.3.5b). Equivocal cases are upstaged. The extent of ECS (either in millimetres or by reference to tissues/structures involved) may be stated as an optional detail.
- Other optional extras include presence of embolization/permeation of perinodal lymphatics, presence of evidence of response of tumour to previous therapy (keratin debris/granulomas).
- A radical neck dissection yields an average of 20–30 nodes (and occasionally up to 100) in the absence of previous chemo- or radiotherapy. Salvage neck dissections may yield fewer than ten nodes.

Table 4.3.1 Example of a selective levels I–III dissection

Nodal level	Total number of nodes examined	Number with metastatic tumour. Specify if isolated tumour cells (ITC) (<0.2 mm) or micrometastasis (0.2–2 mm)	Extracapsular spread: not detected/present
IA	*6*	*3*	*Not detected*
IB	*2*	*0*	
IIA	*8*	*2*	*Not detected*
IIB	*6*	*0*	
III	*5*	*1 – micrometastasis*	*Not detected*
IV			
V			
VI			
Other			
Total number of nodes	*27*		
Total number of positive nodes	*6*		
Size of largest metastasis	*12 mm*		
Extracapsular spread	*Not detected*/present at level I, II, III, IV, V, VI, other (delete as appropriate)		

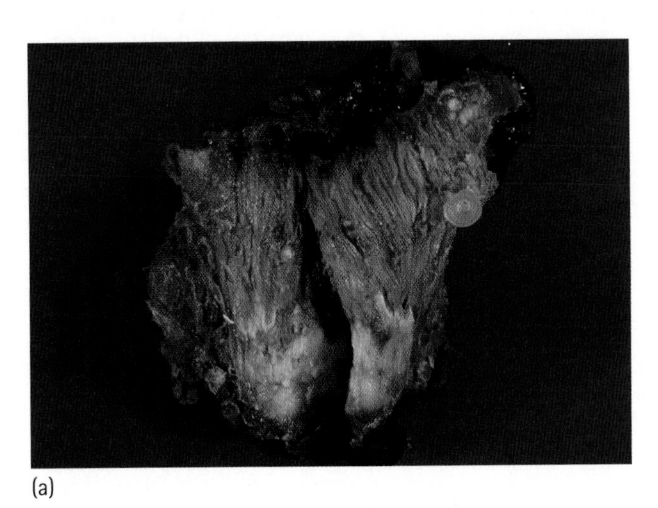

(a)

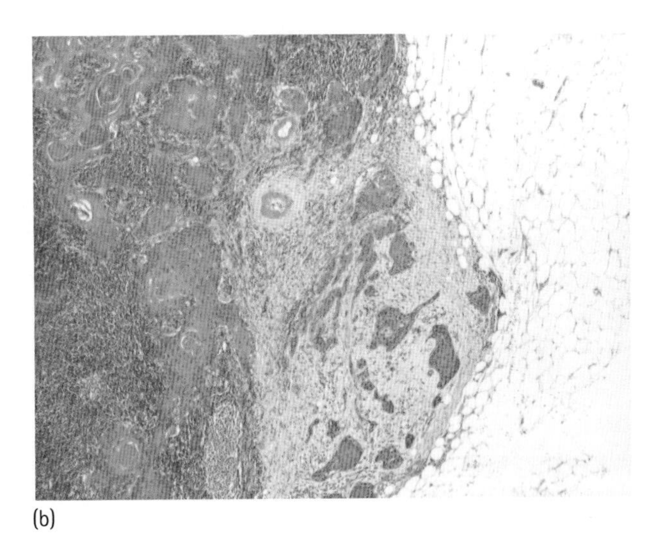

(b)

4.3.5 Extracapsular spread varies widely in extent. Panel (a) shows involvement of the sternocleidomastoid muscle; (b) shows focal invasion of perinodal adipose tissue with a fibrous stromal reaction.

Pathological data: Right neck dissection

Yes/no
If yes, as for left neck.

Summary of pathological data

Tumour site: (state with ICD reference)
New primary/recurrence/not known (delete as appropriate)
Histological type (SCC or list subtype)
Pathological stage:
pT …..; pN …..; pM …..; TNM stage grouping …..
Status of resection margin: clear/close/involved

Note: The UICC TNM clinical and pathological stage categorization criteria are similar.

POTENTIAL INACCURACIES IN PATHOLOGICAL STAGING

- Labelling errors and specimen mix up. Special care is needed when specimen pots have been labelled during preparation of the clinic. Any unused pots must be disposed of to ensure specimens are not placed in incorrectly identified pots.
- Sampling errors:
  - surgical (failure to clear all nodes within the drainage area)
  - laboratory (incomplete harvesting of nodes from fixed specimen, inadequate sectioning of individual nodes)
  - inaccuracies in histological detection (failure to notice).
- Errors in histological interpretation.
- Inherent errors, such as loss of tissue when cutting thin sections.
- Laboratory technical errors and machine malfunction resulting in specimen mix-up or poor quality slides.
- Inadequacies in the written report.
- Secretarial/clerical errors.
- Shortcomings in the UICC TNM staging system, such as the use of tumour diameter not thickness, omission of ECS.

Top tips

Accurate pathological assessment of surgical resection specimens requires strict adherence to agreed protocols at each stage:

- Presentation of the specimen and transport to the laboratory.
- Submission of an accurate, detailed pathology request form.
- Laboratory assessment and dissection of the gross specimen.
- Processing and preparation of histological slides.
- Histopathological examination.
- Presentation of histological findings (core dataset, UICC pathological TNM stage).
- Regular 'risk assessment' of potential inaccuracies and review/revision of protocols.

FURTHER READING

Woolgar JA. Histopathological prognosticators in oral and oropharyngeal squamous cell carcinoma. *Oral Oncology* 2006; **42**: 229–39.

Woolgar J, Triantafyllou A. Neck dissections: A practical guide for the reporting pathologist. *Current Diagnostic Pathology* 2007; **13**: 499–511.

Woolgar JA. Triantafyllou A. A histopathological appraisal of surgical margins in oral and oropharyngeal cancer resection specimens. *Oral Oncology* 2005; **41**: 1034–43.

4.4

Access surgery

BARRIE T EVANS, DOROTHY A LANG

INTRODUCTION

The excellent blood supply of the craniofacial skeleton allows pedicled or free bone fragments to be moved so gaining access to the skull base and adjacent areas. Tooth-bearing maxillary or mandibular bone segments must retain their blood supply and if post-operative radiotherapy is planned, pedicled osteotomies are preferable.

BICORONAL SCALP FLAP

Indications

The bicoronal flap provides access to the frontal bone, upper mid-face, anterior and middle cranial fossa, orbit, temporal and infratemporal fossae in a range of clinical situations.

Applied anatomy

The scalp has five layers (Figure 4.4.1):

- skin
- connective tissue (subcutaneous)
- aponeurosis (galea) connecting the paired frontalis muscle anteriorly and occipitalis muscle posteriorly
- loose areolar connective tissue (subgaleal plane)
- pericranium.

Over the temporalis muscle, the galea is termed the temporoparietal fascia. The subgaleal plane continues laterally over the temporalis fascia.

The temporal branch(es) of the facial nerve supplying frontalis are at risk as they run on or within the deep surface of the temporoparietal fascia. The landmarks of the temporal branch(es) are as follows:

- at least 8 mm in front of the cartilaginous meatus at the zygomatic arch;
- at least 1 cm anterior to the upper anterior attachment of the helix;
- no higher than 2 cm above the frontozygomatic suture (lateral edge of the eyebrow).

Nerve damage is prevented with dissection deep to the temporal fascia beyond these limits (Figures 4.4.2 and 4.4.3).

Surgical technique

Along the line of the incision, the hair is either strip-shaved or parted. The scalp above the galea is infiltrated with lignocaine and 1:200 000 adrenaline.

If a parting is used, the angle of the incision is parallel to the hair follicles to avoid later scar alopecia (Figure 4.4.4). Alternatively, a zigzag incision is used to prevent parting of the hair along the incision line.

The incision commences at the upper anterior attachment of the helix and is carried over the vault of the skull to the opposite side behind the hairline. The incision is through the galea – the first three layers of the scalp lifting as a unit (Figure 4.4.5).

The incision is made with a scalpel or Colorado needle and haemostasis achieved with bipolar diathermy. Dissection is carried forward in the subgaleal plane. Approximately 3 cm above the superior orbital rim, the pericranium is incised and the dissection continued subperiosteally. Resistance is then met at three points: (1) the frontozygomatic suture; (2) the supraorbital neurovascular bundle (freed from its bony canal with an osteotome); (3) the frontonasal suture (Figures 4.4.6 and 4.4.7).

A midline vertical incision in the periosteum aids exposure of the nasal bones and frontal process of the maxilla. Detachment of the medial canthal tendon from the anterior lacrimal crest gives unrestricted exposure of the medial orbit to the optic canal, and the orbital floor to the infraorbital nerve. The medial canthal tendon may be 'tagged' through the periosteum with a suture for later

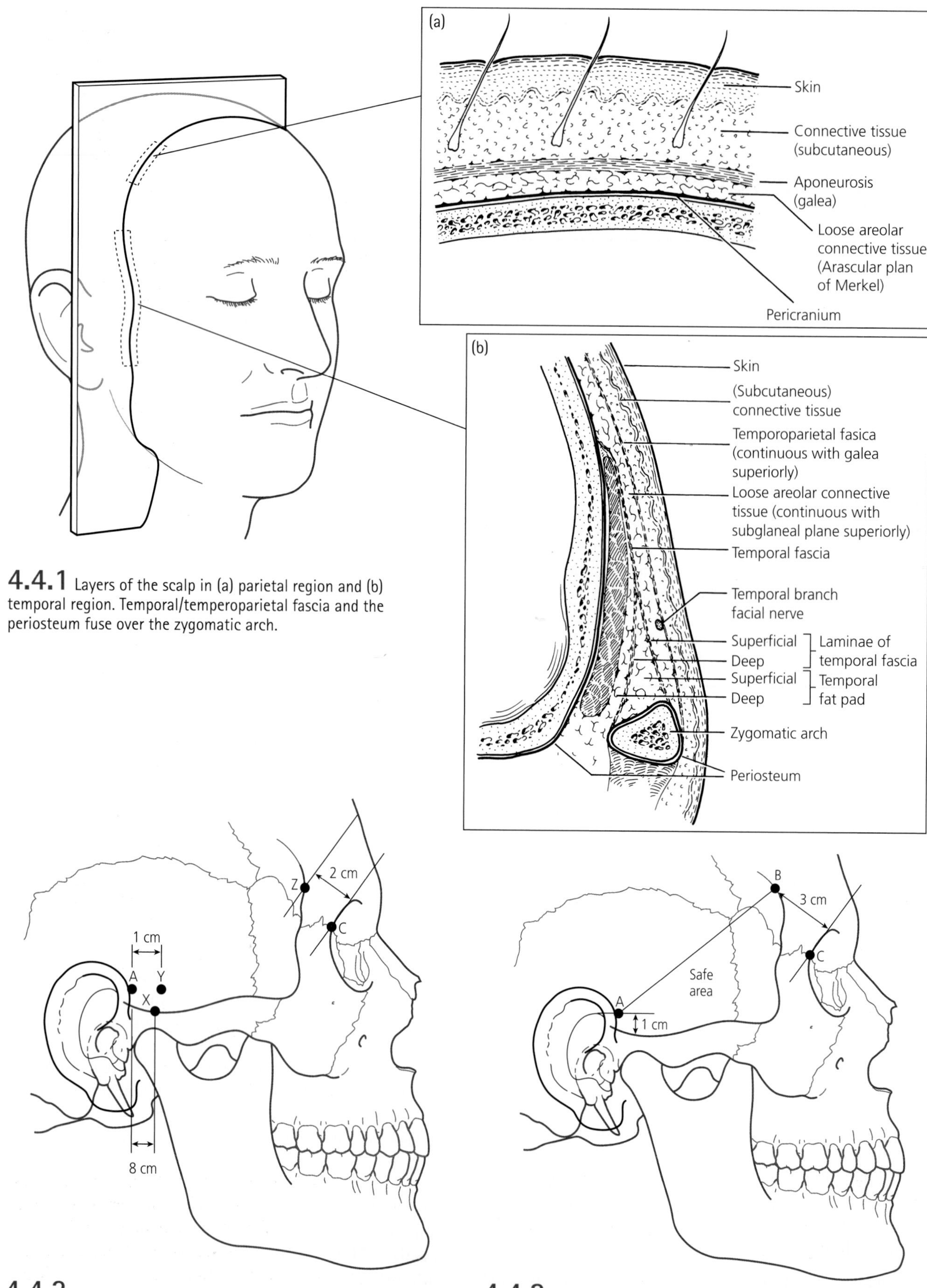

4.4.1 Layers of the scalp in (a) parietal region and (b) temporal region. Temporal/temperoparietal fascia and the periosteum fuse over the zygomatic arch.

4.4.2 The outer limits of the temporal branch(es) of the facial nerve.

4.4.3 The temporal branch of the facial nerve is deep to the temporal fascia anterior to line A–B.

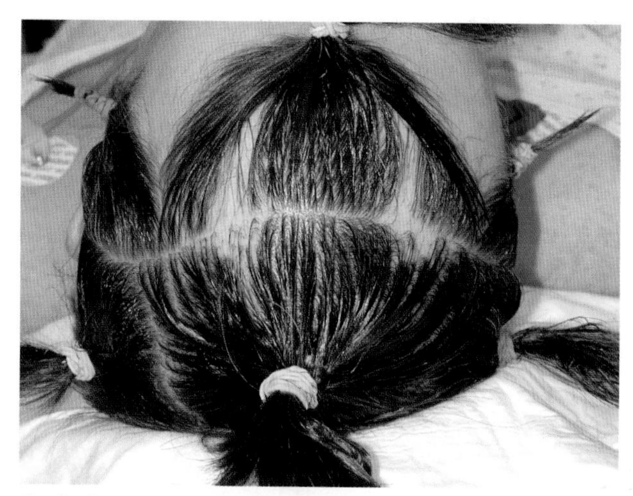

4.4.4 With the hair parted the incision is parallel to the hair follicles.

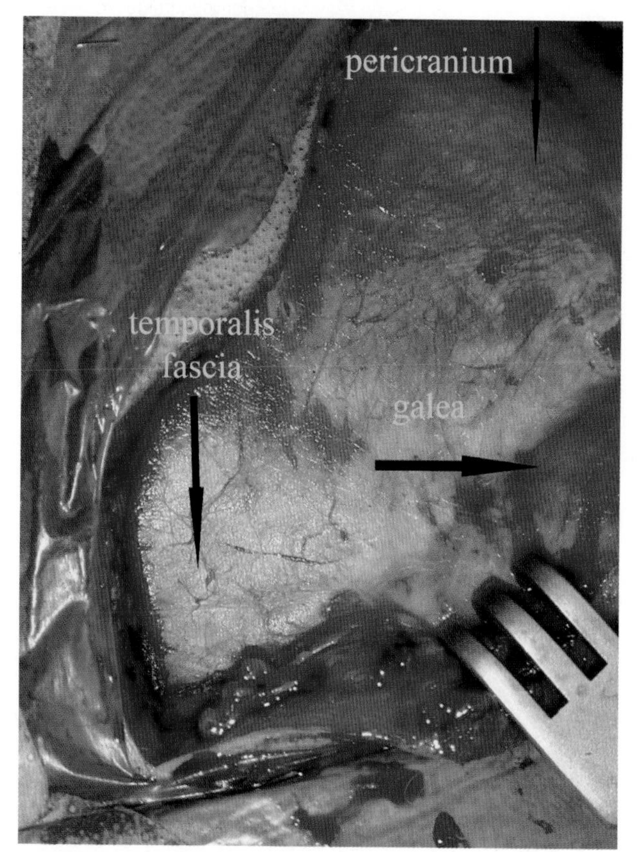

4.4.5 The first 3 layers of the scalp lift as single unit.

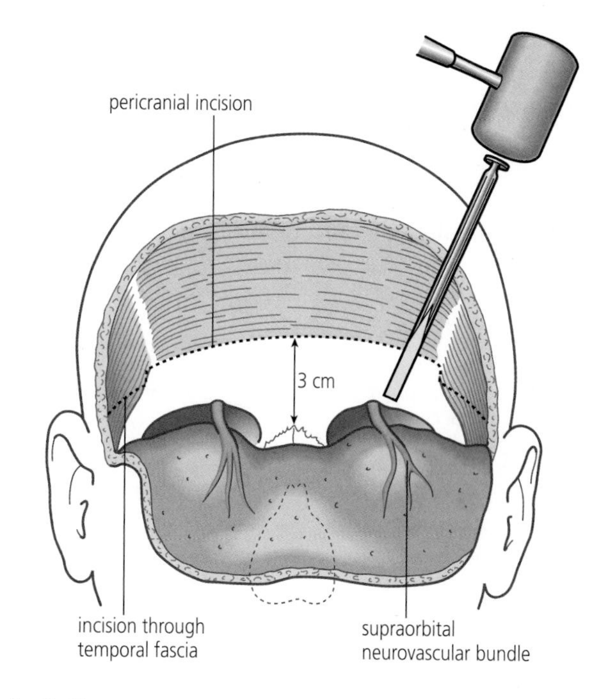

4.4.6 Supraorbital neurovascular bundle freed with osteotome.

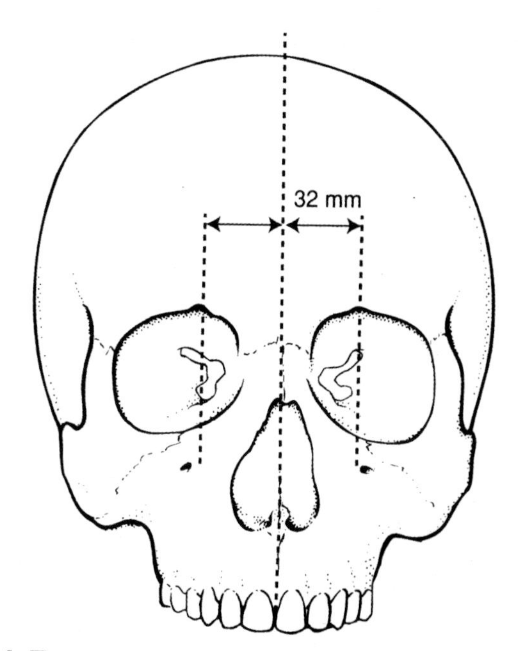

4.4.7 Average distance supraorbital notch/foramen from midline 32 mm (range, 15–38 mm).

reattachment to a microplate (Figure 4.4.8). Subperiosteal dissection medially is now possible as far as the floor of the nose. To expose the temporomandibular joint, zygoma and lateral orbit, the skin incision is extended inferiorly to just below the cartilaginous meatus either in a naturally occurring preauricular skin crease or endaurally around the tragus (Figure 4.4.9a,b). The dissection is taken forwards and medially following the cartilaginous meatus. Superiorly, the skin flap is elevated off the temporalis fascia by blunt dissection. At the upper attachment of the helix, the temporalis fascia is incised about 1 cm above the zygomatic arch, and angled forwards to connect with the supraorbital periosteal incision 3 cm above the superior orbital rim (Figure 4.4.10). The incision in the temporalis fascia is then taken vertically down to the level of the zygomatic arch – easily palpated immediately above the cartilaginous meatus. The periosteum over the zygomatic arch is incised and turned forwards with the temporalis fascia, temporoparietal fascia containing the temporal branch(es) of the facial nerve, and the skin – as a single flap. Subperiosteal dissection is continued anteriorly to expose the zygomatic arch, the body of the zygoma and the lateral orbital rim. The periosteum is freed over the lateral and inferior orbital rim, detaching the lateral canthal ligament. Deep circumferential subperiosteal exposure is now easily achieved. The extent of subperiosteal exposure possible with the bicoronal scalp flap is demonstrated in Figure 4.4.11. Closure of the galea is essential.

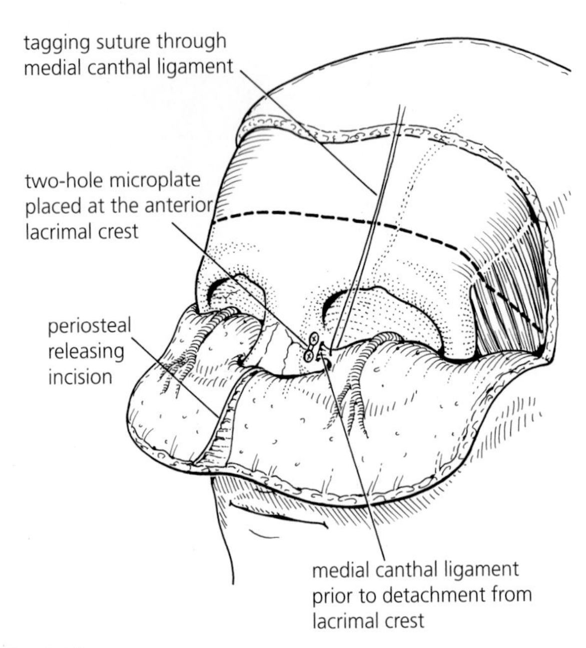

4.4.8 Midline vertical releasing periosteal incision to aid exposure nasal bones. Medial canthus 'tagged' with a suture for later reattachment to microplate.

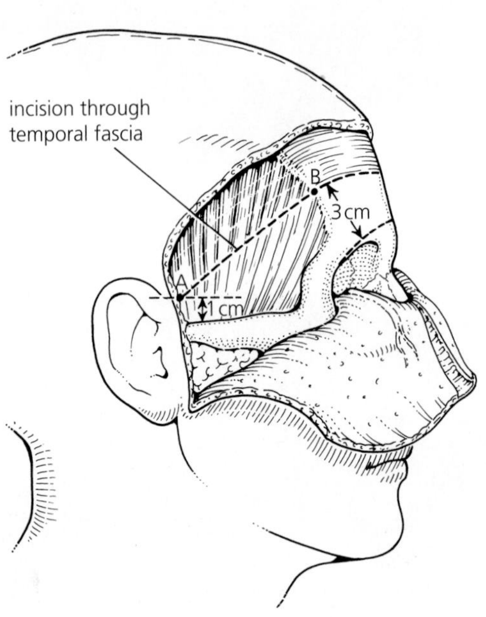

4.4.10 The incision through the temporal fascia is made along line A–B (see Figure 4.4.3) to ensure preservation of the temporal branch of the facial nerve. Complete the exposure of the TMJ and entire zygoma is possible without damage to the temporal branch of the facial nerve.

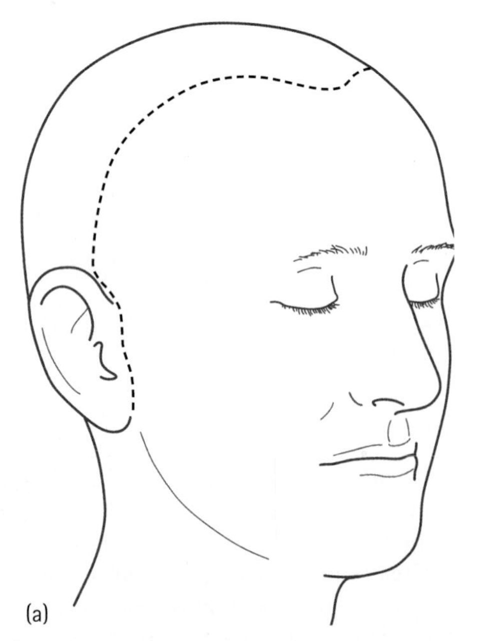

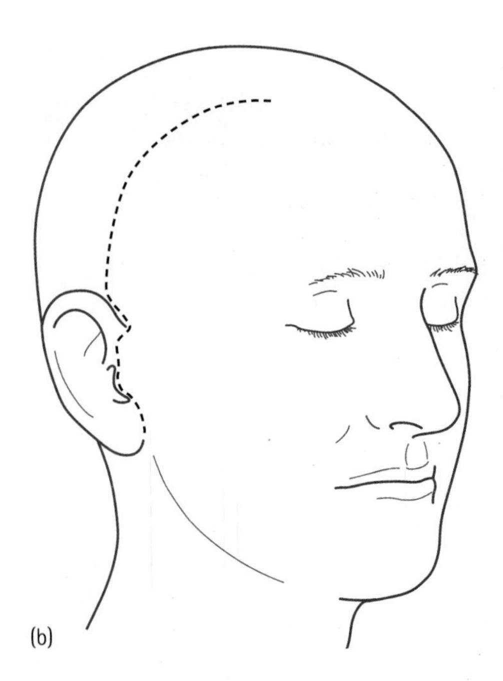

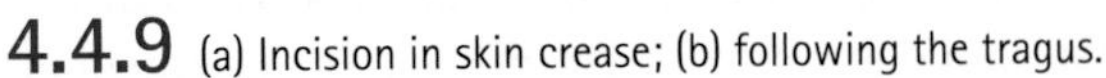

4.4.9 (a) Incision in skin crease; (b) following the tragus.

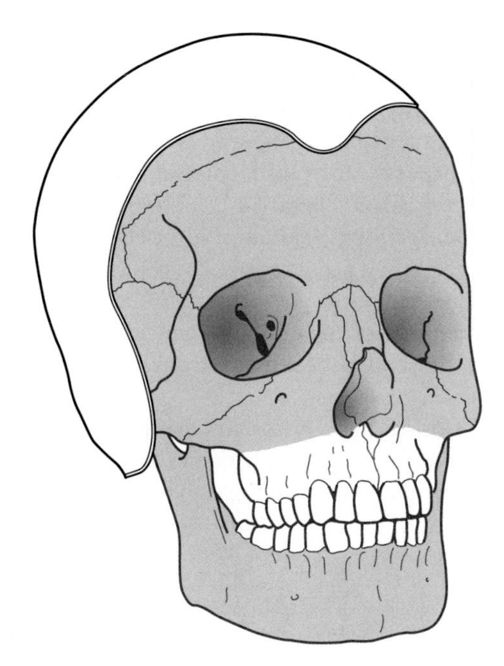

4.4.11 Exposure possible with bicoronal flap.

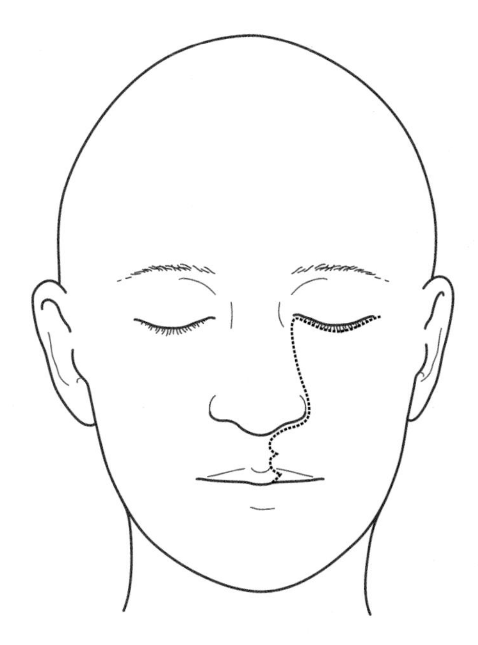

4.4.12 Facial incision for maxillary swing.

MID-FACE PROCEDURES

There are two possible approaches: (1) transfacial approaches and (2) the transoral (Le Fort I) approach. The latter is familiar to all orthognathic surgeons and the surgical technique will therefore not be discussed here.

Transfacial approaches

These approaches mobilize the mid-facial skeleton via a facial incision – ideally pedicled to the soft tissues. The maxillary and nasal swing procedures are the standard approaches – they can be combined, modified or extended.

These approaches access the (1) nasal cavity, maxillary, ethmoid and sphenoid sinuses, (2) soft palate and nasopharynx and (3) infratemporal fossa/parapharyngeal space. The maxillary swing is the gold standard approach – the nasal swing is merely a simple variation.

MAXILLARY SWING: PEDICLED OSTEOTOMY OF THE MAXILLA/HARD PALATE

Incision

A Weber–Fergusson incision is used with a lateral extension along the lower eyelid; the eyelid incision is made within a natural skin crease, 1–2 mm from the lid margin. Subperiosteal stripping is minimized to retain the maximum blood supply to the bone segments. A V-shaped notch made in the upper lip and the vermilion incision, to aid closure and mask scarring (Figure 4.4.12). The incision is made vertically through the alveolar mucosa and attached gingiva between the upper central incisors. The palatal incision is in the mid line extended laterally at the junction of the hard and soft palate behind the maxillary tuberosity (Figure 4.4.13a,b).

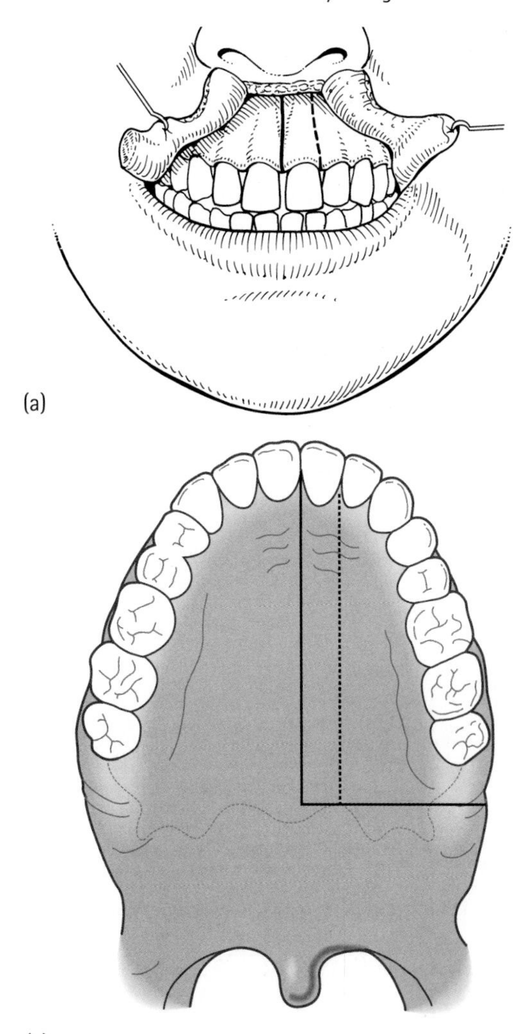

4.4.13 a,b Stepped soft tissue and bone cuts avoids later wound dehiscence/fistulae.

The author's preferred approach is to make the incision around the gingival margins of the teeth, extending from the canine tooth on the opposite side to the pterygoid hamulus, deliberately sectioning the greater palatine neurovascular bundle on the side of the osteotomy. The nasopalatine bundle is preserved if the bone cut is between the central and lateral incisor teeth. The palatal soft tissues are elevated to the opposite side (Figure 4.4.14). This incision avoids the risk of palatal fistulae.

Bone cuts

The bone cuts are made with fine saws or a fissure burr and completed with osteotomes.

The mucoperiosteum of the floor/lateral wall of the nose is elevated and the bone cuts made (1) between the central and lateral incisor teeth, continued paramedially through the length of hard palate into the nasal floor; (2) laterally from the piriform fossa, below the inferior turbinate (preserving the nasolacrimal duct) through the anterior maxilla inferior to the infraorbital nerve through the zygomatic buttress back to the pterygoid plates. The infraorbital nerve is sectioned at the infraorbital foramen as it prevents lateral retraction of the maxilla. The nerve ends may be tagged for later anastomosis.

The bone cut posterior to the zygomatic buttress is angled downwards and may be made either with a fine osteotome or reciprocating saw, to reduce soft tissue stripping.

The maxilla is prelocalized with bone plates (1) above the incisor teeth anteriorly; (2) at the frontal process of the maxilla; (3) on the zygomatic buttress.

The maxilla and pterygoid plates are separated with a curved pterygoid chisel placed through a small vertical buccal incision (Figure 4.4.15). The maxilla is then outfractured, pedicled to the soft tissues of the cheek. The maxilla can be secured to the soft tissues with 0-silk sutures over a gauze swab (Figure 4.4.16).

Following nerve division, wide lateral retraction of the maxilla exposes the soft palate, nasopharynx and infratemporal fossa (Figure 4.4.17). The buccal pad of fat is within the operative field and immediately available for reconstruction as a pedicled flap. The coronoid process and the attached temporalis tendon may impede access to the infratemporal fossa. A coronoidectomy will improve access and has the added benefit of reducing post-operative trismus.

When closing, an occlusal splint may be used if the bite is not 'positive'. The palatal soft tissues are covered with an acrylic cover plate wired to the standing teeth. Closure of

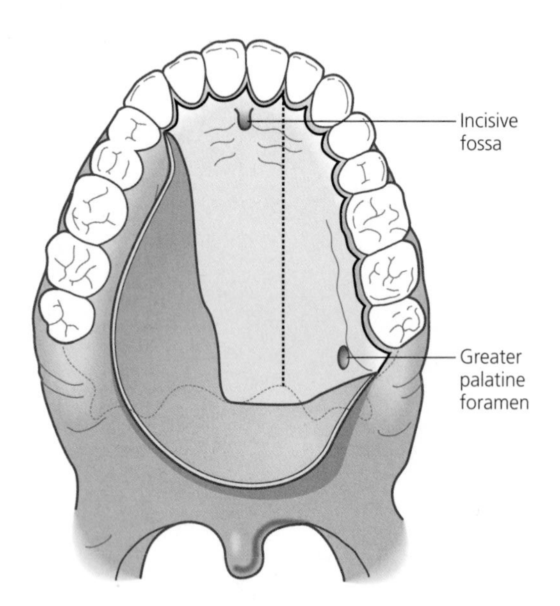

4.4.14 Alternative (favoured) palatal incision. Lines indicate nasopalatine and greater palatine foramina.

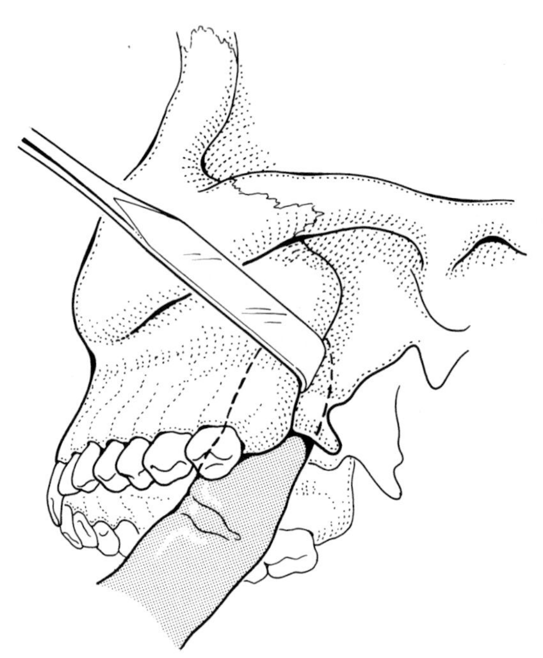

4.4.15 Separation of the pterygoid plates with curved chisel.

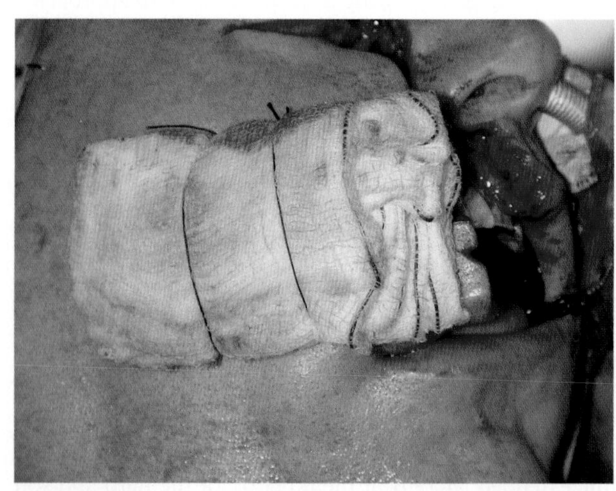

4.4.16 Mobilised maxilla secured to facial skin with sutures

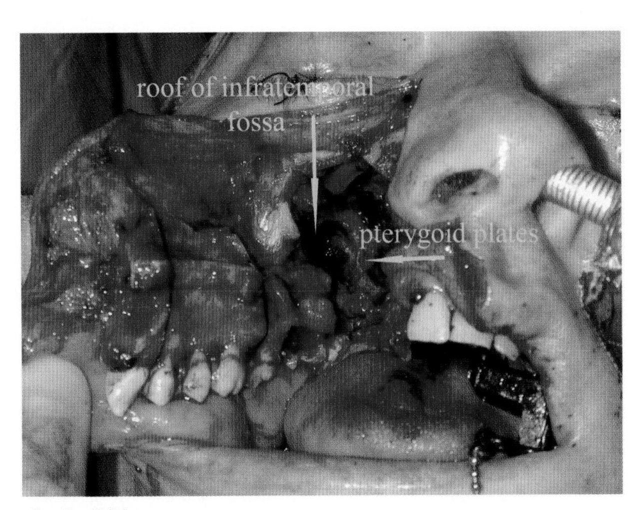

4.4.17 Maxilla swung laterally to access infratemporal fossa.

the palatal tissues is therefore not needed. The plates and screws are reapplied.

The maxilla is frequently mobile to a degree at the completion of surgery. The palatal cover plate can be left *in situ* for 6–8 weeks or until maxillary stability is achieved.

NASAL SWING: PEDICLED OSTEOTOMY OF THE NASAL BONES AND FRONTAL PROCESS OF THE MAXILLA

The nasal swing provides access to lesions in the nose, ethmoid and sphenoid sinuses. Unlike the lateral rhinotomy, it has the advantage of avoiding bone resection.

Incision

The skin incision is as for a Weber–Fergusson incision. Subperiosteal stripping is minimized. The lip split is not always necessary. On the side opposite the skin incision, subperiosteal dissection is achieved by tunnelling. The soft tissue incisions and the bone cuts are stepped. The nasal bones are prelocalized with low profile bone plates (Figure 4.4.18).

The nasal septum restricts complete lateral retraction. A damp tonsillar swab is placed in the opposite nostril and the cartilaginous nasal septum divided vertically in line with the osteotomy bone cuts. The septal cartilage is divided with a cutting diathermy set on 'coagulation' – the damp swab in the opposite nostril prevents accidental trauma to the mucosa of the contralateral lateral nasal wall and the facial skin on the opposite side. The strut of nasal cartilage in the distal nose prevents later nasal collapse. The nasal bones and the nasal soft tissues are retracted to the opposite side (Figure 4.4.19).

The nasal swing links readily with a frontal craniotomy for resection of pathology that also involves the central compartment of the anterior cranial fossa. The transfacial approaches may also be combined with either a Le Fort I osteotomy or mandibular osteotomies for further access.

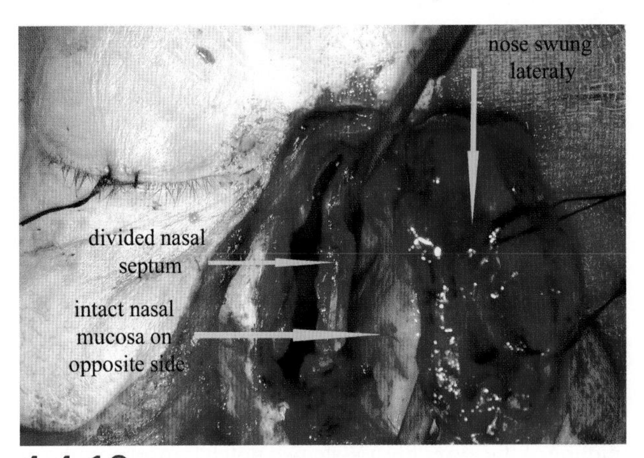

4.4.19 Nasal swing incorporating frontal process of maxilla and nasal bones.

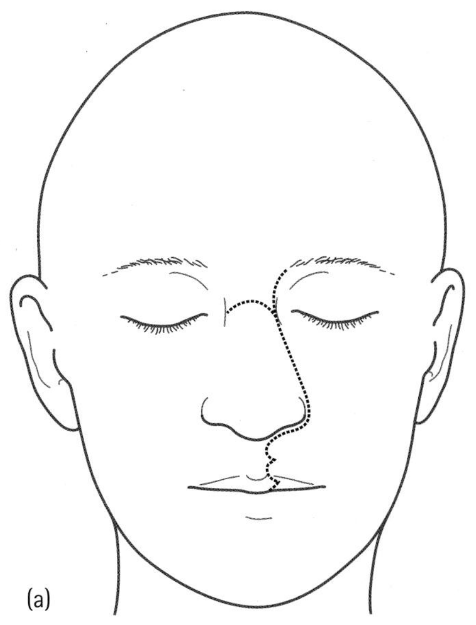

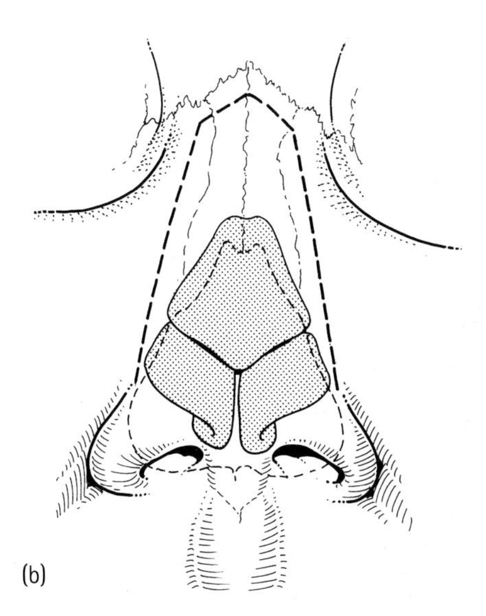

4.4.18 (a) Soft tissue incision; (b) nasal osteotomy bone cuts.

TRANSMANDIBULAR APPROACHES

When accessing the oral cavity, the osteotomy bone cut is in the incisor region. A straight bone cut is used. No incision is made through the lingual mucoperiosteum – the soft tissues are simply elevated off the lingual aspect of the mandible adjacent to the osteotomy. For combined access to the oral cavity and infratemporal fossa, an extended mandibular swing is appropriate; a lip split is necessary. For wide access to the infratemporal fossa/parapharyngeal space without the need to involve the mouth, a lip split is avoided.

Mandibular swing

The technique provides excellent access to the floor of the mouth, mid and posterior third of tongue, tonsillar fossa, soft palate, oropharynx including the posterior pharyngeal wall, supraglottic larynx and medial aspect of the mandibular ramus. Extended posteriorly, it provides equally good access to the infratemporal fossa, and the parapharyngeal space with vascular control.

There are three separate elements:

1 Division of the lower lip and chin
2 Division of the mandible in the incisor region
3 Elevation of the soft tissues off the lingual aspect of the mandible.

Mandibular continuity is restored on completion.

Surgical technique

A full thickness vertical incision is made through the midline of the lower lip; a V-shaped notch is incorporated in the midline lip incision and the vermilion incision for precise closure and to mask scarring. The incision curves around the chin with the concavity of the incision towards the side of the lesion, reducing the risk of chin necrosis. This incision links with the submandibular incision.

The skin incision curves down from the chin to the level of the hyoid bone – extended if necessary to the tip of the mastoid process (Figure 4.4.20).

Intraorally, the incision through the labial mucosa and the attached gingiva is stepped so as not to lie directly over the subsequent osteotomy bone cut. Periosteal elevation and mentalis muscle stripping should be sufficient only for the application of bone plates and screws. The mucoperiosteal flaps are pedicled on the side opposite to the lesion as a precaution against ischaemic necrosis of the flap edges (Figure 4.4.21).

No incision is made through the lingual mucoperiosteum – the soft tissues are simply elevated off the lingual aspect of the mandible adjacent to the osteotomy. A full thickness lingual mucoperiosteal flap is subsequently elevated off the lingual aspect of the mandible when the mandible is retracted laterally. The incision through the oral tissues is

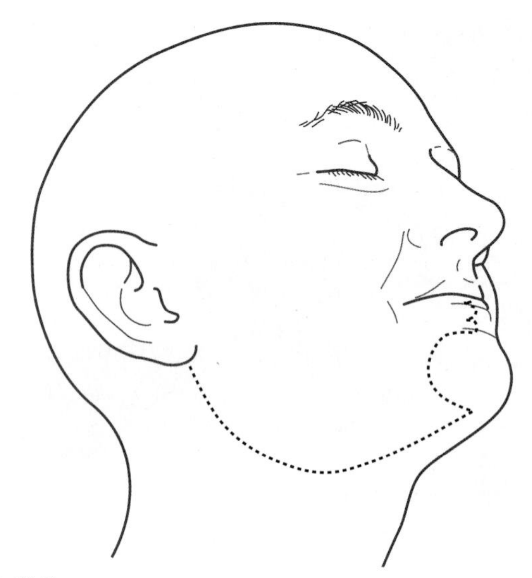

4.4.20 Mandibular swing incision.

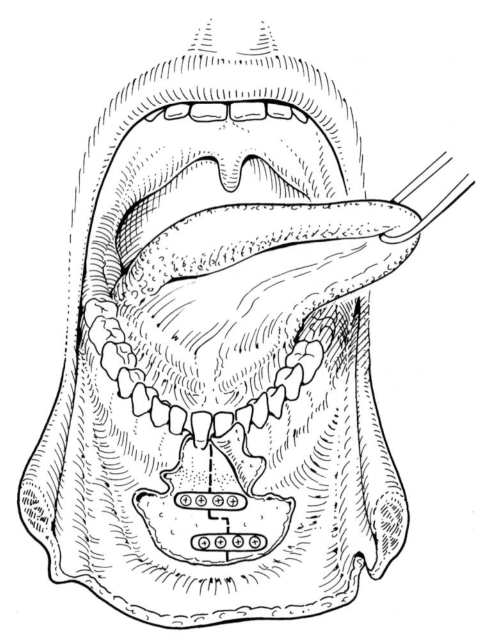

4.4.21 Stepped soft tissue incision and bone cuts. Soft tissue pedicled to opposite side. A stepped osteotomy cut as shown in the figure is not necessary – see text.

adjacent to the pathology – allowing for sufficient tumour clearance.

The osteotomy is always performed in the incisor region for tumours involving the oral cavity. Non-union is rare at this site even with post-operative radiotherapy. Osteotomy in the premolar region anterior to the mental foramen is only employed by the authors to access tumours in the infratemporal fossa/parapharyngeal space when avoiding a lip split incision (see below under Angle osteotomy and double mandibular osteotomy avoiding lip split).

The mandible is divided with a fine saw blade between the roots of the incisor teeth. Occasionally, an incisor tooth is removed if there is insufficient room between the dental roots for the bone cut. Prior to division, the mandible is prelocalized with bone plates acrosss the osteotomy bone cut. These are removed and replaced on closure.

The osteotomy bone cut is a simple straight line in all cases as opposed to the stepped cut demonstrated in Figure 4.4.21. A stepped bone cut aids neither fixation nor bone union.

Following division, the mandible is gently retracted laterally and the lingual soft tissues, including the mylohyoid muscle, are stripped off the mandible (Figures 4.4.22 and 4.4.23).

The extended mandibular swing

By stripping the medial pterygoid off the medial aspect of the mandible, further lateral and superior mandibular retraction is possible and provides wide access to the infratemporal fossa and parapharyngeal space.

Angle osteotomy and double mandibular osteotomy avoiding lip split

For tumours confined to the infratemporal fossa/ parapharyngeal space without the need to involve the oral cavity, the approach is determined by the size of the tumour and the need to preserve lower lip sensation.

For smaller tumours, very limited access is provided by simply elevating the mandibular angle or by detaching the stylomandibular ligament at the angle of the mandible and dislocating the mandibular condyle anteriorly (Figure 4.4.24a,b).

If greater access is needed, then one of the procedures below is used.

1 For larger tumours, if lower lip sensation is already lost or will be lost in the resection, a simple angle osteotomy sectioning the inferior dental (ID) bundle is satisfactory (Figure 4.4.25).

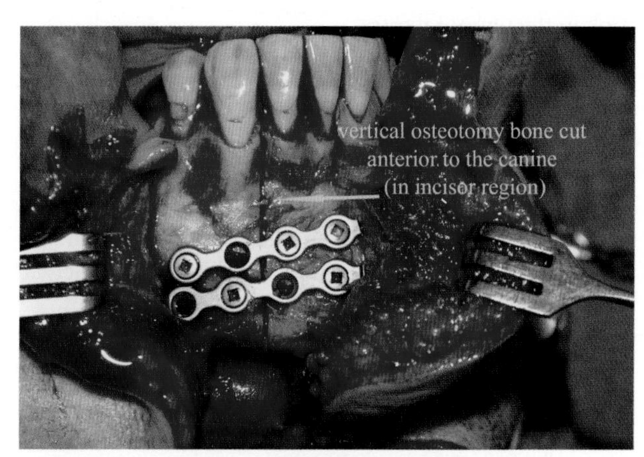

4.4.22 Vertical osteotomy cut in the incisor region – stepped osteotomy not necessary.

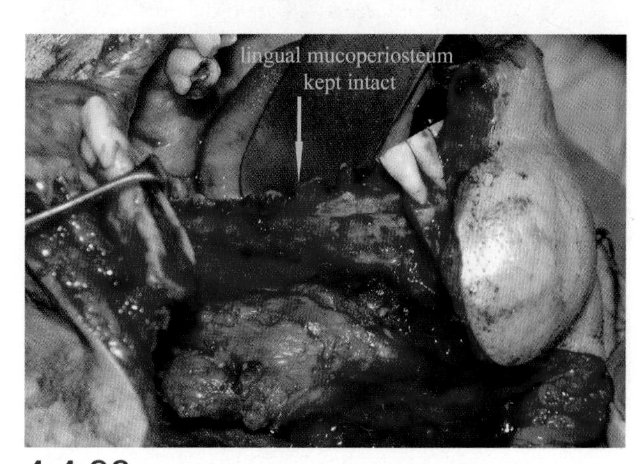

4.4.23 Mandible swung laterally – intact lingual mucoperiosteum.

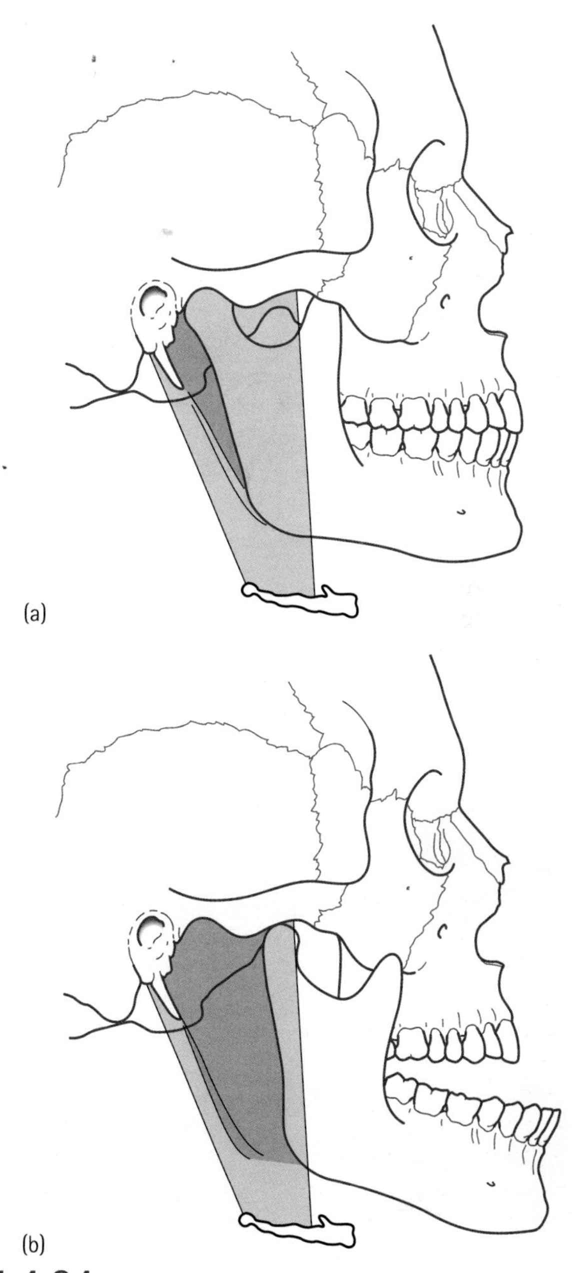

4.4.24 a,b Limited access to parapharyngeal space by anterior mandibular dislocation and division stylomandibular ligament.

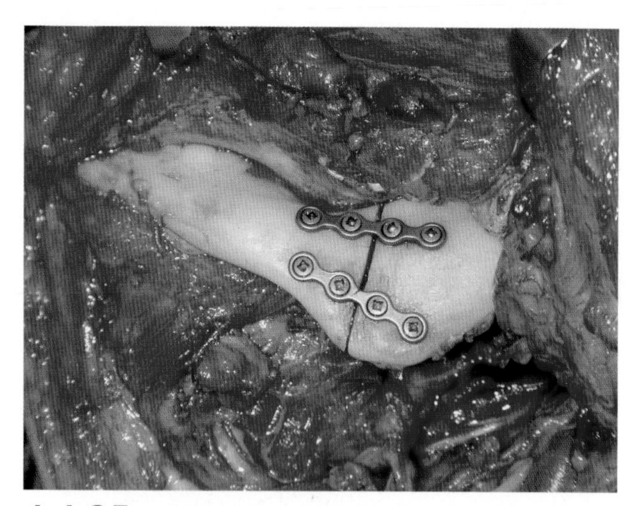

4.4.25 Osteotomy through angle and inferior dental (ID) bundle.

2 If lower lip sensation is to be preserved, a lip split can be avoided by combining a vertical ramus osteotomy behind the lingula with an additional osteotomy anterior to the mental foramen (usually between the canine and the first premolar) (Figures 4.4.26a,b).

In each case, the mandible is prelocalized with bone plates. With both approaches, it is possible to trace the internal carotid artery to the skull base adequately. A horizontal osteotomy of the mandibular ramus is avoided as the area of bone contact is limited with this technique. If resection of the floor of the middle fossa is required in skull base procedures, additional superior access is easily achieved by mobilising the zygoma (see below under Transzygomatic approaches).

TRANSZYGOMATIC APPROACHES

The zygoma links the orbit and the temporal and infratemporal fossae. Its disarticulation inferiorly pedicled to the masseter provides simultaneous exposure of the orbit, temporal fossa and superior aspect of the infratemporal fossa. A frontotemporal craniotomy links the middle and anterior cranial fossae. The site of the pathology determines the extent of the zygoma mobilized and whether the temporalis muscle is reflected inferiorly or superiorly, as follows:

- for subcranial lesions (orbit/temporal and infratemporal fossae), the temporalis is reflected superiorly after dividing the coronoid process;
- for combined exposure of the middle/anterior fossae, the orbit and/or the temporal and infratemporal fossa, the temporalis is reflected inferiorly.

The blood supply of the temporalis is potentially compromised with both superior and inferior reflection.

Standard zygomatic osteotomy

The zygomatic arch and body are exposed with a bicoronal flap. When exposing the orbit, as well as the temporal and infratemporal fossae, limited subperiosteal dissection is carried out in the lateral orbit to protect the orbital contents. The temporalis is reflected off the lateral orbit. The lateral limit of the inferior orbital fissure is identified with a blunt hook in the temporal fossa.

The bone cuts are as follows:

- Superiorly at the frontozygomatic suture.
- Through the body of the zygoma, extending laterally from the inferior orbital fissure. The anterior limit of the inferior orbital fissure is first identified in the orbit with a blunt hook. The cut is in an inferolateral direction.
- The posterior bone cut is just anterior to the articular eminence of the temporomandibular joint.
- The bone cut in the lateral orbit extends from the superior bone cut to the lateral aspect of the inferior orbital fissure – identified earlier in the temporal fossa (Figure 4.4.27a,b).

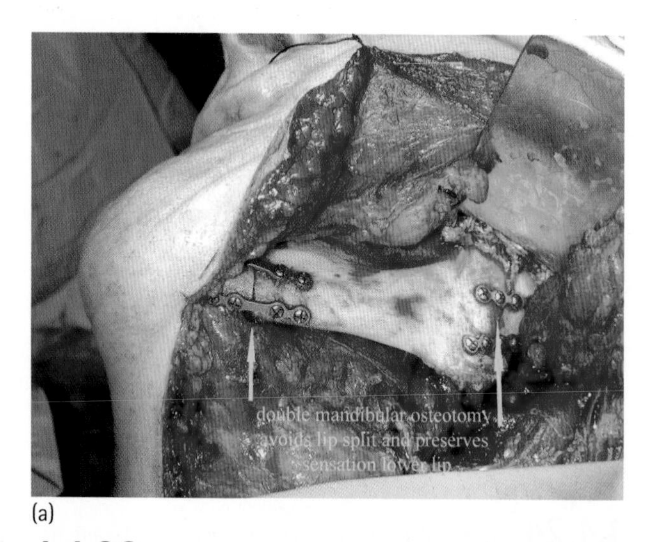

(a)

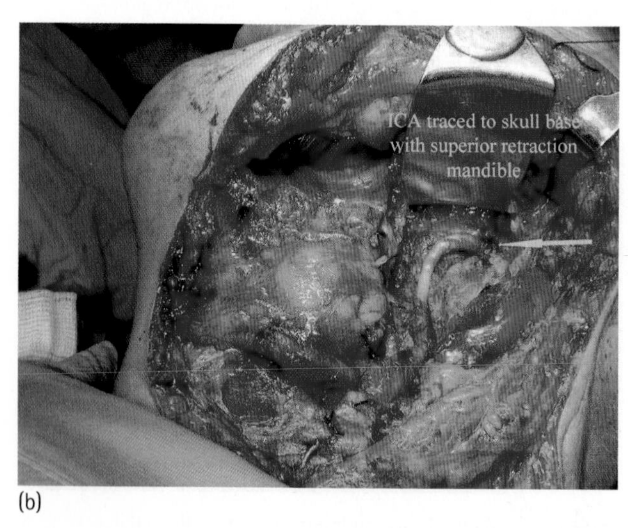

(b)

4.4.26 (a) Double mandibular osteotomy; (b) Superior retraction of ramus and body of mandible. Case courtesy Professor P Brennan.

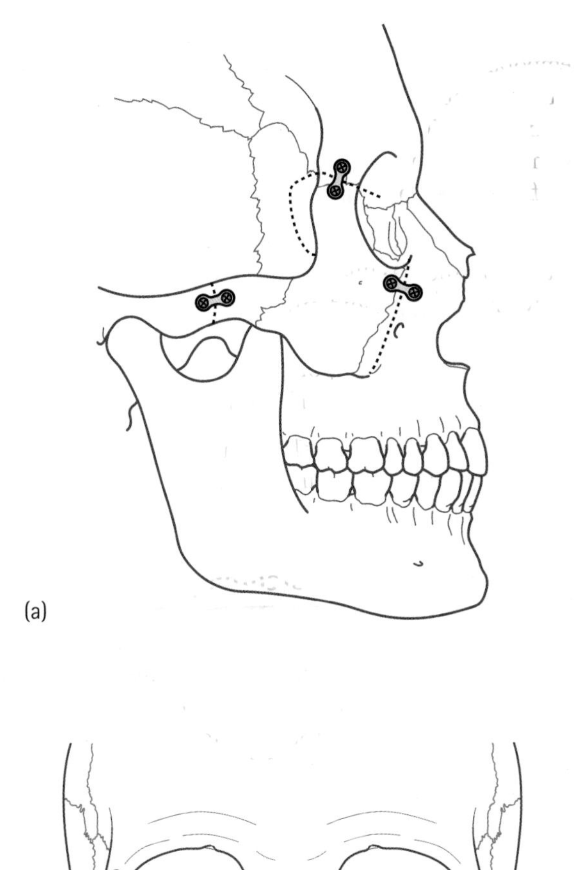

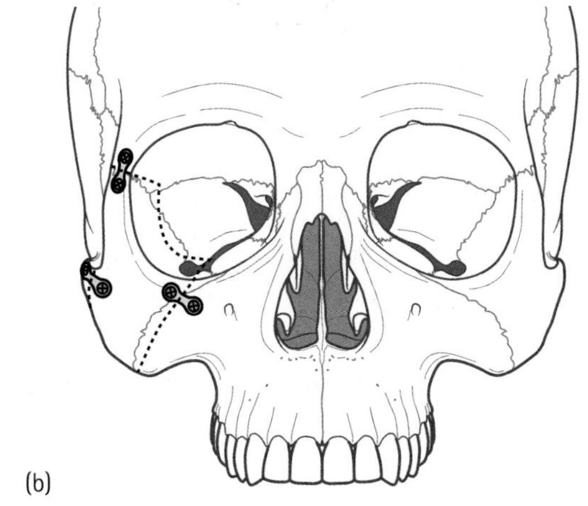

4.4.27 a,b Osteotomy bone cuts.

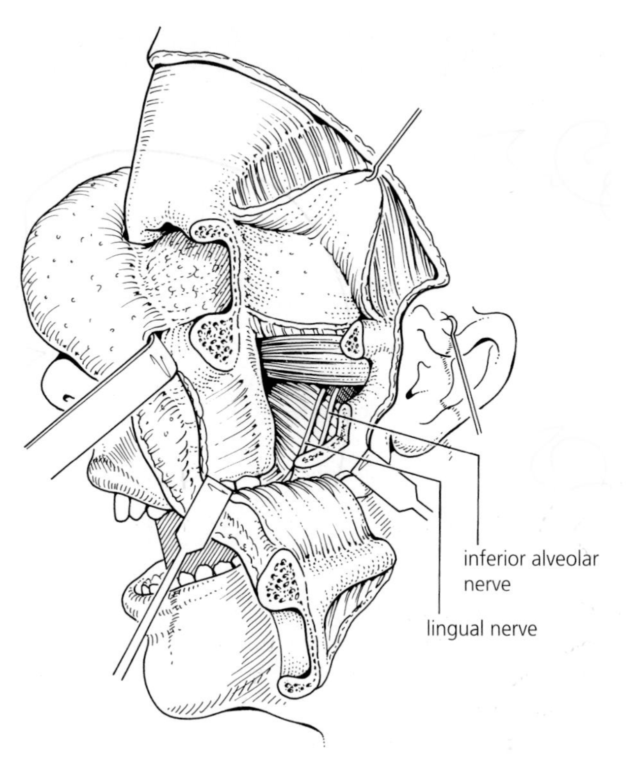

4.4.28 Zygoma displaced inferiorly, temporalis superiorly and mouth opened widely. Lingual (anterior) and inferior dental (posterior) nerves identified after resection of the coronoid.

If orbital exposure is unnecessary, the lateral orbital rim is left intact. A vertical bone cut through the body of the zygoma lateral to the orbital rim is made. The posterior bone cut is the same.

The zygoma is prelocalized with bone plates and screws (1.7-mm plates are satisfactory). With gentle taps, the osteotomy is completed with an osteotome and the zygoma displaced inferiorly. The temporalis is reflected superiorly after a coronoidectomy. The mandible is opened widely with a mouth prop increasing vertical exposure. The lingual and inferior alveolar nerves can be identified in the lateral infratemporal fossa (Figure 4.4.28).

For correction of a malunion of the zygoma, the coronoidectomy and superior reflection of the temporalis are unnecessary.

The extent of exposure of the infratemporal fossa extends inferiorly to the maxillary teeth and medially to the lateral wall of the nasopharynx, following resection of the lateral and medial pterygoid muscles.

Medial exposure is restricted, which limits the approach to treatment of benign pathology in the infratemporal fossa if it is used as the sole means of access. Malignant disease in the infratemporal fossa is better accessed with a transmandibular and/or transfacial approach.

For exposure of the lateral orbit to the apex, a frontotemporal craniotomy is necessary. This allows the safe removal of the greater wing of the sphenoid under direct vision and the exposure of the contents of the superior orbital fissure and the optic nerve.

Top tips

Bicoronal scalp flap

- The first three layers of the scalp lift as one unit in an avascular plane.
- Knowledge of surgical landmarks prevents damage to the temporal branches of the facial nerve.
- Closure of the galea is the most important element in wound closure.

Maxillary swing: Pedicled osteotomy of the maxilla/hard palate

- Step soft tissue and bone cuts so that the wounds lie on sound bone.
- Modified soft tissue incision on the palate around the gingival margins prevents palatal fistulae.
- Secure mobilized maxilla to cheek soft tissues with gauze swab and 0-silk sutures.
- Palatal splint ± occlusal splint, which simplifies fixation of the maxilla on completion.

Nasal swing: Pedicled osteotomy of the nasal bones and frontal process of the maxilla

- Both the frontal process of maxilla and nasal bones are moved.
- Extend soft tissue incision slightly laterally on the face to prevent the bone/soft tissue cuts being in line.
- Place a moist tonsillar swab in the opposite nostril when completing the cut through the cartilaginous nasal septum.

Transmandibular approaches

- When accessing the oral cavity, the osteotomy bone cut is in the incisor region.
- A straight bone cut is used.
- No incision is made through the lingual mucoperiosteum; the soft tissues are simply elevated off the lingual aspect of the mandible adjacent to the osteotomy.
- For combined access to the oral cavity and infratemporal fossa an extended mandibular swing is appropriate; a lip split is necessary.
- For wide access to the infratemporal fossa/parapharyngeal space without the need to involve the mouth, a lip split is avoided.

Transzygomatic approaches

- The lateral aspect of the inferior orbital fissure both within the temporal fossa and the orbit is the key anatomical landmark.
- The temporalis muscle is reflected superiorly for subcranial pathology.
- Trismus is expected post-operatively and is prevented with jaw exercises.

FURTHER READING

BICORONAL FLAP

Feynas DW. Landmarks for the trunk and temporofacial division of the facial nerve. *British Journal of Surgery* 1965; **52**: 694–6.

Shepherd DE, Ward-Booth RP, Moos KF. The morbity of bicoronal flaps in maxillofacial surgery. *British Journal of Oral and Maxillofacial Surgery* 1985; **23**: 1–8.

TRANSFACIAL APPROACHES

Altemir FH. Transfacial access to the retromaxillary area. *Journal of Maxillofacial Surgery* 1986; **14**: 165–70.

Brown AMS, Lavery K, Miller BG. The transfacial approach to the postnasal space and the retromaxillary structures. *British Journal of Oral and Maxillofacial Surgery* 1991; **29**: 230–6.

Curioni C, Padula E, Toscano P, Maraggia A. Gli angiofibrorni del rinofaringe. *Chirugia della Testa e del Colla* 1984; **1**: 47–56.

Wei WL, Lam KH, Sham JST. New approach to the nasopharynx: The maxillary swing approach. *Head and Neck Surgery* 1991; **13** 200–207.

MANDIBULAR ACCESS OSTEOTOMIES

Attia EL, Bentley KC, Head T, Mulder D. A new external approach to the pterygomaxillary fossa and the parapharyngeal space. *Head and Neck Surgery* 1984; **6**: 884–9.

Biedlingnaier JF, Ord R. Modified double mandibular osteotomy for tumours of the parapharyngeal space. *Journal of Oral and Maxillofacial Surgery* 1994; **52**: 348–52.

Smith GI, Brennan PA, Webb AA, Ilankovan V. Vertical ramus osteotomy combined with a parasymphyseal mandibulotomy for improved access to the parapharyngeal space. *Head and Neck* 2003; **25**: 1000–1003.

LATERAL ZYGOMATIC OSTEOTOMIES

Obwegesser HL. Temporal approach to the TMJ, the orbit, and the retromaxillary-infracranial region. *Journal of Head and Neck Surgery* 1985; **7**: 185–99.

Shahinian H, Dornier MD, Fisch U. Parapharyngeal space tumours: The infratemporal fossa approach. *Skull Base Surgery* 1995; **5**: 73–81.

Evans BT, Wiesenfeld D, Clauser L, Curioni C. Surgical approaches to the infratemporal fossa. In: Langdon J, Berkovitz BKB, Moxham BJ (eds). *Surgical anatomy of the infratemporal fossa.* London: Martin Dunitz, 2003: 141–80.

4.5

Excision of skin lesions and orbital and nasal reconstruction

BRUCE B HORSWELL

GENERAL PRINCIPLES

Mohs' surgery

Most facial skin cancers are basal cell carcinomas (BCCs) which are well demarcated and do not extend below the deep dermis. These lesions can be excised with a margin of 5 mm and the depth of incision is located at the level of the muscle fascia. The lesion is excised as an ellipse placed parallel to the natural expression lines (Figure 4.5.1) and closed without tension or distorting structures, such as the eyebrow. The skin incision is made perpendicular to the surface and the wound is closed in layers. The wound edges are undermined as necessary.

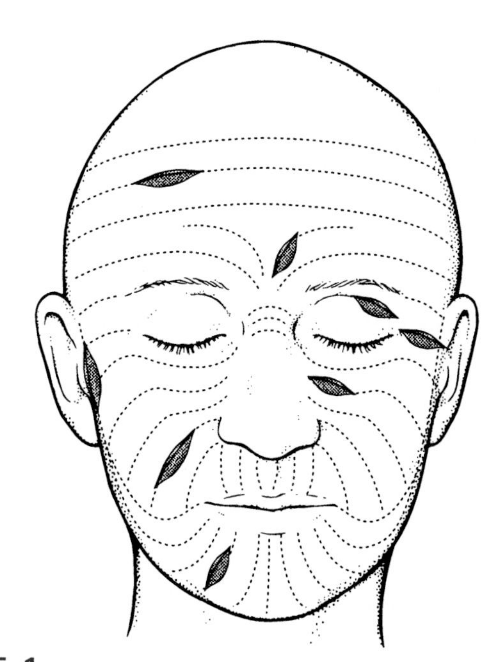

4.5.1 Various elliptical excisions of lesions are demonstrated. Generally, these should be placed parallel to the relaxed skin tension lines (RSTLs) to avoid tension.

Recurrent lesions, post-radiation tumours, morphoeic (sclerosing) BCC and tumours in lines of embryonic fusion require special consideration. These tumours are poorly demarkated; therefore, microscopic controlled surgery (Mohs' technique) may be required to ensure tumour extirpation. Mohs' technique is also indicated where minimal removal of normal tissue is indicated, e.g. the eyelids. The technique relies on accurate mapping of the specimen with microscopic examination of the deep surface to ensure complete removal of the tumour.

Figure 4.5.2 shows a basal carcinoma at the medial canthus (an embryonic fusion line). The excision margin is marked out as shown in Figure 4.5.2a (dotted line).

The tumour is excised with the knife blade held at 45° to the surface (incision A–A′ in Figure 4.5.2b), and a second clearance slice of tissue 1–2-mm thick is excised from the tumour bed (incision B–B′). This thin slice of tissue is turned over on to a slide with the deep surface uppermost and is divided into sections (usually four) like slices of pizza. At least one edge is stained with Indian ink or another dye to accurately orient ('map') the position of residual tumour. In Figure 4.5.2c, slices 1 and 4, which correspond to the nasal portion of the tumour, are seen to contain residual tumour.

Further slices of tissue (5 and 6 in Figure 4.5.2d) will be removed in the area corresponding to specimens 1 and 4 and the process is continued until all slices are tumour free. Many Mohs' surgeons prepare frozen sections from the deep surface and, after reviewing the slides themselves, continue the serial excision on the same day. An alternative method is to fix the slices of tissue for permanent section. Slides will be ready in 24–48 hours. The wound is left open and dressed with mupirocin (Bactroban) cream. Further, excision is carried out in the areas indicated. An important component of this technique is review of the sections by the surgeon to ensure accurate mapping.

When the defect is tumour free, it may be closed with flaps or in some sites allowed to granulate.

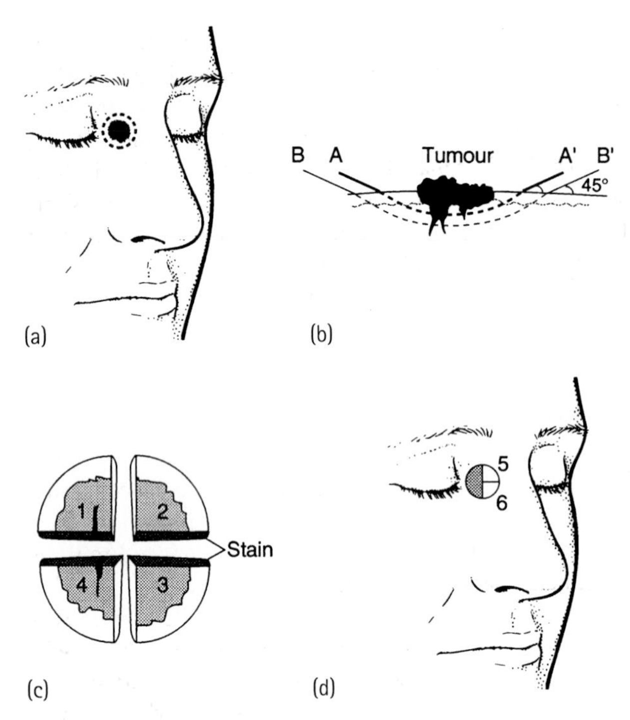

4.5.2 (a) Medial canthal lesion, ideal for Mohs' technique in order to preserve tissue and prevent distortion of adjacent structure after definitive repair; (b) tumour excision with blade at 45° (A–A′); (c) deep disc partitioned into four slices to be stained, analysed and mapped to correspond to the tumour bed; residual tumour is observed in slices 1–4; (d) residual tumour slices 1 and 4 correspond to tumour bed slices 5 and 6; in turn, these will be stained and mapped until the margins are clear of tumour.

FACIAL RESECTION

Principles

Primary closure is the procedure of choice for small (<1 cm) defects where tissue laxity allows. In the brow and temple regions, care should be exercised not to displace the hair-bearing margins.

For larger defects (>1 cm) or where scar contracture has altered tissue character, local flaps may be used. Local tissue flaps can be designed as V-Y advancement, rotational or transposition flaps which will be applicable at different facial sites. Where there has been loss of hair in the scalp region, a combination of staged tissue expansion with local scalp flaps can be undertaken. Temporary resurfacing of avulsion scalp wounds may be performed with free skin grafts (allografts or autografts). At a later date, tissue expansion, with eventual scalp flap advancement or rotation to restore scalp integrity, is performed. Total or near-total brow loss is generally reconstructed with a free tissue graft from the scalp. For smaller brow defects, punch grafts can be placed.

FOREHEAD DEFECT OPERATIONS

V-Y advancement flap

The V-Y advancement flap is used for small and moderately sized midline defects, the limiting factor being the area of tissue laxity. These flaps are particularly useful in resurfacing glabellar, nasal and medial canthal regions. The colour and texture match is excellent. The V-Y midline or glabellar flap is nourished by supratrochlear and canthal arteries and random-pattern facial artery distribution. Care must be taken to preserve the arteries, if possible, when the flap is elevated. Design of the flap (Figure 4.5.3) must take into consideration the pivotal point of the flap located at the flap base opposite the defect. The inferior incision on the pivotal side should not extend below the medial canthal level in order to maintain vascularity.

The length of the vertical limbs of the flap will be dictated by the defect length and laxity of glabellar tissue. The base of the flap (B–C) should be half to two-thirds of the entire base (A–C) which also includes the defect (AB). Dissection of the flap is carried out in the areolar plane to preserve subdermal plexus.

Once the flap has been elevated and turned into the defect, the flap's leading edge should be sutured to the defect margin with clear nylon or polygalactin suture in a buried fashion. Closure of the V-Y segment (Figure 4.5.4) begins superiorly and continues inferiorly, the last sutures being placed at the pivotal area of the flap base. A standing cone (dog ear) usually occurs at the pivotal area, which may resolve over time, or require secondary z-plasties and/or dermabrasion.

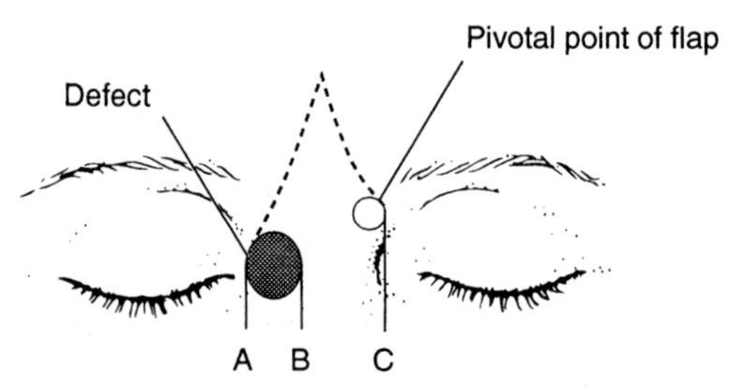

4.5.3 Glabellar V-Y advancement flap. Distance A–B should be no more than half the distance A–C in order to ensure vascular integrity through the area of pivotal point C.

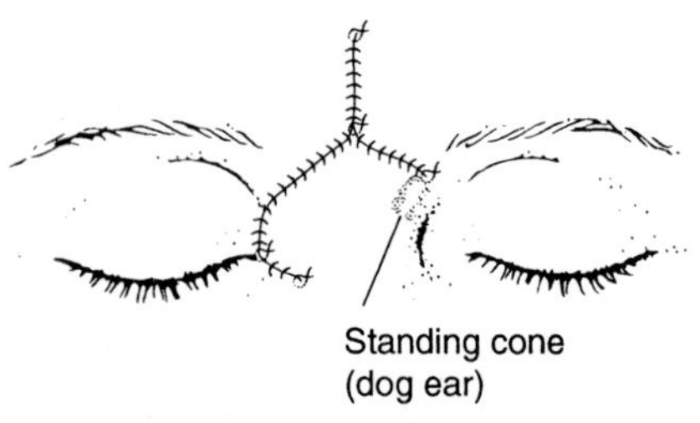

4.5.4 Transposition and closure of glabellar V-Y flap. The leading edge should be sutured first. The standing cone (dog ear) at the pivotal point will settle with time.

Horizontal or 'H' sliding flap

With lateral forehead defects, a transposed median forehead flap (Figure 4.5.5) may be used, however, animation of the frontalis is adversely affected. For small forehead defects, sliding horizontal advancement flaps with incisions hidden neatly in existing frontalis relaxation lines and small Burow's triangles to facilitate closure work well. If tissue loss or resection encompasses the supraorbital nerve in its first 3–4 cm, then microneural repair should be undertaken, with a cable graft using the greater auricular nerve. A vein graft or a polyglycolic 'sleeve' may also be micro-anastomosed to serve as a conduit for the regenerating nerve.

Rotational forehead flap

Rotational forehead flaps are primarily utilized for the closure of large midline defects. They have a semi-circular design with an arc of rotation near the middle of the flap. At times, bilateral rotation flaps may be necessary. The midline defect is triangulated with the base at the hairline, and the apex angle may approach 50°. When the flap is designed, the leading edge should be made long enough to allow adequate rotation of the flap and coverage of the defect.

First, mark out the proposed excision and then a triangulated defect may be constructed (Figure 4.5.6). If a defect is located cephalad (near the hairline), the leading edge (A–C, B–C) should be longer than the defect margin to ensure adequate rotation of the tip (A or B). In order to achieve rotation, a back cut can be performed at the flap pedicle (D or E). Also, wide undermining of the pedicle and surrounding tissue may be undertaken; however, extensive undermining may disrupt vascular perforators.

Rotation of the flap into the defect typically leaves a secondary defect at the flap margin (BB′, DD′, or AA′, EE′). If the defect is a narrow gap at the hairline, this can be closed by simple vertical advancement of both margins (B to B′, etc). The hairline may be temporarily displaced inferiorly in such cases. Other gaps may be closed by extending incisions to allow more rotation and distributing tension during closure along the whole of the wound margin. Rarely, free full-thickness skin grafts may need to be placed in a secondary defect caused by flap rotation.

Tissue expansion

Large forehead defects which cannot be closed with rotational flaps require staged reconstruction with tissue expansion in order to avoid displacement of the brows or asymmetric hairline margins. Typically, these defects involve some element of the hair-bearing scalp. Placement of two or three 200–300 ml saline expanders of various shapes will increase the tissue reservoir in the desired location. The author favours crescent-shaped expanders which fit the contours of the forehead region (Figure 4.5.7).

The expanders are placed in a subgaleal pocket with the access incisions and injection ports placed distant from the area of intended expansion. Expansion proceeds 2 weeks after placement to allow sufficient time for incision healing and proceeds on a weekly basis as the patient tolerates. Usually, the overlying skin blanches when maximal expansion is achieved and a small amount of solution is removed in order to avoid skin ischaemia.

After several weeks, the second stage can be undertaken to remove expanders and rotate or transpose the expanded tissue into the defect. The capsule which forms around the expander should be excised prior to flap mobilization and closure. Drains and a firm supportive dressing are placed to reduce dead space and inhibit haematoma formation.

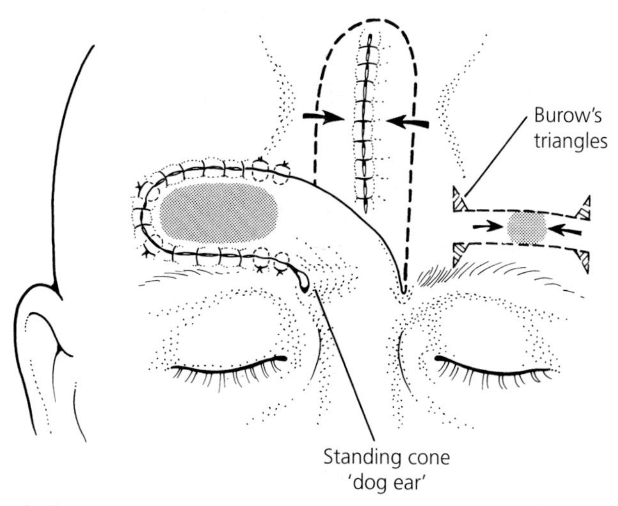

4.5.5 Diagram of median forehead flap to resurface a right forehead defect. The same principles apply as in a turned down forehead flap to the nasal region as described for Figure 4.5.3. A smaller left forehead defect is shown repaired with a sliding 'H' flap. Burow's triangles correct the standing cones at the corners.

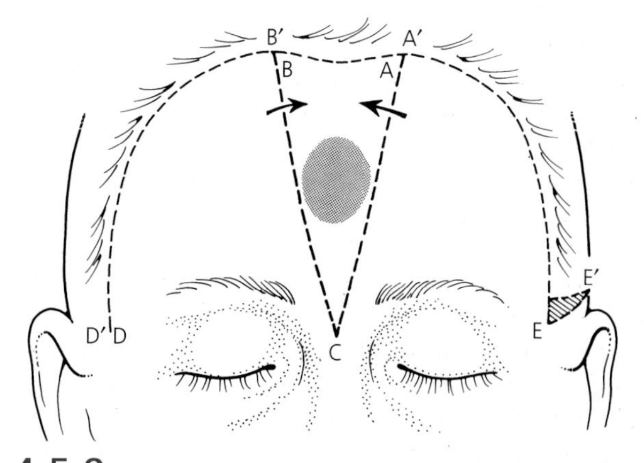

4.5.6 Midline defect repaired with a rotational forehead flap. The leading edges (AC, BC) should be longer than the defect in order to gain enough tip (points A and B) rotation. Back cuts at the flap base (DD′, EE′) are necessary to gain adequate rotation. Areas of incomplete closure (AA′, BB′, DD′, EE′) will usually close with advancement of the cephalad and caudal margins.

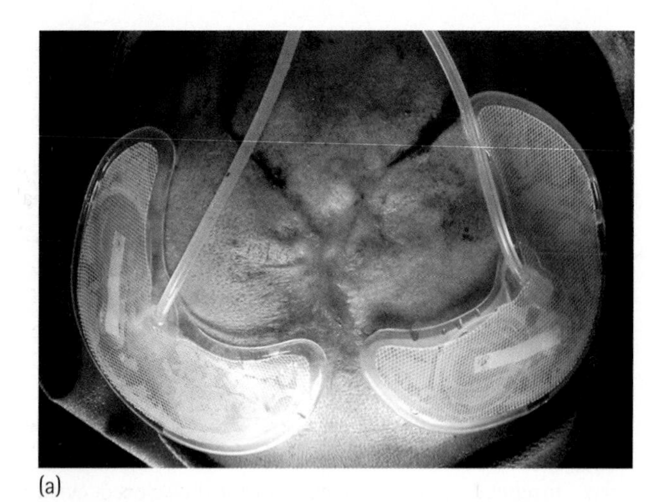

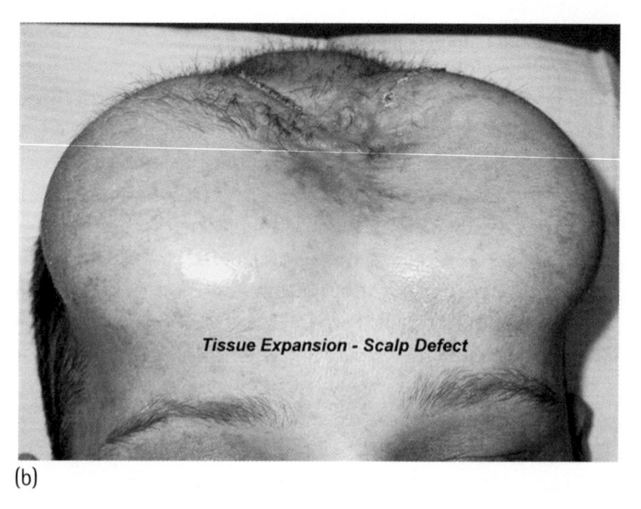

(a) (b)

4.5.7 (a) Crescent-shaped expanders for forehead and scalp tissue expansion for a central defect measuring 10×7 cm. (b) Scalp and forehead expansion several weeks after placement. After removal of the expanders, bilateral rotational flaps will correct the defect in the hair-bearing scalp and forehead skin.

TEMPLE AND CHEEK DEFECT OPERATIONS

Rhombic flaps

Temple and cheek area defects are closed with local tissue flaps which offer laxity, good texture and colour matches. Transposition flaps (rhombic, Dufourmental, bilobed flaps, etc.) offer excellent repairs for small and moderately sized defects, designed and sited such that the incisions fall into relaxed skin tension lines and the transposed tissue does not distort adjacent structures. There are four possible rhombic flaps for each defect; however, usually two are more favourable owing to relaxed skin tension line topography. The correct donor flap extends from lax tissue and the sides of the flap, particularly the leading edge, should be slightly longer than the defect side to compensate for pivotal restraint. If the recipient skin tissue is lax, then surrounding structures, such as eyelids or eyebrow, will move towards the flap.

A rhombus is drawn around the proposed area of excision (see Figure 4.5.8). Two defect sides (A–B and C–D) are drawn perpendicular to relaxed skin lines and extended to encompass the defect. These are then connected with parallel lines and the short link diagonal (B–C) is extended to create one edge of the donor flap. As noted above, the transposed edge (B–F or C–E) and back-cuts may need to be slightly oversized to accommodate the necessary rotation and closure.

Adequate recipient site and pivotal area (flap) undermining is critical for ease of transposition and minimizing tension (and consequent ischaemia). Closure (Figure 4.5.9) begins first at the leading edge corner (IC) followed by a suture at the near corner (BG).

Several buried sutures in the deep dermis plus 'corner sutures' and mattress sutures will assist in distributing tension. The transposed flap tip (2A) should require minimal suturing, thereby reducing tissue ischaemia and necrosis.

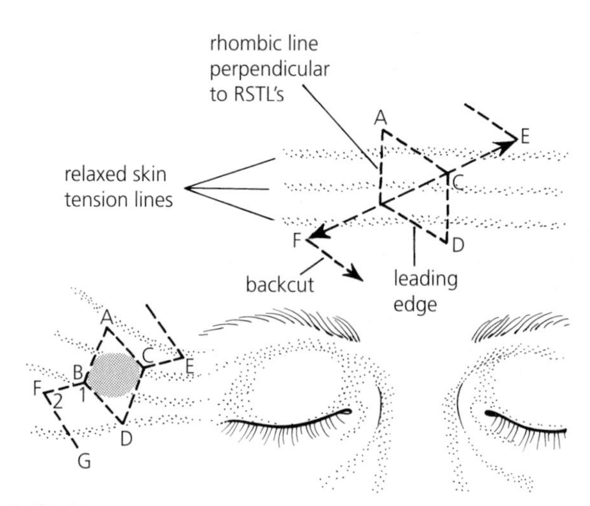

4.5.8 Rhombic flaps incorporate 60° and 120° angles in the design. For flap BDFG, incision FB is equal to BC, and FG is parallel to BD. The leading edge (AC for flap ACEH or BD for flap BDFG) lies perpendicular to relaxed skin tension lines (RSTLs). The more favourable rhombic flap is that which distorts surrounding tissue the least. In the temple region, this is usually the caudally based flap as shown.

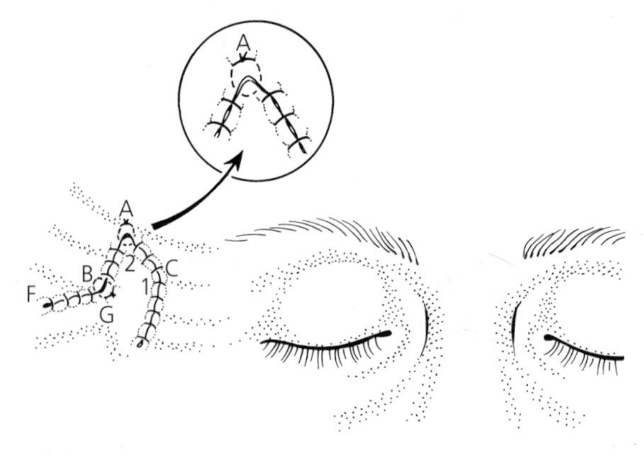

4.5.9 Closure of the rhombic flap begins first at 1C, then corner stitches are placed at the areas BG and 2A. If flap tip ischaemia is evident after suturing, either too much tension exists or improper suture placement is to blame.

Dufourmental flap

The Dufourmental flap (Figure 4.5.10) is a variation of the rhombic design. Its application is in areas of limited tissue reservoir necessary for advancement or transposition of the flap. With the construction of a bisector (BG) of the angle (EBF) created by extension of the short diagonal (A–B) and defect margin (B–C), a more obtuse leading edge margin is created. The back-cut is generally parallel to the long diagonal (C–D) of the rhomboid defect. This design diminishes the degree of vertical tension on the transposed flap.

A wider base is created in the Dufourmental design and this may contribute to difficulty in flap transposition. However, tension at the tip is placed more lateral (not as vertical as in the rhombic design), thereby creating a more stable flap.

Bilobed flap

Bilobed flaps are a combination of transpositional and rotational flap manoeuvres. The key design involves construction of sufficiently long limbs to accommodate the restraint at the flap base which inevitably results from the distance necessary for transposition. A pivotal angle of >30° will usually result in 'standing cones' at the flap base. If cones persist, they may be excised secondarily.

Orientation of the lobed flap is determined by the reservoir of tissue in the area of the defect – from the cheek area for transposition superiorly into the temple region if the defect is high, and inferiorly as shown in Figure 4.5.11 if the defect is low. The incision lines should lie in relaxed skin lines.

ORBITAL DEFECTS AND RECONSTRUCTION

Lateral rhinotomy approach

Access to the medial orbit and ethmoid sinuses for resection of extensive tumours usually involves a combined craniofacial approach from above and access through the naso-orbital region. Craniofacial approaches are discussed elsewhere (see Chapter 4.4). For smaller tumours confined to the ethmoid air cells, the lateral rhinotomy approach may be used. Typically, the orbit is not entered and the eye is preserved.

The incision is carried superiorly from the alar (as in a Weber–Fergusson approach) midway between the medial canthus and mid-nasal point. Greater postero-superior access can be gained through extension of the incision into the supraorbital recess. If a margin can be safely obtained without involvement of the lacrimal crests, then the medial canthus may remain attached. Wider exposure may be obtained with canthal detachment. Osteotomizing a portion of the crestal insertion facilitates canthal re-attachment with microplate fixation. Exposure of the entire medial orbital wall is permitted. After delineation of tumour extent, a 1-cm bony margin is planned. Removal of the lamina papyracea may assist in determining tumour extent and bony margins.

To facilitate tumour exposure, the nasal bones may be osteotomized (Figure 4.5.12). Microplates are placed first. If encroachment on the lacrimal canaliculi or sac is anticipated, cannulation is undertaken for identification purposes and repair.

After resection, the cavity is lightly packed with gauze strips impregnated with antibiotic ointment. If resection has involved the superomedial orbital wall or cribriform plate, the defect should be lined with transposed pericranial flaps or split calvarial grafts. Such a defect may also communicate with the frontal sinus in which case a pericranial flap will serve as a barrier. Fibrin sealant is applied to secure a watertight seal (Figure 4.5.13). If the frontonasal duct is implicated or frontal sinus disease is present, sinus obliteration is performed via mucosal stripping and autogenous (calvarial cortical chips and dust) bone graft placement. (Dual access for extended resection into the superior orbit or frontal sinus region is necessary via coronal and rhinotomy approaches.)

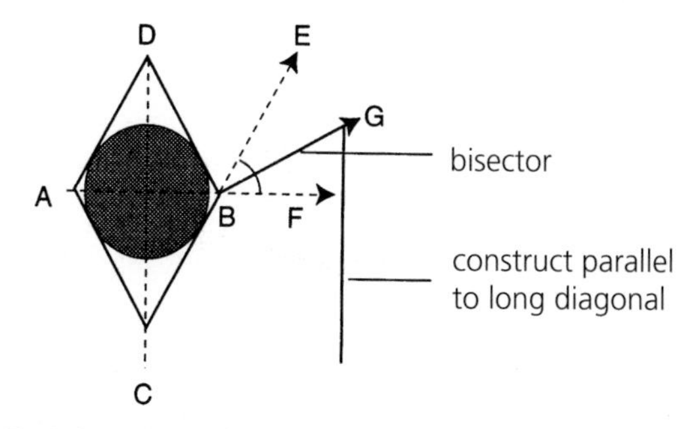

4.5.10 Dufourmental flap design is a type of rhombic and involves constructing a bisect or incision of the angle EBF, then dropping a vertical limb parallel to the long diagonal CD.

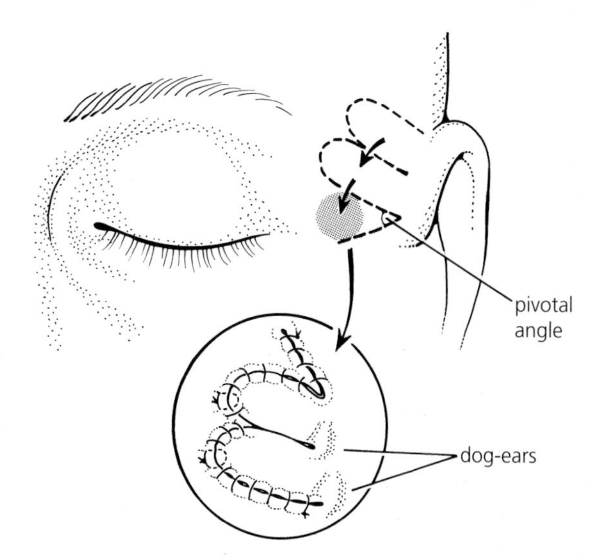

4.5.11 Bilobed flaps should have bases in fairly lax tissue and the incisions made parallel to relaxed skin tension lines (RSTLs), if possible, for cosmesis and stability. Pivotal angles should be 30° or less to avoid standing cones.

Lateral orbital masses and defects

Lateral orbital masses, usually epidermoid or dermoid cysts or tumours arising from the lacrimal gland, are approached through brow, eyelid (with or without lateral canthotomy) or coronal access incisions. Computed tomography (CT) and magnetic resonance imaging (MRI) delineate the mass size, location and vascularity. A coronal approach will allow better access for malignant lesions, particularly with skull base involvement. Transconjunctival incisions with lateral canthotomy give sufficient access for biopsy of large masses or removal of small lateral orbital tumours (Figure 4.5.14).

A coronal approach is performed, exposing the supraorbital and lateral orbital rims. If CT or MRI has indicated the posterior extent of the mass to be more than one-half of the orbit, fronto-orbital craniotomy is indicated. Anterior masses can be approached via an orbital rim osteotomy which is planned to allow sufficient margins of bony and periorbital tissue for malignant tumours of the lacrimal gland. The inferior limb of the osteotomy can be taken to the orbital floor and posterior to the sphenozygomatic suture. Before the lateral canthus is detached, it is identified with a suture or it can be osteotomized with a small (6–8 mm) portion of lateral rim bone to allow precise re-attachment with wire or microscrew fixation. The orbital rim and wall are put aside (with miniplates attached) for later placement.

Rongeur nibbling (Figure 4.5.14) of the orbital wall will also create more posteroinferior access to the retro-orbital region. Superior access, as noted above, is best gained through a fronto-orbital craniotomy.

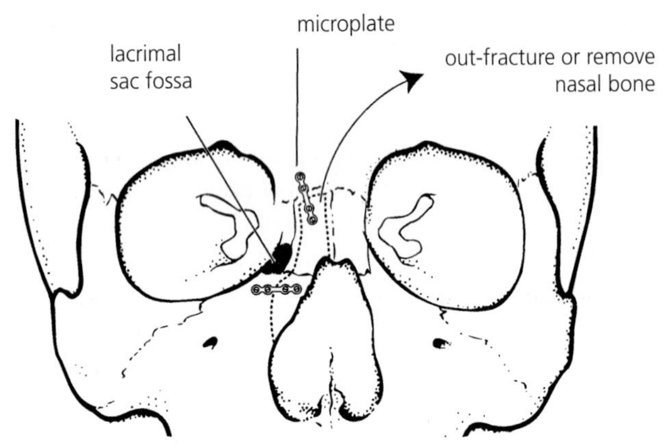

4.5.12 Diagram illustrates nasal osteotomy for access to the superior nasal and ethmoid regions. Fixation plates should be placed initially *in situ* which facilitates replacement after resection.

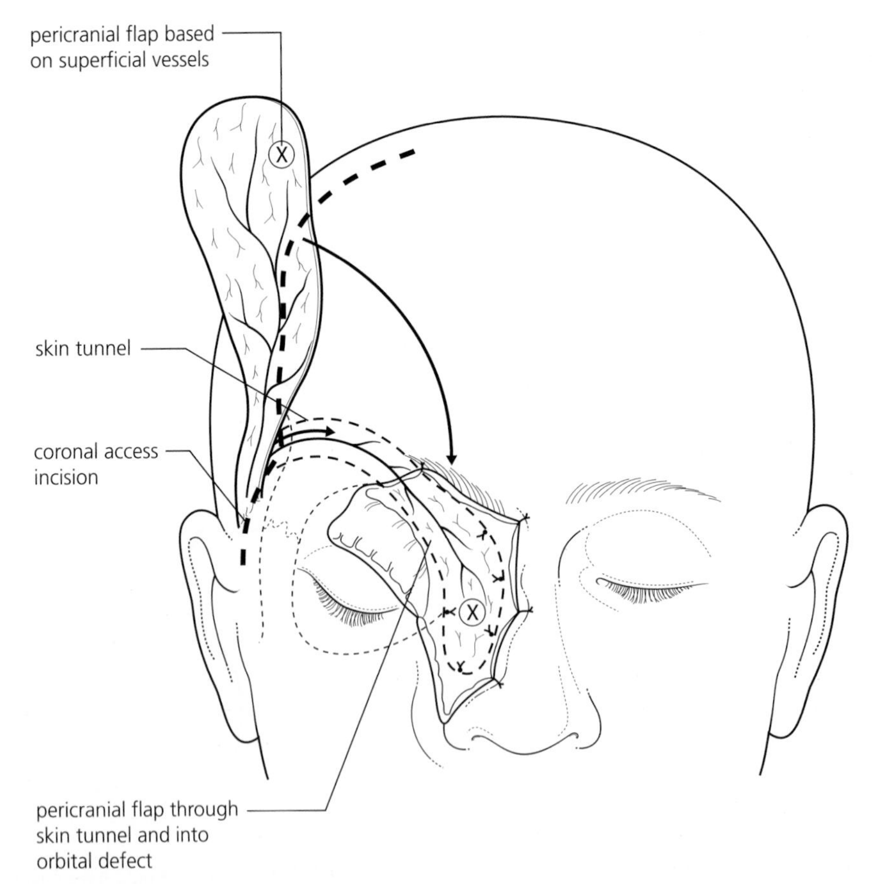

4.5.13 A pericranial or galeal flap may be made to cover a resection defect and provide vascularity for bone grafts. Retention of the flap to the recipient bed is facilitated by placing holes in the bony margins, suturing the flap in place and sealing with fibrin glue. A portion of the outer calvarium may be ostectomized as a pedicled myo-osseous flap for reconstruction of the bony orbit.

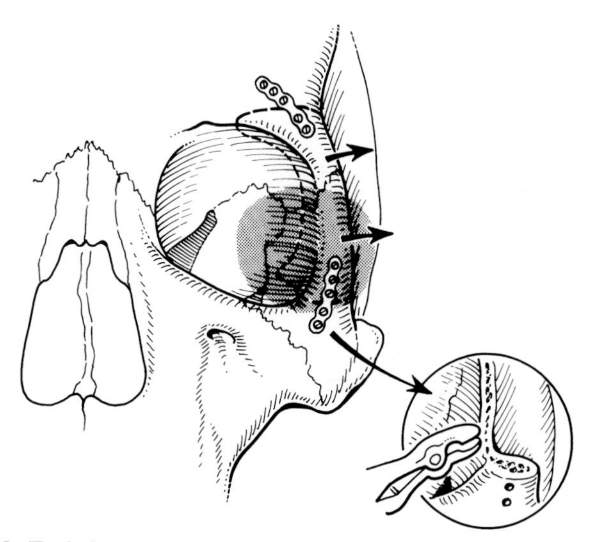

4.5.14 Lateral orbital osteotomies for lateral, superior or deep orbital lesions. The lateral orbital bone can be removed with rongeurs to facilitate access to the retro-orbital region.

Combined approaches

Some posterior masses may require combined approaches to the orbit. A lateral orbitotomy (Figure 4.5.15a) with outward displacement of the globe combined with a medial approach will allow this freedom. An extended lateral canthotomy incision gives good exposure of the lateral rim. The anterior third of the lateral orbital wall is osteotomized and the rim is cut above and well below the frontozygomatic suture. Out-fracture (Figure 4.5.15b) of the lateral wall preserves the attached periosteum as a vascular pedicle.

A Lynch incision to the medial wall or lateral rhinotomy is performed. The medial canthus is identified and either tagged or osteotomized with attached bone. The medial orbital wall is removed and an ethmoidectomy performed. After detachment of the medial rectus muscle, the globe can be gently retracted laterally, thus exposing the posterior intraconal region. If access is still limited, a superior approach through the orbital roof is necessary. After tumour resection, the medial canthus is re-attached with light polydiaxonone sutures or 28-G wire. A gauze pack with antibiotic ointment is placed in the ethmoid resection and a small Penrose drain placed. The lateral wall and rim are affixed with miniplates.

For intraconal lesions, Tenon's capsule (bulbar fascia) may need to be incised (Figure 4.5.15c) lateral to the limbus with dissection over the globe to the muscle insertions. Dissection here is a little more difficult and tedious, therefore the muscle insertion is identified, incised and tagged for later reinsertion. After reflection of the muscle, dissection to the posterior intraconal region is possible.

To reconstruct lateral or inferior wall defects after orbitotomy and resection, a temporal pericranial flap may be mobilized and turned into the defect (Figure 4.5.13). To provide bony support for a resected orbital site, the outer table of calvarium can be harvested ('guitar pick' size), with its pericranial pedicle and tunnelled into the orbit. The subcutaneous tunnel needs to be sufficiently undermined to accommodate the flap and prevent constriction of the pericranial vessels.

Orbital floor or inferior rim reconstruction can also be accomplished by an intraoral coronoidectomy with temporalis insertion preserved, then tunnelling the coronoid to the orbit (Figure 4.5.16) where it is fixed to the surrounding bone with titanium miniplates. This manoeuvre will provide support to the periorbital tissues, as well as a buttress for the lower eyelid retractors and supportive tarsal structures.

EYELID RESECTION AND RECONSTRUCTION

Principles

A variety of benign and malignant lesions are found on the eyelids. Benign lesions include naevi, keratoses, cysts (sebaceous, meibomian), papillomas, etc. Benign lesions are excised with immediate reconstruction. The most common malignancy is BCC followed by squamous cell carcinoma, sebaceous gland carcinoma and melanoma. These lesions should be biopsied for diagnosis, then resection performed with Mohs' technique or frozen section guidance.

BCCs require a 3–4-mm margin, while squamous carcinomas and melanomas should have at least 1 cm of lid margin. Deeply invading tumours affixed to bone or involving the scleral conjunctiva may necessitate exenteration. Reconstruction of the lid may involve lid remnants, local periorbital or opposite lid tissue, local flaps, distant flaps and cartilaginous or banked tissue grafts (allografts). Eyelid reconstruction involves three types of defects: skin only, skin and orbicularis, and full-thickness with the tarsoconjunctival layer. Repair may also require reestablishment of the canalicular and nasolacrimal ducts. Large defects need some structural support for the reconstructed lid.

Partial defects

Partial thickness defects are repaired by advancing local skin and muscle, or with a full thickness skin graft. Skin grafts are harvested from the opposite lid, post-auricular region or supraclavicular area. These areas provide excellent tissue match for thickness, colour and texture. Small lid defects (<2 cm) are easily repaired with opposite lid skin, while larger areas require post-auricular or supraclavicular grafts.

The defect is measured. The donor area is 'ballooned' with local anaesthetic and a vasoconstrictor. The graft is obtained, the donor area closed primarily and the donor skin is thinned by trimming subcutaneous tissue. The graft is fashioned to the defect, taking care to allow sufficient, loose coverage of the defect. The lid should be under full stretch to allow correct fit of the graft to the defect.

The graft is sutured in place with 6/0 black silk interrupted sutures with long tails for a tie-over bolster. For larger grafts,

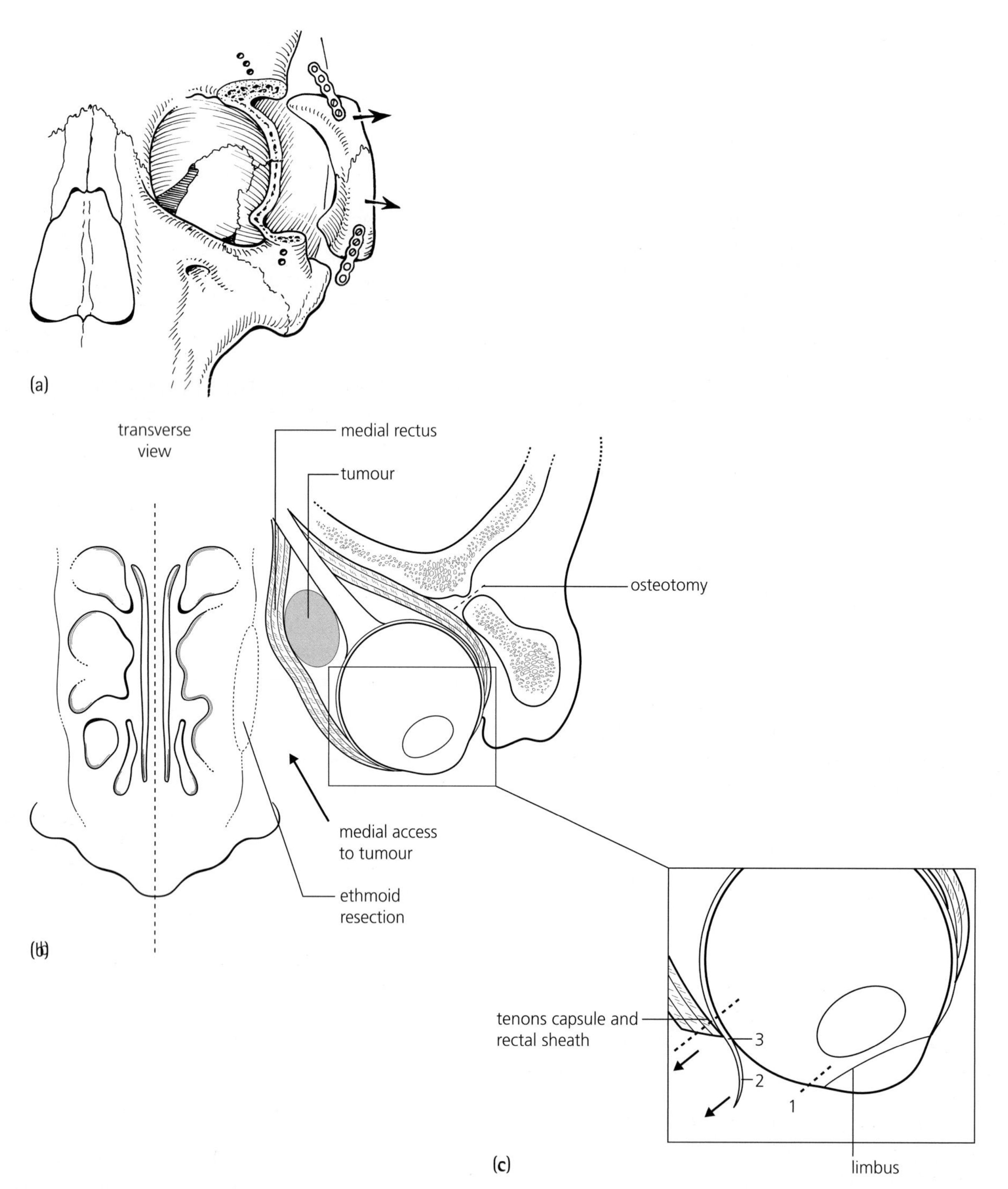

4.5.15 (a) Lateral orbitotomy may be performed to outfracture the lateral orbit pedicled upon its musculoperiosteal attachment. The globe can then be mobilized laterally to provide access for medial and paranasal lesions. (b) Axial view demonstrating outfracture of the lateral orbital wall which then provides improved medial access. (c) Enlargement demonstrating incision lateral to the limbus (1) and dissection of Tenon's capsule over the globe (2). The rectal muscle insertion (3) is incised to gain intraconal access to the lesion.

6/0 chromic gut suture is placed in the mid-portion to assist in graft adaptation to the recipient area. Good haemostasis of the recipient bed is critical to the success of the graft. A non-stick dressing with cotton wool is used as a bolster. The bolster sutures are removed 7 days later.

Local skin or skin muscle advancements can also be undertaken for partial defects. A 'lid-switch' from the opposite lid (usually upper to lower lid) may be performed (Figure 4.5.17). The donor can be transferred as a 'bucket handle' or one end pedicled which allows more flap mobility. 'Pinching' the upper lid skin with a forceps, similar to a blepharoplasty, will assist in determining the amount of tissue available for transfer. These flaps are normally indicated for smaller, narrower defects. Both peripheral and

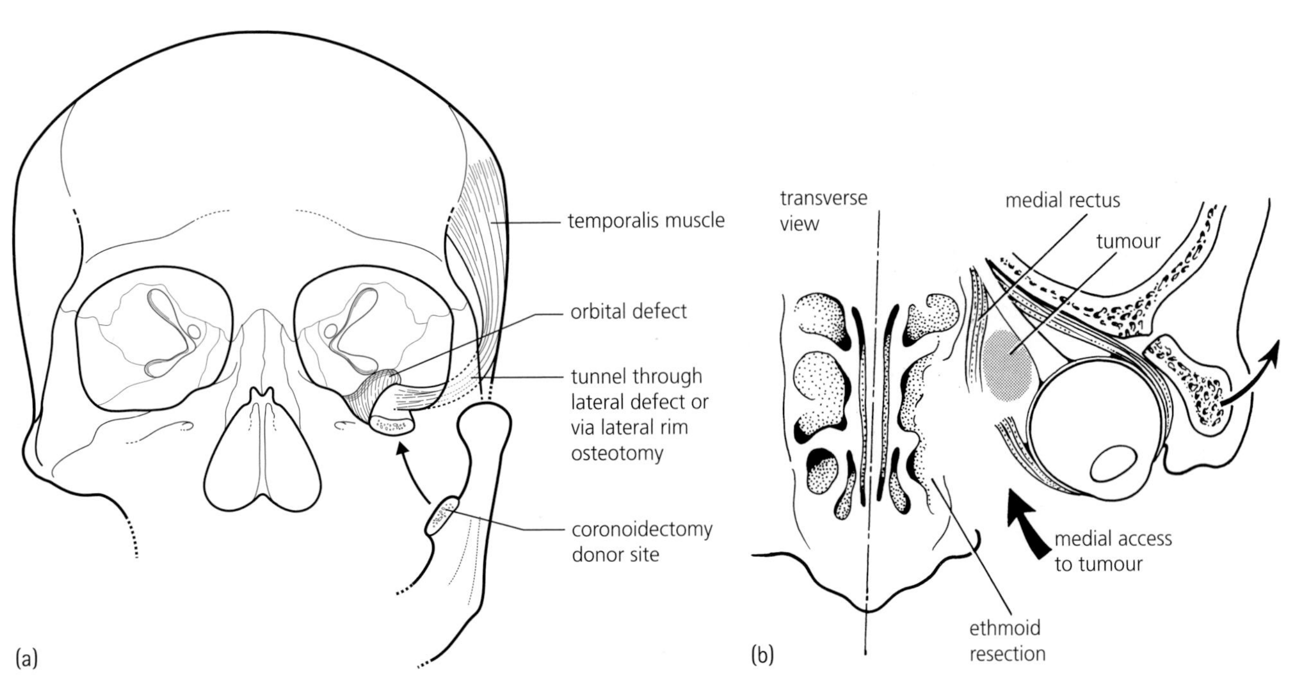

4.5.16 This demonstrates reconstruction of an orbital rim/floor defect with the coronoid process hinged on the temporalis muscle.

central sutures using light resorbable suture should be placed to affix the flap to the defect bed. Frost sutures should be placed for several days to reduce tension on the flap. The flap is divided 7–10 days after surgery.

FULL-THICKNESS DEFECTS

Eyelid flaps

Full-thickness defects <1 cm can usually be closed primarily by performing a wedge excision (Figure 4.5.18). The tarsal margins are coapted with 5/0 chromic or polygalactin suture under loop magnification in order to avoid suture placement through the conjunctiva and subsequent irritation. The lid margin is approximated by placement of a 6/0 or 7/0 silk or polypropylene suture in the lash grey-line. This suture can be left long to incorporate into the dressing at the end. Skin closure is performed with 6/0 or 7/0 interrupted nylon or polypropylene sutures. A tape dressing (Steri-Strip) is placed to support the wound. Ophthalmic antibiotic ointment is applied to the wound twice daily for 2–3 days. The lid margin stitch and tape dressing are removed at 3–4 days and the nylon sutures at 7 days.

Extended temporal flaps

Larger full-thickness defects (>2 cm) require a lateral advancement flap which is a lateral canthotomy incision carried laterally to the hairline, if necessary. The key to flap success is for the lateral incision to be gently curved in an upward arc for lower lid flaps and downwards for upper lid

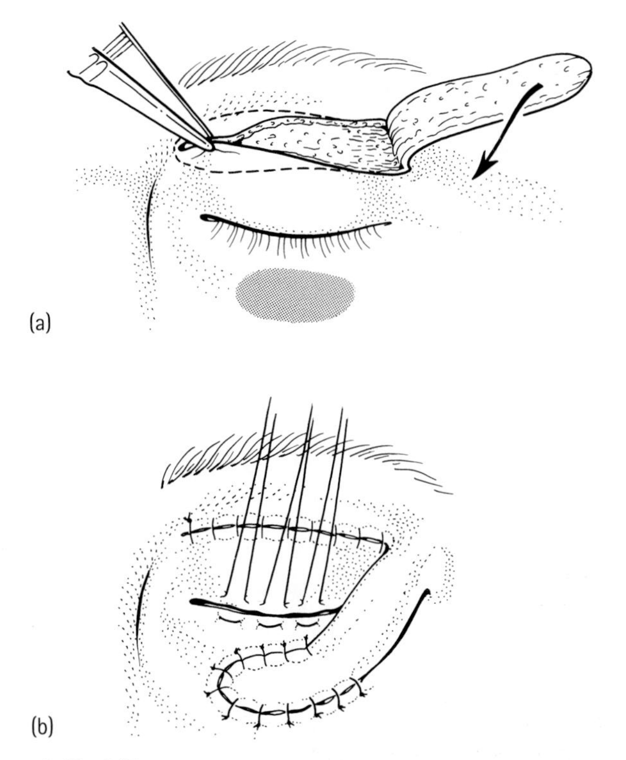

4.5.17 (a) Restoration of a lower lid defect may be performed with redundant upper eyelid. A 'finger flap' is created leaving one end pedicled, then transposing to the lower defect. (b) Transposed 'lid-switch' flap is secured with interrupted suture. Frost sutures should be placed to immobilize the lid for several days. The flap is divided at 7–10 days.

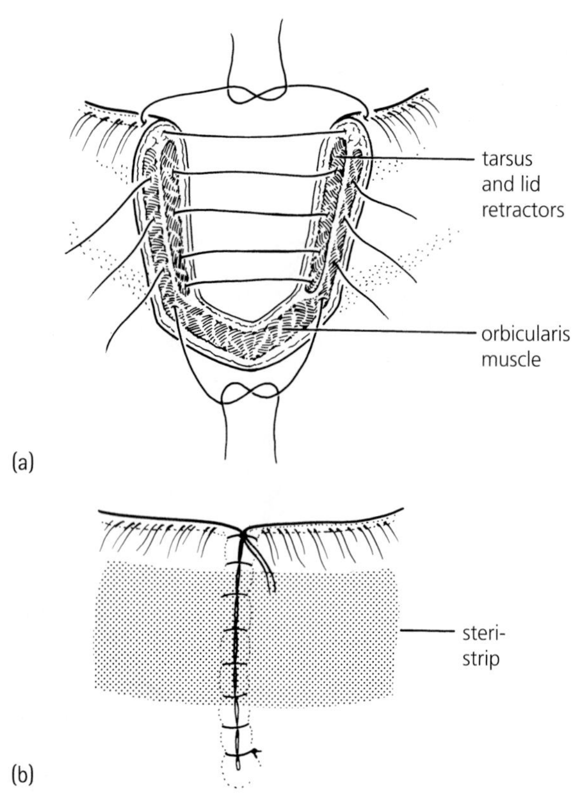

4.5.18 (a) Full-thickness lower lid defects <1 cm can be primarily closed with sutures placed in the tarsal plate (6-0 resorbable suture) with 6-0 or 7-0 nylon or silk at the grey line and skin. (b) The lid margin suture is left long in order to tape the tails inferiorly and avoid irritation of the eye.

flaps. This provides adequate vertical length to the flap, as well as resistance to lagophthalmos of the reconstructed lid. Flap mobilization is carried above the musculoaponeurosis, but includes the orbicularis muscle in the advanced lid to lend some support.

As the flap is mobilized and advanced medially, the conjunctiva will freely follow. A Burow's triangle is placed at the lateral-most extent of the incision to ease tension, McGregor incorporated a Z-plasty at the lateral margin. The lower limb of the 'Z' roughly parallels the defect margin. Closure begins with placement of a 4/0 clear nylon suture at the canthal region to tack the lid subcutaneous tissue to the rim periosteum. The defect and lid layers are repaired as described above for a smaller defect. The transposed Z-plasty triangles may require future mobilization and trimming to fit properly. The wound is taped for 1 week to provide flap support.

For defects too large to provide tarsus in the advanced lid, a septal or conchal cartilage support may be required. The best cartilage is harvested from the scaphoid cartilage of the ear as it is usually sufficiently thin and pliable to prevent lid distortion.

Conjunctival coverage is provided by a turn-down flap (Figure 4.5.19) from the opposite lid or a free palatal or buccal mucosal graft. Both tissues must be secured with direct and tie-over bolsters to immobilize the flap or graft until healing has occurred. This is accomplished with fast-absorbing direct sutures as shown in the figure, making sure the knots are buried, or with full thickness horizontal mattress sutures with or without bolsters. Frost sutures are placed to facilitate lid immobilization. The flap is divided 2–3 weeks later.

Lid defects, particularly with an element of symblepharon, may also be reconstructed with a strip of temporalis muscle

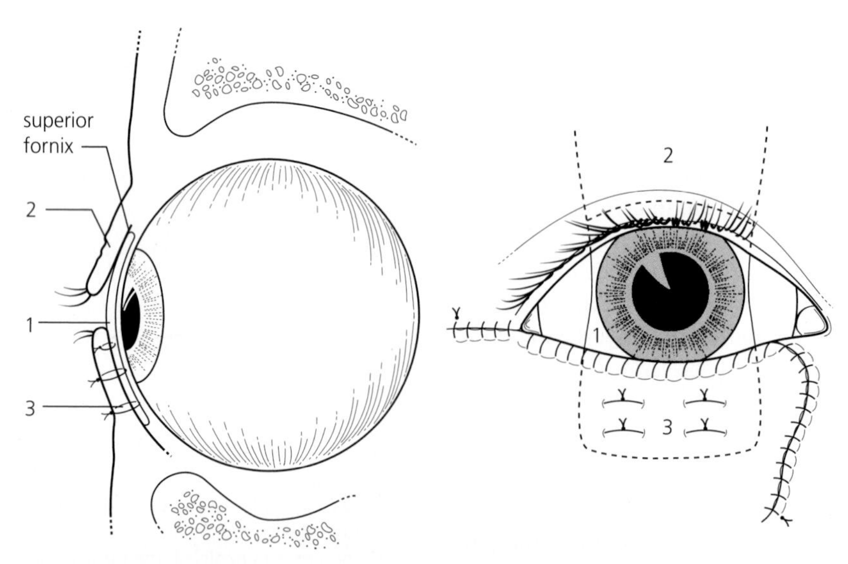

4.5.19 Conjunctival flap from upper eyelid to reconstruct the lower lid defect: (1) The conjunctival flap is seen lying over the cornea. (2) The extent of dissection is high into the fornix. (3) The flap is sutured into the recipient bed of the reconstructed lower lid which, in this case, is on the advanced cheek flap and secured with mattress sutures.

and fascia with its attendant vascular supply. Figure 4.5.20 demonstrates clinical application of this flap. The flap is dissected on its anterior superficial temporal vessels and then tunnelled over the zygomatic arch to the orbital rim. The distal margin of temporalis is introduced via a pull-out suture into a subcutaneous pocket. The flap traverses the whole of the eyelid to its medial extent. It is secured with multiple small bolsters. Deep to the flap and superficial to the eyelid conjunctiva, a free cartilage graft should be placed to restore lid support and competency. A temporary bulge of temporalis muscle over the zygomatic arch will atrophy and flatten with time. The superoposterior 'pull' of the temporalis will naturally assist in tightening and lifting the newly reconstructed eyelid.

Cheek flaps

Total lid defects are reconstructed with cheek rotational flaps (Figure 4.5.21). A lateral canthotomy approach is performed with extension to the hairline laterally and then inferiorly in the pre-auricular region. The flap is elevated above the musculo-aponeurosis and carried as far medially as necessary. A small back-cut at the inferior limb will allow more superior rotation of the flap. A chondral-perichondral graft is placed and sutured into the defect with buried 5/0 resorbable suture. A pull-out light nylon suture may also be placed to assist in stabilizing the cartilage graft. These flaps have a tendency to migrate inferiorly after healing, resulting in some element of cicatricial ectropion and dystopia. If the malar fat pad is present, then superior 'lifting' of the pad with 2/0 clear nylon or polydiaxone sutures pexed to the lateral rim periosteum will help to resist the inferior gravitational pull of the cheek flap. Conjunctival reconstruction is undertaken as previously described. Care must be exercised to avoid sutures piercing the remnant of conjunctiva which will result in abrasion and irritation. Tape dressing is placed for 1 week and ophthalmic antibiotic ointment applied for 3 days.

NASAL DEFECTS

Nasal skin is thick, sebaceous and relatively inelastic, which makes reconstruction with nasal tissue challenging. In nasal reconstruction, the surgeon should approach the nasal subunits separately – the dorsum, tip and alar regions. Each has its own characteristics which define repair. The nasal area has a blood supply from two sources: a rich terminal network of the facial artery which spreads on to the nose as angular and alar branches. These anastomose superiorly on the dorsum with terminals of the ophthalmic artery – the medial palpebral and dorsal nasal. Usually flaps from the glabella and radix can be planned based upon these latter two vessels.

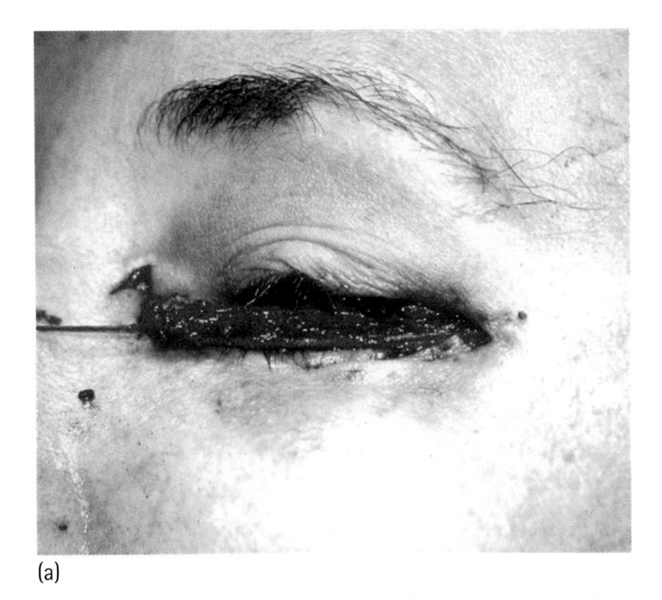

(a)

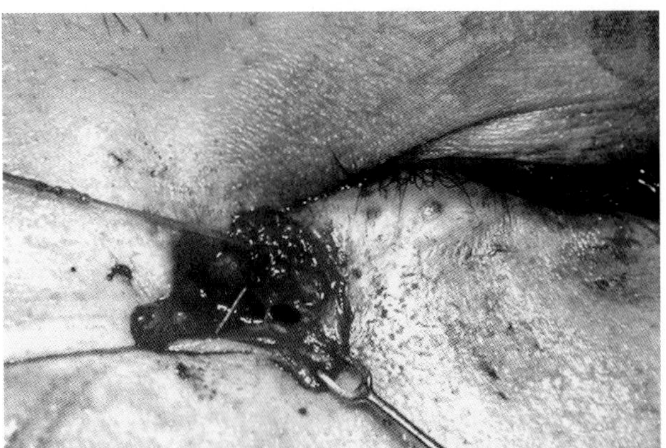

(b)

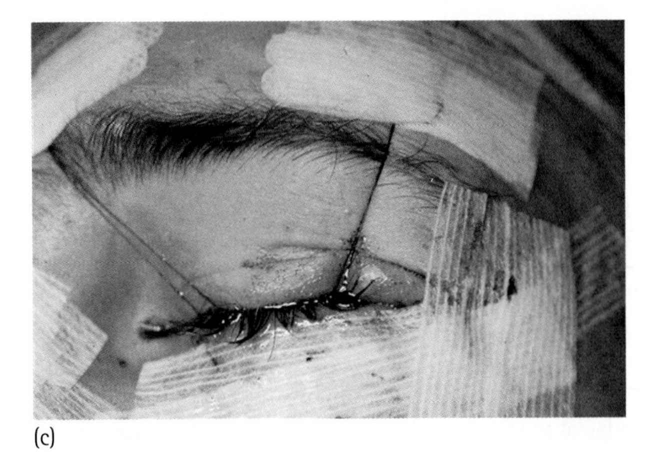

(c)

4.5.20 (a) Clinical photograph of a temporalis myofascial sleeve for lower eyelid reconstruction. (b) Photograph of temporalis sleeve introduced laterally through an extended canthotomy incision and placed in a subcutaneous pocket. Note the distal pull-out sutures which assist in flap placement. (c) Photograph of reconstructed lower eyelid and post-operative Frost sutures to immobilize and support the lower lid.

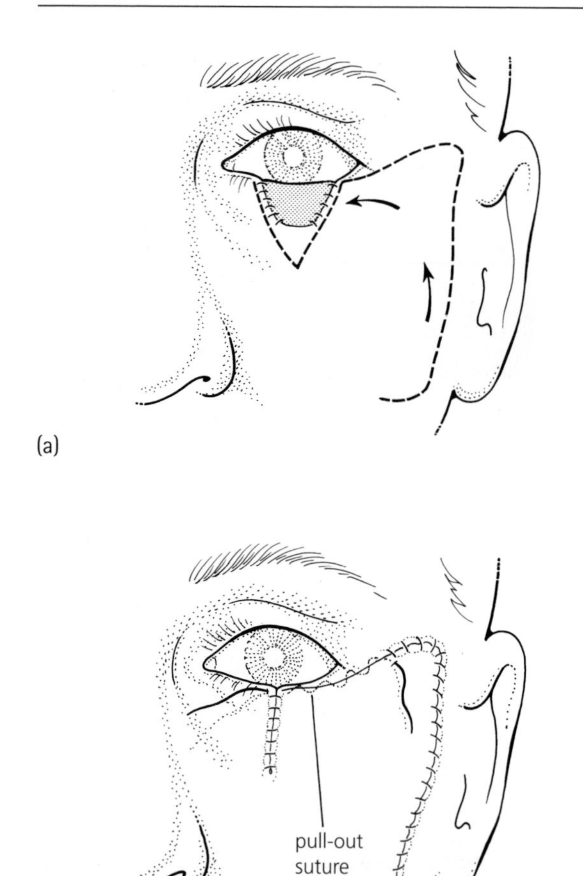

4.5.21 (a) Large lid defect is reconstructed with a cheek advancement flap as outlined. A free chondral-perichondral graft is placed and secured to the conjunctival margins with buried 5-6 chromic suture. (b) Closure of cheek advancement flap. Eyelid margins are closed with a running or subcutaneous 6/0 nylon suture.

Nasal dorsum defects

Defects of the dorsum may be resurfaced with either a glabellar flap (superior defects) or dorsal nasal flap (inferior defects). The glabellar flap (Figure 4.5.22) may be modified to cover defects up to half of the upper dorsum of the nose. The limiting factor in flap transposition is the pivotal area where the nutrient supra-trochlear vessel enters the flap. Suturing is in two layers with buried 4/0 polygalactin suture subcutaneously and 5/0 or 6/0 nylon for skin. The leading edge of the flap is under the most tension, therefore vertical mattress sutures may be helpful in maintaining flap position and viability.

The dorsal nasal flap is pedicled on the medial palpebral vessel. As long as this artery is preserved, a large flap can be raised off the upper dorsal surface and extended into the glabellar region. The flap rotates around the pedicle, thus kinking of the vessel must be prevented. Also, a dog ear remains at this pivotal region, but should be corrected secondarily.

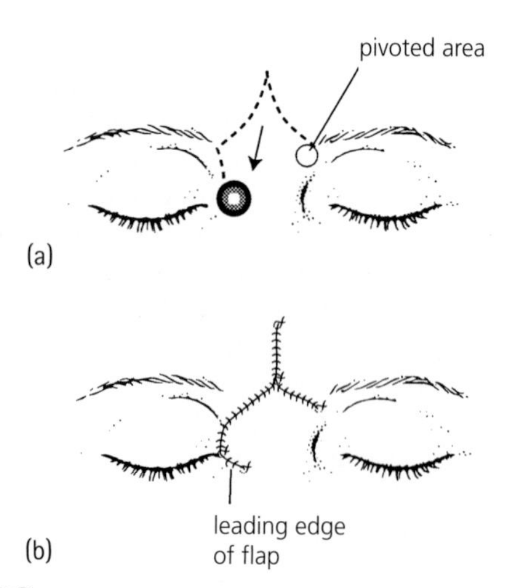

4.5.22 (a,b) Diagram of glabellar flap to cover a small nasal dorsal defect. The pivotal area includes the nutrient vessel (supratrochlear).

Large nasal defects

The paramedian or midline forehead flap is used for resurfacing large nasal dorsal and tip defects. This is a staged procedure: the first stage for placing the flap and a second stage 2–3 weeks later to divide the pedicle. The flap offers a fair tissue match for the nose, particularly in thicker-skinned individuals.

Vascularity to the flap is via the supratrochlear vessels (Figure 4.5.23), which allows the total vertical dimension of the forehead to be incorporated in the flap. The contralateral vessel is selected upon which the flap base will pivot to prevent kinking of the vessels with subsequent failure and necrosis.

Two vertical limbs extending from the nasal root area are inscribed and these may taper to the hairline or run parallel to be joined by a horizontal limb at the hairline. Doppler flow can be used to confirm supratrochlear artery location. Prior to the incision, the precise defect size and shape should be traced as a template and transferred to the donor site. Verification of flap length is confirmed with a gauze strip extending from the pivotal base to the donor site plus about 10 per cent extra to allow for adequate tissue when turning the flap inferiorly. The incision is carried down to periosteum and a subgaleal dissection performed. Periodic Doppler assessment will confirm vessel viability. If tissue blanching disappears, this is usually due to vasospasm which will resolve after several minutes.

The flap is trimmed to fit the recipient site and sutured in place with polygalactin suture in the deep dermis and fine suture for the skin. A drain or gauze wick may be placed under the tissue bridge.

The donor site is closed (Figure 4.5.24) by first widely undermining the forehead tissue with fine, vertical galeal incisions to gain laxity. Next, heavy (2/0 or 3/0) sutures are placed in the galea to gain tissue approximation. Periodic vertical mattress sutures can be placed for skin approximation in conjunction with a running suture.

The flap is divided 2–3 weeks later. Usually the flap base can be discarded; however, if the brows have been displaced too far medially, then return of the flap base in the glabellar region will correct it. Persistent lymphoedema often accompanies these flaps for several months and manual massage may be helpful in resolving oedema of the reconstructed nasal tip.

Nasal tip defects

Nasal tip lesions usually require full thickness skin excision and if there is tumour extension to the deep dermis, cartilage should also be included in the resection. Full thickness skin defects of the nasal tip can be resurfaced with local nasal flaps or nasolabial flaps. Local flaps are optimal for tissue colour, texture and thickness match.

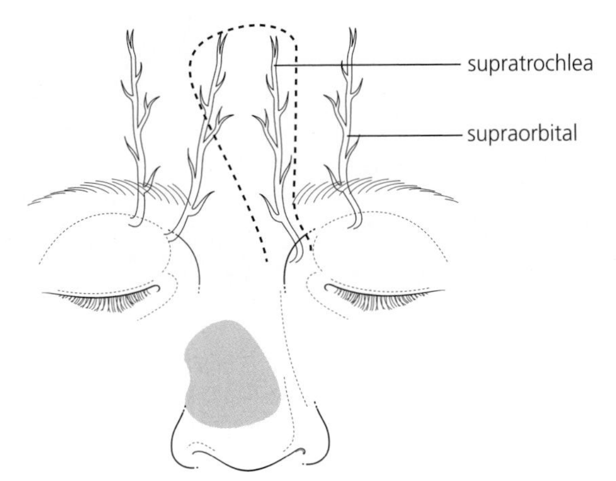

4.5.23 Diagram illustrating pattern of vascular supply to the forehead region. The contralateral vessel is selected as the nutrient pedicle to the flap.

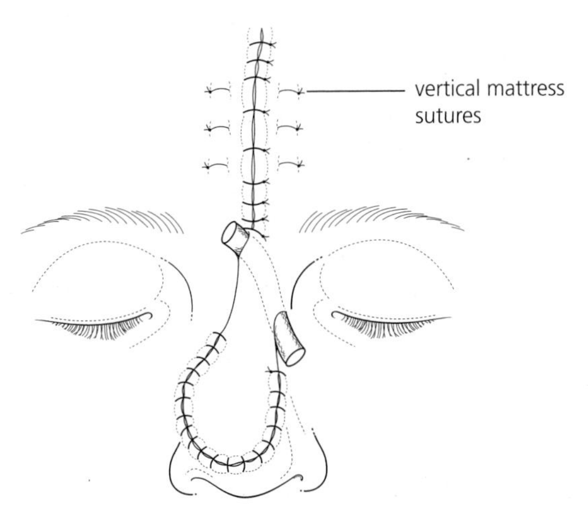

4.5.24 Closure of defect and donor site. A gauze wick should be placed under the bridge of tissue to maintain hygiene until the undersurface heals sufficiently.

Lobed flaps are popular for small nasal tip defects of the midline. After excision, a decision must be made as to whether a one- or two-lobed flap is required. Generally, the larger the defect and the closer to the midline, the more lobes are required (Figure 4.5.25). Lobes derived from the nasal side wall do not transpose easily, but those from the nasolabial area are more mobile and therefore they can be narrower as the donor sites are easily closed.

Tip defects just off the midline may result in some distortion when resurfaced from lobes nearby. The alar rim is particularly affected; however, this usually settles with time. The leading edge is under the most tension, so a two-layered closure with an occasional vertical mattress suture is done.

Central tip defects are best restored with tissue transposed from a more distant flap, such as the dorsal nasal flap or forehead finger flap as previously discussed (Figure 4.5.26). The nasolabial flap can also be used if thickness and colour are similar. Persistent tip lymphoedema will be most pronounced and enduring, and ultimate nasal tip form will not be attained until at least one year post-operatively.

Alar rim defects

Lesions of the nasal ala usually require excision that includes cartilage or results in total rim resection. Restoration of the alar contour requires enough tissue to fold over, e.g. a nasolabial flap, or a free composite graft from the ear.

Nasolabial flaps can be pedicled superiorly, rotated medially and turned in on itself to restore rim contour and bulk (Figure 4.5.27). The distal portion of the flap is at risk for ischaemia because kinking of the small vessels typically occurs at the fold area. suturing should be enough to hold the flap in place as there is little tension on the flap.

Alar rim defects up to 2 cm can be repaired with auricular composite grafts of skin and cartilage (Figure 4.5.28). The outer helix provides an acceptable contour and bulk for restoration of the rim. Since these are free grafts, it is important to stabilize the graft in order to allow capillary

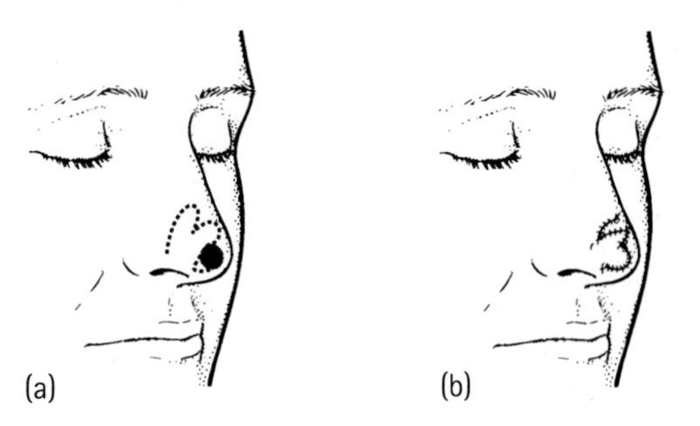

4.5.25 (a,b) Nasal alar or domal defects may be restored with a transposed bilobed flap. These local flaps offer good texture and colour matches. More lobes are created for larger defects closer to the nasal midline.

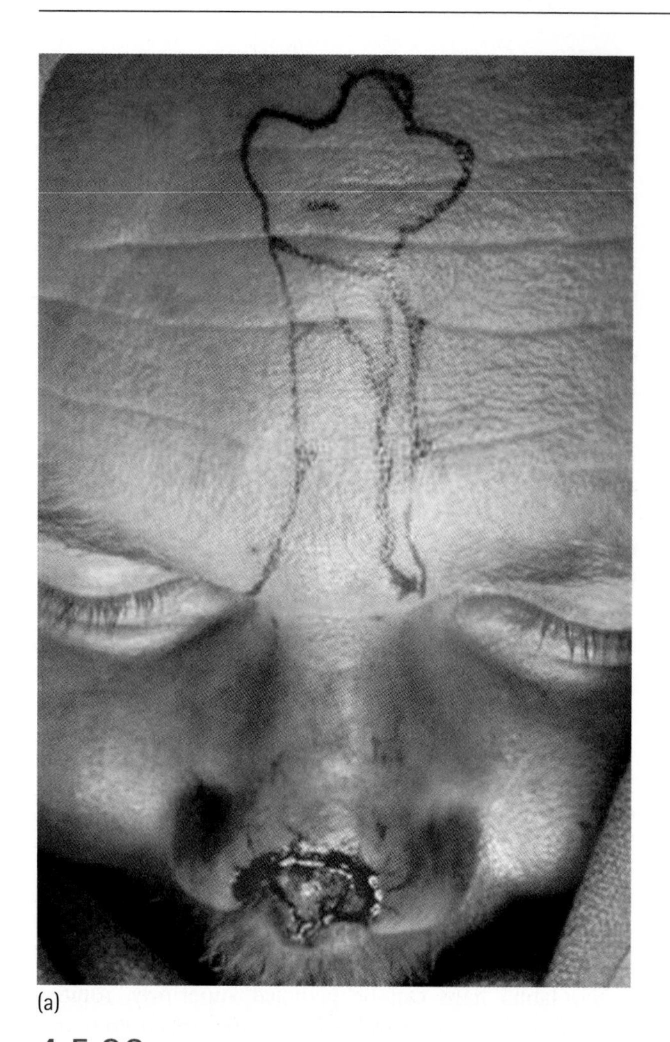

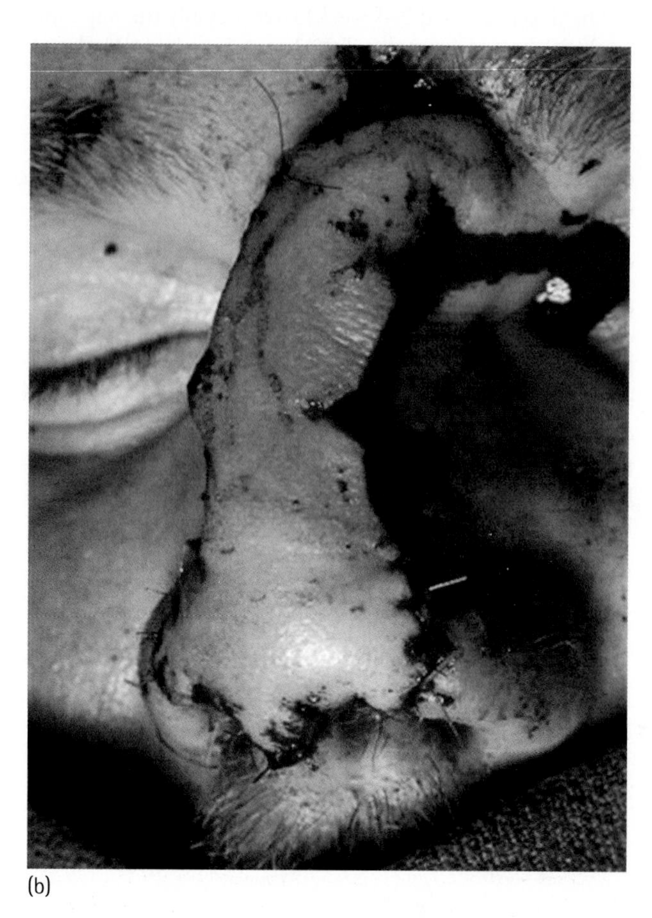

(a) (b)

4.5.26 Clinical photographs demonstrating application of the forehead flap for reconstruction of a nasal tip defect. (a) The flap is marked after confirmation of the supratrochlear vessel and the defect size and length of flap is verified. (b) The flap is sutured into place with buried 4/0 or 5/0 resorbable sutures and 5/0 nylon sutures. A gauze wick dressing is placed under the tissue bridge.

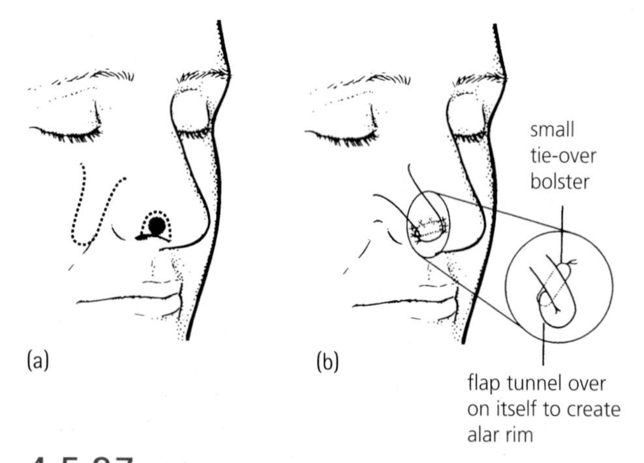

4.5.27 (a,b) Alar rim defect is restored with a local nasolabial flap. The flap may be turned over on to itself to restore the rim margin with lined tissue. A through and through tie-over bolster is then applied to provide form and stability of the flap.

ingrowth and tissue survival. The size and depth of the defect dictates what portion of the helix provides an appropriate match. The outer helix is good for long but shallow defects where a rigid span is required; however, the more fleshy lower helix or that portion next to the superior crus provides more bulk and depth when required. The longer the graft, the greater the risk of necrosis.

A template of the rim defect is taken to the helix and drawn carefully in place. 'Foot extensions' should be incorporated in the graft. These will insert into medial and lateral pockets in the defect.

Prior to graft placement, soft tissue pockets are created in each defect margin where the cartilage feet will be inserted and sutured to remnant rim cartilage and tissue. One 3-0 nylon suture is placed through each defect from out to in, piercing each 'foot' (Figure 4.5.28b). This is then brought back up through the graft and nasal skin from the inside. Antibiotic gauze pledgets 3–4 mm in diameter are placed

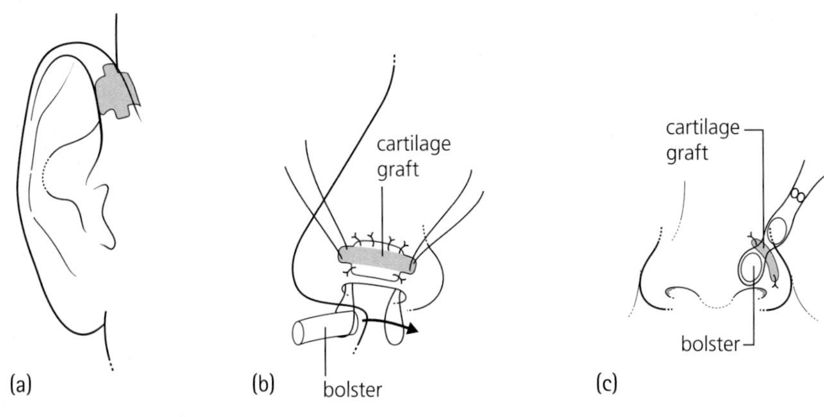

4.5.28 (a) Composite skin-cartilage free graft from the outer helix is demonstrated. Extended cartilaginous 'feet' are harvested to insert on either side of the defect and provide additional support and form to the rim. The donor site is closed primarily. (b) Retention of the free graft is obtained with through and through sutures to secure the graft. (c) Intra- and extranasal bolsters are placed through the sutures to assist in flap stabilization.

intra- and extranasally through each nylon suture loop to serve as a bolster for the graft (Figure 4.5.28c); 4/0 and 5/0 nylon is placed to secure the remainder of the graft to its recipient site. The graft typically appears dusky for the first 48 hours after which vascular ingrowth will be evident. If hyperbaric oxygen is available, this has served well in 'resurrecting' or enhancing the 'take' of large free composite grafts. The bolster and sutures are removed after a week and the graft stabilized with tape dressings for another week. Some free grafts lose their pigmentation or do not have as much vascularity as surrounding tissue so that they are readily noticeable. Cosmetic tattooing can be done if the colour match is not acceptable.

Total nasal defects

Total nasal reconstructions are performed in several stages. The first stage provides adequate soft tissue coverage, both extranasally through the forehead flap and intranasally with local mucosal flaps. Free mucosal flaps harvested from the buccal mucosa may be necessary to provide a physiologic intranasal covering and prevent cicatrization of the raw flap under the surface. Intranasal stents and bolsters are necessary to maintain nasal patency and function.

Once adequate soft tissue is in place, cartilaginous struts and framework harvested from the nasal septum, conchal bowl and crestal regions can be undertaken. Overgrafting is usually necessary as cicatrization and retraction generally ensue over the next several months after graft placement.

Final stage reconstruction involves soft tissue adjustments to the nasal base (dermabrasion or excision of scar), tip (thinning thickened transplanted forehead skin) and alar rim areas (selective thinning of cartilage or skin). Great care should be exercised to avoid compromise of the lining mucosa and nasal vestibular area.

Top tips

Flap design in the facial region should consider these essentials:

- Optimum colour, texture and skin appendage match
- Minimal distortion of donor or recipient site landmarks (e.g. brow, lid, lips, ala)
- Plan for flaps with minimal tension.

Posterior orbital tumours can be accessed through:

- Lateral rhinotomy with medial canthotomy
- Lateral orbitotomy and orbital wall resection.

Dissection of Tenon's capsule and disinsertion of the rectus muscle for intraconal lesions

- Fronto-orbital osteotomy (craniofacial approach) for postero-superior masses.

Eyelid reconstruction must address the following:

- Skin coverage of good match from upper or contralateral lid or post-auricular skin
- Adequate length, laxity and support of flaps to avoid post-operative cicatrization and lid incompetency in conjunction with judicial use of cartilaginous grafts and tarsal fixation techniques
- Sufficient inner (conjunctival) lining to provide a physiologic covering for the globe.

Nasal reconstruction of the dorsum and tip is optimally accomplished through:

- Forehead (paramedian) flaps
- Deferred correction of standing cones ('dog ears') – these often settle with time
- Inform the patient of prolonged tip lymphoedema.

All properly selected and placed flaps will improve in appearance with simple massage, skin support dressings (silastic) and *time* – the patient must be informed of this beforehand.

FURTHER READING

Conley J, Patow C. *Primary regional flaps, flaps in head and neck surgery.* New York: Georg Thieme Verlag, 1989.

Jackson LT. *Local flaps in head and neck reconstruction.* St Louis: CV Mosby, 1985.

Jackson IT. Craniofacial tumours. In: Georgiade N, Georgiade G, Riefkohl R, Barwich W (eds). *Essentials in plastic, maxillofacial and reconstructive surgery*, vol. 1. Baltimore: Willams & Wilkins, 1992.

4.6

Local resection and reconstruction of oral carcinomas and lip cancer

ROBERT A ORD

PRINCIPLES AND JUSTIFICATION

Primary surgery is still regarded as the standard of care for most lip and oral cavity cancers, although radiation therapy may be equally effective in early lesions and is used where the patient is unfit, unresectable or refuses surgery. The major guiding principle is excision of the cancer with negative margins usually regarded as 5 mm or more of histologically normal tissue around the tumour for oral cavity squamous cell carcinomas. In order to achieve this, the surgeon will usually make his excision 1+ cm around the palpable defined margin of the cancer. In the tongue, which has aggressive infiltrative spread, 1.5–2 cm may be justified and in the lower lip 3–5 mm.

INDICATIONS

Any surgically resectable malignant tumour of the lip and oral cavity may be regarded as an indication for wide local resection which may be combined with a neck dissection or adjuvant radiation ± chemotherapy depending on the TNM stage of the lesion.

PRE-OPERATIVE

Anaesthesia

Operations are undertaken using general anaesthesia via a naso-endotracheal tube. In oral squamous cell carcinoma in smokers and drinkers, pan-endoscopy is undertaken first.

OPERATION

Carcinoma of the lower lip

Resection of the lip and repair can be divided into lesions requiring one-third of the lip or less to be resected, one-third to two-thirds of the lip to be resected and those tumours which require more than two-thirds of the lip to be resected.

In lesions less than one-third of the lip, the natural elasticity of the lip, especially in elderly patients, will allow primary closure. In very small lesions a shield-shaped incision (Figure 4.6.1) gives the greatest diameter at the vermillion border and reproduces the natural 'pout' and avoids the flattening seen with simple 'V' excision. Methylene blue may be used as a temporary tattoo to accurately reposition the skin–vermilion interface during closure. The lower lip is held tightly and compressed between finger and thumb by the assistant who everts the lip. The initial incision through skin is made with a 15-blade. The excision is continued with a needle tipped cautery through the obicularis muscle on both sides, taking care to identify the labial artery superiorly as the mucosal surface is approached. The artery is clipped or ligated and the

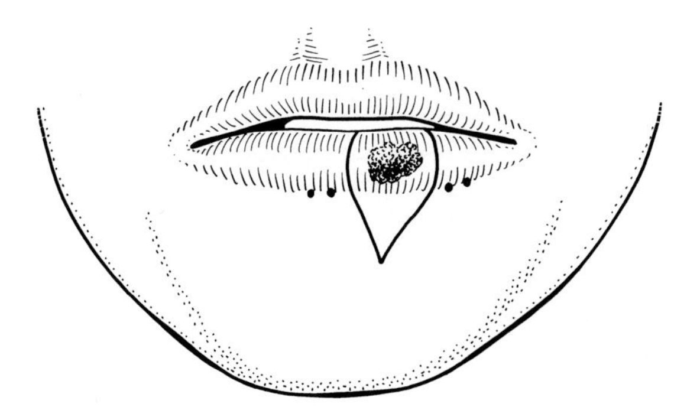

4.6.1 The tumour is marked with a 5mm margin and the vermilion skin junction on each side temporarily tattooed with two dots using methylene blue. This allows accurate suture and alignment post resection.

excision completed through mucosa. Frozen sections may be taken at the vermilion margins. The incision is closed in layers with 4/0 vicryl to mucosa, 3/0 vicryl through muscle and 5/0 nylon to skin with the vermilion border suture being placed first.

In slightly larger and deeper lesions, vertical incisions 3–5 mm from the tumour edge may be oncologically preferable to sloping incisions and a 'W' pattern of excision may be utilized (Figure 4.6.2). The method of excision and layered closure is identical. The wound is closed as a 'W to Y'.

Actinic damage affects the whole lip and in actinic keratosis or multifocal dysplasia/superficially invasive cancer vermilionectomy is indicated. This procedure can be combined with any of the other excisional techniques described in this section. The entire vermilion from the wet line to the skin is marked out with a surgical marking pen. The lower lip is stretched between skin hooks placed in the commissures and starting at one end, an 11-blade is used to transfix the width of the vermilion. Using a sawing motion, the blade is advanced across the lip to excise the entire vemilion (Figure 4.6.3a). The depth of excision will depend upon the depth of the lesion(s) being removed and local control of tumours with up to 3 mm maximum depth of invasion is reported. Multiple irritating bleeding points are coagulated. Closure is usually by an advancement flap of the labial mucosa which is mobilized with sharp scissors or fine mosquitoes dissecting submucosally in the layer between the mucosa and obicularis (Figure 4.6.3b). This simple reconstruction may cause thinning of the vermilion and eversion of beard bristles. Where more bulk is required, a tongue flap can be used. A variety of designs are available, but the bipedicled flap will resurface the entire vermillion (Figure 4.6.4a,b). Two parallel incisions, approximately 1 cm apart, are made with a needle point cautery transversely across the dorsum of the tongue. The bipedicled strip is dissected to a depth of 5 mm of muscle and raised as a bipedicle 'bucket handle'. The bases of the flap at the lateral sides of the tongue diverge to increase blood supply. The flap is passed forward and under the tongue tip and the tongue closed primarily. The central portion of the bipedicled flap is sutured to the lip and the flap pedicles divided 2–3 weeks later and inset to form the lateral portion of the lip vermilion. An alternative is the use of mucosal facial artery musculomucosal flaps (FAMM flaps), which will be discussed later in this chapter. In the office for superficial lesions and dysplasias, vermilionectomy with the carbon dioxide laser is an alternative.

In lesions that require resection of one-third to two-thirds of the lip, the author finds the 'stepladder' reconstruction gives the best results. The excision is marked as a rectangle with appropriate margins (Figure 4.6.5a). The flap design divides the length of the rectangle into A + B and the horizontal extension 'a' equals the length of A and 'b' the length of B. The vertical steps are 8–10 mm in height and the cross-hatched areas show the estimated areas of skin to be removed. (The author does not usually excise these areas until the end of the surgery when the flaps a and b are advanced and enough skin can be removed to avoid 'bunching'.) Incison through skin with a 15-blade and through obicularis with a needle point cautery is carried out,

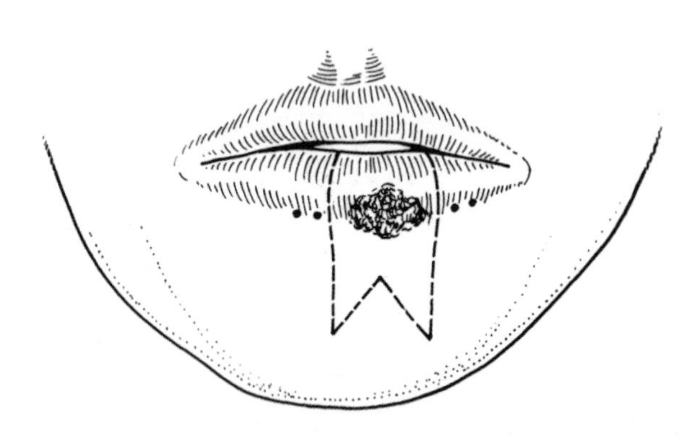

4.6.2 In a larger tumour the 'V' excision may compromise oncologic margins. Parallel excision as in this 'W' excision is preferred.

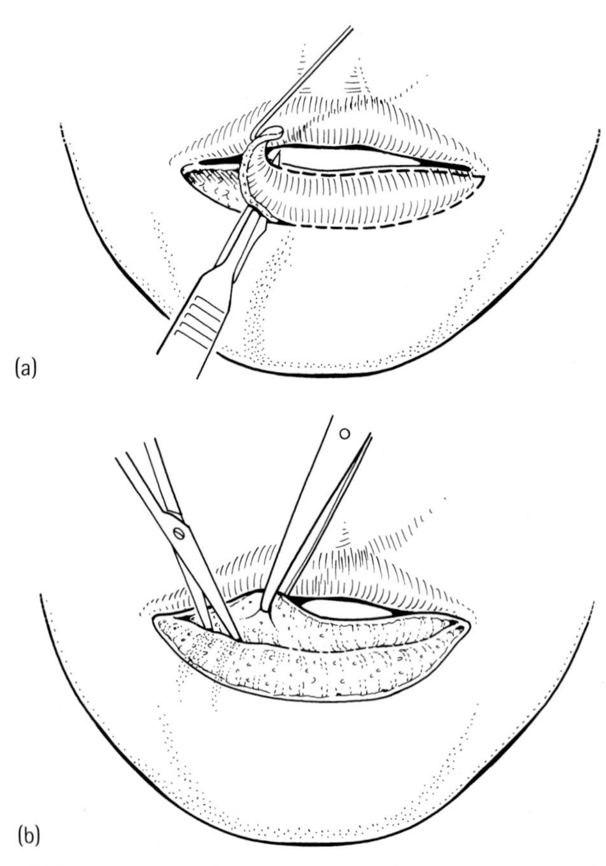

4.6.3 (a) The vermilion is excised in toto from wet line to vermilion-skin margin using a blade (a needle tipped cautery may also be used). (b) Undermining the oral mucosa with scissors to the depth of the sulcus to allow tension free advancement to reconstruct the vermillion.

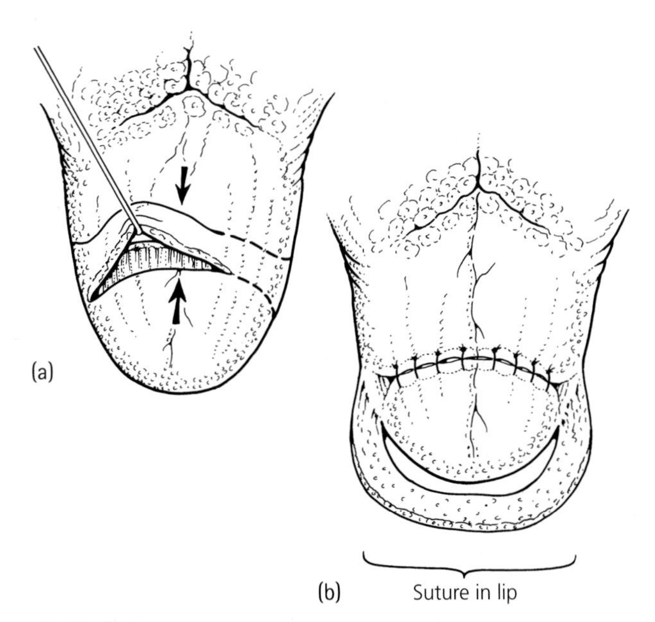

4.6.4 (a) Raising the bipediclled flap from the dorsal tongue. (b) The bipediclled flap is passed anteriorly like a 'bucket handle' to be sutured to the vermillion defect. The tongue is primarilly closed.

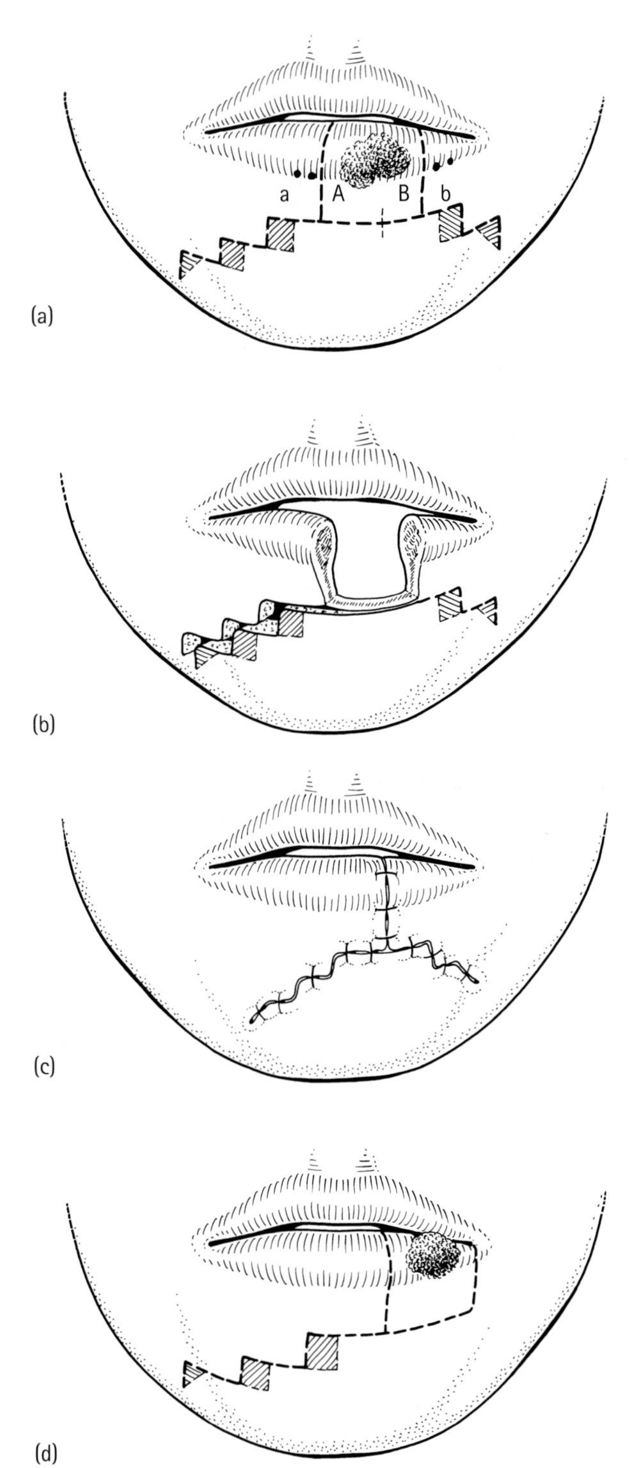

4.6.5 (a) Markings for flap, see text for explanation. (b) The tumour has been excised and the flap raised full thickness through skin and muscle. The mucosa can be left intact. Excess skin is removed in shaded areas to prevent 'dog ears'. (c) Closure. (d) Unilateral flap for lateral lesion.

the mucosa is left intact and does not need to be cut to mobilize the flaps (Figure 4.6.5b). The flaps are closed in layers, as previously described (Figure 4.6.5c). Unilateral flaps can be used for more lateral tumours (Figure 4.6.5d). The sutured incision should lie in the submental fold and the obicularis fibres maintain their natural orientation to maximize function.

When cancers involve the commissure and up to half the lip, the author prefers the geometric design of the McGregor variation of the fan flap. Three equal squares are outlined with a surgical marker as illustrated (Figure 4.6.6a). The tumour is excised as square A. The two other squares are raised as one large full thickness rectangle, the dotted line between B and C being purely for design purposes. The isthmus at the commissure, point X, must be carefully preserved as the pedicle with the superior labial artery is contained within this narrow strip of tissue. Square B is now rotated to reconstruct the lip and square C fills the defect from B (Figure 4.6.6b). The resultant defect is closed by the natural laxity of the cheek in the line of the nasolabial fold (Figure 4.6.6c). The vermilion is reconstructed by advancing the mucosa on the oral side of the flap.

In lesions requiring two-thirds to total lip excision, there are a number of options. The author prefers the Fries's modification of the Bernard flap. The tumour is excised as a rectangle and the flaps are designed as shown (Figure 4.6.7a). The full thickness flaps marked X and Y from the cheeks will be advanced to reconstruct the lip. The two cross-hatched triangles in the nasolabial fold and in the submental areas are Burow's triangles, where excess skin is removed to allow the flaps to advance. The tumour is excised full thickness and the skin incision from the commissure to the nasolabial fold made with a 15-blade sloping gently upward. The muscles are cut with the needle point cautery to the submucosal layer. The mucosa is undermined superiorly in the buccal area and cut superior to the skin

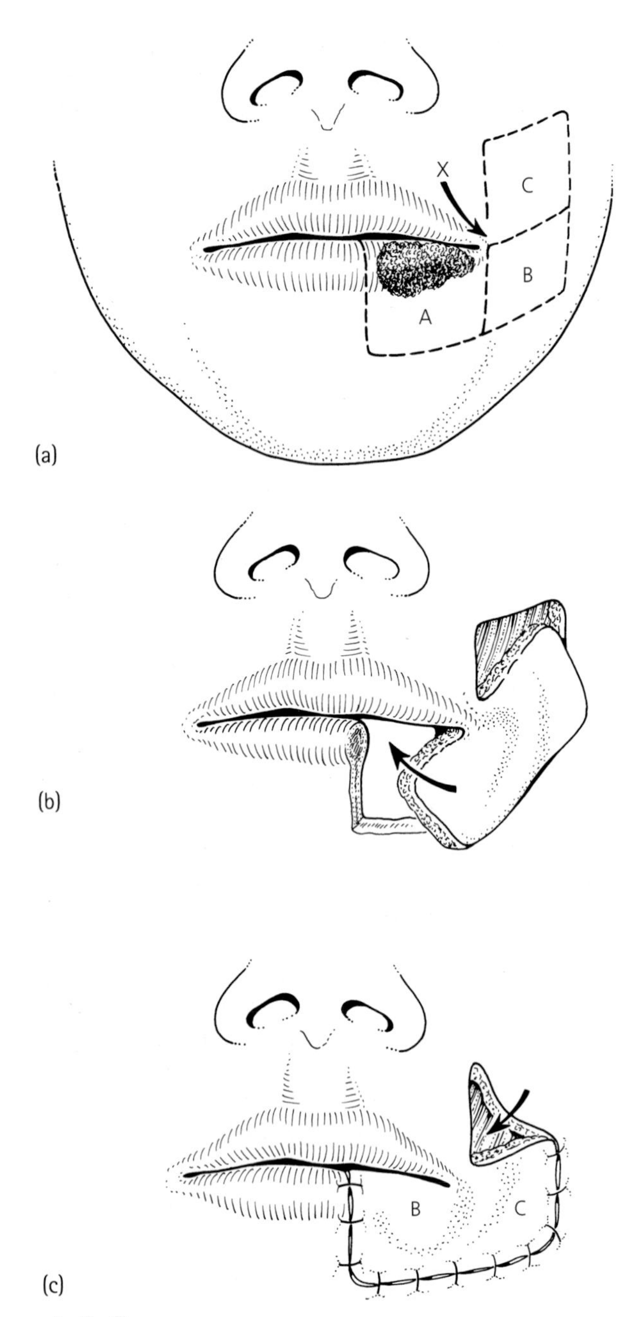

4.6.6 (a) Flaps drawn out, blood supply enters at point X. (b) Following tumour excision, square B is rotated to the defect and replaced in position by square C. (c) The loose cheek tissue superior to square C closes the defect in the nasolabial area.

incision to allow some excess mucosa to be advanced to reconstruct the vermilion. The inferior incision follows the labiomental fold into the submental region. This is a full thickness incision down to bone with an incision running back along the mucosa of the buccal vestibular sulcus to allow the flap to advance. The flaps are advanced with skin hook traction (Figure 4.6.7b). The Burow's triangles are excised as necessary to eliminate dog ears. The lip is closed in layers as previously described and care is taken to mobilize muscle from the upper lip and cheek flap to recreate the commissural sphincter at point Z. The commissure is recreated bilaterally with 0 non-resorbing sutures to prevent drooling (Figure 4.6.7c). This is a good reconstruction in an elderly person with lax cheeks, but may be tight with the lower lip inside the upper in a large total lip defect where local flaps may not give enough tissue, and free flaps should be considered.

Carcinoma of the floor of the mouth

In carcinomas of the floor of mouth, the elasticity of the mucosa can be deceiving and retraction of the tongue to mark out a 1-cm margin can stretch the mucosa giving a false idea of where to place the surgical excision margin. As much as possible, the margin should be marked with the tissues relaxed without retraction. In tumours that approach the mandible in the dentate patient, intraoral access can be difficult, particularly with lingually inclined teeth. Sometimes, a pull-through procedure is useful when neck dissection is also being carried out for adequate access. When an intraoral resection is planned in these circumstances, the surgeon should incise the mucosa on the mandible first down to bone (point x–y marks the level of incision) and lift a subperiosteal flap (Figure 4.6.8). If the periosteum is intact and the bone totally uninvolved, this is a good surgical margin. The periosteum is now incised horizontally deep in the sulcus (indicated by an arrow on Figure 4.6.8). This is similar to the buccal advancement flaps for oro-antral fistula closure which allows the specimen to be moved medially away from the lingual side of the mandible with better visualization and access to the tumour. Most floor of the mouth cancers are found anteriorly near the midline and, when neck dissection is not being performed simultaneously, Wharton's duct must be identified and preserved. When dissecting through the area of the sublingual gland, Wharton's duct will be located on the medial side of the gland and will lie increasingly deeply, the more posterior the surgical margin lies. Sharp dissection with scissors rather than a cautery is used to dissect through the submucosal tissue and the sublingual gland to find the duct. The proximal end of the duct is tagged with a 6/0 nylon suture to prevent retraction once the duct is sectioned. Once the duct is cut, milking the submandibular gland with subsequent salivary flow will confirm the identity of the duct. At this point, the resection is completed with a needle point cautery maintaining a centimetre margin (dashed line on Figure 4.6.9a). The specimen is oriented with sutures for the pathologist and frozen sections are sent. Submucosal dissection with a fine mosquito to a point 1 cm behind the resection margin is undertaken (point x on Figure 4.6.9a) and an opening through mucosa made at this point with a No. 15 blade (Figure 4.6.9a). A fine mosquito is passed through this opening from the mucosal surface and picks up the 6/0 nylon suture tagging the duct. Gentle traction brings the duct through the opening to its new proximal location. One point of the scissors is inserted into the lumen of the duct (using Loupes if necessary) and a 1-cm cut made

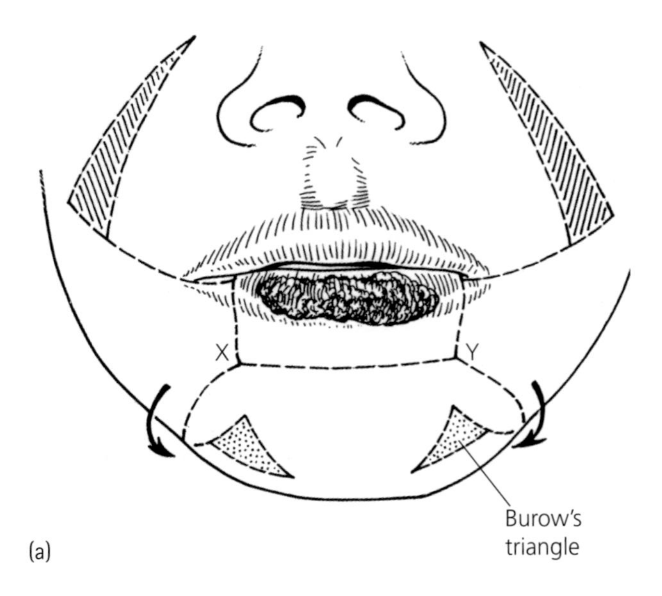

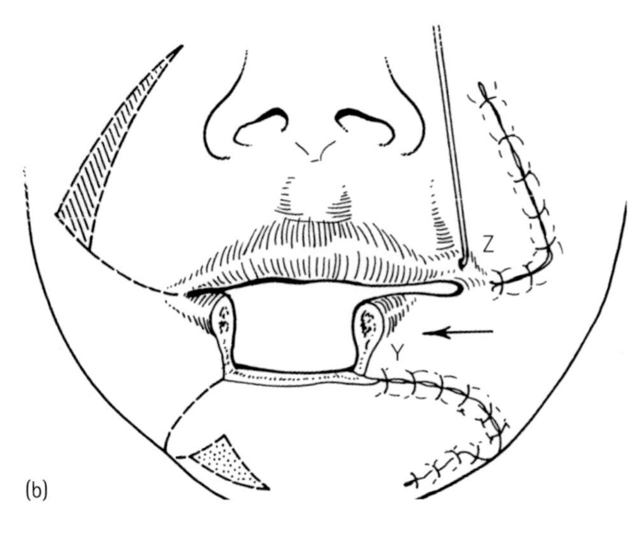

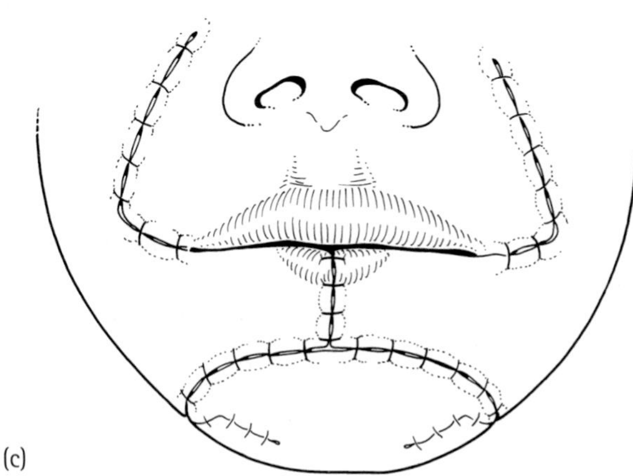

4.6.7 (a) Planned rectangular excision, with shaded areas representing Burow's triangles where skin will be excised in the nasolabial and submental regions to allow flaps X and Y to advance without 'bunching and dog ears'. (b) Flaps X and Y advanced to reconstruct the lip. Large '0' Prolene nonresobable suture is placed to suture upper lip and lower lip obicularis muscles together to reconstruct commissure and prevent drooling. (c) Flaps sutured in layers.

along the line of the duct (marked x Figure 4.6.9b). The duct is then opened as a fish tail and sutured to the mucosa which allows easy fixation and less potential stricture formation (Figure 4.6.9c).

Tumours of the palate

The majority of these tumours are of salivary gland origin and fortunately most are low grade. They usually occur at the junction of the hard and soft palate and will frequently involve the area of the greater palatine foramen and the greater palatine artery. When the periosteum is intact and there is no bone involvement, a soft tissue resection only can be performed. (Obviously, this is not the case in high-grade tumours, such as adenoidcystic carcinoma where maxillectomy will be required.) In planning excision, a 1-cm margin is marked and then developed through mucosa only, with a needle point cautery. First, the thin mucosa of the middle of the palate is incised down to bone with the cautery (margin 'a' on Figure 4.6.10). Next, margin 'b' is cut down to bone. Here, the mucosa is thicker and some oozing may be encountered. Before completing the anterior margin 'c', a periosteal elevator is used to raise the periosteum for a few millimetres along margins 'a' and 'b'. Then the anterior cut 'c' is completed carefully and hopefully the greater palatine artery can be identified and coagulated or clipped before it retracts under the thick mucosa. If this is not the case, the cut can be completed down to bone and joined to 'a' and 'b' to allow rapid mobilization and raising of the anterior portion of the specimen with easier identification of the bleeding vessel. Occasionally, the distal end of the artery will retract into the anterior portion of the palatal tissue and prove difficult to control. In these circumstances, a large 2/0 black silk haemostatic suture is

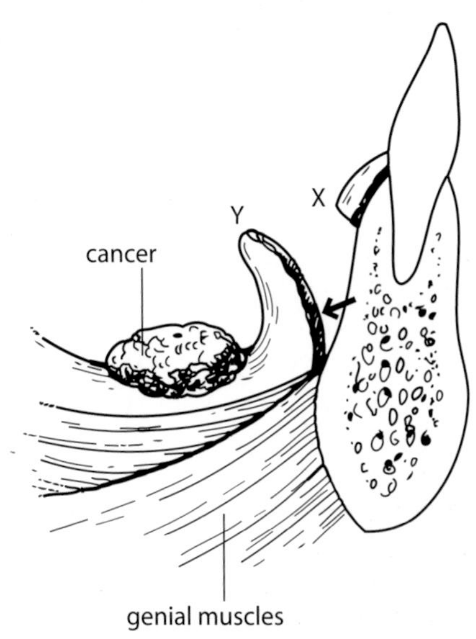

4.6.8 Shows lingual incision of mucosa (point X) and then of periosteum at site of arrow to allow mobilization of the floor of mouth and visualization of a floor of mouth cancer close to the lingual mandible.

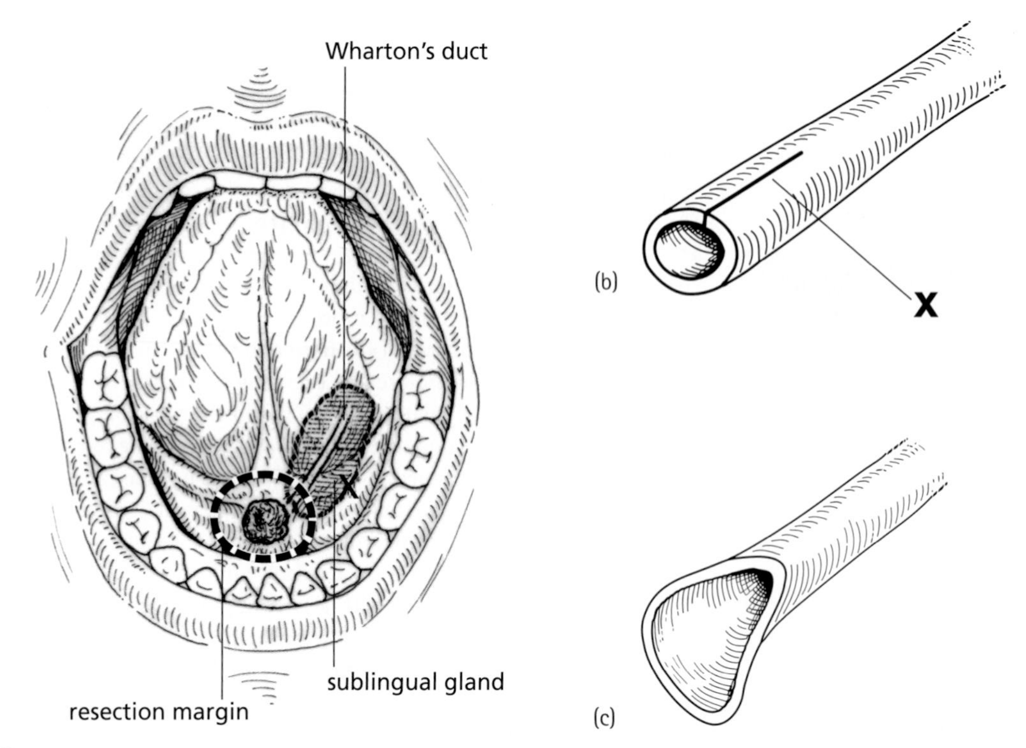

4.6.9 (a) Proposed resection will transect Wharton's duct which will require repositioning. (b) and (c) illustrate 'fish tail' sialodochoplasty.

passed full thickness through the mucosa down to the bone on the medial side of the bleeding and brought up on the lateral side. When tied tightly, the vessel is occluded. The specimen is now mobilized off the bony hard palate with a periosteal elevator until the greater palatine vessel is seen entering its foramen. In very thick palates, this can be a difficult dissection and completing cut 'd' through the soft palate mucosa allows more mobility and visualization.

Usually a right angle can be passed behind the greater palatine artery to pick up a tie and ligate the vessel or a medium clip can be used. If the vessel should be cut and retract into the foramen when not ligated, cautery may not be successful and bone wax is used. It is rare to need a full thickness resection through the soft palate and the musculo-aponeurosis usually defines the depth of dissection at this site. The resection is completed and the specimen oriented for the pathologist with sutures.

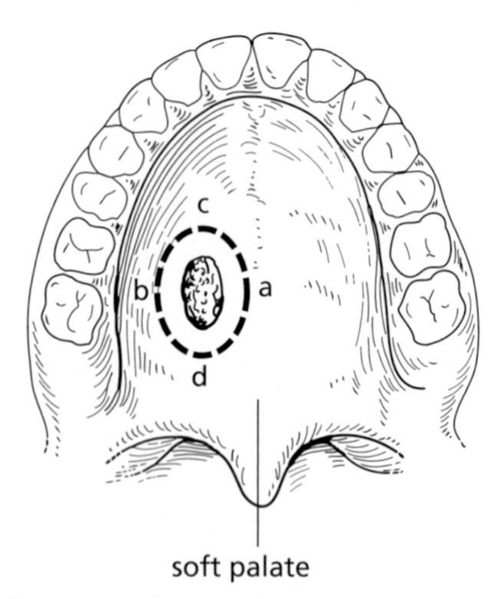

4.6.10 Excision of palatal tumour. See text for details.

Tumours of the tongue

Tongue cancer is the most common oral cancer and behaves aggressively with early muscle invasion. Wide margins of 1.5 cm are justified and an adequate depth of excision is required. Tumours on the anterior and middle third of the oral tongue are usually resectable from an intraoral approach. Those more posteriorly sited may require a mandibulotomy or 'pull through'. It is important after using a surgical marker to delineate the margin of resection to always cut away from the tumour by angling the needle point cautery (as shown by A in Figure 4.6.11). Retraction of the tongue or spreading of the muscle with clamps prior to cutting with the cautery tends to stretch the muscles and subsequent retraction may reduce the safe margin. Angling away from the tumour will reduce this tendency. The surgeon should aim to have a depth of 1-cm muscle deep to the tumour and, for most T2 tumours, the depth will involve the midline septum. In small lesions where primary closure is used, it is important to close the tongue parallel to its length to maintain the length of the tongue for speech. Deep muscle sutures in layers and horizontal everting mattress sutures through the mucosa may help prevent wound dehiscence, which is common in glossectomy due to muscle pull opening the suture line.

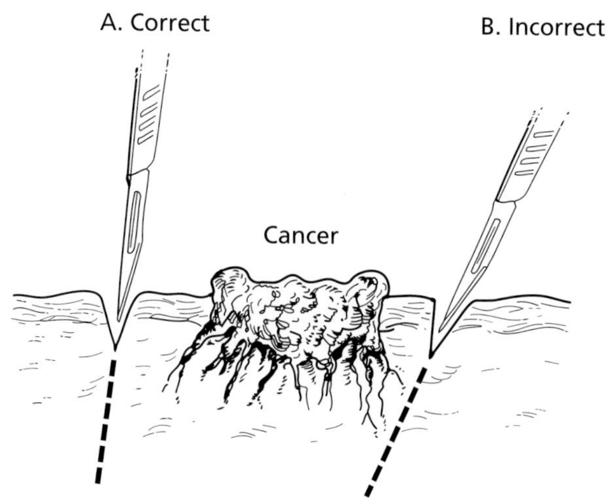

4.6.11 Shows correct A and incorrect B angulation for tumour excision.

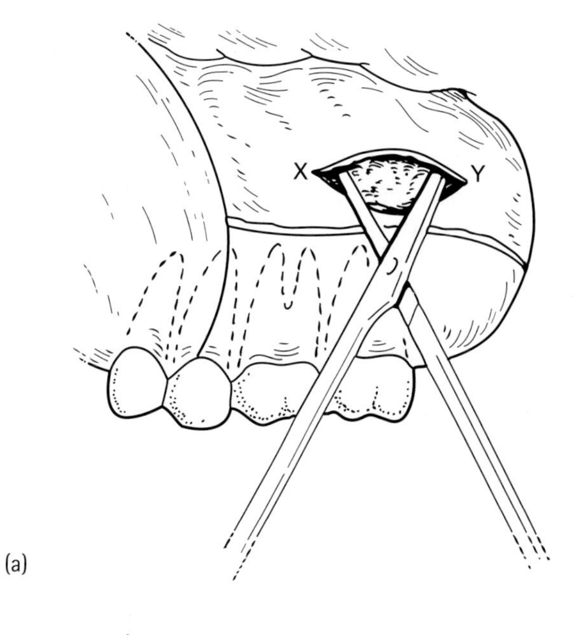

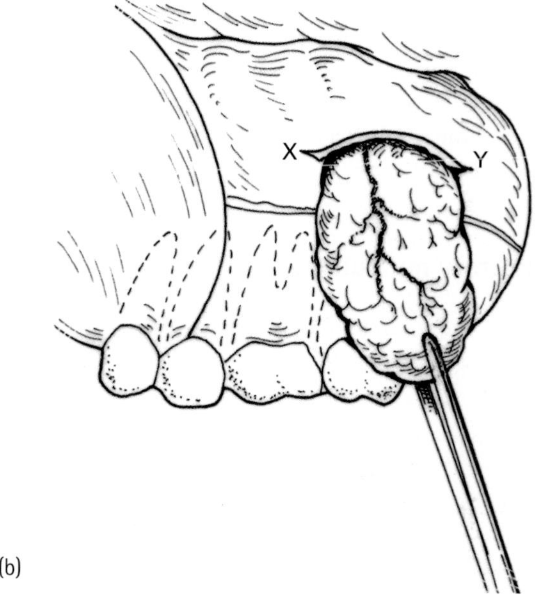

4.6.12 (a) Mucoperiosteal flap reflected and horizontal incision X–Y through the periosteum opposite the maxillary second molar allows access to the buccal fat pad. (b) Using a clamp or scissors to spread the tissues around the fascia of the buccal fat pad flap allows the pad to be mobilised or prolapsed into the mouth.

RECONSTRUCTION

In considering the ladder of reconstruction, many small oral defects may be satisfactorily dealt with by primary closure, skin grafting or local flaps. In larger cases where microvascular-free flaps are not being utilized but imported tissue is required, there are a number of useful local pedicled flaps available to the surgeon. This section will review the buccal fat pad, sebmental island and facial artery musculomucosal flaps.

Buccal fat pad flap

This flap is simple, quick and convenient for the surgeon and can be used to reconstruct defects of the maxillary alveolus (including oro-antral fistulas), the hard palate, soft palate, cheek and retromolar region. The flap is accessed via an incision through the periosteum opposite the second maxillary molar after raising a buccal mucoperiosteal flap (Figure 4.6.12a). The buccal fat pad may prolapse into the wound and be immediately available or may require blunt dissection with clamps or McIndoes around the capsule to release fibrous bands. The buccal fat pad is recognizable as it does not have the small lobules seen in the adjacent adipose tissue. Once the buccal fat pad has been mobilized, it is teased free of the surrounding tissues maintaining its thin fibrous capsule and rotated into the defect using gentle traction with non-toothed forceps (Figure 4.6.12b). The surgeon may see the vessels giving the flap its vascularity entering from superiorly. The flap is sutured to the defect margins with 4/0 vicryl sutures. No skin grafting is necessary and the flap will mucosalize over a 3–4-week period.

Submental island flap

This flap is based on the submental branches of the facial artery and anterior facial vein, and provides a thin pliable skin paddle for reconstruction of the lower two-thirds of the face and the entire oral cavity. Its use in malignant tumours of the anterior oral cavity, where a sound dissection of the submental triangle is oncologically necessary, is contraindicated. In elderly patients with lax submental skin, a large skin paddle up to 15×7 cm is available. The pinch test can be used to assess the ease of closure. The skin paddle is marked in the submental region crossing the midline (Figure 4.6.13a). The upper incision 'a' is made 1–1.5 cm below the chin sloping away and two fingers breadth below the mandible at the angle. This incision can of course be incorporated into a neck dissection incision. The dissection is carried down through subcutaneous fat and platysma muscle and the marginal branch of the facial nerve should be identified crossing the anterior facial vein and preserved bilaterally. The lower incision 'b' is carried out in the same manner. The skin paddle is dissected in a subplatysmal plane. At this point, the flap can be raised from distally back towards the vascular pedicle or from the vascular pedicle forward. We usually identify the facial artery and vein as they run on the posterior and medial side of the submandibular gland. Small branches passing into the gland are clipped. The submental artery and vein are identified running horizontally superficial to the mylohyoid muscle close to the inferior border of the mandible (Figure 4.6.13b) branches to the mylohyoid and lingual periosteum are clipped and any cutaneous perforators passing through platysma identified and preserved. The vessels pass to the angle where the anterior belly of the digastric muscle inserts to the mandible. As 70 per cent of these vessels pass below the digastric muscle and send perforators through the muscle belly, it is necessary to detach the muscle from the hyoid and the mandible and include it in the flap in the majority of cases. The skin paddle can now be rotated to its required site. The arc of rotation can be improved by proximal dissection of the facial artery and veins ligating any branches (Figure 4.6.14a–c).

Facial artery musculomucosal flap

The facial artery runs obliquely across the cheek from where it crosses the mandible just anterior to the masseter muscle to the area of the alar nasi. The artery runs lateral to the buccinator muscle. Although the vein accompanies the artery as they cross the mandible, the two vessels diverge as they ascend with the vein lying posterior to the artery up to 15 mm at the alar. The vein is usually not incorporated in the flap and venous drainage is by multiple small veins that form the buccal plexus. The flap can be based superiorly or inferiorly, although the inferior based flaps are more reliable. These long thin axial flaps can be used to reconstruct the palate, alveolus, lips and nasal fistulae. As originally described, the facial artery is identified with a laser Doppler and marked on the buccal mucosa. In inferiorly based flaps, an incision is made through mucosa fat and buccinator at the level of the alar and the facial artery identified, tied and cut. A full thickness strip of mucosa, fat and buccinator 1–2 cm wide is raised incorporating the facial artery on the surface of the muscle for the whole length of the flap. At the base, the facial vein may be seen and also included, but this is not essential. This 'finger' flap can be transposed with its mucosal pedicle intact or the mucosa only can be cut leaving a good soft tissue base for vascular supply as an island flap. The defect is closed primarily. One of the disadvantages is the vulnerability of the pedicle to trauma from the teeth if the flap is used to reconstruct the tongue or floor of the mouth and crosses the occlusal plane. However, if a selective neck dissection has been carried out with preservation of the facial artery and anterior facial vein, these vessels can be

(a)

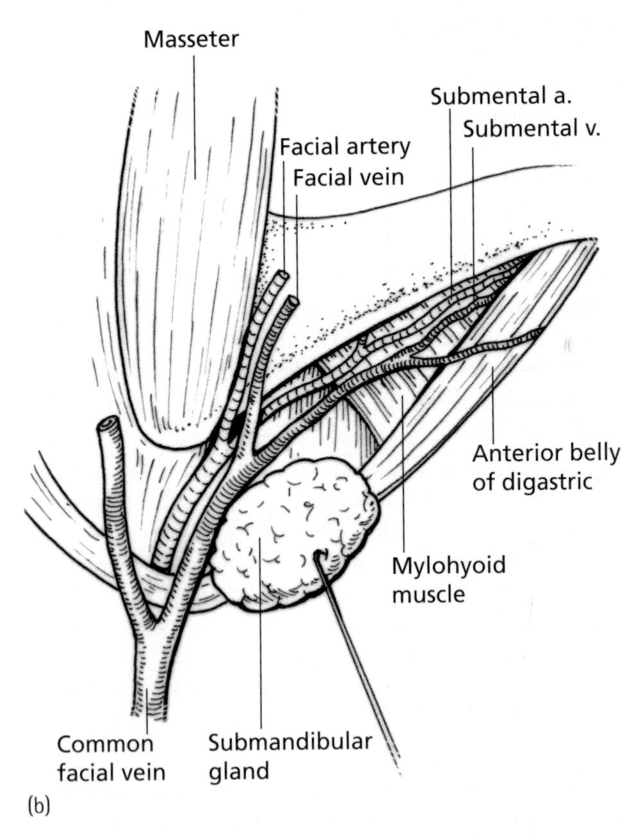

(b)

4.6.13 (a) Skin flap marked in submental region (see text for details). (b) Usual anatomical distrubution of submental vessels.

dissected superiorly to connect with the intraoral dissection, as described above. Taking care not to damage branches of the facial nerve running superficial to the vessels, the flap can be brought into the neck and transferred to the mouth via a tunnel lingual to the mandible (Figure 4.6.15) to reconstruct the floor of the mouth and tongue.

POST-OPERATIVE CARE

In resections of the floor of the mouth and tongue, adequate monitoring of the airway must be undertaken as swelling may cause breathing difficulty. In cases where considerable swelling is anticipated, the airway will have been secured by leaving the endotracheal tube in place or by tracheotomy. All flaps should be monitored for congestion or ischaemia. The author dislikes dressings on lip reconstructions, although Neomycin ointment may be used on the suture line.

COMPLICATIONS

Complications, such as bleeding, may be seen especially in tongue resections and time taken to obtain a dry field at the end of the case is well spent. Also wound dehiscence in primary closure of the tongue or floor of the mouth is not uncommon. Usually, resuturing is not productive and the wound is kept clean and allowed to granulate. In floor of mouth and lip resections, mucocoeles may occur and are treated by removing the underlying minor salivary glands. Scarring and tethering are dealt with secondarily after six months of healing.

(a)

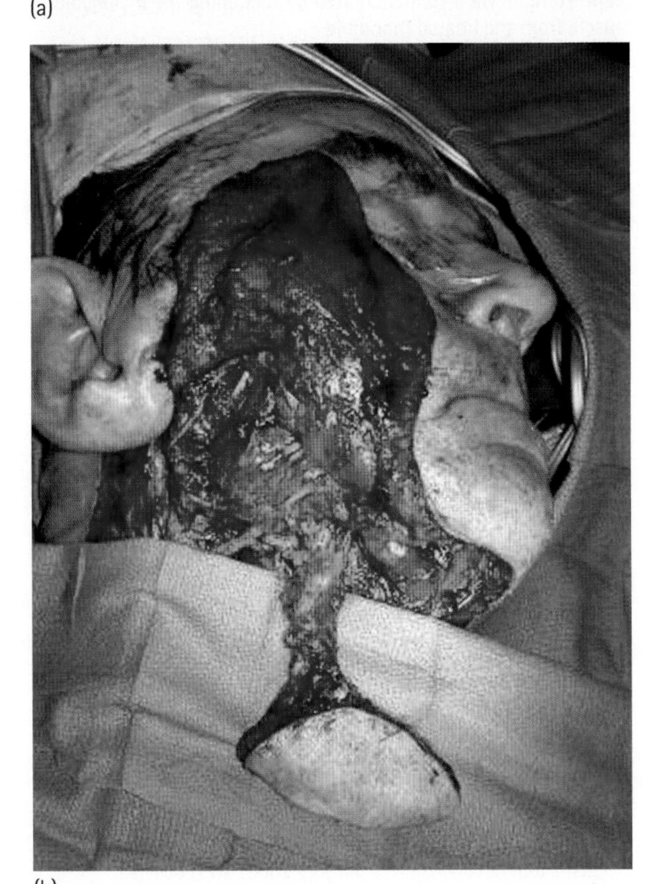

(b)

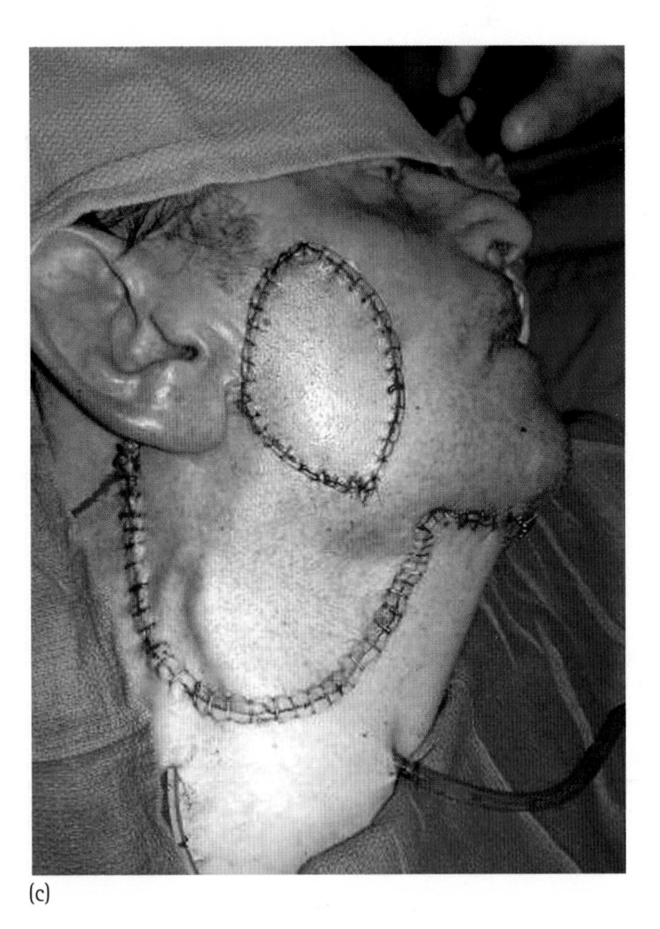

(c)

4.6.14 (a) Patient with desmoplastic melanoma of the parotid for sentinel node biopsy + selctive neck, parotidectomy with skin resection and submental flap marked out; (b) island flap based on submental vessels; (c) flap inset to show good arc of rotation for lower face.

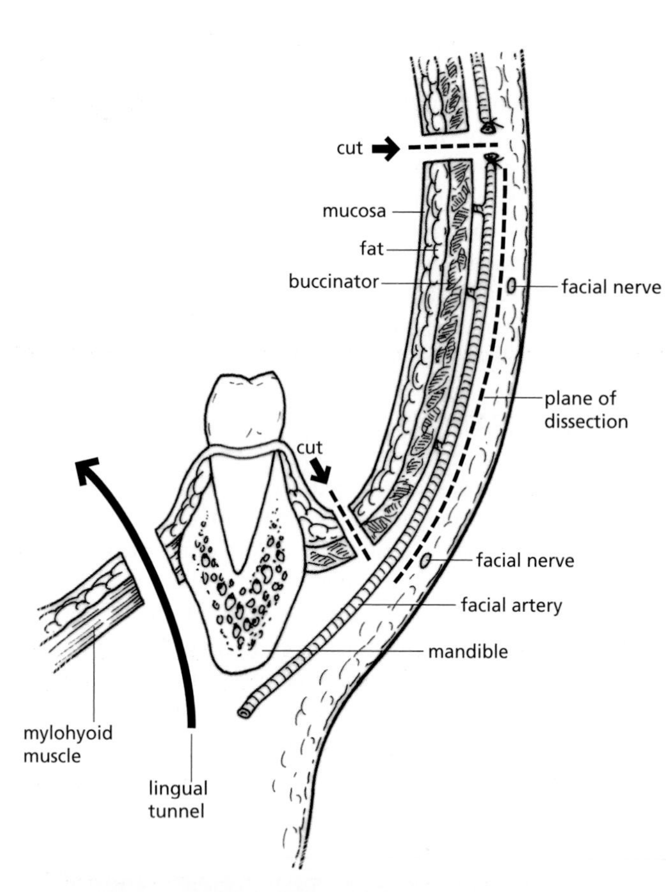

4.6.15 Section through cheek in premolar region to illustrate anatomy of FAMM flap. Dotted line is deep margin lateral to buccinator and facial artery. The two small arrows show full thickness incision superiorly with ligation of the facial artery. The inferior incision is through mucosa and muscle only preserving the vessels and developing a mucosal island flap. The flap is mobilised into the neck and transposed to the floor of mouth/tongue via a tunnel created by sectioning the mylohyoid muscle from the lingual mandible.

Top tips

- Spend time to accurately align the skin–vermilion line in lip closure. Even small malalignments are very obvious to the observer.
- Recreate the muscular commissure with obicularis from the upper and lower lip sutured with a large non-resorbable suture to avoid drooling.
- Section the lingual periosteum low down to allow better access to the floor of the mouth cancer close to, but not involving, the mandibular lingual plate.
- Use a haemostatic suture full thickness for bleeding from the palatine artery that retracts into the palatal tissue.
- Use bone wax for bleeding from the greater palatine artery that has retracted into the bony foramen.
- Although lateral tongue defects can be closed primarily, when they are close to or involve the floor of the mouth, a flap reconstruction will prevent tethering and allow better function.
- In the tongue, it is the deep margin which is most deceptive and the worst site to have a recurrence, usually resecting more muscle than you might think is better.

FURTHER READING

Dupoirieux L, Plane CL, Gard C, Penneau M. Anatomical basis and results of the facial artery musculomucosal flap for oral reconstruction. *British Journal of Oral and Maxillofacial Surgery* 1999; **37**: 25–8.

Faltous AA, Yetman RJ. The submental artery flap: An anatomic study. *Plastic and Reconstructive Surgery* 1996; **97**: 56–62.

Johanson B, Aspelund E, Breine U, Holmstrom H. Surgical treatment of non-traumatic lower lip lesions with special reference to the step technique. *Scandanavian Journal Plastic Reconstructive Surgery* 1974; **8**: 232–40.

Langdon JD, Ord RA. The surgical management of lip cancer. *Journal of Cranio-maxillofacial Surgery* 1987; **15**: 281–7.

Martin AD, Pascal JF, Baudet J *et al.* The submental island flap: A new donor site. Anatomy and clinical applications as a free or pedicled flap. *Plastic and Reconstructive Surgery* 1993; **92**: 867–73.

Pribaz J, Stephens W, Crespo L, Gifford G. A new intraoral flap: Facial artery musculomucosal (FAMM) flap. *Plastic and Reconstructive Surgery* 1992; **90**: 421–9.

Pribaz JJ, Meara JG, Wright S *et al.* Lip and vermilion reconstruction with the facial artery musculomucosal flap. *Plastic and Reconstructive Surgery* 2000; **105**: 864–72.

van der Wal JE, de Viisscher JGAM, Baart JA, Van der Waal I. Oncologic aspects of vermilionectomy in microinvasive squamous cell carcinoma of the lower lip. *International Journal Oral Maxillofacial Surgery* 1996; **25**: 446–8.

4.7

Jaw resection

JAMES S BROWN

RESECTION OF THE MANDIBLE AND MAXILLA

General principles

This chapter concentrates on the resection of squamous cell carcinoma arising in the oral cavity or the midface. A similar approach is required for the resection of bone invaded by malignant salivary tumours, but the points on the patterns of tumour invasion and entry may be different. The principles of the resection techniques may be appropriate to the management of odontogenic tumours, especially if these are recurrent. Resection of the jaws for osteoradionecrosis or osteonecrosis is more of a debridement requiring the resection of bone back to a bleeding base prior to reconstruction. Bone resection for osteosarcoma or primary intraosseous carcinoma requires a more radical removal of bone as the tumour will invade the bone preferentially.

Applied anatomy

MANDIBLE

The mandible provides a bony framework to hold the teeth and sensation to the lip and chin is provided by the inferior alveolar nerve which enters at the mandibular foramen and exits at the mental foramen. Although there are often attempts to preserve this nerve in the treatment of benign disease, the loss of sensation to the lip and chin is an acceptable morbidity for most patients. The relationship of the teeth to the bone varies with patients and the molars run from a buccal position to a more lingual position posteriorly. The temporomandibular joint articulates with the skull base and in some cases the condylar head may require resection. The loss of teeth results in the loss of the supporting alveolar bone. The inferior alveolar nerve will come to lie on the alveolar ridge and the relationship of the floor of mouth muscle insertions will alter with the loss of bone (Figure 4.7.1).

MAXILLA

The maxilla is a complex structure which provides bone for the upper dental arch, supporting the alar base and facial curtain, as well as providing the orbital floor, malar buttress and lateral nasal wall. It is important to understand the articulation with the rest of the skeleton in tumour resection.

Medially, the lateral nasal wall is the least important structure, but care is required in maintaining the lacrimal system. The frontal process of the maxilla and the nasal bones articulate with the frontal bone and immediately behind these structures is the ethmoid sinus and then the sphenoid sinus. The cranium lies directly above these bones and experience in skull base resections is required to safely resect these structures. The lamina papyracea of the medial wall often requires resection and care must be taken to identify the anterior ethmoidal artery in particular. The

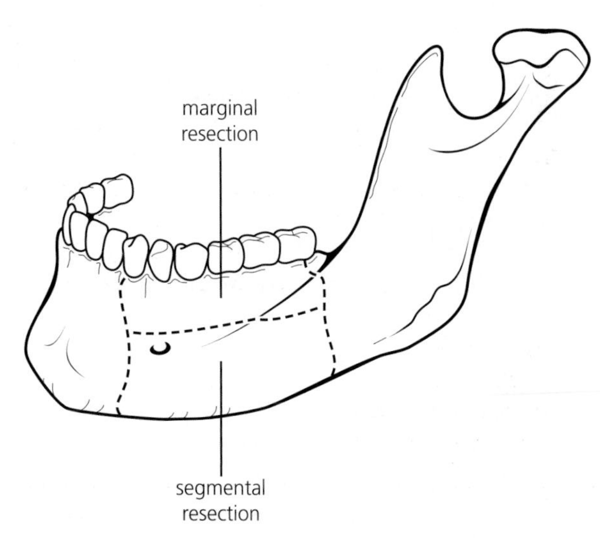

4.7.1 A rim or marginal resection maintains the lower border and a segment requires the full thickness of the mandible to be resected.

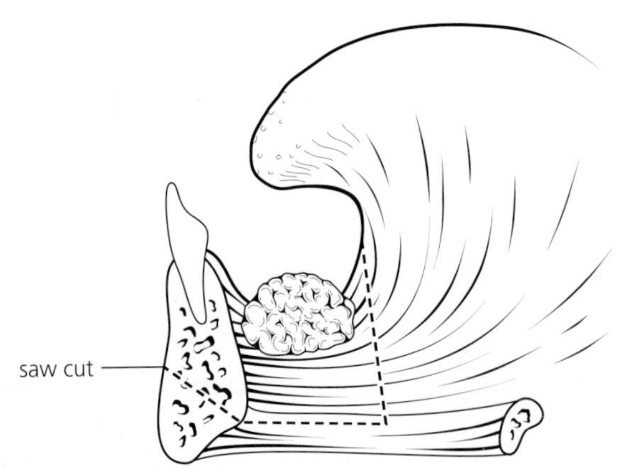

4.7.2 The most common form of rim resection is coronal. This figure illustrates the method used to enter the floor of the mouth deep to the tumour to obtain a clear margin, even though the bone is not invaded.

maxilla provides much of the orbital floor as far as the inferior orbital fissure, and more laterally the lateral wall is made up of the greater wing of the sphenoid and the malar.

MANDIBULAR RESECTION FOR ORAL SQUAMOUS CELL CARCINOMA

Patterns of invasion and routes of tumour entry

Early or shallow invasion of the mandible from the oral cavity will often show an erosive pattern with a pushing front and a connective tissue layer separating the bone from the tumour. The more infiltrative pattern is related to deeper invasion in which the connective tissue layer is lost and separate islands of tumour infiltrate in a less favourable manner. It is not possible to predict the pattern of invasion, so the judgement on how much bone to resect remains clinical and based on imaging.

Various theories of the route of tumour entry to the mandible have been suggested, but it seems most likely that the tumour enters the mandible at the point of contact. In the dentate mandible, this tends to be at the junction of the attached and reflected mucosa and in the edentulous mandible this is more likely at the crest of the ridge due to the lowering of the floor of the mouth due to the loss of teeth. These are important issues if a marginal or more conservative resection of the mandible is being considered.

Pre-operative assessment

There are multiple papers looking at pre-operative imaging techniques and their accuracy in predicting the presence of tumour invasion of the mandible. A recent review article has summarized the findings which are included in Table 4.7.1.

A widely accepted standard is to use magnetic resonance imaging (MRI) as a standard image of the primary tumour and the neck nodes. This will usually provide 5-mm slices and will include T_1, T_2 and fat suppression sequences, as well as gadolinium enhancement. The fat suppression sequence is the most sensitive in indicating tumour invasion of the mandible. The only additional image would be an orthopantomogram if there is clear invasion of the mandible or in which the mandible is unlikely to be invaded. For tumours in which it is unclear if the mandible is invaded, a SPECT (single photon emission computed tomography) scan is included to get a further sensitive imaging of the mandible. The combination of an image with a high specificity with one with a high sensitivity can provide a reasonably accurate prediction of the extent of mandibular invasion and therefore the most appropriate method of resection. A widely accepted classification of the mandible following the loss of teeth has been published and it is clear that in class V and VI mandibles (Figure 4.7.2), there is insufficient height of bone to safely perform a marginal resection for malignant disease. As a result, a guide to mandibular resection has been published which relates to the size of the mandible and the results of the investigations predicting bone invasion (Table 4.7.2).

Table 4.7.1 Summary and comparison of the imaging techniques and clinical examination.

Imaging technique	No. reports	Specificity (mean)	Sensitivity (mean)
Clinical examination	9	66	81
Plain radiography	18	81	76
Bone scintigraphy	15	74	93
SPECT	3	65	97
Computed tomography	7	88	78
DentaScan	3	–	–
Magnetic resonance imaging	4	86	81
Ultrasound	2	93	86

SPECT, single photo emission computed tomography.

Table 4.7.2 The results of the investigations predicting bone invasion.

Mandible classification OPG–, MRI–, BS–	no invasion/periosteal invasion OPG– MRI or BS+	early invasion (<5 mm) OPG+, MRI+, BS+	late invasion (>5 mm)
1–2 (dentate)	Rim	Rim	Rim/segment
3–4 (>20 mm mandibular height)	Rim	Rim/segment	Segment
5–6 (<20 mm mandibular height)	Rim/segment	Segment	Segment

BS, bone scan; MRI, magnetic resonance imaging; OPG, orthopantomogram.

Methods of mandibular resection

In the past the 'commando' operation in which the body of the mandible was sacrificed to remove potential lymphatics containing tumour and to facilitate the soft tissue reconstruction has now been discontinued and yet there are series published in which only 29 per cent of the resected mandibles were invaded by tumour. As in all oncological surgery, the aim is to cure the patient of disease through adequate resection. At the same time, the skilled surgeon should be trying to reduce the morbidity of the operation to a minimum and maintain the best possible function. Good functional results for patients depend more on the tissue left behind than the method of reconstruction.

There are two basic methods of mandibular resection. In the marginal or rim resection, the integrity of the lower or upper border of the mandible is kept intact (Figure 4.7.1). In the full or segmental resection of the mandible, both the upper and lower border are included in the resection so that there is a loss of continuity of the mandible. There is clear evidence to show that functional and aesthetic results are poor if the continuity of the mandible is not restored. The need to reconstruct the mandible to achieve the best functional and aesthetic result will often involve composite free tissue transfers for malignant disease, which will add to the donor site morbidity and increase the risk of flap failure.

MARGINAL OR RIM RESECTION

In the treatment of infective or osteonecrotic disorders, this is a general debridement of dead or infected tissue leaving the lower border intact. As such, there is no special technique to be adopted. If a margin of normal tissue is required in the treatment of odontogenic tumours or a wider margin in malignant disease then there are important anatomical factors that come into the equation.

A marginal resection of the mandible can be performed in the coronal or the sagittal plane. In the majority of cases, a coronal marginal resection is used (Figure 4.7.2). This is the standard method for tumours in which a margin of normal bone is required. It can be used for smaller odontogenic tumours in which there is sufficient residual bone to maintain the lower border. A sagittal marginal resection cannot be used for bone pathology as obtaining any kind of margin is not possible. It has been used for floor of the mouth squamous cell carcinomas to obtain a clear margin when tumour is abutting the mandible, but not obviously invading. This is a high risk strategy as any invasion through the cortex will be reported as an involved margin. In addition, the angle of the mandible in the body region is difficult to judge (Figure 4.7.3). In this situation, it is a safer oncological approach to perform a segmental resection of the mandible. Rim resections that involve the ramus of the mandible can only be done in the coronal plane as the ramus is too thin to split for oncological reasons and it is best to include the coronoid process, as this may reduce trismus post-operatively.

If the lower border of the mandible is to be preserved, then 10 mm of the depth of bone will be necessary for jaw continuity to be reliably maintained.

For marginal resections involving malignant disease except osteosarcomas and primary intraosseous carcinomas, it is possible to assess the extent of tumour invasion into the mandible from the surrounding soft tissues and estimate the extent of the resection required. This technique is illustrated in Figure 4.7.4. Note that periosteal stripping to assess the presence of mandibular invasion and its extent has been used. The use of periosteal stripping is an essential part of the technique in the decision-making process for mandibular resection. It has been shown to be a reliable technique and, in a large series from the unit in Liverpool, the involved bone margin rate is very low compared to the soft tissue margin rate.

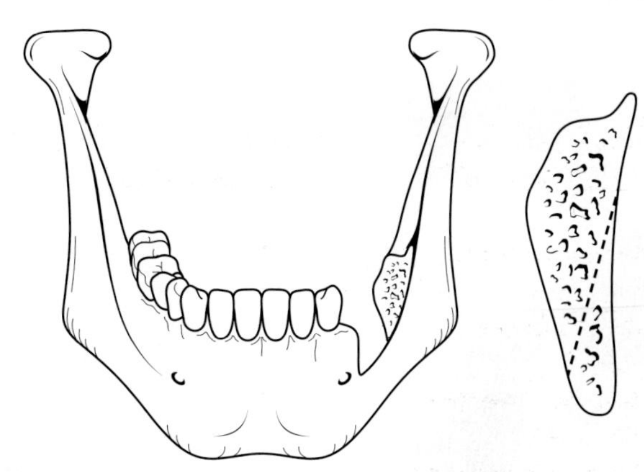

4.7.3 This is a partial sagittal rim resection, but this diagram illustrates the angle of the body of the mandible from medial to lateral if the full sagittal rim is required.

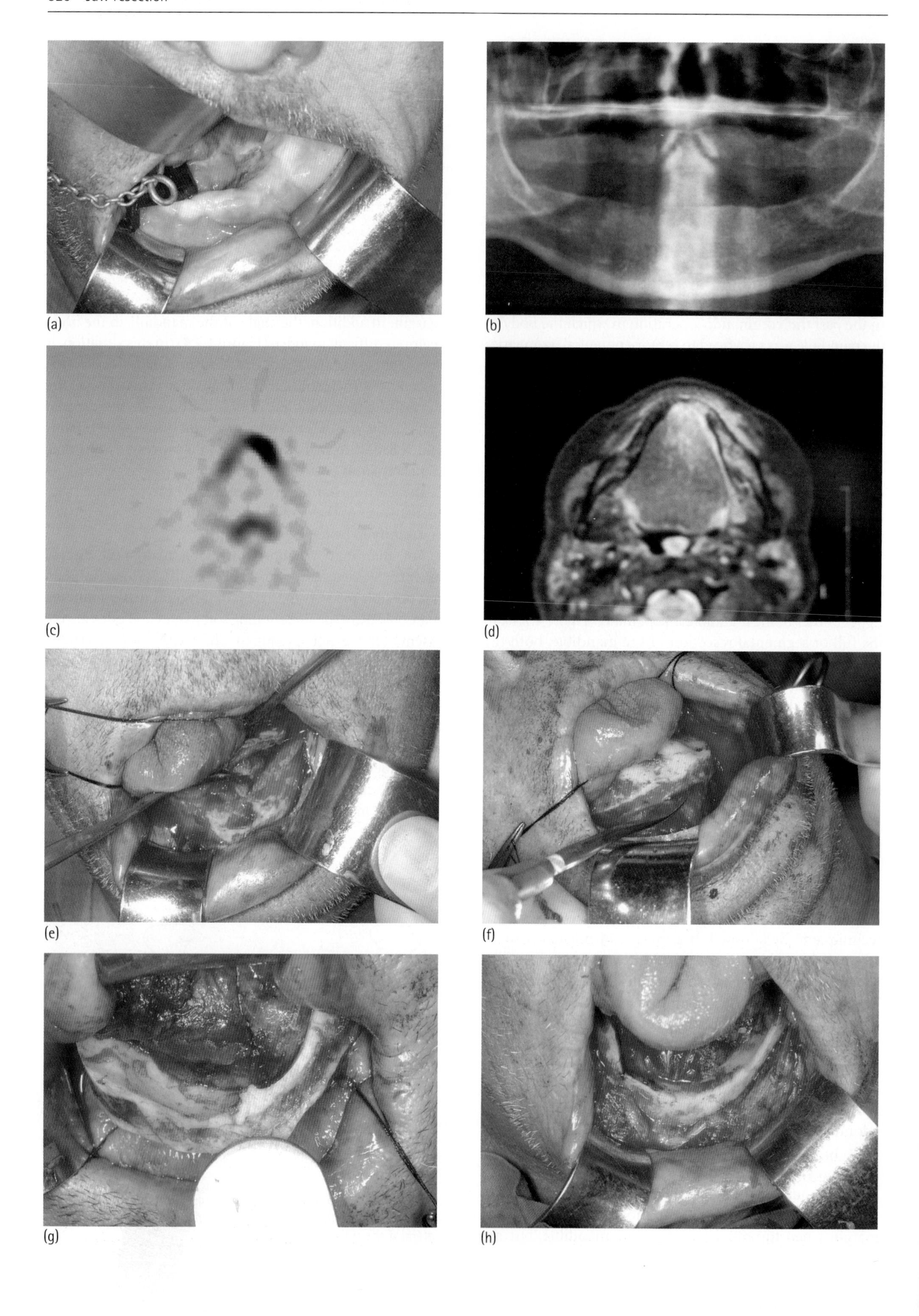
(a)
(b)
(c)
(d)
(e)
(f)
(g)
(h)

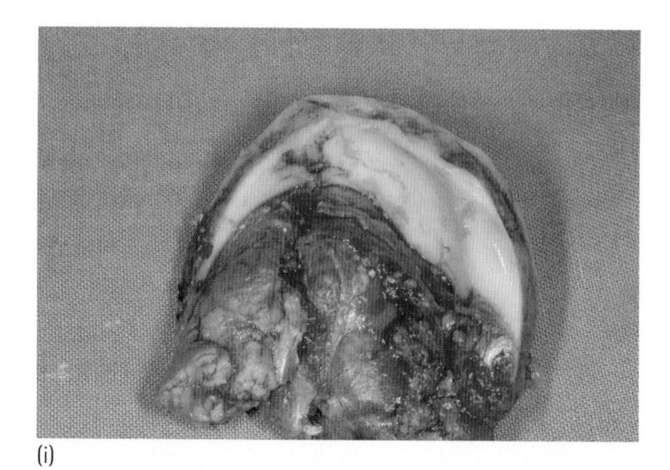
(i)

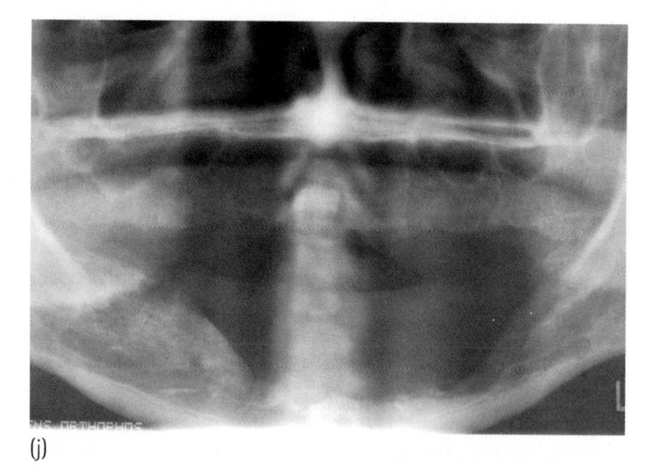
(j)

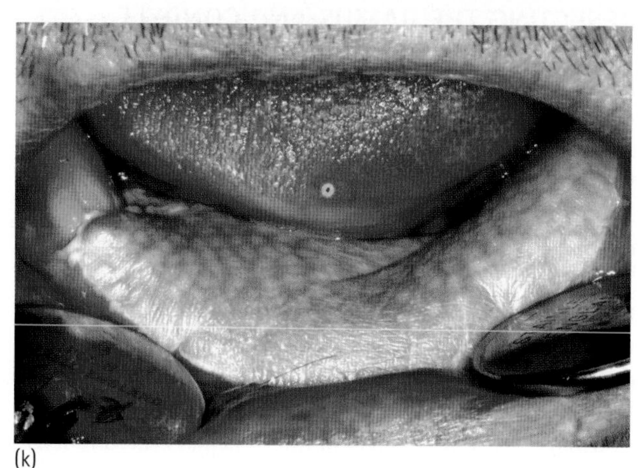
(k)

4.7.4 (a–d) Pre-operative clinical photograph, orthopantomogram (OPG), single photon emission computed tomography (SPECT) scan and magnetic resonance (MR) scan showing early tumour invasion of the mandible. (e) The resection of the buccal side of the mandible. (f) Completion of the planned coronal rim resection. (g) Turning the bone over to inspect the lingual side of the rim resection and ensure clearance of invaded mandible. (h) The resulting defect post-resection. (i) The specimen with lingual periosteal stripping to confirm clearance of resection. (j,k) Post-operative OPG and clinical photograph of anterolateral thigh flap reconstruction.

SEGMENTAL RESECTION OF THE MANDIBLE

This is a basic procedure in the management of malignant disease once the decision has been made not to preserve any part of the involved mandible. The decision as to where the bone cuts are made will depend on the assessment of mandibular invasion and the entry and exit points of the inferior alveolar nerve. In benign disease, it is often possible to keep the nerve intact and allow it to lie in the soft tissues overlying the reconstructed bone.

Periosteal stripping is also an important factor in the segmental resection of the mandible in malignant disease. The periosteum can be stripped back from the undamaged bone until it becomes adherent or the tumour is seen entering the bone. Once this is established, the margin can be decided and the bone cuts planned. It is also important to examine the specimen to ensure that the bone margins are clear of disease by direct inspection (Figure 4.7.5). This is much less reliable in a malignant tumour arising in bone, such as a primary intraosseous carcinoma or an osteosarcoma. In these cases, the periosteum and the cortex of the bone may look clear of invasion as the tumour spreads along the marrow space. As a result, it is necessary to be much more aggressive in mandibular resection and frozen sections should be performed if possible.

It may be necessary to excise the overlying skin in mandibular resection. In most cases, it is possible to preserve the skin cover but care must be taken in the buccal aspect of

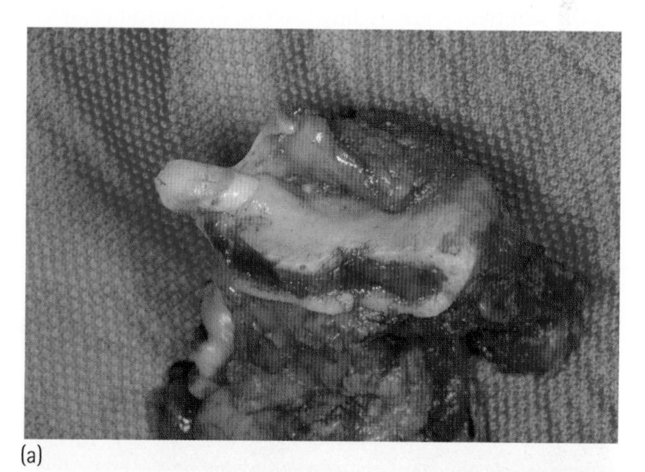
(a)

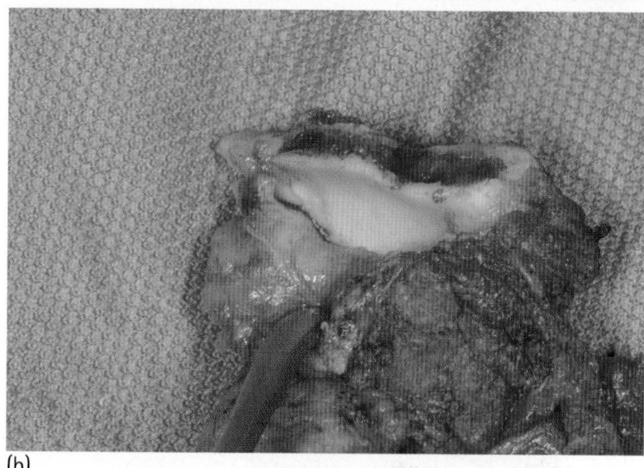
(b)

4.7.5 (a,b) Periosteal stripping post-resection to ensure that the buccal and lingual surfaces are clear of tumour in the distal part of the resection in the region of the lower right canine.

the resection to take sufficient tissue. It is seldom necessary to use an access procedure with segmental mandibular resection. The overlying skin is raised or excised depending on the needs of the oncological ablation and once the bone cuts have been made the mandible can be delivered into the neck and any further resection lingual to the jaw can be undertaken as the last part of the resection prior to the delivery of the specimen (Figure 4.7.6).

Maintaining the occlusion in mandibular resection

There are various methods used to maintain the occlusion prior to mandibular reconstruction. Some surgeons will use a form of external fixation of the non-resected part of the mandible, but this is very cumbersome and the device impedes accurate oncological resection. Templates have been devised using stereolithographic models, but again these are often impractical in surgery for malignant disease. The simplest technique is to pre-bend a plate if the tumour does not involve the buccal aspect of the mandible. In this way, the harvested bone can be grafted into position with the plate already in place. The plate is usually moved back by a screw-hole in the edentulous situation to take the pressure off the soft tissues and reduce the risk of dehiscence. If the use of a pre-bent plate is not possible then the condylar position can be fixed with a miniplate from the part of the ramus that dose not require resection to the maxilla prior to the resection with the mandible in occlusion. Once the mandible has been resected, the position of the ipsilateral condyle remains fixed and the collateral mandible can be located with the residual occlusion. A plate can then be bent into position prior to the placement of the graft. This can be carried out bilaterally for extensive mandibular resections. The length of the plate may need to be estimated, but at least the condyles will be in the correct position relative to each other.

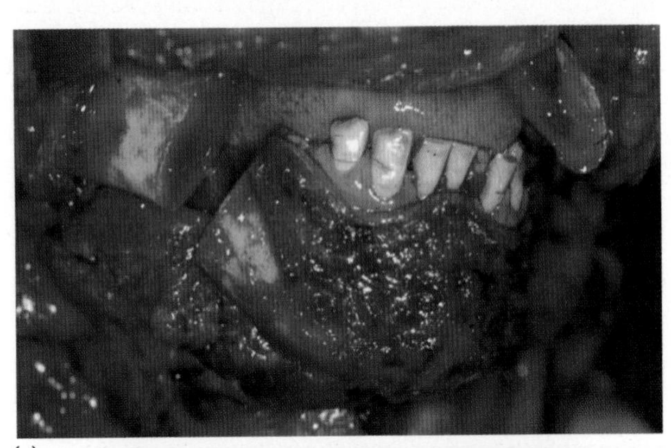

(a)

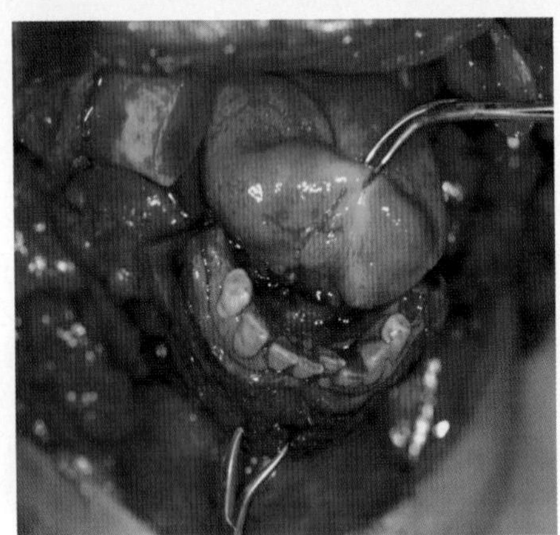

(b)

4.7.6 (a,b) There is no need for access surgery, such as a lip split in segmental surgery, as the tumour can be delivered into the neck to complete the resection.

RESECTING THE RAMUS AND CONDYLE

In most cases of squamous cell carcinoma, it is possible to maintain the condyle and the condylar neck sufficiently to maintain a plate so that this important part of the joint is left in function. The need to resect the condyle makes the subsequent reconstruction more difficult as the condyle cannot be fixed and it is not possible to pre-bend a plate. The resection of the condyle with the ramus and body of the mandible is relatively straightforward, but care must be taken to protect or tie off the maxillary artery and avoid damage to the facial nerve. The facial nerve can be damaged by inappropriate retraction in this region. It is often necessary to use some form of intermaxillary fixation if the patient is dentate to help the patient maintain a functioning occlusion in the post-operative period. Stereolithographic models are much more useful in this situation as the condyle cannot be fixed.

RESECTING THE MAXILLA

Pathology and pre-operative imaging

There is much less controversy over the more conservative approach to maxillary resection than the mandible. It is possible to preserve the bone of the maxilla with a limited resection of the palatal or alveolar mucosa, place a dressing plate and await the pathology report. If there is an involved or close margin, then bone can be resected at a second procedure. This process is also possible in more extensive resections of the maxilla in which an obturator can be placed and again the margins checked and more tissue taken at the time of the obturator change.

There is little discussion on the role of pathology either in terms of the pattern of spread in the bone or the pathway of entry. Most accept that the route of entry in the maxilla is at the point of contact and thus the maxillary resection is guided by the extent of the soft tissue mass.

For the assessment of bone invasion in the maxilla, most prefer a computed tomography (CT) scan. In the author's practice, both an MRI and CT scan are used to fully assess the tumour when there is concern over the involvement of the skull base or the pterygoid fossa. The surgeon wishes to know whether there is extension of the tumour into the orbit, the skull base or the infratemporal fossa. The CT scan is probably best for the skull base, and the MRI to assess the infratemporal fossa and both contribute equally to the invasion of the orbital contents.

The methods of resection are based on the classification illustrated in Figure 4.7.7.

CLASS 1 (ALVEOLECTOMY)

For class 1 defects (Figure 4.7.8), there is no need to use an access procedure as the tumour can usually be visualized with ease. This classification includes a medial maxillectomy often used for inverted papillomas, but resection for this pathology is not included in this chapter.

CLASS 2 (LOW LEVEL MAXILLECTOMY)

In this situation, the orbital floor is not involved with the resection and if the lesion is below the level of the infraorbital nerve then no access procedure may be required. Either a lip-split combined with a lateral rhinotomy or a midfacial degloving procedure may be used for access with equal effect. There are four osteotomies required to deliver the low level maxilla in ablative surgery:

1 Vertical alveolar (Figure 4.7.9a): In the dentate maxilla, it is best to remove a tooth in the line of the osteotomy which is continued to the floor of the nose. Maintaining bone adjacent to the remaining tooth helps the stability of the adjacent tooth to the bone cut for obturated cases. There must be sufficient soft tissue to cover the exposed bone.
2 Le Fort 1 level: A further osteotomy is required at the required height which may include the infraorbital nerve if required. This is carried through to the pterygoid plates.
3 Pterygoid plates: If the tumour is contained in the antrum, the pterygoid plates can be split from the maxilla with a chisel. If the tumour is through the antrum posteriorly, it is essential to make a bone cut through the pterygoid plates superior to the position of the tumour and then resect the infratemporal fossa as required to obtain a margin of resection.
4 Palatal: The alveolar osteotomy is continued into the palate. If possible, the soft tissue incision should allow some of the redundant mucoperiosteum to cover the bone cut, especially if obturation is the method of rehabilitation.

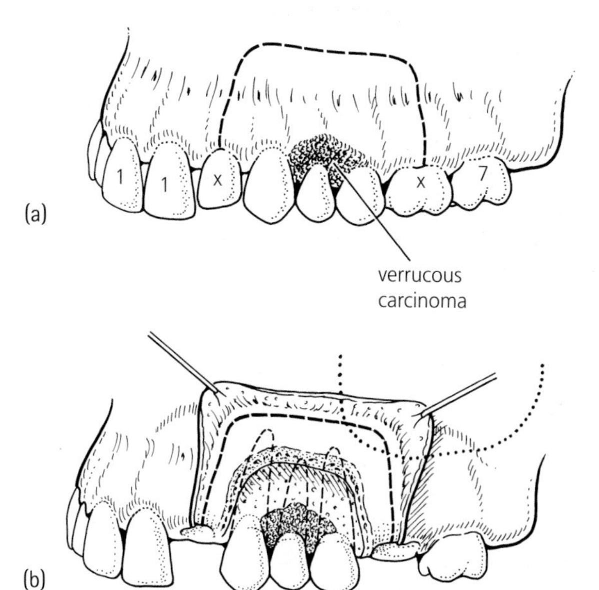

4.7.8 An example of a class 1 type of resection without causing an oro-antral fistula. Healing by secondary intention with the use of a dressing plate may be all that is required.

Once these osteotomies have been carried out, the hemi-maxilla can be mobilized and any soft tissue attachments released.

CLASS 3 (HIGH LEVEL MAXILLECTOMY MAINTAINING THE ORBIT)

The midfacial degloving technique reaches its limit if the orbital floor requires resection or there is extension into the

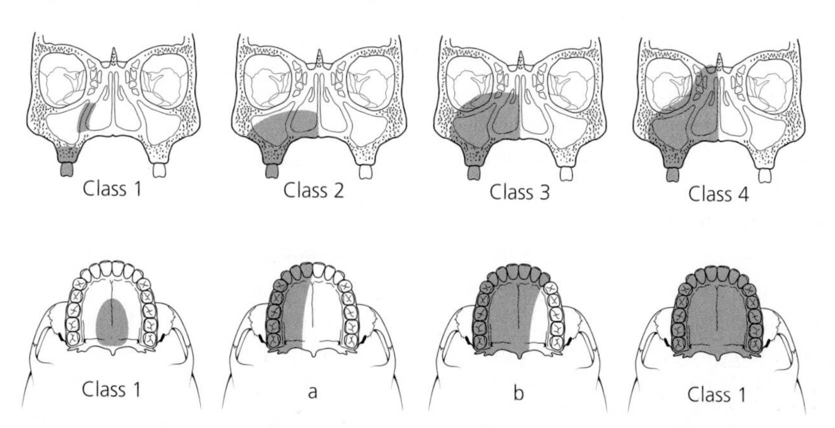

4.7.7 Classification of the maxillectomy defect. The need for reconstructive options increase from class 1 to 4.

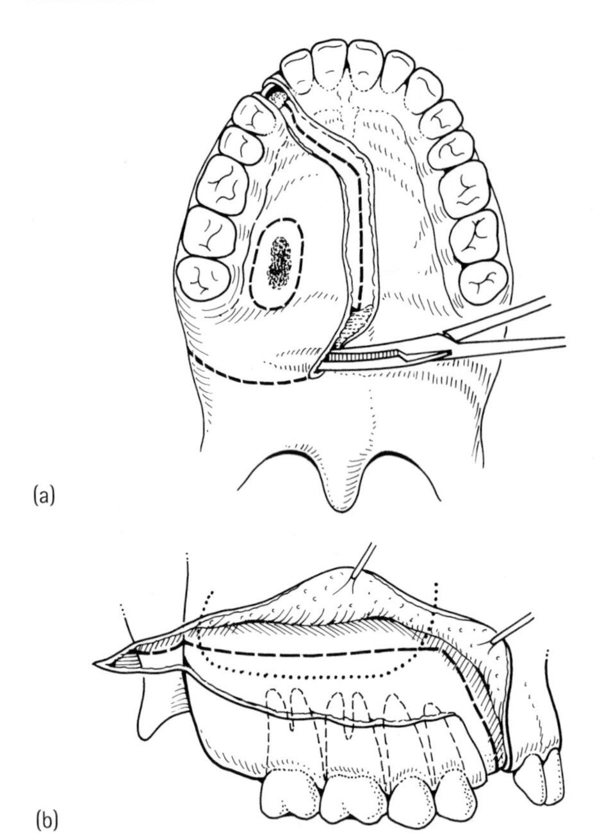

4.7.9 (a) This shows the palatal bone cut. It is usually best to remain on one side or other of the nasal septum depending on the extent of resection required. It is also important to ensure there is sufficient redundant mucoperiosteum to cover the bone cuts for obturated cases. (b) The vertical, Le Fort 1 level and pterygoid plate resection is shown.

medial orbital region of the ethmoids. In this situation, the lip-split and lateral rhinotomy may be sufficient or it may be necessary to extend the incision as a blepheroplasty incision or subciliary incision (Weber–Fergusson). In most situations, it is possible to reach the lateral orbital wall and malar without this extension reducing the risk of ectropion. This is the most complex resection because of the need to preserve the orbit and the lacrimal apparatus. A guide to the osteotomies is as follows (Figure 4.7.10):

- Vertical alveolar and nasal: The previously described vertical alveolar bone cut is extended to include the nasal piriforms and extended to the level of the lacrimal crest. Care must be taken to expose the lacrimal sac and to preserve this structure.
- Orbital: In this situation, the orbital floor is included as far as the inferior orbital fissure. This horizontal bone cut can be extended to the lateral orbital wall or the frontal process of the malar bone, as required.
- Malar: The orbital bone cut is linked to the malar buttress cut which is made lateral to the position of the tumour.
- Pterygoid plates: This often requires the plates to be sectioned higher than in the low maxillectomy close to the skull base. A chisel can be used to fracture off the pterygoid plates with a tumour contained within the antrum.

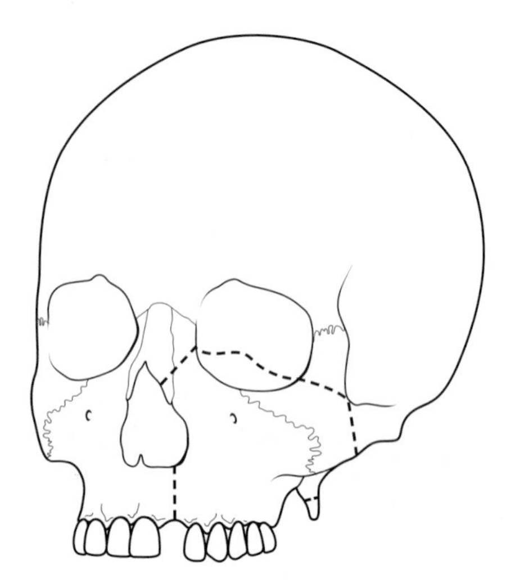

4.7.10 This shows the higher bone cuts required if the orbital floor and/or medial orbital wall require resection.

In these more extensive tumours, this part of the maxillectomy can be delivered intact. In most situations there will be extension into the ethmoid sinuses or superior to the lacrimal sac which will make delivery of the en bloc specimen more difficult. It is still essential to attempt to deliver the main part of the maxillectomy intact and carry out further resection of the medial orbital wall, and ethmoid and sphenoid sinuses as required. If it has not been possible to maintain the lacrimal system, the puncta are stented with silastic tubes and delivered into the nose and tied off. The silastic tube can be cut between the upper and lower puncta at about 3 weeks. It may be possible to repair parts of the lacrimal sac and duct at the time of the resection, but the placement of silastic tubes is still important to guide the tear flow as healing takes place.

CLASS 4 (RADICAL MAXILLECTOMY WITH ORBITAL EXENTERATION)

If the orbit requires resection with the maxilla, then the approach includes the upper and lower lids if there is no attempt to reconstruct the defect with a prosthetic eye. This operation is much easier to perform as no orbital structures need to be preserved.

In this operation, it is better to release the orbital nerve after exenterating the superior part of the orbit after the access procedure.

The same vertical bone cuts are made in the alveolus and nasal bones, but no special attention is required regarding the medial canthal ligament and the lacrimal apparatus. The lateral bone cut is made from the inferior oblique fissure to the malar buttress prior to the release of the pterygoid plates. The palatal bone cuts link with the vertical alveolar and nasal cuts and at this stage the specimen can be mobilized. The soft tissue resection at the base of the orbit is completed and now it should be possible to deliver the specimen. Tumour extending into the skull base, the ethmoids and sphenoid sinuses requires removal after the delivery of the main specimen.

Tumours involving the skull base require a multidisciplinary team approach. In this situation, a coronal flap, craniotomy and frontal bar osteotomy may be required to obtain adequate access to the anterior skull base.

Top tips

Resection of the mandible

- Pre-operative imaging should include a sensitive (bone scan, MRI) and specific (orthopantomogram) technique.
- Pre-operative imaging, clinical examination and the use of peri-operative periosteal stripping all help to decide the type and extent of resection.
- Remember that the tumour will invade the mandible at the point of contact, which may be below the dental line or the crest of the ridge.
- Early invasion is more likely to be the erosive pattern and late invasion infiltrative, requiring a wider margin.
- The option of a rim resection decreases with the extent of mandibular resorption following the loss of teeth (class V and VI).

Resection of the maxilla

- Pre-operative imaging will include an orthopantomogram (OPG) and a CT scan and often an additional MRI will be useful to assess the skull base.
- The main issues in maxillary resection involve the removal of the orbit and the extent of the disease into the infratemporal fossa.
- Using a saw to resect the pterygoid plates above the tumour will ensure a safer resection at the posterior maxilla.
- Close cooperation with the restorative dentist is essential in the planning of maxillary resection.

FURTHER READING

Brown JS, Griffith JF, Phelps PD, Browne RM. A comparison of different imaging modalities and direct inspection after periosteal stripping in predicting the invasion of the mandible by oral squamous cell carcinoma. *British Journal of Oral and Maxillofacial Surgery* 1994; **32**: 347–59.

Brown JS, Kalavrezos N, D'Souza J *et al.* Factors that influence the method of mandibular resection in the management of oral squamous cell carcinoma. *British Journal of Oral and Maxillofacial Surgery* 2002; **40**: 275–84.

Brown JS, Lewis-Jones H. Evidence for imaging the mandible in the management of oral squamous cell carcinoma: A review. *British Journal of Oral and Maxillofacial Surgery* 2001; **39**: 411–18.

Brown JS, Lowe D, Kalavrezos N *et al.* Patterns of invasion and routes of tumor entry into the mandible by oral squamous cell carcinoma. *Head and Neck* 2002; **24**: 370–83.

Brown JS, Magennis P, Rogers SN *et al.* Trends in head and neck microvascular reconstructive surgery in Liverpool (1992–2001). *British Journal of Oral and Maxillofacial Surgery* 2006; **44**: 364–70.

Brown JS, Rogers SN, McNally DN, Boyle M. A modified classification for the maxillectomy defect. *Head and Neck* 2000; **22**: 17–26.

Casson PR, Bonanno PC, Converse JM *et al.* The midface degloving procedure. *Plastic and Reconstructive Surgery* 1974; **53**: 102–103.

Kroll SS, Schusterman MA, Reece GP *et al.* Choice of flap and incidence of free flap success. *Plastic and Reconstructive Surgery* 1996; **98**: 459–63.

McGregor AD, MacDonald DG. Routes of entry of squamous cell carcinoma to the mandible. *Head and Neck Surgery* 1988; **10**: 294–301.

Price JC, Holliday MJ, Johns ME *et al.* The versatile midface degloving approach. *Laryngoscope* 1988; **98**: 291–5.

Shaw RJ, Brown JS, Woolgar JA *et al.* The influence of the pattern of mandibular invasion on recurrence and survival in oral squamous cell carcinoma. *Head and Neck* 2004; **26**: 861–9.

Urken ML, Buchbinder D, Weinberg H *et al.* Functional evaluation following microvascular oromandibular reconstruction of the oral cancer patient: A comparative study of reconstructed and nonreconstructed patients. *Laryngoscope* 1991; **101**: 935–50.

4.8

Orbital resection and reconstruction

ALEXANDER D RAPIDIS

INTRODUCTION

Orbital tumours pose numerous challenges in terms of diagnosis, imaging and management. They can be classified into three main groups according to their origin: (1) primary lesions, which originate from the orbit itself; (2) secondary lesions, which extend into the orbit from neighbouring structures (intracranial tumours and tumours of the paranasal sinuses); and (3) metastatic tumours. Orbital tumours are also divided according to their anatomical site into intraconal and extraconal.

ORBITAL ANATOMY

The orbit is a pear-shaped bony chamber with an anterior opening measuring approximately 40 and 35 mm in horizontal and vertical diameters, respectively. Its volume expands approximately 1 cm posterior to the bony orbital rim and then gradually decreases toward the apex, which consists of the optic canal at its narrowest diameter. In the axial plane, the medial wall measures approximately 45–50 mm from the anterior lacrimal crest to the optic canal. Posteriorly, the lateral wall is bordered with the superior orbital fissure, situated between the greater and lesser wings of the sphenoid bone. This foramen transmits the third, fourth and sixth cranial nerves and the ophthalmic branch of the fifth cranial nerve, the superior orbital vein and sympathetic nerves.

The periorbita is important because it acts as a barrier to the extension of neoplastic growth.

ORBITAL PATHOLOGY

Orbital tumours can derive from tumours of epithelial, mesenchymal, haematologic and nervous origin: vascular tumours, fibrohystiotic tumours, fibro-osseous and cartilaginous tumours, peripheral nerve tumours, hematologic tumours, lacrimal gland tumours, tumours of the lacrimal drainage system, eyelid and peri-ocular skin tumours, conjuctival tumours, ocular tumours, tumours of the cranial and nasal cavities, brain tumours and metastatic tumours.

Orbital lymphoma is the most common malignant tumour of the eyes. It can occur either as the primary site of disease or rarely as a secondary site of systemic non-Hodgkin lymphoma (NHL). Orbital lymphoma typically is a disease of the elderly as the majority are non-Hodgkin's type and are seen primarily in adults in the 50–70-year age group.

Malignancies of the ocular adnexa are the most common reason for orbital exenteration and include squamous cell carcinoma (SCC), sebaceous cell carcinoma and basal cell carcinoma (BCC). Other less common tumours include conjunctival malignant melanoma, adenoid cystic carcinoma of the lacrimal gland and uveal melanoma with extrascleral extension.

Lacrimal gland lesions can be classified as epithelial and non-epithelial lesions. Epithelial tumours can be benign (e.g. pleomorphic adenoma) or malignant (e.g. adenoid cystic carcinoma). Conjunctival melanoma is a rare but aggressive ocular tumour. The most common primary malignant intraocular tumour in adults is uveal melanoma, whereas in children it is retinoblastoma. Rarely, intraocular tumours extend transclerally and invade the periocular tissues and the orbit. The uveal melanoma originates from the monocytes of the uvea and has the capacity to invade the adjacent tissue structures aggressively and metastasize systemically.

A variety of pathologies can involve the preseptal space. Frequently these tumours are benign, for example, xanthelasmas and tumours of limited malignancy. Rare tumours include capillary haemangiomas, lymphomas and orbital metastases from distant sites.

CLINICAL SIGNS AND SYMPTOMS

The most important feature is proptosis. Slowly growing masses of the orbit usually do not alter the anatomic relationship of the eyelids to the globe and extraocular motility is affected only at extreme gazes (Figure 4.8.1).

Lacrimal gland tumours typically present with upper eyelid fullness, alteration of eyelid contour, and downward and nasal displacement of the globe.

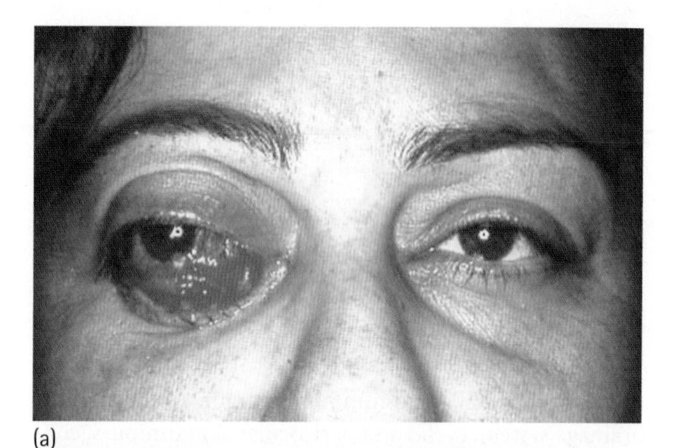

(a)

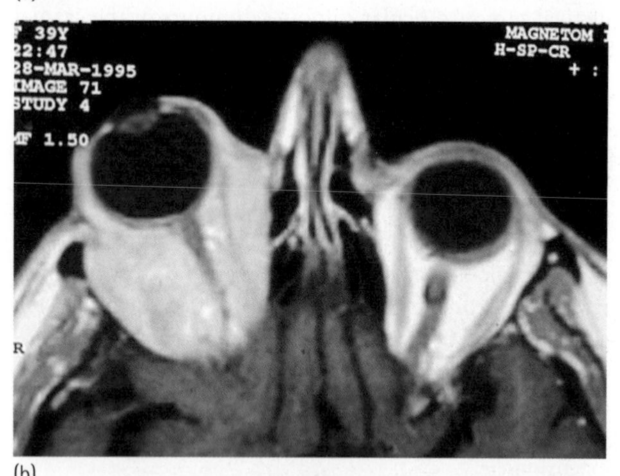

(b)

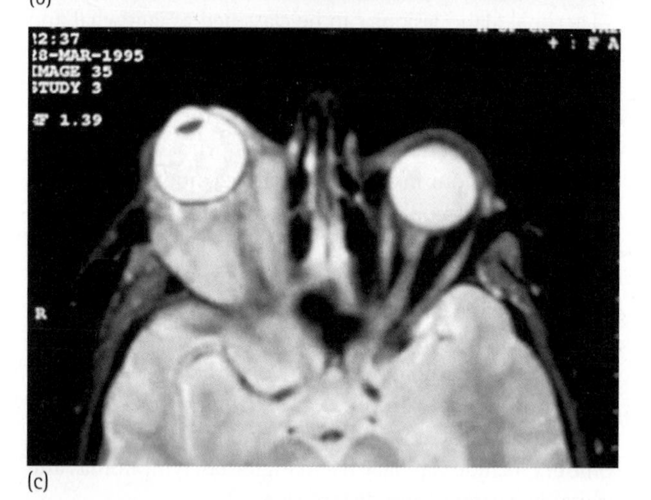

(c)

4.8.1 (a) Clinical photograph of a patient with orbital lymphoma. There is marked proptosis with chemosis of the conjuctiva. (b) Magnetic resonance imaging (MRI) (T_2 weighting) showing diffuse infiltration of the occulomotor muscles from the lymphoid tissue. (c) MRI (T_1 weighting) depicting the same radiological findings. There is marked enlargement of the rectus muscles.

There are two mechanisms by which a tumour can cause diplopia: first, by infiltrating the nerves supplying the extraocular muscles, as seen with malignant tumours, and second, by restricting the normal extraocular motility function and/or deviating the axis of the eye.

Infiltrating tumours have a tendency to 'freeze' the eye in the primary position of gaze because of their indiscriminate infiltration into the muscles and the soft tissues of the orbit (Figure 4.8.2).

Uveal melanomas have as an early sign impairment of visual acuity (Figure 4.8.3).

Primary lacrimal sac lesions, or those affecting the lacrimal sac as part of a systemic process, present with epiphora, dacryocystitis or a hard, fixed mass arising above the medial canthal tendon, sometimes with serosanguinous tears.

Intracranial tumours may rarely extend into the orbit. Orbital extension may produce ophthalmoplegia, optic neuropathy and proptosis.

RADIOLOGICAL DIAGNOSIS OF ORBITAL TUMOURS

Orbital imaging serves for three distinct purposes: (1) to confirm that the signs and symptoms are due to an orbital tumour; (2) to identify the nature of the tumour, its malignant potential, tissue type and extension into other neighbouring tissues; and (3) to monitor treatment effectiveness and the early identification of recurrence.

The main radiographic modalities used in orbital imaging are: computed tomography (CT), magnetic resonance imaging (MRI), ultrasonography, positron emission tomography, digital angiography and radionuclear scintigraphy.

Digital angiography should be considered for any patient with pulsatile exophthalmos.

HISTOPATHOLOGICAL DIAGNOSIS OF ORBITAL TUMOURS

Orbital biopsy techniques include excisional, incisional, core and aspiration biopsies and intraoperative biopsy with frozen section and Mohs' methods. Sentinel node biopsy is also utilized occasionally for staging purposes of certain tumours.

SURGICAL TECHNIQUES

Enucleation is removal of the globe alone, whereas orbital exenteration refers to enucleation combined with removal of the entire orbital contents, including the globe, optic nerve, extraocular muscles, lacrimal gland and lacrimal drainage system, as well as the orbital fibroconnective and adipose tissues.

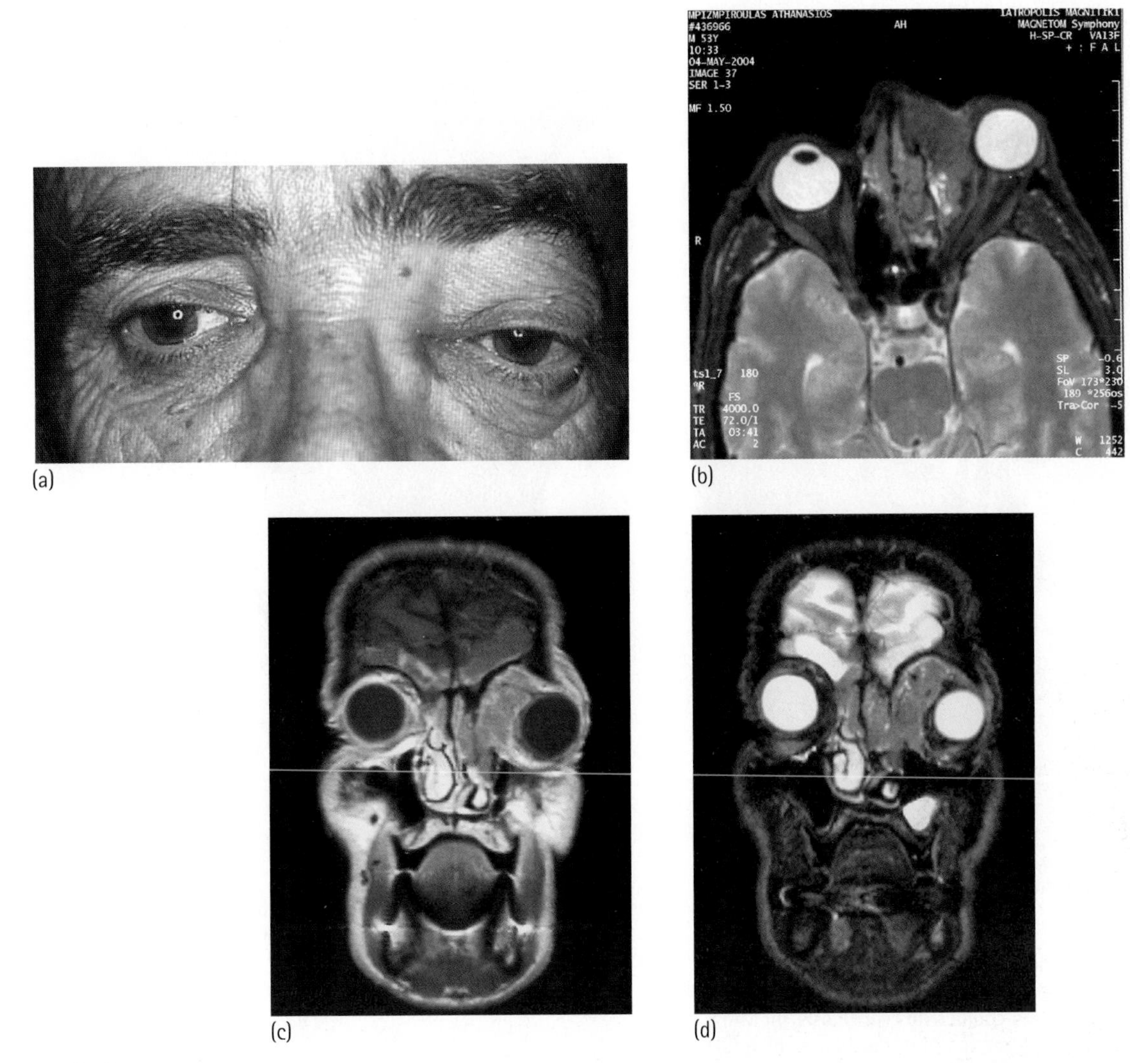

4.8.2 (a) Clinical photograph of a patient with squamous cell carcinoma of the ethmoids with extension into the left orbital cavity. The tumour produces marked proptosis to the left eye with outer displacement and 'freezing' of the eye due to extensive infiltration of the occulomotor muscles. (b) The magnetic resonance imaging (MRI) (T_2 weighting) shows the extension of the tumour of the anterior ethmoids and the nasal cavity into the orbit. There is direct invasion of the globe by the tumour which is confined into the anteriolateral compartment of the orbit. (c) Coronal plane of the MRI (T_1 weighting). The tumour mass is depicted invading the orbit having destroyed the inner lateral thin bony wall. (d) Coronal plane of the MRI (T_2 weighting). The tumour is confined in the naso-ethmoidal area with extension into the orbit without invading the base of the skull and the anterior cranial fossa.

Individualization of exenteration cases should take into account the location, size and aggressiveness of the pathology, as well as the reconstruction plan. If the bones of the orbit are involved with malignancy, bone resection should be performed at the time of initial orbitotomy, even if that procedure is not an exenteration. Orbital exenteration may be subtotal, total and extended.

SUBTOTAL ORBITAL EXENTERATION

In eyelid-sparing exenteration, one may need to spare either the entire eyelid structure or just the eyelid skin. If the eyelid skin is to be spared, the skin incision is placed approximately 2–3 mm above and beyond the lash lines. The skin is dissected until the orbital rim is reached, then the periosteum is cut 360° 2 mm beyond the orbital rim, to continue the exenteration. If the entire eyelid anatomy is to be preserved, the operation is similar to an extended enucleation in which the eye with the bulbar conjunctival lining and the other orbital tissues are removed en bloc (Figure 4.8.4).

TOTAL ORBITAL EXENTERATION

In total orbital exenteration, the eyelids are closed with silk sutures. The bony landmarks are palpated and the line of the desired incision marked out. A circumferential skin incision is made overlying the orbital rim (Figure 4.8.5a). Unless the

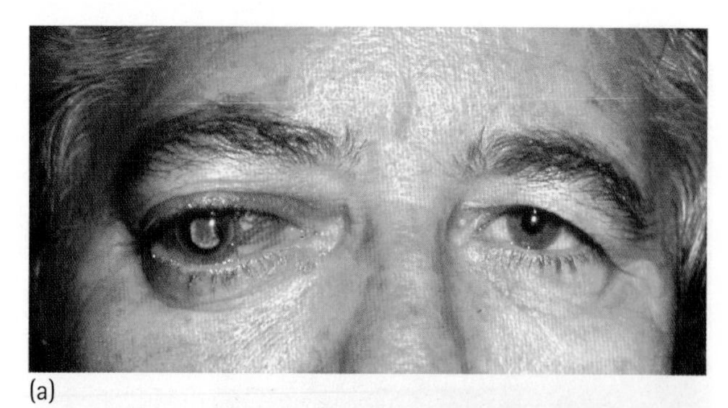

(a)

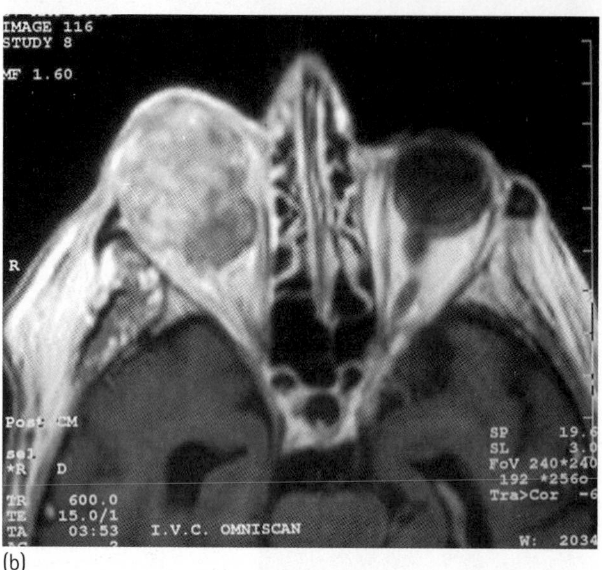

(b)

4.8.3 (a) Clinical photograph of a patient with orbital extension of a uveal melanoma. The intraocular extension of the tumour produces proptosis and conjuctival ecchemosis. (b) MRI (T_2 weighting) showing the distraction of intraocular architecture of the globe by an ill-defined mass with irregular periphery and a mixed consistency. The lesion does not invade the periorbita.

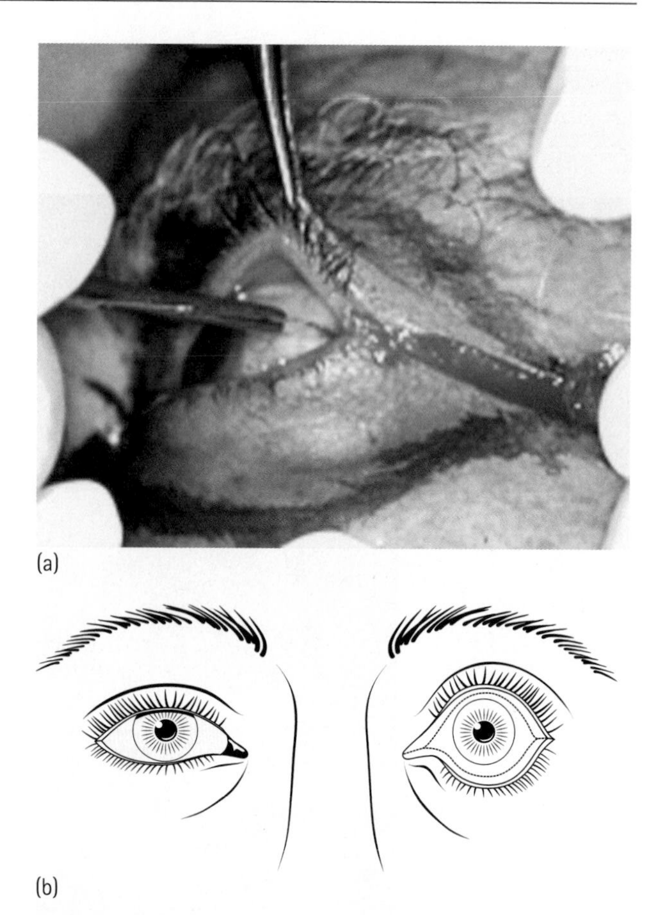

(a)

(b)

4.8.4 Schematic representation of the eyelid-sparing incision for subtotal orbital exenteration: (a) lateral view, (b) front view).

extent of the disease makes it necessary to do otherwise, the line of the incision lies just inside the orbital rim. Medially, it lies on the anterior lacrimal crest and laterally it passes close to the outer canthus. On the nasal wall of the orbit, the periosteum must be raised gently, because the orbital plate of the ethmoid is very fragile and a sinus may result if the ethmoid air cells are opened. When the underlying soft tissues have been reached the incision is continued, usually with the use of unipolar cautery with a fine needle tip (a Colorado tip). To minimize bleeding, an incision is made in the upper quadrant, at the 12 o'clock position, which then proceeds clockwise, leaving dissection of the vascular nasal quadrant to the end. The periorbita is best incised a few millimetres outside the orbit, rather than on the orbital margin, as the blade of the knife can then be used perpendicularly to the bone (Figure 4.8.5b). Although the periorbita here is firmly adhered to the bone, it is thick and does not tear when raised. It is elevated with a sharp periosteal elevator (Figure 4.8.5c). When the periosteum of the orbital rim is reached, it is elevated and the dissection is swiftly continued beyond the rim into the orbit, to complete the procedure as quickly as possible (Figure 4.8.5d). In the region of the anterior lacrimal crest, the lacrimal sac is reflected laterally with the orbital contents when the periosteum is separated from the nasal wall. The nasolacrimal duct is identified as the dissection proceeds from the nasal wall to the floor of the orbit. Ligation of the duct prevents ascending infection from the nose and prevents blood running down into the nasopharynx. During dissection, bleeding is ignored unless haemorrhage is so profuse that it interferes with the view of the surgical field. Laterally, the temporal and malar branches of the lacrimal artery enter the malar bone and medially the anterior ethmoidal artery passes from the orbit into the anterior ethmoidal foramen. These vessels are exposed and are clamped and coagulated with diathermy to avoid bleeding in the depths of the wound. When the soft tissue dissection is complete, haemostasis with cautery is achieved (Figure 4.8.5e). When the dissection toward the apex is completed, the apical bundle of soft tissues, including extraocular muscles, blood vessels and nerves, is reached. These tissues cannot be clamped or cut with one move. The bundle is approached from its nasal aspect, a strong curved haemostat is placed and the pedicle is cut with unipolar cautery or a curved pair of scissors above the haemostat. The same manoeuvre is repeated laterally and inferiorly to free the apex from orbital soft tissues. The bleeding sources of the apex (ophthalmic artery and vein) should be identified, clamped and tied after the removal of the bulk of the soft tissues (Figure 4.8.5f). Excessive application of electrocautery at the apex may create damage in the proximal portion of the optic nerve, which may extend into the optic chiasm. During orbital exenteration, most of the bleeding originates from the supraorbital and infraorbital vessels, the anterior and posterior ethmoidal arteries and the ophthalmic artery when the dissection reaches the apex. Although the posterior bleeding is the most significant, it is easier to control, since by the time the apex of the orbit is reached, all soft tissues have been freed and there is better visibility (Figure 4.8.5g). After removal of the orbital contents it may be possible to apply clamps behind those previously used to reduce the size of the stump by the removal of more tissue. The pedicle is transfixed and ligated.

EXTENDED EXENTERATION WITH RESECTION OF THE OSSEOUS ORBIT

After total orbital exenteration, the orbital walls are examined for any evidence of neoplastic involvement. If there is any diseased bone it is chiselled away, cutting

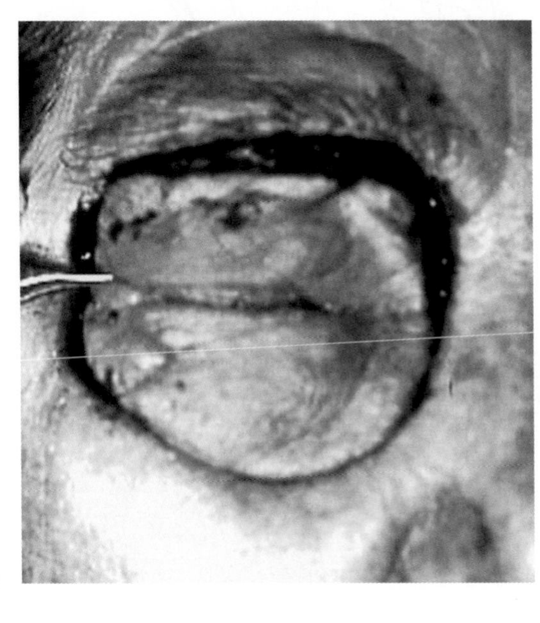
(a)

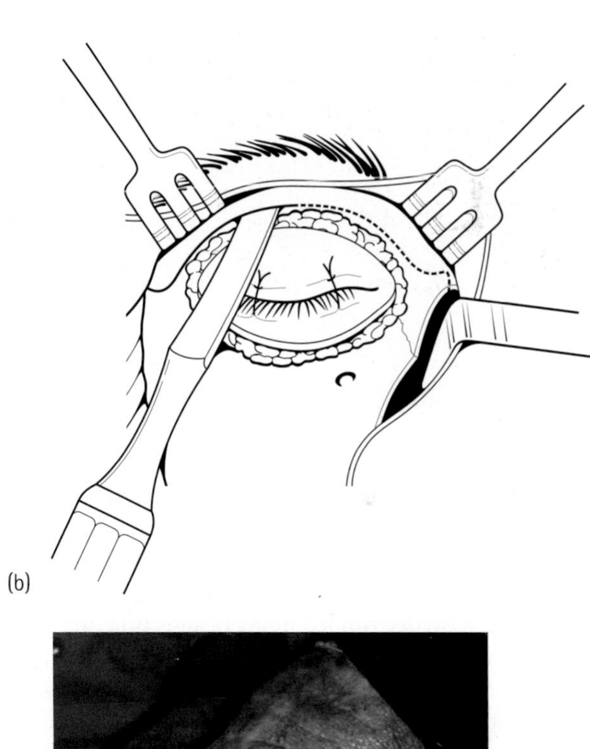
(b)

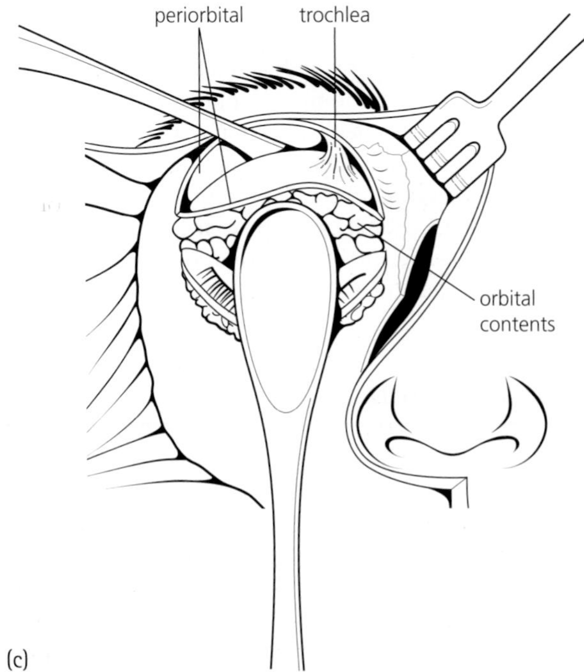

(c)

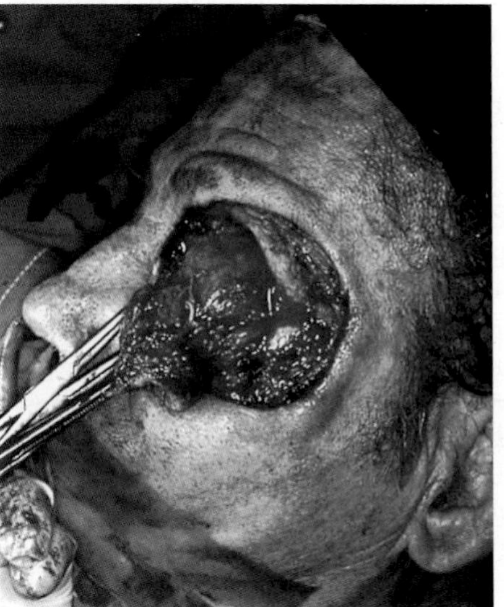
(d)

4.8.5 Schematic representation of total orbital exenteration in stages (see text for explanation of panels (a) to (g)). *continued*

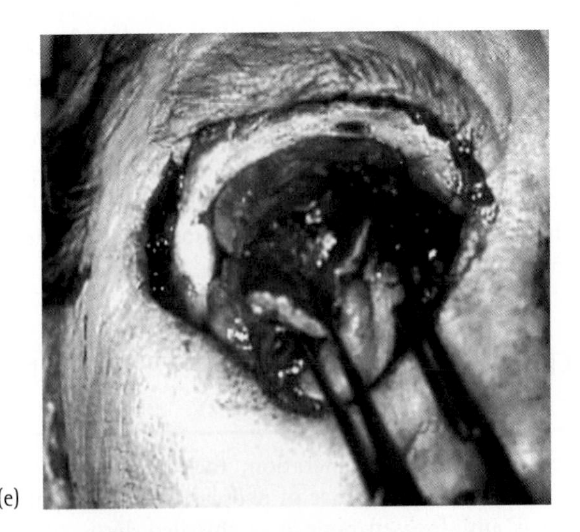

(e)

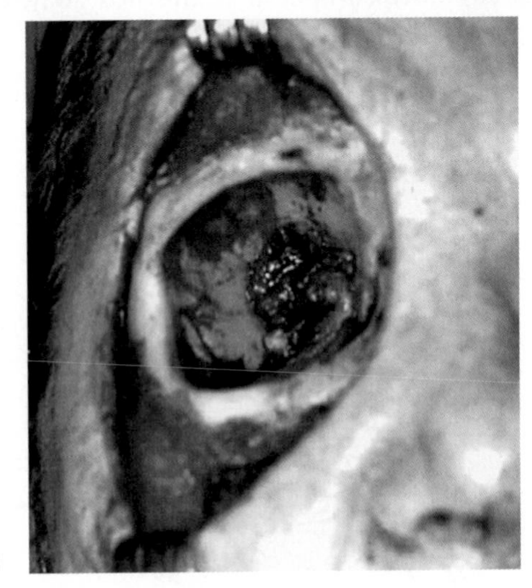

(f)

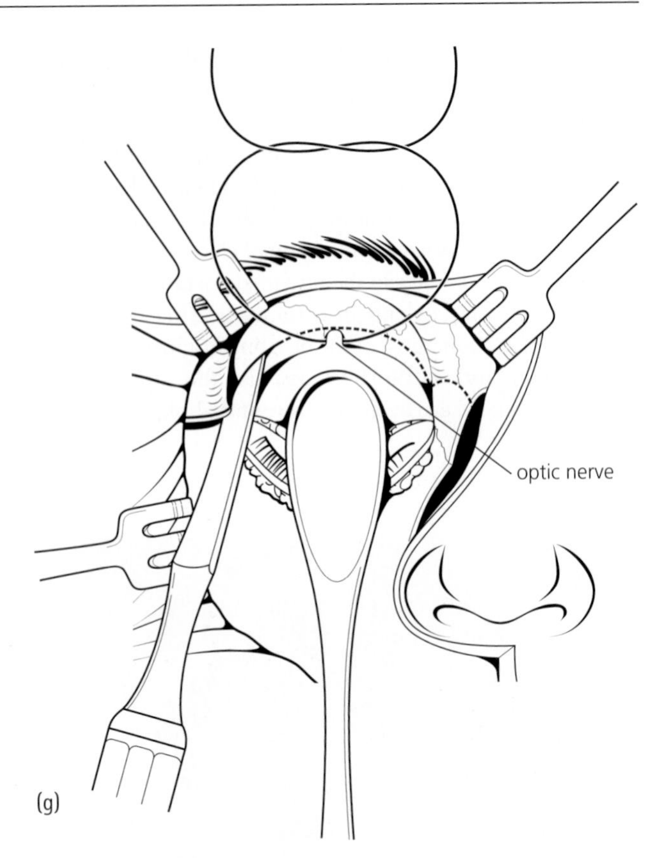

4.8.5 *continued* Schematic representation of total orbital exenteration in stages (see text for explanation of panels (a) to (g)).

through healthy bone. There are no standard techniques for bone resection. In most cases, removal depends on the extent and location of the bony invasion. In most areas of the orbit, it is preferable to score the bone with an oscillating saw along the predetermined limits of resection and then fracture the bone en bloc with a strong rongeur. In some sites, a sharp osteotome and a mallet may be needed to remove pathologic bone (Figure 4.8.6).

EXTENDED EXENTERATION WITH RESECTION OF THE PARANASAL SINUSES

Extensive primary paranasal and skull base malignancies can infiltrate the orbital content. There are four grades of orbital involvement through the paranasal sinuses: (1) tumour adjacent to the orbit, without infiltration of the orbital wall; (2) tumour eroding the orbital wall without ocular bulb displacement; (3) tumour eroding and infiltrating the orbital wall, displacing the orbital content, without periorbital involvement; (4) tumour invading the orbit with periorbital invasion. In cases of obvious bony orbital tumour involvement, the orbit with the adjacent bone and sinuses should be removed. The conventional treatment of the sinonasal malignancies with orbital extension is maxillectomy with orbital exenteration. This extended hemimaxillectomy is approached through a Weber–Fergusson–Dieffenbach skin incision (Figures 4.8.7 and 4.8.8). Ethmoidal malignancies invade the orbit in over 80 per cent of cases. The anatomy of the area and the separation of the orbital cavity from the ethmoids by the lamina papyracea favours the invasion of tumour into the orbit (see also Chapter 4.7).

RECONSTRUCTION

An essential part of the decision-making process is reconstruction and rehabilitation of the exenterated orbital socket. A decision should be made pre-operatively whether the patient will wear a patch or a prosthesis.

Primary surgical closure of the orbital cavity is advantageous with respect to both function and aesthetic outcome, and makes early post-operative radiotherapy possible. With CT and MRI, early local recurrence can be identified.

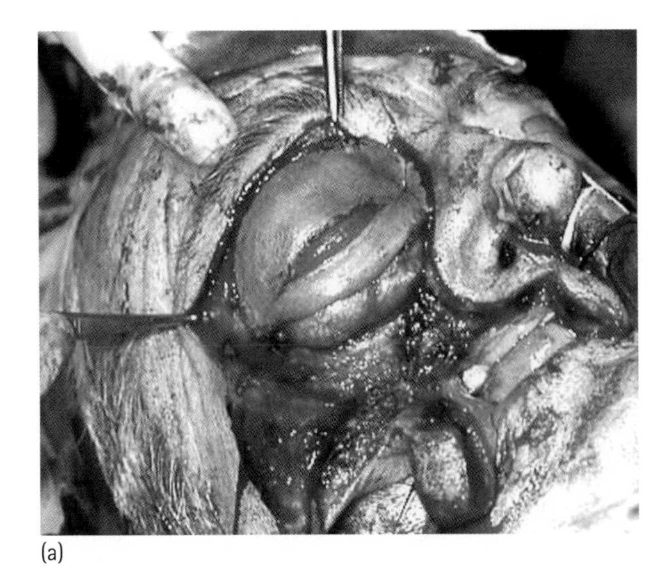

(a)

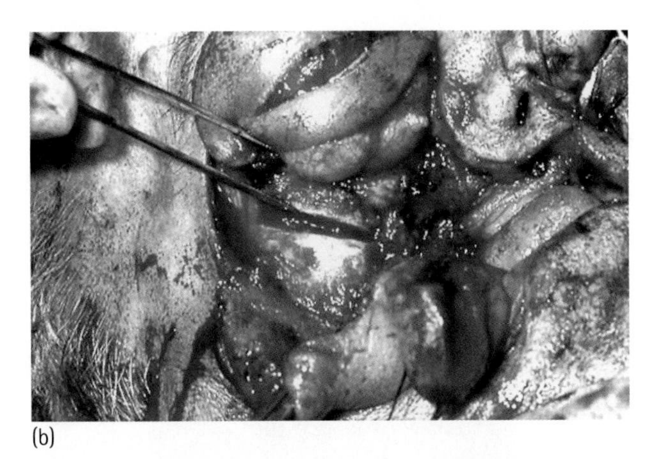

(b)

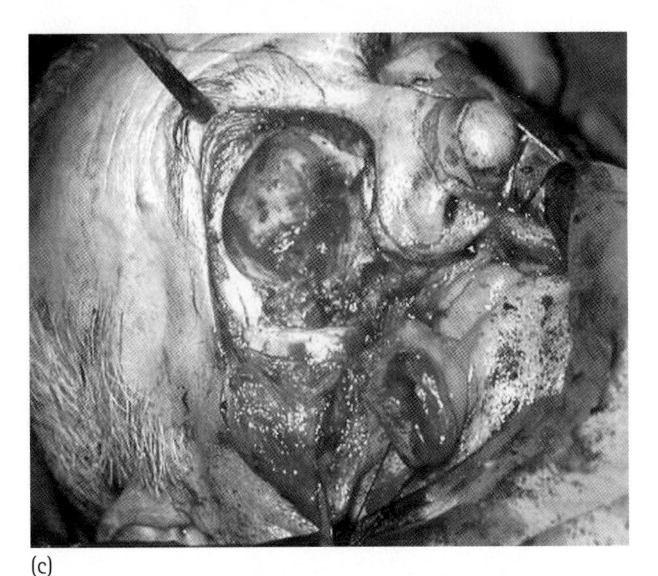

(c)

4.8.6 Extended orbital exenteration with resection of the osseous orbit. (a) Incision lines resemble those of the total orbital exenteration. If needed a lateral rhinotomy extension is performed to facilitate resection of the orbital floor. (b) An osteotomy is performed to include parts of the lateral orbital wall and the bony floor of the orbit. (c) The surgical bed after the extended orbital exenteration.

Orbital exenteration results in significant deformity. The primary goal of reconstruction is the restoration of boundaries between the orbit and surrounding cavities and an acceptable aesthetic outcome.

Orbital reconstructive techniques can be divided in three groups: (1) local reconstructive options (healing by secondary intention, split skin graft or dermis–fat graft); (2) regional reconstructive options (temporalis muscle transfer, frontalis rotational flap or a variant of these procedures); and (3) distant reconstructive options (pedicle musculocutaneous flaps or free vasculized flaps).

Local reconstructive options

SPONTANEOUS GRANULATION

The simplest approach is to pack the orbit with iodine-impregnated gauze and allow the socket to granulate. When the eyelids are entirely removed, the free skin margin is tacked to the orbital rim with interrupted silk sutures and the socket is lined with antibiotic-soaked vaseline or Xeroform gauze.

Healing may take 8–10 weeks. By the time granulation is complete, the orbit is covered with a very thin epithelium, which has the advantage of allowing the detection of recurrent tumour at an early stage. The resulting cavity is deep, but can be fitted with a silicone oculofacial prosthesis. The need for regular dressing changes must be weighed against the potential benefits of healing by secondary intention.

Significant numbers of patients develop sino-orbital fistulas from perforation sinuses occurring pre-operatively (Figure 4.8.9, p. 336).

EYELID SPARING TECHNIQUE

Because the eyelids and conjunctiva are supplied by an extensive vascular network, these tissues remain viable after loss of the posterior orbital circulation. Eyelid-sparing, subtotal exenteration offers significant advantages in terms of reconstruction of the orbit and cosmesis. When it is consistent with the complete removal of all malignant disease, the lids are preserved, and either turned into the cavity as a lining or used to retain a prosthesis (Figure 4.8.10, p. 336).

FREE SKIN GRAFTING

The socket may be lined on completion of the exenteration with split-thickness skin graft. There are a number of advantages for this technique. It is a technically simple procedure which takes little time and it provides a socket that is easily accessible for clinical examination. While split skin grafts provide a reliable lining, they take time to heal and stabilize.

The graft must be free of hair follicles. A graft measuring 8 cm at its widest point is sufficient to line the orbital cavity and a graft of this size can be obtained from the anterior thigh. When the skin graft has been inserted into the orbit, it is important to ensure close approximation of the graft to the bony wall. It is sutured to the margins of the skin with

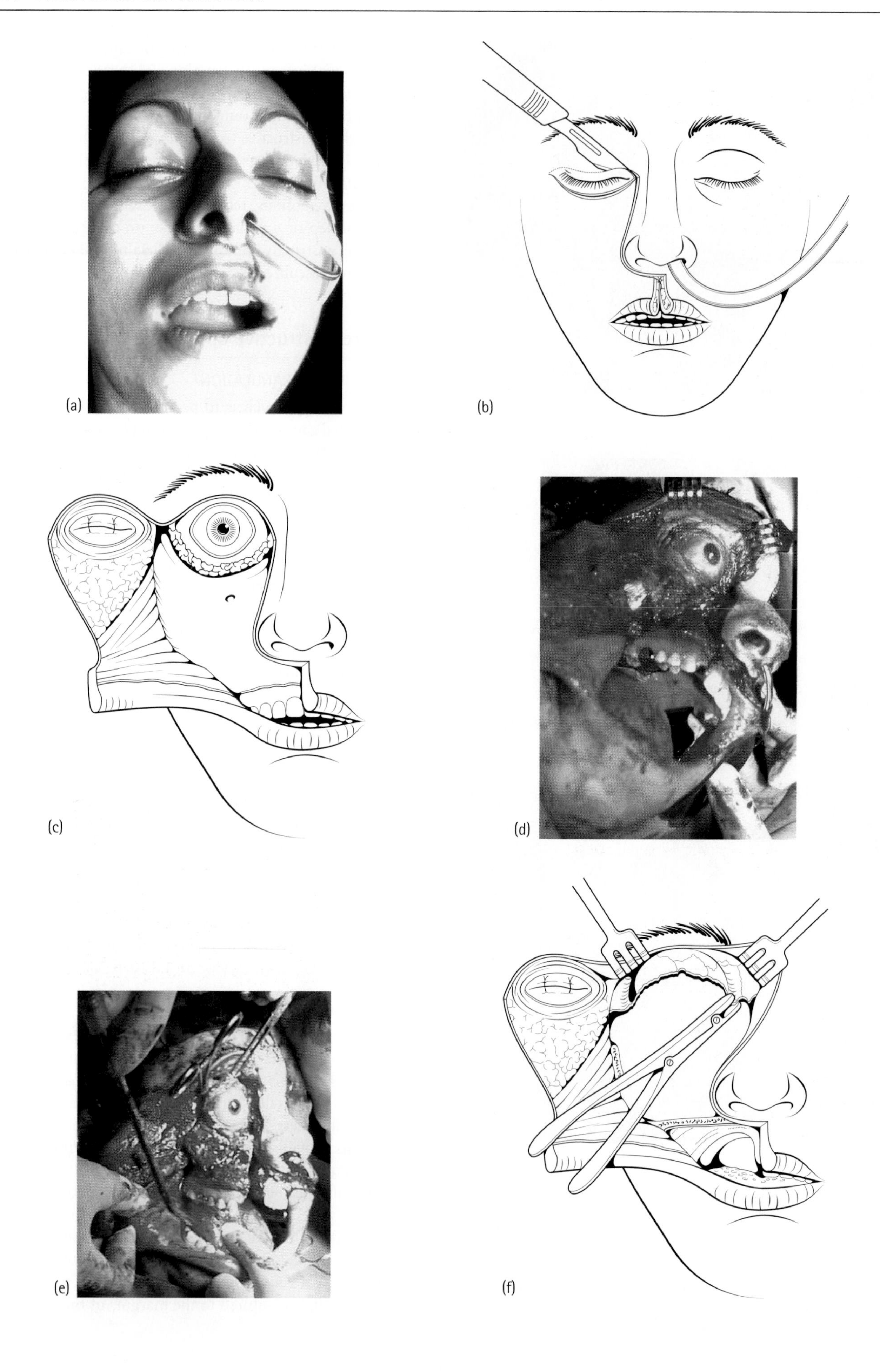
(a)
(b)
(c)
(d)
(e)
(f)

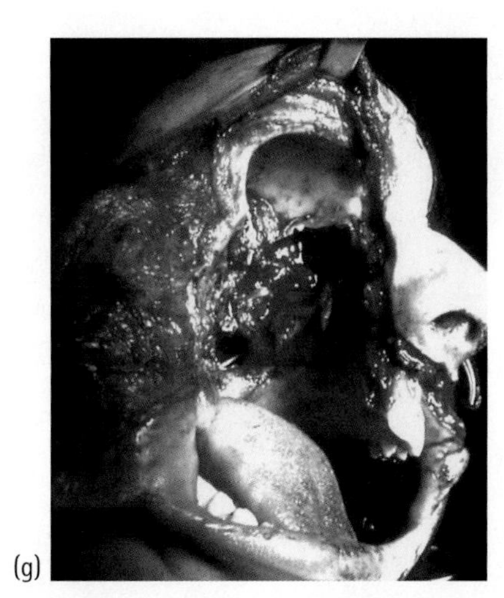
(g)

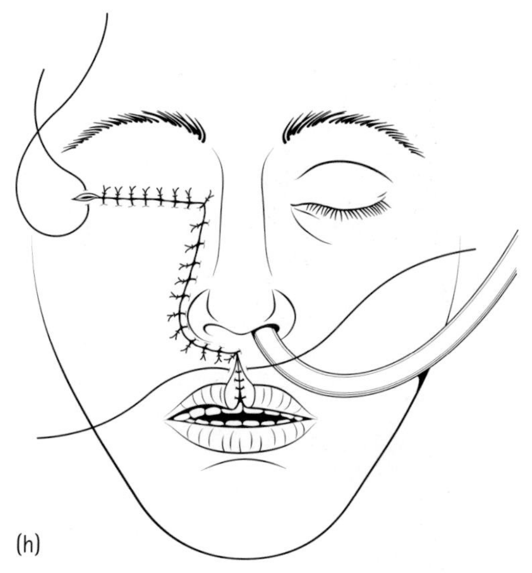
(h)

4.8.7 Schematic representation of extended orbital exenteration with resection of the paranasal sinuses. (a,b) The incision line when a lid-sparing procedure is favoured. (c,d) The cheek flap is reflected and the anterior and lateral walls of the maxillary sinus and the orbit are visualized. (e) Osteotomies are performed to separate the lateral middle third of the face from the facial skeleton. Transection of the zygomatic arch and bone are necessary for the mobilization of the osseous part of the skeleton containing the tumour. (f,g) After the resection of the specimen additional fragments of the facial skeleton may be necessary to be removed. (h) The skin closure lines.

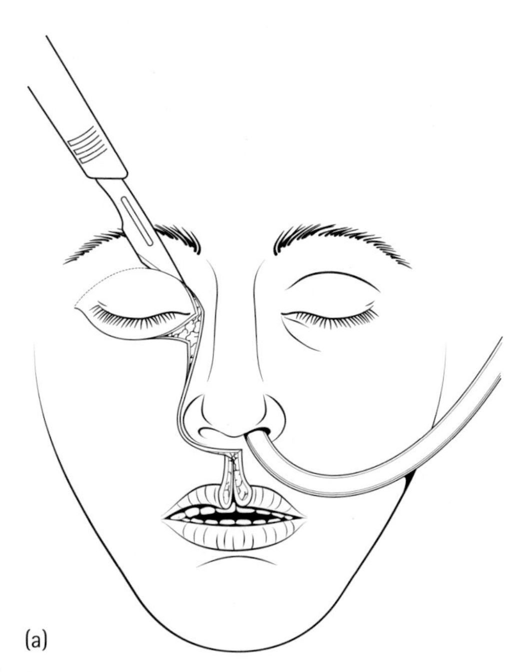
(a)

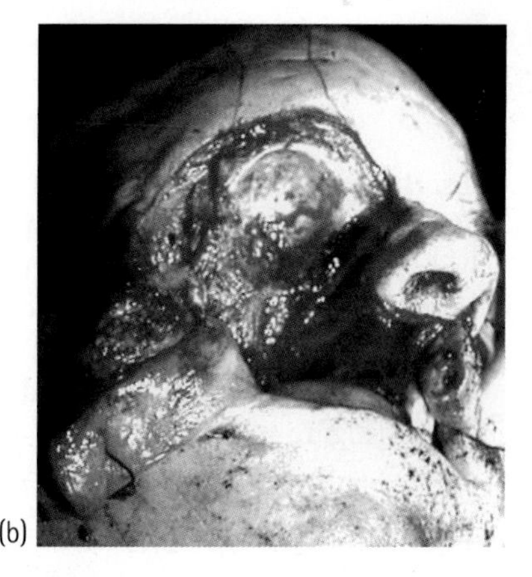
(b)

4.8.8 (a) Schematic representation of extended orbital exenteration with resection of the paranasal sinuses when the lids must be resected with the tumour. (b) The surgical defect after tumour resection.

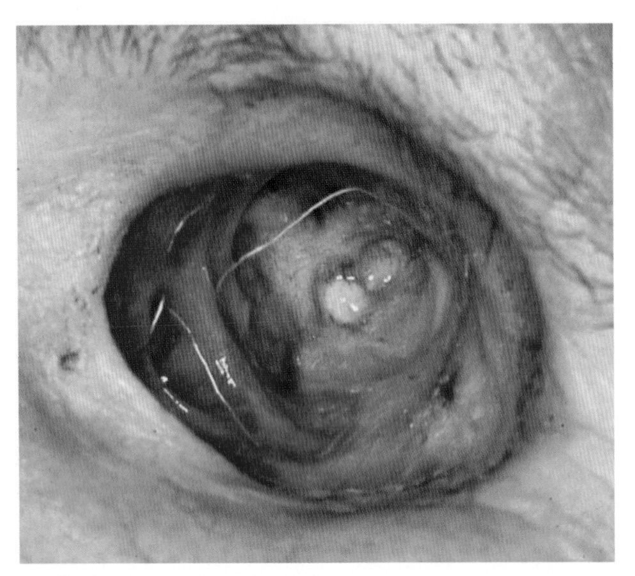

4.8.9 Clinical photograph of a left exenterated orbit after spontaneous granulation. The stub of the optic nerve with its adjacent vessels can be seen. A sino-orbital fistula has been created resulting in an orbito-ethmoidal communication.

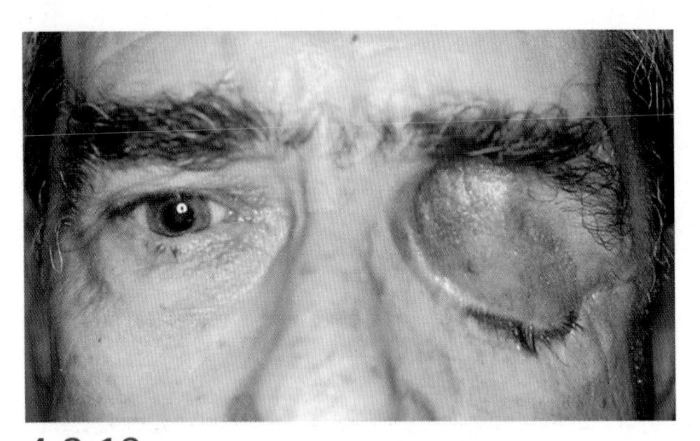

4.8.10 Clinical photograph of a left exenterated orbit with lid-sparing technique.

interrupted absorbable sutures, and the orbit is packed with Xeroform gauze as a mould to provide firm apposition of the graft to the bone. Success depends on the entire surface being held in contact with the bone by firm even pressure.

Although orbits lined by skin grafts heal faster than ungrafted ones, they do not have the advantage of developing fibrosis (Figure 4.8.11).

Regional reconstructive options

MEDIAN FOREHEAD FLAPS

Because forehead flaps are designed with an intact major blood vessel, they provide healing and do not require specialized microvascular surgery. Forehead flaps provide ample tissue for the repair of nasal and maxillary defects that often accompany the resection of orbital and periorbital tumours.

The forehead flap results in aesthetic morbidity at the donor site, a common complaint of patients who undergo such procedures.

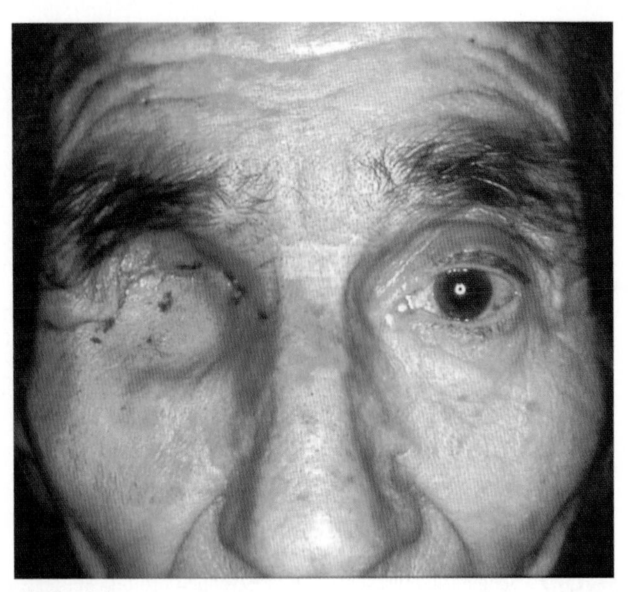

4.8.11 Clinical photograph of a right exenterated orbit lined with split thickness skin graft.

SURGICAL TECHNIQUE

The median forehead flap is outlined on the skin (Figure 4.8.12a) An incision in the natural horizontal furrow of the forehead or parallel to it is made down to the frontal bone periosteum (Figure 4.8.12b). The flap is dissected from its apex toward the base. The subdermal dissection is performed with care taken to leave subdermal vascular territory to maintain the blood supply of the remaining skin, and also with care taken to leave sufficient tissue, including muscle, at the level of the brow to fit the bulk of the flap and to protect hair follicles (Figure 4.8.12c). When the subperiosteal dissection is made toward the level of the orbital rim, the supratrochlear and supraorbital vessel vascular pedicles and supraorbital nerve should be identified. After that, the base of the flap can be undermined sufficiently to permit its easy adaptation (Figure 4.8.12d). Based on its pedicle, the flap is rotated 90°, with a rotation point at the level of the orbital rim (Figure 4.8.12e). After the flap is adapted as a turnover to the defect, it is sutured to the edges of the skin of the orbital defect with 5/0 Vicryl sutures (Figure 4.8.12f). The defect in the forehead, depending on the size of the elevated median forehead flap, is either primarily sutured or can be covered with a full-thickness free skin graft (Figure 4.8.12g). The grafted full thickness skin can be harvested from the supraclavical area or when in the form of a split-thickness skin graft can be taken from the thigh. A tie-over dressing is applied and is left in place for 10 days (Figure 4.8.12h,i). The entire middle third of the forehead will survive elevation on the basis of the dominant vascular pedicle and its height can reach the hairline. The 90° twist needed to reach the exenterated orbital cavity does not usually impair the blood supply. A potential complication is transfer of eyebrow hair to the socket.

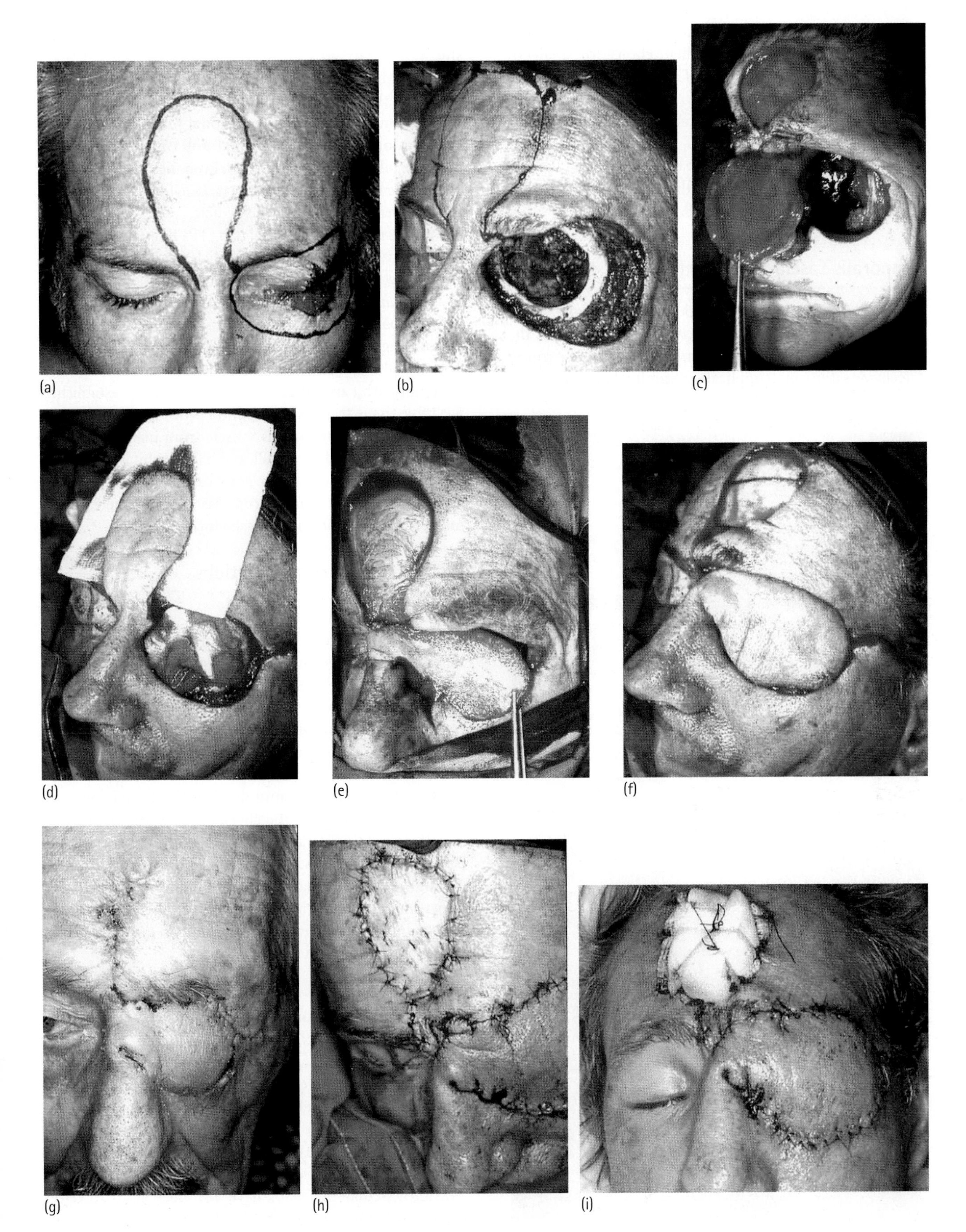

4.8.12 Schematic representation of the use of median forehead flap to cover a total exenteration surgical defect (see text for explanation of panels (a) to (i)).

From a functional and an aesthetic standpoint, the median forehead flap is an excellent choice for small- or medium-sized orbital defects. The forehead skin more closely matches the pigmentation and structure of the periocular tissue. Forehead flaps can be used in conjunction with other local and regional flaps to repair larger orbitofacial defects. The relative ease of harvesting the flap minimizes operative time and the robust blood supply decreases failure rates (Figures 4.8.13 and 4.8.14).

Temporalis fascia and muscle flaps

Among the advantages of the temporalis muscle flap (TMF), one can include easy surgical technique, reliability of the vascular pedicle, sufficient volume to cover large surgical defects, versatility in its application, minimal post-operative complications and freedom from dysfunction at the donor site.

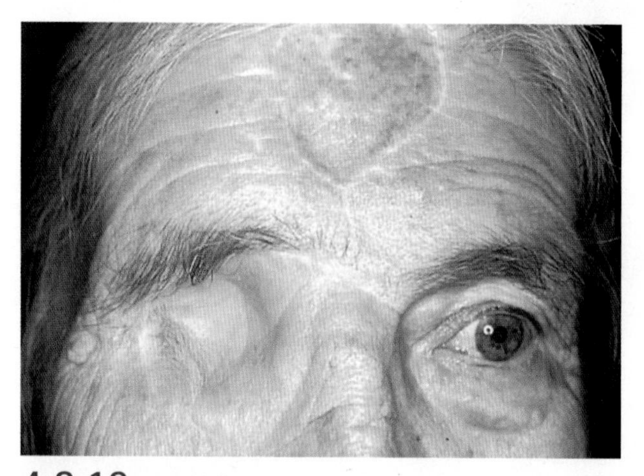

4.8.13 Clinical photograph of a female patient with a right total orbital exenteration and a median forehead flap to reconstruct the orbital defect.

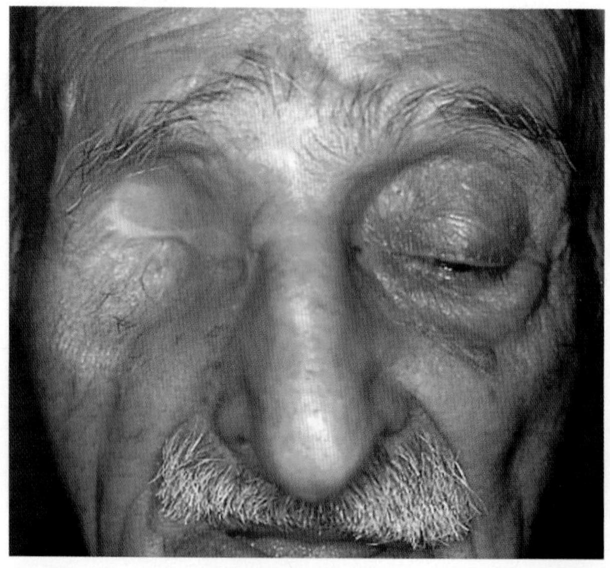

4.8.14 Clinical photograph of a male patient with a right total orbital exenteration reconstructed with a median forehead flap.

The TMF is one of the most frequently used flaps to obliterate the orbital cavity, but only a small portion of the muscle can be used unless additional procedures, such as fenestration of the lateral orbital wall or resection of the lateral orbital rim, are performed. Even these procedures do not enable the entire mass of the muscle to be used, because most of the muscle acts as the pedicle.

The temporoparietal fascial flap (TPFF) is the only fascial flap that can be harvested as a pedicled flap for periorbital and socket reconstruction. Its thin width (average width 2–3 mm) and need for grafting are the main disadvantages.

Small paranasal sinus or brain fistulas are obliterated by performing locoregional flaps transposed through the lateral orbital wall. In more extensive cases, the boundaries between the empty orbit and adjacent cavities must be re-established with free tissue transfer. A common procedure is to borrow a portion of the temporalis muscle from its anterior half, pass it through the lateral wall, and fill the orbital cavity with the bulk of this graft. Skin graft can be placed over the muscle flap. In most instances, this procedure effectively makes the exenteration cavity shallow.

Distant reconstructive options

PEDICLED FLAPS

Regional flaps are used frequently for reconstruction following exenteration, but these flaps can cover only the anterior orbit and leave potential dead space posteriorly.

Use of the pectoralis major myocutaneous flap for orbital reconstruction is limited, due to the distance the muscle pedicle has to travel from the anterior thoracic wall to the orbit. There have been attempts to use the sternocleido-mastoid, trapezius, lattisimus dorsi and platysma flap.

Other local flaps like the cheek flap, the submental and the retroauricular island flap can also be used to reconstruct periorbital defects. They provide superior cosmetic results through enhanced matching of skin colour, texture and structural characteristics, have a rich vascular supply and a low complication rate, and do not require complex microvascular surgery.

MICROVASCULAR FREE FLAPS

Surgical reconstruction of the orbital cavity after orbital exenteration with maxillectomy is technically challenging. The reconstruction of such defects obliterates any communication between the orbit and the nasopharynx, reconstructs the palatal surface and the nasal airway, and provides an acceptable cosmetic result. Ideally, the selected tissue should facilitate this and provide a well-vascularized bed to withstand post-operative radiotherapy.

Microvascular free flaps have also been used to cover defects following extended orbital exenteration. Facial or temporal vessels may be suitable for microvascular anastomoses. A wide selection of free flaps can be used in orbital and orbitomaxillary defects.

Primary reconstruction of orbit and maxillary defects with free microvascular rectus abdominis flaps has numerous advantages. In contrast with procedures that use the temporalis or the pectoralis major as a pedicled flap, the rectus abdominis free flap permits reconstruction with larger volumes of well-vascularized tissue and greater flexibility in placement without associated orientation problems.

Maintaining the nasal airways is often the most difficult problem in this particular group of patients, and a second skin island to address lateral nasal wall reconstruction is often helpful (Figure 4.8.15).

Ocular and oculofacial prosthetics

Orbital prosthetics are never completely lifelike, because vital eye movements are absent. Spectacles can camouflage this aesthetic deficiency and protect the uninvolved eye at the same time.

The key decision to be made when approaching an orbital exenteration defect is whether to leave the cavity open or closed. An open cavity requires less sophisticated surgery, may permit better tumour surveillance and allows the use of a prosthesis. However, an open cavity can lead to surrounding tissue contracture with inferior displacement of the brow and distortion of the cheek.

Despite recent advances in contemporary oculofacial prosthetics, the aesthetic results after a standard orbital exenteration remain poor and unacceptable for many patients. Although traditional exenteration with a spectacle-mounted, osseointegrated or adhesive-secured prosthesis may achieve acceptable cosmesis, many patients have difficulty in obtaining good prosthetic care. Many patients prefer to wear an eye patch to cover the surgical site.

The basic requirements for an exenterated socket that can maintain an ocular prosthesis are (1) orbital tissue volume to support the prosthesis, (2) a mucous membrane surface with fornices to accommodate the prosthesis and (3) eyelids to hold the prosthesis within the socket. The limiting factor in most exenteration cases is the preservation of a mucosal surface, which is essential if the prosthetic shell is to be comfortable. Unless significant portions of the conjunctiva can be retained, an ocular prosthesis is not a rehabilitative option after orbital exenteration, and the surgical plan should take this into account.

Osseointegrated implants have helped overcome a number of the problems associated with facial prostheses. They provide reliable anchorage for large and heavy prostheses and facilitate their rapid placement and removal. Modern magnetic capped implants are very simple to use.

COMPLICATIONS

The most serious post-operative complication in orbital surgery is haemorrhage, which can happen immediately post-operatively or weeks later, but generally occurs in the 4–6 days after the operation. Because the orbit is small and closed, any haematoma may be significant. Wound infection and dehiscence, as well as orbital cellulitis, are unusual post-operative complications following tumour resection.

Orbital exenteration defects left to granulate spontaneously can be complicated by a prolonged healing phase, chronic hygiene problems, orbitosinus or orbitonasal fistula formation, dural exposure and cerebrospinal fluid leaks. The high rate of sino-orbital fistulas following spontaneous granulation of exenterated orbital cavities can be avoided by formal surgical closure and reconstruction.

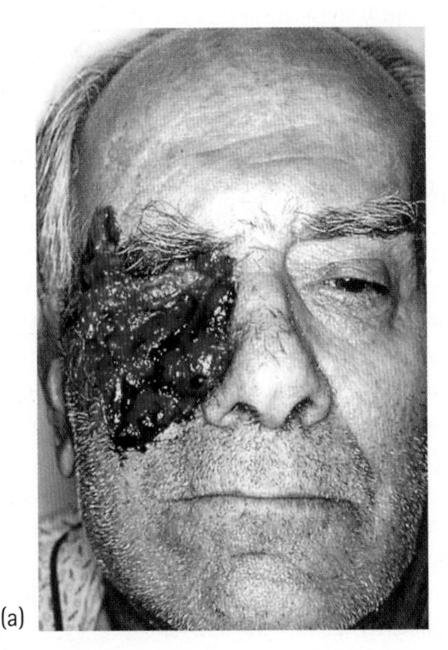

(a)

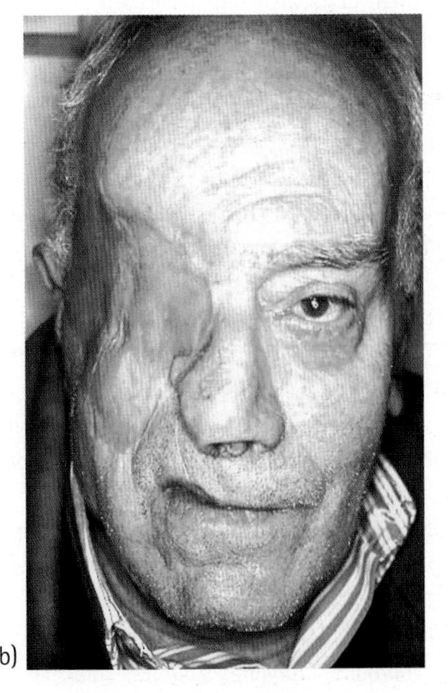

(b)

4.8.15 (a) Clinical photograph of a patient with extensive basal cell carcinoma of the eyelids which extends to the periorbital skin tissues. (b) The extended orbital exenteration defect has been reconstructed with the use of a rectus abdominis muscle free flap covered with split thickness skin graft.

Top tips

- Use magnetic resonance imaging for the delineation of the orbital tumour.
- Use computed tomography for the identification of osseous extensions of the orbital mass.
- Use unipolar cautery (Colorado tip) to delineate the orbital incision.
- Use periosteal elevator to dissect the periorbita from the orbital walls.
- Use curved scissors to cut the optic nerve, and ophthalmic artery and vein.
- Ligate the ophthalmic vessels.
- Start the reconstruction after the extirpation of the tumour as you may need to change the reconstructive plan according to intra-operative findings.

FURTHER READING

Ben Simon GJ, Schwarcz RM, Douglas R *et al.* Orbital exenteration: One size does not fit all. *American Journal of Ophthalmology* 2005; **139**: 11–17.

Callender DL, Frankenthaler RA, Weber RS *et al.* Carcinomas of the lacrimal drainage system. *Head and Neck* 1993; **15**: 313–19.

Chepeha DB, Wang SJ, Marentette LJ *et al.* Restoration of the orbital aesthetic subunit in complex midface defects. *Laryngoscope* 2004; **114**: 1706–13.

Cook BE Jr, Bartley GB. Epidemiologic characteristics and clinical course of patients with malignant eyelid tumors in an incidence cohort in Olmsted County, Minnesota. *Ophthalmology* 1999; **106**: 746–50.

Cook BE Jr, Bartley GB. Treatment options and future prospects for the management of eyelid malignancies: An evidence-based update. *Ophthalmology* 2001; **108**: 2088–98.

Esmaeli B, Ahmadi MA, Youssef A *et al.* Outcomes in patients with adenoid cystic carcinoma of the lacrimal gland. *Ophthalmic Plastic and Reconstructive Surgery* 2004; **20**: 22–26.

Esmaeli B, Golio D, Kies M, DeMonte F. Surgical management of locally advanced adenoid cystic carcinoma of the lacrimal gland. *Ophthalmic Plastic and Reconstructive Surgery* 2006; **22**: 366–70.

Fan J. A new technique of scarless expanded forehead flap for reconstructive surgery. *Plastic and Reconstructive Surgery* 2000; **106**: 777–85.

Gil Z, Abergel A, Leider-Trejo L *et al.* A comprehensive algorithm for anterior skull base reconstruction after oncological resections. *Skull Base* 2007; **17**: 25–37.

Goldberg RA, Kim JW, Shorr N. Orbital exenteration: Results of an individualized approach. *Ophthalmic Plastic and Reconstructive Surgery* 2003; **19**: 229–36.

Iannetti G, Valentini V, Rinna C et al. Ethmoido-orbital tumors: Our experience. *Journal of Craniofacial Surgery* 2005; **16**: 1085–91.

Imola MJ, Schramm VL Jr. Orbital preservation in surgical management of sinonasal malignancy. *Laryngoscope* 2002; **112**: 1357–65.

Jackson IT. Midline forehead flaps in nasal reconstruction. *European Journal of Plastic Surgery* 2004; **27**: 105–13.

Jung WS, Ahn KJ, Park MR *et al.* The radiological spectrum of orbital pathologies that involve the lacrimal gland and the lacrimal fossa. *Korean Journal of Radiology* 2007; **8**: 336–42.

Karcioglu ZA. *Orbital tumors. Diagnosis and treatment.* Berlin: Springer Science + Business Media, Inc, 2005

Leibovitch I, McNab A, Sullivan T *et al.* Orbital invasion by periocular basal cell carcinoma. *Ophthalmology* 2005; **112**: 717–23.

Liarikos S, Rapidis AD, Roumeliotis A, Angelopoulos AP. Secondary orbital melanomas: Analysis of 15 cases. *Journal of Craniomaxillofacial Surgery* 2000; **28**: 148–52.

Menick F. Nasal reconstruction: Forehead flap. *Plastic and Reconstrive Surgery* 2004; **113**: 100e–11e.

Menon NG, Girotto JA, Goldberg NH, Silverman RP. Orbital reconstruction after exenteration: Use of a transorbital temporal muscle flap. *Annals of Plastic Surgery* 2003; **50**: 38–42.

Nassab RS, Thomas SS, Murray D. Orbital exenteration for advanced periorbital skin cancers: 20 years experience. *Journal of Plastic and Reconstrive Aesthetic Surgery* 2007; **60**: 1103–109.

Park SS. The single stage forehead flap in nasal reconstruction. An alternative with advantages. *Archives of Facial and Plastic Surgery* 2002; **4**: 32–36.

Perez DEC, Pires FR, Almeida OP, Kowalski LP. Epithelial lacrimal gland tumors: A clinicopathological study of 18 cases. *Otolaryngology–Head and Neck Surgery* 2006; **134**: 321–5.

Price DL, Sherris DA, Bartley GB, Garrity JA. Forehead flap periorbital reconstruction. *Archives of Facial Plastic Surgery* 2004; **6**: 222–7.

Pryor SG, Moore EJ, Kasperbauer JL. Orbital exenteration reconstruction with rectus abdominis microvascular free flap. *Laryngoscope* 2005; 115: 1912–6.

Rapidis AD, Liarikos S. Malignant orbital and orbitomaxillary tumors: Surgical considerations. *Orbit* 1998; **17**: 77–88.

Santamaria E, Cordeiro PG. Reconstruction of maxillectomy and midfacial defects with free tissue transfer. *Journal of Surgical Oncology* 2006; **94**: 522–31.

Shields JA, Shields CL, Demirci H *et al.* Experience with eyelid-sparing orbital exenteration: The 2000 Tullos O. Coston Lecture. *Ophthalmic Plastic and Reconstructive Surgery* 2001; **17**: 355–61.

Shields JA, Shields CL, Gündüz K, Cater J. Clinical features predictive of orbital exenteration for conjunctival melanoma. *Ophthalmic Plastic and Reconstructive Surgery* 2000; **16**: 173–8.

Shields JA, Shields CL, Scartozzi R. Survey of 1264 patients with orbital tumors and simulating lesions: The 2002 Montgomery Lecture, part 1. *Ophthalmology* 2004; **111**: 997–1008.

Sturgis CD, Silverman JF, Kennerdell JS, Raab SS. Fine-needle aspiration for the diagnosis of primary epithelial tumors of the lacrimal gland and ocular adnexa. *Diagnostic Cytopathology* 2001; **24**: 86–9.

Yeatts RP. The esthetics of orbital exenteration. *American Journal of Ophthalmology* 2005; **139**: 152–3.

Zwahlen RA, Gratz KW, Obwegeser JA. The galea fascia flap in orbital reconstruction: Innovative harvest technique. *European Journal of Surgical Oncology* 2006; **32**: 804–807.

4.9

Neck dissection

PETER A BRENNAN

INTRODUCTION

Many of the surgical principles described in this chapter have not changed significantly since 1906, when Crile published his classic paper describing 132 neck dissections (36 radical and 96 more selective procedures). Only two years later, Sir Henry Butlin described a procedure that is essentially the same as a modern day supra-omohyoid neck dissection (SOHND). Despite this publication of a 'selective' neck dissection, most elective treatment of even the clinically negative (N0) neck during the first half of the twentieth century consisted mainly of radical neck dissection (RND). Over the last 20 years, there has been an increasing trend towards selective neck dissection (SND) for the initial management of patients with no clinical evidence of neck metastasis, and in carefully selected patients with nodal metastasis (although its use in the latter remains controversial).

While SND preserves many vital structures (such as the accessory nerve), the functional results after these procedures are not as good as expected. Shoulder function and pain scores are worse in patients who undergo posterior triangle dissection, which may not recover despite preservation of the accessory nerve. A study has found that the variables that contribute most to quality of life scores relating to the neck were age and weight, radiotherapy to the neck and neck dissection type.

NECK DISSECTION CLASSIFICATION

The nomenclature of neck dissection can be confusing. It can be simplified as follows:

- Radical neck dissection. This refers to removal of lymph nodes in levels I–V en bloc with the sternomastoid muscle, internal jugular vein and spinal accessory nerve. This operation is both cosmetically and functionally mutilating and is used in gross metastatic disease, involving multiple levels of the neck and when preservation of the above structures would compromise surgical clearance. Although this operation has been regarded as the 'gold standard' for the surgical treatment of metastatic neck disease, it has largely been replaced by more selective surgery.
- Modified radical neck dissection (MRND). This refers to dissection of levels I–V, but with the preservation of one or more of the following structures: internal jugular vein, spinal accessory nerve and sternomastoid. The nomenclature refers to the number of structures preserved (so MRND type I is preservation of one of these structures, MRND type II is preservation of two structures and so on). Both RND and MRND are used when the neck has evidence of nodal metastasis (N+), although there is growing evidence to suggest that the more selective neck dissection (see below) has a role to play not only in staging but in the management of the N+ neck as well. The reader is referred to an excellent recent view of this subject.
- Selective neck dissection. In 1991, the Committee for Head and Neck Surgery and Oncology of the American Academy of Otolaryngology and Head and Neck Surgery indicated that 'in all SND, the internal jugular vein, spinal accessory nerve and sternomastoid muscle are routinely preserved. If removal of one or more of these structures is necessary, the structure should be listed after the appropriate term for the neck dissection.' As a result, SND can easily be confused with MRND and indeed some surgeons use the terms interchangeably. However, SND should refer to the dissection of one or more levels of the neck (with careful preservation of the anatomical structures listed above, as well as other nerves, such as the marginal mandibular branch of the facial nerve) rather than all five levels. Examples include the supra-omohyoid neck dissection (levels I–III), lateral compartment neck dissection (levels II–IV) and levels I–IV neck dissection.

TERMINOLOGY OF NECK LEVELS

The most significant change to the well-known Robbins classification was the publication of an updated system in 2002. In addition to the five standard levels, nodal levels were subdivided into levels IA and B, IIA and B (below and above the accessory nerve), and VA and B (above and below the accessory nerve in the posterior triangle) (Figure 4.9.1). The concept of sublevels is clinically relevant since metastasis to level IIB from anterior oral cavity tumours is uncommon and metastases to level VA is rarer still, with studies advocating that the dissection of these levels is not usually necessary.

PRINCIPLES OF SURGERY

The rationale for neck dissection is based on predictable patterns of lymphatic spread from the primary tumour site and the relative risk of nodal metastatic disease. Over 30 years ago, Lindberg's clinical study found that the jugulodigastric and mid-cervical nodes (levels II and III) were the most frequently involved in metastatic disease from the oral cavity. Tumours of the lip, anterior two-thirds of the tongue, floor of the mouth and buccal mucosa also metastasize to the level I nodes (submental and submandibular triangles), often bilaterally. Lindberg described the possibility of skip metastasis, avoiding the first echelon nodes and spreading directly to the level III area. More recent studies have found that when levels I–IV are negative, level V is never node positive, supporting the use of the SND for the clinically negative (N0) neck. Despite many published studies, there is still controversy about neck dissection surgery and the reader should refer to specialist textbooks for a full discussion.

When taking trainees through a neck dissection, the author makes the analogy of walking through a jungle. Some structures in the neck (such as the digastric and omohyoid muscles) will help to delineate the path – these are your trusted guides. However, you will also come across many dangers which if not treated with respect could take you by surprise, sometimes when you least expect it! These include structures such as the phrenic, hypoglossal and marginal mandibular nerves.

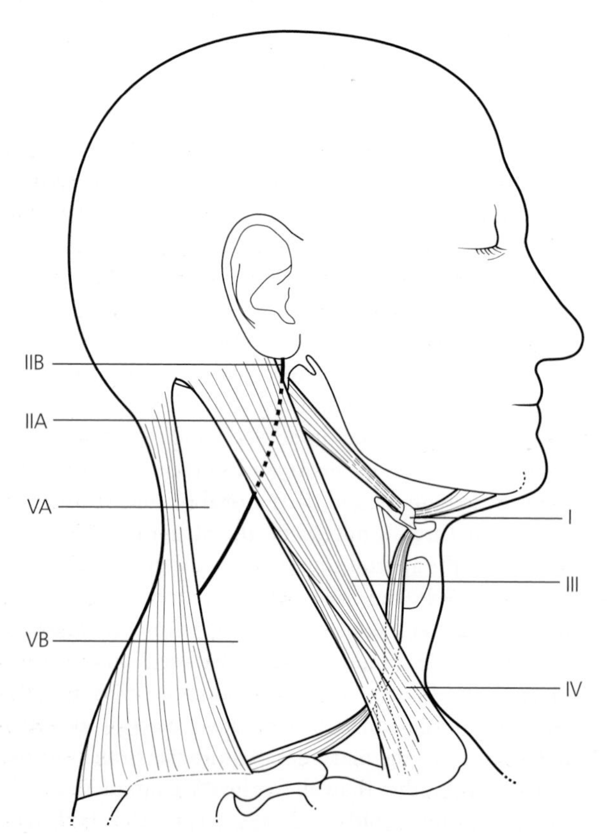

4.9.1 Levels of the neck. Level is divided into 1A (submental) and IB (submandibular triangles).

TECHNIQUE

Patient position

- For all neck dissections, the fully anaesthetized (but unparalysed) patient should be placed supine on the operating table with the head turned away from the side being operated. A sandbag can be used if required to elevate the shoulder. It is sensible to expose the neck from the sternum and lateral clavicle to the ear and lips. Following skin preparation, the drapes need to be secured in place using adhesive strips, sutures or skin clips. It is useful to keep the lower lip exposed (to check for marginal mandibular nerve function).
- Choice of incision. This depends on the type of neck dissection being undertaken. Ideally, skin incisions should be placed in natural skin creases, following Langer's lines. The lower border of the mandible, sternomastoid and clavicle can be marked to assist placement of the incision. For an SND, an incision running from the mastoid to submental area 3 cm below the mandible is usually adequate. When levels IV and V are being dissected, it may be necessary to place a second incision to gain access to these areas. The author routinely uses a Schobinger-type incision for MRND (Figure 4.9.2), except in the previously radiotherapy treated neck, where a MacFee incision is preferred (to reduce the risk of wound dehiscence). When a Schobinger incision is used, it is important not to place the tri-radiate part of the incision over the great vessels, especially if the sternomastoid is removed, as there is a risk of wound infection and vascular compromise. If a MacFee incision is used (this is the correct spelling of the author who described it in 1960, whereas some spell it McFee), an adequate bridge of skin between the incisions (of at least 4 cm) is essential to minimize the risk of skin necrosis (Figure 4.9.3). It is important to mark either side of the incisions (using needle and Bonney's blue, or superficially scoring the skin with the back of a scalpel blade) to facilitate subsequent skin closure.

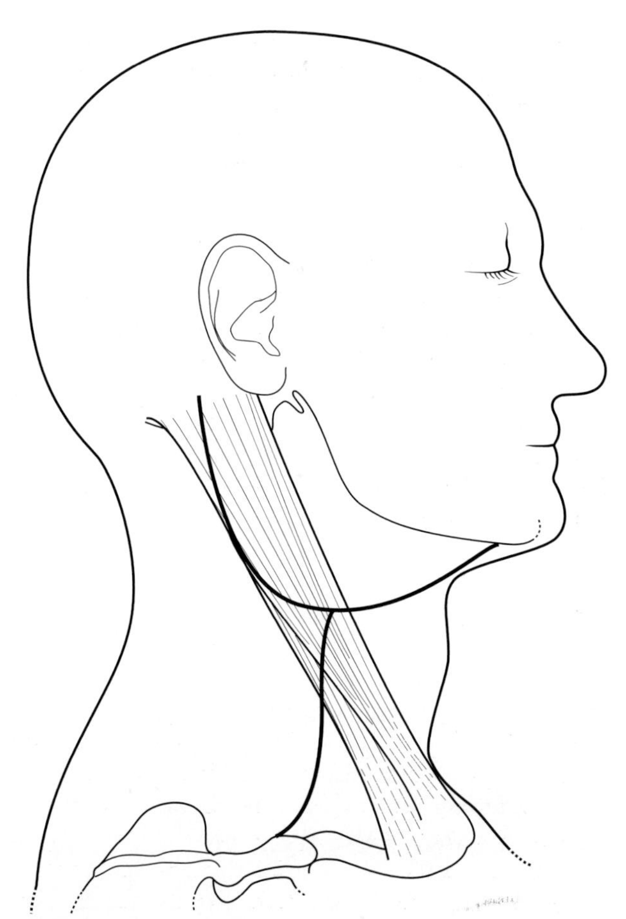

4.9.2 Schobinger incision for modified radical neck dissection.

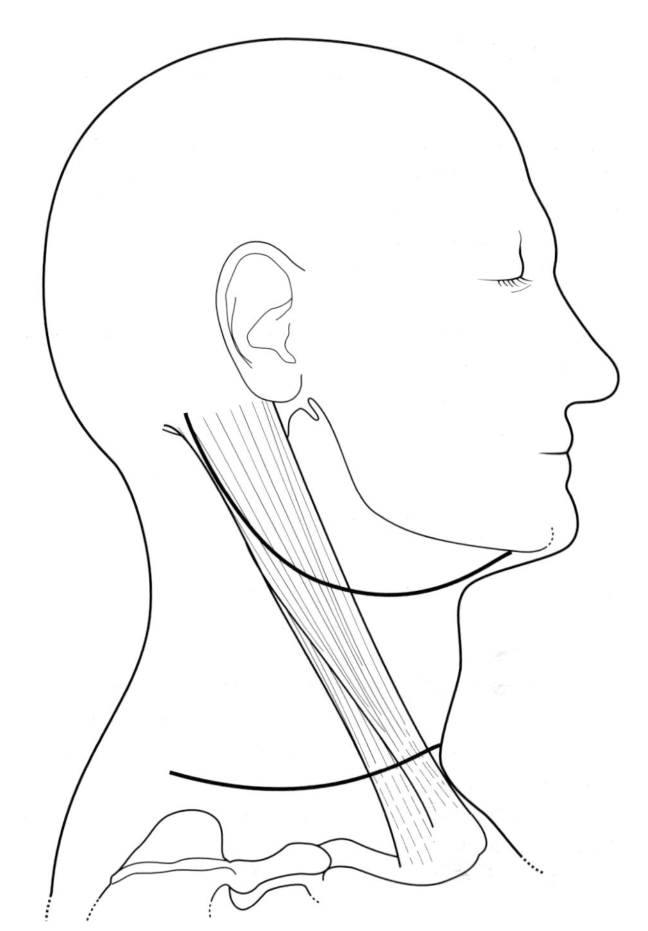

4.9.3 MacFee incision. Distance between incisions should be at least 4 cm.

- Development of skin flaps. It is usual to raise skin flaps in a subplatysmal plane. Local anaesthestic solution may be injected to facilitate this process. The flaps can be raised using monopolar diathermy (Colorado needle), scalpel or scissor dissection. With all of these techniques, but particularly when diathermy is used, care should be taken in the upper skin flap to minimize damage to the marginal mandibular nerve, which lies just deep to the playtsma muscle in the deep cervical fascia. It can be readily identified as it crosses the facial vessels and great care should be taken to preserve this nerve. It is sometimes possible to preserve the great auricular nerve as it crosses the sternomastoid muscle, although the roots (C2,3) are often transacted later on in the dissection. In both the submental and posterior triangles, the platysma muscle often fades away and care should be taken to ensure that the skin flap does not become too thick or thin in these areas. It is sometimes surprising just how superficial the accessory nerve can be! The external jugular vein is easily damaged when the inferior skin flap is being raised as it lies immediately deep to the platysma muscle and may need to be ligated. The flaps should be developed beyond the boundaries of the neck dissection to be performed. For a MRND, the flap should be extended to the trapezius muscle in the posterior triangle. The muscle can be brought into view by having an assistant pushing it upwards and forwards. In bulky disease, it may be necessary to leave the platysma on the metastatic nodes, or even include skin in the resection if clinically indicated. In these cases, it is important to plan skin incisions to facilitate subsequent closure.

Start of neck dissection proper: I–IV SND

Where should I start the neck dissection? This is a question often asked by newcomers to this procedure. There are many ways to perform the procedure (inferiorly to superiorly, posterior to anterior, etc.) and it is often good to try different methods and to vary these on separate occasions to find a way that works for each operator. Even then, one's routine procedure may need to be modified when, for example, a large metastasis is present in level II, in which case it is often wise to start somewhere else. Also, if one particular area is proving difficult, move on to another region and come back to it. The procedure described below is for a level I–IV SND. The RND and MRND variations are discussed subsequently.

Mobilization of the sternocleidomastoid muscle

The fascia overlying the sternocleidomastoid muscle (SCM) is incised along the whole posterior margin length of the muscle and lifted anteriorly. The dissection is continued close to the muscle in a broad front inferiorly and superiorly around its anterior border. Superiorly, the tail of the parotid and the posterior digastric muscle will come into view on its way to the mastoid process. The SCM is then retracted posteriorly, and the carotid sheath will come into view, initially with the internal jugular vein (IJV) (Figure 4.9.4). By maintaining a broad front, the SCM can be skeletonized away from the underlying deep structures. It can then be retracted with vascular slings. The omohyoid muscle will be seen inferiorly, the tendon of which passes superficial to the IJV. This muscle arbitrarily divides the 'surgical neck' into levels III and IV, although the position of the muscle varies with neck position. For a level IV dissection, the omohyoid is dissected free from the IJV, whereas in a SOHND, the dissection commences superiorly to the upper border of this muscle. As one dissects superiorly, the accessory nerve will be found deep to the posterior digastric, passing in a medial to lateral direction into the anterior border of the upper third of the SCM. It can often be felt as a cord-like structure. By hugging the anterior border of the SCM in a broad front, this important nerve is easily identified. It is worth noting that this nerve has many anatomical variations (one can be seen in Figure 4.9.5) and it can pass superficial, deep or even through the IJV.

Clearance down to pre-vertebral fascia

The fatty tissue containing nodes posterior to the IJV is carefully incised at the inferior extent of the dissection in a horizontal direction. This is done in stages, so as to not inadvertently go through the thin pre-vertebral fascia. The use of scissor dissection combined with the intermittent use of a wet swab to sweep this tissue off the pre-vertebral fascia enables easy identification of this fascia. The phrenic nerve will be seen under the pre-vertebral fascia passing from lateral to medial on the scalenus anterior muscle (Figure 4.9.6). More laterally at the root of the neck, the upper trunks of the brachial plexus may also be visualized, again under the fascia. The author routinely extends this dissection laterally to the area over which lies the posterior border of the SCM (effectively including the anterior border of level V in the dissection). Once the correct depth has been established, it is quite easy to carry the posterolateral part of this dissection in a superior direction. This can be facilitated by appropriate retraction and countertraction.

As the dissection proceeds in this way, one will come across cervical nerves that have pierced the pre-vertebral fascia. These can be cut as long as they are superficial to it and the phrenic nerve has been identified. In some cases it is possible to preserve some of these nerves, thereby

4.9.4 Dissection around sternomastoid muscle (SCM) to reveal internal jugular vein (IJV). The accessory nerve is just coming into view (arrowed).

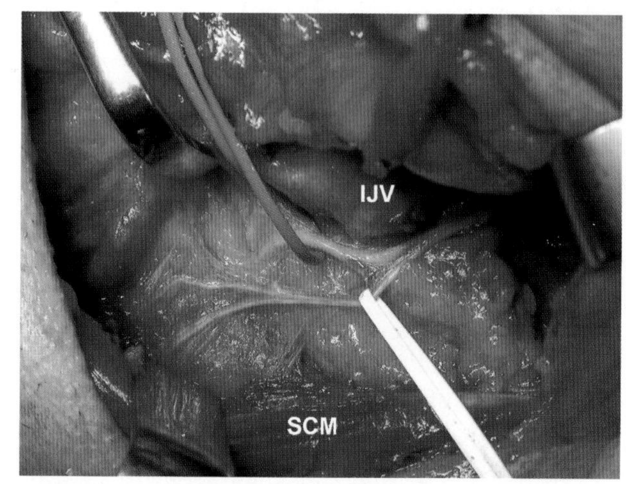

4.9.5 Identification of the accessory nerve. In this case, a variant with innervation from a cervical plexus nerve.

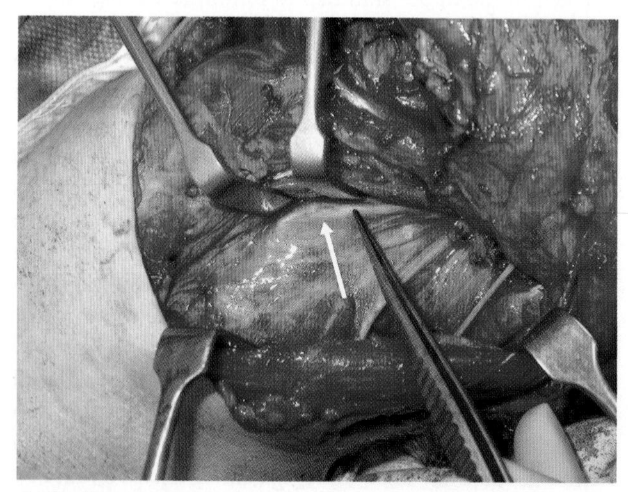

4.9.6 Clearance in level IV. The phrenic nerve under the pre-vertebral fascia is arrowed.

maintaining sensation to the skin in the dermatomes supplied by them. As one reaches the accessory nerve superiorly, the sternomastoid is retracted fully, and the level IIB can be cleared down to the muscular floor. The anatomical variations of this nerve should be remembered (it can be anterior (most common) or posterior to the IJV, or even pass through the vein). Level IIB contains the occipital artery, which runs postero-inferior to the posterior digastric muscle. Once cleared, the fatty tissue can be passed under the accessory nerve in continuity with the neck dissection specimen.

Dissection and clearance around the great vessels

The dissection now proceeds anteriorly on to and around the IJV. The fascia overlying the posterior aspect of the IJV is incised in a broad front (superiorly and inferiorly) and dissection is carried around the IJV itself. With a left-sided neck dissection and when approaching the IJV inferiorly in level IV, an attempt should be made to identify the thoracic duct on its posterior surface. It is also vital to identify the vagus nerve (Figure 4.9.7), which usually lies between the IJV and common carotid artery. Superiorly, the hypoglossal nerve will be seen crossing the internal and external carotids. It gives a descending branch (C1) which joins with C2,3 to form the ansa cervicalis. This nerve usually lies anterolateral to the IJV and should be preserved if possible (if only to show off one's technical expertise!). The sympathetic chain can sometimes be seen on the pre-vertebral fascia deep to the carotid artery, although the dissection itself should not be deeper than the IJV.

Anterior dissection

The limits of the anterior dissection are the anterior border of the omohyoid, and the midline of the neck in the submental triangle. The dissection can proceed quite quickly up the omohyoid muscle. Occasionally, a large vein is identified (sometimes after it has been cut!), but this is readily ligated. As the dissection reaches the inferior part of the hyoid bone, care should be taken to re-identify the hypoglossal nerve as it passes into the submandibular triangle. The dissection can now continue from the midline along the lower border of the mandible. The mandibular periosteum can be incised to create a sharp plane of dissection. The submental area is usually quite vascular, due to many branches of the submental vessels. The bleeding is usually controlled with diathermy.

Submandibular triangle

As the dissection passes along the mandible, the mylohyoid muscle will come into view. The marginal mandibular branch of the facial nerve should be identified (if this has not already been done) and retracted. The facial vessels can be ligated and retracted superiorly to assist retraction of this nerve (Figure 4.9.8). Having dealt with these structures, it is easy to retract the mylohyoid, exposing the floor of the mouth and enabling easy removal of the submandibular gland (Figure 4.9.9). The lingual (superiorly) and hypoglossal nerves (inferiorly) should be identified in the floor of the mouth and the submandibular ganglion and duct ligated and divided. At the posterior aspect of the gland lies the facial artery, which loops over the posterior digastric. This requires division. If possible, when a microvascular reconstruction is taking place, this artery should be left as long as possible to facilitate subsequent anastomosis. All that remains is to join up the posterior part of the submandibular triangle with the level II dissection. The tail of the parotid can be included here and the retromandibular vein will need to be ligated. The specimen should be suitably orientated for the pathologist (see Chapter 4.3).

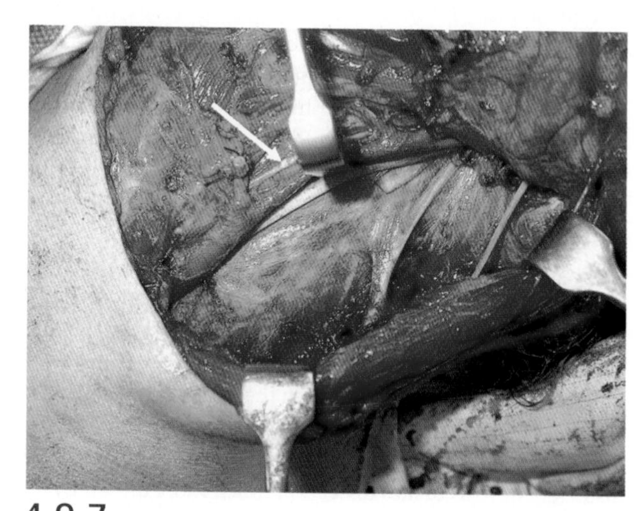

4.9.7 Further dissection reveals the vagus nerve and ansa cervicalis (arrowed).

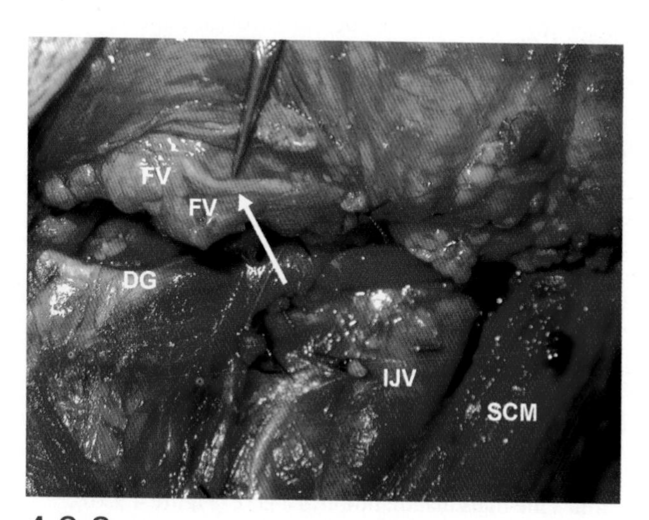

4.9.8 Marginal mandibular branch of facial nerve. The facial vessels (FV) have been ligated. DG, digastric tendon.

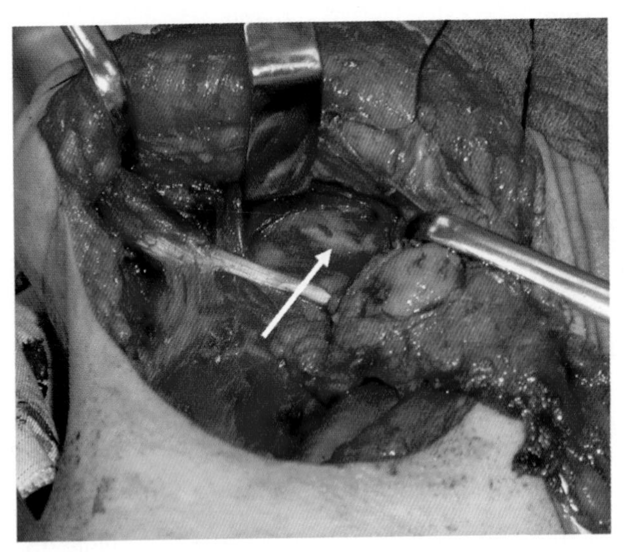

4.9.9 Level I clearance. The lingual nerve is arrowed.

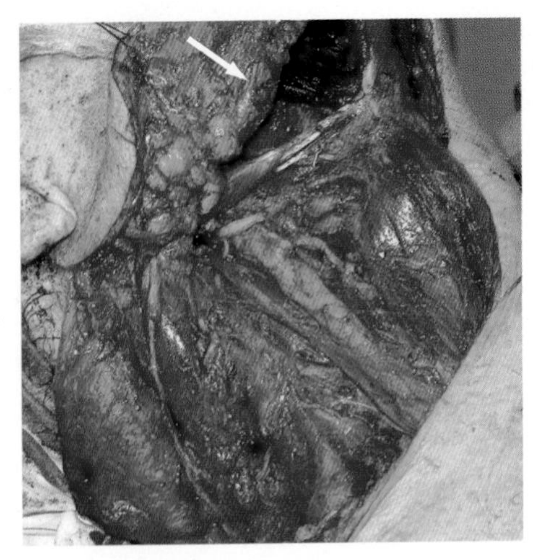

4.9.10 Completed modified radical neck dissection type I with preservation of accessory and marginal mandibular nerve (arrowed).

Drains and closure

Meticulous haemostasis is paramount for this procedure – the patient should be positioned head down to increase venous pressure to visualize bleeding points. A Valsalva manoeuvre given by the anaesthetist to further increase venous pressure is also often helpful. Two large drains (size 16) should be placed. The author routinely uses 4/0 maxon to close platysma, with either 5/0 prolene or skin clips to close the skin itself.

Variations: MRND and RND

In many respects, the removal of the SCM makes the neck dissection much easier, although adds morbidity for the patient. With a RND or MRND (when the SCM and IJV are included), the SCM can be cut through superiorly and inferiorly using monopolar diathermy. The IJV itself requires careful ligation both superiorly and inferiorly. The author places two 2/0 linen ties with a 3/0 silk transfixation suture between them on the IJV being left. On the part of the vein being removed, it is wise to place a transfixation suture as well, since the ties sometimes come off during the dissection giving an unexpected shock. Since there is low pressure in the IJV, any bleeding can be temporarily arrested with pressure. If a tie comes off superiorly at the skull base, it should still be possible to control bleeding with pressure (even suturing packs in place). Once the SCM and IJV are divided, it is easy to use the cut omohyoid muscle belly to rapidly progress the dissection anteriorly. Ideally, if possible, the accessory nerve should be preserved in a MRND, as should the marginal mandibular nerve (Figure 4.9.10).

Level V can be cleared starting initially inferiorly along the clavicle, again down to the level of the pre-vertebral fascia. Large clips (e.g. Roberts) can be used to clamp the fat (and transverse cervical vessels). These are ligated as one proceeds with the dissection. At this point, care should be taken not to inadvertently pull up the subclavian vessels! This can be prevented by initially dissecting straight down through the fat on to the pre-vertebral fascia. It is also possible to damage the lung apex resulting in a pneumothorax, although this is rare. The accessory nerve can be dissected free and skeletonized from the fat if this nerve is being preserved. The cervical nerves will need to be cut to enable removal of level V, but remember that these should only be cut when they are superficial to the pre-vertebral fascia. It may be necessary to cut the inferior belly of the omohyoid.

SUPRA-OMOHYOID NECK DISSECTION

The principles of a more selective procedure are the same as for the I–IV neck dissection described above, although it can be technically more challenging. The dissection usually starts inferiorly over the omohyoid muscle and proceeds superiorly as before. As with a level I–IV neck dissection, it is important to mobilize the SCM muscle and take the dissection posterior to the IJV to sample as many nodes as possible.

EFFECTS OF RADIOTHERAPY

Surgery becomes more difficult in the irradiated neck and it is often more difficult to preserve structures, particularly nerves such as the accessory nerve. Tissue planes are distorted, fibrosis makes dissection much more difficult, and bleeding from small vessels can also be a problem. Furthermore, there is a greater chance of wound breakdown.

Table 4.9.1 Complications of neck dissection

	Complication	Treatment
Immediate	Bleeding	Packing, identify vessel, repair if appropriate (involve vascular surgeons if common or internal carotid (rare)
	Pneumothorax	Chest drain
	Damage to thoracic duct	Oversew with 3/0 silk, use sternomastoid or omohyoid plug
	Inadvertent transaction of nerve	Microneural repair
	Gross swelling (if both IJV compromised)	May need tracheostomy
Early	Chylous leak	Exploration and/or medium chain triglyceride (dietician support)
	Haematoma	Evacuate depending on size
	Infection	Systemic antibiotics/drain if collection
	Wound breakdown	Minimize risk with initial choice of incision and two-layer closure Re-suturing in theatre
Late	Shoulder pain/dysfunction	Physiotherapy
	Contractures	Physiotherapy

Top tips

- Meticulous haemostasis.
- Traction and countertraction.
- Dissection on a broad front.
- Beware of anatomical variations.
- If you get stuck, start dissecting elsewhere and come back.
- Position patient head down at completion to raise venous pressure and identify bleeding points.

FURTHER READING

Butlin HT. *On the results of operations for carcinoma of the tongue. With an analysis of 197 cases.* London: Adlard & Son, 1908.

Crile GW. Excision of cancer of the head and neck. With special reference to the plan of dissection based on one and hundred and thirty two operations. *Journal of the American Medical Association* 1906; **47**: 1780–6.

Ferlito A, Rinaldo A, Silver CE *et al.* Elective and therapeutic neck dissection. *Oral Oncology* 2006; **42**: 14–25.

Hamoir M, Shah JP, Desuter G *et al.* Prevalence of lymph nodes in the apex of level V: A plea against the necessity to dissect the apex of level V in mucosal head and neck cancer. *Head and Neck* 2005; **27**: 963–9.

Lindberg R. Distribution of cervical lymph node metastases of the upper respiratory and digestive tracts. Cancer 1972; **29**: 1446–9.

Macfee WF. Transverse incisions for neck dissection. *Annals of Surgery* 1960; **151**: 279–84.

Robbins KT, Clayman G, Levine PA *et al.* American Head and Neck Society, American Academy of Otolaryngology–Head and Neck Surgery. Neck dissection classification update: Revisions proposed by the American Head and Neck Society and the American Academy of Otolaryngology–Head and Neck Surgery. *Archives of Otolaryngology Head and Neck Surgery* 2002; **128**: 751–8.

Robbins KT, Medina JE, Wolfe GT *et al.* Standardizing neck dissection terminology. Official report of the Academy's Committee for Head and Neck Surgery and Oncology. *Archives of Otolaryngology Head and Neck Surgery* 1991; **117**: 601–605.

Shah JP. Patterns of cervical lymph node metastasis squamous carcinomas of the upper aerodigestive tract. *American Journal of Surgery* 1990; **160**: 405–409.

Taylor RJ, Chepeha JC, Teknos TN *et al.* Development and validation of the neck dissection impairment index: A quality of life measure. *Archives of Otolaryngology Head and Neck Surgery* 2002; **128**: 44–9.

4.10

Sentinel node biopsy

MONI ABRAHAM KURIAKOSE, NIRAV PRAVIN TRIVEDI

BACKGROUND

Lymphatic metastasis generally follows an orderly and predictable pattern of progression beginning with the sentinel lymph node. It has been demonstrated that the status of the sentinel node predicts the presence of metastasis in the remainder of the nodal basin. Lymphoscintigraphy is now established as a reliable and minimally invasive technique of identifying the sentinel nodes in solid tumours. Since the original description to stage patients with cutaneous melanoma, biopsy of the sentinel lymph node has replaced routine elective lymph node dissection in many anatomical regions, including that of the head and neck. Initial attempts at lymph node mapping using the vital dye, isosulfan blue, failed to localize the sentinel nodes in about 20 per cent of cases. The introduction of the hand-held gamma probe has improved sensitivity to over 93 per cent. This technique is now being increasingly used to evaluate cancer of the breast, colon and vulva, and is redefining the standard of care for these treatment sites.

Head and neck squamous cell carcinomas (SCC) are considered to have a predictable pattern of metastasis to cervical lymph nodes in previously untreated patients. However, clinical experience may not provide failsafe information with which to direct therapy for individual patients. It has been reported that 16 per cent of patients with SCC of the oral tongue had 'skip metastases' which bypassed what was considered to be the first echelon nodal basin. This highlights the need for individualized localization of sentinel lymph nodes.

CONCEPT OF SENTINEL NODE

Sentinel lymph node is the first echelon node of the nodal basin. Presence of metastasis to the sentinel node defines the status of the rest of the nodes in the nodal basin (Figure 4.10.1).

DETECTION OF SENTINEL NODE

Sentinel lymph nodes can be identified by three techniques:

1 Isosulphan blue dye
2 Static lymphoscintigraphy
3 Dynamic lymphoscintigraphy.

Isosulphan blue dye technique involves injection of the dye submucously around the tumour. The sentinel lymph nodes are those which are stained blue. As the technique needs visualization, it is necessary to expose the entire nodal basin, thereby increasing the invasiveness of the procedure. Moreover, the isosulphan blue dye has been proven to have lower reliability than lymphoscintigraphy (Figure 4.10.2).

Dynamic lymphoscintigraphy involves injection of Tc^{99}-labelled filtered sulphur colloid at the periphery of the tumour. The flow of radiolabelled dye from the primary tumour to the sentinel nodes can be visualized in real-time using a gamma camera operating in a continuous mode. The position of the nodes where the radioactivity localizes can be marked on the skin using a pen (Figure 4.10.3).

Static lymphoscintigraphy involves identifying the nodes with increased radioactivity using a hand-held gamma probe (Figure 4.10.4). The sentinel node, which is surgically removed, is submitted for various histopathological, immunohistochemistry and molecular marker examination for the detection of micrometastasis.

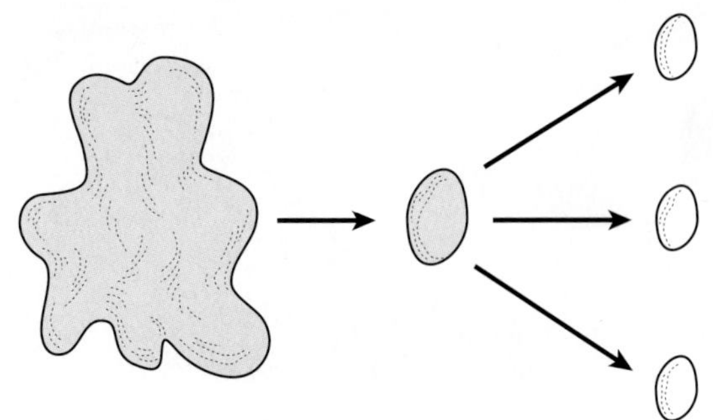

4.10.1 Concept of sentinel node.

INDICATION

Sentinel node biopsy is indicated for early stage (T1, T2) oral cavity squamous cell carcinoma of oral cavity with clinically N0 neck.

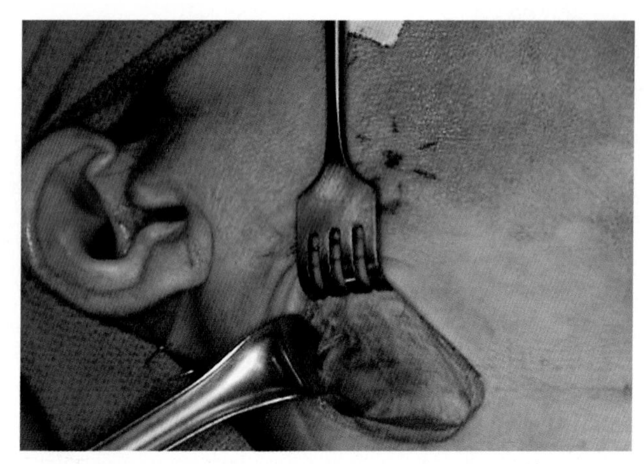

4.10.2 Blue dye technique. We acknowledge Mark Delacure for providing this figure.

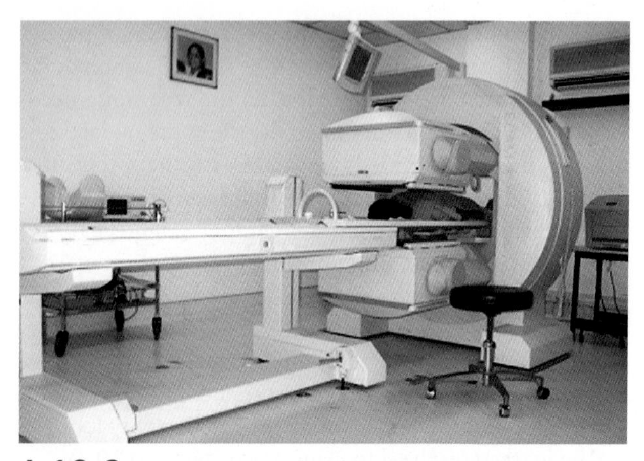

4.10.3 Dynamic lymphoscintigraphy under gamma camera.

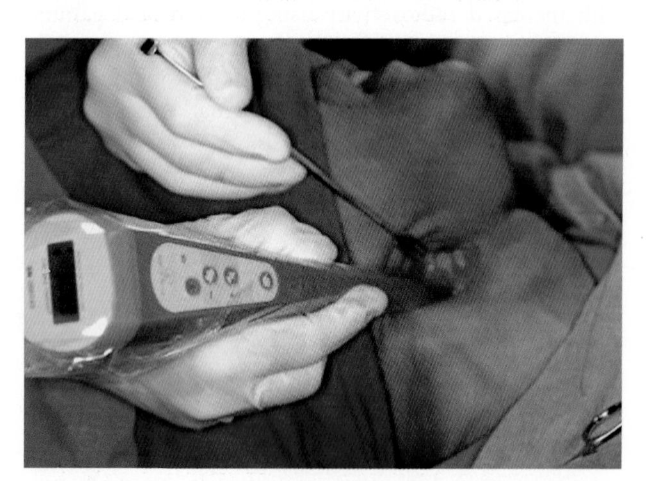

4.10.4 Static lymphoscintigraphy with hand-held gamma camera.

CONTRAINDICATIONS

Sentinel node biopsy is contraindicated in the following:

- advanced stage tumours;
- clinical or radiological evidence of nodal metastasis;
- in cases where the neck needs to be exposed for other reasons (exposure of donor vessels for reconstructive surgery).

LYMPHOSCINTIGRAPHY

Injection of the dye

A total of 5 ml of Tc^{99}-labelled filtered sulphur colloid is loaded in an insulin syringe. Between 1 and 2 ml of the sulphur colloid is injected submucously around the tumour (Figure 4.10.5). This is performed after isolating the tumour with gauze. Care should be taken to avoid spilling of the radioactive material. Should it happen, it should be wiped away with the gauze. Allow the patient to rinse the mouth with saline several times to remove any salivary contamination. It is necessary to instruct the patients to avoid swallowing of saliva contaminated with the radioactive material to avoid misleading images in the gamma camera. All the radioactive material and contaminant should be disposed of according to the institutional radioactive material disposal guidelines.

POSITION OF PATIENT UNDER THE GAMMA CAMERA

Position the patient on the gamma camera table similar to that in the operation table, using shoulder bag and head ring. This is important as the position of skin marking can change with neck extension in the operating table.

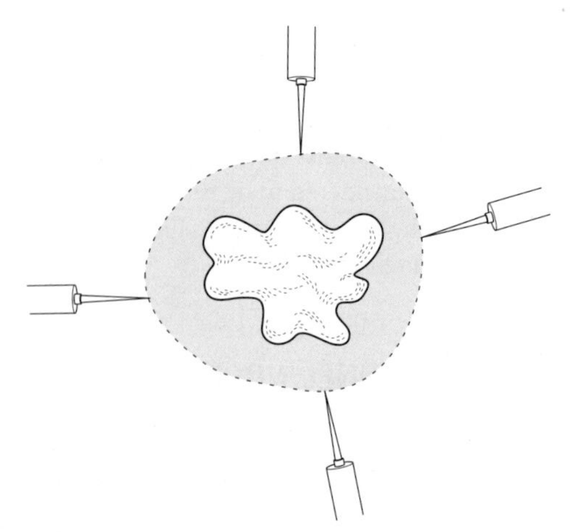

4.10.5 Injection of dye into periphery of tumour.

DYNAMIC IMAGING

Beginning immediately after the injections, the patient is positioned with the injection site centred under a large field-of-view dual-head gamma camera. A large field of view, set at 20 per cent window centred on the 140-keV technetium energy peak and fitted with a low-energy, high-resolution parallel hole collimator, is used to follow the disbursement of the radionuclide from the primary site to the cervical lymphatic. Initially, images are captured in an anteroposterior plane to determine the laterality of the sentinel nodes, following which the images are captured in the lateral view (Figure 4.10.6). The images are captured in a continuous mode. The transit time for drainage of the sentinel node in oral cavity cancer is less than 5 minutes. It is a continuous process where tracking of dye into sentinel nodes can be seen on screen. The primary tumour is seen as a large shadow, while a sentinel node is seen as a smaller shadow. The number of sentinel lymph nodes can vary from two to three in head and neck cancer.

MARKING OF SENTINEL NODES

The position of the sentinel node is marked externally on the neck (Figure 4.10.7). This serves as a landmark for incision in the neck during the surgery. The location of the sentinel node is marked with the guide of a pointer with radioactive tip under gamma camera in a continuous mode. The location where the 'hotspot' of the pen and that of the sentinel node coincide is marked on the skin with an indelible pen.

ANAESTHESIA

The operation is performed under general anaesthesia. Nasal intubation is preferred to avoid interference in dealing with the primary tumour in the oral cavity.

OPERATION

Position of the patient

The neck must be hyperextended with the shoulders and occiput supported with a head ring. The neck is rotated to the contralateral side. The operating table is tipped with a head-up tilt. The head and neck region is prepared and draped in the standard fashion to expose the neck and oral cavity (Figure 4.10.8).

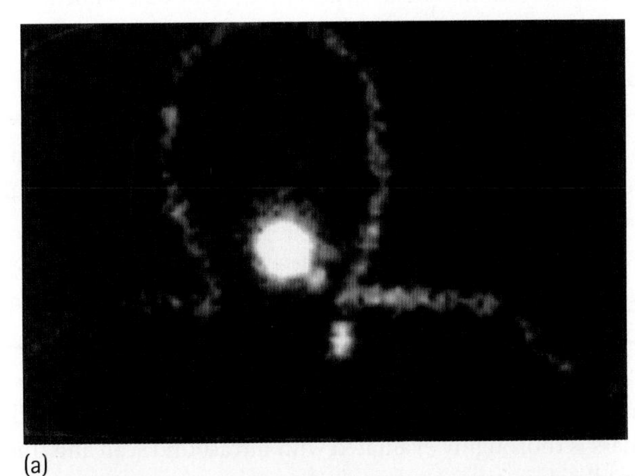

(a)

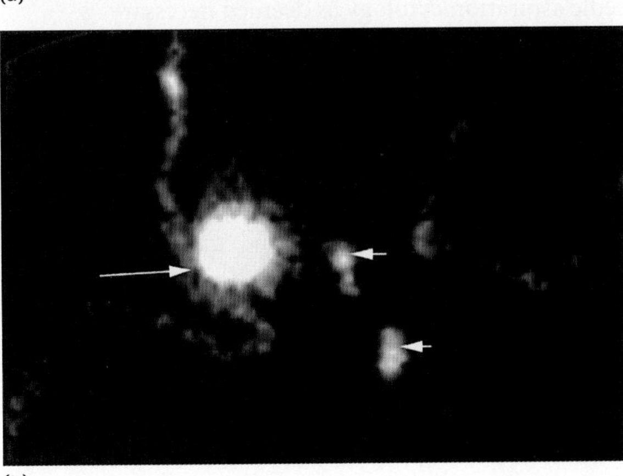

(b)

4.10.6 Nuclear scan images.

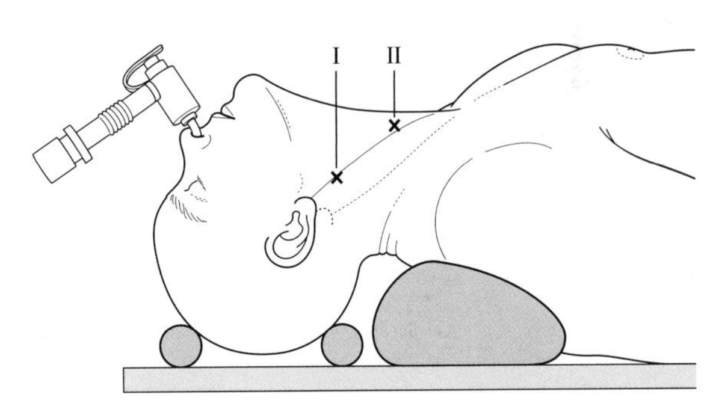

4.10.7 Marking of sentinel node externally on neck.

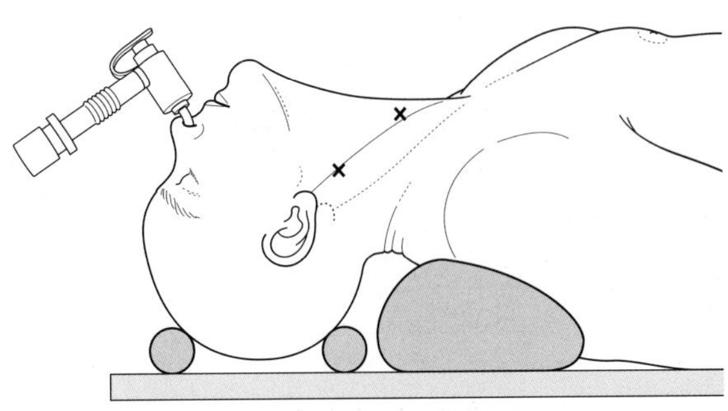

4.10.8 Positioning of patient on operation table.

Surgery of the primary lesion

Emission of radiation from the primary lesion interferes with detection of the sentinel node using the gamma probe, particularly if the node is situated in the region of level I. Excision of the primary lesion in the oral cavity before performing sentinel node biopsy in the neck helps in eliminating this radiation interference.

Neck incision

A transverse neck incision is marked on the neck as in a standard neck dissection. An incision of about 4 cm in length is placed along this marking so as to access the marked sentinel nodes. Occasionally, it may be necessary to make more than one incision. However, all the incisions should be placed in such a way that these incisions should be later extended to perform neck dissection, should it be necessary (Figure 4.10.9).

Raising flaps

Upper and lower skin flaps are raised in the subplatysmal plane over the the region of the marked sentinel nodes (Figure 4.10.10).

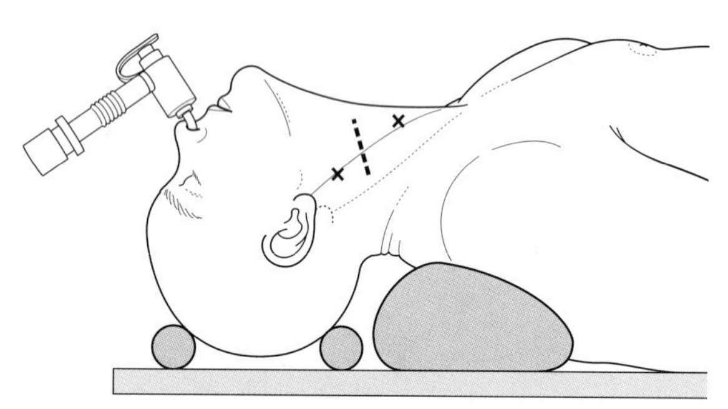

4.10.9 Incision in neck.

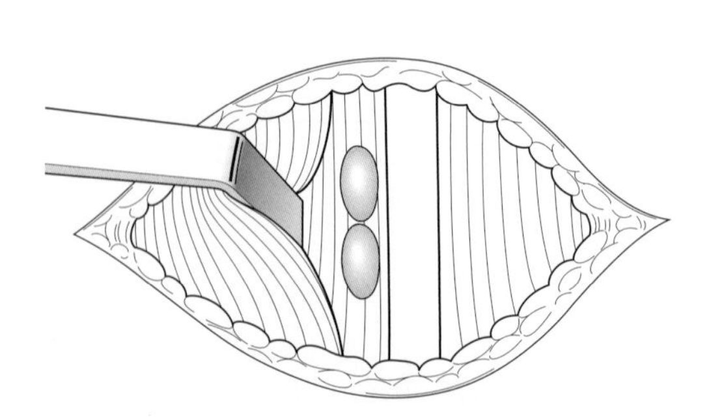

4.10.10 Raising of flaps, exposing lymph node groups.

Identification of sentinel nodes

Using a hand-held gamma camera, the background radiation level is noted in the neck in a position away from the sentinel nodes and primary tumour. Using the skin marking and the hand-held gamma probe as a guide, the region of the sentinel node is explored (Figure 4.10.11). An increase in count of more than three-fold the background is considered significant. This count is noted as an *in-vivo* count. That particular node is removed and the *ex-vivo* count is obtained outside the body to confirm it as a sentinel node. Count of node-bed is noted, which should confirm that the identified node is removed. The procedure is repeated to remove all the marked sentinel nodes. The wound is closed in layers. Drains are not usually required.

SENTINEL NODE PATHOLOGIC EVALUATION

The excised sentinel nodes are sent for histopathological evaluation. Step-sections of the nodes are obtained along the hilum of the node at 3–4-mm intervals. The tissue is processed by haematoxylin and eosin staining. Immunohistochemistry with pancytokeratin antibody or CK-14 polymerase chain reaction may be performed to identify submicroscopic metastasis. The clinical relevance of such lesions is yet to be determined. The feasibility of determining metastatic status by frozen section evaluation also needs to be determined.

POST-OPERATIVE CARE

Sutures are removed on day 7. The final histopathological report is evaluated and if any node shows metastasis, formal neck dissection is carried out.

FOLLOW UP

Regular follow up every month for a year and every two months for the second year is done. Any suspicious neck mass is thoroughly evaluated with ultrasound scan and fine needle aspiration cytology as deemed necessary.

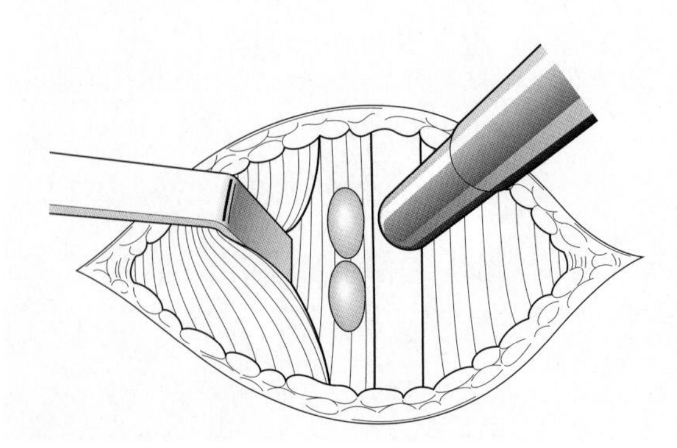

4.10.11 Identification of sentinel lymph node with gamma probe.

CONCLUSION

At present, there are no clear guidelines for the management of clinically N0 neck. Lymphoscintigraphy and sentinel node biopsy offers the possibility of minimal invasive management of the N0 neck, avoiding undue morbidity of surgery or radiation, as well as eliminating the risk of regional recurrence. However, efficacy of the procedure and long-term results need to be assessed before implementing it in clinical practice.

Top tips

- Sentinel node biopsy should be performed in a previously untreated patient.
- Care should be taken to avoid spillage of the dye while injecting around the tumour.
- Instruct the patient not to swallow during injection to prevent ingestion of the dye.
- The position of the patient under the gamma camera should be similar to the position to be adopted in the operating room to increase the accuracy of sentinel node marking.
- If the sentinel node is identified in level I, consider removing the primary tumour first to avoid background radiation.

FURTHER READING

Byers RM, Weber RS, Andrews T *et al.* Frequency and therapeutic implications of 'skip metastases' in the neck from squamous cell carcinoma of the oral tongue. *Head and Neck* 1997; **19**: 14–19.

Giuliano AE, Dale PS, Turner RR *et al.* Improved axillary staging of breast cancer with sentinal lymphadenectomy. Annals of Surgery 1985; **222**: 394–401.

Hamy A, Curtet C, Paineau J *et al.* Feasibility of radioimmunoguided surgery of colorectal carcinoma using indium 111 CEA specific antibody and simulation with a phantom using 2 step targeting with bispecific antibody. *Tumori* 1995; **81**: 103–106.

Levenback C, Burke TW, Morris M *et al.* Potential application of intraoperative lymphatic mapping in vulval cancer. *Gynecologic Oncology* 1995; **59**: 216–20.

Lindberg R. Distribution of cervical lymph node metastases from squamous cell carcinoma of the upper respiratory and digestive tracts. *Cancer* 1972; **29**: 1446–50.

Morton DL, Wen DR, Wong JH *et al.* Technical details of intraoperative lymphatic mapping for early stage melanoma. *Archives of Surgery* 1992; **127**: 392–9.

Pijpers R, Collet GJ, Meijer S *et al.* The impact of dynamic lymphoscintigraphy and gamma probe guidance on sentinel node biopsy in melanoma. *European Journal of Nuclear Medicine* 1995; **22**: 1238–41.

4.11

Tumours of the skull base

DOROTHY A LANG, BARRIE T EVANS

INTRODUCTION

Skull base surgery developed principally throughout the 1990s to become an established and clearly defined surgical subspecialty. The service is consultant delivered, multi-professional and team based. In general, the surgical team will include neurosurgeons, oral and maxillofacial surgeons and/or plastic surgeons. Ophthalmology, ENT (ear, nose and throat) and neurovascular expertise may also be required. The team will also include neurointensivists, neuroanaesthetists and neuroradiologists. Neurosurgical and critical care nursing expertise and a team co-ordinator are essential.

Skull base tumours generally have neural, vascular or meningeal origins. They may also arise from bone, cartilage and extracranial tissues. Although a vast range of different pathological entities is included within the definition, common biological tendencies are observed because of their anatomical location. Management of patients harbouring skull base pathology is complex and surgeons require in-depth anatomical knowledge – usually obtained by cadaveric dissection, and expertise may be required in microvascular anastomosis and neural reanimation.

CLINICAL PRESENTATION

- Neural compression
- Special sense problems
- Cranial nerve dysfunction
- Endocrine dysfunction
- Problems with facial form and function.

In general terms, patients harbouring skull base pathology will present with symptoms that for convenience can be classified as above. The onset and development of clinical features may be insidious because of the relatively slow rate of progression of the majority of tumours. It is crucial to be able to identify and document the pace of progression to ensure timely intervention and pre-empt critical neural decompensation.

Tumours affecting the skull base may be primary or secondary lesions. Metastatic disease in the skull base is not uncommon and biopsy may be required prior to major surgery being undertaken in cases where there is diagnostic doubt. The source of the primary tumour may not be known until after the result of the biopsy.

PATHOLOGY – BROADLY CLASSIFIED

- Benign, e.g. fibrous dysplasia, meningioma
- Low-grade 'malignant', e.g. chordoma, olfactory neuroblastoma
- Malignant, e.g. squamous and adenoid cystic carcinomas, chondrosarcoma, rhabdomyosarcoma, secondary tumours (primary source widespread).

LOCATION

For convenience, skull base tumours can be classified according to primary location, e.g. anterior cranial fossa (ACF), middle cranial fossa (MCF), posterior fossa (PF) and those arising from the paranasal sinuses, orbit, infratemporal fossa and post-nasal space.

CLINICAL CONSIDERATIONS

A number of factors need to be considered in the setting of a multidisciplinary team (MDT) meeting, in order to establish appropriate treatment pathways for these patients. Guidelines issued by NICE (National Institute of Clinical Excellence) indicate the required expertise. Factors to consider include:

- age
- natural history
- pathology and tumour biology
- pre-existing neurology
- quality of life considerations.

An extensive pre-operative work up is required:

- Comprehensive systems review and documentation of neurological deficits.
- Visual function (including acuity and fields as a minimum) will be necessary.
- Formal ophthmological review may be needed and visual evoked potentials may help assess potential for stabilization/recovery of visual function as well as identify 'subclinical' optic nerve failure.
- Olfactory function should be documented.
- Where the lateral skull base is involved, hearing, balance and vestibular function will need to be accurately assessed and noted.

Co-morbidity factors require careful evaluation. In general terms, complications occur in up to 20 per cent of patients undergoing major skull base surgery. Those patients with significant co-morbidity have a higher risk of complications and will be less likely to recover from peri-operative sytems compromise. In patients with established or anticipated lower cranial nerve or bulbar dysfunction, tracheostomy and gastrostomy will be required at an early stage to avoid aspiration pneumonitis and ensure safe adequate nutrition.

IMAGING

Detailed imaging is essential for treatment planning. As a minimum this will include computed tomography (CT) and magnetic resonance imaging (MRI). Three-dimensional CT may be required to evaluate bone involvement. Precise delineation of the tumour is required and critical evaluation of anatomically inaccessible areas is required to identify patients who may not fulfil criteria for surgery, e.g. invasion of the cavernous sinus. In some tumours, or in those patients requiring post-operative evaluation, positron emission tomography (PET) scanning may be required to distinguish tumour tissue from post-operative scarring/flaps used in reconstruction and regions displaying post-operative hyperaemia. Angiography will delineate blood supply and identify patients who may need pre-operative embolization.

MANAGEMENT

In determining options for management, it is important to be able to assess the impact of management on the natural history of the pathology. Where treatment benefits are marginal, conservative management may be in the patient's best interests. In general, neurological deficits are unlikely to recover with treatment and stabilization will be a more rational objective.

The impact of treatment on the patient's quality of life is a further important consideration. In general, surgery may dramatically alter quality of life adversely in the short and medium term. This is less evident with radiotherapy, nonetheless the long-term impact of the latter may need evaluation.

MANAGEMENT OPTIONS

- Conservative treatment
- Surgery
- Radiotherapy/STR (stereotactic radiosurgery)/gamma knife
- Combination/sequential.

It is important to recognize that 'cure' of this type of pathology may be elusive and this needs to be emphasized in discussions held with the patient and carers. Tumour control in the vast majority of cases will prove to be a more realistic option.

KEY ISSUES

- Complex
- High-risk
- 'High tech'
- Resource implications.

In addition to an experienced and multi-professional workforce, adequate theatre time, expensive 'high tech' equipment and the support of a highly trained theatre team is required. Access to neurointensive or critical care facilities is mandatory.

ANAESTHESIA

Fundamental aspects of anaesthesia in skull base surgery include maintenance of haemodynamic stability, control of intracranial pressure (ICP), cerebral protection and cranial nerve monitoring. This latter may preclude the use of long-term muscle relaxants. Intermittent pneumatic compression is used in conjunction with an agreed policy to reduce the incidence of deep vein thrombosis (DVT) and potential traumatic events (PTE). Careful positioning of the head is essential to avoid compromise of the neck veins.

EQUIPMENT

Standard equipment will include an operating chair and neurosurgical microscope. Micro-instruments and non-stick bipolar forceps are essential. Image guidance is helpful, but must not be used by the inexperienced to compensate for a lack of anatomical knowledge and surgical expertise. High-speed drills and ultrasonic aspirators complete the list of essential equipment. Some services have access to intra-operative MRI.

KEY TECHNICAL PRINCIPLES

- Anatomy
- Access (see Chapter 4.4)
- Resection
- Reconstruction.

Anatomy

In planning surgical treatment, a clear understanding of the pathological anatomy is required. While the operating surgeons may be familiar with normal skull base anatomy, the pathological process may distort this. This facilitates planning of the access surgery, tumour resection and reconstruction of the skull base.

Access

It is fundamental that adequate access to the pathology is realized. This may involve the use of craniofacial osteotomies, although with experience their use is rationalized and tailored to the individual patient. A short straight line of sight to the pathology is necessary to create space for surgical manoeuvres and avoid brain retraction. Access should not compromise reconstructive options, e.g. preservation of the superficial temporal and supraorbital vessels. Damage to the temporal muscle should be avoided unless its resection is mandatory. Ideally, osteotomies should be pedicled if post-operative radiotherapy is planned (see Chapter 4.4).

Resection

In the planning process, the overall strategic approach to the tumour must be determined. The following need to be considered.

- The need for staged surgery.
- Possible multiple access routes.
- The requirement for temporary vascular occlusion, e.g. internal carotid artery intra-operative mini-Doppler may assist in confirming post-manipulation patency and identify vessels in spasm.
- Microvascular anastomosis or intracranial bypass.
- Spinal drainage – a spinal drain may enhance brain relaxation, but the amount of cerebrospinal fluid (CSF) drainage must be carefully controlled by the anaesthetist.
- Steroids, mannitol and withdrawal of CSF from the basal cisterns and ventricles may also assist with brain relaxation.
- Minimize brain retraction – craniofacial access may assist.

Exposed brain surfaces must be kept moist and, where retractors are used, non-stick patties or equivalent should protect the brain. Meningiomas and schwannomas adjacent to the brain will usually have an arachnoidal plane within which the dissection should be carried out. Damage to the pia should be avoided. Vascular structures are generally dissected parallel to the encased structure and should only be divided after dissection has confirmed that they supply the tumour. Tumour adherent to perforators should be left *in situ* – tumour eradication should not be preferred to preservation of neurovascular structures.

Dissection en bloc is the ideal with high-grade tumours to avoid tumour spillage. With larger tumours, this may not be possible due to anatomical constraints. In this situation, a so-called modified en bloc resection is performed. The use of the operating microscope is essential in critical areas such as the optic chiasm and cavernous sinus.

Reconstruction

Reconstruction of the skull base is critical to avoid post-operative infection and CSF leak.

- Primary dural closure if possible.
- Repair basal dural defects with vascularized convexity dura or a vascularized pericranial or galeal-pericranial flap passed via a 'letterbox' approach through the convexity dura.
- Tissue glue is helpful to control suture holes and reinforce suture lines, but will not secure a shoddy repair.
- Small bone defects do not generally need reconstruction but larger defects, particularly over the orbital roof, may need a bone graft or free tissue transfer to support the dural repair and prevent pulsating exophthalmos.
- The majority of middle fossa defects can be reconstructed with a pedicled temporalis muscle graft. Extensive defects may require free tissue, e.g. rectus abdominis, particularly if the temporalis muscle is devascularized in the resection.

KEY AREAS

- Frontal sinus, if entry is usually cranialized.
- Central skull base – bone not required in isolated central skull base defects. In more posterior defects, particularly in older patients, reliance cannot be placed on pericranial flaps; galeal pericranial flaps are preferred.
- Orbit – orbital roof reconstruction prevents pulsating exophthalmos. Isolated lateral wall defects may not need reconstruction.
- 'Dead space' may allow accumulation of post-operative clot and may be a focus for infection and allow brain herniation. In the central skull base, this may cause traction injury to the optic apparatus. Free tissue reconstruction is usually required in extensive defects.

INDICATIONS FOR FREE TISSUE TRANSFER

It is relatively unusual to require free tissue to reconstruct the skull base. The relative indications include:

- previous adjuvant radiotherapy/operation
- complex defects (jugum resected)
- coverage non-vascularized dural flaps
- failure of a loco-regional flap.

There are a number of options that can be considered. The choice of flap will depend on the requirement for bulk to obliterate dead space or lining to close a basal defect without altering the intracranial volume. For the former, a wide variety of muscle or musculocutaneous flaps are suitable, e.g. rectus abdominis/latissimus dorsi. For the latter, in the authors' practice, the most frequently used flap is radial forearm for central skull base defects. This versatile flap is used without the cutaneous component to produce a thin fascial flap on a long vascular pedicle.

COMPLICATIONS

Infection is the most dreaded complication of skull base surgery. When this occurs in the setting of an inadequate primary repair, control will only be possible when vascularized tissue is introduced to create a barrier between the intra- and subcranial regions.

Cerebrospinal fluid pathway problems are the next most frequent complication. While the majority settle with temporary CSF drainage, a persistent CSF leak will require further surgery and hydrocephalus may necessitate placement of a shunt.

General medical complications including respiratory tract infection, pulmonary thrombo-embolism (PTE), urinary tract infection and poor nutrition are not uncommon. These are best treated after prompt recognition in a neurointensive care or critical care unit.

ILLUSTRATIVE CASES

The three cases discussed have been selected to illustrate different tumour sites, pathology and reconstructive techniques. They make the point that skull base tumour surgery is not simply the resection and reconstruction of malignant paranasal sinus tumours.

Sphenoid wing meningioma en plaque

This is a difficult tumour to control. The ideal is total resection (Simpson grade 1), but around the skull base this may be precluded by extensive basal dural involvement and proximity to critical neurovascular structures. In general, patients with visual failure and those with proptosis resulting in ophthalmological complications will require craniofacial resection and reconstruction. In our series of patients, the majority (92 per cent) presented with proptosis and the orbit and MCF were involved in 71 per cent. While technically benign, there is a propensity for this tumour to cross anatomical barriers, invade adjacent structures and recur despite initial surgery considered to be complete.

The conventional surgical strategy includes preservation of vision, improvement of aesthetic issues and prevention of the inevitable ophthalmological complications of the untreated primary process.

In most cases, a frontotemporal or pterional craniotomy will be required and orbito-zygomatic (O-Z) osteotomies may enhance access to the middle fossa floor. It is probable that invaded bone in the vault and skull base will require removal. In cases where the temporalis muscle is invaded, this will require resection. Imaging findings may dictate that the superior orbital fissure is decompressed together with the foramina rotunda and ovale. Infiltrated periorbita will then be resected. The optic canal will usually require radical bony decompression and soft tissue compressing the optic nerve will require removal. In patients who have required resection of more than one orbital wall, an orbital reconstruction will be required. This is usually done with split calvarium or other autologous bone graft (Figures 4.11.1–4.11.5).

Olfactory neuroblastoma

This is a relatively rare tumour thought to arise from crest cells of the nasal vault in close proximity to the cribriform plate. Intracranial invasion is not uncommon. The tumour grows slowly and symptoms are late in onset and usually consist of nasal obstruction, epistaxis, headache, visual failure and proptosis. Biopsy is usually required prior to definitive treatment and the neuropathologist requires fresh tissue for conventional staining, immunocytochemistry and possibly electron microscopy. The rarity of the tumour precludes any service having a standard protocol and each individual case will need evaluation and a treatment plan.

Cross-sectional imaging will allow staging into one of three groups:

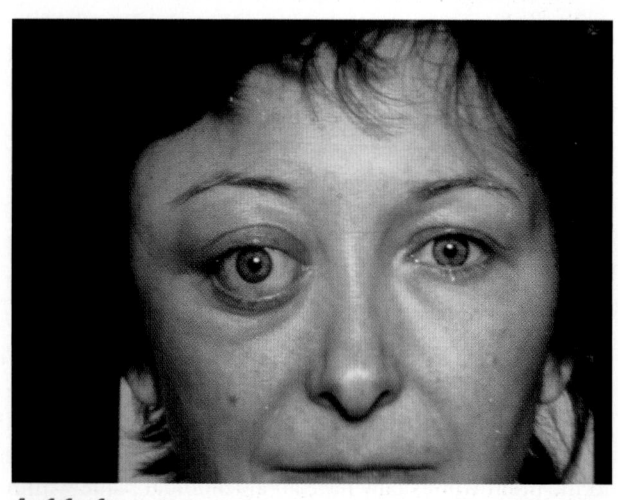

4.11.1 Meningioma en plaque.

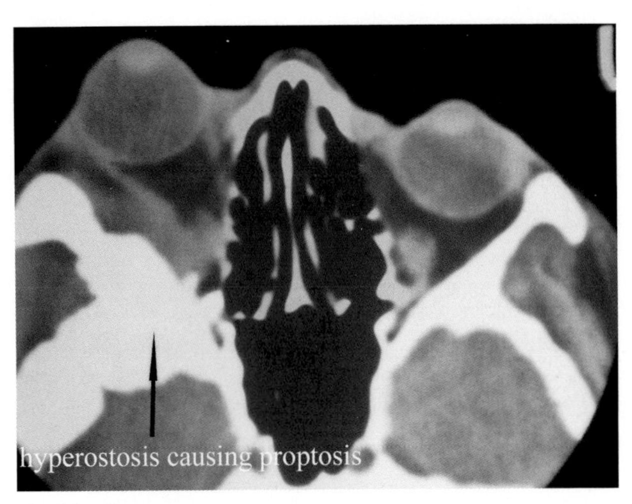

4.11.2 Meningioma en plaque.

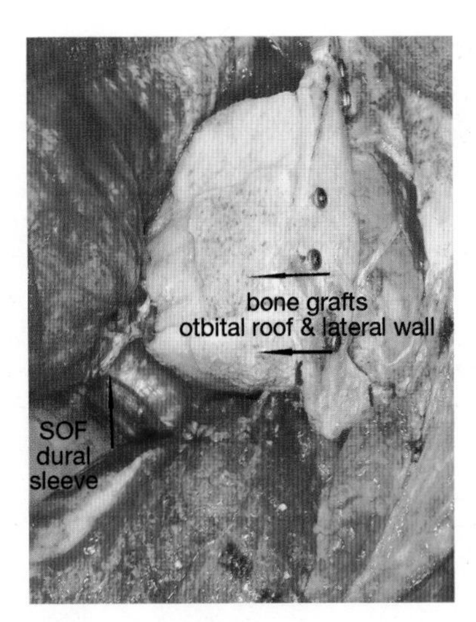

4.11.4 Orbital reconstruction.

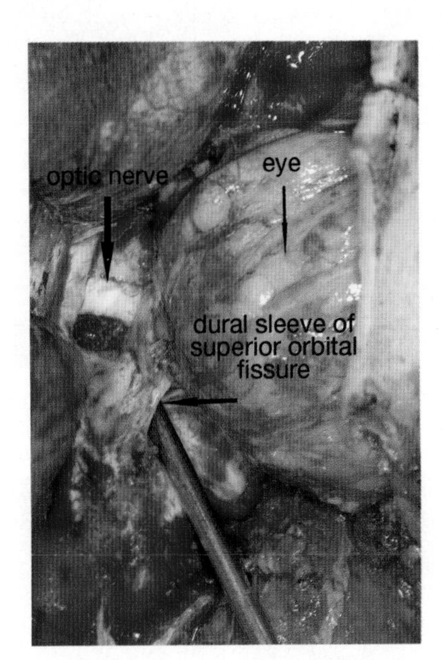

4.11.3 Orbital contents following resection of orbital roof/lateral wall and decompression optic nerve.

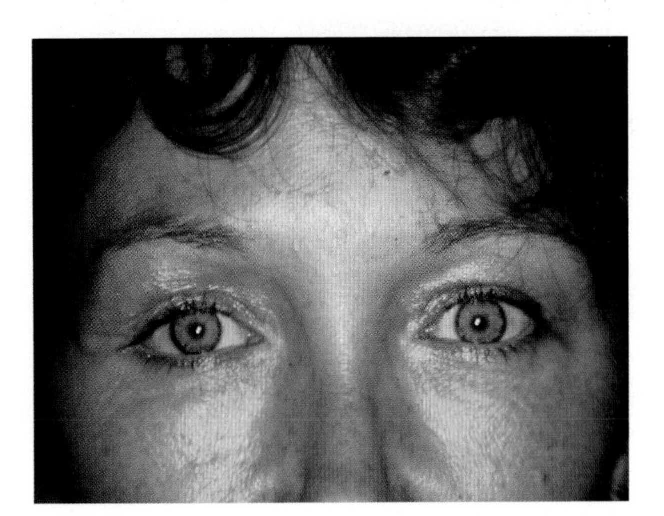

4.11.5 Post-operative result.

1 lesions confined to the nasal cavity
2 lesions extending into the paranasal sinuses
3 lesions involving the skull base, orbit, intracranial cavity or cervical nodes.

Bone scanning and imaging of the chest and abdomen will be required to exclude distant metastases.

The illustrative patient required a bifrontal craniotomy and extended transbasal approach (removal of the orbitofrontal bandeau, orbital roofs and nasal skeleton en bloc). The lesion was then mobilized and excised en bloc. The resected specimen included tumour from the nasal cavity, paranasal sinuses, orbit and dura. A vascularized pericranial-galeal flap was then used to reconstruct the central skull base. The flap was secured with 'parachute sutures' using drill holes in the central skull base. Inner table calvarium was used for the medial orbital reconstruction. The convexity dura was repaired with a non-vascularized graft and the bifrontal craniotomy flap relocated and secured. The repair was protected by a lumbar drain for 5 days post-operatively. There were no post-operative complications. Adjuvant fractionated radiotherapy was used. The patient is now five years post-surgery and remains well without evidence of recurrence on MRI. Vision is stable. In general terms with extensive disease such as illustrated here, 60 per cent five-year survival may be anticipated while this would be 100 per cent were the disease confined to the nasal cavity (Figures 4.11.6–4.11.9).

Recurrent chondrosarcoma

This patient presented with a recurrent high-grade spindle cell sarcoma. Excision was deemed appropriate and required a bifrontal craniotomy in conjunction with a radical maxillectomy, coronoidectomy, zygomectomy and orbital

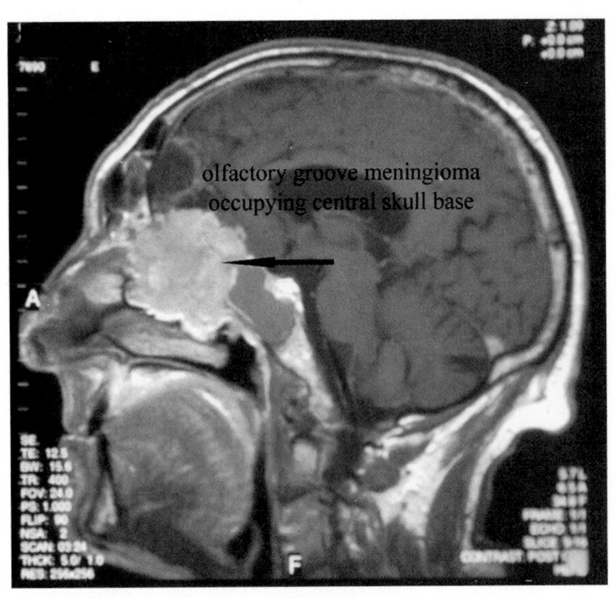

4.11.6 Pre-operative sagittal MRI scan.

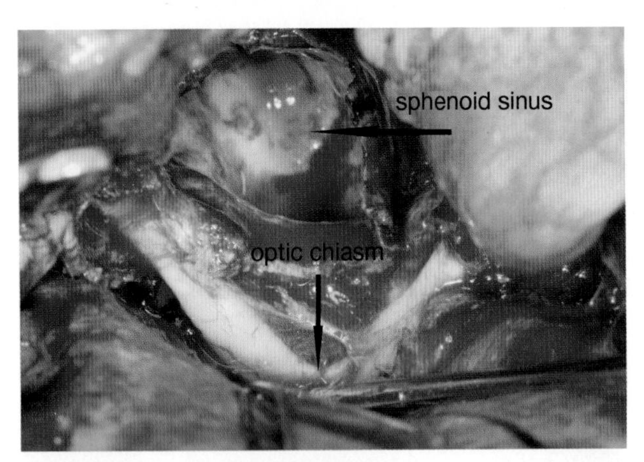

4.11.7 Posterior limit resection.

exenteration. The coronoidectomy facilitated identification of the lingual nerve on the medial aspect of the mandible and this was then traced to the main trunk and foramen ovale. V2 was divided at foramen rotundum. The lesion was removed en bloc dividing the structures of the superior orbital fissure and excising the ACF and MCF floor with preservation of V3. Infiltrated dura was removed and replaced with temporal fascia. The skull base was reconstructed with galea-pericranium (ACF) and temporalis muscle (MCF). A three-paddle rectus abdominis flap was then used to repair the roof of the mouth, the lateral wall of the nose and provide skin cover over the orbit. Post-operative chemotherapy was employed, but the patient died of metastatic disease eight months after surgery.

This patient highlights the difficulties in deciding appropriate treatment in advanced cases – balancing surgical morbidity versus quality of life, which in this case was enhanced despite the limited post-operative course (Figures 4.11.10–4.11.13).

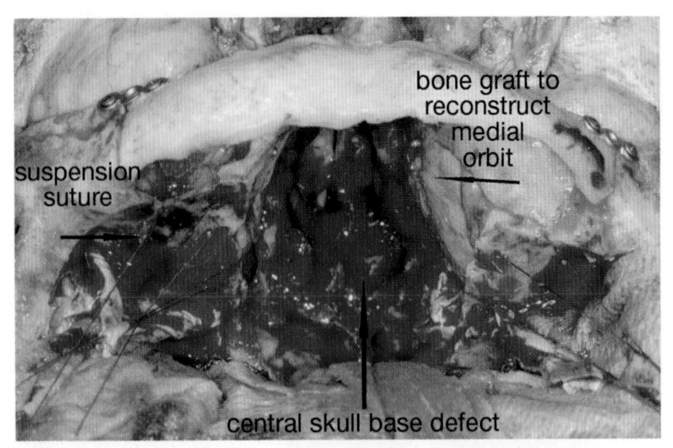

4.11.8 Central skull base defect after tumour resection.

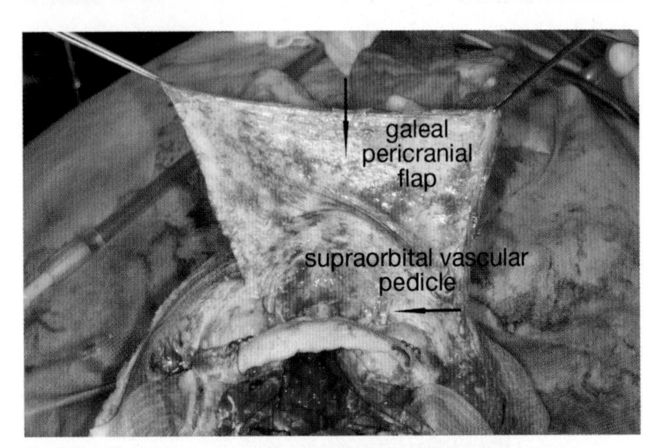

4.11.9 Anterior fossa reconstruction.

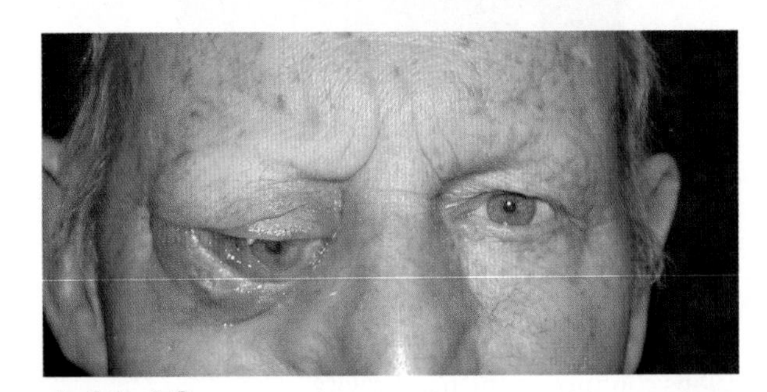

4.11.10 Pre-operative appearance.

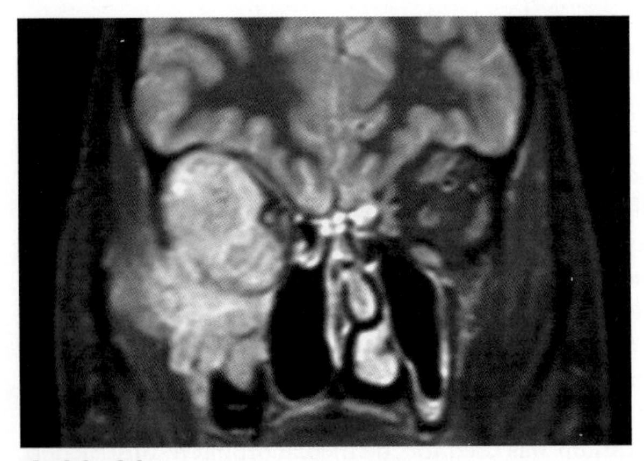

4.11.11 Pre-operative coronal MRI scan.

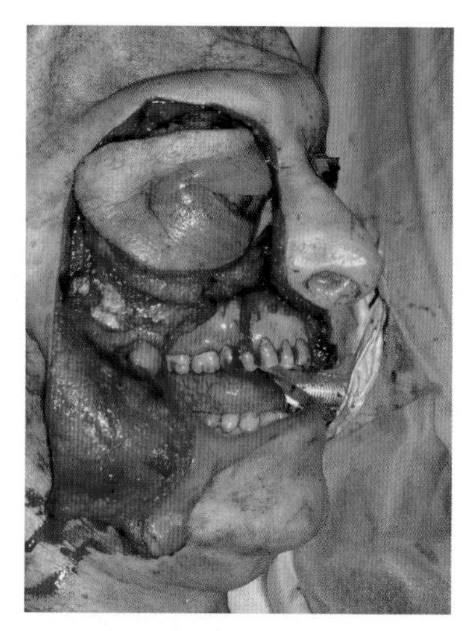

4.11.12 Superficial margins of resection.

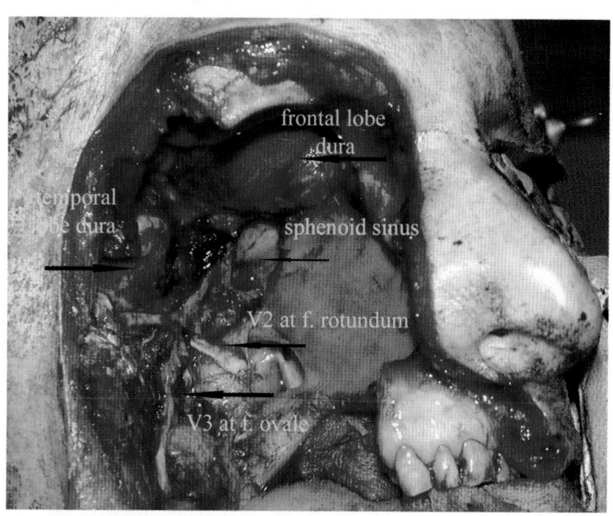

4.11.13 Extent of facial and skull base defect.

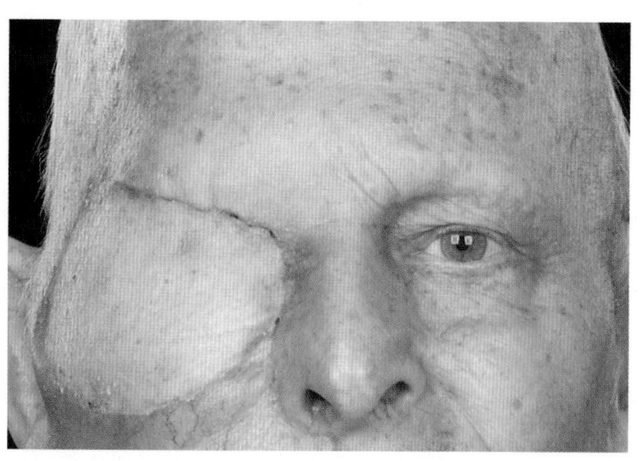

4.11.14 Rectus abdominus flap reconstruction. Postoperative appearance at 6 weeks.

STEREOTACTIC RADIOSURGERY AND GAMMA KNIFE

Patients are becoming aware of these treatments and frequently request their use in preference to surgery. Surgeons must be able to provide reasoned argument for the pros and cons of these forms of irradiation in tumour control:

- control tumour growth
- control not equivalent to cure
- no validated comparison with natural history.

Advantages

- single outpatient treatment
- no operation.

Disadvantages

- total eradication exceptional
- long-term uncertainty in biological behaviour
- lifetime follow up required
- not favoured by a majority of surgeons
- options need to be fully and openly discussed.

Top tips

Skull base surgery should only be contemplated with the appropriate skill mix in a multidisciplinary team.

- Many skull-base tumours are slow growing, and clinical and imaging surveillance play a key role in patient management.
- Sound applied anatomical knowledge is essential to link subcranial with intracranial dissection.
- The use of appropriate access osteotomies may facilitate cerebral protection by minimizing brain retraction, while maintaining a wide corridor of access to the pathology.
- Subtotal tumour resection, particularly in benign and low-grade malignant tumours, will frequently provide adequate tumour control, provide relief from symptoms and minimize morbidity.
- The key elements in reconstruction are the isolation of intracranial contents from the nasal cavity and paranasal sinuses and appropriate support for the frontal and temporal lobes if required. Autologous tissue is the preferred reconstructive option.
- Follow-up protocols will depend on tumour biology – recurrence is expected with certain tumours, including chordoma and meningioma.
- Management recommendations are based on accurate and unbiased information.
- Surgeon's objectives and technical achievement need to be aligned with the expectations of patients and their carers.

FURTHER READING

Evans HL, Ayala AG, Romsdahl MM. Prognostic factors in chondrosarcoma of bone. A clinic-pathologic analysis with emphasis on histological grading. *Cancer* 1977; **40**: 818–31.

Gushing H, Eisenhardt L. *Meningiomas. Their classification, regional behaviour, life history and surgical results.* Springfield, IL: Charles C Thomas, 1938.

Honeybul S, Neil-Dwyer G, Lang DA *et al.* Sphenoid wing meningioma en plaque: a clinical review. *Acta Neurochirurgica* 2001; **143**: 749–58.

Honeybul S, Neil-Dwyer G, Lang DA *et al.* The extended transbasal approach: a quantitative anatomical and histological study. *Acta Neurochirurgica* 1999; **141**: 251–9.

Kleihues P, Burger PC, Scheithauer BW. The new WHO classification of brain tumours. *Brain Pathology* 1993; **3**: 255–68.

National Institute for Health and Clinical Excellence. Improving outcomes for people with brain and other CNS tumours – the manual. London: National Institute for Health & Clinical Excellence, www.nice.org.uk, 2006.

Ringel F, Cedzich C, Schramm J. Microsurgical technique and results of a series of 63 spheno-orbital meningioma-en-plaque. *Neurosurgery* 2007; **60**: 214–22.

PART 5

SALIVARY AND THYROID SURGERY

5.1

Submandibular, sublingual and minor salivary gland surgery

JOHN D LANGDON

PRINCIPLES AND JUSTIFICATION

The most frequent indications for excision of the submandibular gland are when a calculus is present within the gland hilum, or when the gland is the site of chronic infection. Only 10 per cent of salivary tumours arise in the submandibular gland and 60 per cent of these will be pleomorphic adenomas. The remaining 40 per cent will be malignant. Except in advanced malignancy, the tumours rarely extend beyond the capsule of the gland and so excision of the submandibular gland is the definitive surgical treatment. For advanced malignant tumours with spread beyond the capsule, more radical clearance of the submandibular triangle is required, often in continuity with a neck dissection.

There are only two indications for the removal of the sublingual gland. The first is in the management of a ranula and the other is when a tumour is present. The sublingual gland is a very rare site of tumour, but almost all of them will be malignant, the majority being adenoid cystic carcinomas. The most frequent reason for operating on the minor salivary glands is for mucocoele. Another is for tumour. Ten per cent of salivary tumours arise in the minor glands and about 50 per cent of these will be malignant.

Investigations

When there is a history suggestive of obstruction, plain x-rays (mandibular occlusal and oblique lateral views) are appropriate as the majority of submandibular stones are calcified. A sialogram should not be performed unless a calculus has been ruled out on plain film as the sialogram itself might displace the stone proximally, making surgery more difficult. For the investigation of chronic infection, a sialogram is invaluable. It will show the extent of the destruction of the acinae and the post-stimulation emptying film will demonstrate residual function. If the gland is not functioning, it should be removed as an elective procedure to prevent further episodes of infection.

When a mass is present either in the submandibular gland or the sublingual gland, a computed tomography (CT) scan or a magnetic resonance (MR) scan is indicated. The scan should include the neck so that any associated lymphadenopathy is also imaged. For suspected minor salivary gland tumours, if they occur within the lips, cheeks or floor of the mouth, simple excision biopsy is the investigation of choice. However, for tumours arising on the hard palate, imaging with a CT or MR scan is mandatory to assess the deep extent of the tumour.

Biopsy

Open surgical biopsy of a suspected submandibular gland tumour is contraindicated. If the tumour is contained within the capsule of the gland, open biopsy will spill tumour cells into the surrounding tissue planes. As the majority will be benign pleomorphic adenomas, their simple excision will be compromised. If the tumour is malignant, then the hope of cure will have been compromised. Fine needle aspiration biopsy appears to be safe but is unreliable in salivary gland pathology, but fine needle core biopsy is useful if available.

For suspected minor gland tumours arising in mobile soft tissues (lips, cheeks and floor of the mouth), excision biopsy will often be the only treatment required. If the tumour proves to be a high-grade malignancy, further more extensive surgery might be required together with post-operative radiotherapy. The situation is different when a tumour arises from the hard palate. In this situation, an incisional biopsy is mandatory as the diagnosis will have a direct influence on the extent of the subsequent surgery.

SURGICAL REMOVAL OF STONES IN THE DISTAL SUBMANDIBULAR DUCT

If the stone lies within the lumen of the duct distal (anterior) to the point where the duct crosses the lingual nerve, it is a safe procedure to open the duct and remove the stone. For stones more proximal, great care must be taken to avoid damage to the lingual nerve and often it is wise to remove the submandibular gland together with the stone from an external approach.

Anaesthesia

In a co-operative patient, the operation is readily performed under local anaesthesia. If co-operation is in doubt, a general anaesthetic should be used. If the operation is to be performed under local anaesthesia, 2 per cent lignocaine hydrochloride with 1:80 000 epinephrine (adrenalin) is used. A lingual nerve block plus local infiltration suffices. Care must be taken not to infiltrate too much solution immediately over the duct as this can easily distend the floor of the mouth and make it difficult to identify the duct. It is also important not to perforate one of the sublingual veins as this will result in a large haematoma.

Operation

The first stage is to pass a suture into the floor of the mouth around the duct proximal to the position of the stone. This prevents the stone from being displaced backwards during the operation. The ends of the suture are left long and should be held in artery forceps. Gentle traction on the suture will then lift the duct upwards making it more accessible in the floor of the mouth (Figure 5.1.1).

An incision is made in the mucosa along the line of the duct and over the stone. The blade is used in a gentle stroking fashion gradually becoming deeper until the wall of the duct is opened. The duct itself is seen as a pale grey structure with an overlying capillary network (Figure 5.1.2).

It is often helpful to steady the duct with dissection forceps while incising longitudinally through its wall. Often the calculus will be seen through the duct wall and the overlying incision immediately releases it. If the stone is large and there has been scarring and fibrosis, it may be adherent to the lining of the duct. In this situation, fine stay sutures can be inserted into the duct wall on each side of the stone and these sutures can be used to retract the walls. The calculus can be gently mobilized and freed with the careful use of a fine artery clip or small dental excavator (Figure 5.1.3).

Once the calculus has been released, cloudy mucinous saliva will often be released from the duct proximally. The duct should be gently irrigated with sterile saline or water both proximally and distally to ensure that any further epithelial casts or gravel are removed. If these are retained, they readily act as foci for further stones to form (Figure 5.1.4).

The stay sutures are removed and the mucous membrane of the floor of the mouth is closed with two or three resorbable sutures. No attempt should be made to close the duct walls as this would result in scarring and stricture formation leading to further obstruction (Figure 5.1.5).

SURGICAL REMOVAL OF STONES IN THE PROXIMAL SUBMANDIBULAR DUCT

Anaesthesia

Access to the posterior floor of the mouth is difficult in the conscious patient and for this reason general anaesthesia is preferred. Once the patient is on the operating table, it is

5.1.1 A silk suture around the submandibular duct is used to lift the duct upwards out of the floor of the mouth.

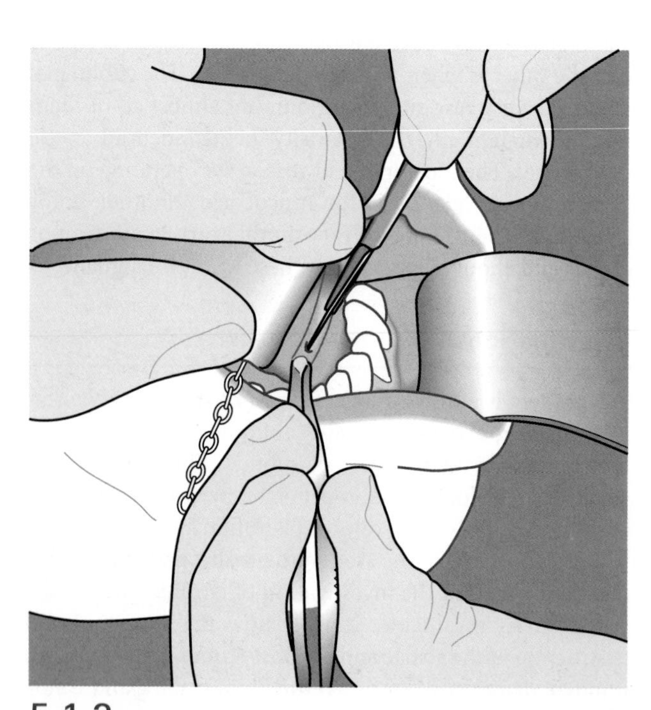

5.1.2 The duct is exposed following an incision in the floor of the mouth.

helpful to infiltrate the floor of the mouth with local anaesthetic containing epinephrine (adrenalin) as this helps to reduce bleeding. Care must be taken not to perforate one of the sublingual veins.

Operation

An assistant is essential. The operator should stand on the contralateral side. A mouth prop is inserted between the molar teeth on the side of the stone. The assistant grasps the tongue with a swab or alternatively a sharp pointed towel clip can be used. The tongue is retracted forward and away from the side of the stone. An incision is made through the mucosa of the floor of the mouth laterally from the third molar region forward and medial to the sublingual gland (Figure 5.1.6).

The sublingual gland is then retracted laterally using one or two stay sutures revealing the submandibular duct on its

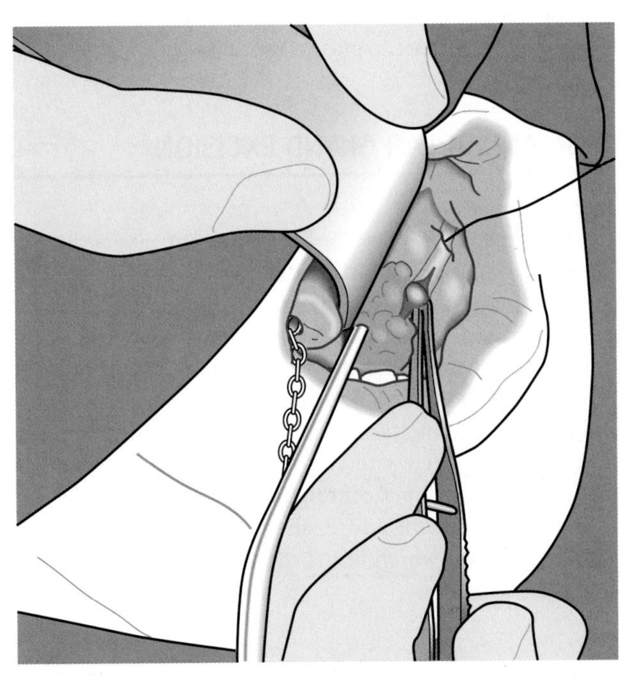

5.1.3 The stone is exposed and gently released.

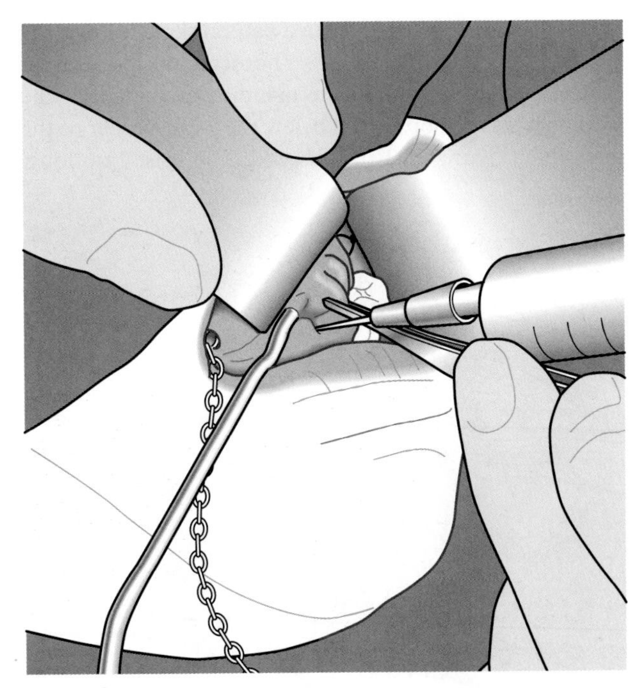

5.1.4 It is important to irrigate the duct proximally and distally to ensure that all 'gravel' is removed.

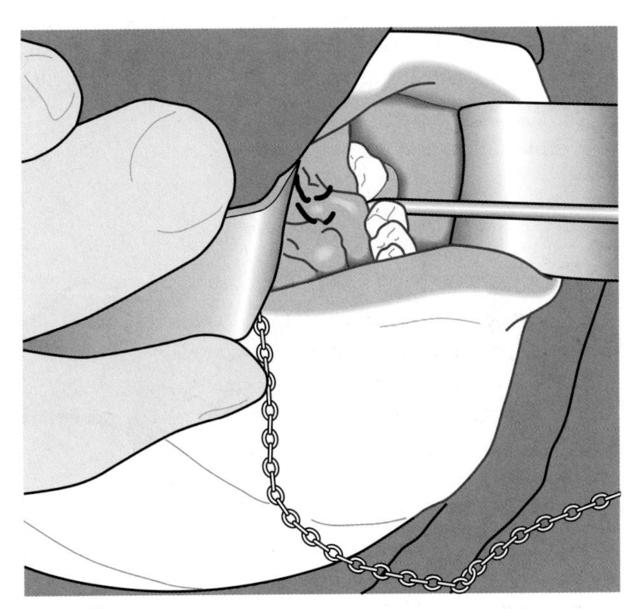

5.1.5 The oral mucosa is closed with sutures.

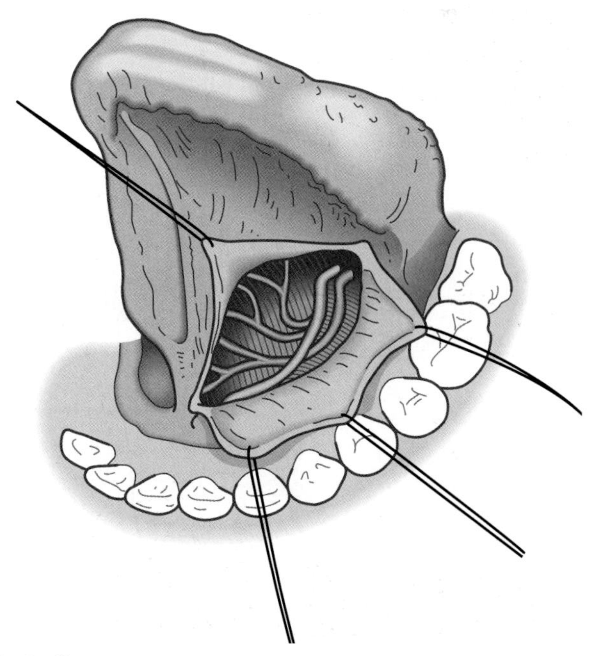

5.1.6 Incision in the floor of the mouth for removal of a stone at the hilum of the submandibular gland.

deep surface. Using careful blunt dissection, the duct is traced posteriorly identifying the lingual nerve passing immediately deep to the duct running from the lateral border of the tongue towards the third molar tooth (Figure 5.1.7).

Once the duct and the lingual nerve have been identified, they must be carefully separated and the duct traced posteriorly into the hilum of the submandibular gland. At this point the lingual nerve lies very superficially and is 'tethered' to the gland itself through the parasympathetic ganglionic fibres (Figure 5.1.8).

At this point, the assistant should apply firm pressure in the submandibular region in order to elevate the hilum of the gland and the proximal duct upwards above the level of the mylohyoid. At this point, the stone is readily palpable. A longitudinal incision is made through the duct wall and the stone is teased out using a small excavator (Figure 5.1.9).

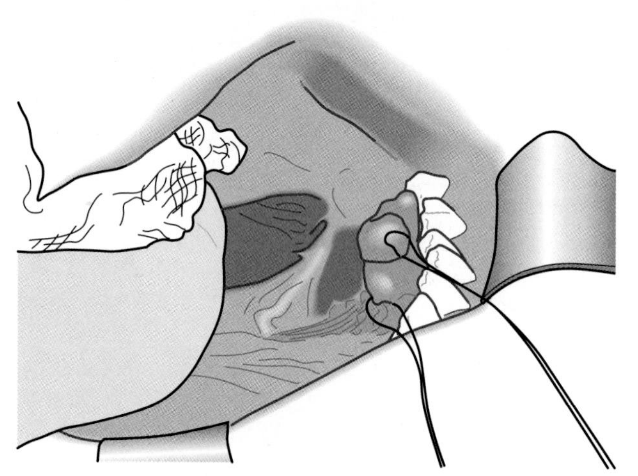

5.1.7 Following retraction of the sublingual gland, the lingual nerve can be seen deep to the submandibular duct.

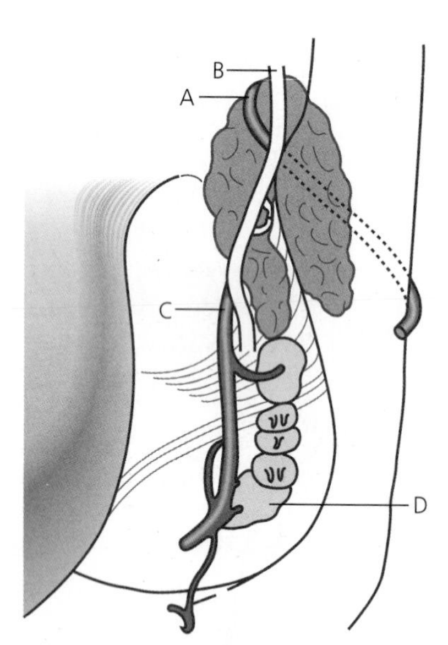

5.1.8 Posteriorly, the lingual nerve ascends towards the skull base crossing the duct as it enters the hilum of the submandibular gland. (a) Facial artery; (b) lingual nerve and submandibular ganglion; (c) submandibular duct; (d) sublingual gland.

The duct is then carefully irrigated in order to wash out any associated 'gravel'. No attempt is made to close the duct wall. Careful use of the diathermy ensures haemostasis. All stay sutures are removed and the mucosa of the floor of the mouth is closed with two or three resorbable sutures.

Post-operative care

As the stone and obstructed gland is likely to be infected, a 3-day course of antibiotics is given. Routine analgesia is used and the patient should be encouraged to eat citrus fruit or to chew gum in order to encourage salivary flow.

SUBMANDIBULAR GLAND EXCISION

Anaesthesia

The operation is performed under general anaesthesia. The patient is placed supine on the operating table with moderate neck extension and the chin rotated to the opposite side. It is helpful to have head-up tilt of the table as this reduces venous engorgement. Following routine skin preparation and draping, the incision is mapped out. The incision line should be infiltrated with conventional dental local anaesthetic containing 2 per cent lignocaine hydrochloride and 1:80 000 epinephrine (adrenaline). This results in some vasoconstriction which limits capillary ooze and helps to define tissue planes.

The incision

The incision should run within a natural skin crease in the neck at least 3 cm below the lower border of the mandible in order to avoid damage to the mandibular branch of the facial nerve as it loops down below the lower border of the mandible (Figure 5.1.10). It should be at least 7 cm long.

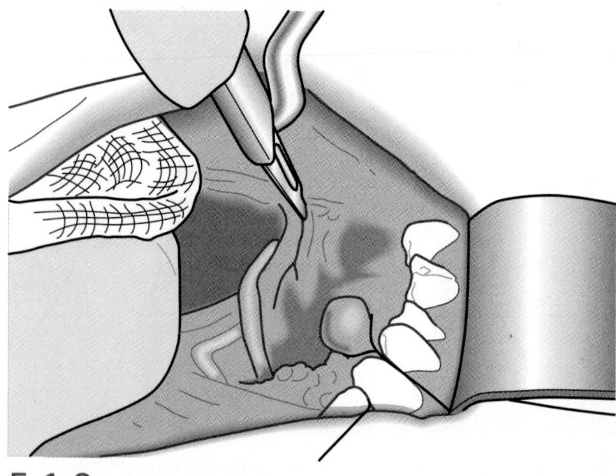

5.1.9 The hilum of the gland is incised to release the stone.

The lower the incision in the neck, the better the post-operative cosmetic result, but incisions lower than 3 cm make the operation slightly more difficult as then the operator must dissect upwards to reach the submandibular triangle.

The incision is made with either a No. 15 blade or with a fine diathermy needle or ceramic blade while the assistant puts tension across the incision line. The incision is made directly down to platysma. The subcutaneous fat is stripped with firm pressure with a swab from the underlying muscle for approximately 1 cm on each side of the incision as this facilitates a layered closure. The underlying platysma is then incised to the full extent of the skin incision, again using either a blade or diathermy (Figure 5.1.11).

The assistant can now retract the wound margins using 'cats paws' or Allis forceps applied to the cut edge of the platysma (*never* the skin edges!). The underlying investing layer of the deep cervical fascia is next divided, preferably with scissors, after the fascia is first tented outwards with toothed forceps. Often the fascia consists of a series of separate laminae like an onion skin, but occasionally it is composed of a single thicker sheet. Again the fascia should be divided along the full length of the incision to avoid the operative field becoming ever smaller (Figure 5.1.11).

Posteriorly, the fascial incision approaches the angular tract where the deep cervical fascia splits to form the investing layer that has just been incised and the deeper layer that forms the floor of the submandibular triangle containing the submandibular gland.

The mandibular branch of the facial nerve normally runs on the deep aspect of the investing layer of fascia, although occasionally it lies between the platysma and the fascia. Great care must be taken to protect this branch. Even with an incision as low as 3 cm below the lower border of the mandible, the nerve may be encountered when the fascia is divided. If it is seen, it should be carefully mobilized and gently retracted with the upper part of the flap.

The delicate capsule overlying the gland is then lifted with toothed dissection forceps and opened with scissors (Figure 5.1.12). The loose connective tissue is separated with scissors to expose the surface of the gland (Figure 5.1.13). The anterior facial vein which lies in the connective tissue overlying the submandibular gland is clamped, divided and tied (Figure 5.1.14).

From now on, the dissection continues as close to the surface of the gland as possible. For chronically infected

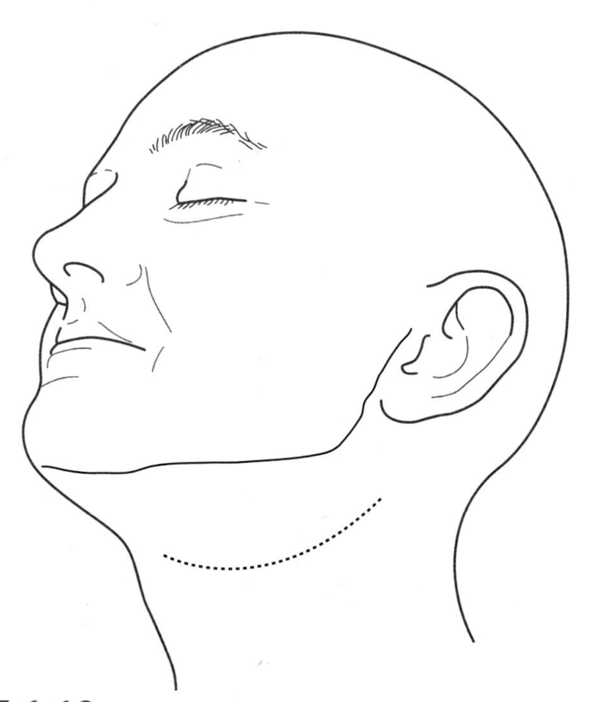

5.1.10 Conventional skin incision for exposure of the submandibular gland.

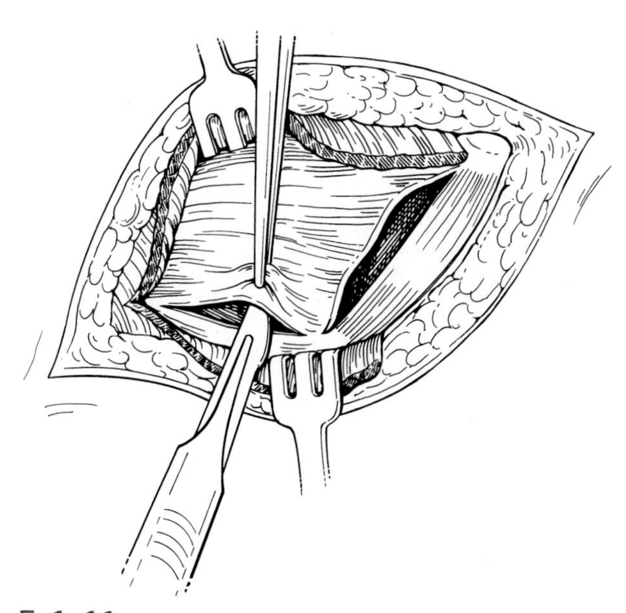

5.1.11 Division of deep cervical fascia following skin incision and division of the platysma.

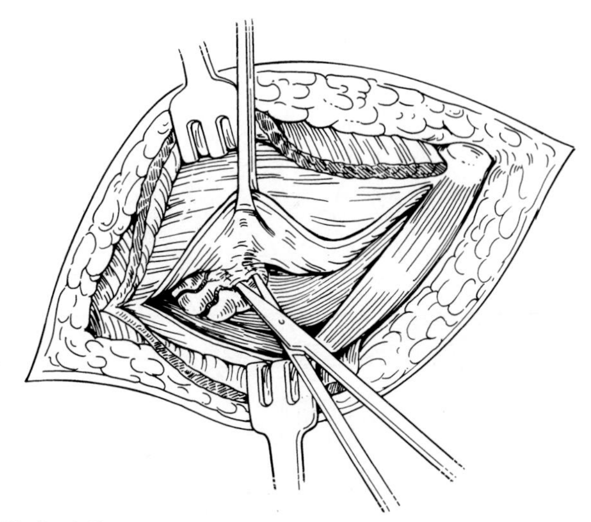

5.1.12 The 'capsule' of the submandibular gland is incised to expose the surface of the gland.

glands, there is frequently extensive fibrosis and care and patience is required to maintain this plane. For all tumours contained within the submandibular gland capsule, the operation should proceed in the plane just superficial to the capsule as it is an effective barrier between the tumour and adjacent structures. For malignant tumours that have extended beyond the capsule, a full submandibular clearance, usually as part of a neck dissection, and often including the periosteum of the lower and inner aspect of the mandible, is needed.

The anterior pole of the superficial lobe of the submandibular gland is first mobilized and retracted upwards with Allis forceps (Figure 5.1.15). This reveals the posterior belly of the digastric which is then gently retracted downwards with a small Langenbeck retractor. This then exposes the facial artery which emerges from behind the stylohyoid muscle and passes upwards and forwards to enter the deep surface of the submandibular gland. The artery is then clamped, divided and tied. Great care must be taken to secure the proximal ligature. As the vessel is divided, it retracts out of site and, if the ligature slips, the bleeding end of the vessel can be very difficult to identify (Figure 5.1.16).

The course of the facial artery is variable. Often it deeply penetrates the substance of the gland to emerge again at its upper border. Sometimes the artery lies in a groove in the deep aspect of the gland. The dissection continues to mobilize the anterior pole of the superficial lobe of the gland which is then gently retracted posteriorly. During this dissection, a number of small arteries and veins will be

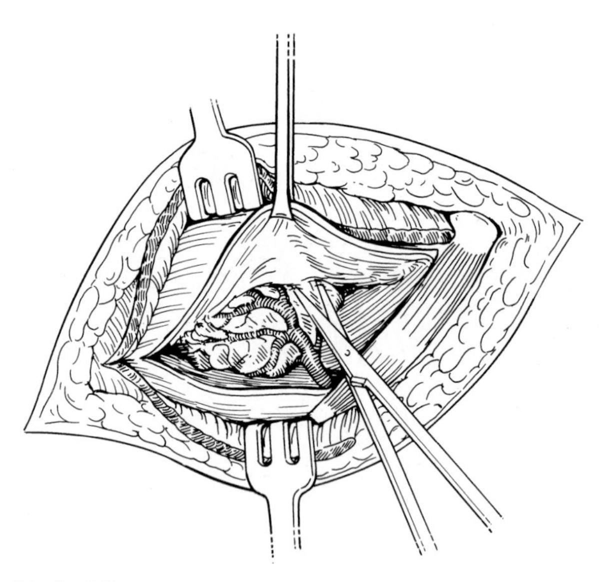

5.1.13 Exposure of the submandibular gland revealing the branches of the facial vessels.

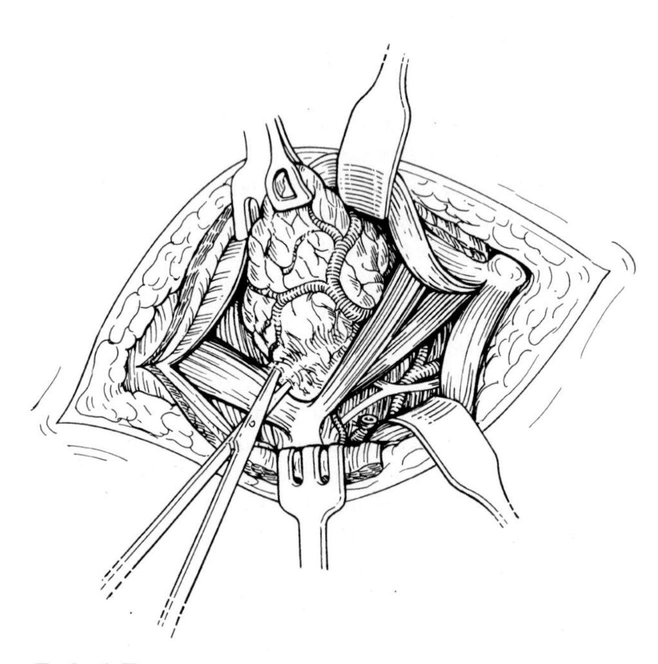

5.1.15 The lower pole of the submandibular gland is mobilized and retracted upwards.

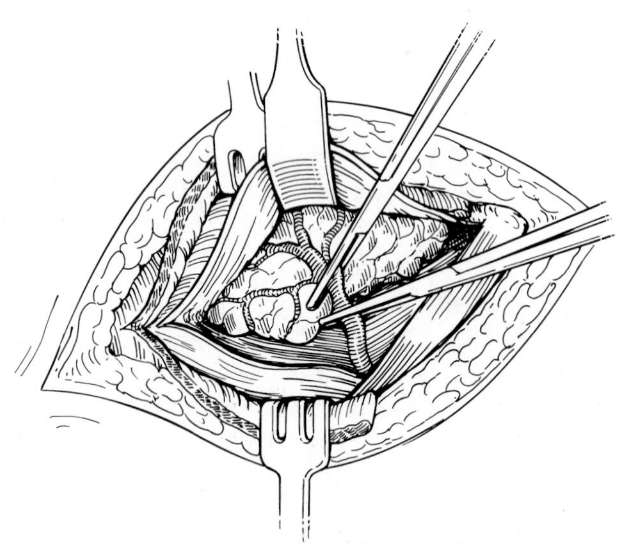

5.1.14 Clamps applied to the vessel prior to division.

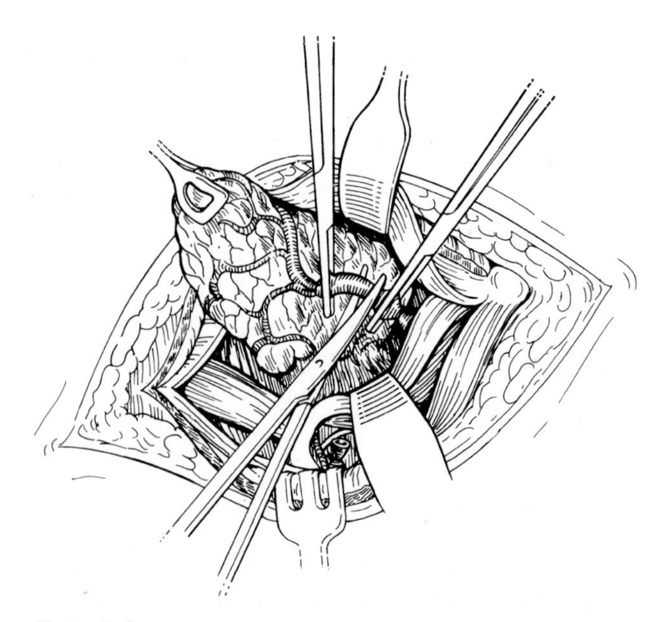

5.1.16 Division of the facial artery as it enters the deep surface of the submandibular gland.

identified entering the gland. These should be carefully clamped, divided and tied or diathermized according to their size. As the dissection continues posteriorly along the lower border of the mandible, the facial artery and anterior facial vein are encountered as they hook around the lower border. These vessels are again clamped, divided and ligated.

Sometimes when the facial artery runs in a groove on the deep aspect of the submandibular gland, it can be preserved without division at the lower edge of the gland and again at the lower border of the mandible. However, although this is technically possible, there is little advantage other than to show off one's technical expertise!

At this stage in the operation, the anterior pole of the superficial lobe of the gland can be retracted posteriorly to reveal the groove between the superficial and deep lobes of the submandibular gland. The posterior border of the mylohyoid lies within this groove. It is gently freed with scissors and then retracted forward with a Langenbeck retractor. The deep lobe of the gland can now be mobilized either with a finger or by opening the blades of the scissors applied to the surface of the gland. On the deep aspect of the deep lobe, one or two small veins may be encountered running from the gland through the underlying hyoglossus muscle into the lingual veins. If these veins are not tied off or adequately diathermized, troublesome bleeding may be encountered.

The submandibular salivary gland can now be pulled downwards revealing the V-shaped lingual nerve (Figure 5.1.17). The apex of the V is the point at which the parasympathetic fibres tether the lingual nerve to the salivary gland. Occasionally, the sublingual ganglion can be identified on the surface of the gland. It is very important to identify the V of the lingual nerve and its paprasympathetic fibres as the latter must be transacted to free the gland. As these fibres are cut, the lingual nerve springs upwards. Finally, the submandibular duct is clamped, divided and ligated as far forward as possible with just enough remaining to drain the sublingual gland. A thin layer of loose connective tissue remains in the gland bed overlying the hypoglossal nerve (Figure 5.1.18).

The wound is inspected for any bleeding points, a vacuum drain inserted and closed in layers using a subcuticular suture to close the skin. The wound edges may be reinforced with skin closure tapes.

Post-operative care

The vacuum drain is removed when drainage has slowed, usually at 24 hours. The subcuticular stitch is removed at about 10 days.

Complications

Three cranial nerves are at risk during removal of the submandibular salivary gland: the mandibular branch of the facial nerve, the lingual nerve (a branch of the third division of the trigeminal nerve) and the hypoglossal nerve. A neck

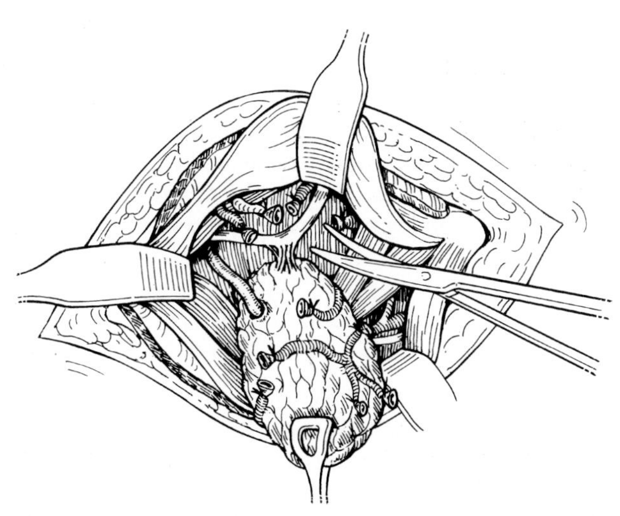

5.1.17 Division of the parasympathetic fibres that anchor the submandibular gland to the lingual nerve.

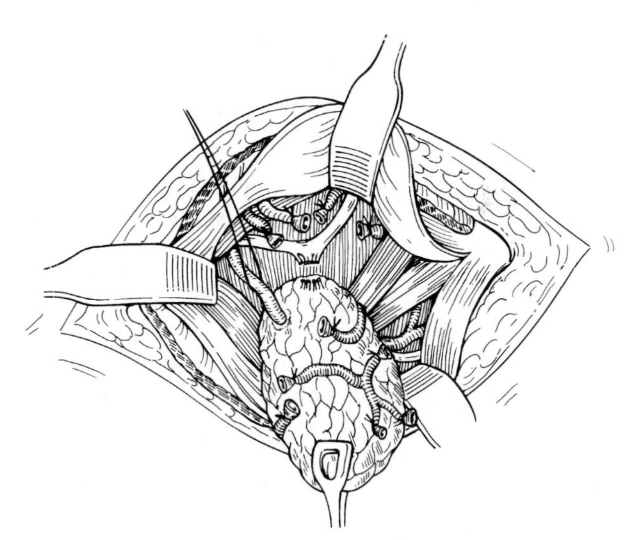

5.1.18 Tie around the submandibular duct prior to removal of the gland.

incision at least 3 cm below the lower border of the mandible and careful surgical technique will avoid damage to the facial nerve.

When chronic infection and subsequent fibrosis have occurred, it is sometimes difficult to identify the lingual nerve and the deep aspect of the deep lobe may be tethered to the hypoglossal nerve. At these stages of the operation, the surgeon must be convinced that these structures have been identified before using any sharp dissection.

Meticulous haemostasis is required throughout the operation as many vessels entering and leaving the submandibular gland are only apparent when the gland is under traction and as soon as they are divided the vessels retract into the adjacent muscle planes. Ligation or disposable titanium vascular clips are safer than diathermy in this situation. Carelessness with these vessels results in extensive haematoma in the neck.

SUBLINGUAL GLAND EXCISION FOR RANULA OR EXCISION BIOPSY

The operation may be performed under general anaesthesia or local anaesthesia. If a general anaesthetic is used, it is helpful to infiltrate the floor of the mouth with a local anaesthetic containing vasoconstrictor before any incision is made.

Incision

For simple excision of the sublingual gland, a linear incision is made in the floor of the mouth parallel to and just lateral to the submandibular duct (Figure 5.1.19). Care must be taken not to extend the incision posteriorly beyond the first molar tooth so as to avoid damage to the lingual nerve. The incision should open the sac of the ranula to allow the mucinous contents to be aspirated.

Isolation of the submandibular duct

The submandibular duct is now carefully identified and retracted medially. Stay sutures passed through the margins of the mucosa are helpful to aid retraction (Figure 5.1.20). Using blunt dissection with scissors, the lingual nerve is identified.

Mobilization of the sublingual gland

The sublingual gland which lies adjacent to the inner cortex of the mandible is then mobilized and its multiple ducts, which drain into the submandibular duct, divided carefully in order not to damage the duct itself (Figure 5.1.21). The anterolateral part of the sublingual gland may be attached to the periosteum of the mandible by fibrous tissue and this too must be divided (Figure 5.1.22). Following removal of the gland, the mucosa of the floor of the mouth is loosely closed with two or three resorbable sutures.

Complications

Damage to the lingual nerve posteriorly or the submandibular duct medially is avoided by careful surgical technique. Meticulous haemostasis is required to avoid a post-operative haematoma in the floor of the mouth.

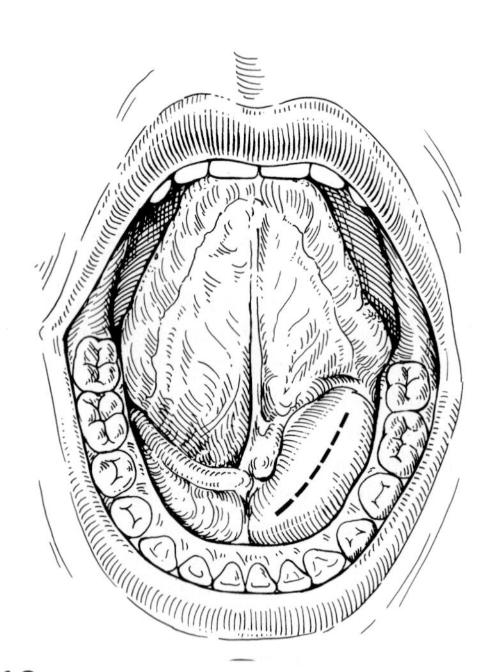

5.1.19 Sublingual incision lateral to the submandibular duct.

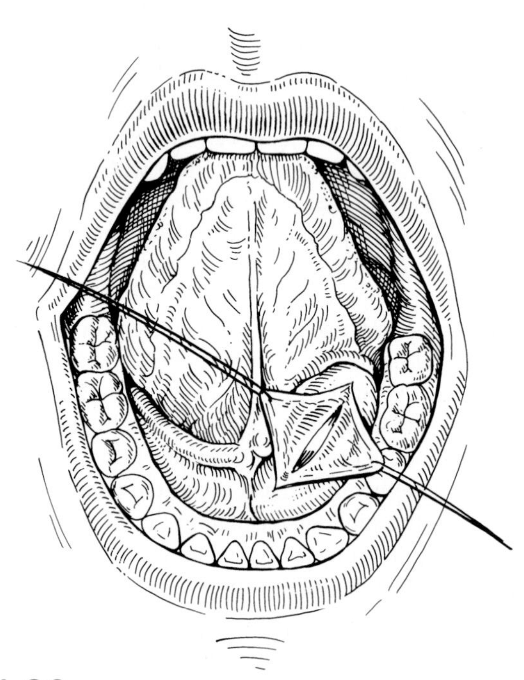

5.1.20 Stay sutures retracting the sublingual mucosa.

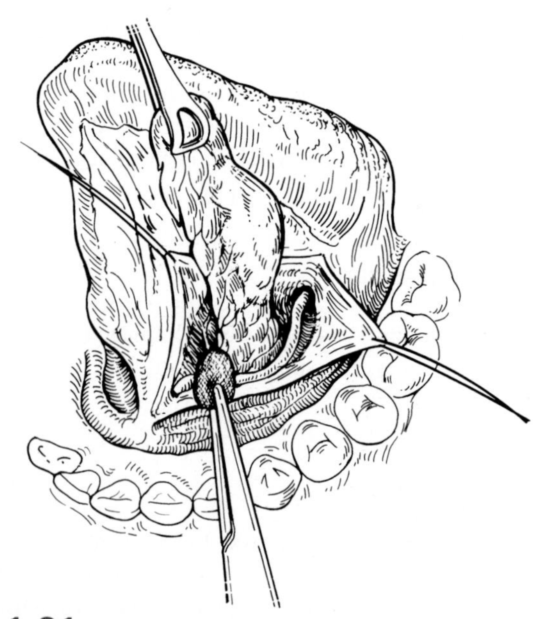

5.1.21 Mobilization of the sublingual gland.

SUBLINGUAL GLAND EXCISION FOR MALIGNANT TUMOUR

Although only a rare site for a salivary gland neoplasm, the majority of such neoplasms will be malignant and therefore removal should encompass a clear margin of normal tissue of at least 1 cm in all dimensions. This normally includes the adjacent floor of the mouth and mylohyoid muscle, a cuff of ventral tongue and a rim resection of the mandible. If the mandible is edentulous, removal of the inner table only is often sufficient. Each tumour should be managed on its merits according to its size and infiltration into adjacent anatomical planes.

The operation

Because of the vascularity of the floor of the mouth, it is helpful to use a cutting diathermy for the soft tissue incisions (Figure 5.1.23). Depending upon the position of the sublingual gland and the size of the tumour, it may be necessary to take a section of the lingual nerve with the specimen.

The mandibular alveolus is approached from the buccal aspect. A bur is used to cut the bone horizontally below the level of the tooth roots. The lingual line of section must lie below the level of the mylohyoid insertion (Figure 5.1.24). Final separation of the alveolus is made with a fine osteotome.

The line of the dissection is then continued across the floor of the mouth deep to the mylohyoid. The mobilized alveolus and sublingual gland within the floor of the mouth must be gently elevated and the hypoglossal nerve, just below the mylohyoid, must be identified and freed. The dissection is then continued to join up with the mucosal incision in the ventral tongue (Figure 5.1.25).

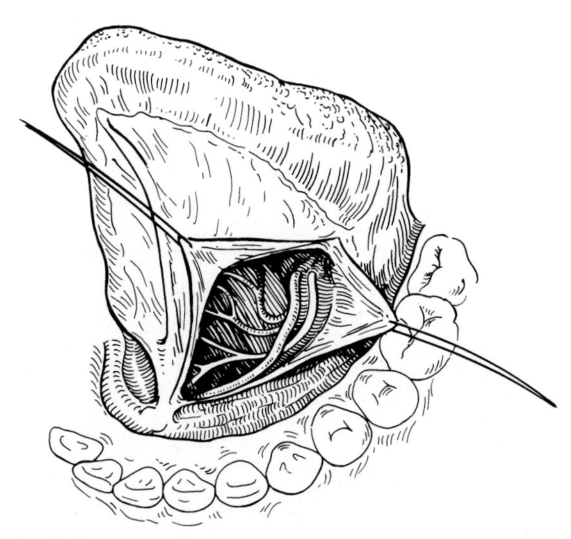

5.1.22 Anatomical features displayed following removal of the sublingual gland.

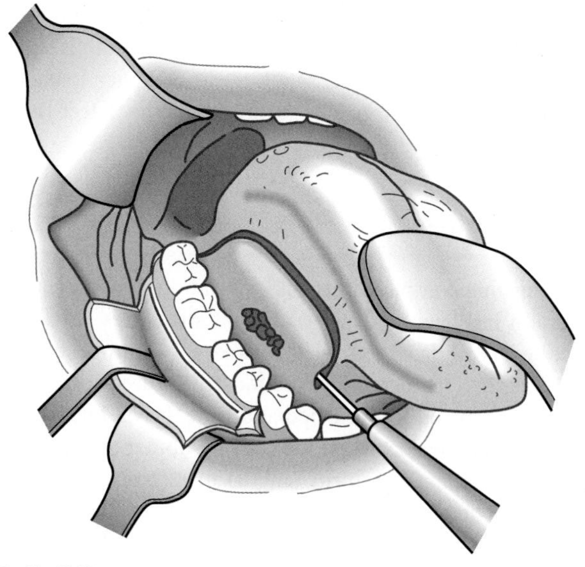

5.1.23 Sublingual tumour excision, necessitating wide excision with a margin of normal tissue.

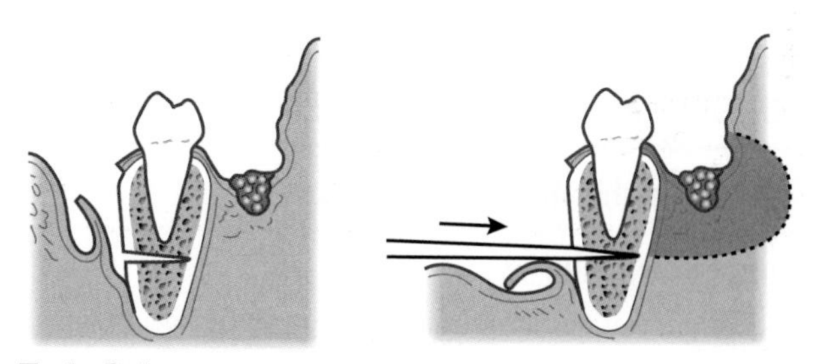

5.1.24 Three-dimensional excision of the sublingual gland including the adjacent alveolar bone.

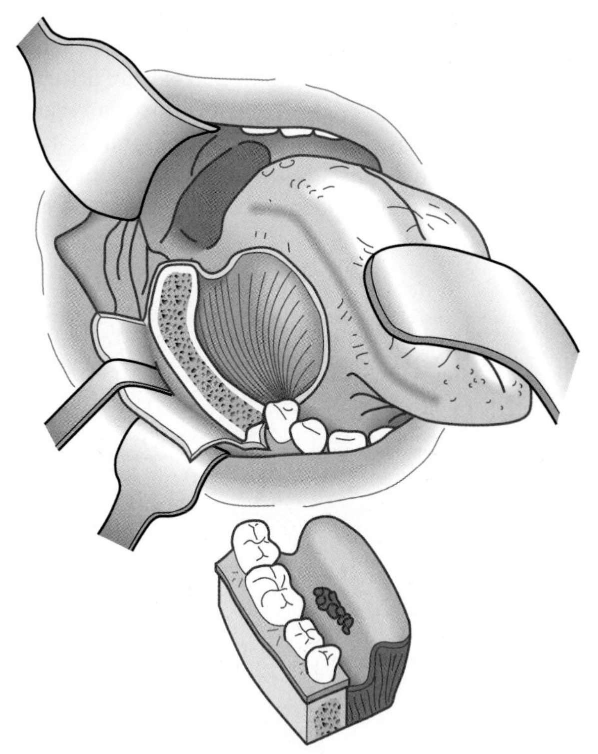

5.1.25 Excised specimen with clear margins and residual defect.

The buccal mucosal flap is used to cover the mandibular bone. The mucosal defect in the floor of the mouth is closed either by mobilizing adjacent soft tissue or a pack soaked in Whitehead's varnish may be sutured over the defect which granulates and epithelializes below the pack.

Complications

The ensuing complications will depend on how radical the excision has been and what adjacent structures have been resected or damaged. The proximal stump of the submandibular duct should be loosely sutured to the oral mucosa at the back of the operation site. It will form a new opening into the floor of the mouth and submandibular gland obstruction is not a problem. Lingual anaesthesia from loss of the lingual nerve and tongue paralysis, if the hypoglossal nerve has been included in the specimen, are major problems. Both of these nerves can be reconstructed by grafting at the time of the tumour excision, although because of the poor prognosis of such tumours, this is often not executed.

SURGERY OF THE MINOR SALIVARY GLANDS

Glands in the mobile soft tissues

MINOR GLAND BIOPSY

The surgeon is sometimes asked to provide specimens of minor glands to confirm the diagnosis of Sjogren's syndrome. The biopsy should be taken from the inner aspect of the lower lip. The incision should be made in the vertical plane just through the mucosa. The lip is then retracted and the assistant places a finger on the outer aspect of the lip, everting the submucosa into the wound (Figure 5.1.26). A minimum of three minor glands are identified and excised. They can be seen as pale yellow glistening 'grains of rice' lying within the connective tissue of the submucosa. Haemostasis is obtained and the mucosa closed with a single resorbable suture.

TUMOUR EXCISION

When a patient presents with a mobile mass in the submucosa of the mobile soft tissues, the assumption should be that it is a neoplasm until proved otherwise. Many of these will be benign pleomorphic adenomas and open incisional biopsy would result in tumour seeding into the adjacent tissues. For this reason, a simple excision biopsy of the minor gland is the appropriate management for all such masses. The excision is performed in the extracapsular plane and even for tumours that prove to be malignant, this will prove to be sufficient as these tumours do not infiltrate the gland capsule until late in their development.

Palatal gland surgery

The detailed pathology of masses and ulcers arising on the hard palate prior to surgery is all important and an incisional biopsy is essential before definitive surgery is undertaken. The differential diagnosis of persistent ulcers arising on the hard palate includes acute necrotizing sialometaplasia (Figure 5.1.27), adenoidcystic carcinoma, squamous cell carcinoma and an antral carcinoma from above. The definitive management of these conditions will all be very different. Even a small adenoidcystic carcinoma will involve at least a partial maxillectomy, whereas a pleomorphic adenoma requires no more than excision with a narrow margin of mucosa and dissection in the subperiosteal plane. Low-grade mucoepidermoid tumours will require a local palatal fenestration and a 1-cm mucosal margin.

OPERATION FOR EXCISION OF BENIGN TUMOURS

This technique is appropriate for such pathology as pleomorphic adenoma, neurofibromas or haemangiomas. Although the operation can be readily performed under local

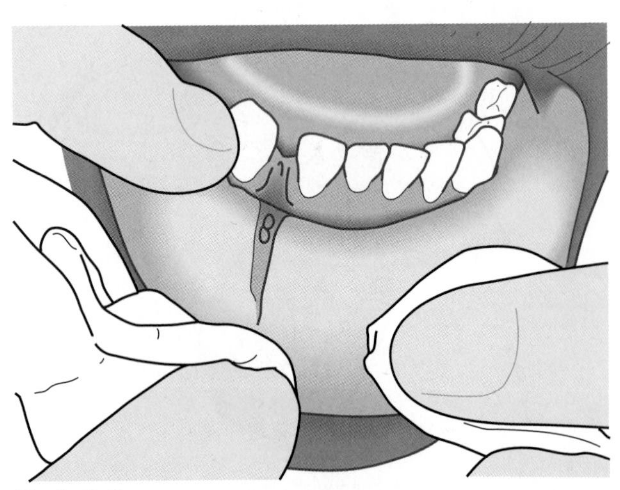

5.1.26 Labial salivary gland biopsy.

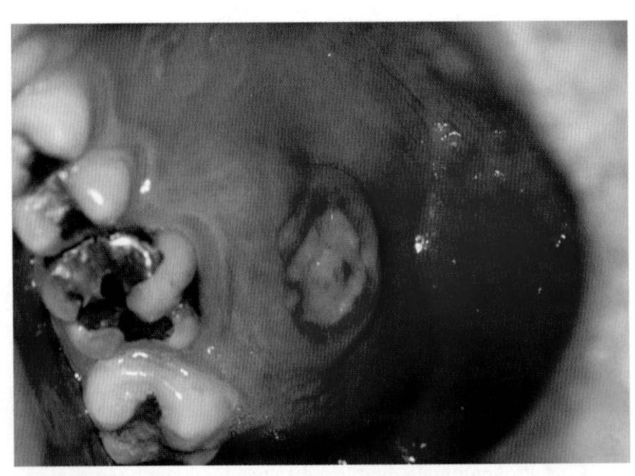

5.1.27 Acute necrotizing sialometaplasia.

anaesthesia, it is often kinder to use a general anaesthetic as bleeding from the hard palate can be distressing for a conscious patient. In this situation, the patient is positioned supine on the operating table with a sand bag under the shoulders and a head down tilt of the table. The surgeon sits at the head of the table. The palate is infiltrated by 2 per cent lignocaine with 1:80 000 epinephrine (adrenalin).

The mucosal margin is mapped out with ink (Figure 5.1.28). A 5-mm margin is adequate. The incision is made down to bone using a fine cutting diathermy needle. The specimen is then freed in the subperiosteal plane with a Howarth's pereosteal elevator or Mitchell's trimmer.

Although benign, long-standing pleomorphic adenomas can result in pressure resorption of the underlying palatal bone and there may be a concavity in the palate (Figure 5.1.29). However, it is important to realize that such benign tumours will never penetrate the periosteum.

The defect may be left to heal by secondary intention, although it should be protected by a Whitehead's varnish pack or by a preformed acrylic appliance which should be relieved over the area of the resection in order to accommodate some periodontal pack as a dressing. The pack or plate should be retained for about 10 days by which time the area will be granulating. Some large defects may take several weeks to heal and in such cases a removable plate should be utilized to protect the area. It must be kept scrupulously clean and removed and rinsed after all meals. A chlorhexidine mouth wash should be used to rinse when the plate is removed for cleaning.

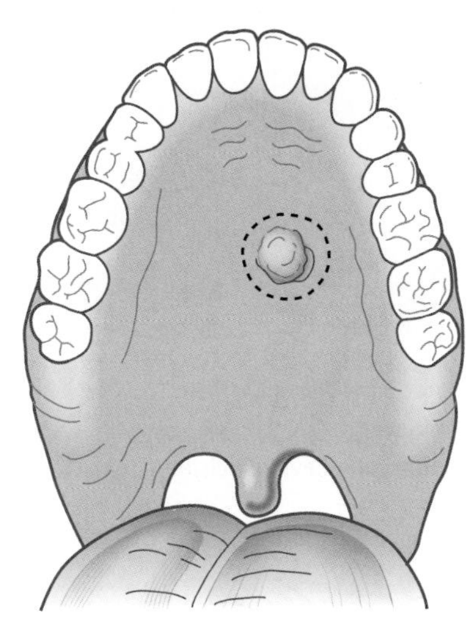

5.1.28 Incision for benign palatal tumour.

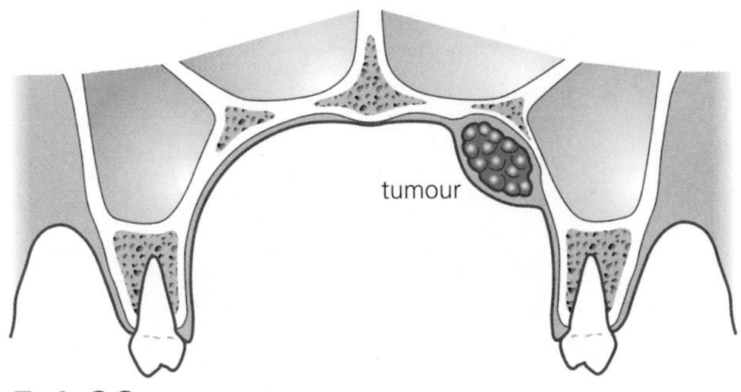

5.1.29 Long-standing pleomorphic adenomas can result in pressure resorption of palatal bone.

OPERATION FOR LOW-GRADE MALIGNANT TUMOURS

For all low-grade malignant tumours, palatal fenestration with a 1-cm mucosal margin is indicated. The operation is performed under general anaesthetic with the patient and surgeon positioned as above.

Following mapping of the 1-cm mucosal margin and the diathermy incision, a dental bur is used to cut through the palatal bone at the margins of the incision. The excision specimen can then be gently elevated and any underlying structures, such as the nasal septum or antral wall, can be divided with heavy scissors.

Whenever possible, an immediate reconstruction should be undertaken. For small defects, a palatal rotation flap may be suitable. The palatal flap should be mapped out parallel to the dental arch and is based on the greater palatine artery. In order to avoid damage to this vessel, the incision should stop 1 cm anterior to the greater palatine foramen (Figure 5.1.30, see also Chapter 3.2).

The flap is raised in the superiosteal plane and rotated to cover the fenestration defect. It needs to be firmly sutured into position with non-resorbable sutures as there is a tendency for the flap to pull back to its anatomical position (Figure 5.1.31). The sutures should be retained for 2 weeks. The donor site defect is covered with a Whitehead's varnish pack.

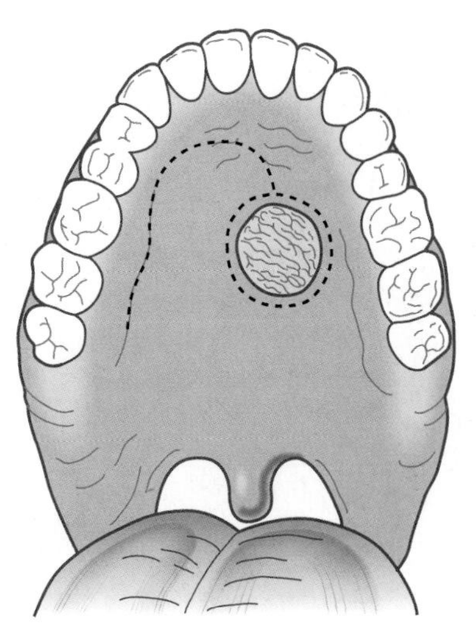

5.1.30 Palatal rotation flap.

For more lateral palatal defects, a buccal advancement flap used to close oroantral communications can be utilized. The flap must be broad based and it should extend to the full depth of the buccal sulcus (Figure 5.1.32).

The periosteum on the deep aspect of the flap is incised with a sharp blade parallel and close to the base of the flap. This relieving incision through the unyielding periosteum allows the flap to be advanced on to the palate (Figure 5.1.33). Great care must be taken not to incise beyond the periosteum as a button hole through the flap will compromise the blood supply. It is also important to ensure that the periosteal relieving incision extends to the full width of the flap. Failure to do this results in the flap failing to advance as it remains tethered by the unyielding periosteum.

The palatal margins of the fenestration defect must be undermined and the mobilized buccal flap is meticulously sutured to the palatal mucosa with everting mattress sutures. Non-resorbable sutures must be used and they should be maintained for 2 weeks to ensure healing (Figure 5.1.34).

Posterior full thickness palatal defects are conveniently closed with buccal fat pad flaps as described in Chapter 3.2. For central palatal defects, bilateral buccal fat pads can be used.

SURGERY FOR HIGH-GRADE MALIGNANT TUMOURS

For all aggressive malignant tumours, particularly adenoidcystic carcinomas, partial or total maxillectomy followed by radiotherapy including the skull base is indicated. When a maxillectomy has been undertaken, the defect is reconstructed with a vascularized hip graft (Chapter 3.13) or a fibular flap (Chapter 3.12). An alternative is to reconstruct the defect with an obturator.

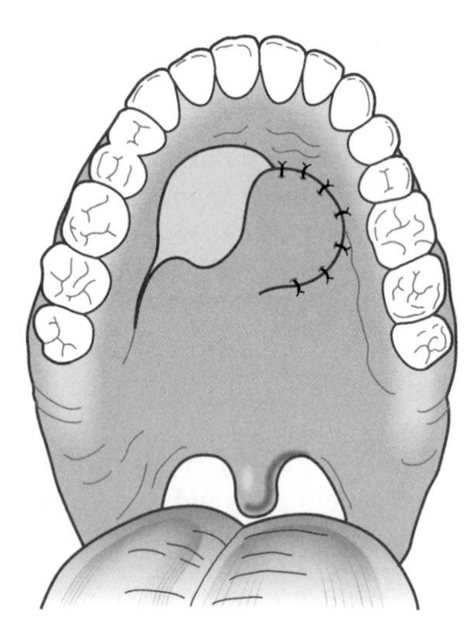

5.1.31 Closure of palatal defect.

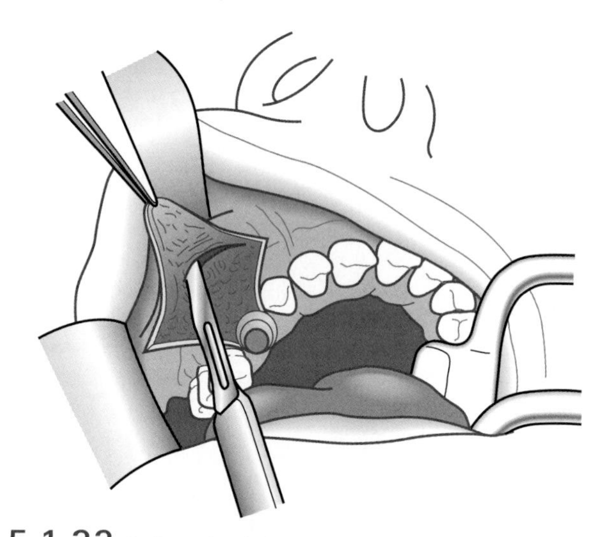

5.1.33 Periosteal relieving incision.

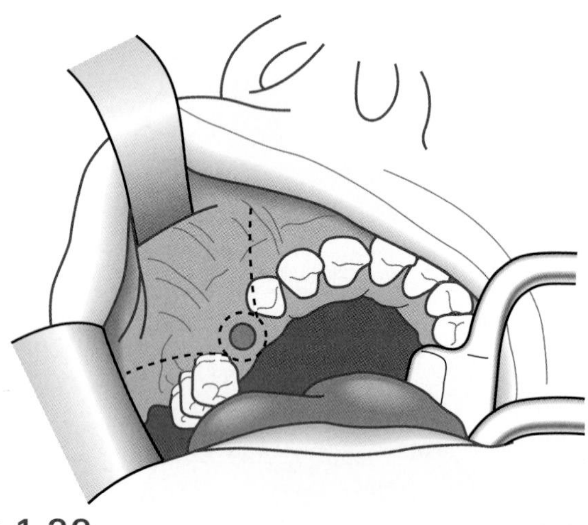

5.1.32 Outline of buccal advancement flap.

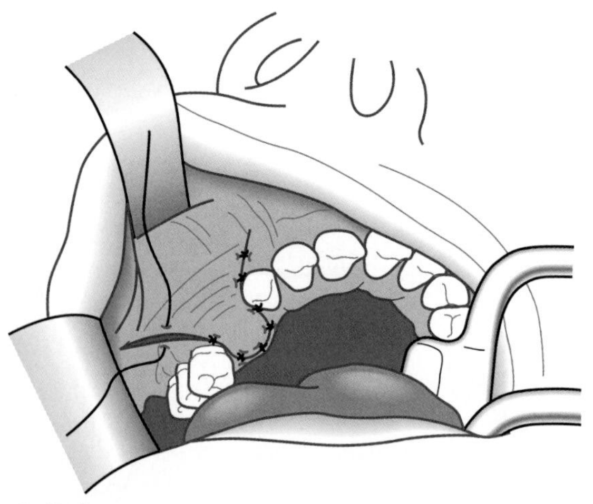

5.1.34 Closure of palatal defect using buccal advancement flap.

Top tips

- When removing submandibular stones, it is important to irrigate the duct in order to remove any 'gravel' remaining in the duct system.
- When excising the submandibular gland, the lingual nerve must be fully visualized and the parasympathetic fibres tethering the nerve to the gland must be severed in order to free the gland.
- The only effective treatment for a ranula is excision of the related gland which is nearly always the sublingual gland. Occasionally, the submandibular gland can be responsible.
- The majority of sublingual gland tumours are malignant and wide surgical excision and post-operative radiotherapy are essential.
- Pre-operative diagnosis of a palatal gland tumour is essential. Benign tumours require local excision with a very narrow cuff of normal mucosa, low-grade tumours require palatal fenestration and high-grade tumours require radical maxillectomy.

FURTHER READING

Cawson RA, Gleeson MJ, Eveson JW. *Pathology and surgery of the salivary glands.* Oxford: Isis, 1997.

McGurk M. Surgical release of a stone from the hilum of the submandibular gland. *International Journal of Oral and Maxillifacial Surgery* 2005; **34**: 208–10.

Seward GR. (1968) Anatomic surgery for salivary gland calculi. *Oral Surgery, Oral Medicine, Oral Pathology,* 1968; **25**: 670–78.

Shaheen OH. Removal of the submandibular gland. In: Carter D, Russell RCG, Pitt HA (eds). *Rob and Smith's Operative Surgery.* London: Butterworths, 1976: 362–8.

5.2

Management of stones and strictures and interventional sialography

MICHAEL P ESCUDIER, JACQUI E BROWN

MANAGEMENT OF STONES AND STRICTURES

Sialolithiasis accounts for approximately 50 per cent of major salivary gland disease. The incidence of symptomatic sialolithiasis is between 27.5 and 59 cases per million population per year.

The presence of a salivary calculus usually results in mechanical obstruction of the salivary duct, causing repeated swelling during meals, which can remain transient or be complicated by bacterial infections. Until recently, recurring episodes necessitated open surgery with calculi that lay in the proximal duct or gland requiring sialoadenectomy despite its attendant risks (see Chapter 5.1).

During the past 18 years, minimally invasive and non-surgical techniques for the removal of salivary calculi have been developed. The basis for this approach resides in the fact that salivary glands have been shown to have significant reparative potential. Scintigraphic studies before and after removal of a submandibular calculus have shown that the gland can recover. In addition, the duration of obstructive symptoms does not influence the amount of recovery observed (Figure 5.2.1a,b).

While a variety of techniques has been investigated, those which have progressed beyond the initial trials and remain in clinical practice include basket retrieval and micro-forceps retrieval, both of which can be performed under either endoscopic or radiological control. Intracorporeal and extracorporeal shock wave lithotripsy have also assumed a continuing role, as has gland-preserving surgery for submandibular calculi and in an endoscopically assisted form for parotid stones.

LITHOTRIPSY

Following the successful introduction of lithotripsy for renal calculi in the 1980s, the technique has been applied to several other areas of the body including, with the development of specialized machines, the salivary glands.

Extracorporeal shock wave lithotripsy

At the present time, the devices which generate the shock wave are either piezoelectric (Piezolith 2501; Richard Wolf, Knittlingen, Germany) or electromagnetic (Minilith; Storz Medical, Switzerland) (Figure 5.2.2).

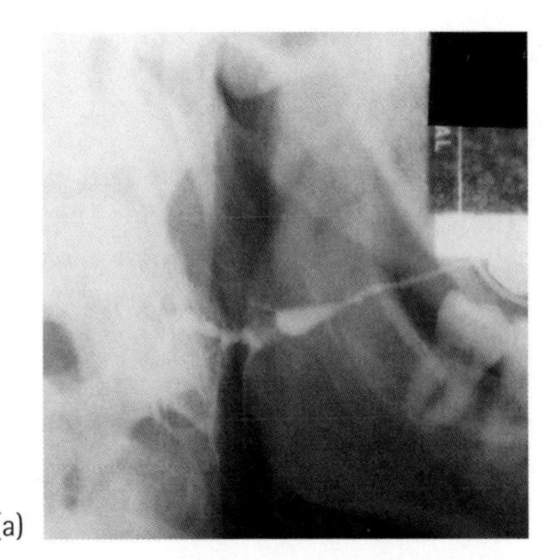

(a)

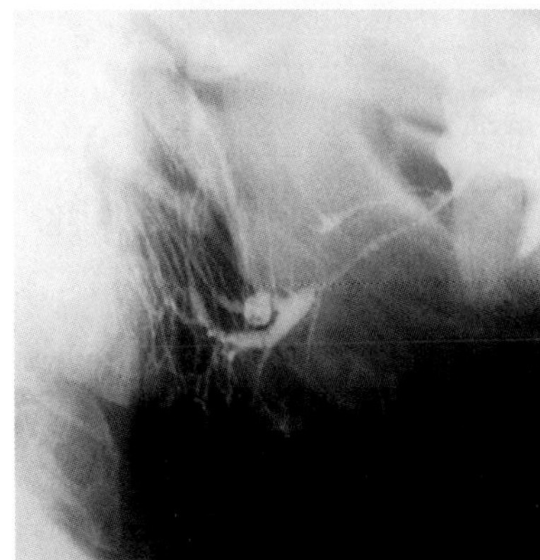

(b)

5.2.1 (a) Pre-treatment sialogram showing presence of obstruction associated with poor ductal architecture. (b) Post-treatment sialogram showing improvement in glandular architecture.

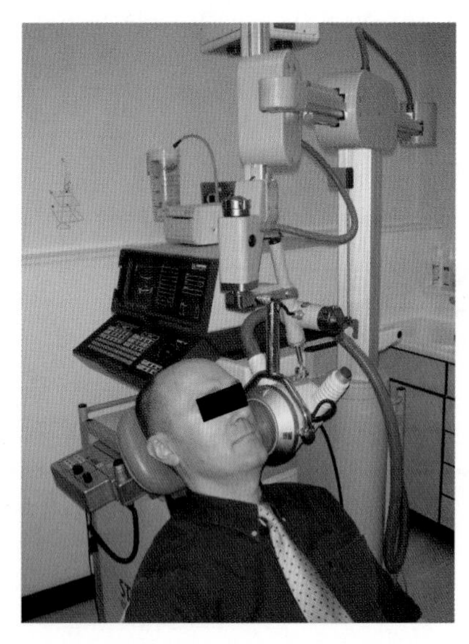

5.2.2 Salivary lithotripter with patient in treatment position for a parotid stone.

PATIENT SELECTION

A number of selection criteria have been developed for this technique (Table 5.2.1), which have led to it principally being used in the management of fixed parotid stones. In addition, where present, acute sialoadenitis must first be treated with antibiotics.

TECHNIQUE

Treatment is performed on an outpatient basis. After ultrasonographic localization of the stone (Figure 5.2.3), shock waves are delivered to a maximum per visit (3000 piezoelectric, 7500 electromagnetic). In general, a series of three sessions separated by 4–12 weeks are required.

Following successful fragmentation, pieces of calculus migrate distally and exit the duct either spontaneously (Figure 5.2.4) or as a result of adjuvant measures (massage, sialogogues) or techniques (dilatation of ostium, papillotomy, endoscopic (Figure 2.5.5) or basket retrieval).

Common, reversible complications include mild swelling of the gland (60–70 per cent), self-limiting ductal haemorrhage (40–55 per cent) and petechial skin haemorrhage (40–55 per cent), while acute sialoadenitis is rare (1.5–5.7 per cent).

OUTCOME

Success rates are generally expressed in terms of cure (stone and symptom free), partial success (residual stone without symptoms) and failure (residual stone and symptoms). In the five published series with over 100 cases, the overall cure rates vary from 29 to 63 per cent, while 56.7–100 per cent are rendered stone or symptom free (Table 5.2.2).

The cure rate is significantly better (34.2–69.3 per cent) for parotid (Table 5.2.3) than for submandibular (29.0–41.1 per cent) stones (Table 5.2.4). Similarly, the percentage of patients with neither stones nor symptoms is higher for parotid cases (68.6–100 per cent) than for submandibular cases (56–100 per cent).

In a long-term (ten-year) follow-up study of submandibular stones, one-third of patients remained stone free,

Table 5.2.1 Selection criteria.

Inclusion criteria	Exclusion criteria
Symptomatic disease	Stones amenable to intra-oral surgery
Exact sonographic location of concretions	Stones amenable to radiologically/endoscopically guided basket retrieval
	Calculi not readily identifiable by ultrasound
	Patients with blood dyscrasias or haemostatic abnormalities
	Patients who are pregnant
	Patients who have undergone stapedectomy or ossicular repair

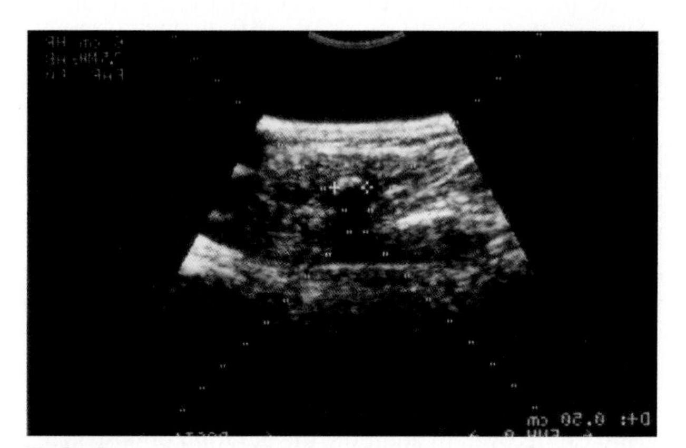

5.2.3 Ultrasound image showing large intraglandular parotid stone with posterior acoustic shadow.

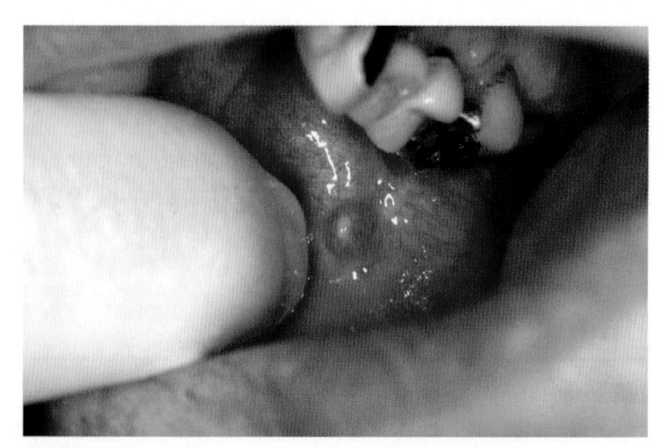

5.2.4 Fragments of parotid calculus at parotid duct ostium following lithotripsy.

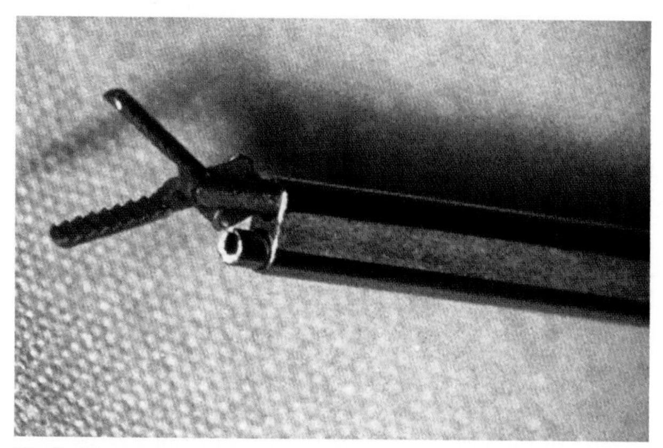

5.2.5 Salivary endoscope with microforcep *in situ*.

one-third still had residual fragments but were symptom free and one-third required additional intervention.

PREDICTIVE FACTORS

As dealt with above, the cure rate for parotid stones is significantly greater than for submandibular stones. Several authors have reported an association between the size of the stone and the stone-free rate, while others have not. This association is not seen repeated in the case of partial success.

Intracorporeal shockwave lithotripsy

The development of micro-endoscopes has enabled sialoendoscopy both for diagnostic and interventional purposes. In intracorporeal shock wave lithotripsy, a lithotripsy probe is passed along the salivary duct, under endoscopic guidance, to be adjacent to or in contact with the stone surface.

Initial studies in this area centred on the use of electrohydraulic and pneumatic lithotripsy. Electrohydraulic intracorporeal lithotripsy (Calcitript; Storz Medical) was successful in fragmenting the calculus in 60–70 per cent of cases. A flexible endoscope together with the shockwave probe were introduced into the duct and advanced until the probe was 1 mm away from the sialolith. The shock waves were generated by a sparkover at the tip of the 600-micron probe. Pneumobalistic lithotripsy used a Lithoclast (Electro Medical Systems, Nyon, Switzerland). This equipment

Table 5.2.2 Overall success rates for salivary lithotripsy (minimum 100 cases).

Study	Year	Lithotripter	No. cases	Cured	Partial success	Failure
Kater	1994	Electromagnetic, Minilith	104	38.4	18.3	43.3
Katz	1998	Electromagnetic, Minilith	200	63.0	34.0	3.0
Escudier	2003	Electromagnetic, Minilith	122	33.0	35.0	32.0
Zenk	2004	Piezoelectric, Piezolith 2500	197	29.0	71.0	0.0
Capaccio	2004	Electromagnetic, Minilith	322	45.0	27.4	27.6

Table 5.2.3 Success rates for parotid stone lithotripsy (minimum 24 cases).

Study	Year	Lithotripter	Parotid cases	Cured	Partial success	Failure
Kater	1994	Electromagnetic, Minilith	29	48.30	10.3	41.4
Ottaviani	1997	Electromagnetic, Minilith	24	58.30	41.7	0
Iro	1998	Piezoelectric, Piezolith 2500	76	50.00	26.3	23.7
Escudier	2003	Electromagnetic, Minilith	38	34.20	44.7	21.1
Capaccio	2004	Electromagnetic, Minilith	88	69.30	27.3	3.4

Table 5.2.4 Success rates for submandibular stone lithotripsy (minimum 75 cases).

Study	Year	Lithotripter	Submandibular cases	Cured	Partial success	Failure
Kater	1993	Electromagnetic, Minilith	75	34.7	21.3	44
Ottaviani	1997	Electromagnetic, Minilith	56	41.1	25	33.9
Escudier	2003	Electromagnetic, Minilith	84	32.1	30.9	37
Zenk	2004	Piezoelectric, Piezolith 2500	197	29.0	71	0
Capaccio	2004	Electromagnetic, Minilith	234	35.9	27.4	36.7

consists of a central unit, connected to a compressed air source, producing a pressure of three bar at the handpiece. The handpiece generated ballistic energy and converted it into shockwaves which were applied directly to the stone via the probe. Using this equipment, in the working channel of a 2.1-mm endoscope, stone-free rates of up to 60 per cent were reported. However, both techniques have been abandoned because of the high risk of unwanted effects such as ductal perforation and nerve damage.

Later studies investigated the use of laser lithotripsy and several systems have been evaluated *in vitro* and *in vivo*. Unfortunately, the Nd-YAG (1064 nm; LASAG-AG, Switzerland) and Alexandrit (755 nm; Dornier Medizintechnik, Germany) lasers were unsuitable because of inadequate fragmentation. In the case of the Eximer laser (308 nm; Technolas Lasertetechnologie, Germany), stone-free rates of up to 91.6 per cent were reported, but were associated with a high rate of ductal perforation and its use in humans is inadvisable. The Rhodamine-6G-Dye-laser (595 nm; Lithoghost, Telemit-Company, Germany), however, proved successful. This had the added advantage of using a novel spectroscopic feedback technique which analyzed the reflected laser light to distinguish between calculi and soft tissue, so minimizing damage to the duct. Its use was associated with complete removal of stones in 46 per cent of cases after between one and three treatment sessions.

All of these techniques required a papillotomy to enable the endoscopically controlled equipment to access the ductal system. In addition to this, the techniques often require expensive equipment and are relatively time consuming for the success rates achieved. As a result, intracorporeal shock wave lithotripsy is currently of limited clinical importance.

ENDOSCOPIC RETRIEVAL

The initial attempts at endoscopically guided stone retrieval used flexible endoscopes. Unfortunately, these were difficult to manoeuvre, fragile, provided only poor images and were difficult to sterilize. This situation improved with the use of semi-rigid endoscopes, although the diameter of the device (relative to the lumen of the duct) resulted in difficulty in progressing along the duct and ductal tears. Rigid endoscopes proved most successful (Figure 5.2.6) and have developed progressively from the initial 2.7-mm diameter arthroscopes, which required a papillotomy to facilitate ductal entry to one (Marchal sialoendoscope; Karl Storz, Tuttlingen, Germany) which measures 1.3 mm in diameter and contains an optic fibre of 6000 pixels, a rinsing channel of 0.25 and a working channel of 0.65 mm for instrumentation.

Clinical and radiographic assessment of prospective cases is essential, as exclusion criteria for the technique include narrow ducts, ductal strictures and intraparenchymal location of stones. In addition, acute sialoadenitis should be treated with antibiotics prior to intervention.

In the technique, the endoscope is introduced into the ductal system and progressed until the sialolith is identified. The stone is then removed with either suction, basket or microforceps. If the stone is large, then fragmentation by microforceps or laser lithotripsy is required to facilitate its removal. Whilst the first is time consuming, the latter is associated with the previously detailed problems associated with laser lithotripsy, although further advances may address these issues. Post-operative antibiotics have been advocated, as have stenting of the duct with a 2-mm polyethylene tube, although the value of the latter is questionable.

Overall success rates of over 80 per cent have been reported. However, the success rates are directly related to the size of the stone with one study reporting a 97 per cent cure rate for stones smaller than 3 mm and 35 per cent for those larger than 3 mm.

INTERVENTIONAL SIALOGRAPHY

Introduction

Radiological techniques have been used to investigate the salivary glands since 1900, when Charpy first described the injection of mercury into the salivary ducts in order to demonstrate salivary gland anatomy. Sialography is still widely practised in the diagnosis of obstruction, sialadenitis and Sjogren's syndrome. It remains the most sensitive method for detecting salivary stones and strictures within the ductal system of the major salivary glands.

In recent years, its role has been developed and extended into interventional radiological techniques in the salivary ducts to treat ductal obstruction. Interventional sialography has thus become one of several new minimally invasive techniques within the armentarium of the clinician seeking to treat one of the most common salivary gland complaints, salivary gland obstruction, without resorting to surgery.

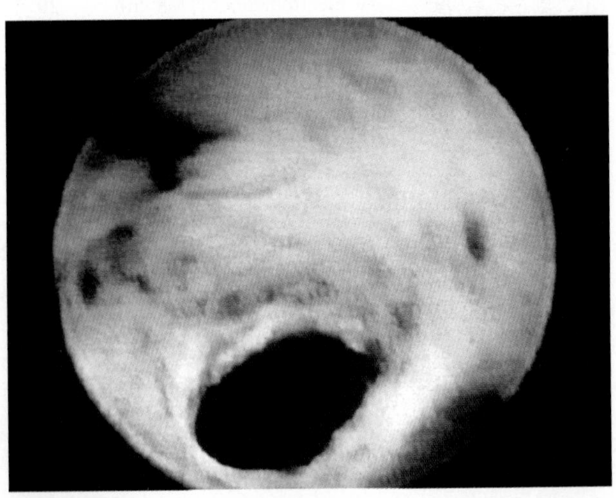

5.2.6 Per-operative endoscopic view of salivary duct.

Salivary gland obstruction may be due to either extraductal or intraductal causes. Intraductal causes are most common and principally include salivary calculi and duct stenoses. A recent analysis of the incidence of salivary ductal obstruction over a series of over 1300 sialograms undertaken for patients with obstructive symptoms showed an obstruction in 64 per cent of the investigated cases, of which 73 per cent has salivary calculi and 23 per cent had a stricture. This highlights the greater incidence of stones (Figure 5.2.7), but also illustrates the very real problem of salivary duct stenosis (Figure 5.2.8). This study also showed that duct strictures were far more common in the parotid glands of middle-aged women and may, in around 7 per cent, be bilateral.

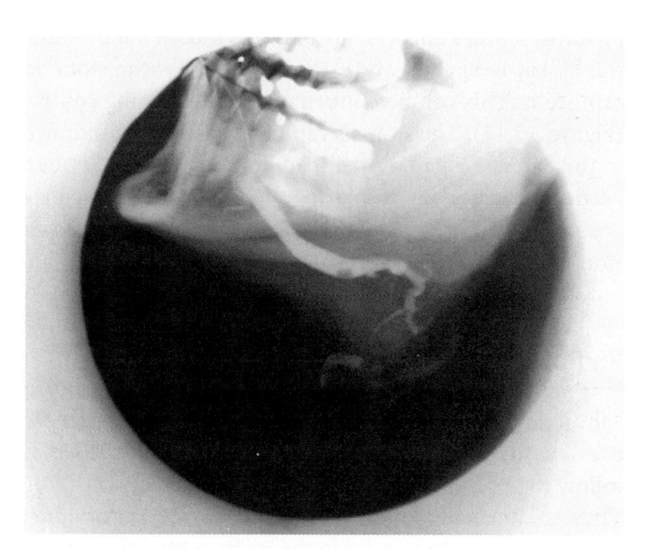

5.2.7 Submandibular sialogram showing a stone in the proximal part of the main duct.

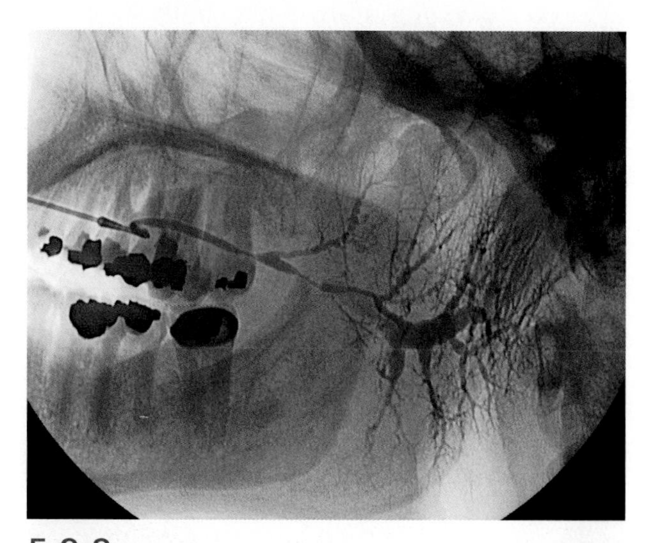

5.2.8 Parotid sialogram showing two diffuse strictures, one at the entry to the hilum of the gland and one more distally placed near the division of the main duct with a secondary branch.

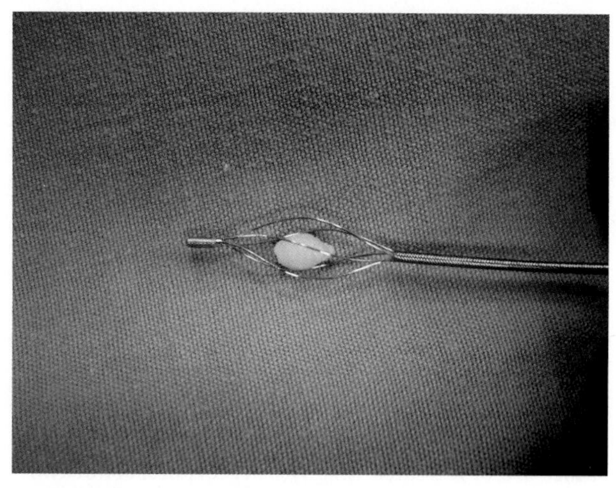

5.2.9 A Dormia basket containing a stone.

Interventional sialography has developed methods for treating both eventualities using ideas taken from other areas of intervention. Ductal calculi may be extracted by capture with devices such as small collapsible Dormia baskets, where these have been employed to extract biliary and ureteric stones (Figure 5.2.9). These are introduced into the ductal system within fine catheters and deployed to capture the stone once they have been positioned around or beyond the stone. Salivary duct strictures are amenable to dilatation by balloon catheters in a similar way to vascular stenoses or strictures developing within the ureteric system or within haemodialysis fistulas.

Case selection and patient preparation for interventional sialography

Sialography and ultrasound examinations form the prerequisite imaging for case assessment prior to intervention in the salivary ducts. Sialography successfully distinguishes salivary calculi from strictures, and ultrasound successfully distinguishes stones from soft mucous plug debris, since a stone will show a bright area within the salivary duct with an acoustic shadow behind it, while soft debris shows a similar appearance but no acoustic shadow.

Sialography and ultrasound also localize a stone or stricture, give its dimensions, identify multiple stones and help to identify if a stone is mobile. Stones within the main parotid and submandibular ducts are amenable to extraction using this technique, but cannot normally reach stones within the submandibular hilum since the Dormia basket cannot pass beyond the genu of the duct. Mobility of the stone on the pre-operative sialogram is a good prognostic factor, since it indicates that the stone is not fixed or fibrosed to the duct wall, which would prevent its extraction. Sialograms also allow assessment of the condition of the proximally placed gland. However, importantly, only sialography allows one to assess the width of the duct running distally from a stone to the duct orifice. This is crucially important if the stone is to be withdrawn down this distal duct, since there must not be too great a mismatch between the size of stone and the duct. It would be sensible to avoid extraction of stones more than 25 per cent greater in width than the width of the narrowest section of the distal salivary duct. Care should be exercised in case selection at this point – if a large stone is captured in a basket but is too large to be withdrawn down the relatively narrow duct, then the basket will become impacted in the proximal duct and will almost certainly require surgical release. This is an important complication, which can be avoided with sensible treatment planning. Larger and very proximal stones are best treated first by extracorporeal shockwave lithotripsy to break down the stone into more manageable pieces. If a stricture is identified distal to the stone to be removed, then planning will be required to dilate this area of duct stenosis prior to stone extraction, using an angioplasty balloon.

Sialography also plays a key role during intervention. During interventional sialography, the pre-operative sialogram is used to confirm the exact nature and location of the obstruction and to guide the placement of the interventional tool in relation to the obstruction.

One noted advantage of minimally invasive techniques has been the ability to carry out treatment under local anaesthesia, avoiding conventional surgery under general anaesthetic and therefore enabling treatment of patients with more complex medical conditions that might otherwise preclude intervention. Treatment under local anaesthesia is additionally more time-efficient, does not require in-patient hospital admission and is generally associated with lower morbidity.

Local anaesthesia is achieved for intervention in the parotid gland by infiltrating the cheek around the Stenson's duct papilla with 2 per cent lignocaine, and by instilling local anaesthetic into the parotid duct to create some topical anaesthesia of the duct wall. For interventional procedures in the submandibular ductal system, an inferior nerve block accompanied by a lingual nerve block is very effective.

Radiologically guided salivary stone extraction

A technique for stone extraction under fluoroscopic radiological guidance was first demonstrated by Briffa and Callum in 1989, and described the extraction of a small stone from the submandibular duct. An angioplasty balloon catheter was inserted into the salivary duct, the balloon slid proximal to the stone and inflated, then withdrawn to the orifice of Wharton's duct, trapping the stone and drawing it up to the orifice. Following this, similar procedures were reported using interventional catheters normally employed for vascular work, such as vascular snares and graspers to trap salivary stones and extract them from the salivary ducts, but most of these subsequent case reports and small case series have reported greatest success with Dormia baskets. In these papers, success rates of between 60 and 100 per cent have been reported.

The technique for stone removal from the parotid and submandibular ducts using a Dormia basket technique under fluoroscopic x-ray guidance and local anaesthesia is a relatively simple procedure with a high success rate and low morbidity. Following treatment planning, on the basis of clinical examination and pre-operative imaging, the patient is given a suitable local anaesthetic and a sialogram is performed. The duct orifice is gently dilated with lachrymal duct and Nettleship dilators to sufficient diameter to receive a 3-French Dormia basket catheter. The Dormia basket catheter is inserted in the closed position and guided into position under radiological control. The catheter tip is normally required to pass beyond the stone, into the proximal salivary duct (Figure 5.2.10). Once in this position, the basket is opened and withdrawn across the stone to capture it. This can be confirmed under imaging control (Figure 5.2.11). The stone is captured and then withdrawn to the papilla, where a small papillotomy incision is often needed to deliver the stone (Figure 5.2.12). An immediate post-operative sialogram is helpful to check for any residual stones.

Radiologically guided balloon ductoplasty

Salivary duct strictures are believed to develop secondary to previous duct wall irritation and inflammation, as may follow the presence of a stone, local trauma or infection. They are normally found within the main excretory duct and 75 per cent are located in the main duct of the parotid

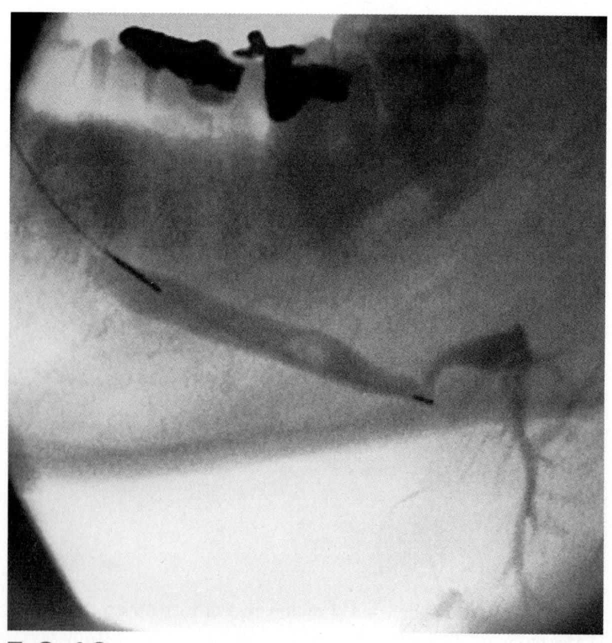

5.2.10 Interoperative submandibular sialogram showing the basket inserted beyond the stone.

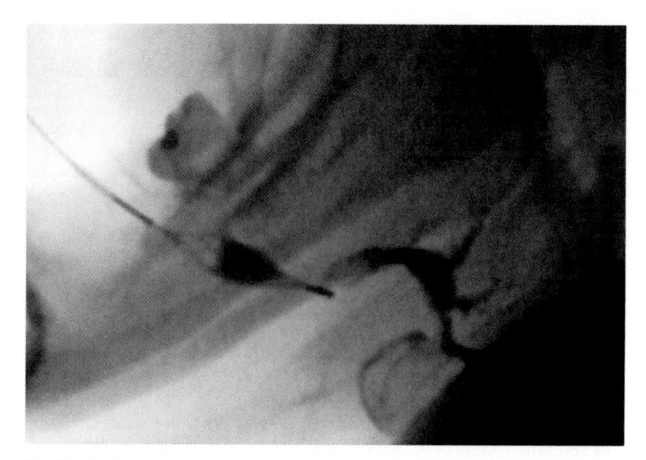

5.2.11 Interoperative sialogram showing the basket, with stone trapped within it, being withdrawn forward to the orifice of Wharton's duct.

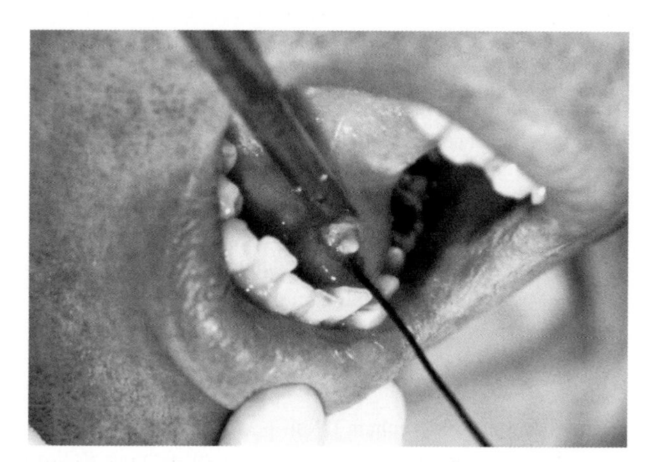

5.2.12 Papillotomy is performed to release a stone, trapped in a Dormia basket, from the submandibular duct.

gland, making these far more common in this situation than in the submandibular system. A recent study also showed these to be more common in middle age and in women.

This technique offers a non-surgical option for those patients developing symptoms of obstruction as a result of duct stenosis, and for relieving strictures distal to a stone prior to stone extraction. Angioplasty balloons are available in widths suitable for dilation of salivary ducts, which normally range in diameter from 1 to 2 mm. The aim of the procedure is to dilate the duct to slightly greater than its normal calibre and to break the circumferential bands of fibrous tissue forming within the duct wall.

The patient is prepared in the same way as for stone extraction, using a pre-operative sialogram to identify the nature and position of the stenosis. A local anaesthetic is given as described previously, the duct orifice dilated manually with dilator instruments and a pre-operative sialogram performed. Immediately, without moving the patient, the balloon catheter is inserted into the duct. The

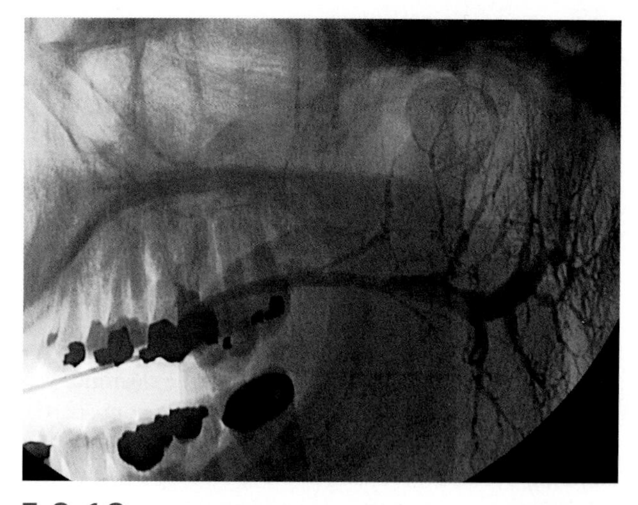

5.2.13 Post-operative view following balloon ductoplasty for two strictures of the parotid duct (see Figure 5.2.7 for pre-operative appearance). Note the filling defect representing mucous plug against the inferior duct wall within the dilated hilum.

lateral sialographic view is used to guide the balloon catheter into position along a guide-wire which, together with the balloon catheter, is inserted into the duct orifice and moved gently but firmly down the duct until it passes through the most proximal area of strictured duct. The balloon is positioned centrally within the stricture and inflated fully for several minutes to ensure good dilation (Figure 5.2.13). Tight stenosis may require several inflations. The balloon is then deflated fully and withdrawn forward to the next, more distal stricture if present. The procedure is repeated, if necessary, until all the stenoses are satisfactorily dilated. A post-operative sialogram is used to check satisfactory duct calibre before the duct is finally irrigated.

Post-operative care

Following a salivary intervention, the patient is advised to keep well hydrated and to stimulate the gland with sialogogues and self-massage to ensure that the operative site remains patent. Intervention in the salivary ducts is normally accompanied by some degree of local oedema, particularly following balloon ductoplasty. The effect of the local oedema may be to cause compression of the duct and a temporary return of gland swelling, especially at meal times. The patient needs to be counselled to expect this for several days. Post-operative antibiotic prophylaxis is not always needed, but may also be appropriate if infection is suspected.

Value of interventional sialography

To date, our experience of this technique at this centre has included 443 interventional radiologically guided salivary gland treatments for benign obstruction; 252 for salivary stone extraction and 194 balloon ductoplasties. Patients included 190 males and 253 females ranging in age from 8 to 85 years, with an average age of 48 years.

In 252 cases of salivary stones, 96 (38 per cent) were in the parotid glands and 156 (62 per cent) in the submandibular glands, which is a rather different distribution to that normally quoted (normally around 80–90 per cent in the submandibular duct system), but probably reflects a different patient group who are keen to avoid surgery, especially a superficial parotidectomy, which carries the risk of facial nerve palsy. Successful stone clearance was achieved in 77 per cent (194/252) of the study group, partial clearance was achieved in 8.3 per cent (that is, some but not all stones were removed) and in the remaining 14.7 per cent (37/252) the procedure failed to remove the intended stone. This was due primarily to an immobile stone (adherent to the duct wall) or to the inability to capture the stone due to an unfavourable position within a secondary duct or side branch.

A total of 194 salivary duct strictures were diagnosed and treated, generally with a higher average age of 51 years and showing a distinct predilection for females (male:female ratio = 1:1.87). Balloon ductoplasty achieved elimination of duct strictures in 78.4 per cent (152/194), while 11.8 per cent (23/194) showed some residual stenosis on post-operative sialogram. The procedure was not completed successfully in 5.2 per cent (10/194) of the group, primarily due to the density of the stenosis which prevented passage of the balloon. Degree of final dilatation was not recorded in nine patients (4.6 per cent).

Conclusion

Increased awareness has led to a demand from the public for less invasive surgical options to treat conditions such as salivary gland obstruction. Conservative management with minimally invasive techniques have come about through technological advances across a range of fields, with many techniques borrowed from other areas of medicine and offers a low-morbidity treatment option. Radiology has followed a similar path and now offers a choice of radiologically guided techniques for treating both salivary stones and strictures. These techniques compliment other new modalities such as extra- and intracorporeal lithotipsy, sialendoscopy and limited-access surgery, such that they may be used in isolation or as part of a combined multimodal approach to treatment.

FURTHER READING

Blaine D, Smith Frable MA. Removal of a parotid duct calculus with an embolectomy catheter. *Otolaryngology – Head and Neck Surgery* 1994; **111**: 312–13.

Briffa NP, Callum KG. Use of an embolectomy catheter to remove a submandibular duct stone. *British Journal of Surgery* 1989; **76**: 814.

Brown A, Shepherd D, Buckenham T. Per oral balloon sialoplasty: Results in the treatment of salivary duct stenosis. *Cardiovascular and Interventional Radiology* 1997; **20**: 337–42.

Brown JE, Drage NA, Escudier MP *et al.* Minimally invasive radiologically guided intervention for the treatment of salivary calculi. *Cardiovascular and Interventional Radiology* 2002; **25**: 352–5.

Brown JE. Interventional sialography and minimally invasive techniques in benign salivary gland obstruction. *Seminars in Ultrasound, CT, and MR* 2006; **27**: 465–75.

Buckenham T, George C, McVicar D *et al.* Digital sialography: imaging and intervention. *British Journal of Radiology* 1994; **67**: 524–9.

Buckenham T, Guest P. Interventional sialography using digital imaging. *Australasian Radiology* 1993; **37**: 76–9.

Capaccio P, Ottaviani F, Manzo R *et al.* Extracorporeal lithotripsy for salivary calculi: A long-term clinical experience. *Laryngoscope* 2004; **114**: 1069–73.

Davies R, Whyte A, Lui C: Interventional sialography: A single center experience. *Cardiovascular and Interventional Radiology* 1997; **20**: 331–336.

Escudier MP, Brown JE, Drage NE, McGurk M. Extracorporeal shockwave lithotripsy in the management of salivary calculi. *British Journal of Surgery* 2003; **90**: 482–5.

Escudier MP, McGurk M. Symptomatic sialoadenitis and sialolithiasis in the English population, an estimate of the cost of hospital treatment. *British Dental Journal* 1999; **186**: 463–66.

Guest P, Maciag A, Buckenham T. Non-operative removal of a parotid duct stone with a balloon angioplasty catheter. *British Journal Oral and Maxillofacial Surgery* 1992; **30**: 197–8.

Iro H, Dlugaiczyk J, Zenk J. Current concepts in diagnosis and treatment of sialolithiasis. *British Journal of Hospital Medicine* 2006; **67**: 24–8.

Iro H, Zenk J, Waldfahrer F *et al.* Extracorporeal shock wave lithotripsy of parotid stones. Results of a prospective clinical trial. *Annals of Otology, Rhinology and Laryngology* 1998; **107**: 860–4.

Isacsson G, Isberg A, Haverling M, Lundquist P. Salivary calculi and chronic sialoadenitis of the submandibular gland: a radiographic and histologic study. *Oral Surgery, Oral Medicine, and Oral Pathology* 1984; **58**: 622–7.

Kelly IMG, Dick R. Technical report: Interventional sialography; dormia basket removal of Wharton's duct calculus. *Clinical Radiology* 1990; **43**: 205–206.

Kim R, Strimling A, Grosch T *et al.* Nonoperative removal of sialoliths and sialodochoplasty of salivary duct strictures. *Archives of Otolaryngology – Head and Neck Surgery* 1996; **122**: 974–6.

Marchal F, Dulguerov P, Becker M *et al.* Specificity of parotid sialendoscopy. *Laryngoscope* 2001; **111**: 264–71.

Marchal F, Dulguerov P. Sialolithiasis management: The state of the art. *Archives of Otolaryngology – Head and Neck Surgery* 2003; **129**: 951–56.

Marchbank N, Buckenham T. Removal of a submandibular duct calculus with a vascular snare. *Dentomaxillofacial Radiology* 1993; **22**: 97–8.

McGurk M, Escudier MP, Brown E. Modern management of obstructive salivary gland disease. *Annals of the Royal Australasian College of Dental Surgeons* 2004; **17**: 45–50.

McGurk M, Escudier MP, Brown JE. Modern management of salivary calculi. *British Journal of Surgery* 2005; **92**: 107–12.

McGurk M, Escudier MP, Brown JE. Modern management of salivary calculi. *British Journal of Surgery* 2005; **92**:107–12.

Nahlieli O, London D, Zagury A, Eliav E. Combined approach to impacted parotid stones. *Journal of Oral and Maxillofacial Surgery* 2002; **60**: 1418–23.

Nahlieli O, Shacham R, Bar T, Eliav E. Endoscopic mechanical retrieval of sialoliths. *Oral Surgery, Oral Medicine, Oral Pathology, Oral Radiology, and Endodontics* 2003; **95**: 396–402.

Ngu RK, Brown JE, Whaites EJ *et al.* Salivary duct strictures: Nature and incidence in benign salivary obstruction. *Dentomaxillofacial Radiology* 2007; **36**: 63–7.

Nixon P, Payne M. Conservative surgical removal of a submandibular duct calculus following interventional sialography. *Clinical Radiology* 1999; **54**: 337–8.

North E. Submandibular sialoplasty for stone removal and treatment of a stricture. *British Journal of Oral Maxillofacial Surgery* 1998; **36**: 213–14.

Ottaviani F, Capaccio P, Rivolta R *et al.* Salivary gland stones: US evaluation in shock wave lithotripsy. *Radiology* 1997; **204**: 437–41.

Poirier P, Charpy A. *In traite d'anatomie humaine*, vol. 4. Paris: Masson et Cie, 1900.

Sharma R, Al-Khalifa S, Paulose K *et al.* Parotid duct stone – removal by a dormia basket. *Journal Laryngology and Otology* 1994; **108**: 699–701.

Yoshino N, Hosokawa A, Sasaki T *et al.* Interventional radiology for the non-surgical removal of sialoliths. *Dentomaxillofacial Radiology* 1996; **25**: 242–6.

Zenk J, Bozzato A, Winter M *et al.* Extracorporeal shock wave lithotripsy of submandibular stones: evaluation after 10 years. *Annals of Otology, Rhinology, and Laryngology* 2004; **113**: 378–83.

Zenk J, Hosemann WG, Iro H. Diameters of the main excretory ducts of the adult human submandibular and parotid gland: A histologic study. *Oral Surgery, Oral Medicine, Oral Pathology, Oral Radiology, and Endodontics* 1998; **85**: 576–80.

5.3

Parotid surgery

JOHN D LANGDON

PRINCIPLES AND JUSTIFICATION

The parotid gland is subject to acute ascending bacterial infection from the oral cavity. Provided the infection is controlled with antibiotics, the gland will usually make a complete functional recovery. In a few cases, the gland becomes chronically infected with recurrent acute flare-ups leading ultimately to sialectasis and duct changes. Chronic infection is particularly common when salivary flow rates are reduced, such as in Sjogren's syndrome or following radiotherapy. In this situation, it is best to remove the superficial lobe of the parotid and to tie off the main duct as far distally as possible. It is not usually necessary to remove the deep lobe, which accounts for only 20 per cent of parotid mass, as this undergoes spontaneous atrophy following superficial lobectomy and duct tie.

Calculi in the parotid duct system are uncommon. The majority impact at the parotid papilla and are readily released by papillary dilatation with lachrymal probes or fine bougies. Failing this, a papillotomy can be performed under local anaesthesia. Calculi in the intraglandular part of the duct are usually located at the junction of the main duct and the first order tributaries, the stone mimicking a stag horn calculus as seen in the renal pelvis (see also Chapter 5.2).

The majority of salivary tumours (75 per cent) are found in the parotid gland. The overwhelming majority present as slow-growing painless masses within the parotid capsule. Of these tumours, 85 per cent will be benign, mostly pleomorphic salivary adenomas. When skin fixation, ulceration or fungation, facial nerve weakness or lymphatic metastasis is present, the tumour is clearly malignant. The abscence of these signs does not exclude malignancy. The majority of malignant parotid tumours are clinically indistinguishable from benign tumours.

PRE-OPERATIVE INVESTIGATIONS

Routine surgical biopsy is not indicated. The majority of intrinsic parotid masses will be pleomorphic adenomas. These tumours are tense and poorly encapsulated. Rupture, either at biopsy or at the time of surgery, leads to widespread spillage of clumps of cells resulting in multiple recurrences which may be very difficult to control. If the tumour remains intrinsic within the parotid at the time of surgery, the exact histological diagnosis is unlikely to influence the definitive surgical procedure. However, if the tumour is obviously malignant and has extended beyond the anatomical boundaries of the parotid, open surgical biopsy is indicated.

Fine needle aspiration biopsy has been widely advocated in the pre-operative diagnosis of parotid masses. Although it is safe, oral pathologists find it difficult to make a definitive diagnosis based on a few aspirated clumps of cells because the architecture of the tumour is lost and many parotid tumours are heterogenous in appearance and the aspirated sample may not be representative. The newer technique of fine needle core biopsy, particularly when performed using ultrasound guidance, offers hope of more accurate diagnosis.

IMAGING

Conventional sialography is the investigation of choice in chronic inflammatory disease, auto-immune disease and duct obstruction. The post-stimulation emptying film is most valuable as it is a good measure of function and will often determine if surgical excision is indicated.

For the imaging of parotid masses, either computed tomography (CT) scanning or magnetic resonance (MR) imaging are equally useful. MR avoids the use of ionizing radiation, but CT is better tolerated by patients. Both techniques give a good anatomical image of the region, but neither can reliably demonstrate the plane of the facial nerve nor distinguish intrinsic malignant tumours from benign.

Ultrasound imaging is indicated in acute parotid swellings as it will reliably demonstrate obstruction and collections of pus. In chronic infection, it will show advanced sialectasis and duct dilatation. It will also characterize calculi if they are calcified. Warthin's tumours are echo poor and show posterior acoustic enhancement whereas pleomorphic adenomas are echogenic.

PAPILLOTOMY

Although readily performed under local anaesthesia, the operation must be performed carefully in order to avoid subsequent stricture formation. A fine metal probe is passed through the papilla into the parotid duct (Figure 5.3.1a). Using the probe as a guide, one blade of a pair of sharp-pointed scissors is inserted into the duct and the wall of the duct is cut open (Figure 5.3.1b). The cut should be extended posteriorly until the point of the scissors enters the dilated part of the duct proximal to the site of obstruction (Figure 5.3.1c). A 6/0 resorbable suture is used to sew the cut edge of the duct lining on to the adjacent mucosa of the cheek (Figure 5.3.1d). This results in the formation of a funnel-like opening of the duct on to the cheek and avoids subsequent stricture formation.

SURGICAL REMOVAL OF PAROTID STONES

Anaesthesia

The operation is performed under general anaesthesia. The patient is positioned supine with moderate neck extension and the head turned away from the operative side. Head up tilt on the table helps to prevent venous congestion and ooze. Some anaesthetists are willing to moderately lower the blood pressure, which reduces arteriolar and capillary bleeding.

The hair in front of the ear is either shaved or gathered into a tuft which can be taped down on to the skin of the cheek. The area is infiltrated with conventional dental local anaesthetic containing 2 per cent lignocaine hydrochloride and 1:80 000 epinephrine (adrenaline). The external auditory meatus is plugged with a small piece of vaseline-impregnated tulle to prevent blood entering the meatus and irritating the drum. The surface markings of the parotid duct are marked on the skin of the face at the start of the operation and can be readily transposed to the surface of the parotid fascia once the flap has been raised. A line is drawn from the lowest point of the alar cartilage to the angle of the mouth. This line is bisected and the midpoint is joined with a straight line to the most posterior point of the tragus. The line is then divided into three equal parts. The middle section corresponds to the position of the parotid duct (Figure 5.3.2).

Incision

The incision starts in the hairline running downwards and backwards to the junction of the pinna and the temple (Figure 5.3.3). The incision then follows the pre-auricular attachment of the pinna skimming across the free edge of the tragus, following the attachment of the lobe posteriorly and then swinging gently down into a neck crease. Alternatively, the incision behind the attachment of the ear lobe may be extended posteriorly into the hairline as with a

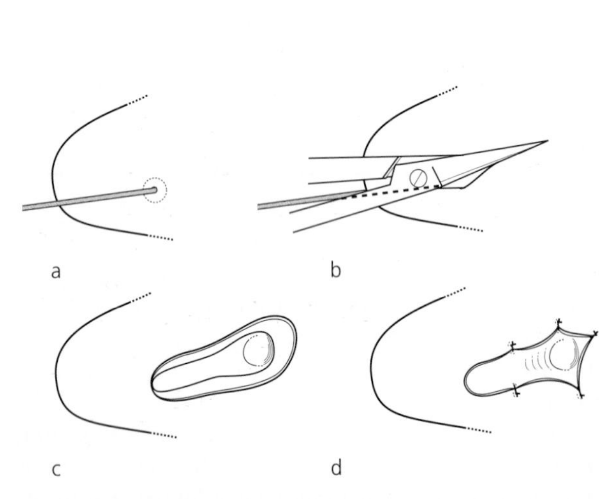

5.3.1 Papillotomy. (a) A probe is passed into the parotid duct. (b) The blade of a sharp-pointed pair of scissors is passed into the lumen and the duct is opened. (c) The duct must be opened as far as the dilated portion proximal to the stricture. (d) The duct lining is tacked on to the adjacent buccal mucosa.

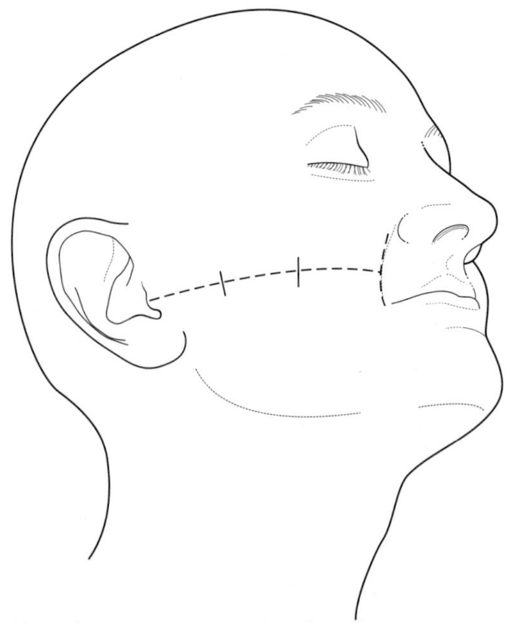

5.3.2 The surface markings of the parotid duct.

face lift incision. This variation results in a less visible scar, but surgical access to the parotid region is slightly more difficult. The incision is made either with a No. 15 blade or preferably with a very fine diathermy needle or ceramic blade. The incision is made through the skin just into the underlying fat.

Exposure of the parotid

The flap is raised either using a scalpel or by blunt dissection with scissors over the surface of the investing layer of the deep cervical fascia which in this region splits to encapsulate the parotid (Figure 5.3.4). In this situation, the dissection can be deep to the superficial musculo-aponeurotic system (SMAS) as this layer will be returned to its anatomical position at the end of the operation. At the superior and anterior margins of the parotid gland, great care must be taken not to damage branches of the facial nerve which in these areas become very superficial. The flap must be raised just beyond the anterior border of the parotid. The flap is held forwards by suturing the flap to the head drapes with mattress sutures.

Identification of the parotid duct

The duct is identified where it emerges from the anterior border of the parotid. The surface marking of the duct is transferred on to the fascia. The fascia is incised along the line of the duct and, by careful blunt dissection, a search is made for the duct which is pinkish-grey and covered with a fine capillary network. The branch of the facial nerve supplying the upper lip runs parallel with the duct either on its surface or a few millimetres superior to the duct. If the duct is not readily identifiable, it is useful to pass a fine IV cannula through the parotid papilla into the duct. This splints the duct and it can be easily palpated within the parotid (Figure 5.3.5).

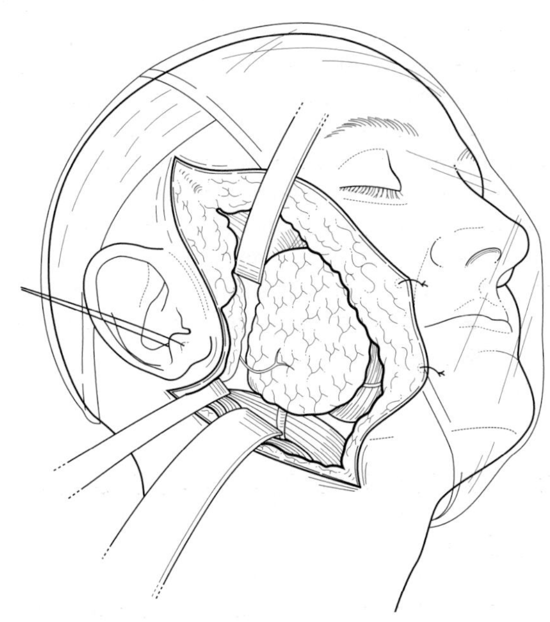

5.3.4 Exposure of the parotid gland and identification of the duct anteriorly.

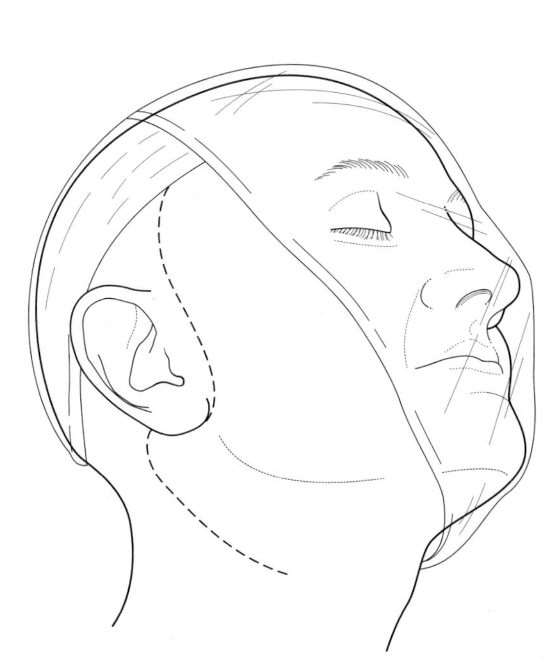

5.3.3 Skin incision for parotid exposure.

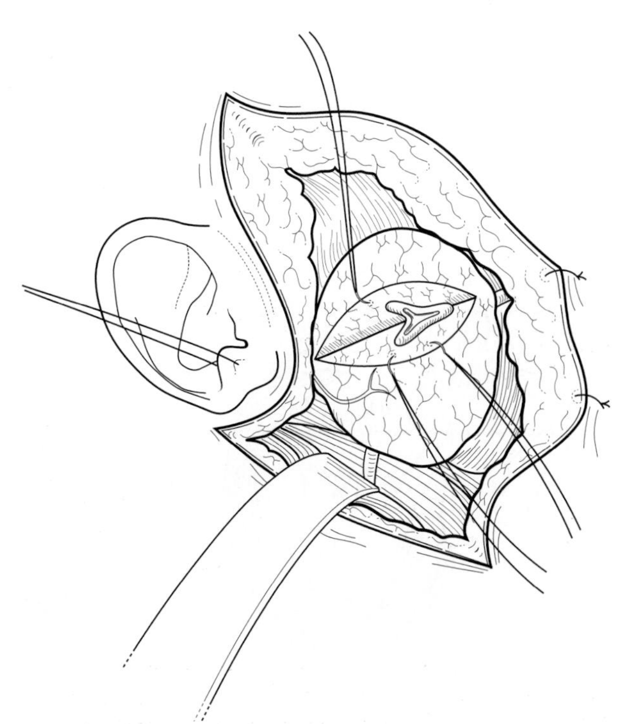

5.3.5 Isolation of the intraglandular parotid duct and identification of the calculus.

Retrieving the stone

Once the duct has been identified at the anterior border of the parotid gland, it is fairly simple and rapid to follow it back into the substance of the gland. With fine scissors, the tissues overlying the duct are progressively separated and divided. Stay sutures through the edges of the dissection are used to retract the parotid. Provided the dissection continues in the plane immediately above the duct and the branch of the facial nerve to the upper lip is kept in sight, there is no risk to other branches which at this point have fanned out (Figure 5.3.6). Any fine intercommunicating branches will be encountered crossing the surface of the duct. Tributaries of the posterior facial vein are carefully clamped, divided and tied.

Once the calculus has been reached, it can be palpated through the duct wall. A longitudinal incision is made in the duct wall and the calculus is carefully teased out of the duct. The duct is then carefully irrigated proximally and distally with sterile saline or water to flush out any associated 'gravel', which if retained acts as a focus for recurrent stone formation.

Closure

No attempt should be made to suture the duct wall as this results in stenosis. The stay sutures are removed and the parotid capsule closed with resorbable sutures. A small vacuum drain is inserted under the skin flap to avoid haematoma formation and the flap is closed in two layers.

Post-operative care

As the parotid gland is likely to be infected proximal to the site of the calculus, antibiotics are administered for 3 days post-operatively. The drain is removed at about 24 hours and the skin sutures are removed at 5 days.

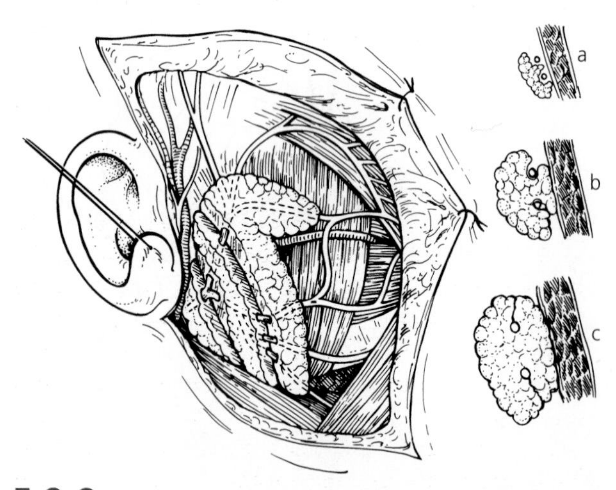

5.3.6 Development of the parotid gland to engulf the facial nerve branches resulting in two lobes united by an isthmus.

Complications

Apart from anaesthesia in the territory of the skin flap, there are few complications. As the fascia forming the capsule of the parotid gland is closed, salivary fistula and Frey's syndrome do not occur. The paraesthesia gradually resolves as the cutaneous sensory fibres regenerate from the periphery. If a face lift incision has been utilized, healing is normally excellent and after six months the scar becomes almost invisible. However, if a conventional lazy-S incision has been used, hypertrophic scarring sometimes occurs in the cervical extension of the incision. For this reason, patients should be carefully followed up for the first six months so that, if hypertrophic changes are seen, the scar can be treated appropriately. Weekly infiltration with triamcinalone acetonide will usually prevent further scarring.

SUPERFICIAL PAROTIDECTOMY

Indications

Treatment of parotid tumours is classically by superficial lobectomy for all tumours within the superficial lobe and total parotidectomy for all tumours within the deep lobe. Such deep lobe tumours should never be approached from the pharyngeal aspect even when they present as lateral pharyngeal masses. The facial nerve, if not macroscopically invaded by malignant tumour, is preserved in all cases.

Surgical anatomy

The key to successful parotid surgery is the observation of two anatomical features (Figure 5.3.6):

1 The parotid gland has two 'lobes' (superficial and deep) united by an isthmus. The parotid gland is not embryologically a bilobed structure, but its developmental relationship to the facial nerve results in the two surgical 'lobes'.
2 The facial nerve and its branches are surrounded by these lobes, invested in loose connective tissue. The facial nerve, except when invaded by tumour, does not enter the substance of the gland.

There are four anatomical landmarks leading to the identification of the trunk of the facial nerve as it leaves the stylomastoid foramen (Figure 5.3.7):

1 The cartilaginous external auditory meatus forms a 'pointer' at its anterior inferior border indicating the direction of the nerve trunk.
2 Just deep to the cartilaginous pointer is a reliable bony landmark formed by the curve of the bony external meatus and its abutment with the mastoid process. This forms a palpable groove leading directly to the stylomastoid foramen. Unfortunately, this groove is

filled with fibrofatty lobules that often mimic the trunk of the facial nerve, which can lie as much as 1 cm deep to this landmark.

3 The anterior superior aspect of the posterior belly of the digastric muscle is inserted just behind the stylomastoid foramen.

4 The styloid process itself can be palpated superficial to the stylomastoid foramen and just superior to it. The nerve is always lateral to this plane and passes obliquely across the styloid process. A branch of the post-auricular artery is usually encountered just lateral to the nerve.

Anaesthesia

The operation is performed under general anaesthesia. The patient is placed supine with a sand bag or pad under the shoulder on the side of the operation. The neck is moderately extended and the head turned to the opposite side. The table is tilted 'head up' to reduce venous engorgement. The anaesthetist should be requested to drop the blood pressure to reduce capillary and arteriolar bleeding. The incision line is infiltrated with lignocaine hydrochloride and 1:80 000 epinephrine (adrenaline).

Incision

The incision starts in the temporal region and passes inferiorly in the pre-auricular crease, crossing the base of the tragus and passing posteriorly behind the lobe of the ear. It then either extends posteriorly into the hairline as in a face lift or alternatively swings down inferiorly from the mastoid to continue in a neck crease. The incision may be made either with a No. 15 blade or with a fine needle diathermy or ceramic blade. The skin flap may be raised in the plane of the preparotid fascia, but if it is raised superficial to the SMAS, this layer can be mobilized as a separate exercise and used to cover the raw surface of the parotid avoiding much of the cosmetic deformity and the incidence of Frey's syndrome (*vide infra*). The flap is held forward by suturing the margins of the flap to the adjacent head drapes (Figures 5.3.3 and 5.3.4).

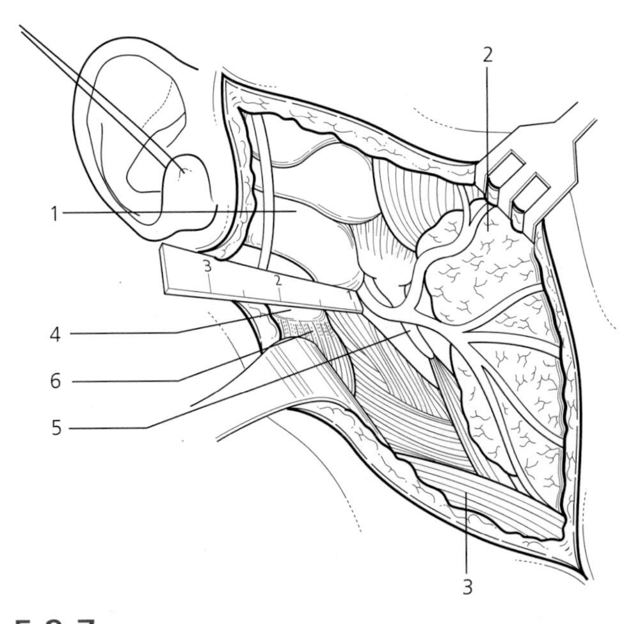

5.3.7 Anatomical landmarks leading to the identification of the trunk of the facial nerve. 1, Cartilagenous external acoustic meatus; 2, parotid gland; 3, sternocleidomastoid muscle; 4, tip of the mastoid process; 5, styloid process; 6, posterior belly of digastric muscle.

Identifying the trunk of the facial nerve

The routine use of a nerve stimulator is not advocated as it may be misleading due to tissue conduction or fatigue of the nerve. The blood-free plane anterior to the cartilaginous meatus is opened up by blunt dissection with scissors. This leads down to the base of the skull just superficial to the styloid process and the stylomastoid foramen and defines the depth of the dissection. This plane is then gently opened up in an inferior direction by blunt dissection until the trunk of the facial nerve is seen. It is usually possible to preserve the posterior branch of the great auricular nerve if care is taken to avoid dissecting too deeply deep to the ear lobe.

With large posterior tumours, this plane may be difficult to open up. In this situation it is helpful to identify the posterior belly of the digastric muscle in the cervical extension of the incision. The anterior border of the sternocleidomastoid muscle is mobilized and retracted inferiorly to display the digastric muscle beneath it. This manoeuvre necessitates sectioning the great auricular nerve. The posterior belly of the digastric muscle is traced upwards and backwards to its insertion on to the mastoid process which lies immediately below the stylomastoid foramen, thus leading the operator to the facial nerve from below (Figure 5.3.8).

Very rarely, most often after recurrent infection with fibrosis or previous radiotherapy, the trunk of the facial nerve cannot be confidently identified. In this situation, the peripheral branches of the nerve at the anterior border of the parotid are identified and traced centrally towards the stylomastoid foramen.

Removal of the superficial lobe

Once the facial nerve trunk has been identified, the superficial lobe of the parotid can be 'exteriorized' by opening up the plane in which the branches of the facial nerve run between the two lobes using blunt dissection. Initially, as it leaves the stylomastoid foramen, the trunk of the facial nerve turns abruptly to become more superficial and also divides into the larger zygomaticofacial trunk and smaller cervicofacial trunk. The five main branches of the nerve are then followed centrifugally through the parotid until the superficial lobe is completely freed. This part of the operation is performed using fine scissors, opened up in the plane of the facial nerve branches, with care always taken to identify the nerve fibre before dividing parotid tissue (Figures 5.3.9, 5.3.10 and 5.3.11). During the lower part of the dissection, branches of the posterior facial vein will be encountered immediately deep to the marginal mandibular branch of the facial nerve. Great care must be taken when vascular clamps are applied to these branches to avoid damaging the facial nerve. If the superficial parotidectomy is being performed for chronic infection, the duct should be tied off as far forward as possible to prevent recurrent ascending infection (Figure 5.3.12).

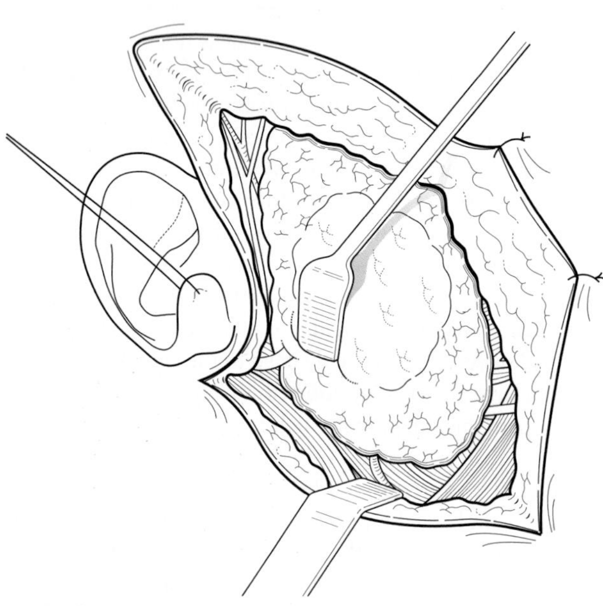

5.3.8 Identification of the facial nerve trunk at the insertion of the digastric muscle on to the mastoid.

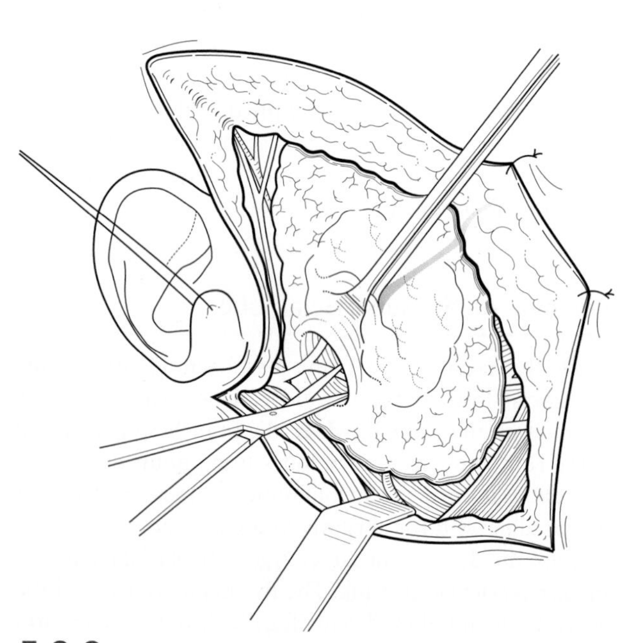

5.3.9 The trunk of the facial nerve turns abruptly to become more superficial.

Partial superficial parotidectomy

When the tumour lies within the tail of the parotid gland, there is no necessity to dissect all the branches of the facial nerve or to remove the entire superficial lobe. Once the main division of the nerve trunk has been identified, only the cervicofacial trunk needs to be followed and the inferior part of the superficial lobe mobilized and ultimately removed.

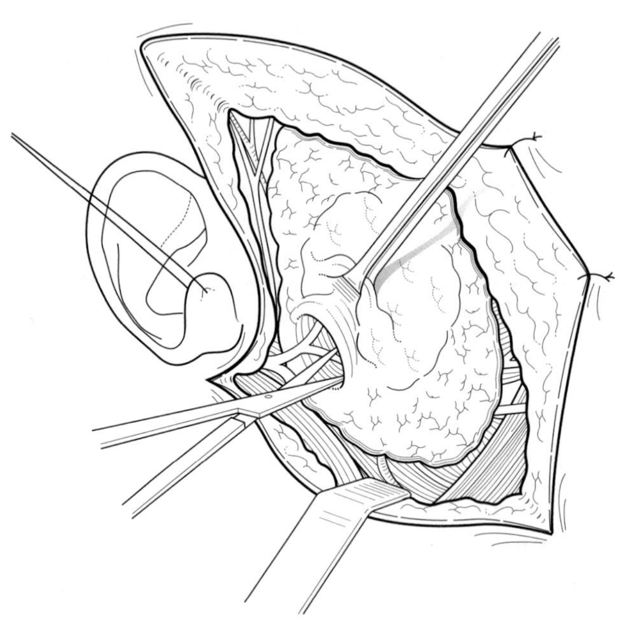

5.3.10 The lobes of the parotid gland are separated using blunt scissors in the plane of the facial nerve.

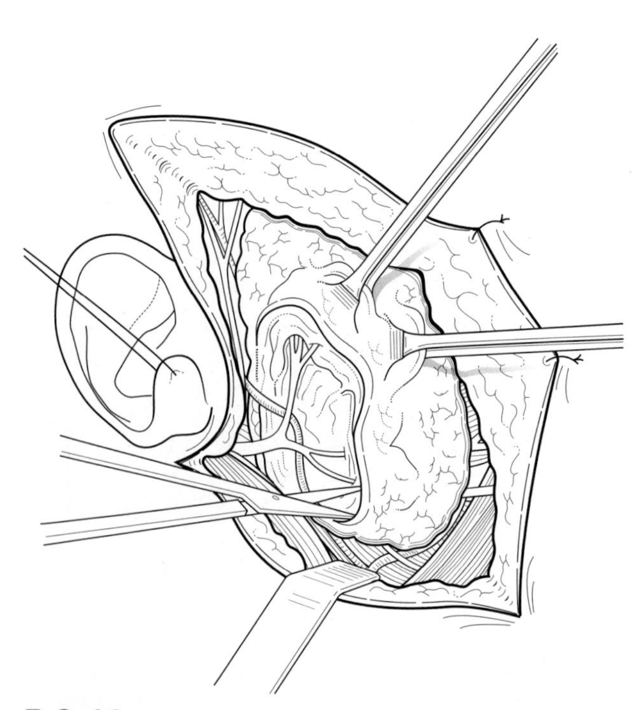

5.3.11 As the dissection progresses, the branches of the facial nerve are exposed to the anterior border of the parotid, 'exteriorizing' the superficial lobe.

Similarly, if the tumour lies above the level of the meatus, only the zygomaticofacial trunk should be dissected and the corresponding part of the superficial lobe removed.

Total parotidectomy

If the tumour lies in the deep lobe of the gland, a conventional superficial parotidectomy is performed as described. Next, the branches of the facial nerve are mobilized and lifted on nylon tapes to enable the deep lobe to be freed around its margins and removed by dropping it downwards (Figure 5.3.13). As this space is wedge-shaped with its apex superiorly, it is almost invariably possible to do this. The deep lobe is covered by a capsule (the deep layer of the deep cervical fascia which splits to envelope the parotid) and is surrounded by the parapharyngeal fat. Thus, it is relatively easy to mobilize the deep lobe by blunt dissection either with scissors or with a finger. Only very rarely is it necessary to perform a mandibulotomy (either vertical subsigmoid or angle) to gain access to the deep lobe (Figure 5.3.14).

Closure

Following removal of the parotid, the blood pressure is returned to normal and the head-up tilt returned to horizontal. All bleeding points must be meticulously controlled. A vacuum drain is inserted under the flap and the wound carefully closed in two layers. A firm pressure dressing will help to prevent any collection of blood or saliva under the flap.

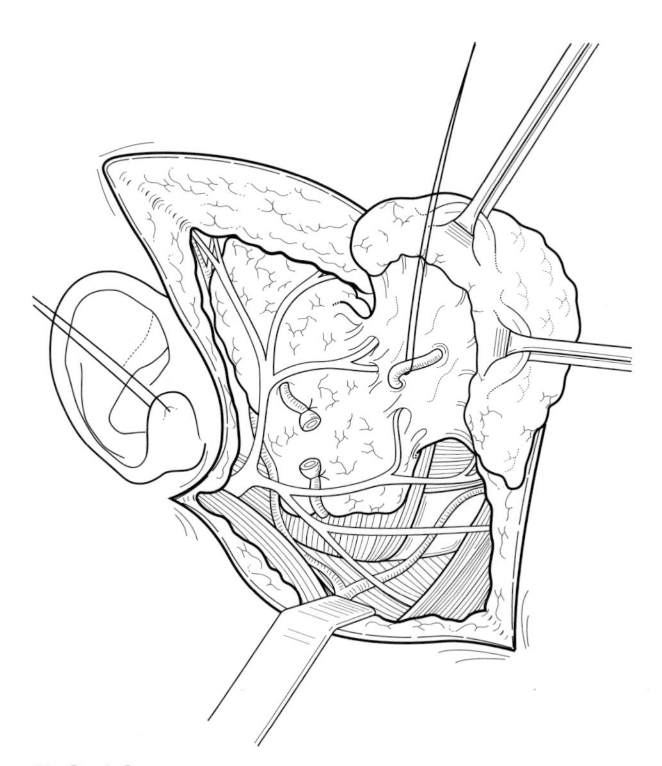

5.3.12 The parotid duct can be identified at the anterior border of the parotid.

Post-operative care

The pressure dressing, if used, is removed at about 12 hours and the vacuum drain at 24 hours if the wound is no longer draining. Skin sutures are removed at 5 days.

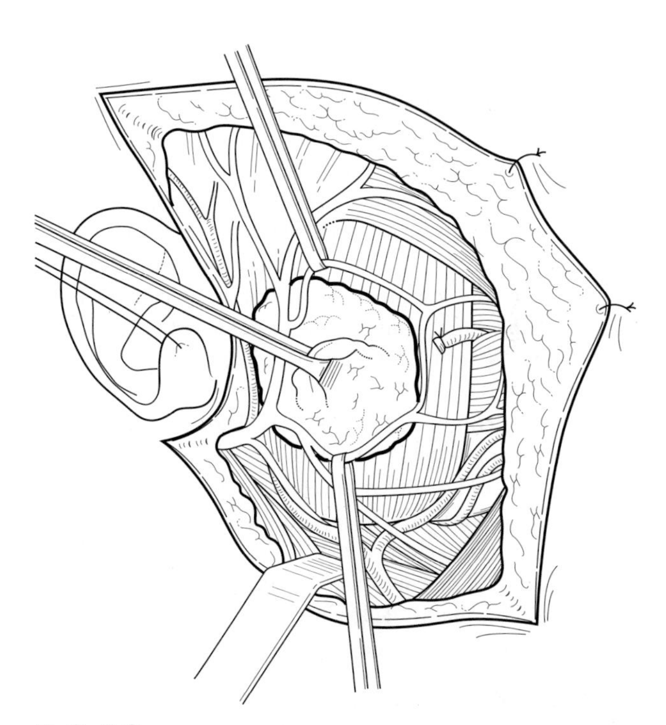

5.3.13 The branches of the facial nerve are gently retracted to give access to the deep lobe of the parotid.

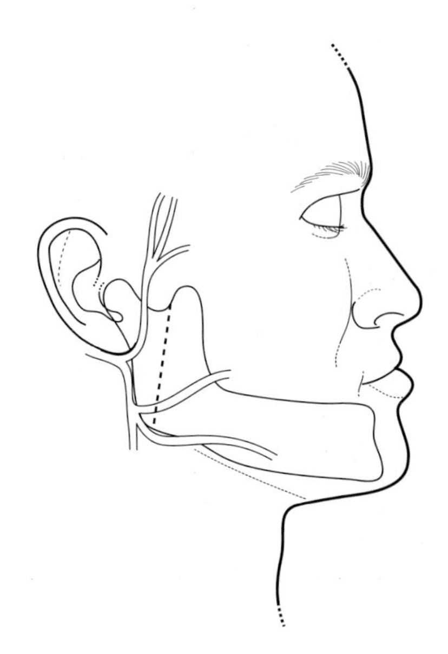

5.3.14 Improved access to the deep lobe can be achieved following a mandibular osteotomy.

Complications

Permanent facial nerve paralysis following superficial or total parotidectomy is very rare, except when branches of the facial nerve have been deliberately sacrificed. When the facial nerve or its branches are sacrificed as a result of macroscopic tumour involvement, an immediate nerve graft may be undertaken using conventional microneural techniques. Temporary weakness due to neuropraxia occurs in approximately 20 per cent of operations, but recovers usually within 6 weeks.

Anaesthesia of the skin flap slowly resolves as the sensory nerves regenerate from the periphery over a four-month period. Anaesthesia of the ear lobe due to sectioning of the great auricular nerve can be troublesome. Recovery can take up to 18 months and may not be complete. Furthermore, a painful amputation neuroma can develop on the stump of the sectioned nerve and requires excision.

Frey's syndrome (gustatory sweating) is a regular sequel to parotidectomy occurring in more than half the patient if looked for carefully. The only effective way to control the symptoms if troublesome is to map out the area of sweating and then infiltrate the subcutaneous plane with botulinum toxin. This will need to be repeated at intervals of four to six months.

Other rare complications, such as sialocoele or salivary fistula, occasionally follow parotidectomy. Both complications are managed conservatively and resolve spontaneously after days or weeks. Very rarely, a parotid fistula persists despite attempts at surgical closure. In this situation, post-operative radiotherapy will destroy any residual functioning glandular tissue and allow the fistula to close.

Parotidectomy can result in a significant cosmetic defect with hollowing of the facial contour behind the mandible. Where this is likely to be a problem, the superficial part of the sternocleidomastoid muscle can be mobilized, transacted inferiorly and swung up to cover the defect (Figure 5.3.15). The flap must be anchored in place with non-absorbable sutures as it tends to pull down into the neck.

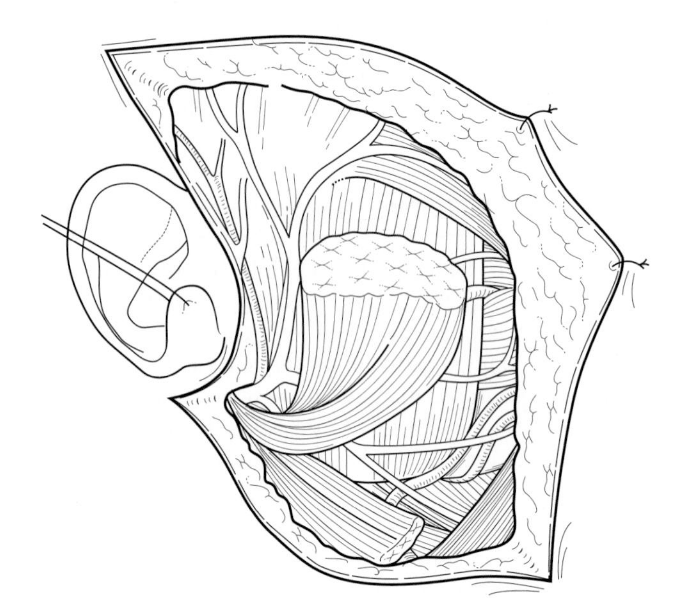

5.3.15 Sternocleidomastoid flap turned up to restore the cosmetic defect following total parotidectomy.

The superficial musculo-aponeurotic system flap

The superficial musculo-aponeurotic system can be elevated as a separate flap if the skin flap is raised in the subcutaneous layer (Figure 5.3.16a). On completion of the parotidectomy, the SMAS layer can be mobilized to cover the defect behind the mandible by suturing its free edge posteriorly to the anterior border of the sternocleidomastoid muscle and periosteum of the zygomatic buttress (Figure 5.3.16b). This will also partially advance the skin flap and excess tissue may need to be trimmed. Great care must be taken when a tumour lies very superficially within the parotid. Mobilizing the SMAS flap can very easily rupture the tumour capsule and it is better to buttonhole the flap overlying the tumour rather than risk rupture. The evidence suggests that not only does the use of the SMAS flap improve the cosmetic result, but it also dramatically reduces the incidence of Frey's syndrome.

Tumour spillage

Spillage of a benign pleomorphic adenoma should not occur if a formal parotidectomy is undertaken. However, there are four circumstances where even with meticulous surgical technique this can happen:

1. Extremely large pleomorphic adenomas occupying the entire superficial lobe making mobilization of the gland difficult. In this circumstance, it may be better to dissect the facial nerve from the periphery.
2. Tumours that are intimately associated with branches of the facial nerve requiring very delicate dissection along the capsule of the tumour to release the nerve.
3. Tumours with lobular extensions extending beneath the mastoid, zygomatic arch or mandible.
4. Some tumours that are abnormally friable with even routine retraction of the superficial lobe resulting in rupture.

If rupture does occur, an extremely careful inspection of the wound must be undertaken and the area thoroughly irrigated. The circumstances should be discussed subsequently at the head and neck cancer multidisciplinary team (MDT) meeting for consideration of prophylactic post-operative radiotherapy to prevent multiple recurrences due to tumour seeding.

ADVANCED MALIGNANT TUMOURS

In a small proportion of cases, the subsequent histopathological diagnosis will be of malignancy. Provided the tumour was intrinsic to the parotid and the tumour was not

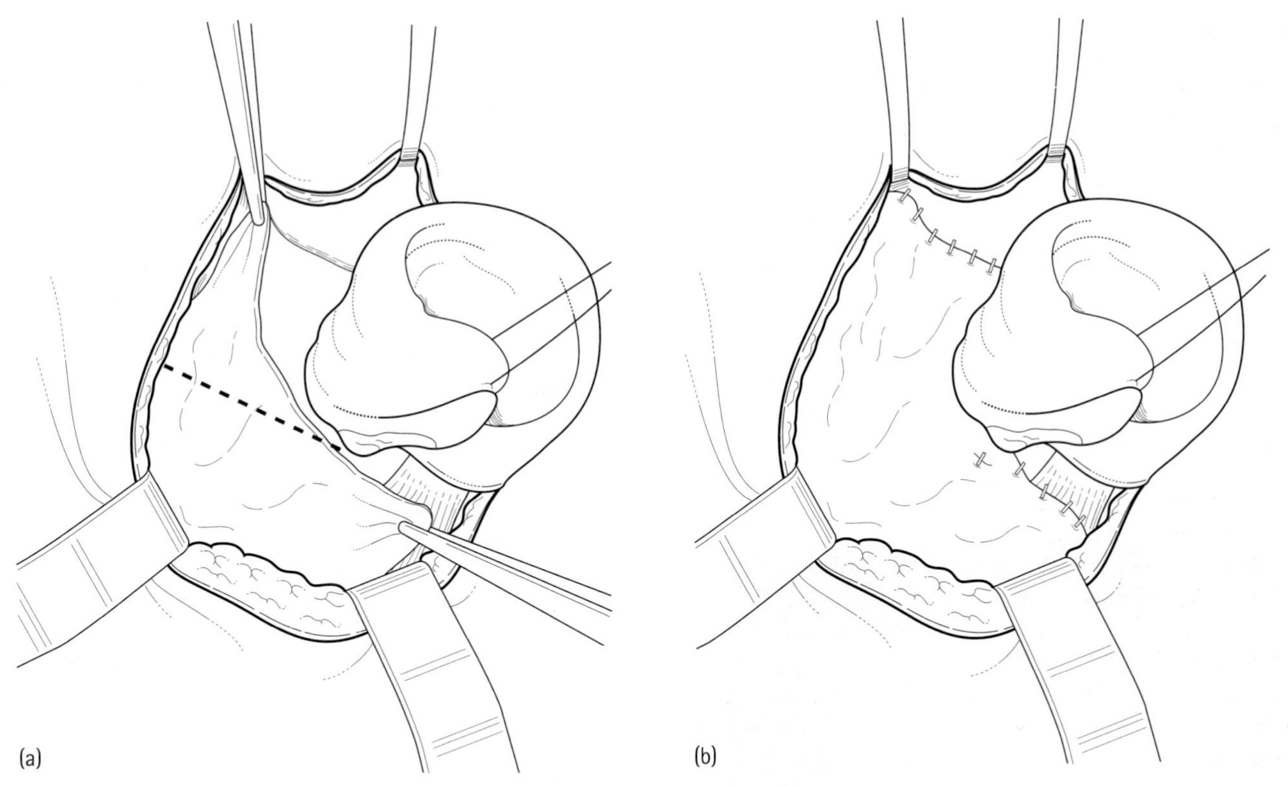

5.3.16 (a) Area of the undermined superficial musculo-aponeurotic system (SMAS) flap. The hinge is indicated by the dotted line. (b) Re-attachment of the SMAS to the zygomatic buttress and sternocleidomastoid muscle.

ruptured during parotidectomy, no other surgery is necessary or desirable. Each case should be discussed at the MDT meeting and considered for post-operative radiotherapy. In general, all high-grade tumours should be treated with radiotherapy and also those where there is any doubt about the margins being clear.

Patients with advanced disease with extension beyond the parotid capsule into adjacent tissues or with lymphatic metastasis should be treated with a sound oncologic technique according to the specific circumstances. Often this will include mandibular resection, clearance of the infratemporal fossa and neck dissection. If any branches of the facial nerve are functioning pre-operatively, they may be preserved as the evidence suggests that radical sacrifice of the facial nerve does not improve survival.

EXTENSIVE DEEP LOBE AND OTHER PARAPHARYNGEAL TUMOURS

On occasion, very extensive deep lobe parotid tumours develop with minimal signs and symptoms. In such circumstances, a transpharyngeal approach using a lower lip split and mandibulotomy with mandibular swing will give adequate access to the deep lobe and infratemporal fossa.

TRANSPHARYNGEAL APPROACH TO THE DEEP LOBE

Although this approach is mostly used for large extraparotid masses, it is occasionally indicated for the exceptional tumour arising in the deep lobe (Figure 5.3.17). After anaesthetic induction, an elective tracheostomy is performed as there can be considerable swelling in the oropharynx post-operatively.

Incision

A skin crease incision is made from the level of the hyoid bone and extended forward towards the chin point. At this point, the incision is continued either around the chin point or vertically in the midline. The decision is dictated according to the local anatomy. In patients with a pronounced chin 'cleft', it is best to use a midline vertical incision and for those with a well-developed chin 'button', it is preferable to incise around this (Figure 5.3.18). The lower lip is split in the midline, but a notch should be incorporated in the incision line at the vermillion border. These helps with the aligning of the vermillion border at skin closure and also acts as a Z-plasty to prevent tethering of the lower lip.

Exposure

After retraction of the sternocleidomastoid muscle posteriorly, the carotid sheath is isolated and traced upwards to the skull base. Vascular slings are placed around the internal and external carotid arteries in case either vessel is ruptured later in the operation and urgent control is required. Often it is sensible to clamp, divide and ligate the external carotid at this stage.

The dissection is then continued forward deep to the submandibular salivary gland. It must be carefully freed from the underlying hyoglossus and mylohyoid muscles, while remaining attached to the lower border of the mandible.

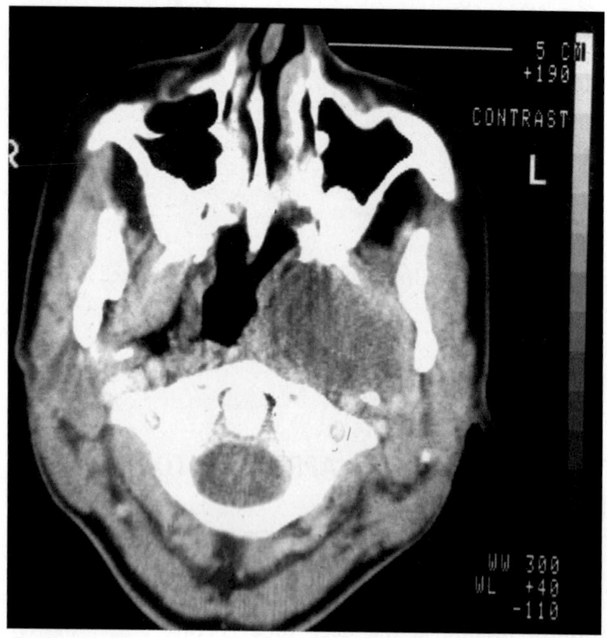

5.3.17 Computed tomography (CT) scan showing an extensive deep lobe tumour excised using a transpharyngeal approach.

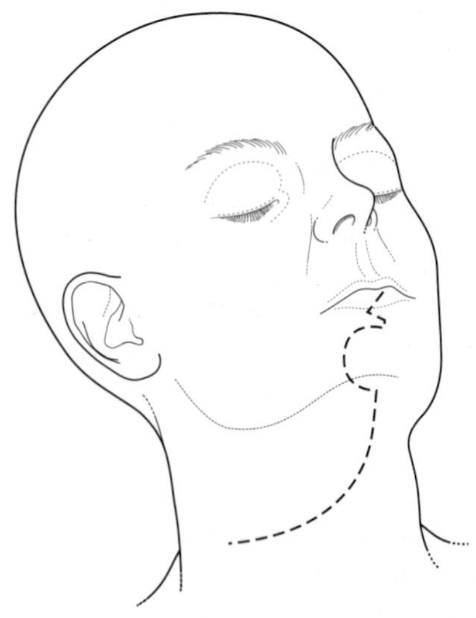

5.3.18 Skin incision for the transpharyngeal approach.

The surgeon should then return to the chin incision and expose the buccal aspect of the mandible from the midline back to the premolar region carefully isolating the mental nerve as it exits the foramen between the premolar roots.

The mandibulotomy is then marked running between the first premolar and canine teeth. Two microplates are then adapted to the buccal aspect of the mandible and the screw holes drilled. The plates are then carefully put aside, care being taken to mark them for position and orientation.

The mandibulotomy cut is then made with a reciprocating saw. Great care must be taken between the two adjacent teeth so as not to damage the roots. It may be wise to cut just through the buccal cortex with a bur and continue the mandibulotomy with a very fine osteotome at this level.

The mandible is then retracted laterally and the mucosal incision extended posteriorly along the floor of the mouth medial to the submandibular duct (Figure 5.3.19). The incision should extend up the anterior pillar of the fauces to the upper pole of the tonsil.

During this stage of the operation, the lingual nerve and the hypoglossal nerve must be identified. The hypoglossal nerve can be readily displaced medially and protected, but it may be difficult to release the lingual nerve sufficiently. In this case, the nerve should be cleanly divided with a blade and the ends tagged, so that an anastamosis can be performed at the end of the operation.

At this stage of the operation, the parapharyngeal space can be opened through the incision and the tumour mobilized and delivered by blunt dissection (Figure 5.3.20).

Closure

Following meticulous haemostasis, a vacuum drain is inserted into the parapharyngeal space. The intraoral

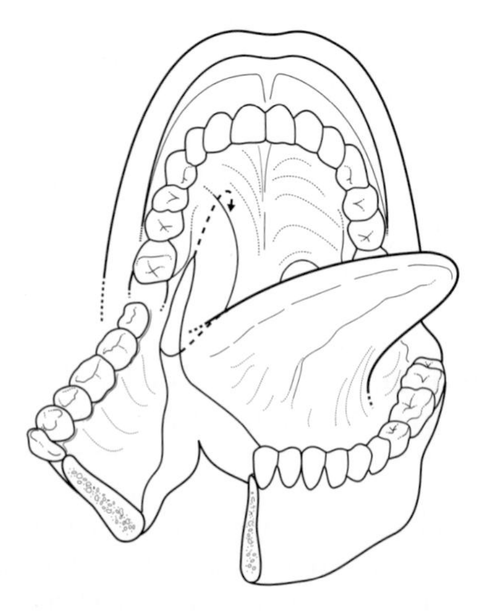

5.3.19 The mandible is divided between the first premolar and canine teeth and retracted laterally.

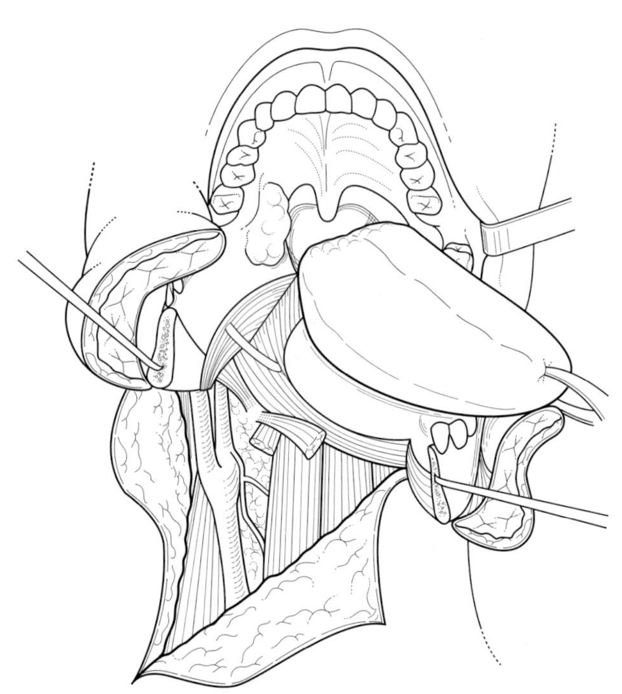

5.3.20 Clearance of the tumour from the infratemporal fossa.

incision is closed in at least two layers with the mucosa being closed with everting mattress sutures as it is important to achieve a watertight closure to prevent the formation of an orocutaneous fistula. At this stage, the lingual nerve should be repaired with microvascular techniques if it has been previously divided. Once the floor of the mouth has been repaired, the previously adapted microplates are screwed into their previously drilled holes and mandibular continuity is restored without any disturbance to the occlusion.

The skin incision is closed in two layers. Great care must be taken with the lip closure. The orbicularis muscle should be repaired with resorbable sutures before commencing a two-layered closure of the skin. It is very important to achieve perfect alignment of the vermillion as failure to achieve this results in a very unsightly scar. The drain is removed usually at 24 hours and the skin sutures at 7 days.

Complications

The greatest risk with this operation is the development of an orocutaneous fistula. Watertight closure of the mucosal incision is vital. Should a fistula develop, it is worth returning the patient to the operating theatre and resuturing the mucosa where it is leaking. If this is done, the drainage through the neck will close spontaneously.

Damage to the teeth adjacent to the mandibulotomy can be prevented by careful technique at the time of the operation. The lingual nerve repair will normally give useful function, but sensation almost never returns completely. The patient should have been warned of this pre-operatively.

Top tips

- Surgical biopsy of an intrinsic parotid tumour carries a severe risk of seeding tumour cells into the adjacent tissues and rarely affects the definitive surgical procedure.
- Although embryologically composed of a single lobe, the parotid gland consists of two surgical lobes separated by the facial nerve which is enclosed in loose connective tissue.
- The trunk of the facial nerve is very constant anatomically. It should be identified before any facial nerve dissection, except when a centripetal approach is to be used. The anatomical landmarks are 100 per cent reliable.
- The great majority of deep lobe tumours may be safely removed without dividing the mandible.
- Preserving the SMAS and re-attaching it at the end of a parotidectomy improves the cosmesis and dramatically reduces the incidence of Frey's syndrome.
- The only reliable way of controlling Frey's syndrome is the subcutaneous infiltration of botulinum toxin into the affected area.

FURTHER READING

Cawson RA, Gleeson MJ, Eveson JW. *Pathology and surgery of the salivary glands.* Oxford: Isis, 1997.

Hobsley M. *A colour atlas of parotidectomy.* London: Wolfe, 1983.

Norman JedeB, McGurk M. *Colour atlas and text of the salivary glands.* London: Mosby-Wolfe, 1995.

Seifert G, Miehlke A, Haubrich J, Chilla R. *Diseases of the salivary glands.* Stuttgart: Georg Thieme Verlag, 1986.

Seward GR. Anatomic surgery for salivary calculi. Part V. Calculi in the extraglandular part of the parotid duct. *Oral Surgery, Oral Medicine, Oral Pathology* 1968; **25**: 810–16.

Seward GR. Anatomic surgery for salivary calculi. Part VI. Calculi in the intraglandular part of the parotid duct. *Oral Surgery, Oral Medicine, Oral Pathology* 1968; **26**: 1–7.

5.4

Extracapsular dissection

MARK MCGURK, LUKE CASCARINI

PRINCIPLES OF JUSTIFICATION

Extracapsular dissection (ECD) is an example of the general move towards minimally invasive procedures. Historically, pleomorphic adenomas in the parotid gland have had a reputation for tumour recurrence. Consequently, an approach was adopted towards superficial or total conservative parotidectomy.

The reputation for pleomorphic ademonas having a propensity to recurrence is largely undeserved. The reason for this is that in the 1930s when the high incidence of recurrence was noticed, these lesions were thought to be hamartomas and not true neoplasms, and they were called 'pathological adenomas'. Consequently, it was acceptable practice to enucleate these lesions after opening the capsule.

It was soon realized that a significant number recurred. In response, a number of surgeons started to develop new techniques to deal with these parotid lumps and subsequently the techniques of superficial and total conservative parotidectomy became the universal standards of care and the incidence of recurrence dropped with this change, so reinforcing the intellectual and scientific bases underpinning these techniques.

In the late 1940s, before the debate had been resolved in favour of conservative parotidectomies, a general surgeon, Alan Nicolson at the Christie Hospital, Manchester, UK was continuing with his own local dissection technique. It was his opinion that the main problem lay with surgical exposure.

By the late 1950s, when the debate was settled in favour of superficial parotidectomy, Nicholson had ten years experience of the extracapsular dissection technique with evidence of very low rates of recurrence. Consequently, he continued with this technique and was followed in turn by his successors and other surgeons both at Guy's Hospital, London and Erlangen, Germany. There are now over 800 reported cases treated by extracapsular dissection, some with a follow up of over 15 years.

In reality, surgeons have been dissecting benign tumours to some extent in an extracapsular plane ever since the conservative parotidectomy technique was conceived.

INDICATION

Extracapsular dissection is suitable for superficial, benign tumours of the parotid gland. It has little or no application in submandibular or intraoral tumours because these tumours sites have a higher propensity towards malignant disease for which extracapsular dissection is inappropriate and the morbidity of the surgery in these sites is not comparable to the parotid gland.

Every effort should be taken to avoid inadvertent extracapsular dissection of a salivary malignancy. This error of patient selection, which has probably delayed general acceptance of the technique of extracapsular dissection, happens extremely rarely with high-grade neoplasms which are easily recognized, but most often with small, low-grade, malignant neoplasms. These small parotid malignancies are challenging as they can be indistinguishable from benign tumours. This is because a small (<1 cm diameter), low-grade neoplasm has not had time to declare itself clinically. It is not attached to local structures and there is the very real risk that it has been misdiagnosed on fine needle aspiration cytology. Therefore, small parotid tumours should be approached with caution and, if ECD is being considered, extra care should be taken to obtain the best possible cytological evidence prior to surgery.

The ideal lesion is a well-defined lump, 2–6 cm in diameter, in the superficial portion of the parotid gland, the circumference of which can be defined by palpation.

PRE-OPERATIVE

Although there is evidence that clinicians can discern benign from malignant tumours in over 90 per cent of cases by clinical examination alone, it is prudent to undertake fine needle aspiration cytology assessment as it is a simple technique that can improve this diagnostic rate even further.

The role of imaging in benign superficial parotid tumours is debatable. However, imaging will confirm that the tumour is indeed superficial and may reveal other hidden neoplasms in the deep lobe or elsewhere.

ANAESTHESIA

Hypotensive anaesthesia is not necessary for extracapsular dissection. If a paralysing agent is used, it should be short acting as it is important that the patient is not paralysed during the surgery.

Aspirin therapy does not need to be stopped prior to surgery, although it may increase the degree of bruising; however, clotting times should be in the normal range to avoid excessive bleeding.

The patient's neck is extended as it makes the parotid gland more prominent; this can be done by placing a small pack beneath the nape of neck. A nasal endotracheal tube is used because an oral endotracheal tube props open the mouth and makes it difficult to draw the mandible forward, which is very important when the tumour is wedged between the ramus of the mandible and the mastoid process.

The patient is supine, the operating surgeon on the same side as the tumour with the head turned away. The drapes are placed to leave the ipsilateral face exposed and, in combination with a nerve monitor, facial twitching is a useful indicator of proximity to the facial nerve. It is important that the surgeon is comfortable, usually sitting with adequate support of the arms. Most surgeons use some degree of magnification for this procedure, such as surgical loupes.

INCISION

A bloodless field is induced by infiltrating the pre-auricular tissues with 20 to 30 ml of 1:200 000 epinephrine solution. This provides a dry surgical field and hydrodissects the subcuticular tissues from the parotid fascia. The solution is injected early in the procedure so it has time to induce adequate vasoconstriction.

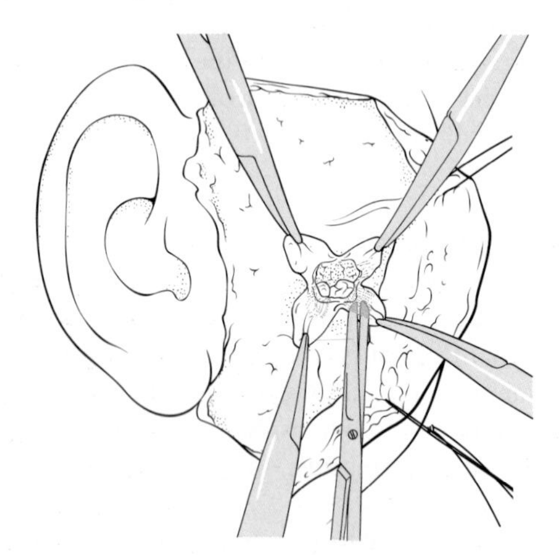

5.4.1 Extracapsular dissection.

The proposed incision should be marked; it is useful to put superficial scratch marks across this incision line in order to relocate the skin flap. The standard approached for extracapsular dissection is a pre-auricular incision with cervical extension. With experience, modifications can be made to this, such as the rhytidectomy incision.

Shaving the patient's hair has no impact on healing. It can be swept back and tied or held in a swimming cap so it is kept out of the surgical field.

DISSECTION

The skin is raised in a plane immediately superficial to the parotid fascia. This is a shining white plane which is easy to identify and follow forward until the fibres of the platysma muscle are encountered. The lobe of the ear should be freed from the mastoid process and both the skin flap and the ear are retracted with sutures. At this point, the greater auricular nerve should be identified as it runs over the sternomastoid muscle and in approximately 60 per cent of cases of ECD it can be preserved.

When the skin flap has been raised, the clinical features of the tumour are checked once more. If the lump is clearly mobile and there are no features of tethering to suggest malignancy, then ECD can proceed.

The periphery of the tumour is marked in ink and a cruciform incision drawn across the surface. It is very important that this incision extends for 1 cm beyond the tumour margin as it improves access to the tumour. Four artery clips are attached to the centre point (Figure 5.4.1) and used to provide upward tension, while the parotid fascia is incised along the cruciform lines.

The key to extracapsular dissection is finding a safe plane in which to dissect. This is done by drawing the normal parotid tissue away from the tumour, revealing loose tissue planes 2 or 3 mm wide of the tumour capsule. It is a common error to pull the tumour away from the parotid tissue, but this may increase the likelihood of capsule rupture and encourages the surgeon to dissect too close to the capsule.

The artery clips are left attached to the parotid fascia and used as retractors. The tumour is moved by gentle finger pressure alone. It cannot be emphasized more strongly that the retraction must be on the normal parotid tissues adjacent to the tumour and never the tumour.

The process of dissection in the safe plane is identical to that used in superficial parotidectomy when exposing the trunk of the facial nerve. The closed end of a pair of blunt-tipped scissors or artery clip is pushed gently through thin sections of parotid tissue and opened with upward pressure to part the parotid tissue. It is imperative that no tissue is cut without seeing the scissors through the fascia. In this way, a facial nerve can be readily identifiable and injury avoided. If a branch of the facial nerve is identified, it is traced forward to reveal its position and if in close contact with the capsule, is dissected from the tumour in the normal way. If it becomes apparent that the tumour arises from the deep lobe of the parotid gland, then the parotid over the tumour is freed by extending the cruciform incision in conjunction with firm traction on the artery clips. Once the full surface of the tumour is exposed, the nerve is freed from the capsule of the tumour. The dissection then continues around the periphery of the lesion until it is free. This situation is no different from that encountered in superficial parotidectomy.

Another important point is to work slowly around the periphery of the tumour. If at any point the dissection becomes difficult, the surgeon should move to another area of the tumour. This should avoid working in the bottom of a hole and as the tissues around the lump are released, areas that previously posed a problem suddenly become accessible and easier to dissect.

It is not necessary to search for the facial nerve. An unseen nerve is a safe nerve. It is the dissection of the nerve that produces facial nerve damage.

Once the tumour is delivered, the parotid fascia is reapproximated along the lines of the cruciform incision and closed with multiple, interrupted, resorbable sutures. This restores the contour of the cheek, eliminates any dead space within the parotid gland, and the closed fascia also minimizes the risk of Frey's syndrome. The skin flaps are closed in two layers over a suction drain and a mastoid-type pressure dressing is applied.

POST-OPERATIVE

The pressure dressing is left *in situ* for 24 hours. It is important that it is taken down the next day in order to check on the perfusion of the helix. The dressing is then reapplied for a further 24 hours. It is often possible to discharge the patient home on the first post-operative day or on occasions on the same day.

COMPLICATIONS

The risk of tumour rupture is the same as superficial parotidectomy (1–3 per cent). If such an event occurs, the operation should be stopped. A clean sucker should be used to suction up any spilt tumour. The sucker should then be discarded. The tear in the tumour capsule should be closed with liga clips or sutures and covered by a small fascial graft, glued into placed to seal the broken capsule. The operation is then recommenced, but the tumour is no longer handled at all. If this routine is followed and contamination is minimal, then the risk of recurrence is about 8 per cent at 15 years. If gross contamination of the wound is encountered, then the risk of recurrence is increased and the possibility of adjuvant radiotherapy should be considered.

HAEMATOMAS

The parotid gland is a vascular structure and the risk of post-operative haematoma is always present. There does not seem to be any greater or lesser risk with ECD. Careful haemostasis should be maintained, patience and a piece of damp gauze are often adequate, bipolar diathermy should be used only carefully and sparingly. A pressure dressing and suction drain will help.

FACIAL NERVE INJURY

With ECD, the incidence of transient facial nerve injury is reduced from 30 to 10 per cent and permanent damage is the same as superficial parotidectomy (1–2 per cent). The management of facial nerve injury applies to all parotid surgery; the transacted nerve should be repaired directly.

PAROTID DUCT INJURY

The transected parotid duct is treated in the same way for any type of parotid surgery. The duct should not be tied in the process of removing a benign parotid tumour unless it is absolutely essential. Tying the parotid duct increases the risk of sialocoele formation.

SIALOCOELE

Pressure dressings are important in reducing the incidence of sialocoeles and also in their management. If it occurs the incision line must not be reopened, it should be managed by regular aspiration and pressure dressings. Initially, it may require aspiration every 2 or 3 days, but gradually the frequency will reduce and the sialocoele will resolve spontaneously over a period of 2–3 weeks. Botulinum toxin-A injections to stop saliva production are seldom required. A combination of external pressure and time is required for the parotid fascia to bind to the overlying skin to eliminate the space for saliva to collect. Once the pressure in the sialocoele is greater than that in the duct system, the saliva will preferentially flow down the duct.

NEUROMA

Traumatic neuromas are more common with superficial parotidectomy than extracapsular dissection. This is due to the limited exposure of the parotid gland with extracapsular dissection; the greater auricular nerve can be avoided in the dissection in over 60 per cent of cases. There are no established ways of avoiding a traumatic neuroma once the nerve is transected. There are numerous anecdotes and suggestions in the literature, but none has proven to be effective.

FREY'S SYNDROME

The incidence of Frey's syndrome is less than 10 per cent following extracapsular dissection because the re-approximated parotid fascia is a barrier to neural infiltration.

Top tips

- Beware the small tumour, it may be low-grade malignancy.
- Have a quick check after the skin flap is raised to ensure that ECD is appropriate.
- Retract the parotid away from the tumour, not the opposite.
- Never use any retractors on the tumour.
- If you can't see through the tissue, don't cut it. If you always do this, you will never cut a nerve.
- Don't work in a hole, if it's getting difficult move around the tumour and comeback later – it will be easier then.
- The Warthin's tumour is an ideal case for surgeons learning this procedure because it is not a true neoplasm, so fear of recurrence is absent and most Warthin's tumours lie in the tail of the parotid, well away from the facial nerve.
- Time spent applying an effective pressure dressing is well spent. It will reduce the likelihood of haematoma and sialocoele formation.
- If during an ECD the surgeon becomes uneasy with the surgical environment, then the operation can be drawn to a close by re-approximating the cruciform incision with three or four simple sutures. The surgeon can revert to the superficial parotidectomy. Nothing is lost in this approach.

THE FACIAL NERVE

The facial nerve is not routinely identified and explored in extracapsular dissection. The act of leaving the nerve untouched within the parotid tissue reduces the incidence of transient nerve injury to 10 per cent or less. Permanent injury is identical to that experienced with superficial parotidectomy at 1–2 per cent.

RECURRENCE

The incidence of recurrent tumour following extracapsular dissection is identical to that for superficial parotidectomy about 1–2 per cent at ten years. The median time to recurrence is seven years.

FURTHER READING

Donovan DT, Conley JJ. 1984. Capsular significance in parotid tumour surgery: Reality and myths in lateral lobectomy. *Laryngoscope* 1984; **94**: 324–9.

Bailey H. Treatment of tumours of the parotid gland with special reference to total parotidectomy. *British Journal of Surgery* 1941; **28**: 337–46.

Janes RM. The treatment of tumours of the salivary gland by radical excision. *Canadian Medical Association Journal* 1940; **43**: 554–9.

McFarland J. Three hundred mixed tumours of the salivary glands, of which sixty-nine recurred. *Surgery, Gynecology and Obstetrics* 1936; **63**: 457–68.

McGurk M, Renehan A (eds). *Controversies in the management of salivary gland disease*. Oxford: Oxford University Press, 2001.

Patey DH, Thackray AC. The treatment of parotid tumours in the light of a pathological study of parotidectomy material. *British Journal of Surgery* 1958; **55**: 447–87.

5.5

Thyroidectomy, cysts of the thyroglossal duct tract and ectopic thyroid

ERIC J DIERKS

THYROIDECTOMY

Thyroidectomy is indicated for a variety of benign, malignant or potentially malignant conditions for which the benefits of removal of part or all of the thyroid gland outweigh the risks of the procedure.

Preparation

It is advisable to perform an assessment of vocal cord mobility prior to thyroid surgery. This is especially important in cases of thyroid malignancy involving the recurrent laryngeal nerve (RLN), where pre-operative documentation of the lack of vocal cord function may enable the surgeon to expeditiously sacrifice the RLN if necessary. Patients requiring revision thyroid surgery, as well as the surgeons that operate these often difficult cases, benefit from pre-operative documentation of vocal cord mobility or the lack thereof. Loupe magnification of 2.5–3.5× is most helpful in dissecting the parathyroid vasculature and recurrent laryngeal nerve.

Pre-operative imaging may be performed by computed tomography (CT) scan or ultrasound examination, although ultrasound may not clearly define the extent of substernal thyroid extension. Radioactive iodine thyroid scan might best be deferred until post-operatively in the patient with thyroid malignancy.

Anaesthesia

General endotracheal anaesthesia utilizing a hypotensive technique is very useful to minimize bleeding. Local anaesthesia is infused into the incision area. A mixture of 1:100 000 epinephrine in saline can be helpful to minimize oozing in the critical dissection adjacent to the RLN. Anaesthesia for the hyperthyroid patient requires high-dose beta-blocker therapy, in addition to other considerations, to avoid thyroid storm.

Positioning

The head and neck are extended either by appropriate positioning on a Mayfield horseshoe headholder or by placing a roll beneath the scapulae (Figure 5.5.1). Women with heavy breasts or obese individuals may require taping the breast area inferiorly to facilitate access to the neck.

Neck incision

The incision extends from the mid-point of the right sternocleidomastoid (SCM) to its counterpoint on the left and is situated roughly one fingerbreadth above the clavicles. If concomitant neck dissection is planned, the thyroidectomy incision is extended superiorly along the posterior border of the SCM to create a bucket-handle or 'hockey-stick' incision (Figures 5.5.2 and 5.5.3). The incision extends through the platysma and a subplatysmal dissection plane is created with scissors or electrocautery to the level of the hyoid superiorly and to the sternum inferiorly. Weitlander or Gelpey

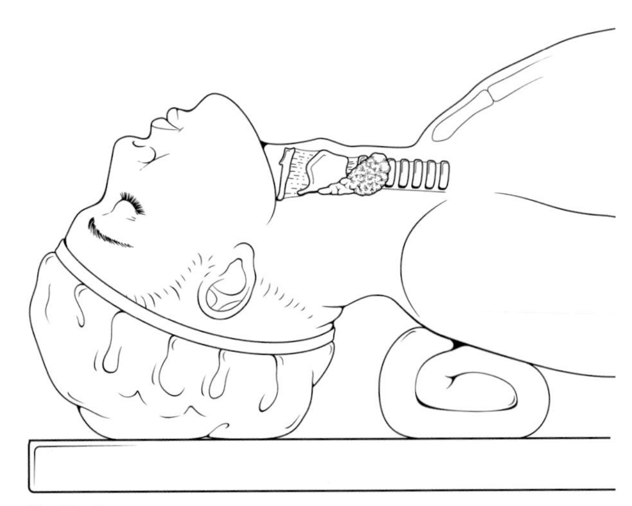

5.5.1 Patient positioning.

retractors are helpful and require occasional repositioning as the dissection continues.

Strap retraction

The superficial layer of the deep cervical fascia is opened vertically in the midline with either electrocautery or sharp dissection along the full vertical extent of the wound (Figure 5.5.4). The strap muscles, principally the sternohyoids, are retracted laterally. The deeper situated sternothyroid muscles are somewhat adherent to the thyroid capsule and can usually be swept off with blunt dissection. Large tumours or goitres may require unilateral or bilateral transverse division of the sternohyoids, as well as the sternothyroids, which can be performed without functional sequelae. If necessary, this is done at or above the cricoid level to preserve innervation of the straps by the ansa cervicalis. If a tumour is adherent to the strap muscles, a portion of the sternothyroid and sternohyoid muscles can be left attached to the mass and excised (Figure 5.5.5).

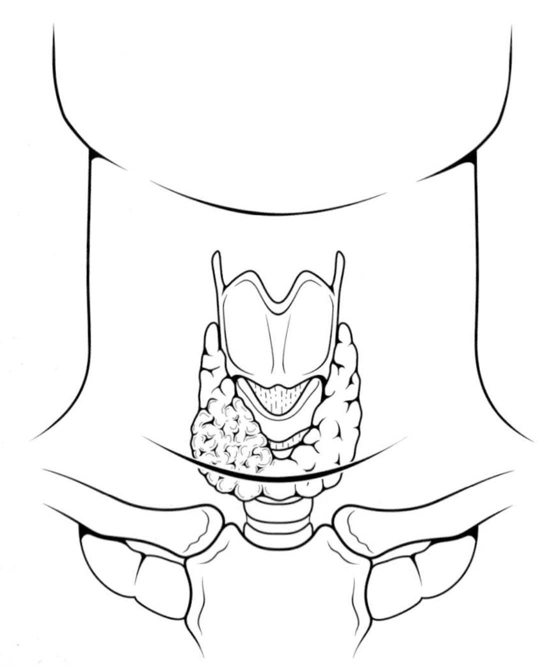

5.5.2 Neck incision.

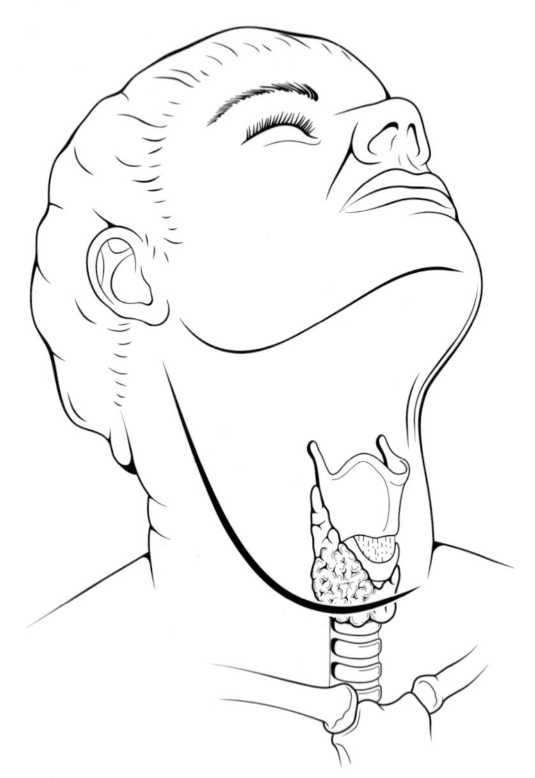

5.5.3 Neck incision with extension for neck dissection.

Inferior pole

The trachea is identified in the midline, beneath the thyroid isthmus. The tracheo-esophageal groove is then entered and the thyroid lobe is retracted laterally and superiorly. A fine dissection instrument or small haemostat is used to spread the tissues to allow careful division of overlying fascial tissues with a No. 12 scalpel blade directed outward and away from the area of the RLN. The right RLN 'recurs' under the subclavian artery, whereas the left RLN 'recurs' under the aortic arch. The course of the RLN relative to the inferior thyroid artery and vein is variable, and retraction of the inferior thyroid artery is helpful in identifying the RLN. On the right side, the RLN courses from inferolateral to superomedial toward the larynx, whereas on the left, its course is straighter and more parallel to the trachea. Bipolar cautery is helpful for haemostasis. Once the RLN has been identified, the overlying inferior thyroid veins can be divided

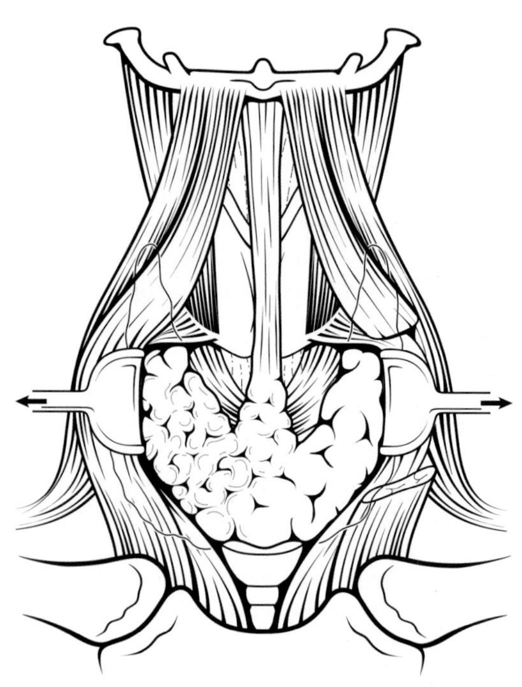

5.5.4 Strap retraction.

between ligatures, surgical clips or radiofrequency coagulation according to the surgeon's preference. The middle thyroid vein is divided as it courses laterally toward the internal jugular vein (Figure 5.5.6).

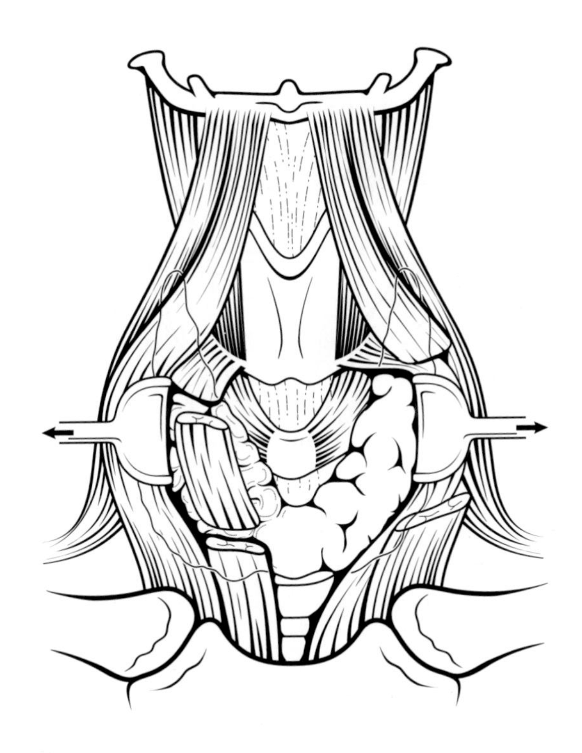

5.5.5 Strap resection with underlying malignancy.

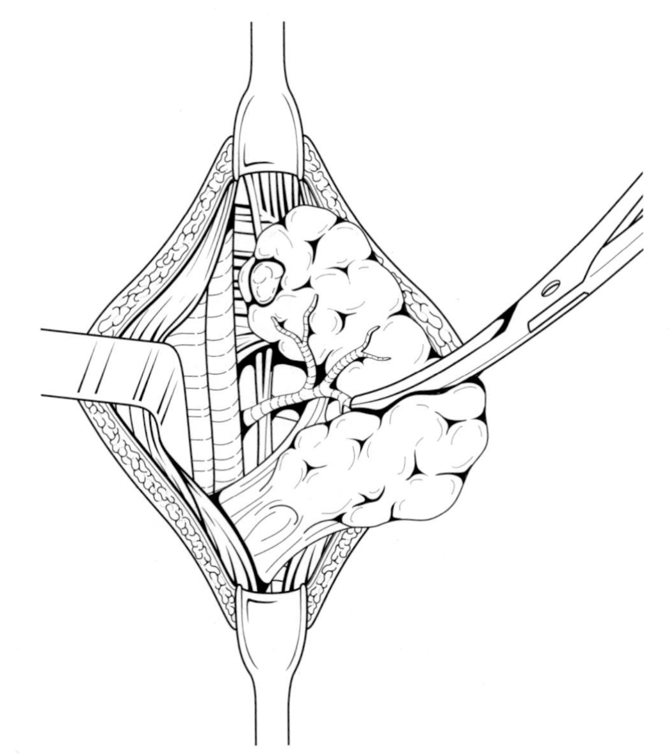

5.5.6 Inferior pole.

The inferior parathyroid is visualized in this area of the dissection. It is caramel brown in colour, generally 5–8 mm in diameter and lies in a more superficial plane than that of the RLN. It is typically seen anteromedial to the RLN in the fatty tissue around the inferior thyroid artery (Figure 5.5.7).

The inferior thyroid artery nourishes the parathyroids and its branches should be divided at the surface of the thyroid capsule only after the inferior parathyroid is identified. If a question arises regarding the parathyroids, frozen section testing of a small piece of the structure can be helpful. On the right side, if the RLN is not identified, further superolateral dissection may identify a non-recurrent RLN, coursing directly from the vagus. This variation is present in about 1 per cent of the population and is associated with a retroesophageal right subclavian artery. Haemostasis must be absolute and ongoing oozing can be minimized with irrigation of a 1:100 000 epinephrine solution. The RLN is traced cephalad as it passes posterior to Berry's suspensory ligament (Figure 5.5.8), posterior to the cricothyroid joint and into its entry zone into the larynx. All tissues overlying the course of the RLN are divided, allowing the thyroid lobe to be gently retracted medially. The RLN may pass through a small portion of thyroid tissue in the area of Berry's ligament.

The assistant must not excessively retract as this can produce a traction injury to the RLN. Branching of the RLN may occur outside the larynx. The superior parathyroid is usually visualized at this stage, lying deep to the course of the RLN, adjacent to the cricoid cartilage. The parathyroid is separated from the thyroid capsule, if necessary, while preserving its attachments to its soft tissue bed. If the parathyroids are not identified, the thyroid capsule should be opened posteriorly and a search conducted for an intracapsular parathyroid. A devascularized parathyroid

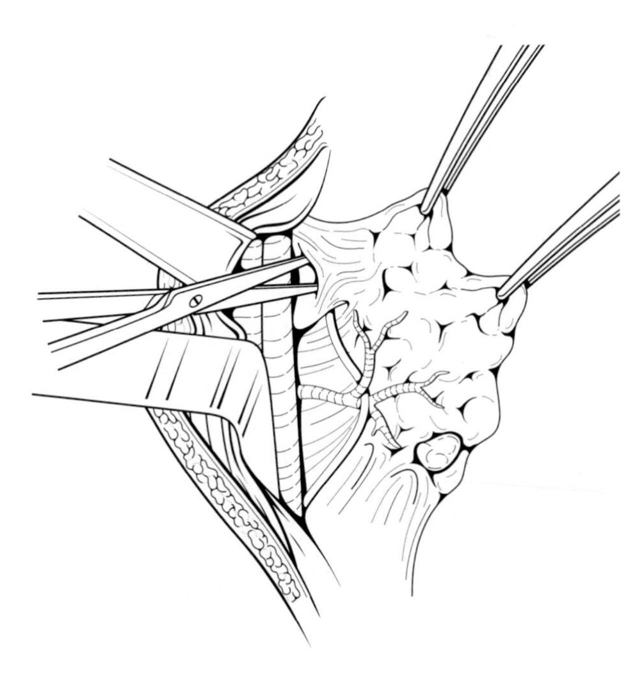

5.5.7 Inferior parathyroid.

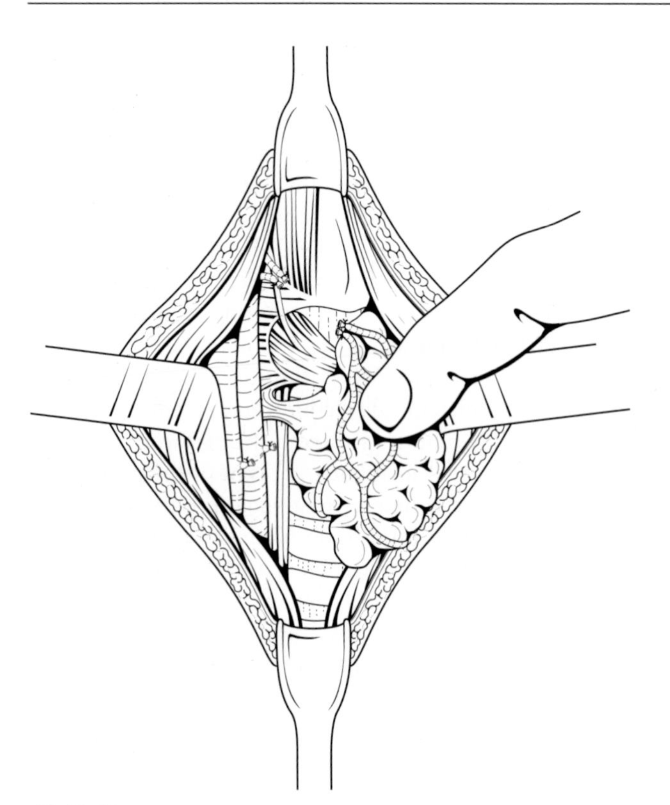

5.5.8 Recurrent laryngeal nerve (RLN) at Berry's ligament.

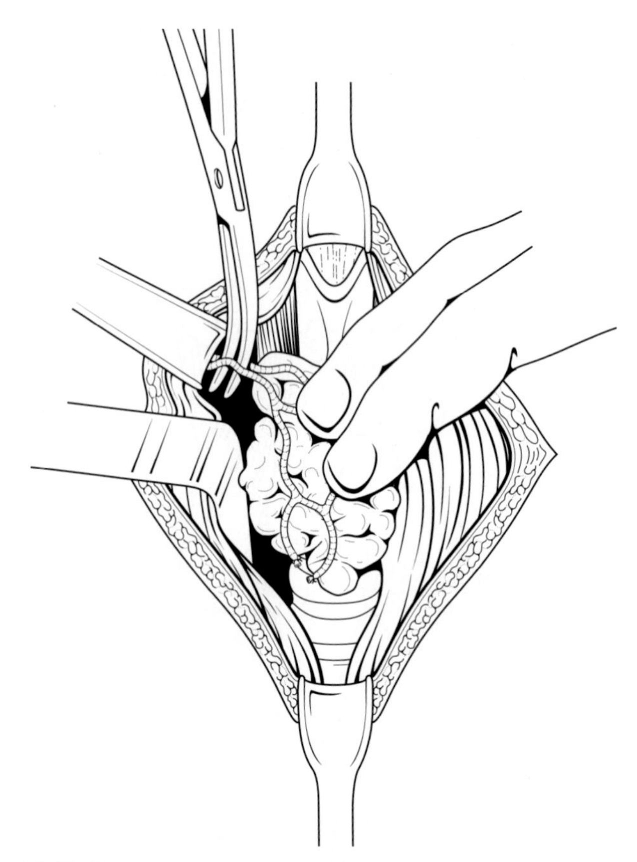

5.5.9 Superior pole.

should be minced and embedded in the SCM, and its site marked with a circle of titanium surgical clips.

Superior pole

The thyroid lobe is retracted inferiorly by the assistant's hand, utilizing a gauze sponge for traction on the capsule. The superior thyroid artery and vein are identified and ligated very close to the tip of the upper pole (Figure 5.5.9). Multiple branches of these vessels are the rule, rather than the exception. The superior laryngeal nerve (SLN) is usually not specifically identified; however, the dissection remains close to the thyroid capsule to avoid damage to this structure. The external branch of the SLN lies in greatest jeopardy, although the internal branch can also be damaged. The superior pole is thus elevated and retracted medially. The RLN is again visualized and further separation of Berry's ligament can be done. With the RLN safely out of the way, the gland is separated from the trachea. If a hemi-thyroidectomy is planned, the isthmus is customarily included up to its junction with the opposite lobe, and the stump suture-ligated. If a total thyroidectomy is planned, the above dissection is repeated on the opposite side.

Closure

Haemostasis is rechecked prior to closure. A suction drain is placed deep to the strap muscles, which are loosely re-approximated in the midline. If horizontal division of the strap muscles has been performed, they are also re-approximated. Platysmal closure is done with a resorbable suture and skin is closed with a resorbable running subcuticular/intradermal suture.

Variations

The safe removal of bulky thyroid tumours or large goitres can be enhanced by preliminary removal of the entire thyroid isthmus, while remaining well away from the RLN (Figure 5.5.10). Removal of a bulky isthmus allows improved medial retraction of each thyroid lobe.

Substernal or retrosternal thyroid tissue can almost always be removed transcervically, despite a worrisome appearance on pre-operative imaging studies. If necessary, a median sternotomy extending to the angle of Lewis, then turning laterally toward the side of the mass and exiting in the second interspace, can be employed for access to the anterior mediastinum. If this approach is necessary, thymic remnants are often encountered and removed prior to removal of anterior mediastinal thyroid tissue (Figure 5.5.11 and 5.5.12).

Subtotal thyroidectomy entails the preservation of an approximately 1.5×2.5-cm strip of thyroid tissue overlying the RLN and tracheo-esophageal groove (Figure 5.5.13).

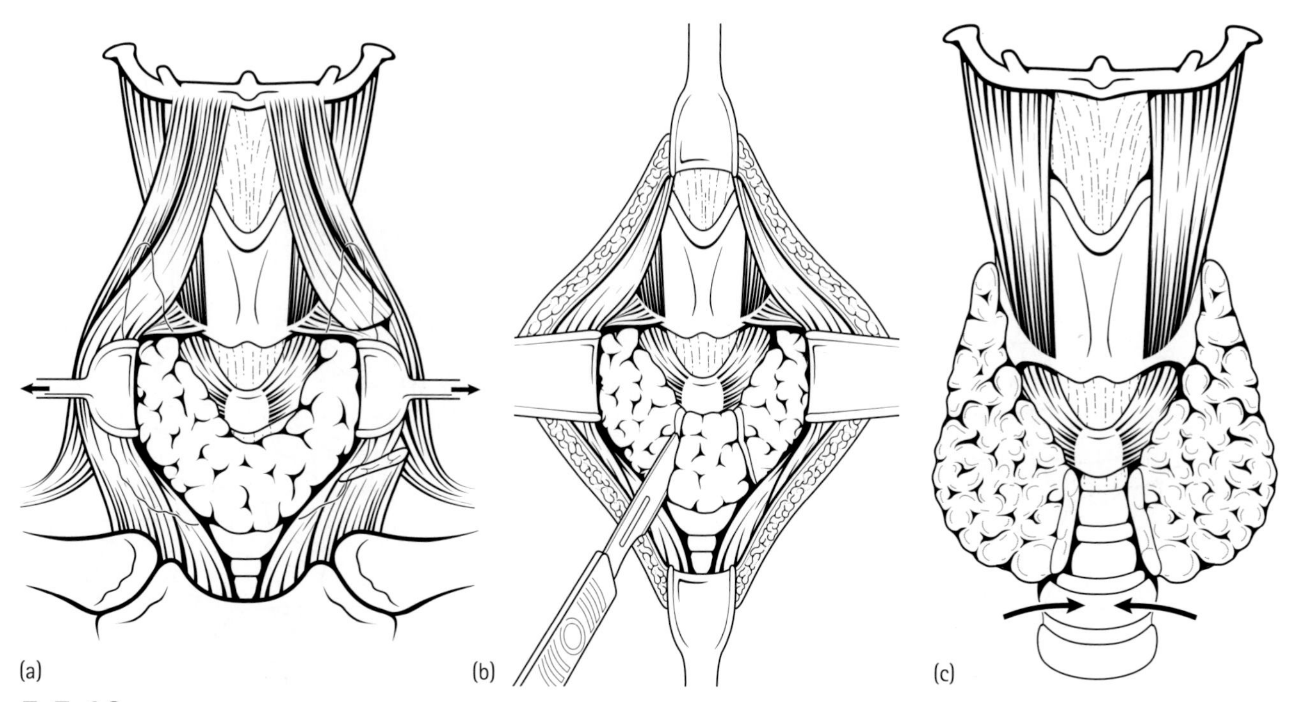

5.5.10 (a) Enlarged isthmus often present with goiter. (b) Resection of enlarged isthmus. (c) Medical retraction of lobes is facilitated by isthmus reaction.

If thyroid hormone replacement therapy is available, subtotal thyroidectomy offers no advantages over total thyroidectomy. In areas where thyroid replacement may not be available to the patient, this operation may be appropriate for hyperthyroidism, multinodular goitre, Grave's disease and Hashimoto's thyroiditis, among others, especially among women of child-bearing age who may not be candidates for radioisotope thyroid ablation therapy.

Concomitant neck dissection may be appropriate for malignant thyroid tumours, but is generally reserved for patients with lymphadenopathy that is palpable or otherwise demonstrable on pre-operative imaging studies. Thyroid malignancy invading the trachea may require a sleeve tracheal resection and anastomosis. Direct involvement of the RLN by thyroid malignancy in a patient with documented paralysis of the ipsilateral vocal cord should be managed by RLN resection without nerve grafting.

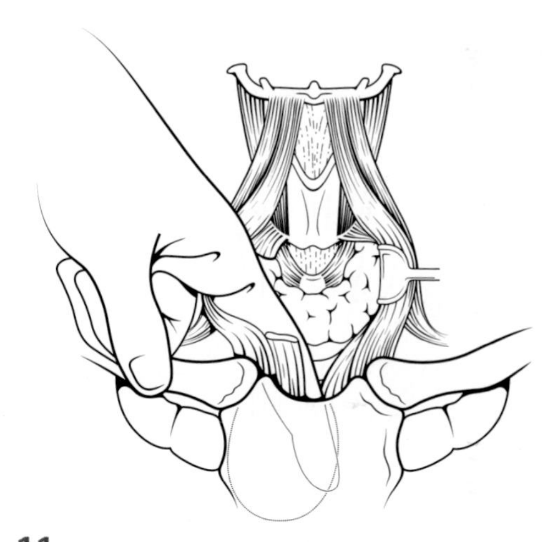

5.5.11 Transcervical removal of substernal thyroid.

Non-recurrent nerve

A non-recurrent right RLN courses directly from the vagus transversely toward the larynx and occurs in approximately 1 per cent of patients.

Complications

HYPOPARATHYROIDISM

A transient post-operative dip in ionized calcium is expected, but sustained hypocalcaemia can produce perioral and stocking-glove hypaesthesia and muscle spasm. Permanent hypoparathyroidism following thyroidectomy occurs with an incidence of approximately 3 per cent.

VOCAL CORD PARALYSIS

Permanent, unplanned RLN injury occurs with an incidence of approximately 2 per cent. Prolonged hoarseness resulting from temporary unilateral RLN injury may require palliative injection of the affected vocal fold with a resorbable material to improve the voice as the RLN recovers. Vocal fold medialization techniques may be required for permanent unilateral vocal cord paralysis. Bilateral vocal cord paralysis produces significant airway compromise and usually requires tracheotomy until one vocal cord regains mobility.

HAEMORRHAGE WITH AIRWAY OBSTRUCTION

A tiny artery feeding an expanding haematoma can exert tremendous pressure on the trachea. A post-operative

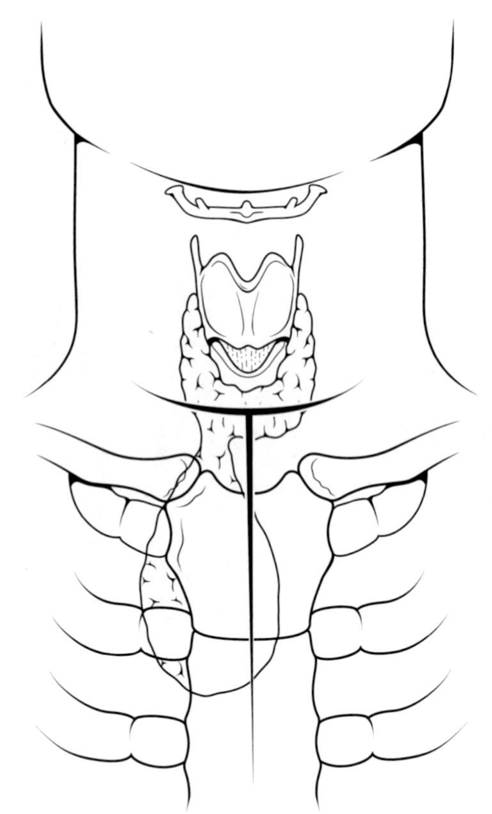

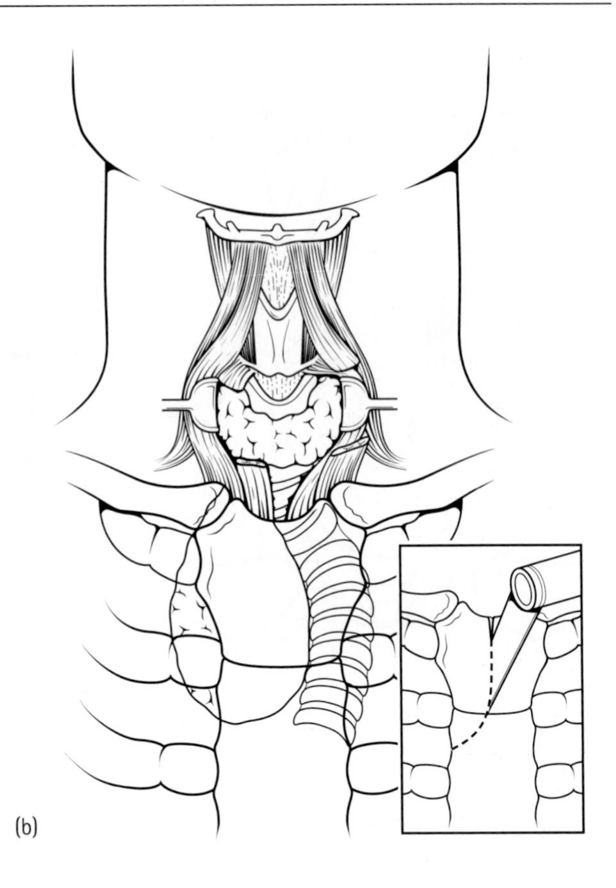

5.5.12 Sternotomy for large substernal goitre or tumour.

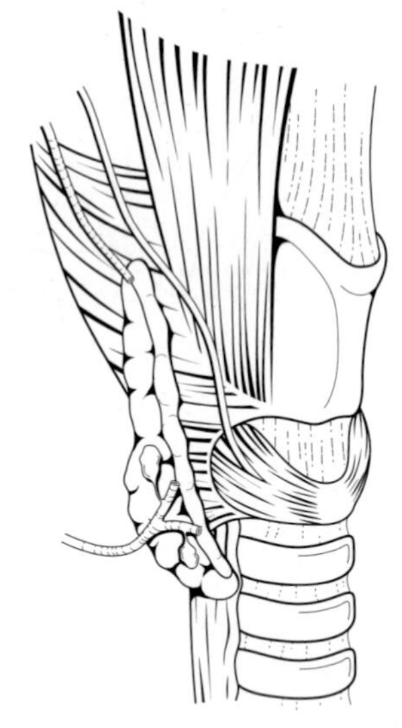

5.5.13 Subtotal thyroidectomy with preservation of strip of residual thyroid.

haematoma with airway obstruction mandates immediate wound opening and haematoma evacuation. This may need to be performed as an emergency at the bedside prior to transport to surgery.

SUBSTERNAL THYROID

Almost all substernal thyroid tissue can be removed transcervically via superior retraction. Preliminary mobilization of the superior poles helps with this retraction. Anticipate difficulty in patients with a history of prior radioactive iodine therapy, especially multiple doses, prior surgery or prior external radiotherapy. Median sternotomy is rarely necessary.

RLN monitoring utilizing a specially designed endotracheal tube, although not routine, may be particularly helpful in cases made difficult by prior surgery or high-dose radioactive iodine therapy.

If anaplastic (undifferentiated) thyroid carcinoma can be identified on pre-operative fine needle aspirate or core biopsy, thyroidectomy is not advised as survival is approximately six months.

CYSTS OF THE THYROGLOSSAL DUCT TRACT

Cysts arising from the thyroglossal tract are generally diagnosed by early adulthood with about two-thirds diagnosed by age 30 and two-thirds occurring as painless masses adjacent to the hyoid bone at or near the midline of the neck. The classic technique of excision including removal of a central portion of the hyoid bone (previously reported by Schlange) plus the excision of the proximal duct was described by Sistrunk in the early twentieth century. This reduced the recurrence rate to about 3 per cent and is still used with minimal modification.

Preparation

A CT scan of the neck generally reveals the site of the thyroglossal duct cyst or cysts. The scan will also demonstrate the presence, or occasional absence, of a thyroid in the normal position. Ultrasound can also be used for pre-operative evaluation of the neck. Pre-operative thyroid scanning is advisable for cases of suspected lingual thyroid, but is optional for routine thyroglossal duct cysts.

Anaesthesia

General endotracheal anaesthesia is employed and epinephrine-containing local anaesthesia is infused into the incision area to help with haemostasis and to provide post-operative analgesia.

Positioning

The head and neck are extended either by appropriate positioning on a Mayfield horseshoe headholder or by placing a transverse roll beneath the scapulae, similar to positioning for a thyroidectomy.

Incision

A transverse incision approximately 3 cm in width is placed over the hyoid bone (Figure 5.5.14). Upper and lower skin and subplatysmal flaps are elevated superiorly half the distance to the mandibular symphysis and inferiorly to the level of the thyroid gland.

Inferior dissection below the hyoid

Only occasionally is a discrete thyroglossal duct clearly visible. A zone of tissue is outlined extending 1.5–2 cm on either side of the midline, extending down to and including the pyramidal lobe of the thyroid, if present. This strip of tissue is dissected away from the strap muscles and off the underling thyroid cartilage and is elevated, maintaining its continuity with the hyoid bone (Figure 5.5.15).

Management of the hyoid bone

The central one-third of the hyoid is removed with the specimen. Electrocautery is used to create an opening over the hyoid, approximately 1.5 cm on either side of the midline (Figure 5.5.16). A right-angled dissector or clamp is insinuated deep to the hyoid and spread, allowing the hyoid to be cut with heavy scissors. The hyoid can be supported during this manoeuvre laterally with an Allis clamp. Care is taken to preserve the continuity of the cyst(s) with the specimen.

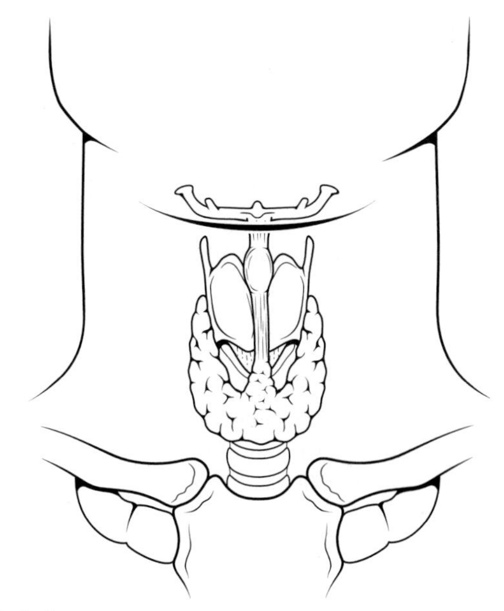

5.5.14 Incision for thyroglossal duct cyst.

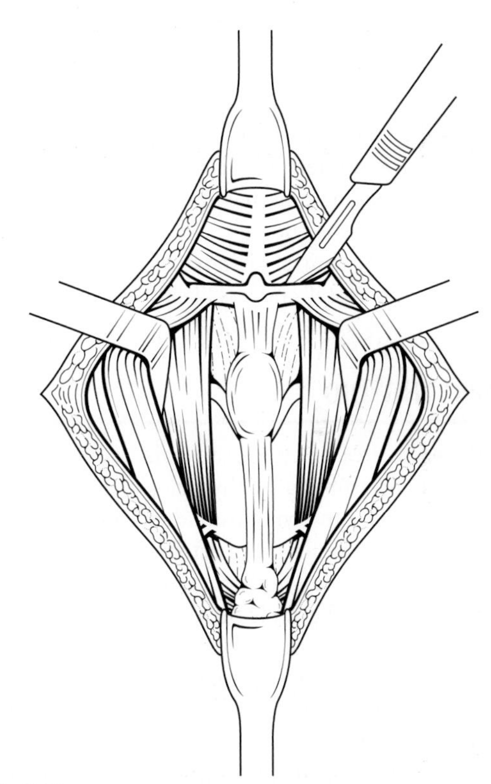

5.5.15 Dissection below the hyoid to the pyramidal lobe, if present.

Management of the tongue

The specimen is gently distracted and dissection of a cone-shaped specimen of tongue musculature is performed as the dissection proceeds the relatively short distance to the area of the foramen caecum (Figure 5.5.17). The tip of the cone should lie just below the foramen caecum at the base of the tongue. A formed thyroglossal duct is rarely seen and an arbitrary zone of tissue is removed. This dissection can be facilitated by placing the finger of the surgeon or assistant into the vallecula to press the base of tongue forward. The specimen is amputated just deep to the surface of the base of the tongue. If a perforation into the pharynx occurs, it is closed in a watertight fashion with a resorbable suture.

Closure

The tongue musculature then closed upon itself with a resorbable suture after haemostasis has been achieved. A 0.25-inch Penrose drain is placed and skin is generally closed with a resorbable subcuticular/intradermal suture.

Complications

Recurrence of a thyroglossal duct cyst occurs at up to 3 per cent after the Sistrunk operation. Re-excision should be preceded by CT scanning and radioactive iodine thyroid scanning. Surgery for recurrent thyroglossal ducts cysts should involve resection of a wide zone of tissue throughout the path of the thryoglossal duct.

Haematoma and infection are rare. Like thyroidectomy, an arterial-fed haematoma has the potential to produce emergent airway obstruction.

Resection of the central cylinder of tongue tissue may damage the hypoglossal, and less likely, the lingual nerves.

ECTOPIC THRYOID

Four potential sites of ectopic thyroid tissue have been described: lingual, sublingual, thyroglossal and laryngotracheal. The path of the thyroglossal duct's descent into the neck is the most common site of ectopic thyroid tissue with lingual thyroid much less likely. Sublingual and laryngotracheal, or intratracheal ectopic thyroid, are exceedingly rare with only ten reported cases of laryngeal thyroglossal tissue. Other sites of ectopic thyroid that are rarely encountered include mediastinal locations, such as the heart and lungs, the pancreas and the adrenal glands.

Congenital lingual thyroid may be associated with otherwise normal descent of the gland into the neck or may be the only functioning thyroid present. In neonates, this can present as an airway-obstructing mass in the base of the tongue. Treatment for this condition is based on the level of symptoms with surgical reduction or excision of the base of tongue mass reserved for relief of obstruction. A significant female predilection has been reported. Lingual thyroid tissue can present in the neonate or infant with swallowing difficulties or partial airway obstruction. Smaller deposits of lingual thyroid tissue may be identified later in life as an incidental finding on routine examination.

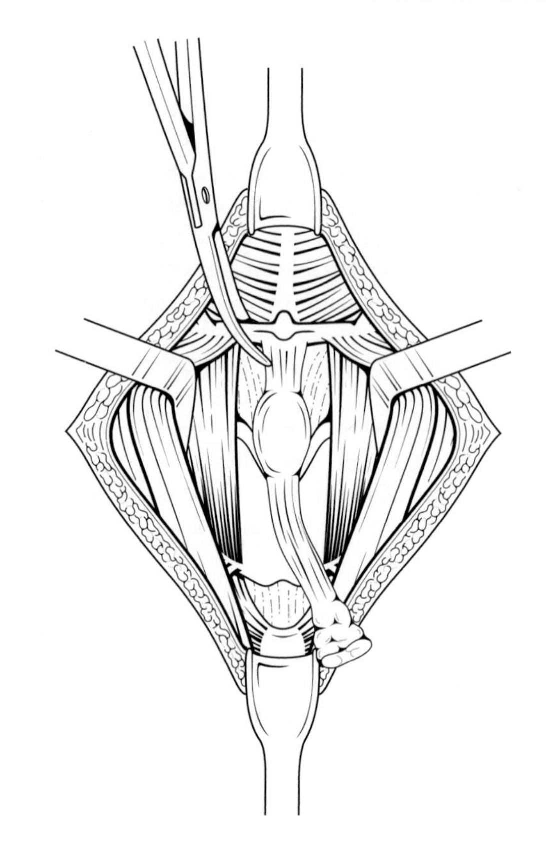

(a)

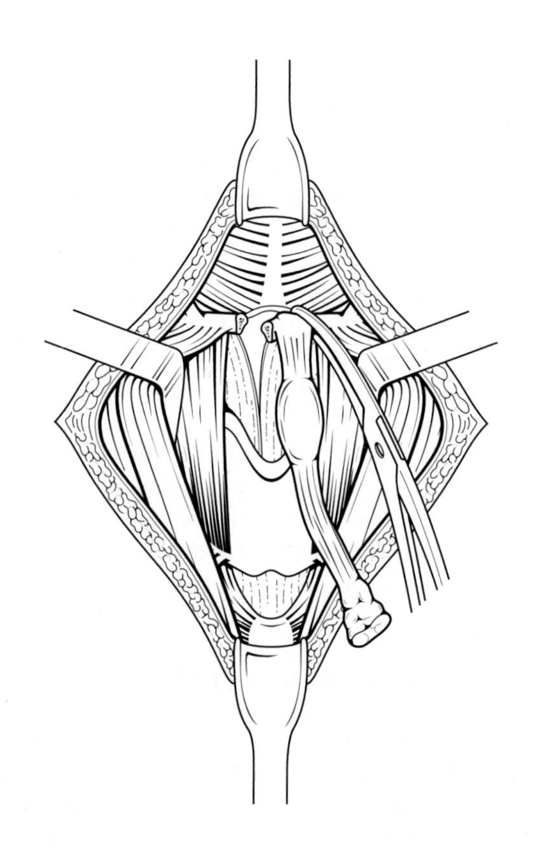

(b)

5.5.16 (a) Division of hyoid with heavy scissors. (b) Central part of hyoid remains attached to tongue following bilateral division.

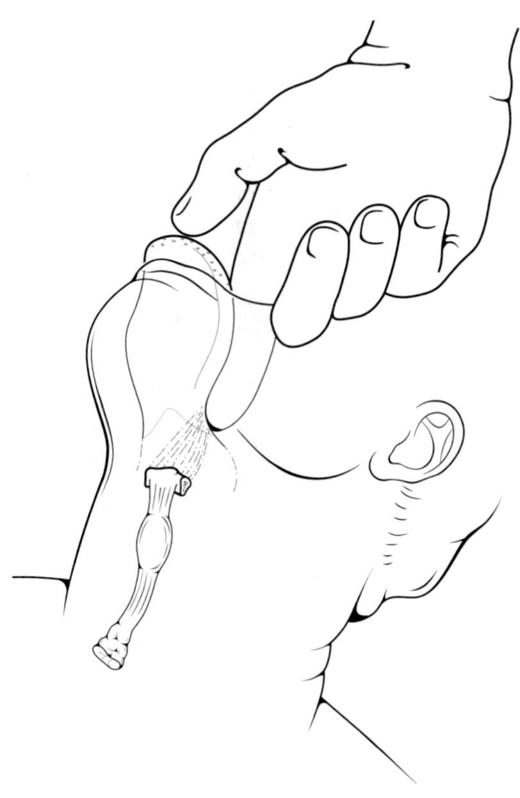

5.5.17 Resection of cone of tongue musculature up to foramen caecum.

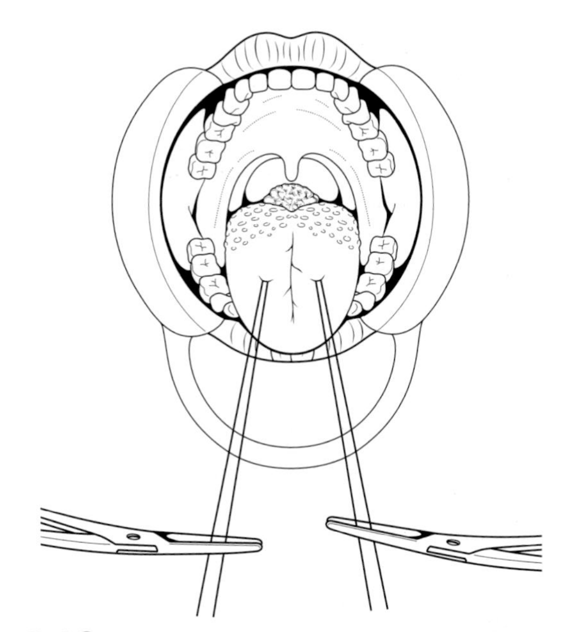

5.5.18 Positioning and retraction for trans-oral resection of lingual thyroid.

Evaluation

Thyroid function testing and thyroid scanning is important for these patients as approximately 70 per cent will have no other functional thyroid tissue. The need for resection of lingual thyroid is based upon symptoms and not on the mere presence of the mass. Thyroid hormone suppression may be all that is needed in asymptomatic cases. Malignancy in lingual thyroid has been reported with follicular carcinoma identified among two of 12 cases in the series of Kamat et al.

Procedure

Lingual thyroid tissue in young children as well as in some older patients can be removed via a transoral route. The patient is placed in a head-back position, similar to that for cleft palate surgery (Figure 5.5.18). A bite block is positioned to maintain an open mouth position and bilateral traction sutures of 2/0 silk are placed on the dorsal surface of the tongue, at the junction of the anterior and posterior halves of the oral tongue. A plastic self-retaining photographic lip retractor can be helpful.

The lingual thyroid is grasped with a DeBakey or other forceps and electrocautery is used to resect the ectopic thyroid tissue. The resulting defect is either closed with resorbable suture or left open to heal by granulation. In 1998, Zitsman *et al.* described the adjunctive use of a cervical incision through which the assistant's finger can press the lingual thyroid into the surgical field.

A midline glossotomy may be necessary to resect lingual thyroid in larger children and adults (Figure 5.5.19). This can be done transorally in edentulous patients and among those that can open the mouth widely. Mandibulotomy may be required to further improve surgical access. Through either approach, the glossotomy is performed with electrocautery through the midline raphe of the tongue,

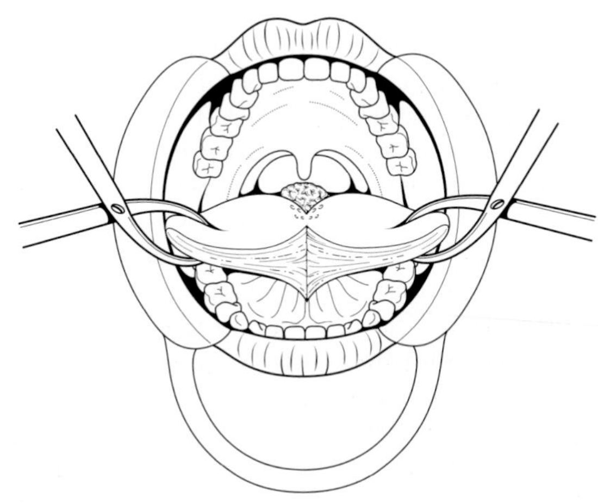

5.5.19 Median glossotomy to approach lingual thyroid.

spreading the tongue halves with a Weitlander retractor or by distracting each hemi-tongue with traction sutures or penetrating towel clips. The ventral surface of the tongue is divided between the sublingual plica, taking care to preserve the submandibular duct orifices. The lingual thyroid is excised and the tongue is closed utilizing multiple deep resorbable sutures, as well as standard mucosal closure. The actual defect of the lingual thyroid may be left to granulate if it cannot be closed.

Complications

- Post-operative haemorrhage usually requires a return to surgery for control.
- Airway obstruction from oedema following median glossotomy.
- Unanticipated permanent hypothyroidism.

Top tips

Thyroidectomy

- It is advisable to document normal vocal cord mobility prior to thyroidectomy, either via direct fibre-optic examination or by indirect mirror laryngoscopy.
- Avoid violation of the thyroid capsule during dissection, as this will encourage bleeding.
- Access to a bulky goitre or large thyroid tumour may require high, horizontal division of the strap muscles.
- Removal of a bulky goitre or tumour can be facilitated by initial removal of the isthmus. This will allow each thyroid lobe to be rotated medially, improving access to the recurrent laryngeal nerve (RLN) area.
- Avoid aggressive medial retraction of the thyroid lobe while dissecting over the RLN to avoid a traction injury on the nerve.
- 0.3 ml of 1:1000 epinephrine mixed into 30 ml saline = 1:100 000 epinephrine solution. Use a tuberculin syringe for greater accuracy and clearly label any container with this mixture to avoid errors. This solution can be a helpful topical vasoconstrictor in the area of the RLN.

Cysts of the thyroglossal duct tract

- An acutely infected thyroglossal duct cyst may require incision and drainage, with definitive removal deferred until the active inflammation has subsided.
- Thyroglossal duct cysts do not always present in the midline and can occasionally occur several centimetres lateral to the classic midline position.
- The dissection of the duct tract to the foramen caecum is rarely an anatomic dissection of a discrete duct. Instead, a cone-shaped excision is performed from the hyoid to the foramen caecum area. The insertion of a finger into the vallecula to press the base of the tongue forward can assist during this dissection.
- In the course of the Sistrunk operation, some surgeons will simply observe the thyroid bed intra-operatively to confirm the presence of a thyroid gland in the neck, to avoid pre-operative thyroid scan or imaging.
- Carcinoma arising from ectopic thyroid tissue is rare, but usually involves papillary adenocarcinoma. The role of subsequent total thyroidectomy is controversial.

Ectopic thryoid

- Intubation of these patients can be difficult and elective tracheotomy or the surgeon's presence at intubation should be considered.
- The excision of a lingual thyroid in a neonate should remove sufficient thyroid tissue to restore the airway. The subsequent administration of thyroid hormone therapy may inhibit regrowth of the lingual mass.
- Median glossotomy closure can be facilitated by the creation of a Z-plasty on the ventral surface of the anterior tongue, to limit scar contracture. Peri-operative steroids or tracheotomy may be necessary to avoid post-operative lingual oedema and airway obstruction.
- Reimplantation of excised lingual thyroid has been reported and may be applicable to those patients who might not have access to life-long thyroid hormone replacement.

FURTHER READING

Al-Samarrai AY, Crankson SJ, Al- Jobori A. Autotransplantation of lingual thyroid into the neck. *British Journal of Surgery* 1988; **75**: 287.

Chanin LR, Greenberg LM. Pediatric airway obstruction due to ectopic thyroid. *Laryngoscope* 1998; **98**: 422–6.

Fish J, Moore RM. Ectopic thyroid tissue and ectopic thyroid carcinoma: A review of the literature and report of a case. *Annals of Surgery* 1963; **157**: 212–18.

Kamat MR, Kulkarni JN, Desai PB, Jussawalla DJ. Lingual thyroid: A review a 12 cases. *British Journal of Surgery* 1979; **63**: 537–9.

Moulton-Barrett R, Crumley R, Jalilie S *et al.* Complications of thyroid surgery. *International Surgery* 1997; **82**: 63–6.

Nicollas R, Mimouni O, Roman S, Triglia JM. Intralaryngeal manifestation of thyroglossal duct cyst. *Otolaryngology – Head and Neck Surgery*, 2007; **137**: 360–61.

Sistrunk WE. The surgical treatment of cysts of the thyroglossal tract, *Annals of Surgery* 1920; **71**: 121.

Sistrunk WE. Techniques of removal of cysts and sinuses of the thyroglossal duct. *Surgery of Gynecology and Obstetrics* 1928; **46**: 109.

Skolnick EM, Newell RC, Rosenthal IM *et al.* Autotransplantation in lingual ectopic of thyroid gland. *Archives of Otolaryngology* 1963; **78**: 187–91.

Zitsman JL, Lala VR, Rao PM. Combined cervical and intraoral approach to lingual thyroid: A case report. *Head and Neck* 1998; **20**: 79–82.

PART 6

VASCULAR LESIONS

6.1

Treatment techniques, surgery and sclerosants

MARIA E PAPADAKI, LEONARD B KABAN

CLASSIFICATION OF VASCULAR ANOMALIES

The management of vascular anomalies has been confusing for surgeons because of an illogical and largely descriptive nomenclature that has reflected a lack of understanding of the biology of these lesions.

In 1982, the clinical behaviour and endothelial cell characteristics of vascular lesions were analyzed and an elegantly simple biologic classification system was proposed (Table 6.1.1). Vascular lesions were categorized as either haemangiomas or vascular malformations. Haemangiomas are tumours of endothelial cell origin and vascular malformations are structural abnormalities of blood vessels lined by normal endothelial cells (Table 6.1.2).

PRINCIPLES OF MANAGEMENT

The first and most crucial step in evaluating a patient with a maxillofacial vascular anomaly is to determine whether the vascular lesion is a tumour or a malformation.

Newborn, infant and childhood photographs are reviewed with the parents to determine if the lesion was present at birth, as well as the rate of growth. History and physical examination provide an accurate diagnosis in more than 90 per cent of patients with vascular lesions.

Magnetic resonance imaging (MRI) with gadolinium is the standard, initial imaging technique for diagnosis of vascular anomalies.

Table 6.1.1 Classification of vascular anomalies.

Tumours	Malformations
Haemangioma (infantile)	**Slow flow:**
Haemangioendothelioma	Capillary (CM)
Angiosarcoma	Lymphatic (LM)
	Venous (VM)
	Combined (CLM, CVM, LVM, CLVM)
	Fast flow:
	Arterial (AM, AVM, AVF)

AVF, arterial venous fistula; CLM, capillary-lymphatic malformation; CVM, capillary venous malformation; LVM, lymphaticovenous malformation; CLVM, capillary lymphaticovenous malformation; AM, arterial malformation; AVM, arteriovenous malformation.

Reproduced with permission from Kaban LB, Mulliken JB. Maxillofacial vascular anomalies. In: Kaban LB, Troulis MJ (eds). *Pediatric Oral and Maxillofacial Surgery*. Philadelphia: WB Saunders, 2004: 260.

INFANTILE HAEMANGIOMA

The standard of management is observation, reassurance of the parents and excision of the fibrofatty tissue and abnormal skin after involution when the child is 8–12 years of age. It may be helpful, in cases where there is family pressure for immediate operation, to show the parents photographs of a similar tumour during proliferation and involution. For psychological reasons, a well-localized, disfiguring haemangioma can be excised, even if not fully involuted, before the child starts school.

Indications for treatment

- Well-localized tumour
- Ulceration
- Bleeding
- Airway obstruction (subglottic)
- Lesion interfering with vision (upper eyelid haemangioma)
- Abnormal skin and fibrofatty tissue
- Distortion of the facial features.

Treatment options

- Intralesional steroids. For haemangiomas less than 2 cm in diameter, serial intralesional steroid injections

Table 6.1.2 Clinical characteristics of vascular anomalies.

	Haemangioma	Vascular malformations
Initial presentation	Usually not present at birth[a]	Present at birth May not be obvious
Growth	Rapid proliferation in the first 4 weeks of life. Proliferating phase may last until 12 months	Grow proportionately with the patient
Involution	Slow regression at 12 months to 12 years (involuting phase)	No regression Persist throughout life
Hue	Superficial: bright red Deep: bluish or no discolouration Involuting phase: the skin becomes pale, particularly in the centre of the lesion Involuted phase: (after 12 years) normal skin is restored in 50% of children. The remainder have some laxity, discolouration, scarring, telangiectasias or a residual fibrofatty mass	Capillary: pink to red Venous: bluish Lymphatic: colorless **Macrocystic**: transilluminate **Microcystic**: irregular surfaces, clear or dark haemorrhagic bullae and vesicles (salmon eggs) AVM: pink or no skin discoloration
Palpation	Firm or rubbery Non-compressible Cannot be emptied of blood with compression No pulsations Involuting phase: softer on palpation	Capillary: flat Venous: soft, compressible, refill rapidly Lymphatic: soft AVM: firm, warm and pulsatile
Intraosseous location	No[b]	Yes
Secondary bone involvement	Bony distortion[c]	35% involve the bone directly Slow-flow: bone overgrowth High flow: bone destruction

[a]A pale spot or telangiectatic or macular stained area may be present at birth at the site where the haemangioma will proliferate.
[b]The intra-osseous lesions called haemangiomas in the oral surgical literature are most commonly low flow venous malformations. However, primary vascular tumours, such as haemangioendothelioma, haemangiopericytoma and angiosarcoma do occur in bone.
[c]For example, depression of the outer cortex, nasal deviation, orbital enlargement and minor hypertrophy of the maxilla or mandible are occasionally noted in the presence of, or after involution of, a large cutaneous facial haemangioma.

(3–5 mg/kg triamcinolone) are performed through a 25-gauge needle. Usually, three to five injections at 6–8-week intervals are required to accelerate involution (Figure 6.1.1). Intralesional injections can be used for upper eyelid haemangiomas with caution.

- Systemic corticosteroids (for destructive, function-impairing or life-threatening lesions). Prednisolone, at a dosage of 2–3 mg/kg per day, is administered once a day for 2 weeks. If there is a response, the drug is continued and slowly tapered and withdrawn at about 10–11 months of age. Haemangiomas in the involuting phase do not respond to steroids.
- Interferon alpha-2a or -2b or vincristine (in cases unresponsive to corticosteroids). Interferon is administered daily, at a dosage of 3 million units/m^2 subcutaneously. Transient side effects of interferon therapy include fever and a flu-like syndrome at the start of treatment (most patients), neutropenia, skin necrosis and skin rash. Interferon can adversely affect the central nervous system in infants, producing spastic diplegia. This is potentially reversible upon cessation of therapy; careful clinical observation is required during treatment.
- Surgical excision (Figure 6.1.2). In 2002, the strategy of circular excision and purse-string closure for haemangiomas was introduced.
- Staged resection is often necessary for labial haemangiomas because they cause distortion in three dimensions. The mass is debulked by excising involved mucosal and submucosal tissue, usually in a transverse axis. Excision at the vermilion–cutaneous junction should be delayed, and vertical incisions on the skin should be avoided.

Complications

- Ulceration is common for infantile haemangiomas, especially for those on the lip. These ulcerated areas should be treated by frequent cleaning and application of topical antibiotic ointment. Occasionally, debridement is required, followed by dressing changes. If the ulcer fails to heal with local measures, treatment with steroids is indicated.
- Bleeding can usually be controlled by local pressure. Embolization is rarely used for uncontrollable bleeding from deep, extensive haemangiomas.

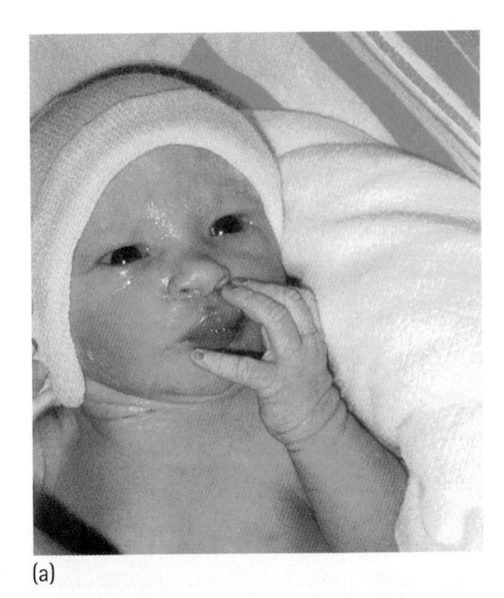
(a)

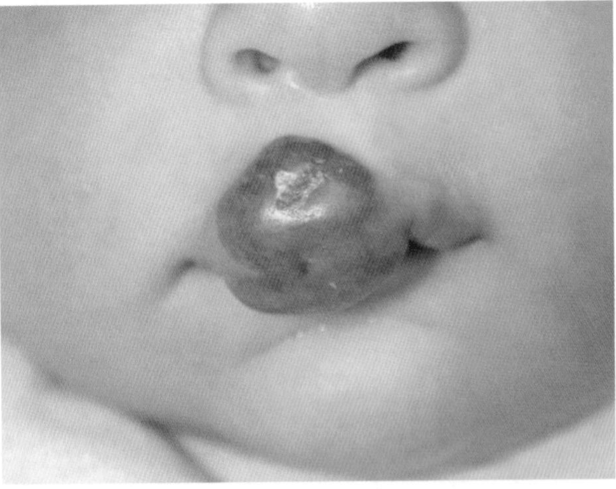
(b)

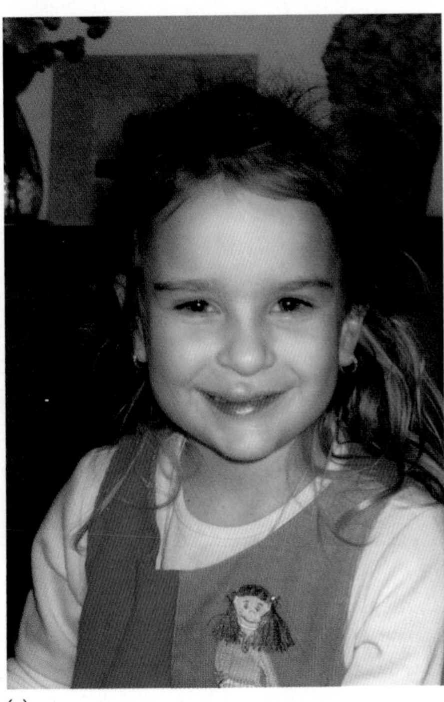
(c)

6.1.1 Infantile haemangioma. (a) A newborn infant with normal facial appearance, except for a small discoloration at the lower end of the philtral column. (b) At four months of age, the lesion shows rapid growth (proliferative-phase haemangioma) and superficial ulceration. (c) Frontal photograph at six years of age after three intralesional triamcinolone injections and excision at the involuting phase. Reproduced with permission from Kaban LB, Mulliken JB. Maxillofacial vascular anomalies. In: Kaban LB, Troulis MJ (eds). *Pediatric Oral and Maxillofacial Surgery.* Philadelphia: WB Saunders, 2004: 263.

- Steroid therapy may cause temporary growth retardation and decreased appetite.
- Large cutaneous haemangiomas can cause life-threatening congestive heart failure and anaemia.
- Thrombocytopenia due to platelet entrapment in large haemangiomas may cause bleeding. This is managed with steroid therapy. Platelet transfusions are not beneficial.

VASCULAR MALFORMATIONS

The first step in the care of a patient with a vascular malformation is to determine whether it is a slow- or fast-flow lesion. Complete resection is not possible in most cases, hence the possibility of uncontrollable bleeding during operation and the likelihood of recurrence. Occasionally, a well-localized, low-flow venous malformation of the jaw can be resected.

When slow-flow malformations without direct intraosseous involvement cause secondary bony distortion, orthodontic treatment and orthognathic surgical procedures can be carried out safely, without fear of excessive bleeding. Fast-flow lesions usually produce bony destruction and extractions or orthognathic surgery are prohibitively dangerous. In combined vascular anomalies, management is based on the characteristics of the predominant, deeper malformation.

Indications for treatment

- Increasing size and swelling
- Pain
- Bleeding
- Infection
- Macroglossia, dysarthria, dysphagia
- Feeding difficulties
- Bone distortion and malocclusion
- Airway obstruction.

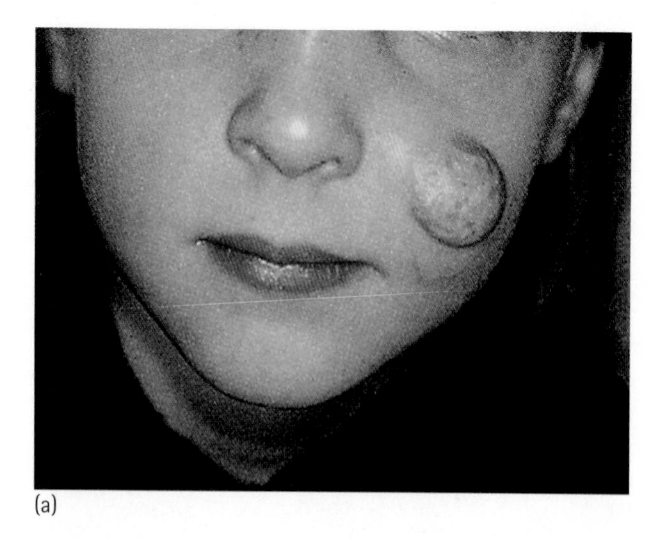

(a)

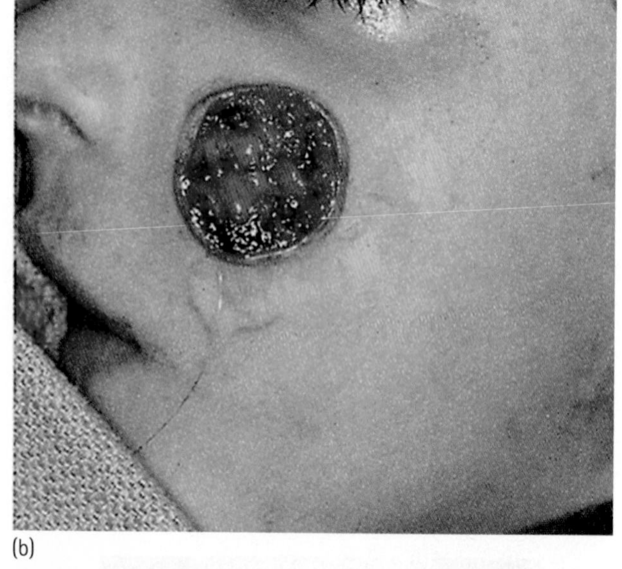

(b)

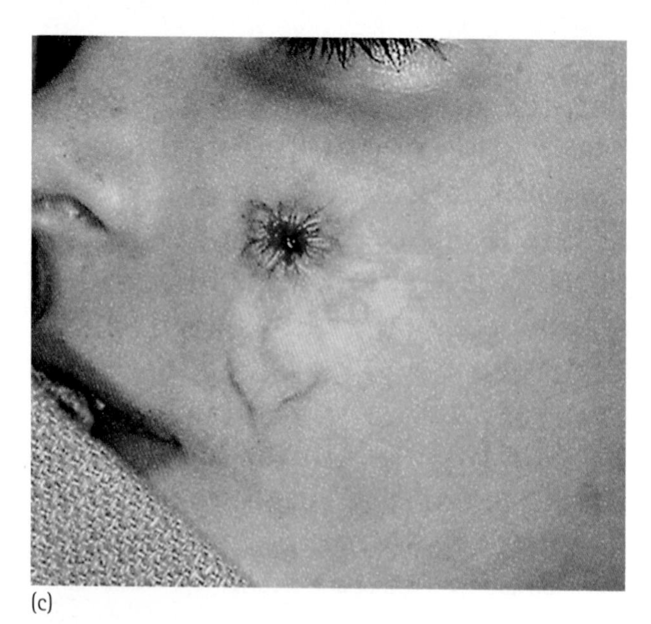

(c)

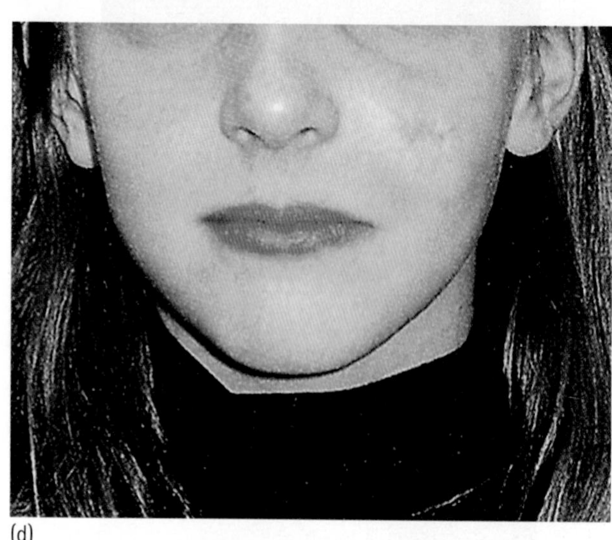

(d)

6.1.2 Circular excision of a haemangioma. (a) Involuting-phase haemangioma of the left cheek. A circular or ovoid incision is planned to include all the altered skin. In the proliferating phase, this includes damaged and ulcerated skin. In the involuted phase (as in this case), it includes atrophic skin and fibrofatty residuum. Minimal subcutaneous undermining is required. (b) A running, intradermal purse-string suture (4-0, 5-0 polydioxanone) is placed along the wound edge. (c) The suture is tightened to gather the edges and appose the wound margin. A gauze wick is placed if a small opening remains. The wound is covered with an absorbent dressing. Alternatively, the edges may be closed with percutaneous sutures in the axis of relaxed skin tension. (d) After several months of healing and remodelling, a decision is made to accept a small circular scar or to revise it. Clinical appearance of the patient three years post-operatively. Reproduced with permission from Kaban LB, Mulliken JB. Maxillofacial vascular anomalies. In: Kaban LB, Troulis MJ (eds). *Pediatric Oral and Maxillofacial Surgery*. Philadelphia: WB Saunders, 2004: 282 and Mulliken JB, Rogers GF, Marler JJ. *Plastic and Reconstructive Surgery* 2002; **109**: 1544–54.

CAPILLARY MALFORMATION

Capillary malformations rarely present major problems for the oral and maxillofacial surgeon (Figure 6.1.3).

Treatment options

- Pulsed dye laser: 50–75 per cent of patients will notice improvement with between two and 20 sequential treatments (lightening of the lesion) under general anaesthesia or local anaesthetic cream.
- Excision and skin grafts or flaps: These are occasionally used in cases where the skin is very thick and the laser is unsuccessful.
- Orthognathic surgery for skeletal overgrowth and distortion. Maxillary and mandibular overgrowth is common when there is staining of the overlying facial skin and mucosal lining. In patients with dentoalveolar distortion, osteotomies can be performed without fear of excessive bleeding (Figure 6.1.3).

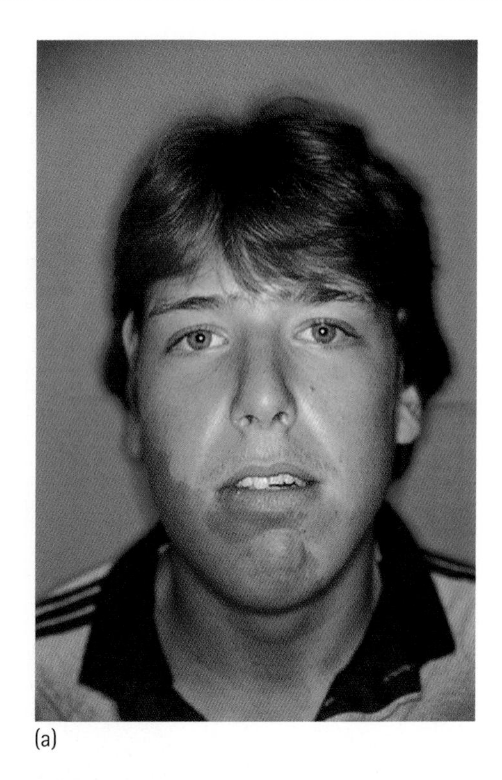

(a)

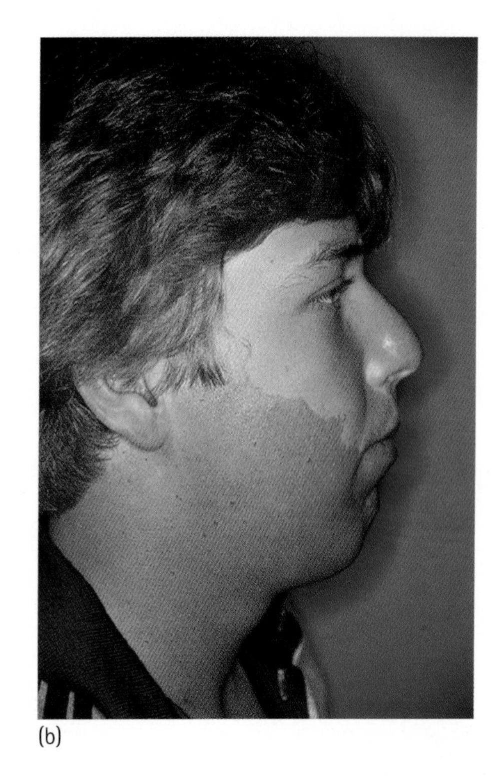

(b)

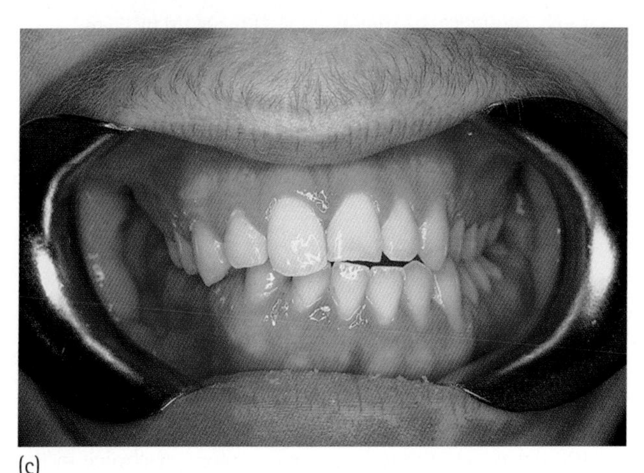

(c)

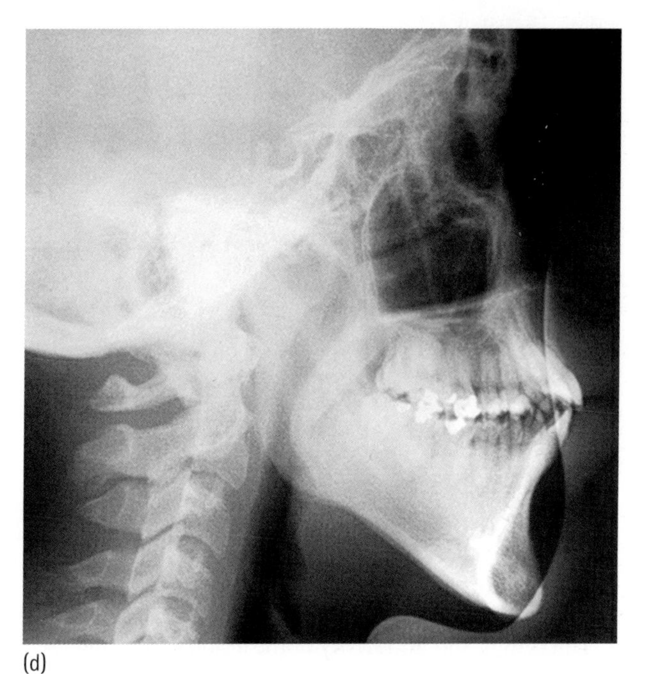

(d)

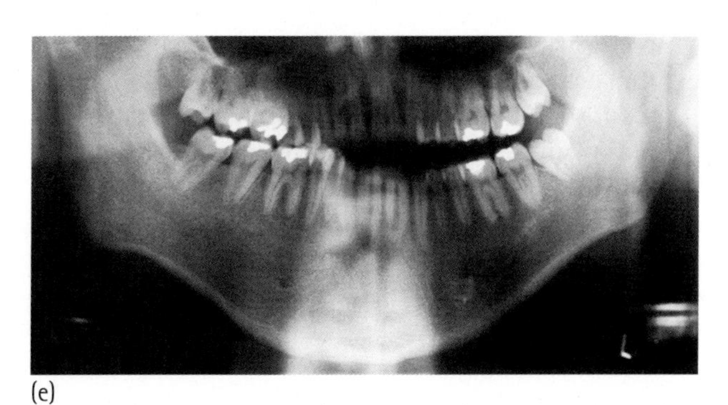

(e)

6.1.3 (a) Frontal and (b) lateral photograph of a teenage boy with dermal capillary malformation in the distribution of the second and third division of the trigeminal nerve. This is also a frequent finding in the Sturge–Weber syndrome that includes a capillary malformation of the V1 or V1–V2 trigeminal areas, choroidal vascular ectasia and leptomeningeal vascular anomalies. (c) Intraoral photograph shows malocclusion due to excessive vertical growth of the maxillary alveolus on the right side. (d) Lateral cephalogram demonstrates the long lower face height and bimaxillary dentoalveolar protrusion. (e) Panoramic radiograph shows the hypertrophy of the mandibular body on the right side. Orthognathic surgery could be performed without risk of bleeding, since the malformation did not extend into the bone. *continued*

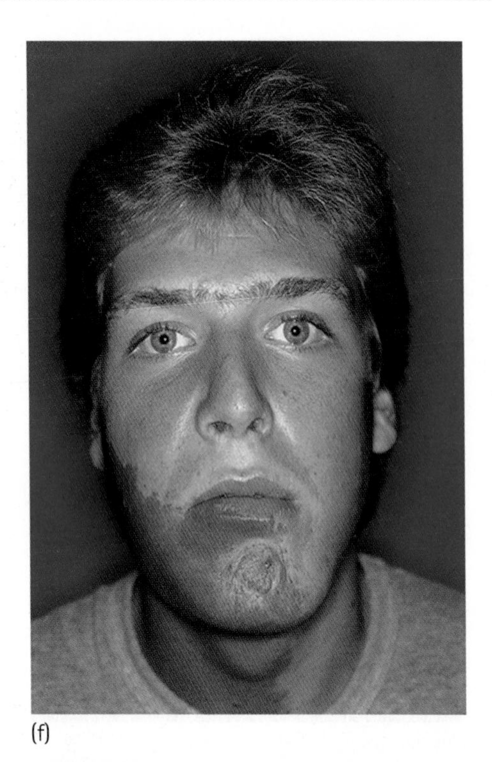

(f)

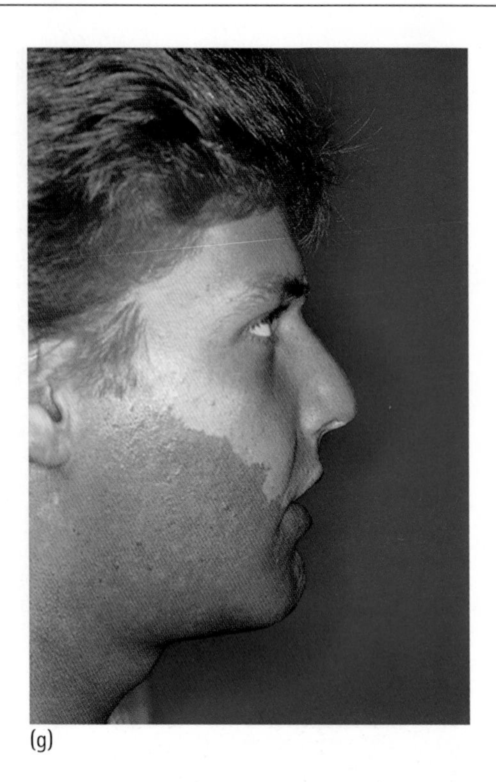

(g)

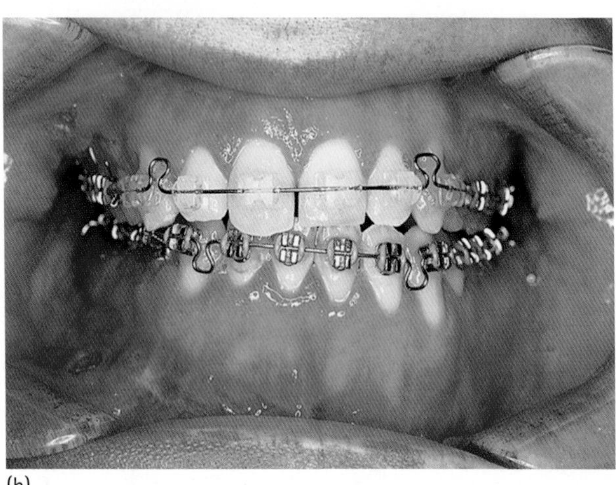

(h)

6.1.3 *continued* (f) Frontal, (g) lateral and (h) intraoral photographs after three-piece Le Fort I osteotomy, bilateral mandibular osteotomies and genioplasty. Reproduced with permission from Kaban LB, Mulliken JB. Maxillofacial vascular anomalies. In: Kaban LB, Troulis MJ (eds). *Pediatric Oral and Maxillofacial Surgery*. Philadelphia: WB Saunders, 2004: 264.

Complications

- Thickening and nodularity of the lesion with aging.
- Impaired vision. Involvement of the eyelids can be associated with elevated intraocular pressure and glaucoma (V1–V2 distribution).
- Recurrence after treatment.

VENOUS MALFORMATION

Venous malformations (VM) are the most common type of vascular anomaly. They occur in a spectrum, from isolated skin or mucosal varicosities to localized spongy masses, to large complex lesions permeated throughout tissue planes.

Treatment options

- Sclerotherapy: For large venous malformations with localized venous 'lakes', direct injection of absolute (100 per cent) ethanol (sclerozing agent of choice in the United States) by an interventional radiologist is indicated. This requires general anaesthesia with real-time fluoroscopic guidance. Usually several sessions are necessary to shrink a large venous malformation. Ethiblock (Ethicon, Hamburg, Germany), a radiopaque mixture of ethanol, contrast agent and amino acids, is also used in Europe. Small oral mucosal venous malformations can be sclerozed with injection of 1 per cent sodium tetradecyl sulphate.
- Well-localized cutaneous VM can be excised.
- Resection marginal or segmental for well-localized bone lesions (Figure 6.1.4).

Complications

- Intermittent swelling, pain and fever are a common problem encountered in venous and combined lymphatic–venous lesions. Such lesions increase in size in

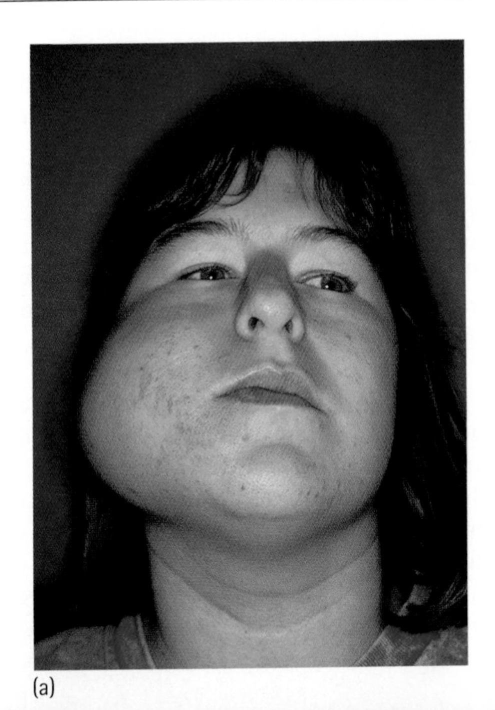

(a)

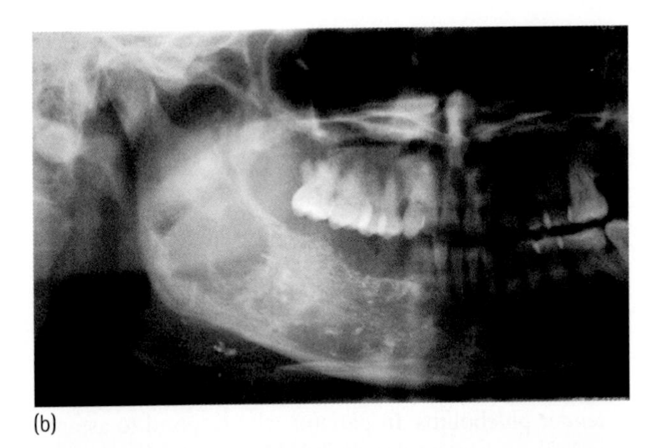

(b)

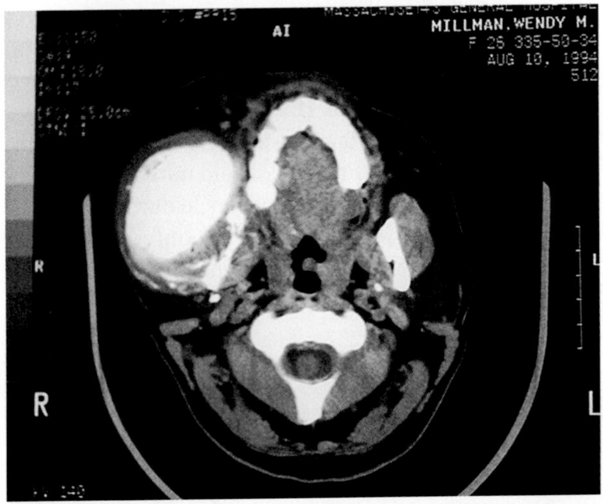

(c)

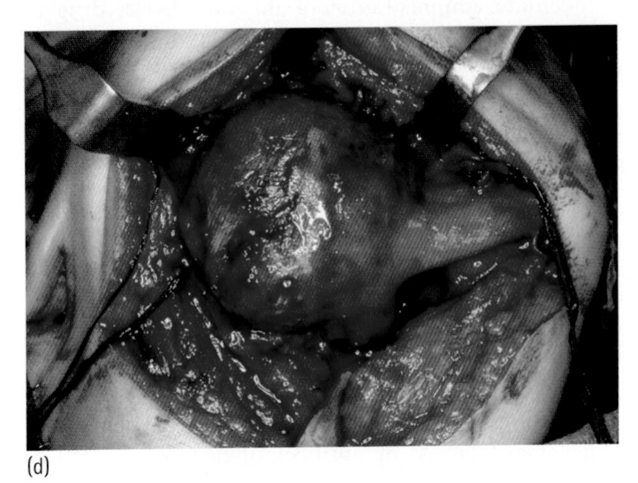

(d)

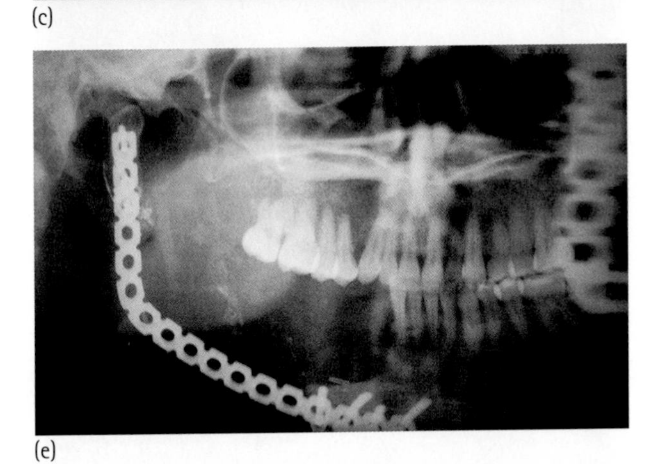

(e)

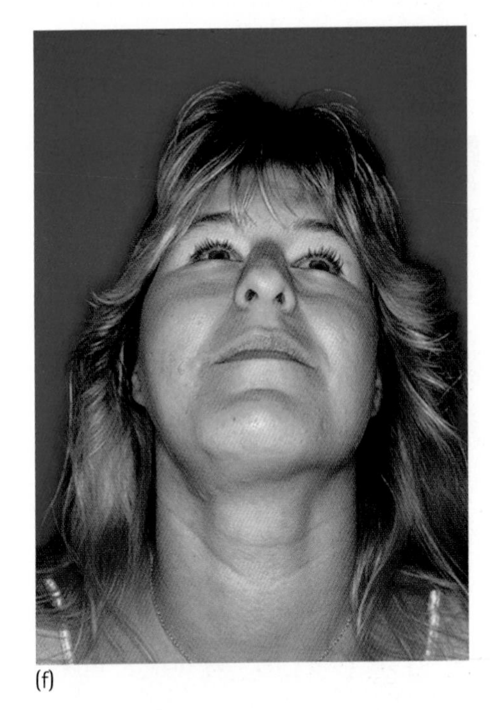

(f)

6.1.4 (a) Frontal ('worm's eye') view of a patient with venous malformation of the mandible. (b) Panoramic radiograph shows lytic changes in the bone. (c) Computed tomographic scan with contrast demonstrates the large malformation extending into the soft tissues. (d) Intraoperative photograph. Well-localized low flow vascular malformations can be treated with resection without the risk of excessive bleeding. (e) Panorex one year post-operatively and (f) submental view of the patient one year post-operatively. Reproduced with permission from: Kaban LB, Mulliken JB. Maxillofacial vascular anomalies. In: Kaban LB, Troulis MJ (eds). *Pediatric Oral and Maxillofacial Surgery*. Philadelphia: WB Saunders, 2004: 277.

relation to viral illness, trauma, adjacent (odontogenic) or intralesional infection and clotting. In these patients, it is difficult to distinguish between cellulitis, intralesional abscess, thrombophlebitis and phlebothrombosis. A local source for infection, such as carious teeth, periapical abscess or pericoronitis must be excluded. Administration of the appropriate antibiotic (usually penicillin or clindamycin in the maxillofacial region) is begun. A drainage procedure is carried out only for an obvious abscess. Aspirin anticoagulation therapy may be useful in cases of venous malformation enlargement, if there are no local or systemic sources of infection and when there are tender phleboliths. In patients who respond to aspirin, indefinite administration of this antiplatelet drug to prevent intralesional clotting should be considered.

- Localized or systemic coagulopathy may result in major haemorrhage spontaneously or during an operation in large VMs. Disseminated intravascular coagulopathy can be caused by stasis and turbulence associated with the venous malformation. This is a consumptive coagulopathy. Prothrombin (PT) and partial thromboplastin times (PTT) are often normal; thrombin time and levels of fibrin split products and fibrinopeptide may be elevated, with decreased fibrinogen and platelet levels. Heparin treatment is instituted when indicated and only when the coagulopathy is corrected are surgical procedures feasible. Another approach is to begin giving heparin, followed by antifibrinolytic therapy with ε-aminocaproic acid. Failure to address this chronic consumptive coagulopathy will result in uncontrollable bleeding during a procedure.
- Systemic sepsis related to local infection with haematogenous spread. In these cases, hospital admission, blood cultures and intravenous antibiotic therapy are necessary.
- Recanalization of extensive venous malformation after sclerotherapy is a recognized occurrence. Repeat of sclerotherapy in this situation can be dangerous and cause local blistering, deep ulceration, full-thickness skin necrosis, nerve damage, haemolysis, haemoglobinuria and potential renal toxicity and cardiac arrest.
- Bleeding after teeth extractions is controlled by packing with pledgets consisting of microfibrillar collagen (Avitene, Davol, Warwick, RI) wrapped in oxidized cellulose sheets (Surgicel, Ethicon, Someville, NJ). These are held in place with 2/0 chromic catgut figure-of-eight sutures across the sockets. Extractions should be performed after sclerotherapy.
- Painful expansion secondary to injury, partial resection or endocrine changes (e.g. puberty, pregnancy, birth control pills). This may be the first evidence of the lesion.

LYMPHATIC MALFORMATION

Lymphatic malformations (LM) are classified as macrocystic or microcystic. Macrocystic (called cystic hygroma in the past) occur below the mylohyoid muscle in the neck most frequently in front of the sternocleidomastoid muscle (Figure 6.1.5). Microcystic commonly involves the tongue, the floor of the mouth, the cheek, the lips and the mandible.

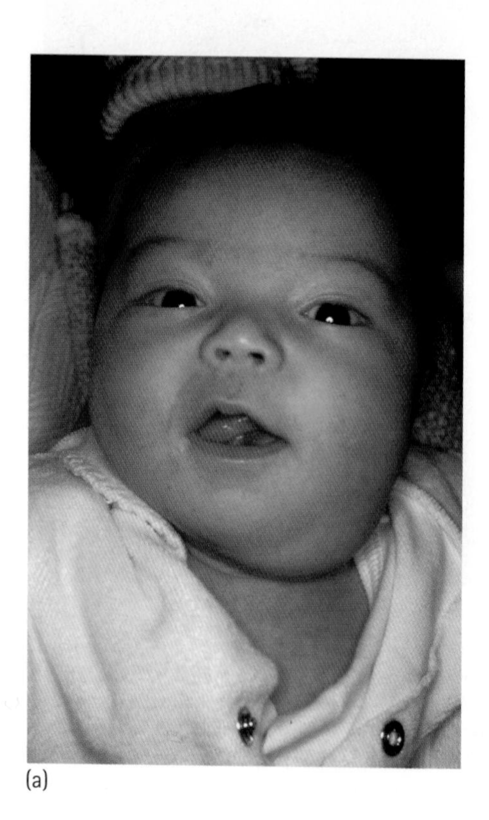

(a)

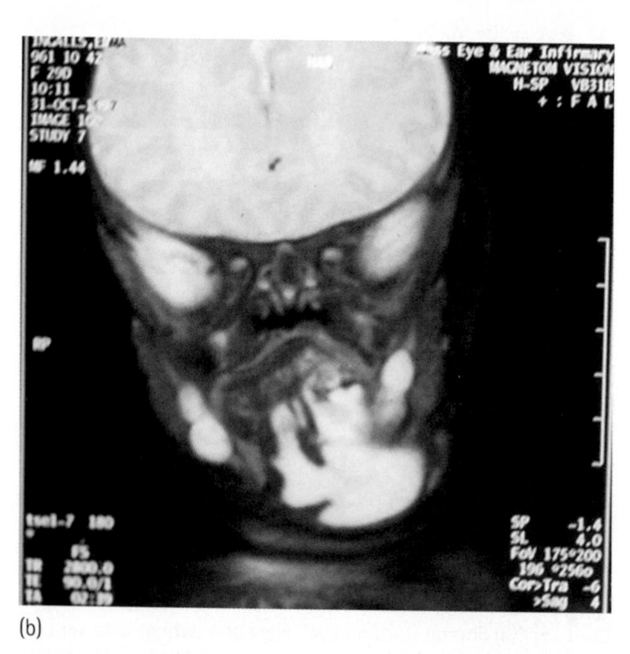

(b)

6.1.5 (a) Infant at 2 weeks of age with a left submandibular lymphatic malformation (LM). (b) MRI T2 with gadolinium shows a macrocystic LM with homogenous enhancement that involves the anterior neck triangle. *continued*

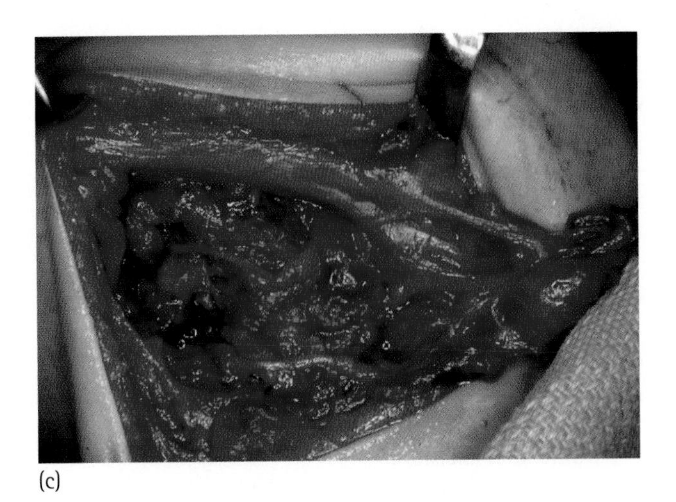

(c)

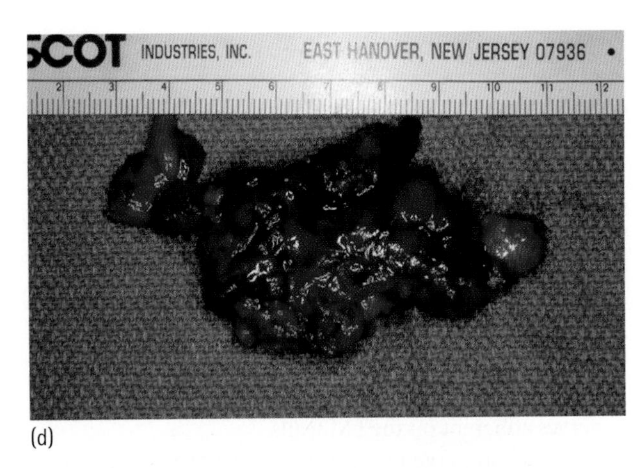

(d)

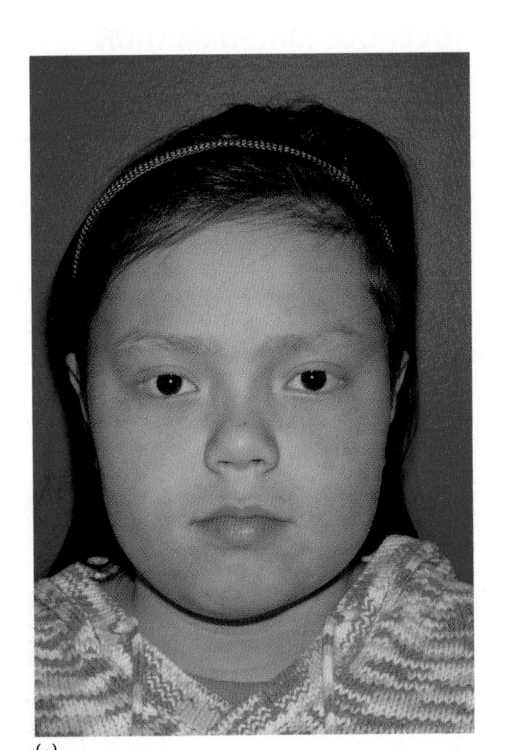

(e)

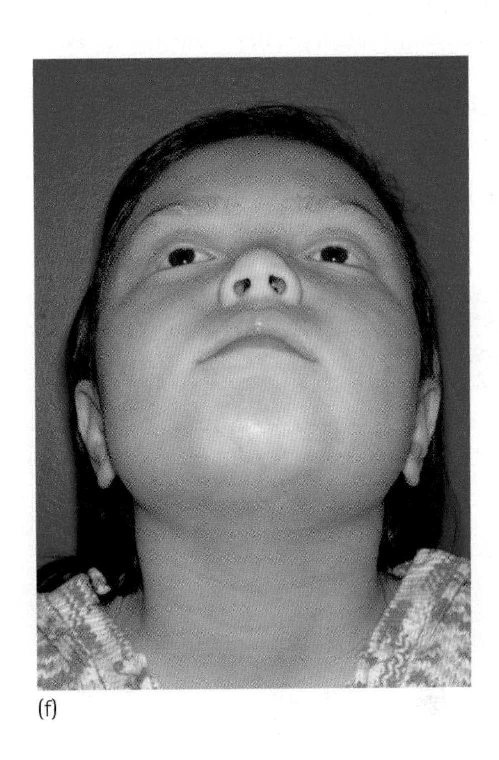

(f)

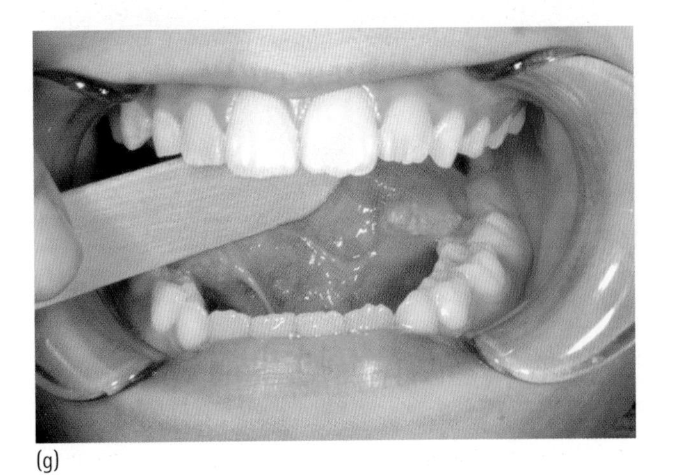

(g)

6.1.5 *continued* (c) Intraoperative photograph. Excision was performed through combined submandibular–intraoral (sublingual) approach. The malformation extended to the floor of the mouth. During the course of the dissection, the lingual and hypoglossal nerves were identified and preserved. (d) Specimen. (e) Frontal; (f) submental and (g) intraoral view at nine years of age.

Treatment options

- Sclerotherapy with ethanol, OK-432 (attenuated *Streptococcus pyogenes*) or 1 per cent sodium tetradecyl sulphate for macrocystic LM.
- Intralesional injections of bleomycin have been described with encouraging results.
- Small well-localized LM can be excised.
- Excision of cervical macrocystic lymphatic malformation with neck dissection approach. Complete excision may not be achieved as typically LMs in the neck extend deep into the parapharyngeal space with carotid artery and nerves adherent on the LM walls.
- Patients with large microcystic cervicofacial LM require serial, staged surgical excisions of the floor of the mouth and submandibular tissues.
- Orthognathic surgery after soft tissue excision to minimize recurrence and manage malocclusion and distortion of the maxillofacial skeleton (Figure 6.1.6).

Complications

- Bacterial infection (cellulitis) can cause sudden expansion of LM.
- Intralesional bleeding or bleeding from the irregular surface of microcystic LM in the morning upon awakening, possibly due to the increased venous pressure of sleeping supine.
- Airway obstruction when LM is located in the floor of the mouth or the tongue.
- Recurrence even years post-operatively.
- Sudden expansion often occurs coincident with upper respiratory tract infection.
- Seroma after excision.

ARTERIOVENOUS MALFORMATION

A clinical staging system for arteriovenous malformations (AVMs) that is helpful in predicting the natural history has been introduced (Table 6.1.3).

The current strategy for management of AVMs is arterial embolization for occlusion of the nidus (centre of the AVM) of the malformation, followed 24–72 hours later by surgical excision. The surgical goal is complete resection of the AVM nidus and involved overlying tissue, although this is often not possible.

(a)

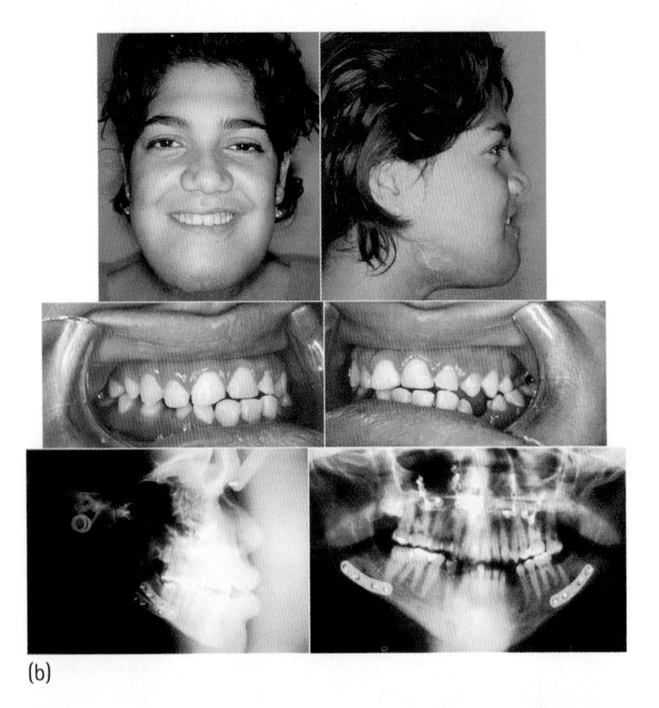

(b)

6.1.6 (a) Frontal, lateral and intraoral photographs of a 13-year-old girl with a cervicofacial lymphatic malformation, mandibular prognathism and open bite, secondary to the progressive mandibular distortion. Lateral cephalogram and panorex show obtuse mandibular plane angle and anterior open bite. (b) Frontal, lateral and intraoral photographs, lateral cephalogram and panorex five years post-treatment. The patient underwent resection of the lymphatic malformation, Le Fort I osteotomy, bilateral mandibular osteotomies and genioplasty. Reproduced with permission from Padwa BL. Orthognathic surgery in the growing child. In: Kaban LB, Troulis MJ (eds). *Pediatric Oral and Maxillofacial Surgery*. Philadelphia: WB Saunders, 2004: 384–5.

Table 6.1.3 Schobinger clinical staging system for arteriovenous malformation.

Stage	Description
I (Quiescence)	Pink-bluish stain, warmth, and arteriovascular shunting by continuous Doppler scanning or 20-MHz colour Doppler scanning
II (Expansion)	Same as stage I plus enlargement, pulsations, thrill, and bruit and tortuous, tense veins
III (Destruction)	Same as stage II plus either dystrophic skin changes, ulceration, bleeding, persistent pain, or tissue necrosis
IV (Decompensation)	Same as stage III plus cardiac failure

Reproduced with permission from Mulliken JB, Fishman SJ, Burrows PE. Vascular anomalies. *Current Problems in Surgery* 2000; **37**: 520.

Treatment options

- Superselective arterial embolization is performed by an interventional radiologist. The principle is to obliterate the nidus of the malformation with embolization materials (Table 6.1.4). Thus, inflow to the AVMs is reduced with low risk of collateral flow development. Superselective embolization may be performed electively and followed by resection or it may be required as a life-saving procedure in the presence of acute bleeding. Proximal vessel embolization is contraindicated because of the rapid development of collateral flow to the nidus of the AVM. Post-embolization angiography is obtained to ensure reduced blood flow in the malformation and the AVM is examined for clinical improvement (skin colour, size, pulsation).
- Intraosseous direct puncture of the AVM with platinum coils or other embolization materials may be used to supplement superselective embolization or in cases where further vessel embolization is not feasible (Figure 6.1.7).
  - A 16-gauge needle trocar is placed directly through the bone or alveolus intraorally using direct fluoroscopy.
  - Placement of the trocar into the AVM nidus is confirmed by an arteriogram.
  - Through the trocar, an 18-gauge catheter is placed using a guide wire.
  - Embolization material is injected directly into the nidus through the catheter.
  - This procedure can be repeated for multiple varices of the AVM.
  - Post-treatment arteriogram is obtained.
- Partial or complete surgical resection of soft tissues or bone is performed 1–3 days after embolization. Embolization does not decreace the extent of resection. Hypervascularity makes haemostasis difficult intraoperatively, even after embolization. Intraoperative embolization must be available. All small arteries that supply the AVM should be ligated except the main, proximal arteries.

Table 6.1.4 Embolization materials.

	Material
Temporary (resorbable)	Gelfoam Collagen Iodine oil
Permanent	Polyvinyl alcohol particles (e.g. ethylene-vinyl-alcoholcopolymer; Onyx, Micro Therapeutics, Irvine, CA, USA) Acrylic glue Silky thread Stainless steel Platinum coils

- Teeth extraction after AVM embolization (Figures 6.1.7 and 6.1.8). In patients with intraosseous malformation in the tooth-bearing portions of the maxilla and mandible, teeth may be removed 24–48 hours after embolization insertion. The sockets are packed with Avitene and surgical pledgets and oversewn. Once the sockets heal and the wounds are completely mucosalized, the malformations often become quiescent and remain in Shobinger stage I. This is probably because the irritant of mobile teeth constantly being compressed by occlusal forces and perhaps chronic low-grade inflammation are eliminated.

Complications

- Massive blood loss during the operation may be life-threatening. Even a single tooth extraction associated with an AVM can result in exsanguinating haemorrhage. Preoperative embolization is performed to prevent this complication. Intraoperative bleeding is managed with urgent embolization or haemostatic materials such as Surgicel, Avitene, suturing and pressure. However, local haemostatic measures may be insufficient to control the bleeding. Prolonged intubation to secure the airway and blood transfusions may be necessary.
- Unfortunately, AVMs are not usually well localized and recurrence with expansion of vessels deep or at the periphery of the resection occurs in a high percentage of patients. For these patients, embolization is palliative and re-operation may not be feasible.
- Development of collateral vessels and flow to the nidus of the malformation occurs especially after proximal ligation or embolization.
- Absorption of embolization materials and recanalization of AVM.
- Extrusion of embolization materials through the mucosa intraorally.
- Embolization of internal carotid branches can cause ischaemic stroke. General risks of angiography and embolization are death, bleeding, coma, damage to blood vessels and infection.
- Bleeding or ulceration of the overlying skin.

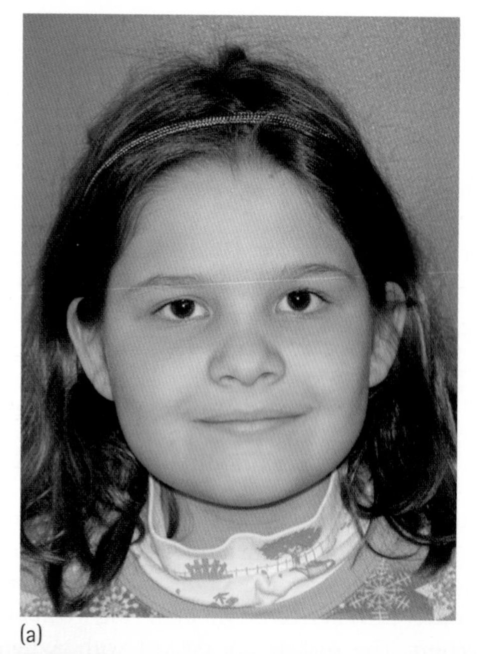

(a)

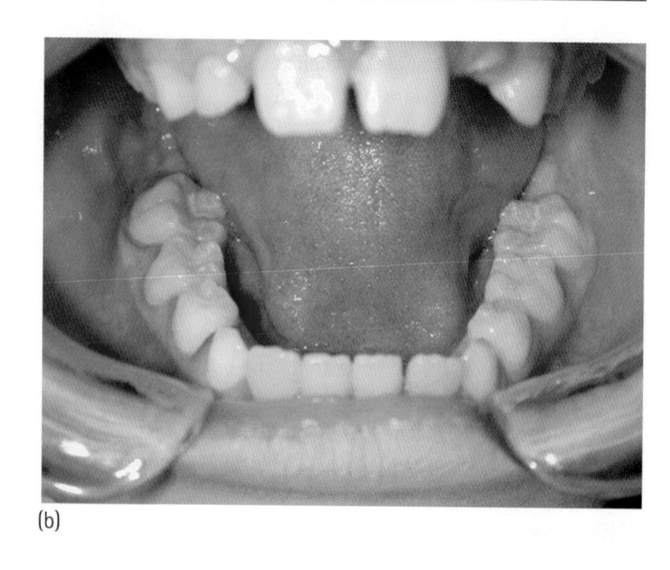

(b)

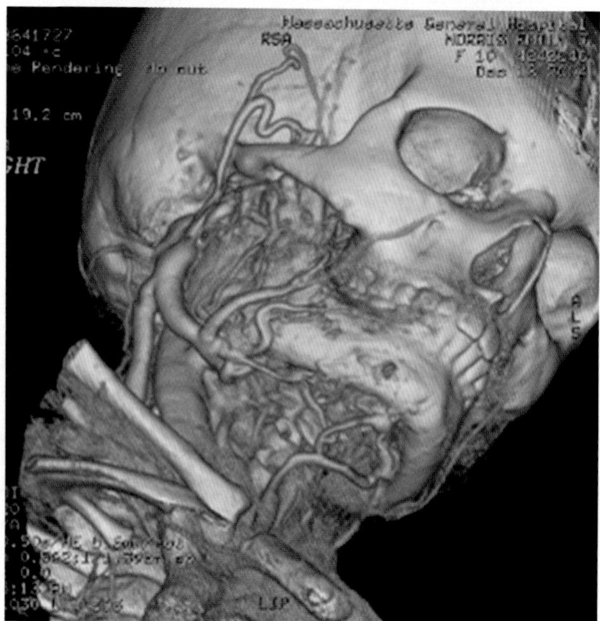

(c)

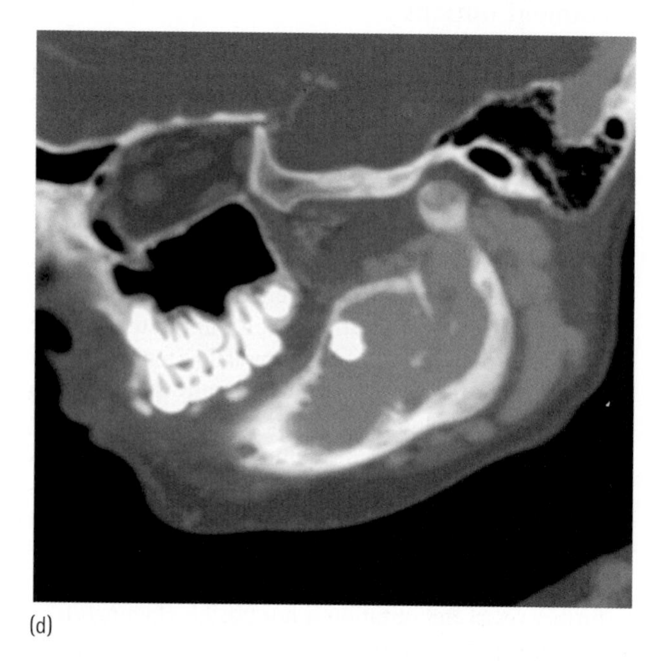

(d)

6.1.7 (a) Frontal and (b) intraoral photographs of a ten-year-old girl with arteriovenous malformation (AVM) of the right hemimandible. The patient had noted swelling and intraoral bleeding at the right mandible two months prior to her initial visit. Physical examination revealed enlargement of the right hemimandible, warmness of the area on palpation, but no tenderness and no discoloration of the overlying skin. A loud bruit was auscultated by stethoscope examination of the right submandibular region and a thrill was palpated. The teeth were mobile and depressible. (c) Three-dimensional computed tomography (CT) angiogram (3D-CTA) demonstrates the supply of the malformation from branches of the enlarged right (R) external carotid artery (R internal maxillary, R facial artery) and the left facial artery. No contribution of the right internal carotid artery is identified. Drainage of AVM (stage II–III) is via innumerable large venous varices that drain into an enlarged right internal jugular vein. (d) Sagittal section of CT scan shows the lytic AVM that involves and expands the right hemimandible including the ascending ramus.

continued

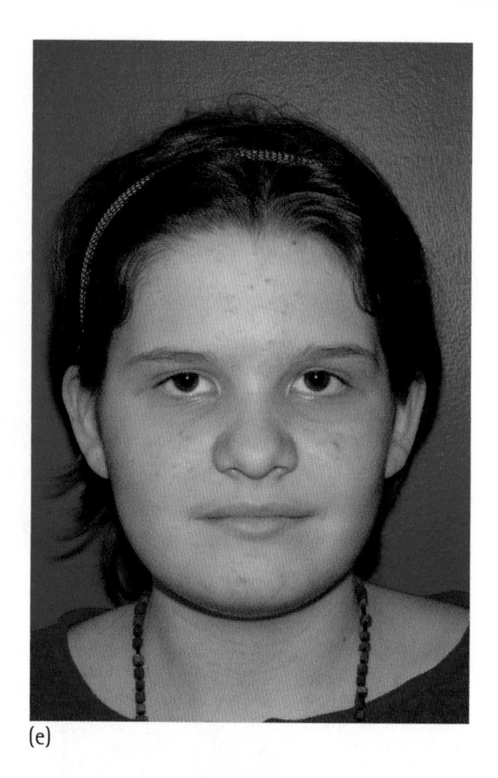
(e)

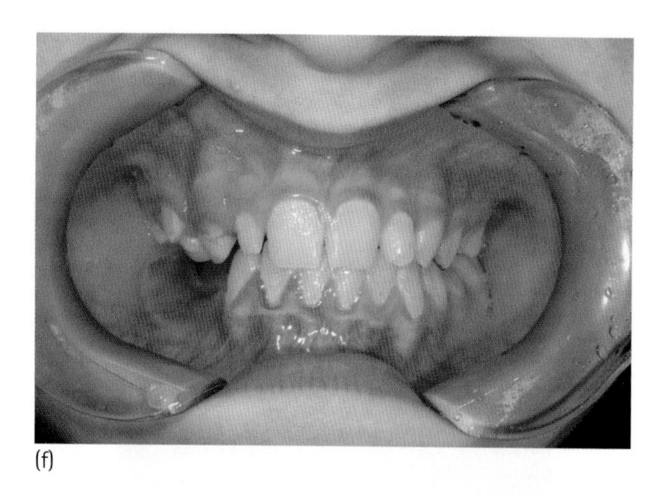
(f)

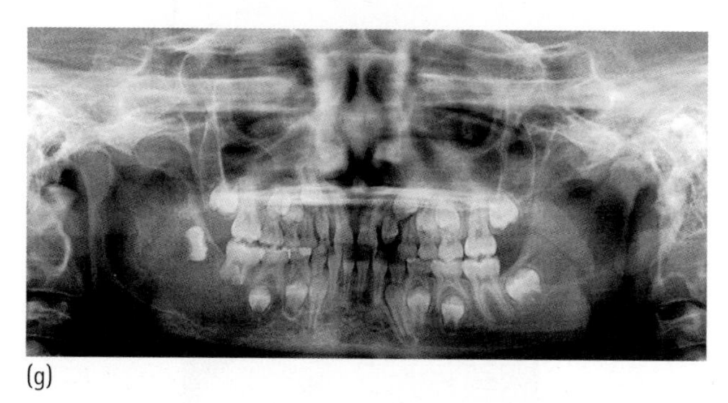
(g)

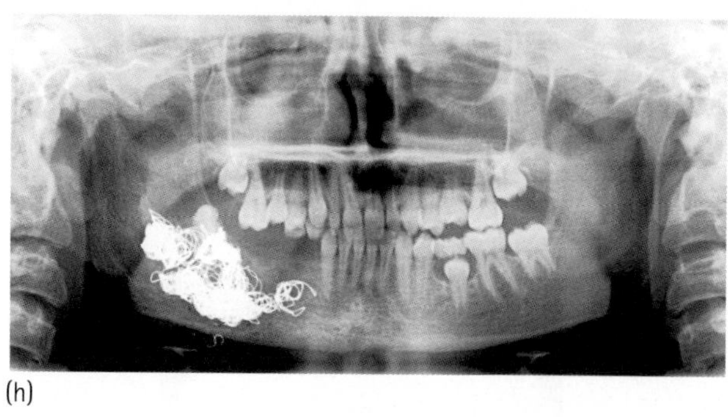
(h)

6.1.7 *continued* (e) Frontal and (f) intraoral photograph three years after the patient's initial visit. She underwent multiple, urgent and scheduled embolizations with platinum coils and extraction of posterior mandibular teeth on the right side. (g) Panorex before intervention shows the large AVM that appears as a multiloculated radiolucent lesion extending from the first premolar to the sigmoid notch. The mandibular 12-year molar is floating in the radiolucency and there is resorption of the six-year molar. The second premolar tooth bud is also displaced and there is thinning of the inferior border cortex. (i) Panorex three years after the initial visit shows the intraosseous coils and the filling of the cavity with bone. After the treatment, the AVM became quiescent (stage I).

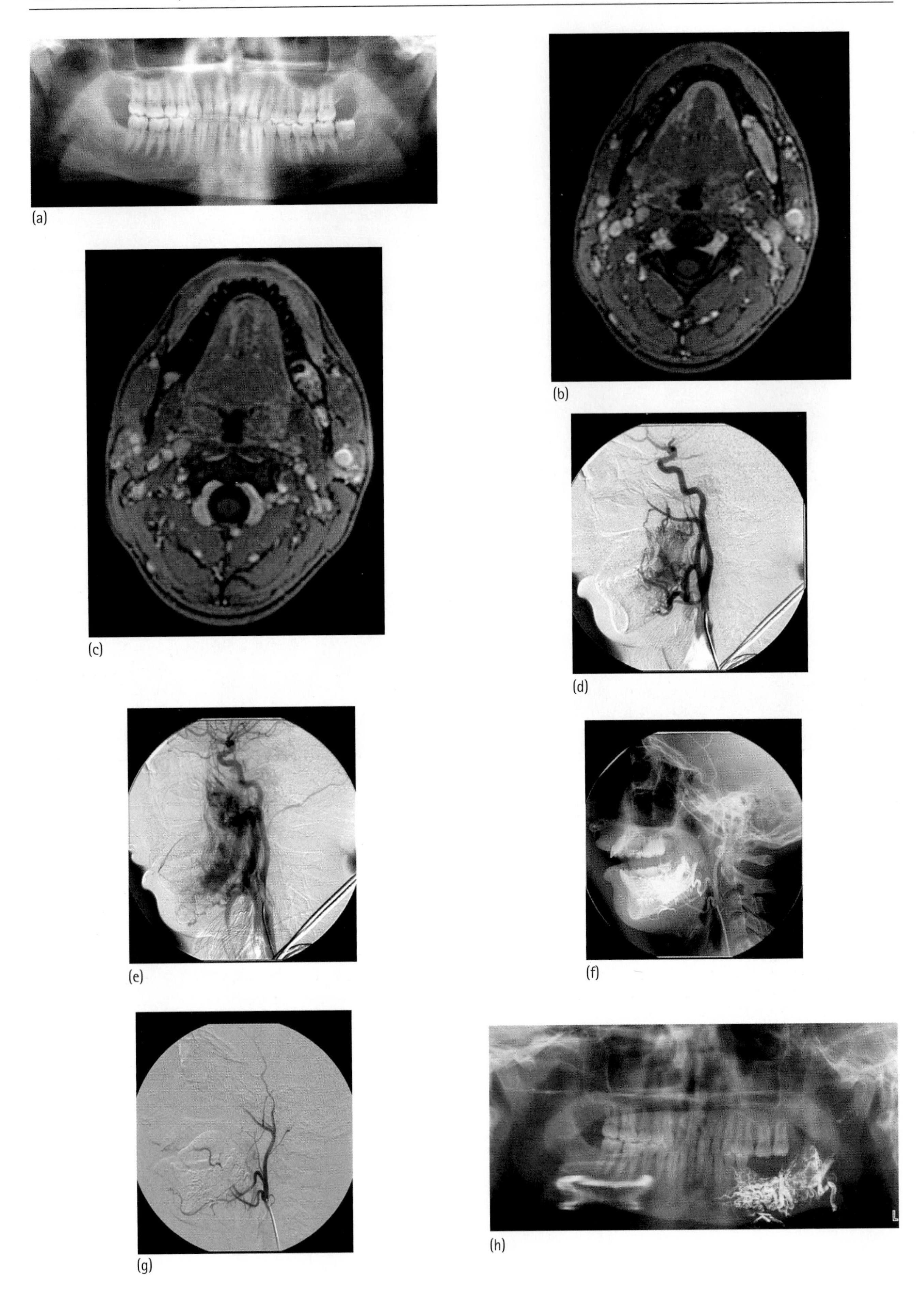
(a)
(b)
(c)
(d)
(e)
(f)
(g)
(h)
L

6.1.8 (a) Panorex of a 17-year-old boy who experienced excessive bleeding after an unsuccessful attempt to extract the left lower wisdom tooth. The procedure was aborted and the patient was referred to hospital. The radiograph shows a radiolucent area in the left mandible extending from the left first molar to the middle of the ramus above the lingula posteriorly. There is resorption of the third and second molar roots and the distal root of the first molar. (b,c) Axial sections of MRI T1 with gadolinium show a 36×12-mm septated lytic area in the left mandible with homogenous enhancement with flow voids indicating high-flow malformation. The patient was scheduled for transfemoral angiography and embolization under general anaesthesia. (d,e) Angiography of the left external carotid shows two large tangles of vessels, one over the angle of the mandible and the other over the condyle that interconnect with each other. Feeding arteries that supply the AVM are the lingual, facial and the first five branches of the internal maxillary artery (inferior alveolar artery, pterygoid artery, messeteric artery, buccinator artery, and posterior superior alveolar artery). There is early venous drainage into the venous compartment of the mandible that drains into the external jugular vein. (f,g) Angiogram after embolization of the AVM nidus with 3.9-cc liquid Onyx (Micro Therapeutics, Irvine, CA, USA). There is an onyx cast seen within the facial artery, the pedicles of the AVM and within the venous saccule of the mandible. Approximately 25 per cent of the AVM has been embolized. During the procedure, excessive intraoral bleeding was controlled with extraction of the lower left second and the third molars, packing the sockets with Avitene and Surgicel, suturing and pressure. Two months later the lower left first molar was also extracted due to tooth mobility, pain and bleeding from its gingival sulcus. (h) Panorex 2.5 years post embolization and extraction of three molars associated with the AVM shows the embolization material in the bony cavity. The malformation became and remains quiescent (Shobinger stage I) after treatment.

Top tips

- First determine if the lesion is an haemangioma or a malformation.
- An intraosseous vascular lesion is most frequently a malformation, not an haemangioma.
- If an haemangioma, determine if proliferating or involuting.
- If malformation, determine slow-flow versus fast-flow.
- Sclerotherapy is effective for slow-flow vascular malformations, especially macrocystic LM and VM with large venous lakes.
- AVMs are treated with embolization and resection when possible, but recurrence rate is high. If dentoalveolar segment is involved, embolization and then removal of the teeth may result in long-term control with the lesion remaining in Shobinger stage I (quiescence).
- Patients with slow-flow lesions adjacent to bone can have skeletal deformity treated. With proper preparation there is little chance of life-endangering haemorrhage.

FURTHER READING

Boon LM, MacDonald DM, Mulliken JB. Complications of systemic corticosteroid therapy for problematic hemangioma. *Plastic and Reconstructive Surgery* 1999; **104**: 1617–23.

Boyd JB, Mulliken JB, Kaban LB *et al.* Skeletal changes associated with vascular malformations. *Plastic and Reconstructive Surgery* 1984; **74**: 789.

Ezekowitz RA, Mulliken JB, Folkman J. Interferon alfa 2a therapy for life-threatening hemangiomas of infancy. *New England Journal of Medicine* 1992; **326**: 1456–63.

Kaban LB, Mulliken JB. Vascular anomalies of the maxillofacial region. *Journal of Oral and Maxillofacial Surgery* 1986; **44**: 203.

Kaban LB, Mulliken JB. Vascular lesions of the maxillofacial region. In: Kaban LB, Troulis MJ (eds). *Pediatric oral and maxillofacial surgery*. Philadelphia: WB Saunders, 2004: 259–84.

Kohout MP, Hansen M, Pribaz JJ, Mulliken JB. Arteriovenous malformations of the head and neck: Natural history and management. *Plastic and Reconstructive Surgery* 1998; **102**: 643–54.

Mulliken JB, Glowacki J. Hemangiomas and vascular malformations in infants and children: A classification based on endothelial characteristics. *Plastic and Reconstructive Surgery* 1982; **69**: 412.

Mulliken JB, Rogers GF, Marler JJ. Circular excision of hemangioma and purse-string closure: The smallest possible scar. *Plastic and Reconstructive Surgery* 2002; **109**: 1544–54.

Padwa BL, Hayward PG, Ferraro NF, Mulliken JB. Cervicofacial lymphatic malformation: Clinical course, surgical intervention, and pathogenesis of skeletal hypertrophy. *Plastic and Reconstructive Surgery* 1997; **95**: 951–60.

Perrott DH, Schmidt B, Dowd CF, Kaban LB. Treatment of a high-flow arteriovenous malformation by direct puncture and coil embolization. *Journal of Oral and Maxillofacial Surgery* 1994; **52**: 1083–6.

Qin Zhong P, Xin ZF, Ren L. Long term results of intratumorous bleomycin A5 injection for head and neck lympangioma. *Oral Surgery, Oral Medicine, Oral Pathology, Oral Radiology, and Endodontics* 1998; **86**: 139–44.

Watson WL, McCarthy WD. Blood and lymphatic vessel tumors: Report of 1056 cases. *Surgery, Gynecology and Obstetrics* 1940; **71**: 569.

6.2

Interventional radiology of the head and neck

JOHN S MILLAR

INTRODUCTION

There has been rapid and widespread development of vascular interventional radiological techniques and devices over the past two decades and this chapter will outline their role in maxillofacial surgery. First, an understanding of the classification and the role of imaging in the diagnosis of head and neck vascular malformations is essential. The various endovascular techniques that are employed in the treatment of these conditions will follow.

The importance of a multidisciplinary team approach to the management of these conditions must be stressed. In addition to oromaxillofacial surgeons and interventional radiologists, the expertise of numerous specialists, drawn from dermatology, diagnostic radiology, ENT ophthalmology, paediatrics, plastic and reconstructive surgery, pathology and neurosurgery, will be required to deal optimally with these complex lesions. It goes without saying that close involvement of the patient in all decision making is essential and psychotherapeutic support may be necessary as curative treatment may not be possible.

CLASSIFICATION

The classification of vascular anomalies of the head and neck, proposed by Mulliken and Glowacki in 1982, is widely employed. They categorized vascular anomalies according to endothelial cell characteristics and, although many more types of vascular lesions are recognized with the aid of modern immunohistochemical techniques, it has stood the test of time and represents a sound basis for the effective understanding and communication of these conditions (Table 6.2.1).

Haemangiomas are characterized histologically by high endothelial cell turnover. They are true neoplasms that usually present in infancy. They enlarge by cellular proliferation and exhibit a clinical life cycle which typically includes phases of proliferation, plateau and subsequent involution. They may be further characterized by cell markers (e.g. GLUT-1, merosin, Lewis Y) that are otherwise found only in human placental tissue. Most other vascular anomalies are properly termed 'malformations', which are characterized by normal endothelial cell turnover and abnormal gross vascular anatomy. These are thought to be present from birth and enlarge as the patient grows. From the therapeutic point of view, it is convenient to separate these into low flow and high flow malformations.

Other indications for endovascular interventional radiology in the head and neck include the pre-operative embolization of various hypervascular tumours including paragangliomas, juvenile angiofibromas, extracranial meningiomas and endolymphatic sac tumours. Uncontrolled, spontaneous epistaxis and oral or nasopharyngeal haemorrhage secondary to malignant tumour, radiotherapy or trauma may require urgent embolization which can be life saving. Traumatic or congenital arteriovenous fistula of the head and neck are now usually dealt with by endovascular techniques.

Table 6.2.1 Vascular anomalies according to endothelial cell characteristics.

Tumours	Vascular malformations	
	High-flow	Low-flow
Juvenile haemangioma	Arteriovenous malformation	Venous malformation
Rapidly involuting congenital haemangioma		Lymphatic malformation
Noninvoluting congenital haemangioma		Lymphatic-venous malformation
Kaposiform haemangioendothelioma		Capillary (or venular) malformation (port wine stain)
Tufted angioma		
Pyogenic granuloma		

Reproduced with permission from Mulliken and Glowacki, revised by the International Society for the Study of Vascular Anomalies, 1996.

IMAGING

Useful information may be obtained from ultrasound and computed tomography (CT), but magnetic resonance imaging (MRI) is the examination of choice. MRI accurately defines the extent and depth of vascular anomalies of the head and neck. It also provides information on whether the lesion appears discrete or invasive which is of fundamental importance in surgical planning. Contrast administration is helpful in defining the full extent of haemangiomas and solid, hypervascular components of vascular anomalies and tumours. Signal void within a lesion raises the possibility of high flow due to arteriovenous shunting which may be further elucidated by magnetic resonance angiography.

Calcification in a phlebolith, a characteristic of venous malformations and gas, may also exhibit signal void on MRI, mimicking high flow. Phleboliths and gas are readily identified on CT and will often be visible on plain x-ray. Doppler ultrasound, particularly colour flow, will often reveal areas of high flow not appreciated on clinical examination, but the full characterization of the angioarchitecture of high flow lesions however, can only reliably be made with selective and superselective catheter, digital subtraction angiography (DSA).

In addition to general neuroradiological catheter skills, training in the various microcatheter techniques and the handling of embolic agents, is required. A thorough understanding of vascular anatomy of the head and neck is essential. There are numerous predictable anastamoses between branches of the external carotid artery (ECA) system and the intracranial circulation in addition to critical supply to the cranial nerves from certain ECA branches. A detailed account of these is beyond the scope of this text and the interested reader is referred to texts listed in the bibliography.

EQUIPMENT

High quality, biplane angiography with fluoroscopy and road map facility is essential for the avoidance of inadvertent penetration of embolic material through dangerous anastamoses, particularly when one is working in the region of the skull base. The success of modern interventional techniques depends in no small measure on the advances that have occurred in microcatheter and guide wire technology. Procedures are carried using a coaxial technique. Typically an external carotid branch is selectively catheterized with a 5F or 6F guide catheter. A 2F microcatheter is passed through the guide catheter and navigated superselectively into the desired vessel. Thromboembolism is the main risk of these procedures. Haemostatic valves permit continuous flushing of catheters with heparinized saline throughout the procedure, in addition to systemic heparinization employing point-of-care assay to monitor clotting.

The list of embolic materials employed is extensive and growing (Table 6.2.2). It includes agents for temporary and permanent occlusion, liquid or particulate agents and coils, which may be pushable or detachable by a variety of mechanisms. These are usually made of platinum and may be bare or covered with Dacron fibres to increase thrombogenicity. A variety of sclerosant agents for the treatment of venolymphatic malformations are available. These are discussed in more detail in Chapter 6.1.

Table 6.2.2 Embolic agents in common use.

Large vessel	Medium vessel	Small vessel
Coils:	Gelatin	Particles
Pushable	Gelfoam sponge/particles	PVA 50–150 micron Embospheres®)
Detachable – electrolytic, thermal, mechanical, etc.	Particles	Liquids
Balloons	Polyvinyl alcohol (PVA) 250–1000 micron	Cyanoacrylate/Lipiodol
	Trisacryl gelatin microspheres (Embospheres®)	Ethylene vinyl alcohol copolymer (EVAL-Onyx®)

PRINCIPLES AND PROCEDURES

Neuroendovascular therapy may be curative in its own right, e.g. coiling of cerebral aneurysms, embolization of dural arteriovenous fistula/brain arteriovenous malformations (AVM), etc., but in the head and neck, it is usually employed to reduce operative blood loss in hypervascular lesions. In some instances, conditional on the appropriate choice of embolic agent, embolization may lead to permanent devascularization of the lesion leading to necrosis and shrinkage or cure, but usually the reduction in vascularity is temporary. Embolization and surgery therefore need to be scheduled with this constraint in mind. The aim of embolization depends on the type of lesion (Table 6.2.3).

Although polyvinyl alcohol (PVA) is nonresorbable and is therefore considered a permanent agent, in practice it acts as a temporary embolic agent because recanalization occurs around the particles. Gelfoam is an example of a truly resorbable, temporary agent. Cyanoacrylate glue is widely used as an embolic agent in Europe, but less often in North America due to licensing issues. It is a highly effective, permanent embolic agent which, because it is a liquid, is capable of distal penetration. It polymerizes rapidly once it comes into contact with ionic solutions, including blood. This process can be delayed by mixing it with Lipiodol which also renders it radio-opaque. Because it is capable of penetrating small branches, the risk of cranial nerve damage

Table 6.2.3 Choice of embolic agent according to target.

Condition	Target	Agent
Tumour/ Haemangioma	Tumour capillary bed	PVA (NBCA)
AVM	Nidus	NBCA, Onyx
AVF	Point occlusion of fistula	Coils, balloon
Epistaxis	Reduce regional arterial pressure	PVA
Venolymphatic malformation	Sac of abnormal vessel	Sclerosant, e.g. alcohol, ethibloc, etc. NBCA

AVM, arteriovenous malformation; AVF, arteriovenous fistula; PVA, polyvinyl alcohol.

and inadvertent intracranial embolization is much greater than with particulate embolization. It is the material of choice for direct, percutaneous embolization.

Ethylene vinyl alcohol copolymer dissolved in dimethyl sulphoxide (DMSO) (Onyx®) is a recently introduced liquid embolic agent which has been found to be extremely useful in the treatment of AVMs of the brain and dural arteriovenous fistula. Its possible role in the management of superficial AVMs has not been established.

Effective treatment of an arteriovenous fistula (AVF) requires point occlusion of the fistula and proximal draining vein. This is not always as straightforward as it may seem, due to problems of access and difficulties accurately identifying the exact site of the fistula. Balloon occlusion of AVF was the earliest type of neuroendovascular procedure and it remains an effective method of treatment. Coil occlusion is, however, generally preferred because it affords a greater degree of control at the fistula site and the risk of migration and distal embolization is reduced.

Thus, although there is commonality of the techniques and the materials employed, the aim of embolization is not the same in every case and an understanding of the natural history of the lesion, before and after treatment is essential. For example, while proximal occlusion of feeding arteries is desirable in epistaxis, it is contraindicated in the treatment of AVMs, as this would lead to angiogenesis and vascular recruitment around the periphery of the lesion making subsequent, curative treatment more difficult.

In the head and neck, particularly in the facial vessels, vascular tortuosity and lack of external support often makes peripheral microcatheter vascular access difficult if not impossible. Conversely, a superficial location lends itself to direct puncture and this is therefore a technique that is frequently employed, not only of necessity for angiographically occult, low flow malformations, but also for peripheral high flow AVMs.

There are some situations where free flow around a microcatheter during embolization is essential, e.g. particulate embolization of a glomus jugulare from the ascending pharyngeal artery and others where a wedged microcatheter position is desirable, e.g. Onyx embolization of an AVM or dural AVF in order to achieve good nidal penetration. In the former, a wedged position risks forcing particles through anastamoses to the vertebral circulation with a consequent risk of stroke or occlusion of the supply to the vasa nervosum of the lower cranial nerves.

ARTERIOVENOUS MALFORMATIONS

The target for AVM embolization is the 'nidus'– the abnormal vessels which represent the level of the shunt. After occlusion of the nidus, it is desirable to occlude the proximal draining vein. The lesion may be a discrete or diffuse collection of anomalous vessels comprising a plexiform network resulting in arteriovenous shunting or may include a larger AVF responsible for the majority of the shunt. In either case, high flow secondary to the AV shunt is a hallmark feature. Over time, this leads to arterial and venous dilatation, tortuosity and occasionally aneurysm formation.

The exception to targeted nidal embolization of an AVM is the occasional requirement for preoperative devascularization of large feeding arteries to high flow AVMs immediately before surgery. In such cases, proximal embolization is acceptable. Preoperative occlusion of surgically inaccessible arterial feeders reduces blood loss and improves visualization of the limits of the lesion making curative excision more likely and, provided surgery is carried out soon after embolization (24–48 hours), peripheral recruitment of feeders should not be a problem.

As with all vascular lesions of the head and neck, close consultation between the surgeon and the interventional radiologist is essential in order to plan the appropriate treatment strategy. Understanding the goal of treatment is crucial. The location of the AVM, angioarchitecture of the nidus, and the feasibility of vascular access defined by angiography merely determine the most effective method of achieving that end. The appropriate choice of embolic agent, the method of access and the target follow from that.

HAEMANGIOMAS

Haemangiomas usually occur in infancy and rarely require active treatment due to the tendency for spontaneous involution. Indications for treatment include threat to vision, airway obstruction, haemorrhage or skin necrosis associated with infection. High output cardiac failure and consumptive coagulopathy (Kasabach–Merritt syndrome) may occur with large visceral haemangiomas, dictating the need for intervention. Embolization may be required before surgery. The technique employed is similar to that for the embolization of a hypervascular tumour.

HYPERVASCULAR TUMOURS

This group of conditions includes paraganglioma (glomus, chemodectoma), meningioma, juvenile angiofibroma, endolymphatic sac tumour and hypervascular metastases (typically, thyroid and renal). Detailed selective and superselective angiography is performed to define the feeding arteries and define any dangerous anastamoses. The largest contributing branch is usually embolized first. With the microcatheter tip in the appropriate vessel, in a condition of free flow around the catheter, a suspension of PVA particles (150–300 μ) in contrast medium is injected under fluoroscopic control until near stasis is achieved. The catheter is then flushed with saline. In some instances, fibred pushable coils will be placed in the pedicle to ensure haemostasis.

The procedure is then repeated in each of the feeding arteries until the tumour is devascularized or the risks of further embolization are judged to outweigh the potential benefit.

Some tumours, particularly paragangliomas, may have arteriovenous shunts within the tumour circulation. These carry the risk of pulmonary embolization of small PVA particles. If suspected on angiography, larger PVA particles may be employed at the outset to occlude this component. Once this has been achieved, switching to smaller particles will achieve a more effective devascularization of the intratumoral vessels.

ARTERIOVENOUS FISTULA

Arteriovenous fistula of the head and neck may arise from the branches of the external carotid artery (ECA) or the vertebral arteries (VA). The latter usually shunt into the adjacent vertebral venous plexus and may be congenital or arise secondary to trauma which can be penetrating or nonpenetrating. AVF of the ECA may occur secondary to trauma, infection, malignant invasion or radiotherapy. They are a feature of hereditary hemorrhagic telangectasia (Osler–Weber–Rendu syndrome).

Vertebro-vertebral fistula can usually be occluded by the endovascular route employing detachable balloons or coils. If the shunt is so large that point occlusion of the fistula is not feasible then 'trapping' the fistula may be necessary. This involves occlusion of the vertebral artery above and below the fistula. Occlusion from above usually requires retrograde navigation of the vertebral artery from the contralateral side via the vertebrobasilar junction.

AVF of the ECA may present with a pulsatile mass or haemorrhage. Embolization with large PVA particles may be possible, but risks pulmonary embolization in large shunts. Occlusion with coils or cyanoacrylate may therefore be necessary.

EPISTAXIS

Spontaneous epistaxis can usually be controlled by anterior and, if necessary, posterior nasal packing. Nasal endoscopy is frequently employed to ligate the sphenopalatine artery and its branches. If, despite these measures, it cannot be controlled, embolization with PVA particles is usually highly effective. Superselective catheterization of the sphenopalatine artery is performed and, under conditions of free flow, 150–300 μ particles suspended in iodinated contrast medium is injected on the side of the epistaxis. Bilateral embolization may be required to control the haemorrhage, but carries an increased risk of tissue necrosis.

The technique is similar to the embolization of hypervascular tumours, but the principle in this case is to reduce the arterial head of pressure to the nasal mucosa rather than occlude the microvasculature of the nasal mucosa. This technique may also be employed in oropharyngeal haemorrhage uncontrolled by other methods. The distressing and life-threatening condition of 'carotid blow-out' requires more drastic therapy. This is usually due to malignant invasion of the common or internal carotid artery in the setting of an open wound, leading to massive haemorrhage. Carotid occlusion (trapping) may be life-saving, but carries a significant risk of stroke even if the collateral circulation of the Circle of Willis appears intact. Stenting of the carotid artery has been successfully employed in some instances avoiding the need to occlude the artery.

VENOLYMPHATIC MALFORMATIONS

These will often be dealt with by sclerosant therapy, but this may not be suitable for very large malformations. They are angiographically occult, which means they cannot be accessed from the arterial route. Venous outflow is exceedingly slow and a retrograde venous approach is usually not possible either. Direct puncture and contrast venography to define the malformation and confirm an intravascular position may allow injection of cyanoacrylate glue as a prelude to excision.

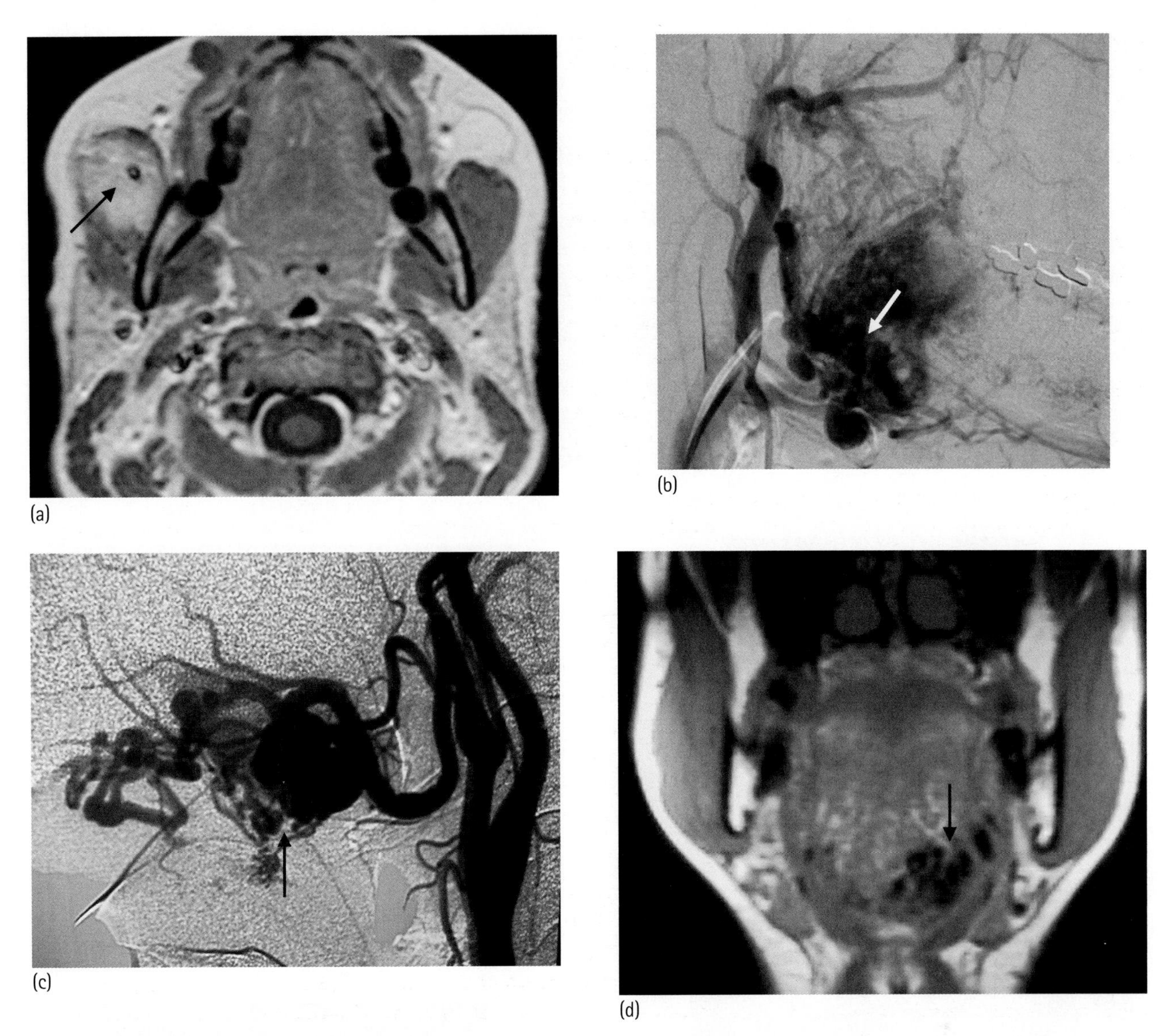

6.2.1 Appearance of vascular lesions of the head and neck on magnetic resonance imaging (MRI). Axial contrast enhanced T1W MRI (a) reveals a solid enhancing component and a region of flow void in a presumed haemangioma of the masseter. Lateral DSA shows corresponding tumour blush and enlarged facial artery (b). In contrast, the submental AVM in panels (c) and (d) illustrate a lesion exhibiting exclusively flow void on coronal T1W MRI corresponding to the AVM nidus revealed on lateral DSA.

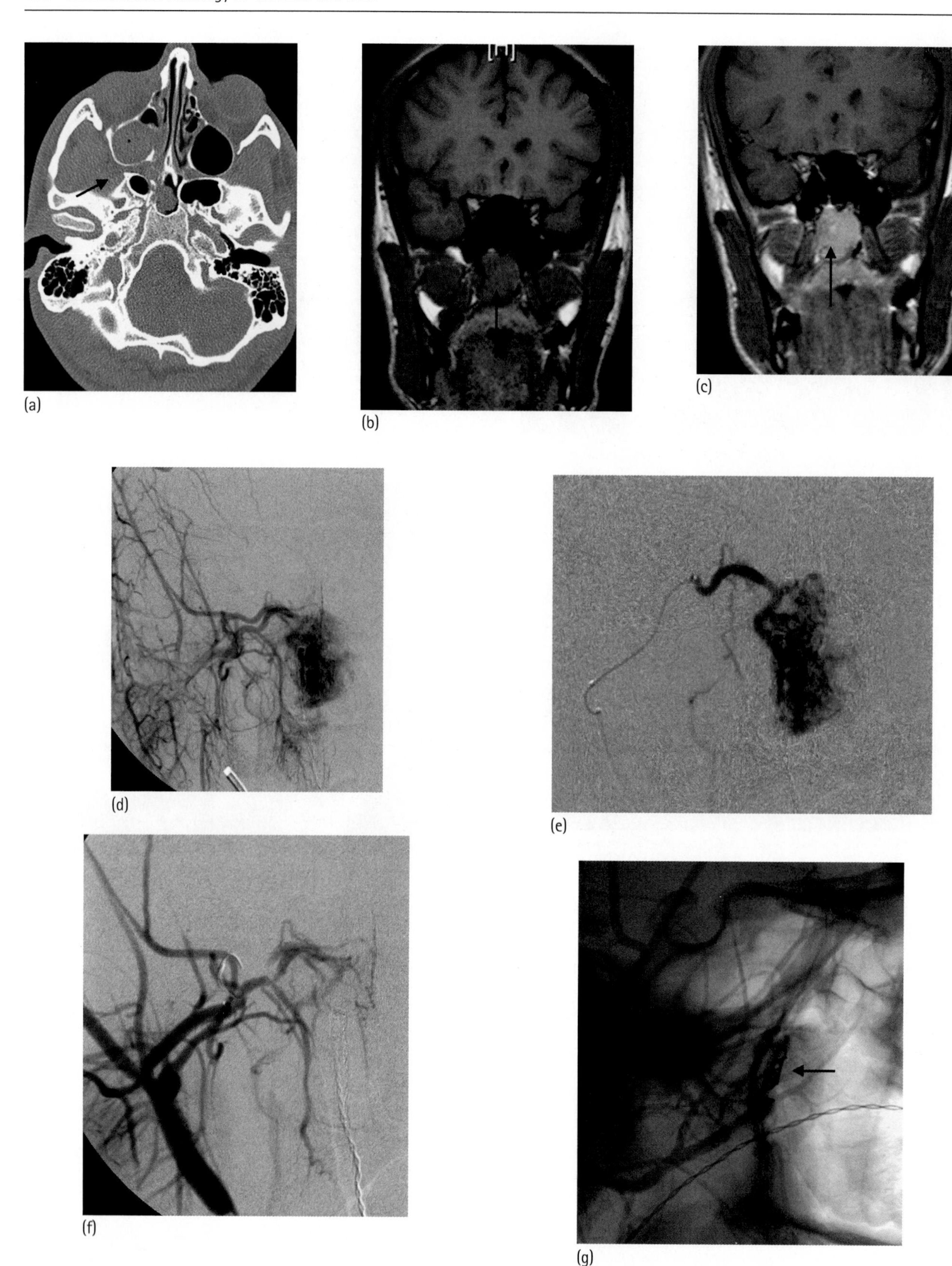

6.2.2 Juvenile angiofibroma. Axial CT (a) reveals characteristic enlargement of pterygomaxillary fissure. Coronal MRI before and after contrast (b,c) delineate a brightly enhancing mass in the posterior nasal space. Frontal selective and superselective DSA (d,e) show typical tumour blush. Pre-operative, superselective embolization of tumour with PVA and coils (f,g). (Photography courtesy of Dr Adam Ditchfield, Wessex Neurological Centre, Southampton, UK).

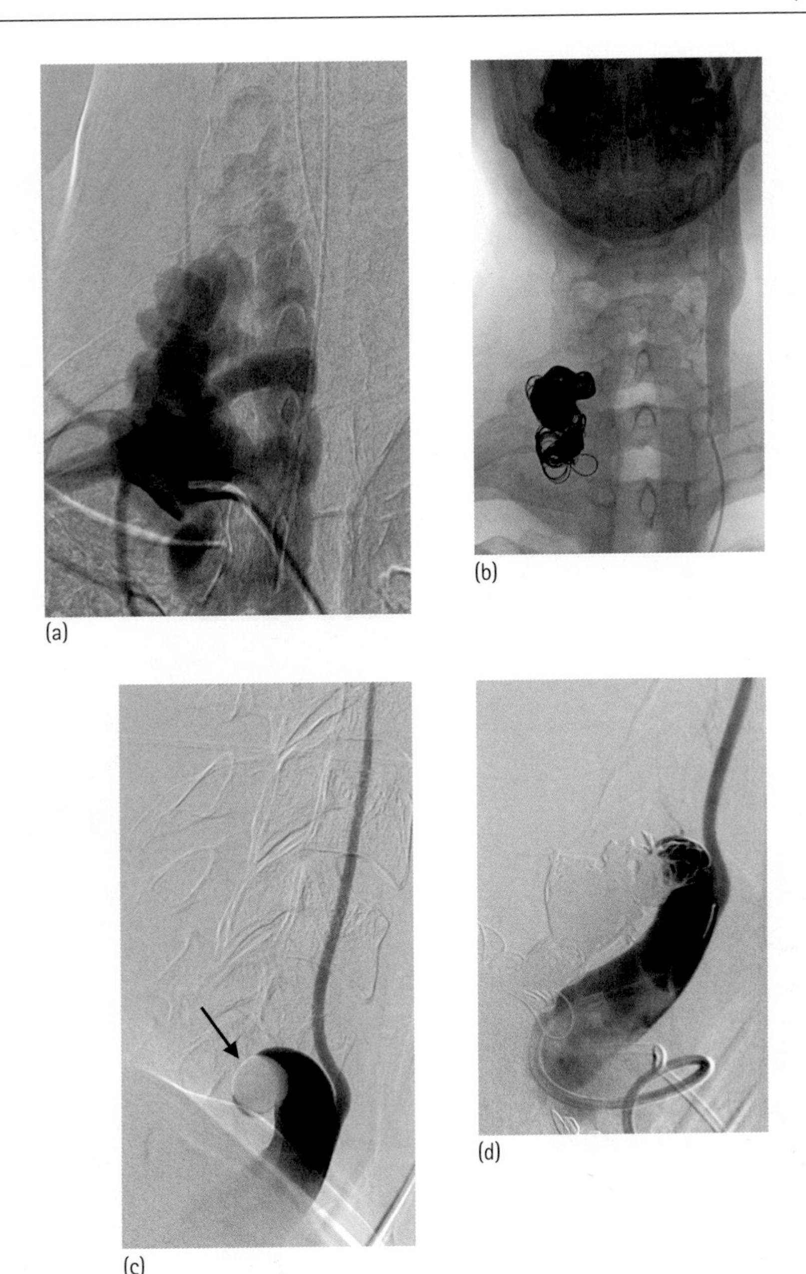

6.2.3 Large hole, congenital vertebro-vertebral arteriovenous fistula (AVF). Frontal DSA before and after (a,b) curative coil embolization with detachable coils. The shunt was so rapid that coil occlusion had to be performed with temporary balloon occlusion (c, arrow) in order to reduce the risk of inadvertent coil embolization to the spinal veins or pulmonary circulation. (d) Fistula occluded by coils (8.5 m), temporary balloon deflated; normal caliber, distal vertebral artery preserved.

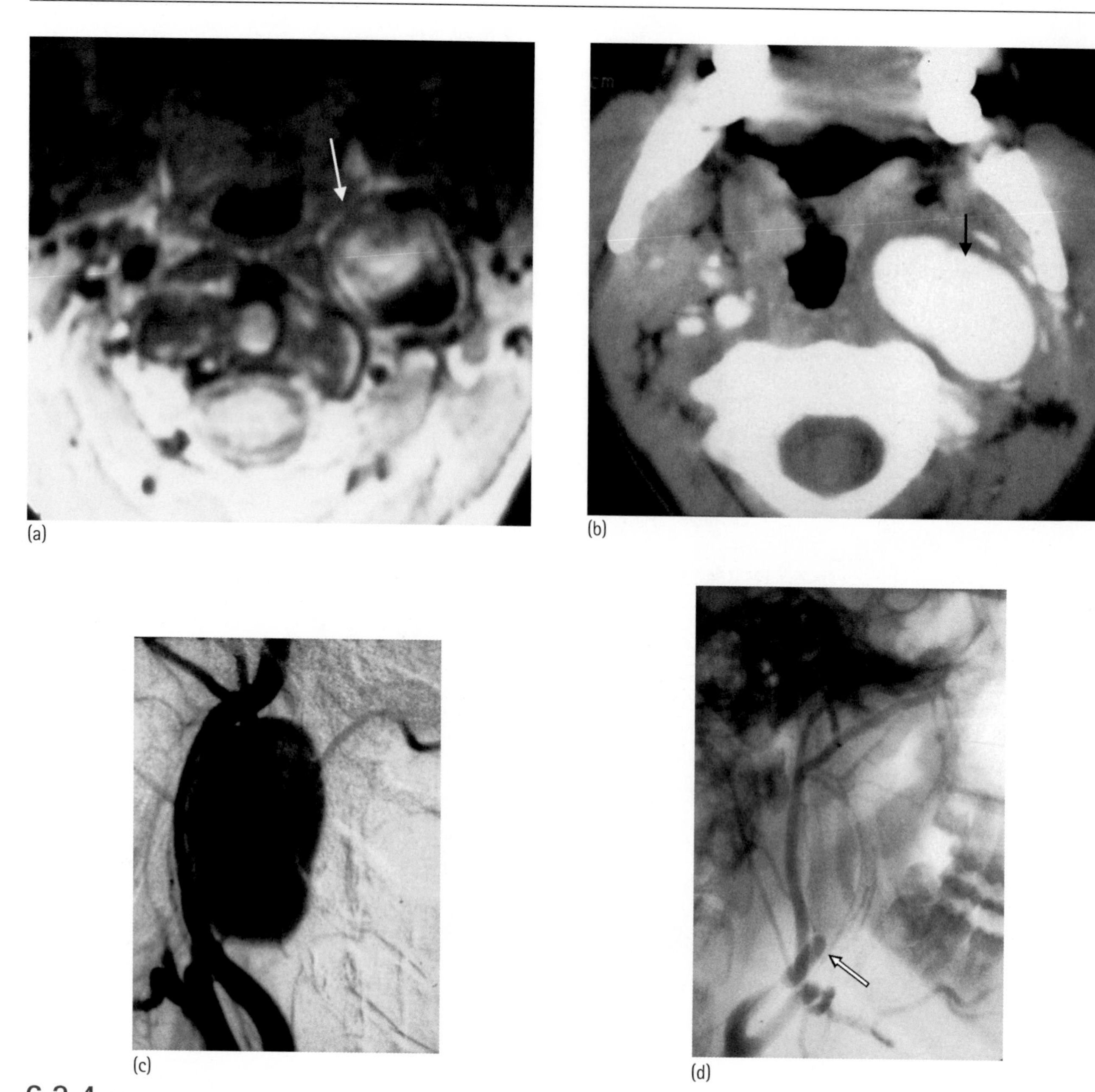

6.2.4 Giant dissecting aneurysm of the cervical internal carotid artery following trauma. Mixed signal intensity mass on axial T1W MRI (a) due to turbulent flow. Bright, uniform enhancement on axial contrast enhanced computed tomography (CECT) (b). Lateral DSA before and after balloon occlusion (c,d, arrow indicates position of balloon following detachment).

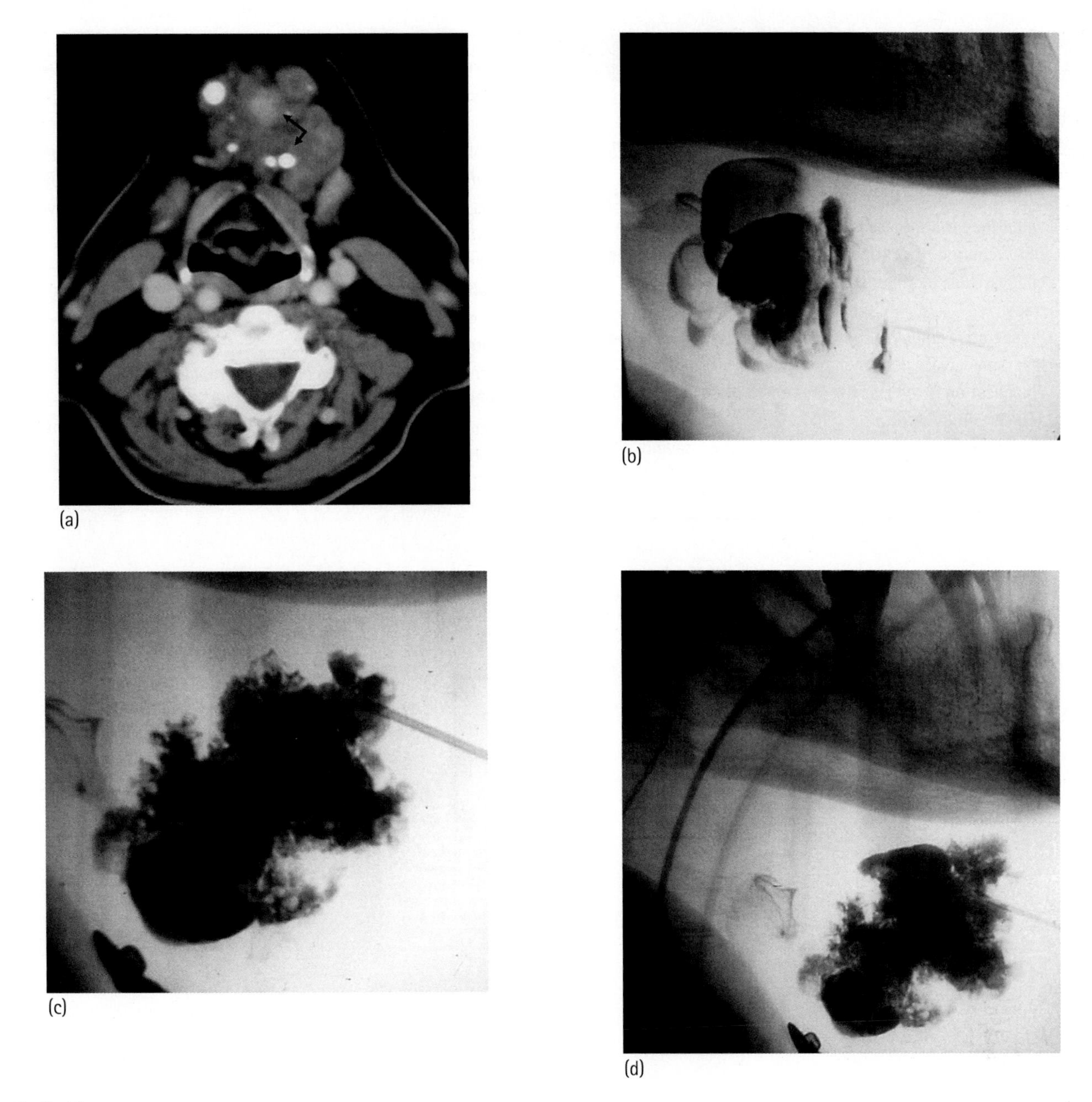

(a)

(b)

(c)

(d)

6.2.5 Large submental, venous malformation. Axial CT reveals characteristic phleboliths and venous lakes (arrows, a). Direct, percutaenous venography confirms slowly emptying venous venous lakes (b). Pre-operative embolization with cyanoacrylate/lipiodol (c,d).

Top tips

Investigation
- Signal void on MRI – consider high flow vascular lesion, calcification or gas.
- CT and contrast enhanced computed tomography (CECT) will differentiate these conditions.
- DSA required to define angioarchitecture and guide endovascular treatment.

Therapy
- Preoperative embolization can significantly reduce blood loss in hypervascular lesions.
- Embolization is the curative treatment of choice for AVF and certain AVMs.
- Emergency embolization may be life saving in uncontrolled haemorrhage.

FURTHER READING

Berenstein A, Lasjaunias P. *Surgical neuro-angiography*, vols 1–5. Berlin: Springer-Verlag, 1987–92.

Connors JJ, Wojak JC. *Interventional neuroradiology: Strategies and practical techniques*. Philadelphia: WB Saunders, 1999.

Morris P. *Interventional and endovascular therapy of the nervous system. A practical guide*. New York: Springer, 2002.

Mulliken JB, Glowacki J. Hemangiomas and vascular malformations in infants and children: A classification based on endothelial characteristics. *Plastic and Reconstructive Surgery* 1982; **69**: 412–22.

Osborn AG. *Diagnostic cerebral angiography*. Philadelphia: Lippincott, 2000.

Yousem DM. *Head and neck imaging (Neuroimaging clinics of North America)*. Philadelphia: WB Saunders, 1996.

PART 7

TRAUMA

7.1

Assessment and initial management

MOHAN F PATEL

INTRODUCTION

The facial soft tissues and underlying facial bony skeleton are at once the most important and most vulnerable portion of the human body. Here the personality is perceived and the senses reside, but it is also here that accident and assault most frequently occur.

Some compensation for this is found in the ready access of the area for examination, and the obvious familiarity of the structures. The facial skeleton is also largely subcutaneous and readily amenable to direct and indirect repair.

The initial temptation to allow spectacular and disfiguring facial injuries to override measured surgical practice must be resisted.

The proactive and comprehensive systems taught on all advanced trauma life support (ATLS) and trauma skills courses are followed with prompt, appropriate and structured assessment and action with constant reappraisal of the patient's condition.

GENERAL ASSESSMENT

The care of the trauma patient arriving in an accident and emergency unit can be broken down into four elements:

1. A primary survey is carried out, in which the so-called ABCs are assessed and if necessary dealt with immediately.
   - A (airway): The oronasal airway is assessed, foreign bodies cleared, blood and inspissated secretions aspirated: a check is made that a potentially unstable cervical spine fracture is not displaced.
   - B (breathing): This is checked to ensure that the apparently clear airway is functioning. At this stage, assisted respiration and ventilation with necessary intubation or tracheal access surgery may be required.
   - C (circulation): The presence of an adequate blood circulation is assessed and any significant haemorrhage is controlled, usually by pressure.
2. The second element is resuscitation of the patient and includes the constant reassessment of problems identified in the primary survey, with continuation of care. Treatment of shock is commenced, including the placement of vascular lines, urinary catheters and nasogastric tubes if appropriate, and ECG monitoring. In the case of multisystem trauma, emergency screening radiography is carried out to include lateral cervical spine, chest and pelvic x-rays.
3. The third element of the trauma patient's care is a consolidation exercise where a thorough total examination of the patient is carried out as a 'secondary survey'.
4. In the fourth element, definitive care will be decided by specialist teams, and it may be necessary to transfer the patient for this (for example, to a maxillofacial or neurosurgical unit). The primary survey is usually carried out by the frontline team in the accident and emergency department, while maxillofacial surgeons will require to undertake a secondary survey prior to the definitive management of maxillofacial injuries.

After the initial care of the trauma and before the patient is passed to specialist maxillofacial assessment and initial management, it is worth considering a number of topics in more detail.

CERVICAL SPINE INJURIES

It should be assumed that any significant maxillofacial injury may be associated with a cervical spine injury. Care, therefore must be taken when the head and neck are manipulated during maintenance of the airway, examination and radiology. A lateral view of the cervical spine showing all cervical vertebrae must be examined and if there is a high index of suspicion, then cervical anterioposterior and open mouth odontoid views should also be taken. Confirmation of a cervical spine injury may require simple tomography or computed tomography (CT) scanning. Where there is doubt, the opinion of a neurosurgeon should be sought, and the use of a semi-rigid cervical collar considered in the interim.

SKULL FRACTURES

Although these fractures are not invariably involved with brain injury, they provide a significant index of suspicion with regard to present or future neurological deficit or the presence of developing haematomas.

Skull vault fractures may be linear when they will often require no direct treatment, or depressed, when they may require elevation. Basal fractures are often diagnosed by a leakage of cerebrospinal fluid, a classic bruising in the mastoid area (Battle's sign) or blood sequestered behind the tympanic membrane. Skull fractures which expose the brain or dura require early surgery. Patients with head injuries require continuous assessment and reassessment of their neurological status and this monitoring may be done by the use of a combination of the Glasgow Coma Scale (GCS), pupillary assessment and extremity weakness. Abnormal and particularly deteriorating results of these assessments should raise suspicion of neurological damage or of a developing space-occupying lesion.

Glasgow Coma Scale

This system of assessment works on the basis of numbers being allocated to a spectrum of grades of neurological responses, including eye opening, best motor response and best verbal response. The scores for the three groups are summated as the GCS. When these assessments are repeated, a trend towards improvement or deterioration can clearly be seen and appropriate action taken.

- Eye opening is graded 1–4 as follows:
  1 = no eye opening;
  2 = opening to pain;
  3 = opening to speech;
  4 = spontaneous opening.
- The best motor response is graded on limb movements from 1 to 6:
  1 = no movement;
  2 = extensor response only;
  3 = abnormal flexion;
  4 = withdrawal from painful stimuli;
  5 = movement towards painful stimuli;
  6 = movement of limb on command.
- Capability of verbal response is graded from 1 to 5:
  1 = no verbal response;
  2 = inarticulate sound;
  3 = recognizable words inappropriately uttered;
  4 = confused conversation;
  5 = fully orientated.

Patients with GCS <8 are in a coma and have a severe head injury. Those with a GCS of 9–12 are considered to have a moderate head injury and a GCS of 13–15 indicates a minor head injury

Pupillary assessment

Pupil size is measured regularly. A unilaterally enlarged pupil may indicate a contralateral space-occupying lesion. It is helpful to know from relatives or friends if the patient had a disparate pupil size before the trauma. Slow light reactions may indicate brain injury.

Extremity weakness

Equal movement of limbs on both sides is looked for, while a lateralizing weakness suggests contralateral brain injury.

The use of GCS, pupillary assessment and extremity weakness assessment together provides a sensitive and easily understood neurological monitoring system.

OCULAR INJURY

The proximity of swelling, bruising, lacerations and facial fractures around the orbits and the type of trauma suffered will give some indication as to the likelihood of eye injury. If there is any doubt, an ophthalmologist must be asked to see the patient, and guidance sought as to whether exploration of the orbit surgically might be required.

The eyelids, conjunctiva, cornea and globe should be grossly examined for damage, and particularly for lacerations. Visual fields in both eyes should be grossly measured, with the patient wearing glasses where appropriate, either counting fingers at a distance or reading newspaper print. The pupils are assessed for normal shape and light response. The eye should be examined with an opthalmoscope for internal derangement. Flaccidity of the globe on palpitation may indicate a laceration.

PREGNANCY

There will be some obvious differences in assessing the pregnant woman. Where x-rays are essential, they should be taken and an obstetrician requested to see the patient as soon as possible.

TRAUMATIZED CHILDREN

It is often difficult to examine a traumatized and distressed child accurately and a history may be impossible to obtain. In view of the child's small size and incompletely calcified skeleton, there is often a higher chance of organ damage, while paradoxically the skeleton is more often spared than in adults. A thorough examination and the advice of a paediatrician is therefore essential and in most hospitals a paediatric team will wish to become closely involved with the child's management. It should be remembered that in view of a child's relatively large surface area in proportion to body volume, loss of heat may occur more rapidly than with an adult, and the smaller blood volume can result in a child becoming shocked with what appears to be a relatively small blood loss in adult terms. It should be remembered that a distressed and terrified child can be severely traumatized psychologically, as well as physically, and sympathetic management should reflect this concern.

ABDOMINAL TRAUMA

It can be easy for occult abdominal damage to remain so until the patient descends into extremis or death, and it is therefore important that the abdomen is examined thoroughly and then reassessed. A history of trauma to, or pain from, the abdomen should be noted and the abdomen inspected for wounds and contusions. A careful auscultation should be carried out to assess the presence of bowel sounds which may be absent, as in an ileus owing to peritoneal irritation by blood or bowel contents, or extra-abdominal injury to the spine. Gentle palpation will elicit pain, and involuntary muscle guarding is a sign of underlying peritoneal irritation. A routine rectal examination may show blood from a bowel perforation or more local damage.

LARYNGOTRACHEAL DISRUPTION

Fractures of the larynx are uncommon and are indicated by emphysema, hoarseness and local crepitus. Loud tracheal breath sounds may indicate partial obstruction of the airway that may be followed by a complete cessation of sounds when total obstruction occurs. Use of endoscopy to assess tracheal damage is often invaluable.

Obstruction in the trachea and upper airway can be overcome with a number of surgical interventions depending on the severity of the obstruction and its level. A needle cricothyroidotomy with jet insufflation of oxygen (Figure 7.1.1) can be a useful emergency measure and allows for formal tracheostomy to be carried out in a less hurried fashion.

Apart from respiratory obstruction, tracheostomy may be indicated in patients where there are flail segments or lung contusion or in severe head injury cases. This procedure, which can be carried out under either local or general anaesthesia, should be in the armamentarium of all surgeons. The technique is fundamentally a simple one. However, for most surgeons who do not perform it regularly, the procedure can be more testing than textbooks suggest. A conscious patient is likely to be distressed and after trauma the neck can be engorged with oedema fluid and blood. Bearing this in mind if a methodical approach is taken, the procedure is usually accomplished successfully.

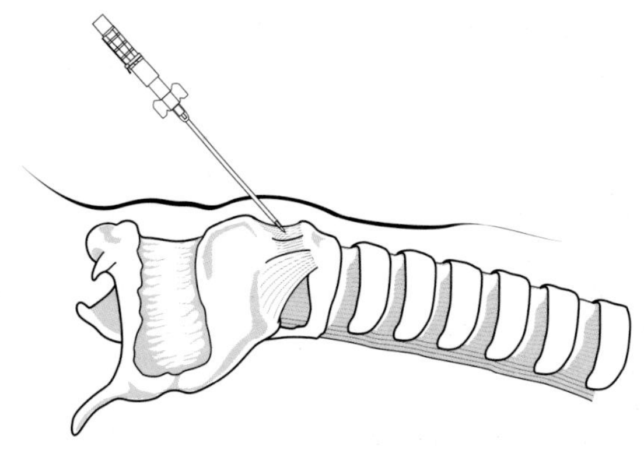

7.1.1 Jet insufflation of oxygen via a needle cricothroidotomy.

MAXILLOFACIAL ASSESSMENT AND INITIAL MANAGEMENT

Maxillofacial injuries often excite considerable anxiety amongst clinical and nursing members of the trauma team, due to the grotesque swelling and bruising with which they are associated. The majority of road trauma and interpersonal violence cases are associated with maxillofacial head injuries to a greater or lesser extent and it is important therefore that these injuries are treated practically and without mystique.

The very real risk to both the nasal and oral airway in severe injuries gives additional concern, and the temptation to employ the aphorism that 'the injury invariably looks worse than it is' should be resisted. Although this is often the case, a careful check using the fundamental ABC system can prove life-saving.

Fractures of the facial bones are often difficult for other clinicians to understand, owing to the close juxtaposition of intricate bony complexes and the need to comprehend these in three dimensions. In addition, the difficulty of obtaining good quality diagnostic radiographs, particularly late at night, of a swollen patient in pain, and often without a specialist radiographer, can make diagnosis yet more fraught.

We have discussed the importance of first identifying collateral injuries before concentrating on the maxillofacial region. However, once potentially life-threatening injuries have been identified and controlled, maxillofacial injuries must be accurately assessed. These may be broadly divided into lacerations of the soft tissues of the scalp, face and neck, and fractures of the facial skeleton. It should be remembered that there is often a direct relationship between an overlying laceration and an underlying fracture.

LACERATIONS OF SOFT TISSUE

These wounds cause a discontinuity in the soft tissue at any level, from superficial skin abrasions to deep cuts, and may open up a number of tissue planes. They may be clean, contused or puncture wounds, or any combination of these three.

Initially, any significant haemorrhage should be controlled with pressure. The presence of foreign bodies or the involvement of important underlying structures and any loss of tissue can then be assessed. The possibility of infection must not be overlooked, and although clean, noncontused wounds may not require antibiotics, old or dirty wounds or those occurring in a medically compromised patient, such as a diabetic, should be 'covered' by antibiotic prophylaxis.

Contused, deep or puncture wounds, especially those occurring in the open air or as part of a multiplicity of injuries, require an assessment of the patient's tetanus immunization status. The use of tetanus immune globulin (TIG) rarely causes adverse reactions and may be considered for individual patients. If the patient has received two or more injections of toxoid in the past, TIG is only indicated if the wound is tetanus-prone or over 24 hours old. The use of equine tetanus antitoxin is potentially hazardous.

Repair of lacerations

Uncomplicated lacerations in cooperative adults and older children are usually treated well and promptly under local analgesia. The use of general anaesthesia may be necessary for complex lacerations, particularly where there is skin loss, or simple lacerations in young uncooperative children.

The wound should first be carefully examined to enable the removal of foreign bodies (soft tissue radiographs may help to locate radio-opaque material). Tissue with poor viability may require clean excision, but a most conservative approach must be taken in the facial region, where every effort should be made to conserve soft tissue.

Dirt should be thoroughly removed from wounds to prevent skin tattooing and a sterile nail brush should be used with dilute chlorhexidine solution to thoroughly remove any such debris, followed by copious irrigation with sterile normal saline.

Haemostasis should be obtained by electrocoagulation for small vessel bleeds and ties used for bleeds from larger vessels.

The cleansed wound is first loosely assembled, in order that an assessment of any tissue loss can be made. If the wound can be brought together with only moderate tension after wide undermining of the adjacent tissue if necessary, then primary closure should be carried out. If an aesthetic and functional primary closure is not possible, consideration of grafting procedures or flap development should be considered, and this is likely to be scheduled as a further elective procedure. This may involve the use of split or full-thickness skin grafts, local rotation flaps, distant pedicled flaps or free flaps with microvascular anastomosis. In these instances, temporary closure of a wound will reduce the possibility of infection or haemorrhage, while arrangements for definitive treatment are made.

When dealing with lacerations in the facial region, it is essential to assess the integrity of the facial nerve, particularly where damage to the parotid gland has occurred. Where nerve division has occurred, the nerve ends may either be repaired immediately or tagged (with a suture) for future repair, including grafting.

Lacerations in the cheek may also damage the parotid duct requiring repair over a fine catheter.

Injuries to the eyelids must be associated with careful examination to rule out damage to the globe and lacrimal duct injuries.

MAXILLOFACIAL FRACTURES

The facial skeleton is arbitrarily divided into the upper third or frontal bone, middle third or bony skeleton, from the frontal bone down to the upper alveolus, and the lower third or mandible.

Upper third fractures are usually linear cracks or bony depressions over the frontal sinuses. Middle third fractures result in detachment of this portion of the facial skeleton to a greater or lesser extent from the rest through the areas of anatomical weakness identified by Le Fort during his cadaver studies, and which are illustrated in Figure 7.1.2.

Severe displacement of the middle third of the facial skeleton can result in the detached portion being thrust backwards down the inclined slope of the base of the skull, causing the classic 'dished-in' facies. There is also a danger that this posterior movement of the midfacial skeleton might close off the nasopharyngeal airway. This should be assessed promptly in the primary survey of the trauma

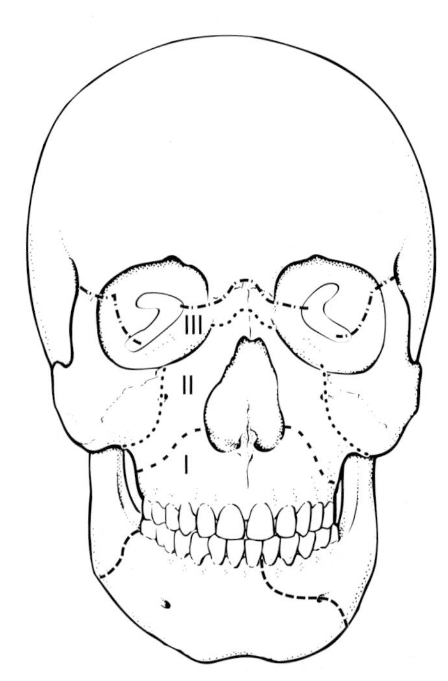

7.1.2 Le Fort low (I), middle (II) and high (III) fracture lines. The mandible exhibits right angle and left parasymphyseal fracture lines.

patient, and can be rectified either by attempting to draw the posteriorly impacted bony complex forward by finger pressure around the hard palate and tuberosities, or by prompt tracheostomy.

Fractures of the middle third of the facial skeleton should be considered as a combination of the major lamella displacements described by Le Fort, and of damage to the specialized bony complexes which we recognize as the dentoalveolar, mid-maxillary, malar, nasal and orbital complexes. Fractures at more than one Le Fort level or at different levels on separate sides are common. Specialized complexes may be damaged in isolation or in any combination.

Mandibular fractures are notated by site, as condylar, ramus, angle, body or parasymphaseal fractures. The combination of parasymphaseal and angle fracture occurs most commonly, and it is wise always to look for more than one mandibular fracture.

Fractures of the maxilla and mandible occur in numerous combinations, often with comminution and, whilst rarely compound in the maxilla, are invariably so in the mandible, along the roots of the teeth into the mouth.

Assessment

A clinical assessment for fractures of the facial skeleton is usually best carried out systematically from above downwards, starting with a careful examination and palpation of the cranium, gently probing through any lacerations, where present, for underlying bony damage.

Next, the orbital rims are examined with the nasal skeleton, malar bodies and zygomatic arches. Tenderness and step deformities or swellings will usually betray underlying fractures.

When the facial skeleton from the front has been viewed, a further examination should be made by the physician standing behind the seated patient: looking down on the facial skeleton from above can be revealing. Nasal deviation or depression and flattening over the malar prominences can be seen, as can 'thumb print' depressions over the zygomatic arch. It is always wise to question the patient with regard to previous nasal fractures that can otherwise be deceptive.

The dentition and alveolus must be carefully checked for fractured or missing teeth and radiographs of lacerated soft tissue or chest and abdominal films used to reveal the presence of avulsed teeth or dental prostheses.

The mandible is carefully examined by palpation, feeling for step defects; intraorally the occlusion is examined for discontinuity. The patient will be able to perceive any small disruption in the occlusion accurately. The presence of lacerations or ecchymosis in the buccal or lingual sulci often indicates underlying mandibular fractures.

Le Fort fractures

The appearance of bilateral orbital ecchymosis and oedema of the soft tissues of the face, with disruption of the nasal skeleton, and the presence of blood in the nostrils is quite characteristic of this type of pan-midface fracture (Figure 7.1.3). The maxilla is often mobile and a cerebrospinal fluid (CSF) rhinorrhoea or otorrhoea should be looked for. If the 'examining' hand grasps the upper alveolus and gently but firmly moves it, whilst the 'watching' hand palpates at Le Fort I, II and III levels in turn, some idea of the extent of the mid-face injuries can be ascertained.

Malar complex

These fractures (Figure 7.1.4) are characterized clinically by a flattening over the malar prominence or zygomatic arch that can be obscured by oedema, and a difficulty in moving the jaw when the coronoid process impinges on a depressed zygomatic arch. Circumorbital and subjunctival ecchymosis may be present, with limitation of eye movements where there has been muscle trapping, often the inferior rectus in fractures of the floor of the orbit. A step defect is usually palpable in the inferior rim of the orbit and there is frequently numbness over the distribution of the inferior orbital nerve ipsilaterally.

There may be diplopia, often owing to oedema or displacement of the orbital complex, but sometimes owing to detachment of suspensory ligaments of the globe. The globe should be examined by an ophthalmologist to rule out internal derangement. Malar complex fractures and those of the orbit are frequently associated with subconjunctival

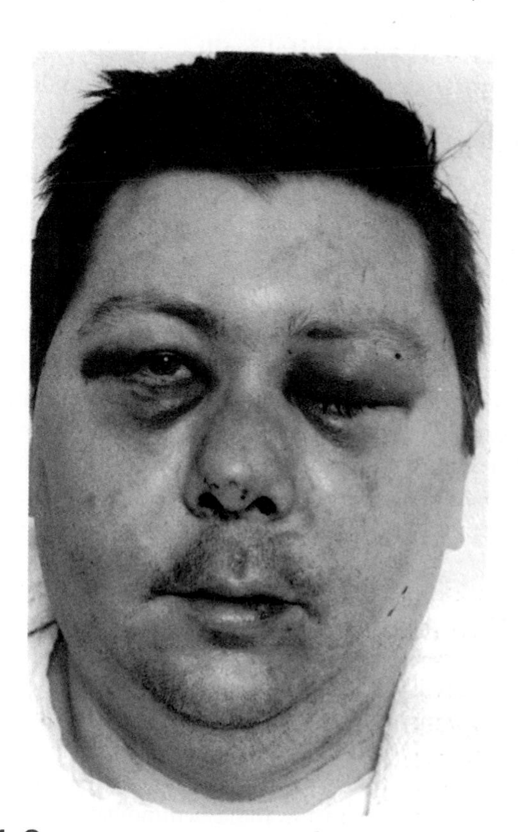

7.1.3 Classic appearance of panfacial fractures (at all Le Fort levels).

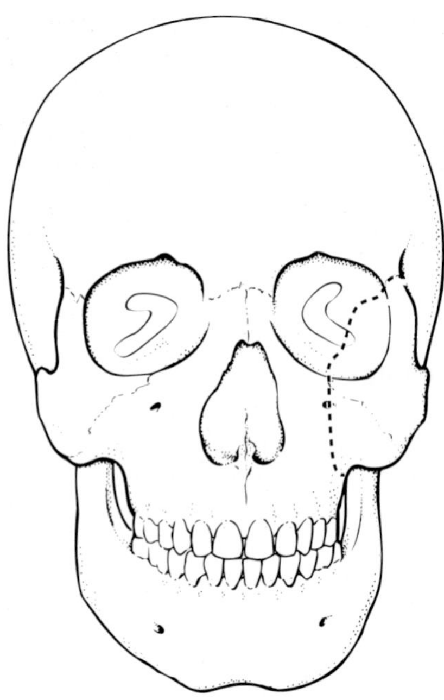

7.1.4 Malar complex fracture.

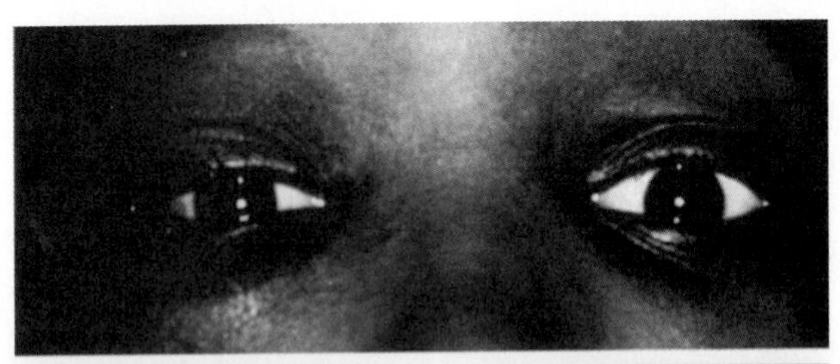
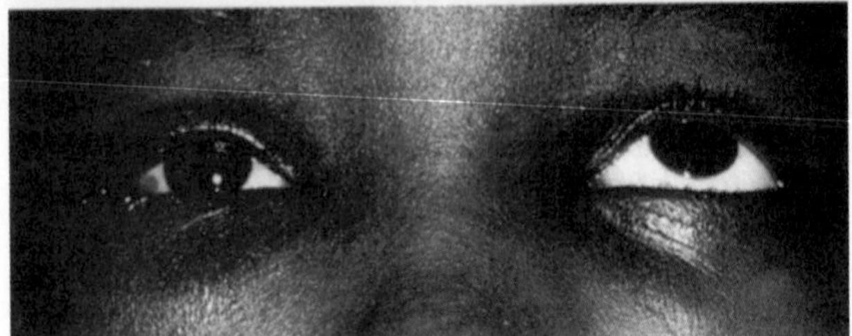

7.1.5 Tethering of inferior rectus muscle on upward gaze after orbital floor 'blow-out' fracture.

ecchymosis, which has no posterior margin extending as it does from the depths of the orbit posteriorly. Punctate subconjunctival ecchymosis occurs when a blow to the eye causes the extravasation of blood below the conjunctiva related locally to the blow.

Fractures of the orbital walls

The paper thin bones of the floor of the orbit also form the roof of the antrum and are in continuity with the zygomatic complex. Fractures to the fragile floor of the orbit also occur in isolation, particularly when there is direct blunt trauma to the globe itself which, by displacement or distortion of the globe, 'blows out' the vulnerable bone of the orbital floor. On these occasions, a herniation of periorbital fat and the inferior rectus muscle may occur, often with a restriction of eye movement, particularly on upward gaze (Figure 7.1.5), and a lowering of pupillary height on the affected side. Enophthalmos can present either early or late. The thin medial wall of the orbit is also prone to being 'blown in', with a commensurate increase in orbital volume and a danger of late enopthalmos.

Nasal skeletal fractures

Bilateral circumorbital ecchymosis is pathognomonic of this type of fracture, along with a deviation of the nose laterally where lateral force has been applied, or resulting in the collapse of the nose where the trauma has occurred anteriorly. Epistaxis occurs invariably. In nasoethmoidal disjunction, the damage must be analysed carefully in order to plan satisfactory reconstruction. In addition, damage involving the cribriform plate may be signalled by cerebrospinal fluid leak, and can result in anosmia.

Fractures of the mandible

These fractures are normally easy to elicit, particularly in the dentate patient. There is an inability to close the teeth into normal occlusion, with commensurate discomfort over the fracture site. Often, and particularly when there has been distraction at the fracture site, there can be anaesthesia of the lower lip on the affected side, from inferior alveolar neuropraxia. Where fractures of the body of the mandible have occurred, this can often be identified by bleeding from tears in the overlying mucosa. Step defects in the occlusion and lower border of the mandible are usually easily identified.

Radiology

This screen of radiographs should provide adequate views for an initial diagnosis to be made:

- submentovertical;
- occipitomental;
- lateral skull;
- orthopantomogram of the mandible or, if not available, the following mandibular views used in isolation or combination:
  - posterioanterior view;
  - lateral oblique views;
  - reverse Townes view.

As we have noted earlier, the possibility of cervical spine injury must first be excluded by clinical examination and, if appropriate, cervical spine views.

The submentovertical view provides a 'skyline' view of the zygomatic arches (Figure 7.1.6) showing the arches and any displacement. The occipitomental views show the integrity of the orbital rim and floor, providing further useful views of the zygomatic arches and will clarify the outline of the antral walls and the presence of fluid levels in the sinuses. The so-called 'hanging drop' sign caused by soft tissue herniating through the floor of the orbit into the antrum below is best seen in this view (Figure 7.1.7).

Fractures of the nasal bones and posterior maxilla can be seen on the lateral skull view. If nasal bone fractures are suspected, a 'soft tissue' lateral will often show these clearly. The orthopantomogram allows fractures of the basal bones of the mandible, the teeth and alveolus to be assessed (Figure 7.1.8). As this latter view is tomographic, remember that there is always a danger of information outside the 'focal trough' not being reproduced.

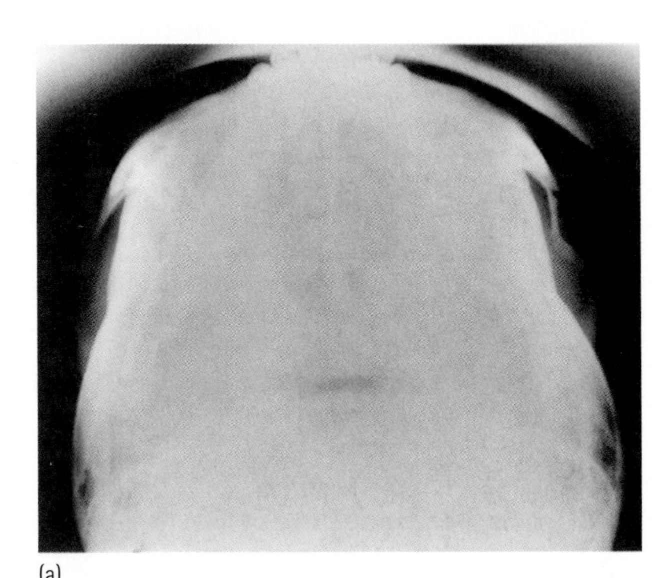

(a)

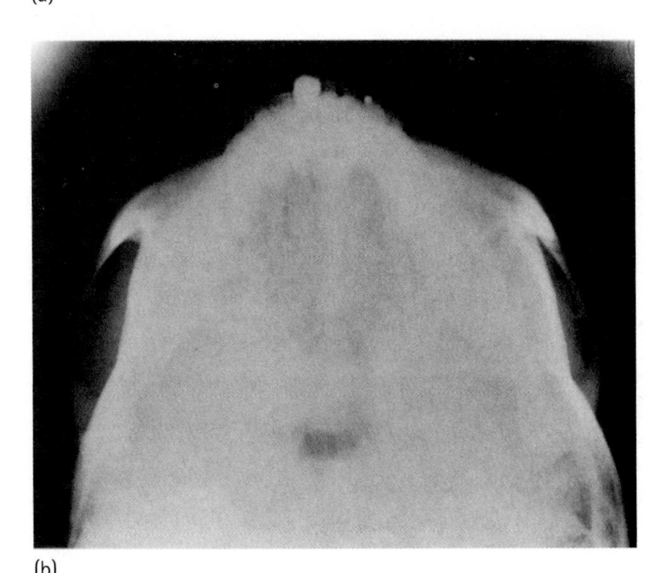

(b)

7.1.6 Submentovertical view clearly showing (a) the pre-operative crumpled and (b) post-operative reduced left zygomatic arch as 'sky-line views'.

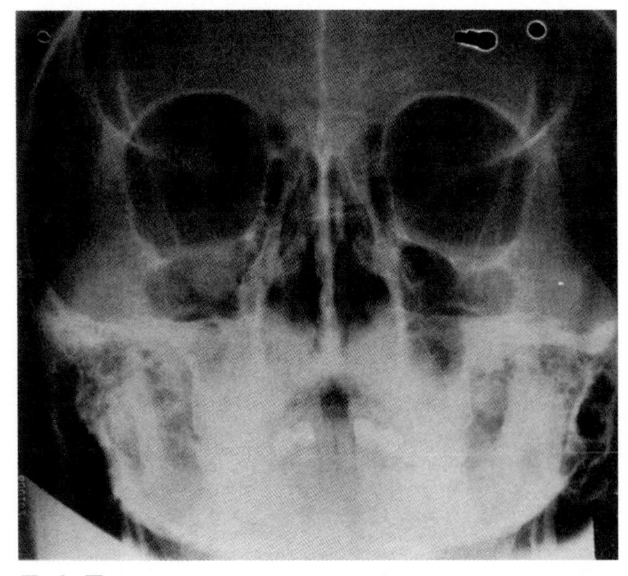

7.1.7 Herniation of fat through fractured right orbital floor, giving the classic 'hanging drop' sign.

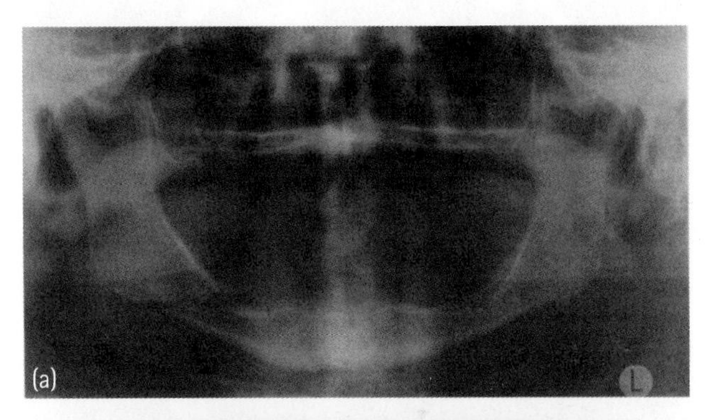

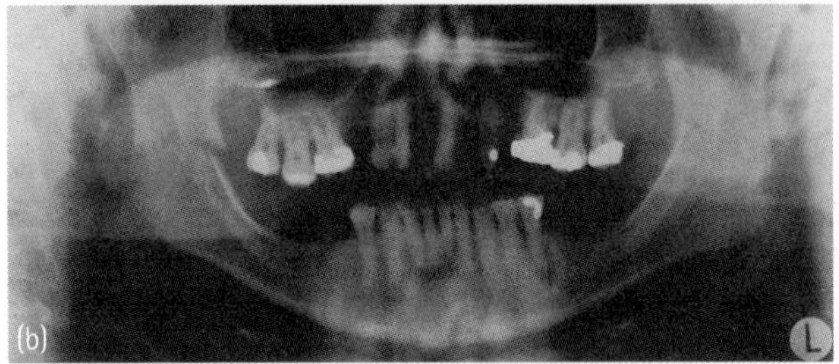

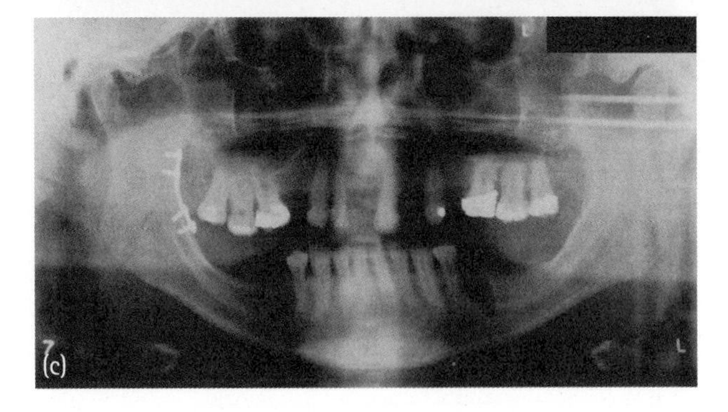

7.1.8 Orthopantomograms illustrating (a) right body fracture in edentulous mandible; (b) right-angle fracture in partially dentate patient; (c) reduction and fixation of fracture in (b) using miniplate osteosynthesis.

The plain films here are important for the diagnosis and localization of fractures of the facial skeleton. In order to examine the three-dimensional relationships of the complex facial fractures, CT scans are invaluable, especially with three-dimensional reformatting. In the case of a fracture of the frontal bone over the frontal sinus, for example, a CT scan will show the extent and severity of the injury to the outer bony table and, in addition, define any involvement of the inner table of the sinus wall (Figure 7.1.9).

The increasing use of CT scanning with three-dimensional reformatting, especially with spiral machines, is providing unparalleled imaging of complex fractures of the facial skeleton with the facility for 'virtual' surgery and with the possibility of utilizing the software to mill prostheses to replace large portions of lost bone.

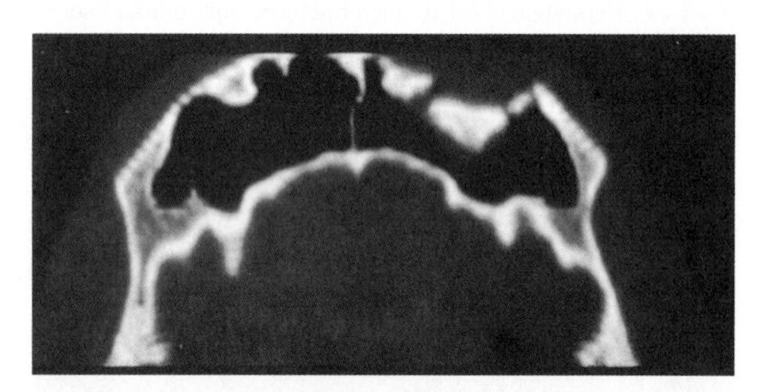

7.1.9 Axial CT scan showing comminution of anterior wall frontal sinus with intact posterior wall.

Top tips

- Remember! Facial lacerations may overlie an underlying fracture.
- Obtaining pretrauma photographs builds empathy with relatives and can act as a useful operating guide.
- Sudden deterioration of an otherwise stable patient prompts reassessment of the primary survey.
- Even severe lacerations are rarely associated with significant tissue loss.
- Check for damage to the lacrimal and parotid ducts and facial nerve branches before closing deep lacerations.

FURTHER READING

Ali T, Shepherd JP. The measurement of injury severity. *British Journal of Oral and Maxillofacial Surgery* 1994; **32**: 13–18.

American College of Surgeons. *Advanced trauma life support for doctors.* Chicago, IL: American College of Surgeons.

Key SJ, Thomas DW, Shepherd JP. The management of soft tissue facial wounds. *British Journal of Oral and Maxillofacial Surgery* 1995; **33**: 76–85.

Marks PV, Lavy CBD. *A practical guide to head injury.* London: WB Saunders, 1992.

Mok D,. Kreel L. *Essential radiology in head injury.* Oxford: Heinemann Medical Books, 1988.

Russell C, Matta B. *Tracheostomy: A multiprofessional handbook.* London: Greenwich Medical Media, 2004.

7.2

Contemporary maxillofacial fixation techniques

DOMENICK P COLETTI

INTRODUCTION

Hippocrates was the first to emphasize the importance of reduction and immobilization of the mandible fracture, with the use of the interdental 'bridal wire'. As time passed, closed reduction and stabilization with maxillomandibular fixation (MMF) was introduced by techniques such as external bandages (i.e. the Barton bandage), internal splints (i.e. Gunning splints), external frame and pin fixation, and various forms of interdental wiring. These techniques rely on secondary bone healing, but have limited application in modern practice, because of the delayed return of function and higher rates of infection, malunion, nonunion and malocclusion. This led to the development of open reduction and internal fixation techniques, which provides anatomical reduction and stabilization, in turn optimizing primary bone healing.

One of the earlier forms of internal fixation was the use of transosseous wires, a semi-rigid form of fixation, which was an effective technique for its time, and is occasionally still employed. In the 1960 and 1970s, this technique was replaced with the advent of plates and screws. These early plating techniques were first adopted from orthopaedic experience with the treatment of long bone fractures. However, large compression plates, which used bicortical screws that were placed along the inferior border of the mandible splayed the superior aspect of the fracture. Compression plates apply force to areas of the mandible which are already under biomechanical compression. Eccentric dynamic compression plates were then developed to attempt to counteract these distaction forces, but were too cumbersome and technique sensitive.

More recent advancements in plating techniques have provided many different forms of plating technology to the surgeon including nonlocking plates, threaded locking plates, tapered locking plates, bicortical and monocortical fixation, rigid and semi-rigid plates. In order to achieve a level of excellence for each patient, today's surgeon must not only understand each type of technique, but also appreciate the advantages and disadvantages of each, as well as their basic principles of management. The goals of treatment should be as follows:

- anatomic reduction and stabilization of fractures;
- preservation of facial dimensions;
- establish and preserve the occlusion;
- early return to function;
- avoidance of infection.

Understanding these goals is paramount and the surgeon must weigh the risks against the benefits of the proposed management. The objective of this chapter is to provide the clinician with an overview of the advancements made in maxillofacial fixation and the types of techniques available.

CLOSED TREATMENT FIXATION

Arch bars

Maxillomandibular fixation is a hallmark principle of maxillofacial trauma which uses the patient's occlusion to establish the proper reduction and stabilization of facial fractures, thus providing a foundation to reconstruct facial form and function. Various forms of MMF have been described in the literature, e.g. eyelet loops, skeletal suspension wires and Erich arch bars. Arch bars are currently the workhorse for MMF, they are applied using circumdental wires (Figure 7.2.1). The patient is placed into his premorbid occlusion upon the final tightening of the intra- and interarch wires. Arch bars are valuable in re-establishing the intra-arch contour when managing dentoalveolar fractures and they also serve as a 'tension band' by resisting the forces along the alveolar level of the mandible. They provide a versatile means of directing vectors of forces with a V–W pattern of crossbracing, to assist in fracture reduction and re-establishment of the premorbid occlusion. While arch bars provide an effective means of MMF, their use is not without consequence.

Increased surgical time both in placement and removal, risk of penetrating injury to the surgeon, trauma to the periodontal soft tissue and compromised oral hygiene are all shortcomings of traditional arch bars. Also, arch bar placement in the paediatric patient can be difficult, depending on the patient's age and stage of tooth eruption. The height of contour position and contacts in the primary dentition may prevent the application of circumdental wires. Second, there is the potential for extrusion of the primary tooth upon tightening the wire, especially in the root resorption stage for exfoliation.

Intermaxillary fixation screws

Recently, the introduction of self-drilling/tapping intermaxillary fixation screws (IMF) screws has eliminated some of the problems associated with arch bars (Figure 7.2.2). Many clinicians elect to use them based on a decreased risk of penetrating injury for the user, ease of placement with shorter operating room time, decreased trauma to the periodontium, convenience of maintaining oral hygiene, and the ability to use them both intra-operatively and post-operatively, such as with guiding elastics. The first generations of IMF screws were simply modified monocortical self-tapping screws. Because they required a drilled hole for placement, there were concerns about suboptimal placement and root damage that occurred during placement. The second generation self-drilling/self-tapping screws improved tactile feedback, limiting the possibility of root damage. Additionally, because power equipment is not needed, the system can be used outside the operating room (i.e. in the intensive care unit or emergency department). The manufacturer recommends placing screws above the root apices; however, the author has found that subapical placement led to mucosal overgrowth complicating their removal. Instead the screws should be placed in a bicortical fashion between the roots at the level of the mucogingival junction. It is recommended, if possible, to obtain a panorex film prior to placement of the screws in order to evaluate the root morphology. When possible, at least one screw should be placed proximal and distal to the fracture. However, multiple screws can be placed to direct the vectors of the interarch wires appropriately, which in turn aids in fracture reduction and stabilization. Since their introduction, they have been met with both enthusiasm and criticism. Recent reports have illustrated several inherent risks and limitations which include root injury, screw loosening, screw shearing and aspiration. The self-drilling feature offers a greater degree of tactile feedback during placement, allowing the operator to change insertion location before root damage occurs. In paediatric patients, the IMF screws should be avoided or used with caution to prevent injury to the tooth buds.

External mandibular fixation

External mandibular fixation has played an important role in the management of comminuted mandible fractures, infected mandible fractures and maintaining continuity defects secondary to infected osteoradionecrosis (Figure 7.2.3). However, through the advancements made with rigid fixation, as well as microvascular reconstructive surgery, this technique has waned in its use. In circumstances which are relative contraindications to internal rigid fixation (i.e. infected hardware) where the surgeon is attempting to optimize soft tissue health, the external fixator functions to maintain the mandibular continuity defect, as well as eliminating any foreign body within the wound bed. Once soft tissue stabilization is achieved, the definitive repair can take place and the external fixation removed.

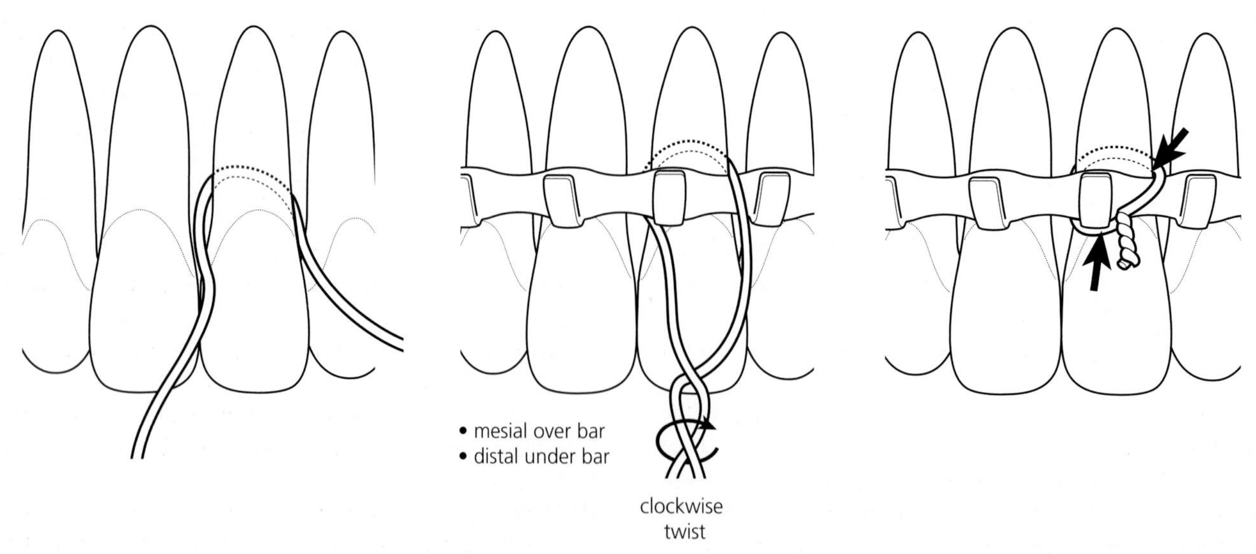

7.2.1 Arch bars.

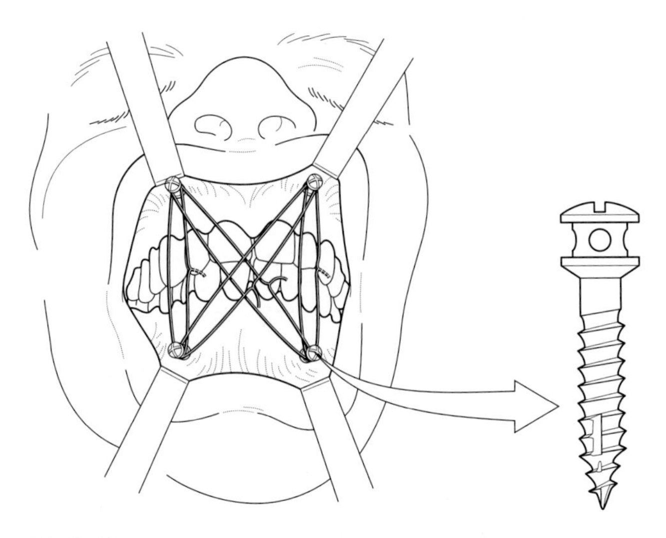

7.2.2 Intermaxillary fixation screws.

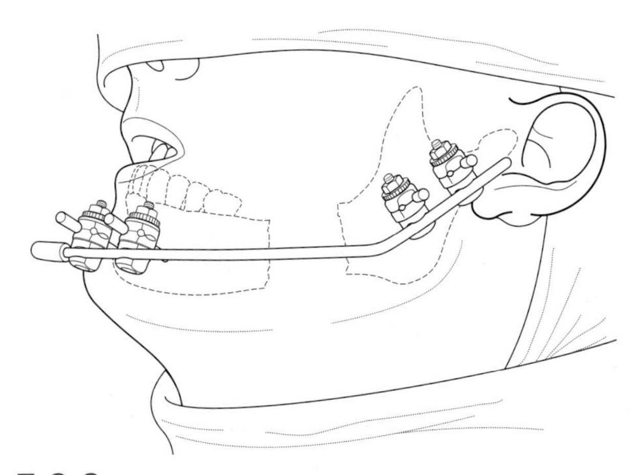

7.2.3 External mandibular fixation.

First-generation external fixators utilized transcutaneous bicortical pins (placed along the inferior border) which were then bridged by filling an endotracheal tube with acrylic resin. Today's second-generation systems still use similar types of pins, but instead use alloy bars or carbon fibre, with locking clamps to finalize the fixation. These fixators are less cumbersome with streamlined instrumentation. One advantage is the ability to perform minor adjustments to address malocclusions, by simply loosening the clamps, placing the patient into MMF and retightening the clamps.

The technique to place the fixator is as follows:

- placement into MMF if indicated;
- palpation of the inferior border proximal and distal to the continuity defect;
- a stab incision with a No. 15 blade where pins are to be placed;
- blunt dissection to the inferior border with a hemostat;
- placement of transcutaneous trocar;
- drill bicortically with appropriate size drill bit;
- measure width of inferior border with depth gauge;
- place appropriate length bicortical pin;
- after all pins are placed, attach clamps and precontoured bar;
- release MMF and verify occlusion.

RIGID INTERNAL FIXATION

Nonlocking plates/screws

Rigid fixation utilizes bicortical screws and rigid plates (2.0–2.4 mm) along the inferior or posterior border of the mandible, with or without a second monocortical plate (typically a miniplate) placed in the subapical region or external oblique ridge. This plate is termed a 'tension band' because of its use in an area of biomechanical tension. Rigid fixation should not require the use of post-operative MMF. Depending upon the circumstance, rigid fixation can be placed either through a transoral/buccal (described below under Miniplate (semi-rigid) fixation) or transcervical approach, the author's approach is as follows:

- Local anaesthesia and muscle relaxation is avoided during this dissection to allow localization and protection of the marginal mandibular branch of the facial nerve.
- A curvilinear incision is based at least 2 cm inferior to the inferior of the mandible within a skin crease.
- The marginal mandibular branch is superior to the inferior border of the mandible once it passes to the anterior facial vessels. However, when it is posterior to these vessels the nerve is within 1 cm below the inferior border 19 per cent of the time.
- Incision is made through the skin and subcutaneous tissue to the level of the platysma.
- Dissection continues through the platysma to the level of the superficial layer of the deep cervical fascia.
- In addition, the external jugular vein and greater auricular nerve are identified overlying the sternocleidomastiod muscle (SCM).
- The superficial layer of the deep cervical fascia is incised, the facial vein is identified and is then clamped, divided and ligated. The distal aspect of the vein is left on a long silk tie and is gently retracted superiorly with this suture. This manoeuvre retracts the nerve (which is superficial to the vein in the cervical fascia) superiorly protecting it from injury.
- The facial artery is identified at the posterior/superior aspect of the submandibular gland. It is then clamped, divided and ligated.
- The fascial plane overlying the SCM is followed to the angle and posterior border of the mandible.
- In the submental region, the fascial plane overlying the anterior belly of the digastric is followed superiorly to its attachment at the symphysis.
- The periosteum and masseteric sling is then incised and a subperiosteal plane of dissection is then performed to expose the mandible.

Almost all the screws manufactured today for use in the mandible are self-tapping in design. A plating system is defined by the diameter of the screws; depending on the manufacturer, the diameters used for mandibular repair will range from 2.0 to 3.0 mm. The nonlocking plates/screws are designed to act as separate units working in conjunction with one another to establish a stabilized fracture. When nonlocking screws are tightened, the heads of the screws exert pressure upon the plate which provides stabilization across the fracture. This design is effective, but is not without potential consequences. The pressure generated by the screws is translated through the plate to the underlying bone (Figure 7.2.4). This has the potential to cause bone resorption beneath the plate. If this occurs prior to the time required for primary bone healing, the hardware can then fail, increasing the risk of nonunion, malunion, malocclusion and infection. In addition, poor technique with plate adaptation and utilizing nonlocking screws can increase the potential for fracture displacement (Figure 7.2.5). This occurs when the screw head comes into contact with the plate during the tightening process. This action pulls the fracture segments to the plate, resulting in displacement of the segments and malalignment. There are specific situations where this feature can be used to the surgeon's advantage, such as reducing the lingual splay of symphyseal fractures caused by muscle pull. In these situations, the plate can be intentionally over-contoured and the use of nonlocking screws will help reduce the lingual cortex (Figure 7.2.6).

Locking plates/screws

The introduction of locking plates/screws has addressed some of the issues discussed above (Figure 7.2.7). The locking plate/screws have two sets of threads, bone threads and plate threads, which are threads in the head of the screw. This second set of threads unifies (locks) the screws to the

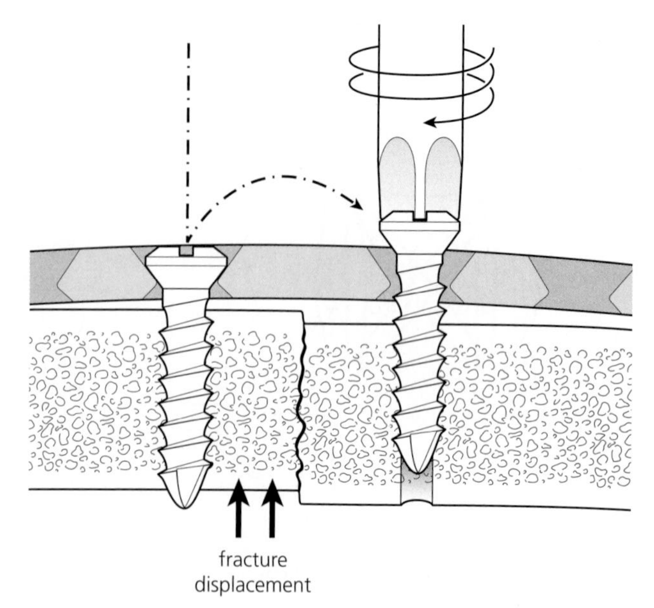

7.2.5 Non-locking plates/screws.

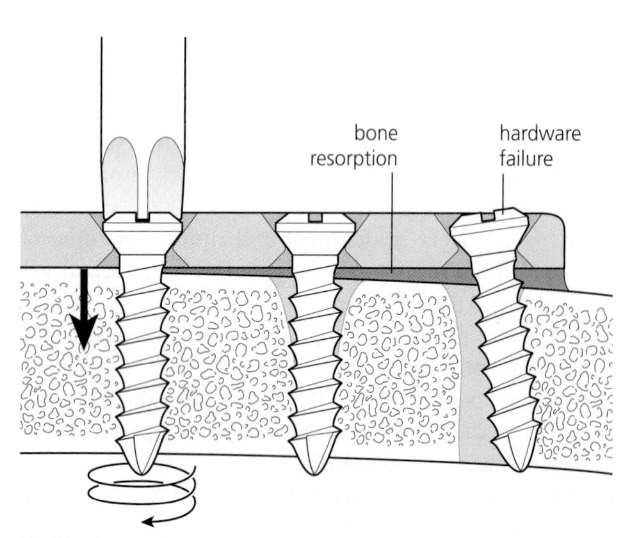

7.2.4 Non-locking plates/screws.

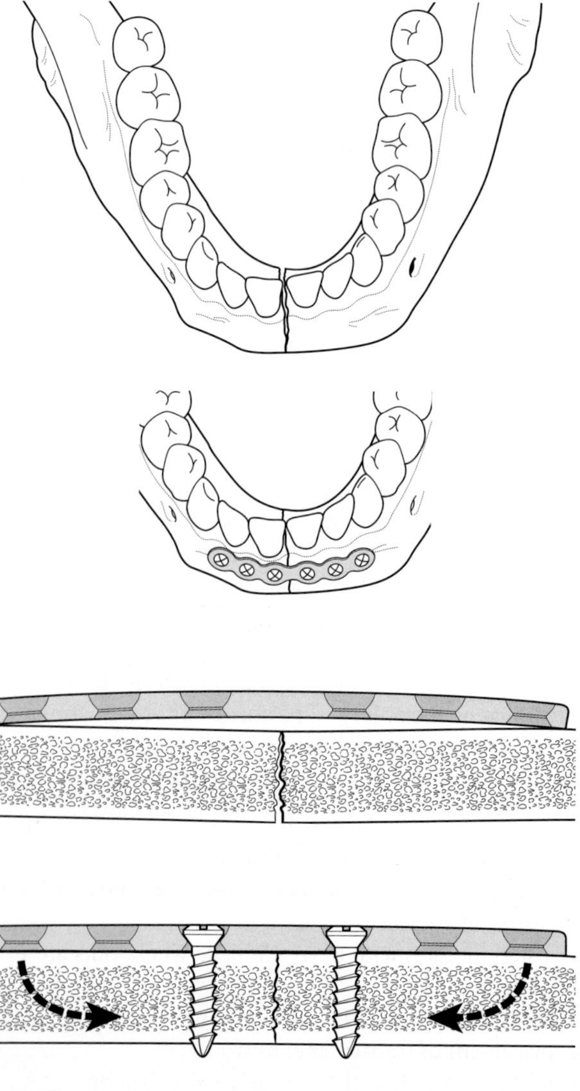

7.2.6 Non-locking plates/screws.

plate creating a single rigid functional unit. Some feel this type of design is more stable and predictable to use. It creates a system which eliminates pressure being translated through the plate and underlying bone, thereby decreasing the likelihood of bone resorption and hardware failure. In addition, should any gaps exist between the plate and bone due to imprecise bending, this system is theoretically more forgiving, with less likelihood of fracture displacement, although studies indicate displacement is still possible with locking plates.

There are two types of locking designs available, the threaded and tapered systems. Each uses the same principle of locking the screw to the plate; however, the actual mechanics vary, giving each a relative advantage and disadvantage. In the threaded design, the plate itself also has machined threads, so that these screws are placed perpendicular to the plate. The second set of screw head threads mesh with the plate threads creating a locking system. When using locking technology in ablative surgery, the manufacturers recommend limiting the number of times the same screw is reinserted to three attempts. In addition, although these screws should be placed perpendicular to allow the threads to mesh appropriately. Some manufacturers state that the screws can be angled in limited access cases, essentially allowing the screw/plate to cross-thread.

Most recently, tapered locking plates/screws have been introduced, where the threads in the head of the screw are tapered and, depending on the manufacturer, there is either a single machined thread within the plate or no machined threads at all. The threads in the head of these screws will either cut its own thread pattern into the plate as the screw is being seated, or upon the last turn of the screw a single thread will engage the plate, providing a locking mechanism. It is suggested that one of the advantages of the tapered locking design is the freedom to place the screws at up to a 10° angulation from the plane perpendicular to the plate. This alleviates the risk of cross-threading and security of the locking mechanism. This may be advantageous when access is limited, although the author rarely finds this to be an issue.

A theoretical advantage of the tapered locking design is its ability to compensate for thread/hole distortion. This potentially occurs during the adaptation and bending process of the plate. To help alleviate this problem with the threaded design, some manufacturers have fabricated bending inserts which are screwed into the plates during the contouring process, and are later removed. In practical application, the amount of distortion remains unknown, because the plates are bent between the screw holes, not directly over them. If, however, thread/hole distortion in the plate is considered a clinical concern, the concept of a tapered screw design might alleviate this issue. In order to prevent the possibility of fracture displacement, the author recommends a modification of the manufacturer-recommended sequence of screw placement (Figures 7.2.8 and 7.2.9).

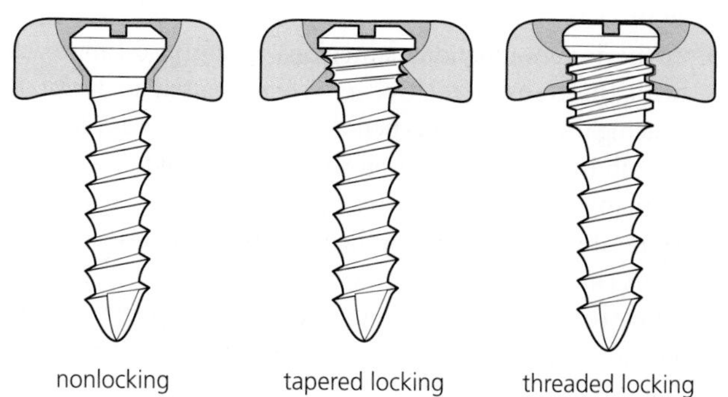

7.2.7 Locking plates/screws.

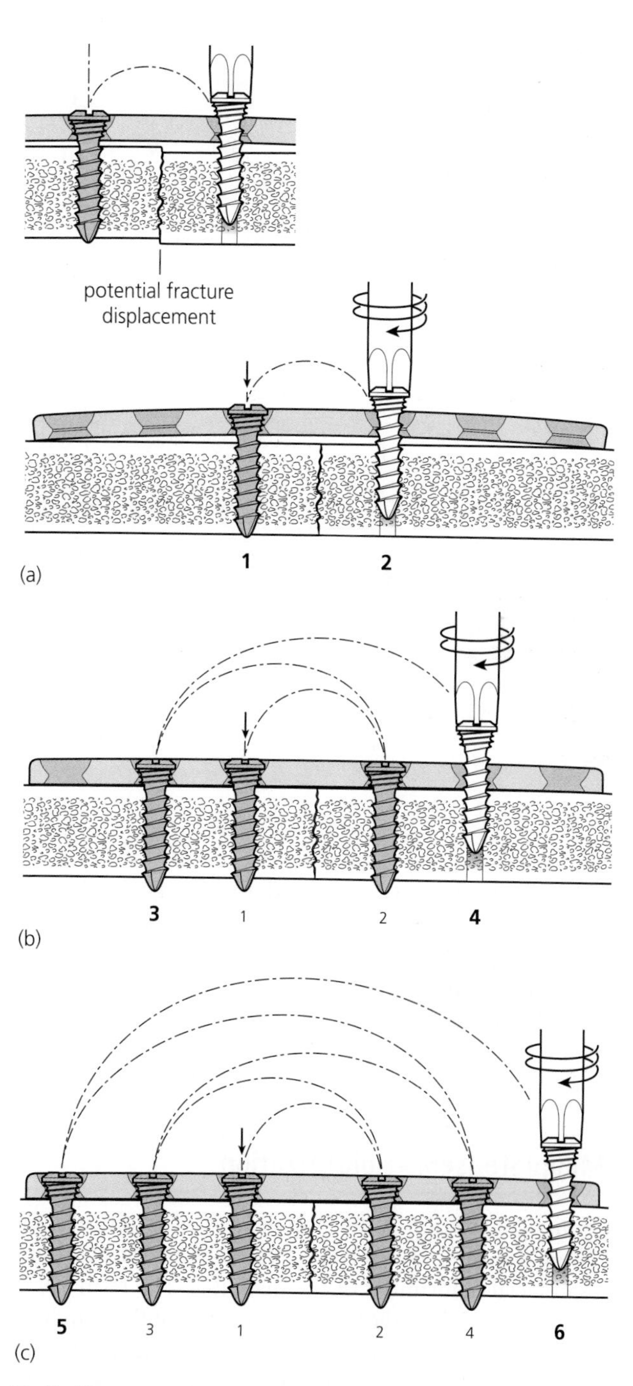

7.2.8 Locking plates/screws.

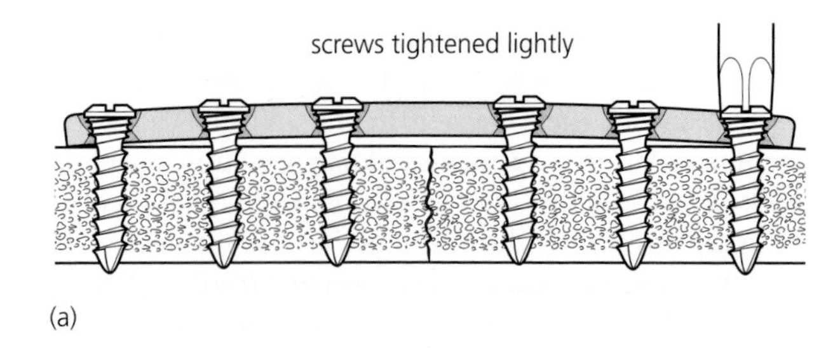

(a)

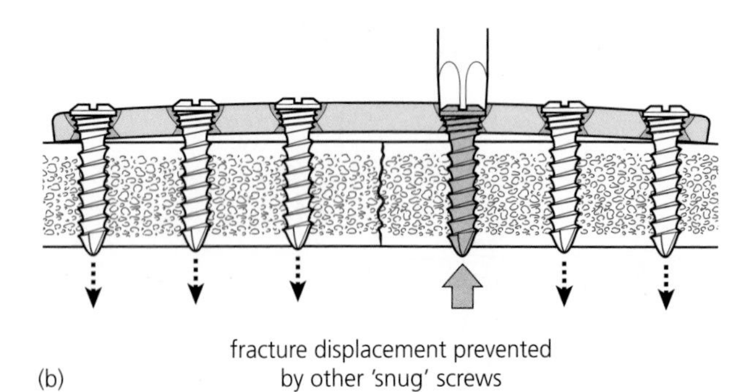

(b)

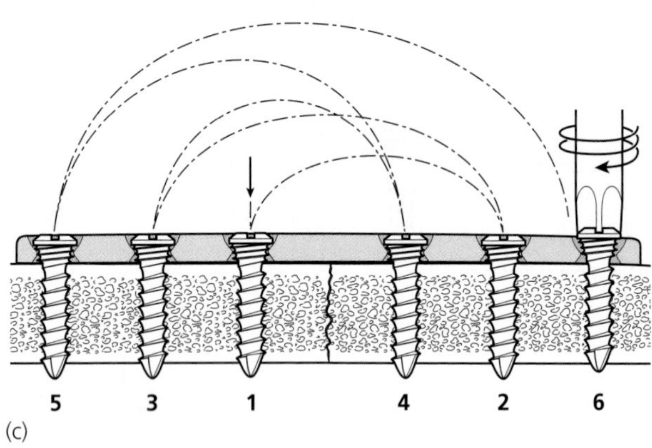

(c)

7.2.9 Locking plates/screws.

Although the theory behind the design of locking plates/screws is plausible, presently there is lack of clinical data to support their superiority to its nonlocking counterpart when used in mandible fracture repair. However, the use of locking technology for mandibular continuity defects has been shown to be of benefit when compared to its nonlocking counterpart.

Miniplate (semi-rigid) fixation

Semi-rigid fixation is the employment of miniplates and monocortical screws for the treatment of fractures and dentofacial deformities of the mandible. The term 'semi-rigid' is reserved for the load-bearing areas of the mandible; however, these miniplates are considered rigid forms of fixation when used for upper and midface trauma because of the nonload-bearing features of these regions. Semi-rigid fixation has been described as an effective form of treatment of mandible fractures when placed along the lines of osteosynthesis. The lines of osteosynthesis are biomechanical points of compression, tension or torsion (depending on the region of the mandible). This technique has undergone modifications since its introduction and it utilizes a transoral and/or transbuccal approach (Figures 7.2.10 and 7.2.11) and can involve a single malleable plate or three-dimensional ('box') plate, with 2.0-mm diameter monocortical screws proximal and distal to the fracture.

Transoral approach

The transoral approach involves the following:

- Local anaesthesia and vasoconstrictor are injected along the planned incision (if not contraindicated).
- Incisions are based in the mandibular vestibule at least 5–7 mm inferior to the mucogingival junction to facilitate ease of closure and prevent dehiscence.
- The dissection is performed through mucosa, submucosa, mentalis or buccinator muscle (depending on the location of the fracture) and periosteum.
- A subperiosteal plane of dissection is then performed to the inferior border of the mandible.
- The mental nerve is identified in the premolar region and the nerve sheath is carefully skeletalized with a scalpel or tenotomy scissors. This is to allow for mobilization of the nerve and to prevent possible avulsion from the foramen by retractors.
- The fractures are mobilized, and any soft tissue entrapped within the fracture is removed, care is taken not to injure the inferior alveolar nerve.
- The patient can then be placed into MMF.
- Bone-reducing forceps can be utilized in the transoral approach to assist in fracture reduction within the parasymphyseal region. They are difficult to use in the angle region due to limited access.

Transbuccal approach

The transbuccal approach involves the following:

- The approach is essentially the same as the transoral approach.
- In the posterior mandibular regions, a transbuccal approach with the transbuccal trocar system is used to facilitate placing the screws as perpendicular to the plate as possible.
- A stab incision is made on the cheek overlying were the anticipated hardware is to be placed.
- Blunt dissection through the masseter and periosteum is performed with a hemostat.
- The trocar system is then placed in a nontraumatic fashion and the cheek retractor is assembled to the trocar handle.
- Fixation is then applied.

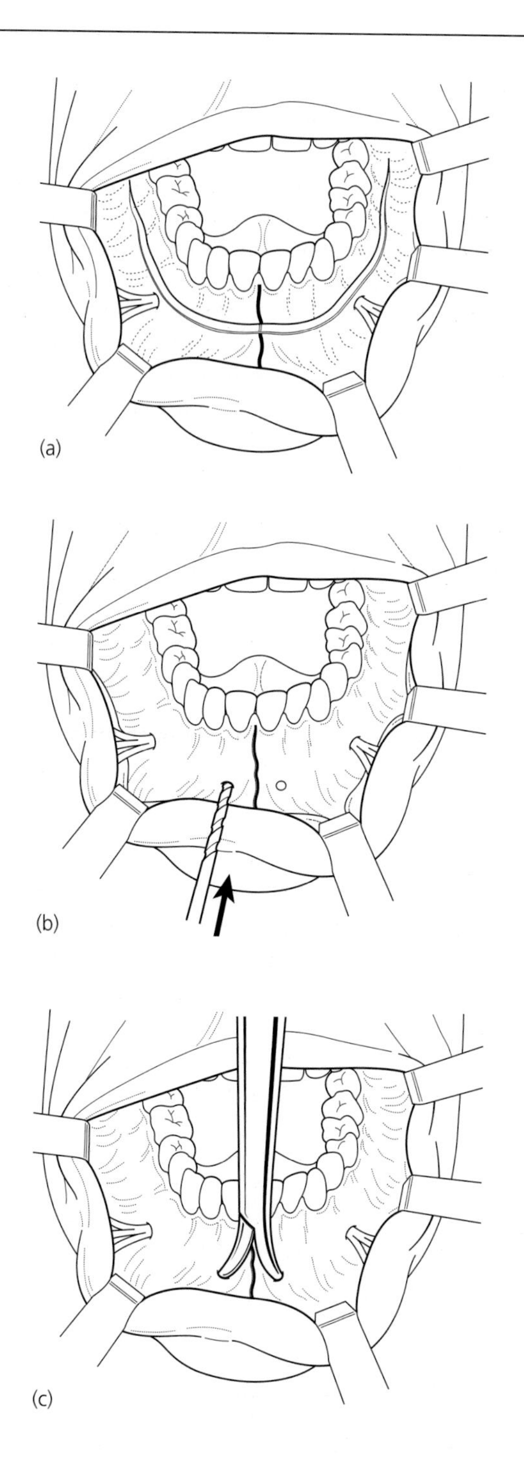

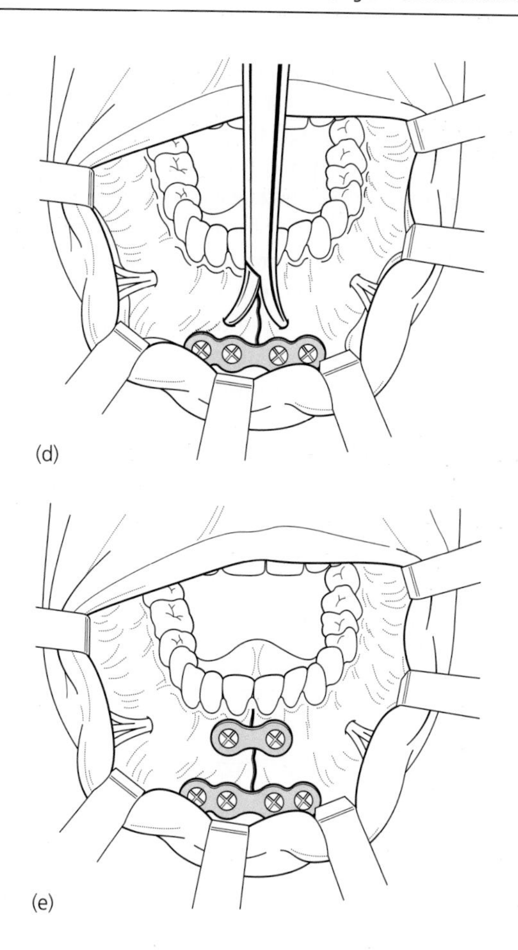

7.2.10 Transoral approach.

In its classic form, the 'Champy technique' uses a single plate in the subapical region or along the external oblique ridge when fractures are posterior to the mental foramen. When treating parasymphyseal fractures (anterior to the mental foramen), two miniplates are used in order to resist the forces of torsion seen in this region. The first plate is placed in the subapical region and the second plate 5 mm inferior to the first. Miniplate fixation is not recommended in cases that lack adequate buttressing of bone or situations were patient compliance is doubtful.

When miniplates are used in the upper and middle facial thirds, the size of the plate/screws used varies from 1.0 to 2.0 mm. This is typically dependent on the region being fixated, as well as the manufacturer of the plating system. The types of screws used for miniplates are either self-tapping (which require predrilling) or self-drilling. Again, the circumstances (i.e. bone quality, pattern of fracture) will determine the type of screws used with the miniplate.

Positioning screws/lag screws

Another form of rigid fixation is the use of positioning or lag screws (Figures 7.2.12 and 7.2.13). This form of fixation is typically used in orthognathic surgery of the mandible, bone grafting procedures and specific patterns of mandible fractures. The lag screw engages the inner cortex of the bone alone, so the head can apply compressive forces along its axial length. Positioning screws engage both cortices and do not apply the same compressive forces seen with lag screws; they fixate the bone in a more neutral position. When utilizing the position screw, the segments of bone are approximated (i.e. sagittal split ramus, bone graft), the bone is predrilled with the appropriate size bit prior to screw placement. Proponents of positioning screws for sagittal split ramus osteotomies feel there is less potential for compression of the inferior alveolar nerve and less torquing of the condyle from the fossa (more likely occurring with flared rami). When fixating these osteotomies, three screws can be placed along the external oblique ridge; or a triangulation technique can be employed with two screws along the external oblique ridge and one at the inferior border. Due to the nature of the positioning screws, one can experience a false sense of security because the screw can appear tight even if it is stripped from one of the cortices. For this reason, the surgeon must be aware of the screw engaging both cortices upon insertion.

There are two different ways to apply lag screws: one requires more bone preparation by the surgeon, the other uses a premanufactured lag screw (which requires less bone preparation). In order to be effective, the screws must be

7.2.11 Transbuccal approach.

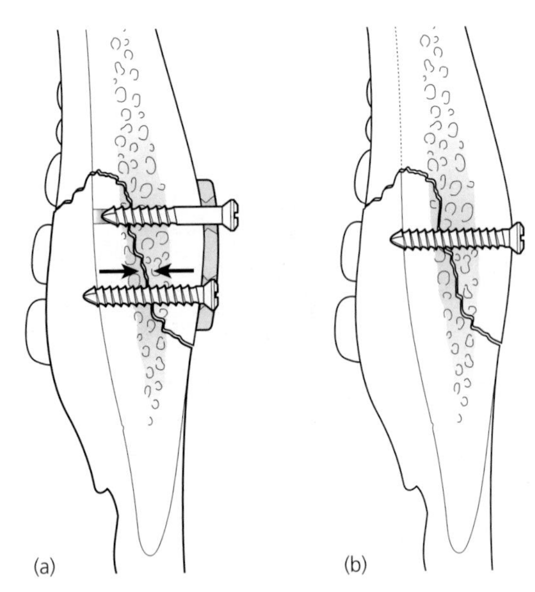

7.2.12 Positioning screws/Lag screws.

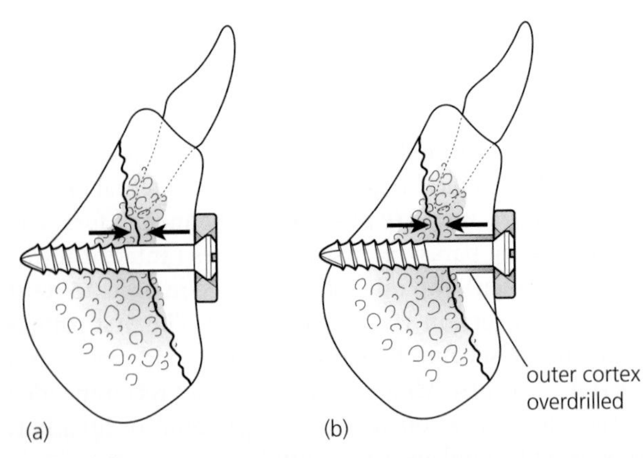

7.2.13 Positioning screws/Lag screws.

placed perpendicular to the fracture line. The diameter of lag screws can range from 2.3 to 3.5 mm and lengths vary depending upon the application. In the first method, both cortices are predrilled, but the proximal cortex is drilled to a larger diameter than the screw. This assures that only the distal cortex is being engaged so the screw head can compress the inner and outer cortices together. The second method relies on a manufactured lag screw which has threads only on the distal half of the shank; the proximal half is smooth. After the bone is predrilled, only the distal half has threads which engage the inner cortex, allowing the head of the screw to apply compressive forces to both cortices.

Lag screws have been described for fracture fixation in every region of the mandible. They are ideal for symphyseal fractures which have stable buttressing. Ideally, two screws are placed parallel to each other and perpendicular to the fracture line, in order to resist the forces of torsion within this area. Countersinking the outer cortex is recommended to allow the screw head to sit flush with the bone. Some manufacturers provide washers to be used under the screw head to prevent the compressive forces from submerging the screw head beyond the lateral cortex into the medullary space. If this occurs, the technique is rendered ineffective and retrieval of the screw is difficult.

FURTHER READING

Coletti D, Caccamese J, Norby J *et al.* Comparative analysis of the threaded and tapered locking reconstruction plates. *Journal of Oral and Maxillofacial Surgery* 2007; **65**: 2587–93.

Coletti D, Salama A, Caccamese J. Application of intermaxillary facial screws in maxillofacial trauma. *Journal of Oral and Maxillofacial Surgery* 2007; **65**: 1746–50.

Collins CP, Pirinjian-Leonard G, Tolas A, Alcalde R. A prospective randomized clinical trial comparing 2.0-mm locking plates to 2.0-mm standard plates in treatment of mandible fractures. *Journal of Oral and Maxillofacial Surgery* 2004; **62**: 1392–5.

Dingman RO, Grabb WC. Surgical anatomy of the mandibular ramus of the facial nerve based on the dissection of 100 facial halves. *Plastic and Reconstructive Surgery* 1962; **29**: 266–72.

Eckelt U, Hlawitschka M. Clinical and radiological evaluation following surgical treatment of condylar neck fractures with lag screws. *Journal of Craniomaxillofacial Surgery* 1999; **27**: 235–42.

Ellis E 3rd. Use of lag screws for fractures of the mandibular body. *Journal of Oral and Maxillofacial Surgery* 1996; **54**: 1314–16.

Gordon KF, Reed JM, Anand VK. Results of intraoral cortical bone screw fixation technique for mandibular fractures. *Otolaryngology, Head and Neck Surgery* 1995; **113**: 248.

Gutwald R, Alpert B, Schmelzeisen R. Principle and stability of locking plates. *Keio Journal of Medicine* 2003; **52**: 21.

Haug RH, Street CC, Goltz M. Does plate adaptation affect stability? A biomechanical comparison of locking and nonlocking plates. *Journal of Oral and Maxillofacial Surgery* 2002; **60**: 1319.

Jones DC. The intermaxillary screw: A dedicated bicortical bone screw for temporary intermaxillary fixation. *British Journal of Oral and Maxillofacial Surgery* 1999; **37**: 115.

Kallela I, Ilzuka T, Laine P, Lindqvist C. Lag-screw fixation of mandibular parasymphyseal and angle fractures. *Oral Surgery, Oral Medicine, Oral Pathology, Oral Radiology, and Endodontics* 1996; **82**: 510–16.

Martin H. Surgery of head and neck tumors. New York: Hoeber-Harper, 1957.

Onishi K, Maruyama Y. Simple intermaxillary fixation for maxillomandibular osteosynthesis. *Journal of Craniofacial Surgery* 1996; **7**: 170–2.

Schneider AM, David LR, DeFranzo AJ *et al.* Use of specialized bone screws for intermaxillary fixation. *Annals of Plastic Surgery* 2000; **44**: 154–7.

Soderholm AL, Lindqvist C, Skutnabb K, Rahn B. Bridging of mandibular defects with two different reconstruction systems: An experimental study. *Journal of Oral and Maxillofacial Surgery* 1991; **49**: 1098–105.

7.3

Soft tissue injuries

SUHAIL K MITHANI, EDUARDO D RODRIGUEZ

PRINCIPLES

The following principles apply to the management of soft tissue injuries:

- Initial management of facial trauma should adhere to Advanced Trauma Life Support (ATLS) guidelines with attention paid to ABCs (airway, breathing and circulation) and identification of concominant injuries prior to addressing facial soft tissue injuries.
- Up to a quarter of facial lacerations suffered through high speed mechanisms have associated facial fractures which should be recognized prior to the repair of soft tissue injuries.
- There are several types of soft tissue injuries that can occur and treatment is dependent upon identification and assessment of the severity of these injuries:
- contusion;
  - abrasion;
  - laceration;
  - puncture with or without associated foreign body inspissation.
- Haemorrhage arising from soft tissue injuries can often be controlled with direct pressure. However, intractable bleeding may require angiography for control.
- Adequate repair of facial soft tissue injuries can often be achieved with delays of up to 24 hours when life-threatening injuries delay access for repair.
- Mucosal and subcutaneous tissues are closed with absorbable sutures, while skin is closed with nonabsorbable suture which is removed 4–6 days after closure.
- Photography of injuries is essential before embarking on repair of injuries for both evaluation of results and for medicolegal reasons. Pretrauma pictures, when available, are extremely helpful in guiding treatment especially in extensive soft tissue injuries.

ANATOMY

The face is comprised of multiple soft tissue layers, reapproximation of which must be considered in planning of repair:

- skin;
- subcutaneous tissue;
- superficial muscular aponeurotic system (SMAS);
- muscle;
- mucosa.

Innervation of the face is provided by cranial nerves V (sensory) and VII (motor). Most motor branches of cranial nerve VII are deep to the muscle, but in the periorbital, perioral and cheek regions, these nerves are superficial. The blood supply of the face is myriad and rich, which aids greatly in prevention of devitalization even in the setting of extensive injury. However, haematoma formation is a common occurrence which may complicate repair and should be considered.

PRE-OPERATIVE

- Thorough evaluation and identification of facial injuries is imperative prior to the institution of therapy.
- Particular attention should be paid to devitalized tissues, as these need to be debrided to prevent a nidus of infection.
- Evaluate the eyelids to identify ocular injuries.
- Radiographic evaluation for associated fractures or foreign bodies may be indicated based upon the mechanism and extent of trauma.
- Facial and scalp hair can be cut or shaved to facilitate visualization and cleansing of wounds; however, it is imperative that eyebrows are not shaved even when they

are involved in the injury. The eyebrow serves as a reference point and should guide reapproximation of tissue. Poor alignment of reapproximation produces a cosmetically undesirable result.
- All wounds should be thoroughly irrigated with saline.
- Extensively contaminated wounds may require surgical debridement or pressure irrigation to clean.
- Presence of foreign materials should be noted and these should be removed either by cleansing or gentle debridement.
- Patients who have not been immunized or whose immunization is not current should receive tetanus toxoid.

ANAESTHESIA

- Soft tissue injuries which are minor in nature can be repaired with local anaesthesia.
- 1 per cent lidocaine with epinephrine (1:100 000) is preferred.
- For significant injuries or those associated with concominant facial skeleton injuries, general anaesthesia is the preferred method of repair.

INJURY TYPES

Abrasion

Thorough cleaning with mild detergent is imperative to ensure a clean wound. Grease, carbon or other embedded particles should be removed from the wound using a lubricant or solvent if necessary. Preventing partial thickness injuries from converting to full thickness injuries necessitates application of a moist, occlusive dressing for the duration of the healing process. Irregular and unsightly scarring can be managed using laser re-surfacing or dermabrasion.

Contusions and haematomas

Bruising injury resulting from trauma is often associated with tissue oedema. Gentle handling is imperative for the reduction of the sequelae of permanent scarring and disfiguration. These injuries are often associated with haematoma, which, if small, is resorbed by the body. A moist, heated compress may aid in reabsorption. Larger haematomas may be selectively incised and drained to prevent subcutaneous scarring.

Avulsion

These injuries result from tangential penetrating forces and the thinned tissue at the leading edge of the avulsion flap is most susceptible to oedema and contracture. If small, an entire area of avulsion can be excised and the tissue reapproximated. If this is not possible, the leading edge of the avulsion should be excised sharply to promote full thickness healing with suture approximation. Due to the excellent vascularization of the face, even avulsive flaps with narrow bases can be viable, so caution must be advised in making the decision to excise tissue, especially in the perioral, nasal and orbital regions. Application of a pressure dressing after wound closure is key to minimizing oedema and venous congestion, promoting better healing and cosmesis.

Bites

Human and animal bites result in extensively contaminated wounds (Figure 7.3.1). Copious irrigation and sharp debridement of devitalized tissue is essential in preventing wound infection. This may result in sacrifice of vital soft tissue components in aesthetically sensitive areas, but cannot be avoided. Often, delayed primary reconstruction with local flaps or free tissue transfer is necessary. Prophylactic antibiotics are important adjunctive therapy, but should not replace thorough cleaning and debridement. Often, wound infection is not preventable. Human bites result in greater degree of wound contamination than animal bites.

Laceration

Laceration is the most common type of facial injury requiring surgical intervention (Figure 7.3.2). Assessment of the depth of injury and reapproximation of transected tissues is undertaken prior to closure of the skin. Irregular edges and devitalized tissues should be excised to provide sharp edges for easier reapproximation when cosmetically possible. Closure should be undertaken in multiple layers with absorbable sutures used for deep layers, and the skin closed with monofilament sutures which should be removed after 3–5 days. Closure may be delayed up to 24 hours if the laceration is appropriately cleaned and dressed. This may be necessary in the setting of concominant life-threatening injuries which require attention.

ANATOMIC CONSIDERATIONS

Eyebrow injury

Injuries to the eyebrow should be managed with minimal debridement and without shaving, since cosmesis is noticeably affected. Tissue loss in this area should be closed primarily when possible with interval hair graft from the posterior scalp. Detection and repair of supraorbital nerve injury should be made at the time of laceration repair.

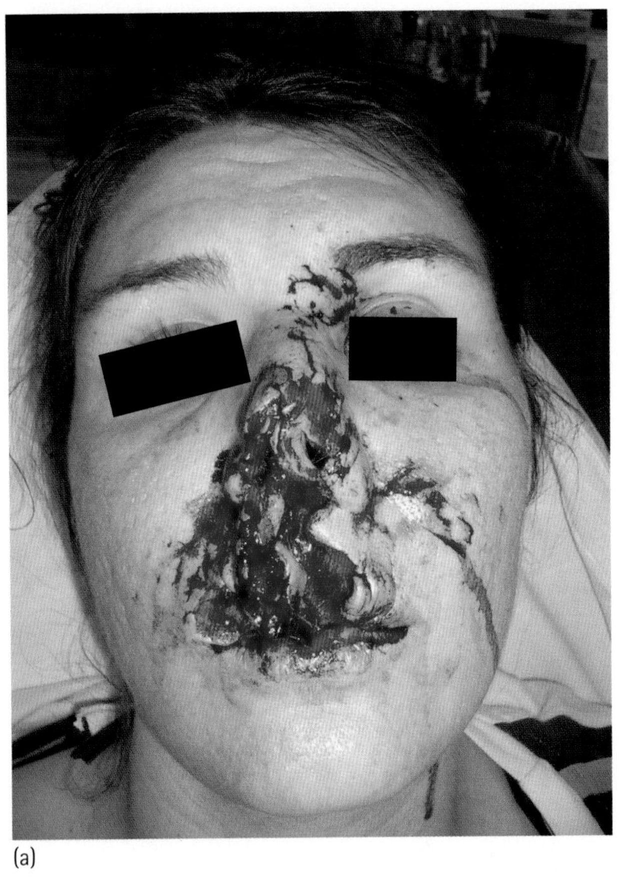

(a)

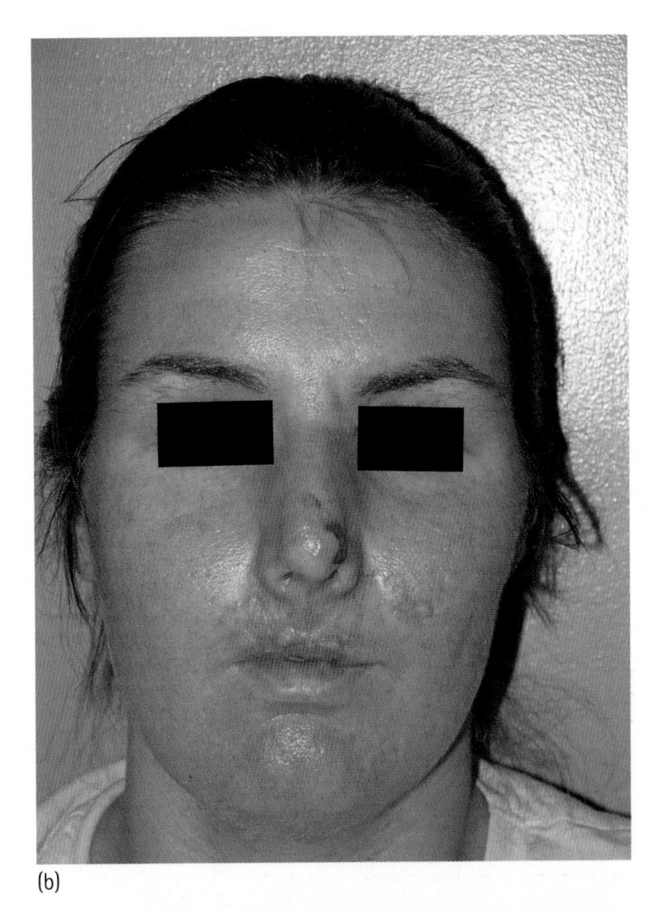

(b)

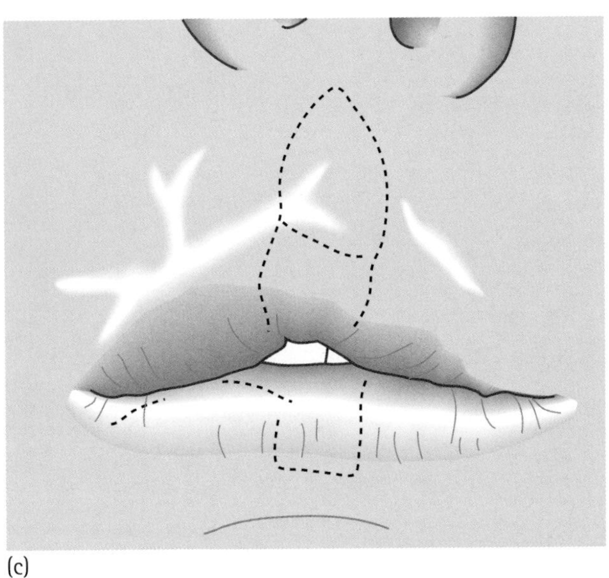

(c)

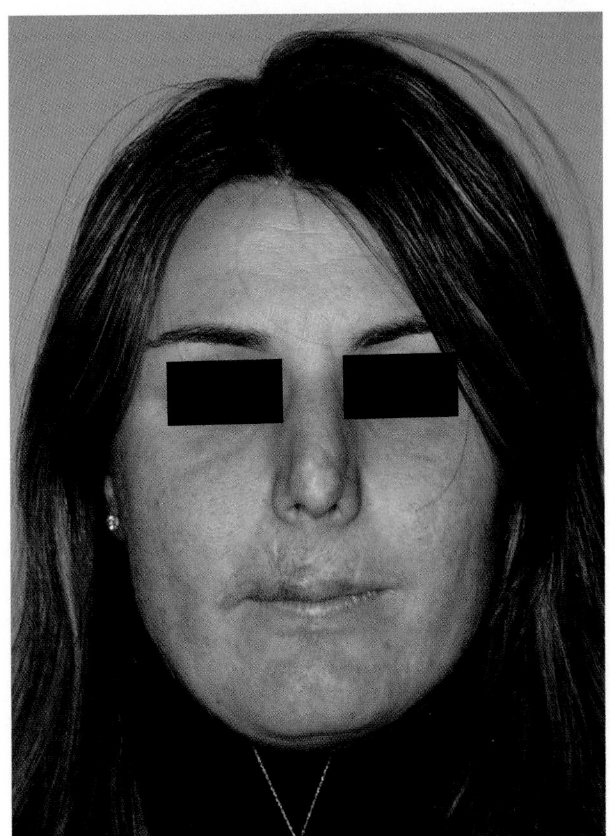

(d)

7.3.1 (a) Extensive canine bite injury involving the mouth and nose. (b) Appearance after initial laceration repair. Note the severe scarring and contracture of the oral vestibule and nasal ala. (c) Abbe flap to augment upper lip and release contracture. (d) Final appearance after multiple procedures to augment soft tissue and release scar contracture.

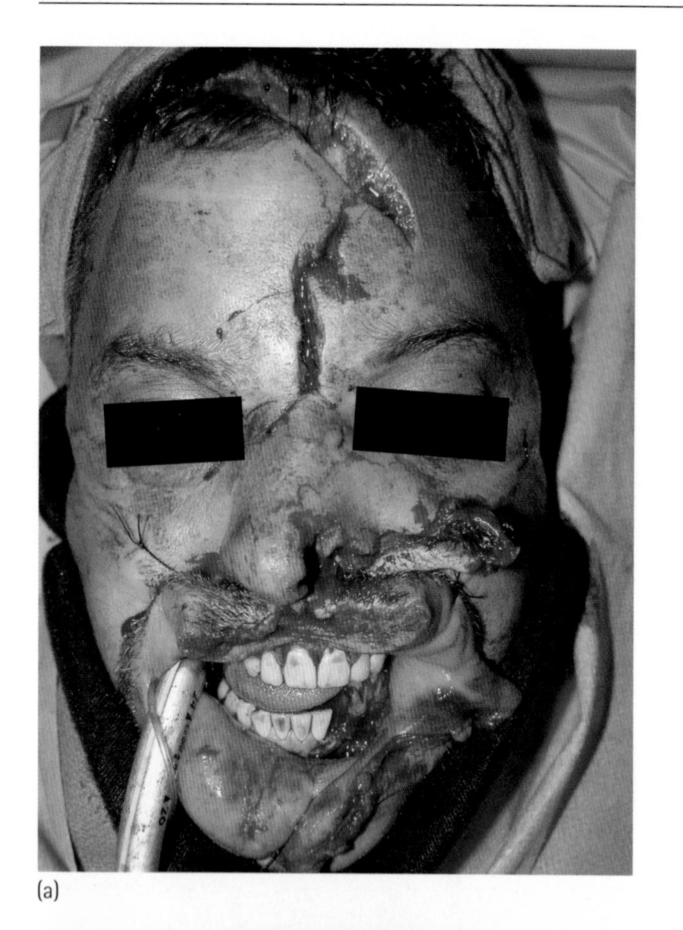
(a)

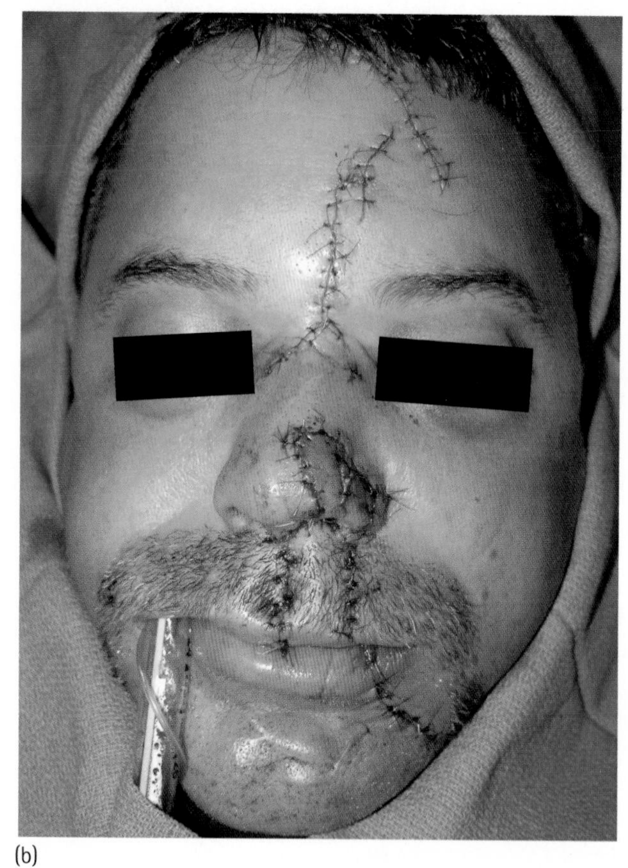
(b)

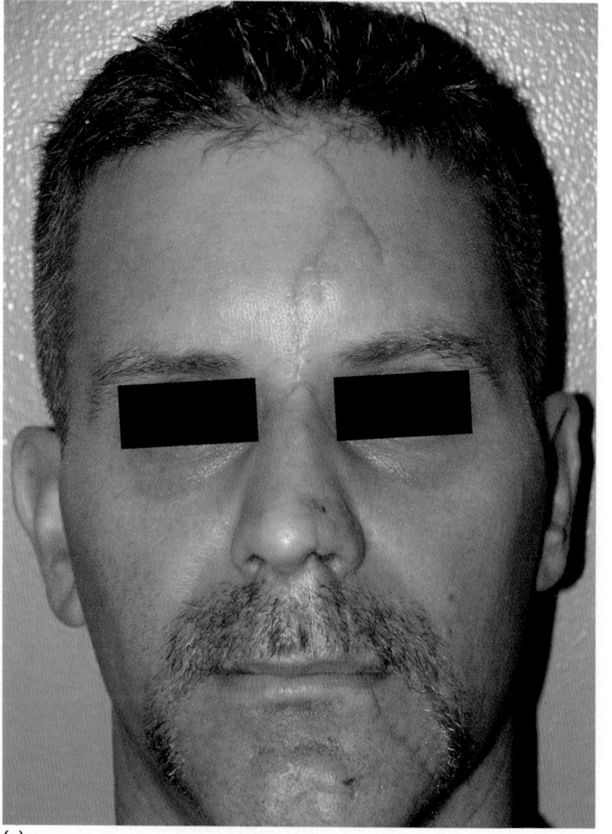
(c)

7.3.2 (a) High speed motor vehicle collision with laceration and avulsion injury to the mouth, nose and lips. (b) Primary reconstruction with careful reapproximation of the vermillion border, philtrum and nasal ala. Note that despite initial venous congestion and severe devitalization of the nasal ala, primary repair was performed. (c) Final appearance with adequate preservation of the nasal contour and lip border following primary hard and soft tissue repair.

Eyelid injury

Patients with eyelid lacerations should be carefully evaluated for globe injury prior to repair. All lacerations should be closed in multiple layers, with careful reapproximation of the muscles, conjunctiva or tarsus, when necessary. Deep sutures must be tied in such a manner as to direct the knot away from the globe when possible. Lacerations extending through the eyelid margin should be closed with attention paid to lining up the cilia. A tissue defect in this setting may require partial lateral canthotomy to mobilize the lid medially in order to facilitate primary closure.

Nasal injury

Nasal injuries are common and often uncomplicated to repair (Figure 7.3.2). Principles of aesthetic reconstruction include minimal debridement when possible and anatomic realignment of the soft tissues, especially the nasal rim. With associated bony injury, restoration of the skeletal framework of the nose is often sufficient to realign the soft tissues, making reapproximation easier. Lacerations of the nose may involve the skin, nasal cartilages and mucosa. Repair of injuries involving all three layers should proceed from deep to superficial with repair of the mucosa, followed by cartilage and then skin. Often the skin and subcutaneous tissues can be closed in a single layer. Thorough evaluation of nasal injuries includes careful speculum examination to diagnose septal haematoma. If seen, this can be evacuated through a small incision in the septal mucosa. Failure to diagnose septal haematoma can result in erosion and loss of septal cartilage and resultant ossification.

Lip injury

Injury to the lip may involve the underlying orbicularis oris muscle, as well as the mucosa, and should be repaired in multiple layers with attention paid to precise alignment of the tissues (Figure 7.3.2). Key to achieving cosmetically suitable repair is alignment of the vermillion borders. This must be done prior to injection of local anesthetic agents with vasoconstrictive properties (e.g. lidocaine with epinephrine). The white roll can either be aligned with suture or tattooed prior to injection of local anaesthetic agent to serve as a landmark for lip repair.

Auricle injury

Injuries of the ear require careful and precise primary reconstruction as secondary reconstruction is often extremely difficult (Figure 7.3.3). Due to the uniqueness of

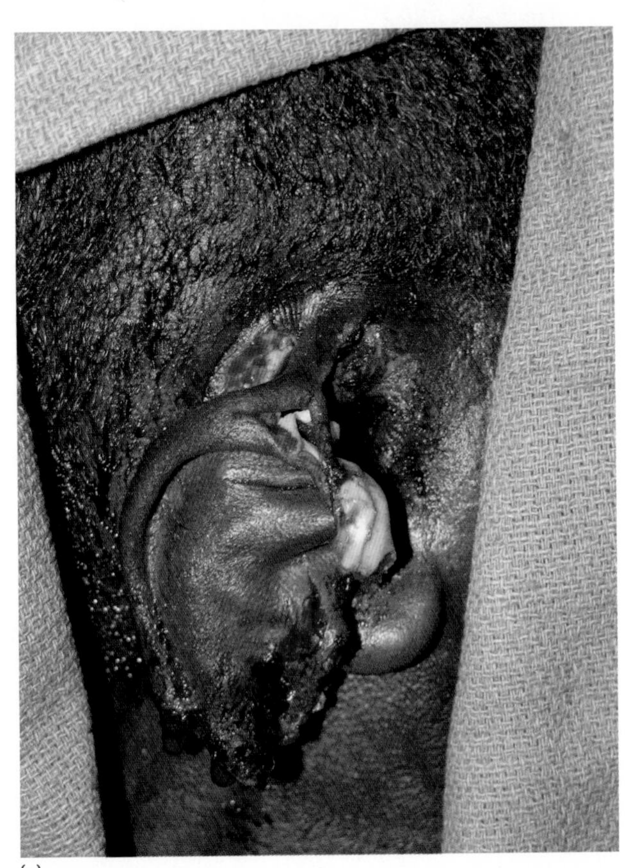
(a)

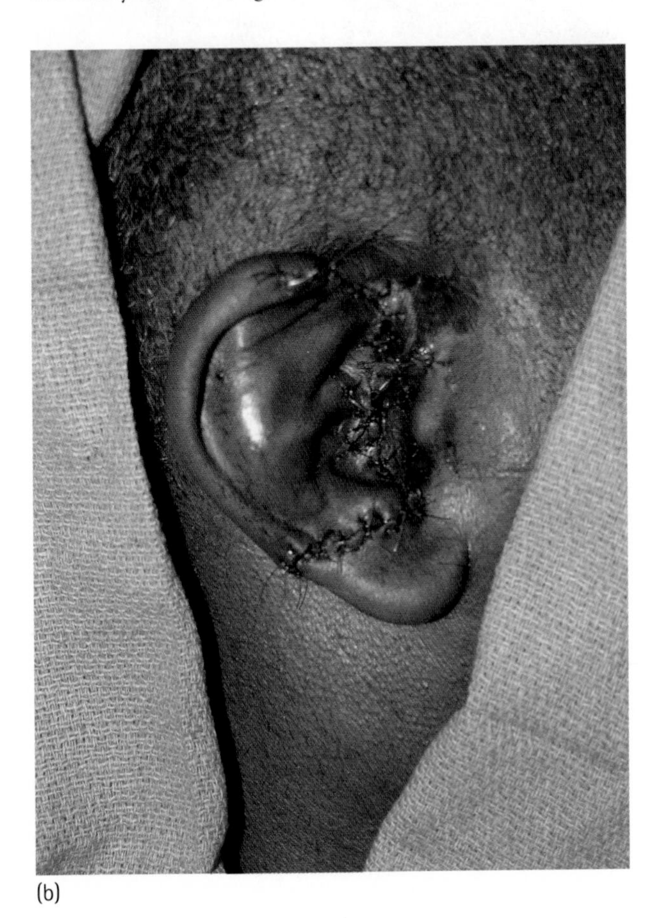
(b)

7.3.3 (a) Ear avulsion involving skin and auricular cartilage. (b) Primary repair with reapproximation of the cartilage and skin.

character and composition of the ear, it is important to salvage as much tissue as possible to aid in repair. Debridement should be kept to a minimum, with no more than 1 mm of tissue removed from wound edges. Due to the excellent vascularity of the ear, pedicles of tissue with a narrow base will often survive with careful reapproximation. Even completely avulsed tissue can be successfully replaced in the anatomic position. Severed tissue should be thoroughly cleansed and placed in cold, sterile saline until reimplantation. This should be attempted in all instances regardless of the volume of lost tissue. Leech therapy may be a useful adjunct to facilitate successful replantation. Through and through lacerations of the ear and underlying cartilage can be repaired with nonabsorbable cutaneous sutures alone, if the cartilaginous skeleton is adequately supported. In extensive lacerations, the cartilage is repaired separately with absorbable suture with care taken to direct the knot towards the medial surface of the ear. Injuries of the ear canal should be repaired similarly with stenting placed in the ear canal. Haematoma formation is of special concern since it can result in failure of primary repair. A bolster should be placed and a pressure dressing applied with circumferential wrapping of the head.

Intraoral injury

Intraoral injuries must be identified and addressed as they are bathed in saliva and exposed to oral flora (Figure 7.3.4). Closure can be performed with absorbable suture. Extensive soft tissue loss in the setting of blast injuries can often be repaired with local flaps. Composite defects often require free tissue transfer for reconstruction, depending upon the extent of defect. Particular attention should be paid to repair of the injury in the setting of post-traumatic hardware placement on the alveolus, since contamination of hardware

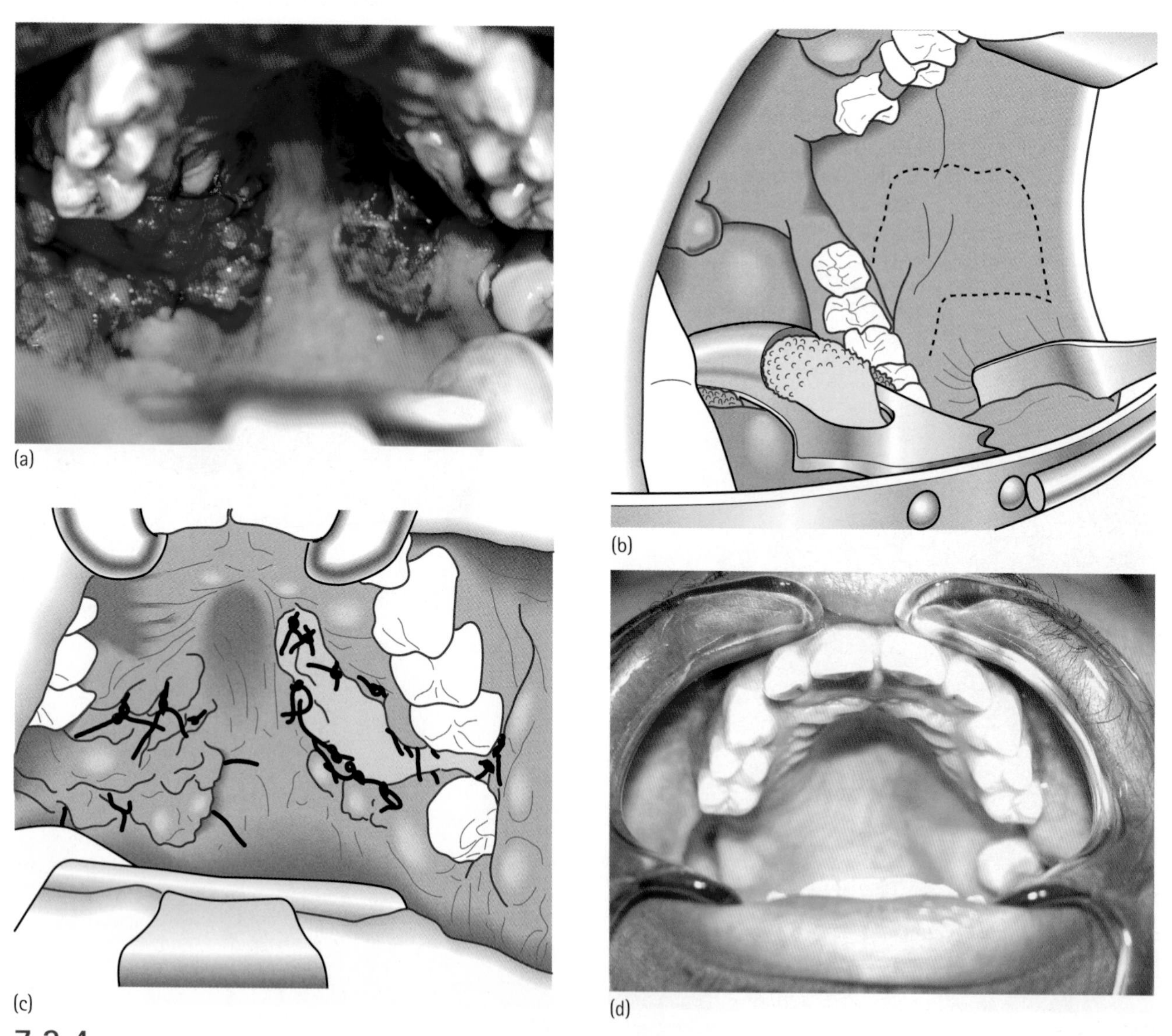

7.3.4 (a) Oroantral fistula resulting from soft tissue defect of the soft palate secondary to gunshot wound. (b) Marked out local facial artery myomucosal rotational flap. (c) Inset of flap. (d) Closure of fistula with satisfactory result.

with oral flora can result in infection. Injuries of the buccal mucosa should be carefully explored to ensure that the papilla of Stensen's duct is not involved, and care should be taken to not occlude it with repair.

REPAIR OF DUCTAL AND NERVE INJURIES

Salivary gland injuries

The parotid gland is superficially located anterior to the ear and superior to the angle of the mandible. Injury to the parotid duct (Stensen's duct) must be considered with deep injuries to the cheek (Figure 7.3.5). The buccal branch of the facial nerve is intimately associated with the parotid duct and injury to either structure necessitates consideration of injury to the other. Injuries to the parotid parenchyma do not require primary repair, but should, however, induce exploration for ductal injury. The duct is located in a line parallel with a line drawn from the tragus to the midpoint of the upper lip. Its papilla is located adjacent to the crown of the second upper molar. The opening of Stensen's duct can be dilated with a lacrimal duct probe and saline, sterile milk or methylene blue can be instilled through the opening and used to identify injury within the wound. The duct should be reapproximated with fine suture over a polyethylene stent which can be introduced in either an anterograde or retrograde direction and sutured securely intraorally. Salivary cutaneous fistula is common, but self-limited, and can be minized by placement of a subcutaneous drain at the time of duct repair.

Injury to the submandibular gland or duct is treated by gland excision and duct ligation.

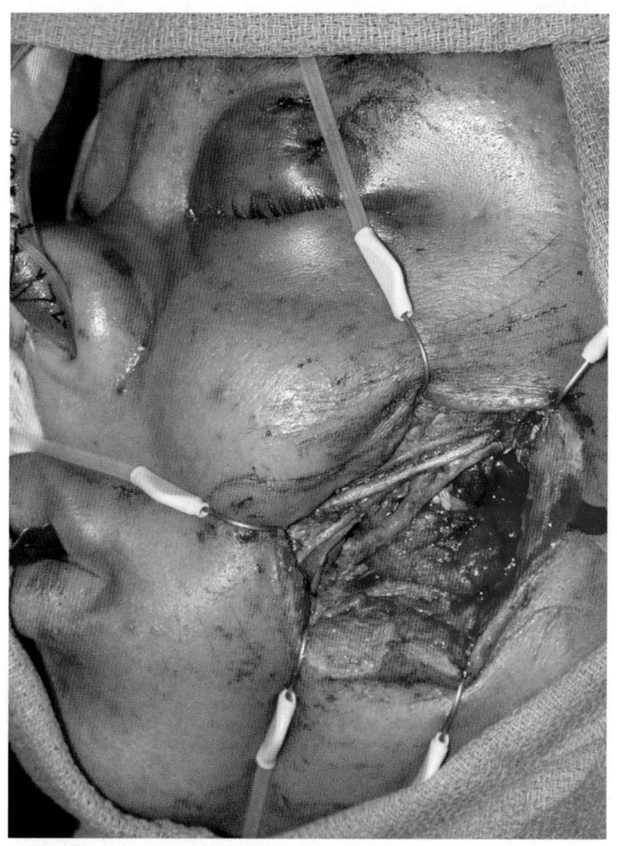

7.3.5 Avulsive cheek defect resulting in transection of the buccal branch of the facial nerve and Stensen's duct. The patient underwent microscopic buccal branch neurolysis/neurorrhapy, as well as repair of Stensen's duct with silastic tube stenting.

Lacrimal duct injury

Lacrimal duct injury should be considered in injuries involving the medial canthus of the eye. Injuries can be indentified using the operative microscope. The lacrimal duct can be repaired with fine suture over a thin silastic catheter. The catheter should extend through the entire lacrimal system and be sutured in place in the nose to provide adequate drainage while the duct heals.

Facial nerve injuries

Deep lacerations of the inferior aspect of the cheek threaten branches of the facial nerve (Figure 7.3.6). Signs and symptoms of motor denervation are readily apparent when injury occurs. Injury to the upper division of the facial nerve is especially debilitating since eye closing is restricted with subsequent sequelae of corneal abrasion and ulceration. Nerve injuries that occur anterior to a line drawn vertically from the lateral canthus do not result in permanent loss of muscle function due to the distal branching of the facial nerve. However, all patients with a facial motor deficit after laceration should undergo exploration with identification of cut ends of the nerve. Once identified, crushed ends should be debrided and the neurorrhapy performed microsurgically. If a gap between cut ends remains, a nerve graft or neural tube may be utilized to restore continuity and promote restoration of function. Muscles injured should also be reapproximated at this time to improve both functional outcomes and to permit some nerve regeneration by muscle neurotization.

POST-OPERATIVE CARE

When identified early and appropriately cleansed and debrided, facial wounds often heal without incident. Perioperative antibiotics may be necessary in the setting of grossly contaminated wounds or with delay in initiation of treatment. Suture lines on the skin can be covered with antibiotic ointment, and intraoral suture lines may be cleansed with oral rinses of antibiotic mouthwash or half strength peroxide. Nonabsorbable sutures can typically be removed in 4–6 days, but may need to remain in place longer in the setting of a patient with impaired wound healing (e.g. diabetic, critically ill, immunocompromise).

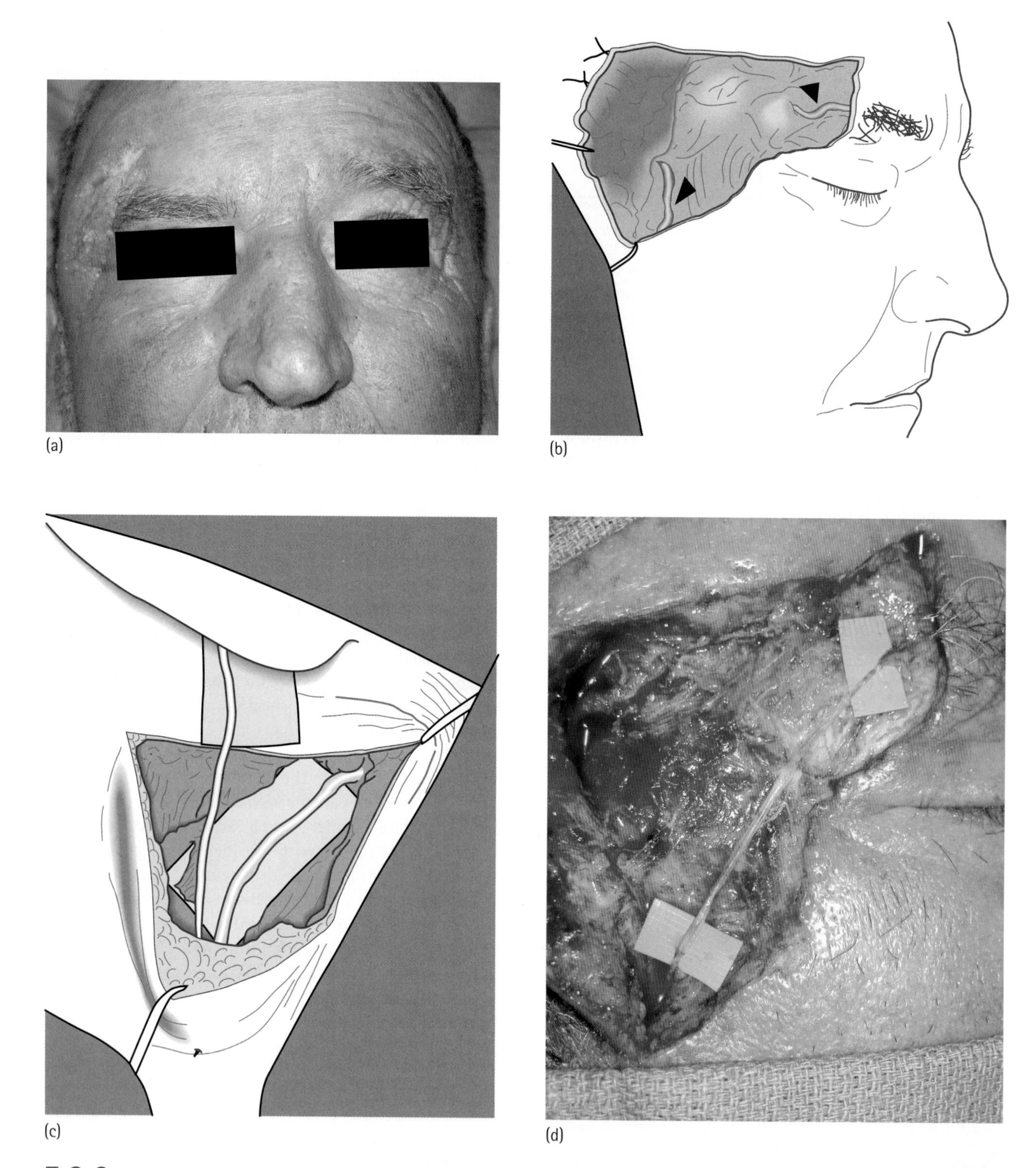

7.3.6 (a) Assymetric elevation of brow resulting from injury to the frontal branch of the facial nerve following a kick from a horse. (b) Initial dissection with identification of transected ends of nerve (blue markers). (c) Dissection and isolation of branch of greater auricular nerve. (d) Neurorrhaphy of frontal nerve branch with nerve graft.

continued

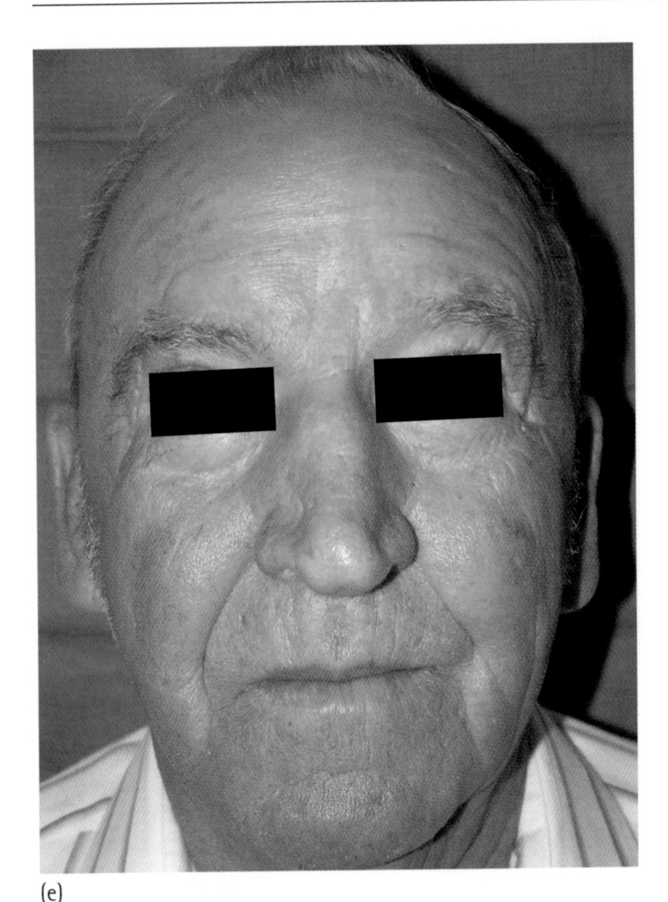

(e)

7.3.6 *continued* (e) Restoration of motor function with adequate elevation of brow at three months' follow up.

COMPLICATIONS

Infection

The robust blood supply of the face and head diminishes the incidence of infection; however, vigilance must be maintained in identifying wound infection early and instituting appropriate therapy as the consequences of missed diagnosis can be severe. Infection impairs the body's ability to heal resulting in undesired cosmesis, but superficial soft tissue infection of the face can rapidly spread through valveless facial veins to the sinuses and subsequently to the brain. Most infections are superficial and commonly treated with a warm compress and antibiotic therapy.

Scars

Wound characteristics and hypertrophic scarring often result in unsightly scar appearance, despite appropriate management and meticulous technique (Figure 7.3.7). It is imperative to prepare patients for this possibility at the time of primary repair. Patients with known keloid tendencies can be treated at the time of initial operation with locally injected steroids to minimize the risk; however, it is not possible to completely eliminate this possibility. Scar revision can be performed using a variety of techniques. It is important to wait for complete healing (often six months to a year) prior to attempting revision. Scars parallel to tension lines may be excised and closed primarily with or without the adjunctive use of tissue expansion. Scars crossing tension lines may be managed by Z- or W-plasty to alter their prominence. Surgical abrasion can often be employed successfully to manage contour irregularities resulting from abrasion and avulsion injuries. These techniques may decrease the prominence of scars, but it is important to make patients aware that they are unlikely to make the scars imperceptible and all interventions carry the risk of further scarring and exacerbation.

INABILITY TO ACHIEVE PRIMARY REPAIR

Soft tissue defects that cannot be closed primarily should be dressed with a bio-occlusive dressing (e.g. allograft) until definitive management can be undertaken. A myriad of advancement and rotational flaps are available to facilitate wound closure. In the absence of a satisfactory local flap, free tissue transfer should be considered to facilitate wound closure.

Top tips

- Initial evaluation of the extent of facial soft tissue injury includes thorough cleansing and removal of wound contaminants (e.g. dirt, glass).
- Lacerations can be repaired with up to 24 hours delay with excellent results.
- A low threshold should be maintained for taking a patient to the operating room for evaluation and repair of soft tissue injuries.
- Photographic documentation of injuries and repair is imperative
- Radiographic evaluation should be performed to rule out fracture or presence of foreign bodies.
- Avoid shaving the eyebrow to facilitate injury evaluation.
- All patients with periorbital injuries should be evaluated for ocular injuries.
- Avulsed or amputated tissue can often be restored successfully to the native.
- Reapproximation of the vermillion border should be performed prior to injection of vasoconstrictive local anaesthetic agent for repair of lip lacerations.

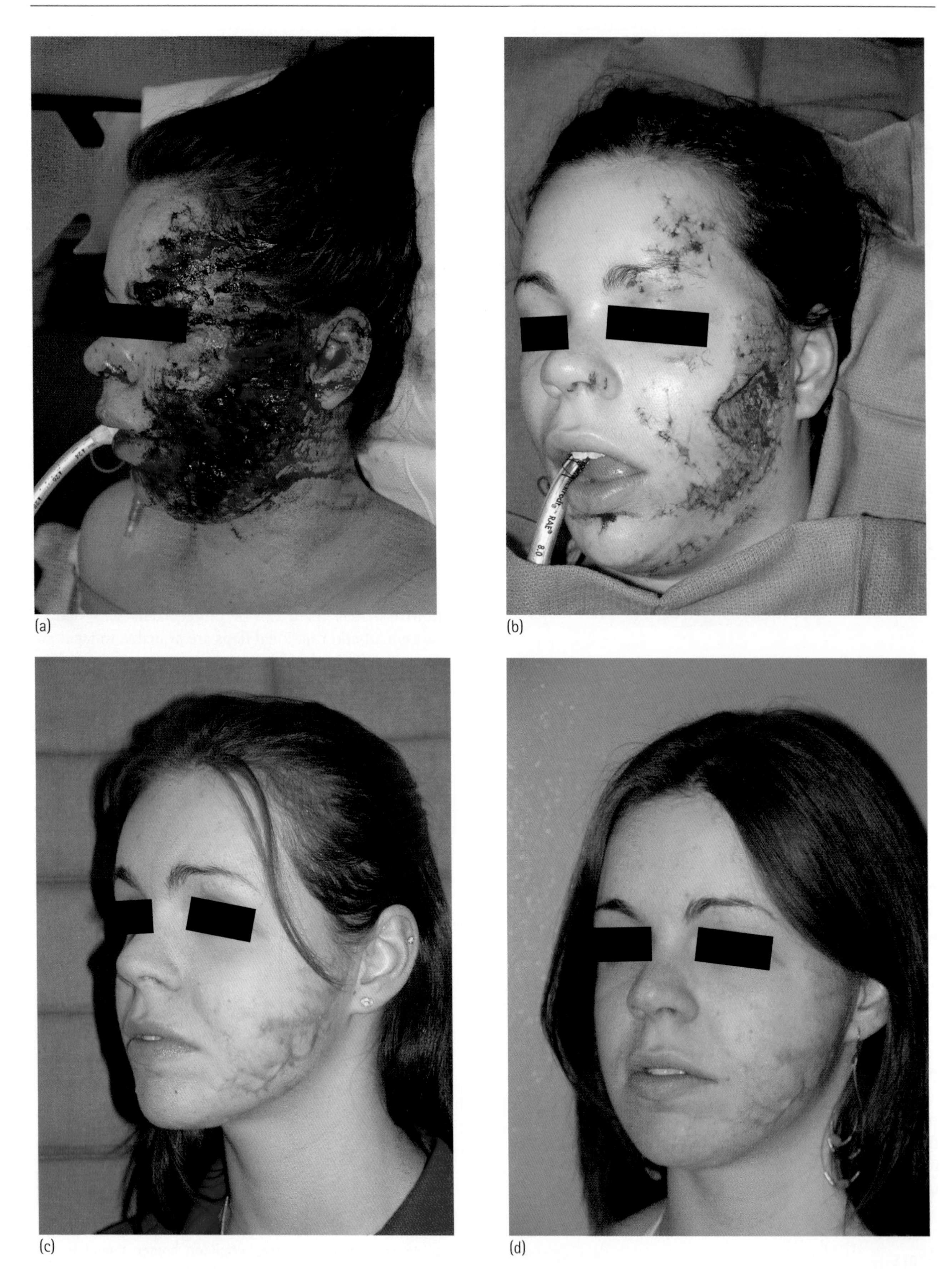

7.3.7 (a) Severe abrasion injury from motor vehicle collision. (b) Appearance after extensive irrigation and debridement of devitalized tissues and primary repair of lacerations. Free tissue transfer was utilized to replace soft tissue deficit. (c) Initial appearance after three months. (d) Scar appearance following dermabrasion at 12 months.

FURTHER READING

Harmon CB, Hadley ML. A cosmetic approach to cutaneous defects. *Atlas of the Oral and Maxillofacial Surgery Clinics of North America* 2004; **12**: 141–62.

Hunter WS. Laceration of the eyelids. *Applied Therapeutics* 1969; **11**: 595–6.

Lee RH, Gamble WB, Robertson B, Manson PN. The MCFONTZL classification system for soft-tissue injuries to the face. *Plastic Reconstructive Surgery* 1999; **103**: 1150–7.

Maxwell GP, Manson PN, Hoopes JE. Reconstruction of traumatic defects utilizing arterialized cutaneous, muscle, myocutaneous and free flaps. *American Surgeon* 1979; **45**: 215–22.

Metzger JT. Immediate reconstruction of simple lacerations. *Annals of Plastic Surgery* 1978; **1**: 450–2.

Myckatyn TM, MacKinnon SE. The surgical management of facial nerve injury. *Clinics in Plastic Surgery* 2003; **30**: 307–18.

Sanders B, Andrews J, Akers P, Lawrence F. Management of wound breakdown after primary repair of a facial laceration. *Journal of Oral Surgery* 1974; **32**: 531–4.

Sclafani AP, Mashkevich G. Aesthetic reconstruction of the auricle. *Facial Plastic Surgery Clinics of North America* 2006; **14**: 103–16, vi.

Silapunt S, Goldberg LH, Peterson SR, Gardner ES. Eyebrow reconstruction: Options for reconstruction of cutaneous defects of the eyebrow. *Dermatologic Surgery* 2004; **30**: 530–5; discussion 535.

7.4

Dentoalveolar trauma

BERNARD J COSTELLO, BRIAN MARTIN

BACKGROUND

Dentoalveolar trauma is common in children and occurs by many aetiologies. In paediatric patients, clinicians must have an awareness of potential child abuse. In addition, timely treatment of traumatic injuries to the alveolar process and dentition is important for positive outcomes.

GENERAL EVALUATION/MANAGEMENT PRINCIPLES

- A complete head and neck examination is important to assess for other injuries.
- A full trauma evaluation should be considered in some instances when the history or mechanism of injury warrants (i.e. motor vehicle crash, falls, assaults).
- A detailed history directed at signs and symptoms of concussion should be completed in many instances where force has been great enough to fracture teeth and bone.
- An evaluation of the occlusion is important to optimize positioning of the fractured segment, and also to rule out maxillary or mandibular fractures. A high degree of suspicion for mandibular condyle fractures in children is appropriate. They are often missed injuries.
- The evaluator should have a high degree of suspicion for mandible and maxillary fractures.
- Teeth and bone segments should undergo a full directed evaluation, including percussion, palpation, inspection and transillumination. Careful assessment for root fracture should be performed.
- Pulp testing can have value after treatment to determine the viability of teeth that may require endodontic therapy, but is usually unreliable in the acute setting. Following a healing period of several weeks, pulp testing can be helpful in determining vitality of the injured teeth.
- Periapical radiographs are often important to obtain a detailed view of the root structures and rule out root fracture when possible. Occlusal views may be helpful in diagnosing root fractures.
- Panoramic tomogram views offer very good overall images, but may not offer the detail that periapical radiographs afford, particularly in the anterior maxilla.
- Computed tomography (CT) in multiple planes offers excellent views of bone and roots. While not indicated for isolated dentoalveolar trauma, if a CT is obtained for evaluation of other facial structures, they can be a valuable asset.
- Cone beam CT may offer additional information in a three-dimensional format that allows for excellent visualization of the injury and post-treatment evaluation.
- The Ellis classification is used to describe tooth fracture:
  - I, Fracture of enamel
  - II, Fracture of enamel and dentin
  - III, Fracture into the pulp chamber within the crown
  - IV, Fracture through the root structure.
- Several key definitions are helpful when describing injury to the dentoalveolar structures and the type of displacement of teeth/bone.
  - *Concussion*: Injury to the tooth structures without significant displacement or loosening. Inflamed periodontal ligament = tender tooth.
  - *Subluxation*: Injury to the tooth structures with mobility, but without significant displacement.
  - *Luxation*: Injury to the tooth structures with displacement in any number of dimensions.
  - *Extrusion*: Injury to the tooth structures with displacement from the alveolar process with some attachment.
  - *Avulsion*: Complete displacement of tooth from socket. Periodontal ligament is severed; fracture of alveolus may occur.
    - Timely intervention is a major outcome factor in successful repositioning and replantation of injured teeth.

- Contraindications to replantation include: immunocompromise, severe uncontrolled seizure disorder, severe uncontrolled diabetes, lack of alveolar integrity.
- Avulsed teeth should be preserved in isotonic solution, saliva or milk.
- Extraction and debridement can be considered if an extended time period has elapsed since avulsion, particularly if the tooth has not been stored in a physiologic medium. Teeth with extraoral dry times of greater than 60 minutes have poor long-term survival rates due to root periodontal ligament cell death.
- Avulsed teeth should be immediately replanted if possible. If the tooth cannot be reimplanted in 5 minutes, it may be stored in Viaspan, Hank's balanced salt solution (tissue culture medium), cold milk, saliva, physiologic saline, or water. If extraoral time is greater than 60 minutes, soak the tooth with fluoride for 20 minutes, rinse with saline, and reimplant.

OPERATIVE MANAGEMENT/PRINCIPLES

- Local anaesthesia with 0.5–2% lidocaine with 1:100 000 or 1:200 000 epinephrine. Appropriate maximum doses should be calculated and respected in children. Consider nerve blocks for comfort when possible. Local infiltration is helpful for hemostasis.
- Thorough debridement of debris, clot and nonviable tissue is important to allow for accurate repositioning of the segments.
- Extract the nonviable, fractured, or grossly carious teeth.
- Extract primary teeth that exhibit gross mobility and consider space maintenance when necessary.
- If soft tissue is available, the surgeon should consider socket preservation for eventual implant placement.
- The segment(s) are repositioned and the occlusion is checked to ensure that the repositioned teeth are not placed in supraocclusion. Teeth can be adjusted with a handpiece to ensure that traumatic occlusion does not occur.
- Obtain a dry field with good suction, gauze and cotton rolls. Good operating conditions, including good lighting and instrumentation, contribute to a successful stabilization procedure.
- Replantation of avulsed teeth and firm repositioning of fractured/displaced segments should achieve the original relationships. Do not attempt to extrude or reposition intruded teeth in the acute phase.
- Stabilization can be accomplished with braided 26- or 28-gauge wire that is positioned passively along the apical one-half to one-third of the crown. Heat-softened (dead soft) 0.016 or 0.018 orthodontic wire can also be utilized. Rectangular orthodontic wire with brackets can also be utilized if available, but these must be placed passively. Ideally, the injured teeth should not be in occlusion.
- Temporization of tooth crown fractures with temporary cement, composite resin 'bandage' and/or pulpotomies can be helpful until definitive endodontic and restorative therapy is possible.
- Dentin fractures without pulp exposure may benefit from placement of a calcium hydroxide base while secondary dentin is developed. This should be then covered with a composite resin bandage. After two months, a more definitive restoration can be performed.
- Dentin fractures with pulp exposure that is still viable may be considered for a direct pulp cap or Cvek pulpotomy with calcium hydroxide. Ideally, this is performed quickly after the injury as time is a significant outcome factor.
- Dentin fractures with pulp exposure and the presence of nonviable pulp should undergo either an apexification procedure (if the apex of the tooth is immature) or formal root canal therapy.
- Crown-root fractures in the vertical dimension usually require extraction. If a fracture is above the cervical margin, then endodontic therapy and restorative measures can be considered.
- Root fractures that are vertical usually require extraction. Root fractures in the apical to middle third of the tooth root can be splinted for 12 weeks and re-evaluated. Root fractures from the middle third and more incisal may be considered for splinting and then orthodontic extrusion.
- Intruded teeth will, in many instances, extrude without significant manipulation. They should be evaluated from an endodontic perspective once initial healing has occurred. Endodontic therapy is necessary at some point in many cases as resorption is common.

POST-OPERATIVE CARE

- Antibiotics may be given for 7 days and should cover most oral pathogens.
- Patients/families should follow up in 1–2 weeks.
- Chlorhexidine solution can be utilized twice a day as directed.
- Oral hygiene instructions should be detailed. Flossing the injured areas should be avoided.
- A soft, nonchew diet is important during the first few weeks to allow for adequate bone healing.
- At some point, a complete endodontic evaluation should be performed to assess whether therapy should be instituted.
- Some initial cosmetic bonding may be helpful for aesthetic reasons and to protect the dentin, but comprehensive restorative and prosthodontic therapy should wait for more complete healing.
- If mild to moderate tooth mobility is being managed with splinting without significant alveolar fracture, then splinting can usually be removed at approximately 7 days.

- Remove the wires and splint material at 3–4 weeks after injury following significant alveolar fractures.
- Orthodontic therapy can be considered at two months for most injuries.
- Bone grafting for implant placement can occur after initial bone healing and remodelling occurs. This is variable based on the degree of injury.

COMPLICATIONS

- Missed injury (tooth, facial fracture, concussion, or other)
- Pulp necrosis
- Discoloration: Remedied with bleaching and/or veneers
- Failure of teeth to replant
  - Consider implants
  - Many patients require bone grafting prior to implant placement due to loss of the facial plate
- Infection may mean the loss of the involved teeth and may require extraction to resolve the infection. In many instances, antibiotics alone will not resolve the infection.
- Ankylosis of repositioned teeth can occur and may significantly compromise orthodontic or prosthodontic therapy.
- Malocclusion of teeth segments that have healed in a malunion may require occlusal adjustment, orthodontic treatment, prosthetic treatment or extraction. Segmental osteotomy is rarely an option, but possible in specific cases.
- Necrosis of bone segments may occur, but this is rare in healthy patients.
- If internal hardware is utilized, then this may become exposed. Treatment involves removal of the hardware.
- A frequent complication in severe trauma is loss of attached gingival and grafting is required for some patients. This is completed once total healing has occurred at the sites.
- Periodontal defects may require long-term interdisciplinary management. A long-term reconstructive and prosthetic plan should be discussed early in the post-operative phase if significant reconstruction is anticipated.

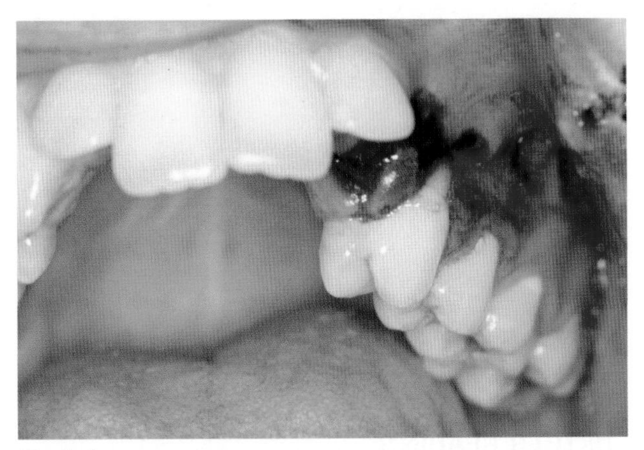

7.4.1 Fractured dentoalveolar segment. Photo courtesy of Dr Peter Guevara, Pittsburgh, PA, USA.

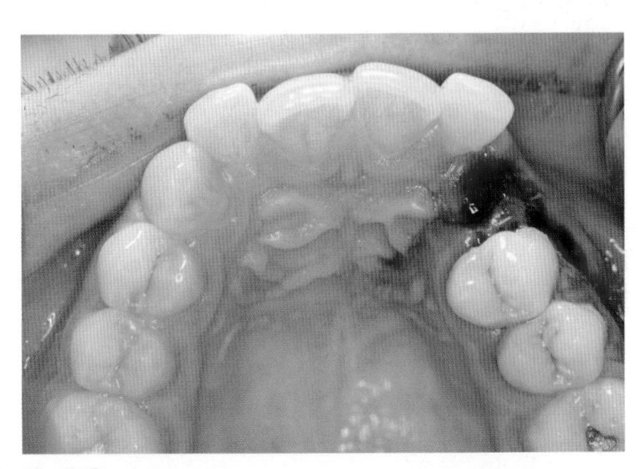

7.4.2 Inferior view. Photo courtesy of Dr Peter Guevara, Pittsburgh, PA, USA.

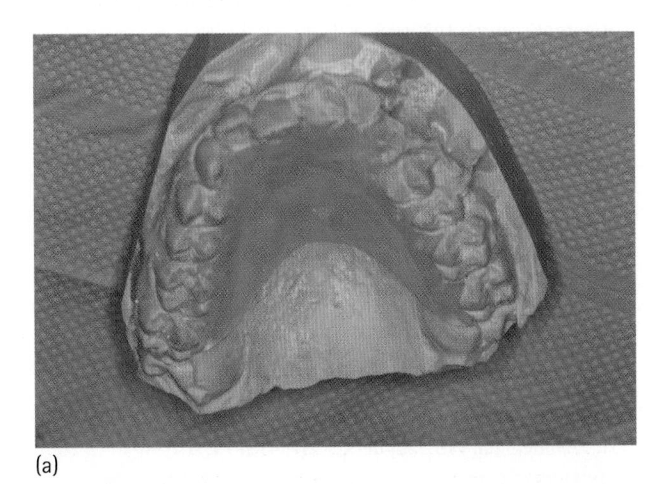

(a)

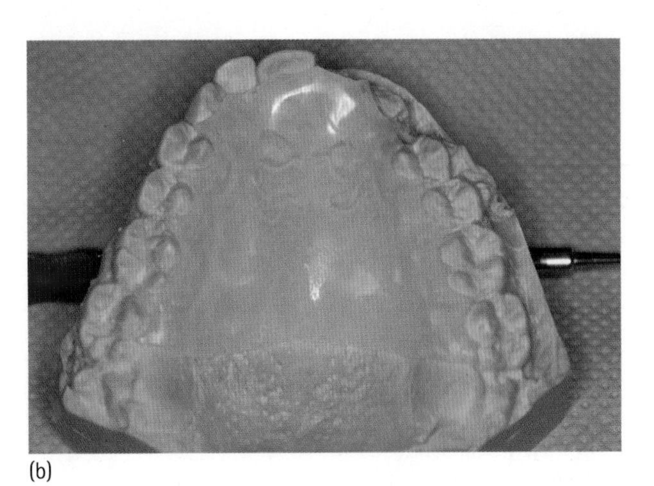

(b)

7.4.3 Cast after model surgery to reposition segment and stabilize with acrylic splint; (b) inferior view. Photo courtesy of Dr Peter Guevara, Pittsburgh, PA, USA.

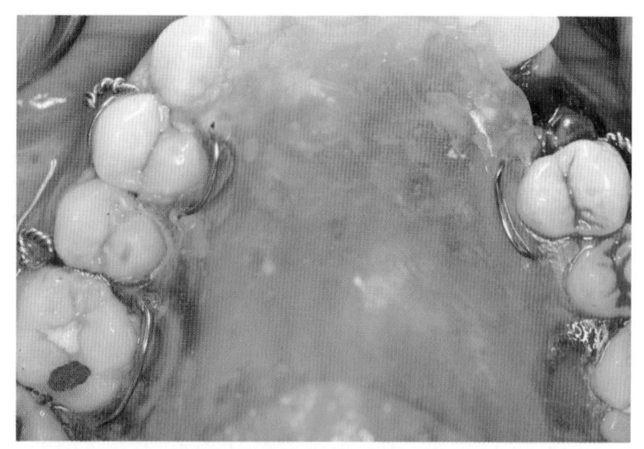

7.4.4 Photo courtesy of Dr Peter Guevara, Pittsburgh, PA, USA.

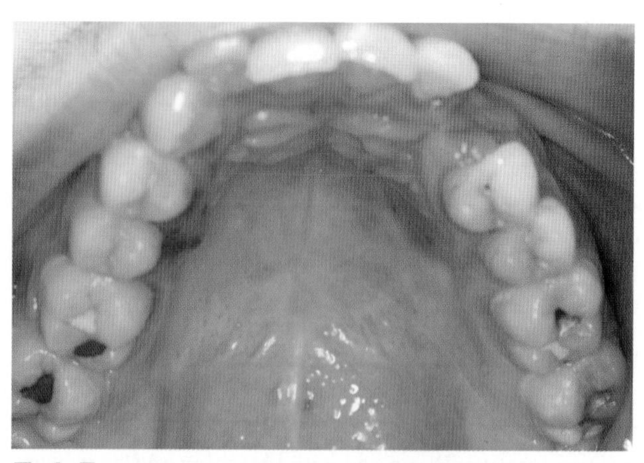

7.4.5 Photo courtesy of Dr Peter Guevara, Pittsburgh, PA, USA.

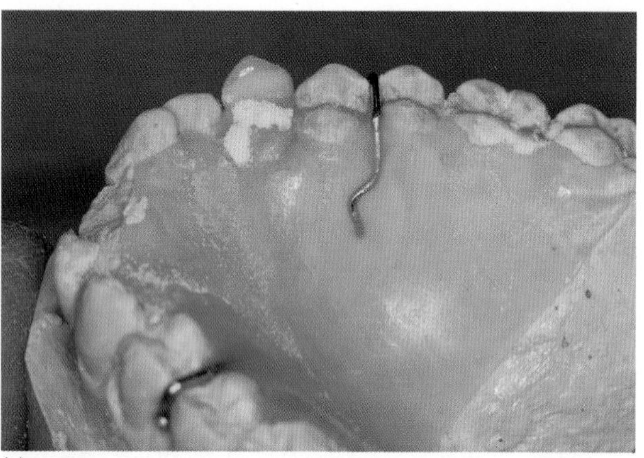

(a)

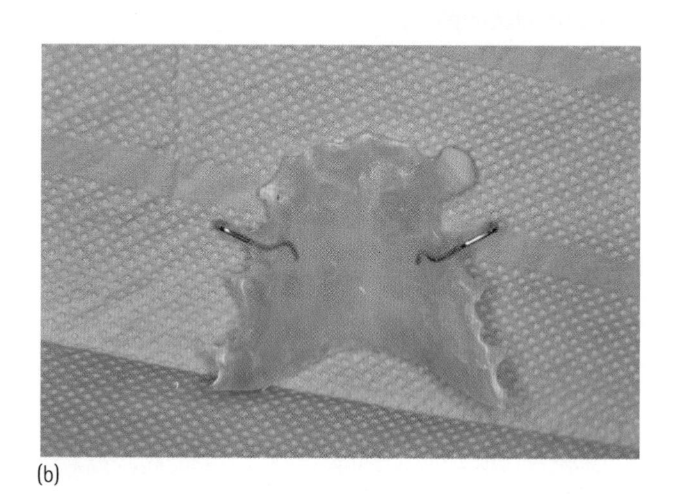

(b)

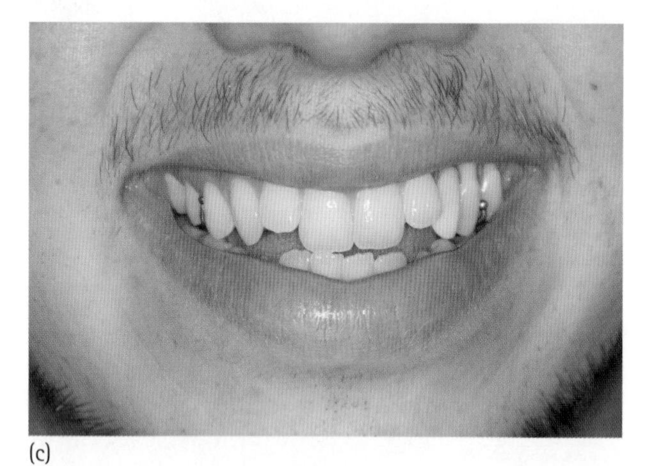

(c)

7.4.6 Photo courtesy of Dr Peter Guevara, Pittsburgh, PA, USA.

Top tips

- Timely treatment.
- Passive splinting.
- Appropriate imaging based on mechanism.

FURTHER READING

Andreasen JO. Etiology and pathogenesis of traumatic dental injuries: A clinical study of 1298 cases. *Scandinavian Journal of Dental Research* 1970; **78**: 329–42.

American Academy of Pediatric Dentistry. *Guidelines on management of acute dental trauma.* Chicago, IL: American Academy of Pediatric Dentistry, 2007.

American Association of Endodontists. *Endodontic considerations in the management of traumatic dental injuries.* Chicago, IL: American Association of Endodontists, 2006.

Ellis RG, Davey KW. *The classification and treatment of injuries to the teeth of children*, 5th edn. Chicago: Year Book Medical Publishers, 1970, 13.

Powers MP, Quereshy FA. Diagnosis and management of dentoalveolar injuries. In: Fonseca JR, Walker RV, Betts NJ, Barber HD (eds). *Oral and maxillofacial trauma*, 2nd edn, vol. 1. Philadelphia, WB Saunders, 1997, 419–72.

Parameters of care. Clinical practice guidelines for oral and maxillofacial surgery (AAOMS ParCare 07); Version 4.0. *Journal of Oral and Maxillofacial Surgery* 2007; (Suppl.).

7.5

Mandibular fractures

MICHAEL PERRY

INTRODUCTION

The mandible is important in airway maintenance, speech, mastication and deglutition. Fractures and injuries to the associated muscles can therefore result in considerable dysfunction and pain. Remember that in some instances – multiple fractures, or associated bleeding, soft tissue swelling, alcohol intoxication and brain injury, and in the supine position (see Advanced Trauma Life Support (ATLS) guidelines) – the airway may be placed at risk and needs careful and repeated evaluation.

Morphologically, the mandible is a U-shaped 'long bone' and can be divided anatomically into:

- symphysis;
- parasymphysis;
- body;
- angle;
- ramus and condyle.

Of particular note are the many muscle insertions (which can either support or displace fractures), the teeth (which together with the periodontal ligament can act as a source of infection), the periosteum (which can assist fracture stability) and the inferior alveolar (inferior dental) nerve (which together with the mental nerve, can be injured at the time of fracture or during their repair) (Figure 7.5.1).

The muscles of mastication and suprahyoid muscles are the principle movers of the mandible. Considerable forces can be generated; hence certain fractures can significantly displace and remain painfully mobile. Conversely, the thick, fleshy masseter and medial pterygoid muscles attach to much of the ramus and therefore splint fractures occurring here. Ramus fractures (as distinct from the condyle) rarely need operative repair. The genioglossus (which forms the bulk of the tongue) and geniohyoid are attached to the midline genial tubercles – mobile fractures in this region may lead to loss of tongue support and airway compromise.

The canine teeth have long roots and the mandibular third molar teeth are often partially erupted. Together with the mental foramen these factors can weaken bone locally and account for the frequency of fractures in these regions. In young patients, the periosteum may resist fracture displacement at the time of impact and in minimally displaced fractures may facilitate nonoperative management. However, once it is torn (by injury or surgical exposure), fracture displacement can occur.

Common fracture sites include (percentages may vary):

- condyle (36 per cent);
- body (21 per cent);
- angle (20 per cent);
- parasymphyseal (14 per cent);
- ramus (3 per cent);
- alveolar (3 per cent);
- coronoid (2 per cent);
- midline symphysis (1 per cent).

ASSESSMENT

'If you leave the patient facing towards heaven, it won't be long before they get there' (paraphrased, original source unknown).

Assessment commonly occurs in one of two scenarios:

1. High velocity injuries, where coexisting torso injuries exist and ATLS principles apply. Of direct relevance here is immobilization of the entire patient and its potential effect on the airway.
2. The 'walking wounded', where other injuries have been ruled out.

In both scenarios, assessment always starts with the airway, while simultaneously protecting the cervical spine until injury can be excluded. Although an appropriate verbal response is encouraging, direct inspection of the oropharynx must be undertaken. Oral bleeding and foreign bodies can be missed, which in the supine patient pose an obvious threat to the airway. In awake, supine patients, blood may

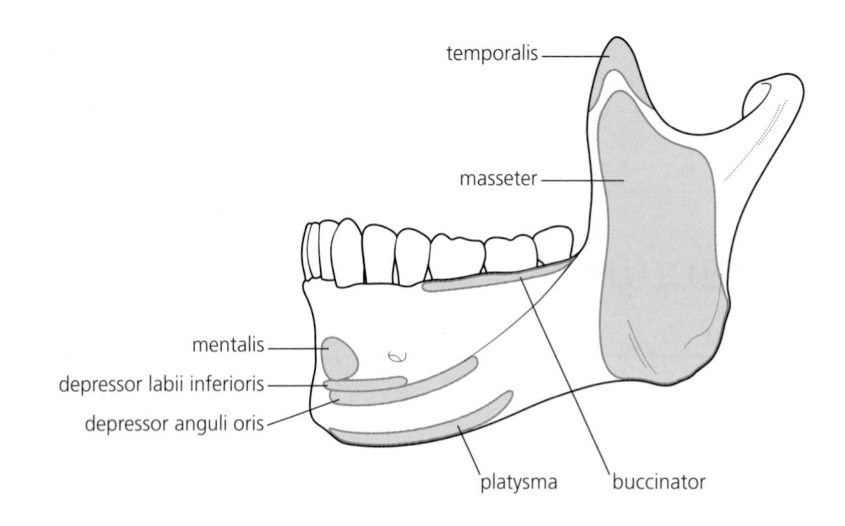

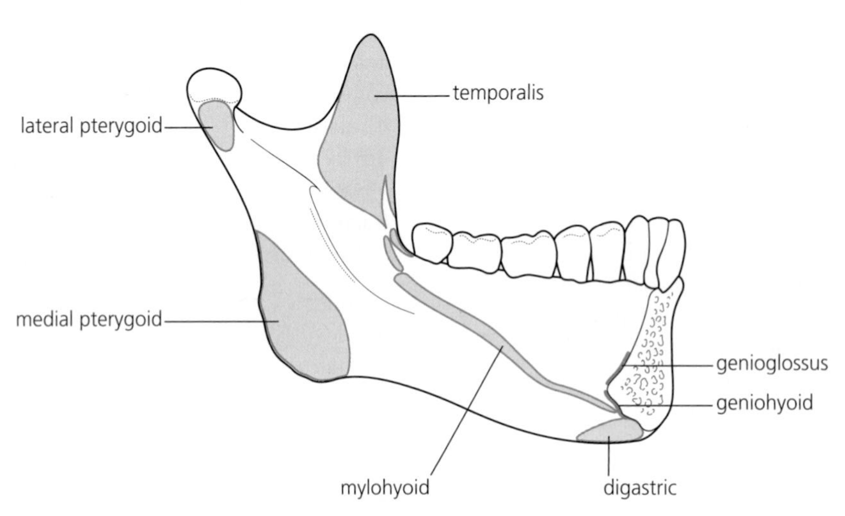

7.5.1 Outer and inner view of the mandible showing muscle attachments.

be swallowed initially, but if it continues places the patient at risk of vomiting later (possibly when they are under less supervision). With mandibular fractures, swallowing may be painful and ineffective. Correctly fitting rigid collars restrict mouth opening and make airway assessment difficult, but in all cases should be sufficiently loosened to enable thorough examination. During this time, manual in-line immobilization of the neck must be correctly performed. Sizing of collars and careful application are also important. Correctly fitting collars can support some mandibular fractures, while poorly fitting ones can compromise the airway and exacerbate ongoing swelling.

In obtunded patients, the jaw thrust and chin lift are commonly performed to maintain the airway, but may be difficult with comminuted fractures. Those patients at high risk of vomiting may require intubation to protect the airway. However, not all patients vomit and the difficulty therefore lies in deciding who should have their airway secured as a precaution. This decision is even more critical if interhospital transfer or imaging (notably computed tomography (CT)) outside the relative safety of the resuscitation room is necessary.

The hallmark of a mandible fracture is a change in the occlusion. However, a normal occlusion does not rule out a mandible fracture. Most fractures occur following blunt injury to the face, commonly following interpersonal violence in many countries. Sports injuries, falls and accidents are other frequent causes. Clinically, the following signs may be elicited to varying degrees:

- pain, especially on talking and swallowing;
- drooling;
- swelling;
- altered bite;
- numbness of the lower lip;
- trismus and difficulty in moving the jaw;

- loosened teeth;
- mobility of fractured segment;
- bleeding from the periodontium;
- sublingual haematoma;
- ipsilateral facial numbness (rare) caused by medial displacement of the condyle resulting from injury to the trigeminal nerve;
- ipsilateral facial weakness (rare) caused by damage to the facial nerve from a direct blow over the ramus.

RADIOGRAPHS

Confirmation and evaluation of a fracture requires imaging. In most cases, plain film radiographs suffice (orthopantomogram (or lateral obliques) plus a posterioanterior view of the mandible). A true lower occlusal view is also very helpful. In selected cases, CT scanning may be necessary.

FIRST AID MEASURES

Pain relief may be achieved by infiltration of local anaesthesia or if possible by an inferior dental nerve block. If the neck is 'clear', a soft collar can be used to support the mandible. Bridal wires (Figure 7.5.2) are the maxillofacial equivalent of a backslab in limb fractures. This is a tightened loop, or figure-of-eight wire, encircling the teeth either side of the fracture. This, and/or intermaxillary fixation (IMF), should be considered when delays in repair (i.e. surgery the next day) are anticipated. Any loose dentoalveolar fractures should also be splinted.

TIMING OF SURGERY

Ideally, all fractures should be repaired as soon as possible, but this rarely happens. For all open fractures (e.g. overlying laceration, or involvement of the periodontium), it is generally assumed that the longer the delay, the more likely infection will occur. However, excessive delay is not clearly defined in the literature. By and large, in the absence of airway problems, active bleeding and excessively mobile (and painful) fragments, most patients can be safely deferred until the next day. General anaesthesia can be risky and is best avoided late at night.

TREATMENT PRINCIPLES

Treatment can be considered as either 'closed' or 'open'. The principles for closed treatment are as follows:

- analgesia;
- antibiotics in open fractures (at 1 week);
- soft diet until a firm callus forms (usually around 4–6 weeks);
- with/without intermaxillary fixation.

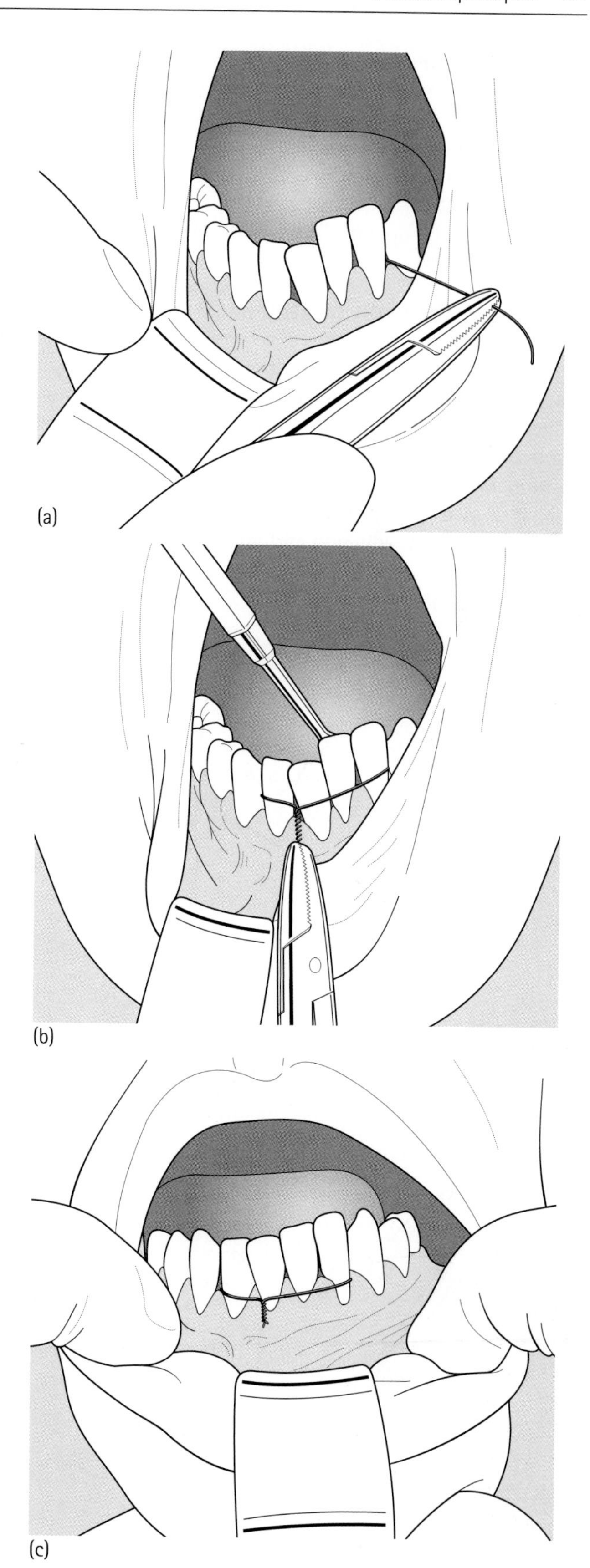

7.5.2 Bridal wires. (a) Pass wire as a figure-of-eight around one or preferably two teeth, either side of the fracture (must be firm). (b) Reduce fracture and tighten wire ends. Ensure wire is below maximum bulbosity of the teeth (in the cervical margin). (c) Wire tightened.

Indications for closed treatment

- No or minimal displacement;
- no or minimal fracture mobility;
- ability to obtain pre-injury occlusion;
- no infection;
- good patient co-operation and follow up.

Indications for open treatment

Open treatment is indicated when closed treatment is inappropriate or has failed. Closed treatment does not reduce fractures anatomically – it is wrong to assume that just because the teeth meet, the fractures are in the correct position. IMF does work, but is required for at least 4 weeks and has its own set of problems – and it is not without risk. Alternatively, open reduction and internal fixation (ORIF) may be undertaken. Both ORIF and IMF have advantages and disadvantages which should be carefully weighed up and if possible discussed with the patient.

With ORIF, surgical exposure of the fracture site and (hopefully) anatomical reduction is carried out. There are two schools of thought:

1 Mandibular fractures need rigid fixation. Dynamic compression osteosynthesis offers this. However, this requires an external approach (scar and risk to the mandibular branch of the facial nerve) (Figure 7.5.3), bicortical screw fixation (risk to the dental roots and inferior alveolar nerve) and a second procedure to remove the metalwork, later. The mandibular curvature makes this technically demanding and there are concerns about stress shielding. Nevertheless, this is reliable treatment and patients return to normal function quickly.

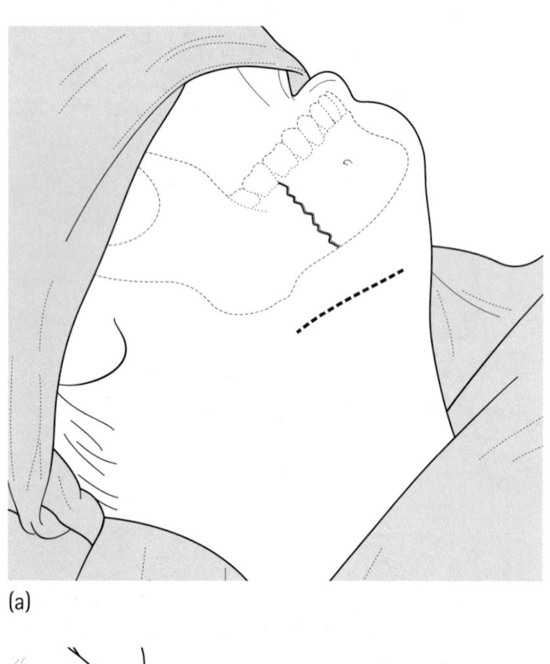

(a)

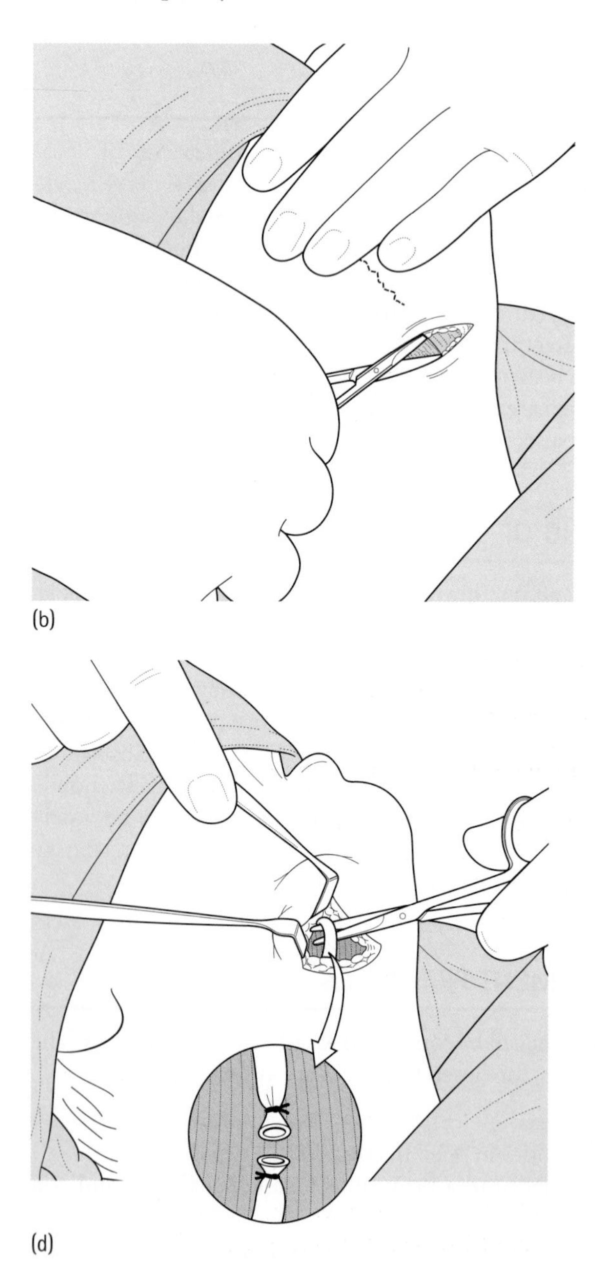

(b)

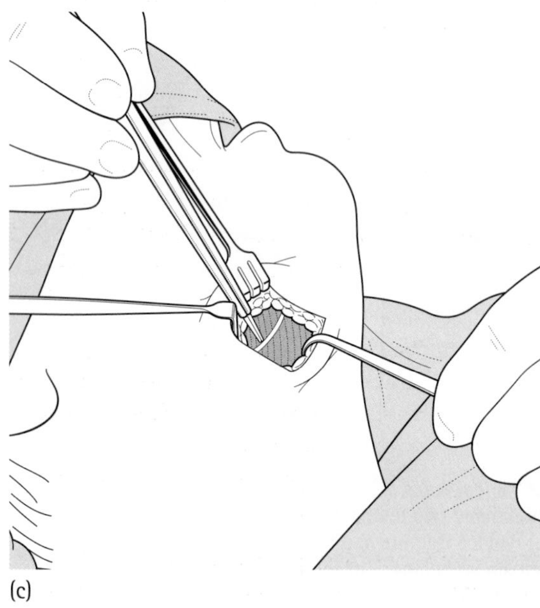

(c)

(d)

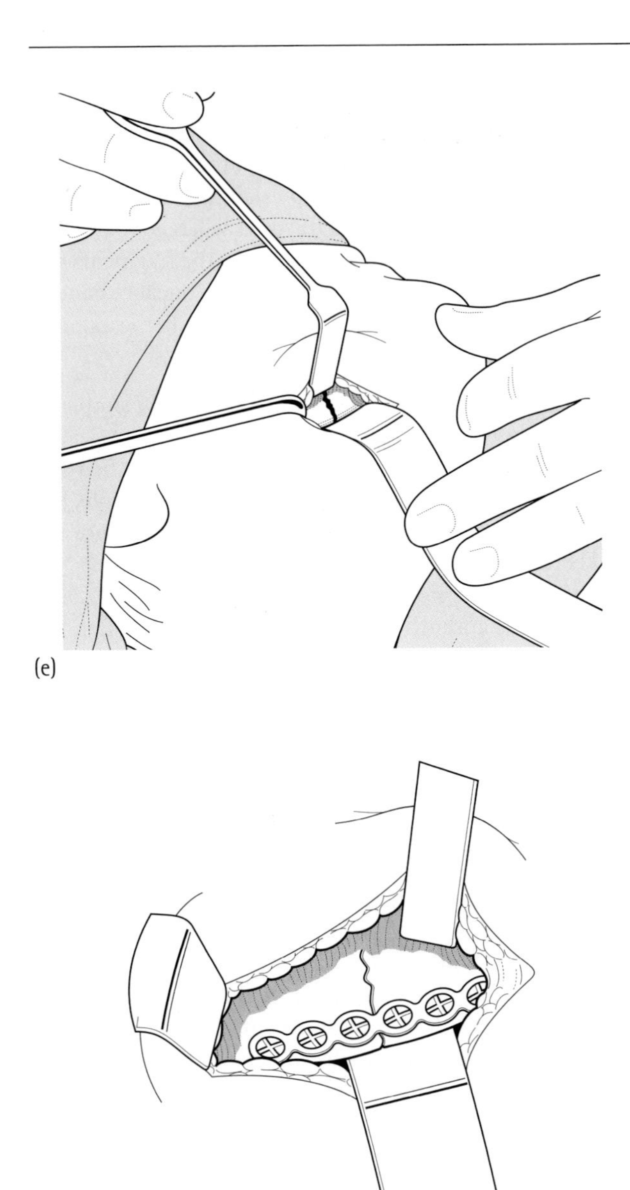

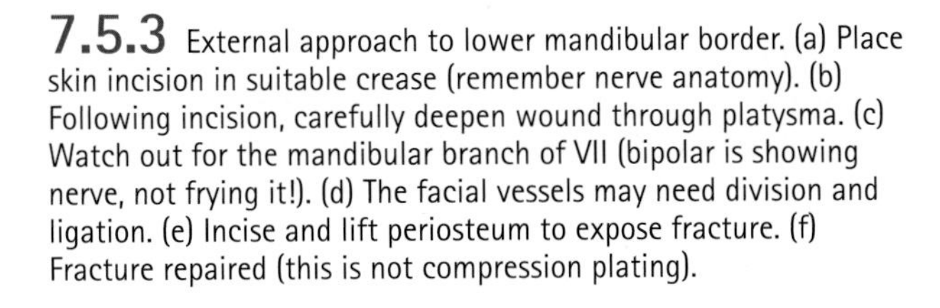

7.5.3 External approach to lower mandibular border. (a) Place skin incision in suitable crease (remember nerve anatomy). (b) Following incision, carefully deepen wound through platysma. (c) Watch out for the mandibular branch of VII (bipolar is showing nerve, not frying it!). (d) The facial vessels may need division and ligation. (e) Incise and lift periosteum to expose fracture. (f) Fracture repaired (this is not compression plating).

2 Mandibular fractures do not need rigid fixation. Studies have shown that micromovement, following semi-rigid fixation, encourages callus formation and healing. Instead of large rigid plates, smaller ones are placed along well-defined 'zones of tension' arising at the fracture site (Figure 7.5.4), effectively converting them into 'zones of compression'. In selected cases, this can be done under local anaesthesia. For this fixation to work, the periosteum needs to be mostly intact with good abutment of the fracture ends. Noncompression miniplates can be placed transorally (or via an overlying laceration) and secured with monocortical screws, thereby avoiding some of the problems associated with the larger compression plates. Fine tuning of the bite is possible with elastic IMF and routine removal of the plates is not necessary. However, plates can get infected and patients still require a soft diet for the same period of time.

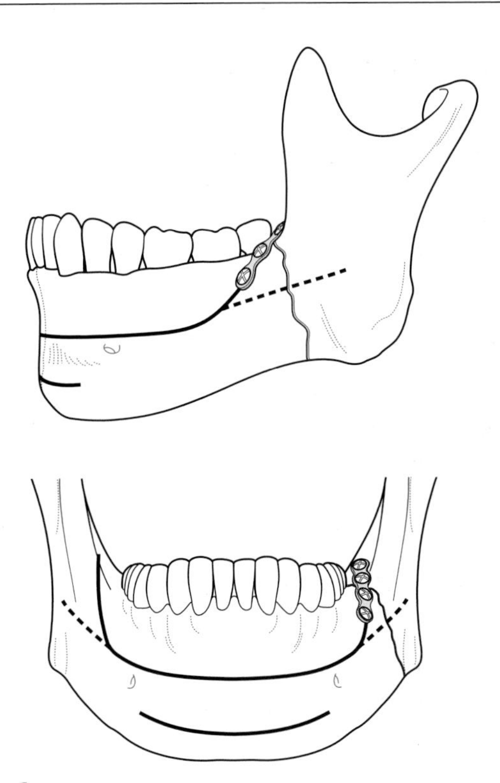

7.5.4 Champy's lines: Zones of tension along which fixation plates may be secured.

EXTERNAL FIXATION

External fixation (Figure 7.5.5) should be regarded as open, even if the fracture is not accessed for inspection. It is used less frequently, but is a useful alternative to IMF in the following circumstances:

- in 'first-aid' stabilization prior to transfers;
- to maintain space and fragment orientation in mandibular continuity defects (e.g. gun shot injuries);
- in severely comminuted fractures;
- in infected/contaminated fractures, at risk of spreading infection and/or osteomyelitis.

External fixation involves inserting rigid pins into the bone fragments via the skin, which are then joined by a system of joints and connecting rods. Fixation can be applied rapidly. Reduction is 'blind', although the fractures can be adjusted post-operatively. Pin insertion may damage the inferior dental nerve or teeth, patient activity is restricted and the pin sites may become infected and scarred. The frames are disliked by patients and they can injure themselves.

SPECIFIC FRACTURES

Condyle fractures

This is covered elsewhere.

Ramus fractures

These rarely need repair. The attached muscles of mastication effectively splint any fractures. If the occlusion is significantly disrupted, elastic IMF may be applied.

Angle fractures

These may be partly splinted by the medial pterygoid and masseteric muscles, but are often displaced and mobile. Fractures have been classified as vertically and horizontally favourable or unfavourable, depending on the orientation of the fracture and tendency for it to displace by the pull of these muscles. This can occur when the periosteum has been ruptured or stripped from the bone allowing displacement to occur.

MINIPLATE PLACEMENT

Access can be made through a variety of incisions, sited along or lateral to the external oblique ridge. As a general principle, surgical wounds should not lie over any metalwork. Either an incision 'down to bone' or a two-layer approach may be used. The fracture is then manipulated, while re-establishing the occlusion (either by IMF or, if experienced 'hand-held'), until it appears anatomically reduced. With simple fractures, a single twisted (propeller) miniplate placed along the external oblique ridge (tension line) is usually sufficient in most cases. More recently, however, there has been interest in the placement of one or two plates, along the buccal surface of the reduced fracture. This approach requires drilling and screw placement via a transbuccal approach, whereby a trochar is passed through the cheek. Each approach has advantages and disadvantages and the final choice is a matter of surgical preference. Certainly in comminuted and very unstable fractures, more than one plate may be necessary. In such cases, a limited external approach to enable lower mandibular border fixation may be required.

Symphyseal and parasymphyseal fractures

With symphyseal (midline) fractures, the mylohyoid and geniohyoid muscles may help stabilize the fracture. However, obliquely orientated fractures will tend to overlap. With bilateral parasymphyseal fractures, the fragments can displace posteroinfeiorly – so-called 'bucket handle' fractures. There are a number of approaches to the anterior mandible:

- Gingival sulcus incision. Although relatively simple, if poorly closed can result in gingival recession.
- Single layer incision at the junction of the attached and nonattached mucosa. This is also relatively simple, but requires a careful and watertight closure to reduce the likelihood of infection or dehiscence.
- A two layer incision placed in the sulcus (Figure 7.5.6). This is this author's preferred approach. Very often the branches of the mental nerve can be seen through the mucosa and protected. A two-layer closure is also usually secure.
- Via any overlying lacerations. Even small ones should be considered – it is surprising how much access you can get once the deeper tissues have been mobilized.

With 'anterior' fractures (usually taken to mean those between the mental foramina), two miniplates are usually required to resist torsional forces following muscle pull. Place the lower along the thick lower border if possible. Care is required with drilling the upper (dental roots). In theory, holes can be drilled over the roots (monocortical screws), although in practice many surgeons place the holes 5 mm or more below the apices, to avoid damage. This principle is often extended to the premolar region, and the number of plates used depends very much on the fracture configurations.

ANTIBIOTICS, STEROIDS AND TETANUS PROPHYLAXIS

Protocols may vary between different units. Antibiotics are usually given for fractures which are open, particularly if there is any delay in repair. Penicillin (or a cephalosporin) and metronidazole is one option, but many exist. Tetanus prophylaxis should be considered, especially in unclean wounds. Some surgeons like to give steroids (dexamethasone/methylprednisolone) to reduce facial swelling, but this is not essential – a stable repair is.

SPECIAL CONSIDERATIONS

Tooth in the fracture site

This is common in angle fractures with associated lower third molars. Removal of the tooth may reduce the risk of infection, but can make repair tricky and unstable. The

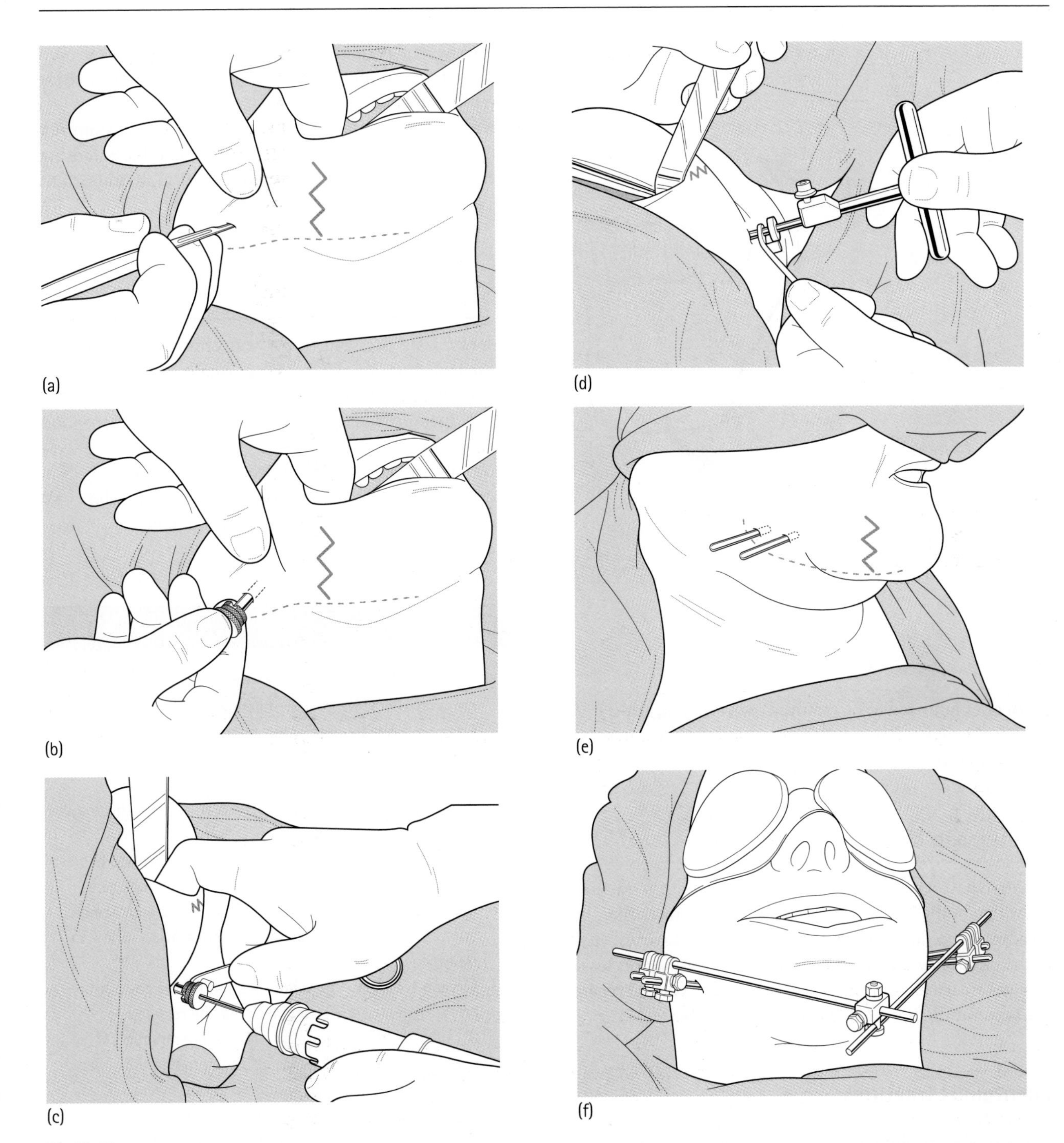

7.5.5 Expose fracture intraorally to precisely define its site and extent. Then: (a) Stab incision for pin placement. (b) Pass pointed trochar down to bone. (c) Replace inner pointed trochar with drill guide and drill bicortical hole. (d) Remove drill guide and place pin (depth gauge may be used). (e) Repeat so that there are two pins either side of fracture. (f) Completed arrangement.

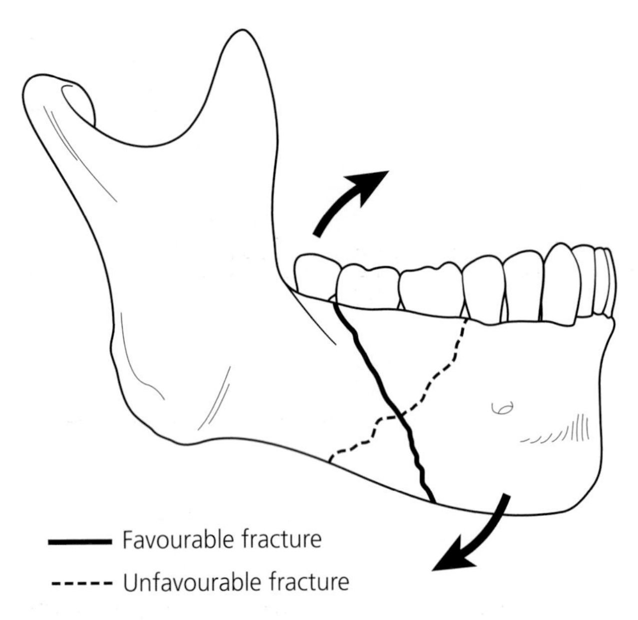

7.5.6 Favourable and unfavourable angle fractures (note tendency to displace).

tooth does not need to be removed in every case, but if it is fractured or has symptoms or signs of infection it may be best to remove it.

Fractures in children

Children have softer bones compared with adults. A fracture anywhere in the body implies relatively more force than in an adult (especially ribs). Mandibular fractures are unusual as the facial skeleton is less prominent. Any minor occlusal changes are usually compensated for with growth and repair is less common. Resorbable plates are often used.

Edentulous fractures

The severely atrophic edentulous mandible often has a poor outcome, especially when the height of the mandible is 10 mm or less. These are characterized by poor blood supply and slow healing, in patients with poor general health and osteoportic bones. IMF is not possible (no teeth) and any periosteal stripping affects the blood supply. Alternatives to ORIF include the following:

- Soft diet and regular review. Fractures may still heal, even if not anatomically. As long as the mucosa is intact, these are not open fractures.
- Wiring the patients dentures (if a good fit) or customized 'Gunning splints', to the maxilla and mandible and using these to provide IMF. Patient selection is important (respiratory diseases, etc.).

POST-OPERATIVE CARE

- Genioplasty dressing to prevent chin ptosis following extensive anterior exposure (optional);
- antibiotics (protocols vary);
- post-operative radiographs may be taken to confirm good repair;
- soft diet and nutritional advice for 4–6 weeks;
- scrupulous oral hygiene (tooth brushing and hot, salt water mouth rinses being the main element);
- regular follow up.

Top tips

- Fractures of the mandible in restrained supine patients is not a good mix. Never leave such patients unattended.
- Comminution implies high energy and the risk of significant airway swelling.
- Check the hyoid and larynx for associated injuries.
- Beware patients who repeatedly ask to sit up – this may indicate airway difficulties.
- Vomiting is best managed by tilting the trolley head down, rather than attempting to log roll the patient.
- Mental paraesthesia is both an important diagnostic sign and an important medicolegal observation prior to treatment.
- Missing teeth must be accounted for. Both a chest x-ray and soft tissue view of the neck may be required.
- A sublingual haematoma is pathognmonic of a mandibular fracture and may also compromise the airway.
- The mandible commonly fractures in two places – if you see one fracture, look for another (as in pelvic fractures).
- Unerupted wisdom teeth can rotate in their sockets and displace angle fractures sufficiently to affect the occlusion.
- If removing an associated tooth, plate the fracture first, take the plate off and remove the tooth. This can help in unstable fractures.

7.6

Management of condylar fractures, including endoscopic reduction

ROGER CURRIE

INTRODUCTION

Condylar fractures are an important subgroup of mandibular fractures both in presentation and management. Fractures may present in isolation or in conjunction with other mandibular fractures, or as a component of a pan-facial injury. The age of the patient is also an important factor in the management of this subgroup of fractures. Various issues have challenged the management of condylar fractures; these have included a variety of classifications, concern in relation to surgical access and the limitations of technology. The contemporary management of condylar fractures exemplifies the advances in technology and surgical access that the last decade has seen in oral and maxillofacial surgery.

INCIDENCE AND CLASSIFICATION

The literature has various figures for the incidence of condylar fractures from 30–50 per cent of all mandibular fractures. The most common cause of presentation in the United Kingdom is a result of interpersonal violence, with at least 50 per cent of patients having an associated mandibular fracture. Over 80 per cent of fractures are unilateral, with the highest incidence in the age range of 20–39 years with at least a 2:1 sex ratio (male:female).

Classification of condylar injuries has been difficult. This is in part due to the types of classification in use. These may relate to anatomical position, i.e. condylar neck, or may relate to displacement of the condylar fragment. Previously, classifications have included Speissl and Schroll, and MacLennan and Lindahl. In 2005, as part of the SORG study, Loukota *et al.* published a subclassification of condylar fractures which is both pragmatic and clinically useful as it aids visualization and consideration of treatment options when combined with degree of overlap (in mm) and angle of displacement.

DEFINITIONS

1. Diacapitular (through the head of the condyle) fracture; the fracture starts in the articular surface and may extend outside the capsule.
2. Fracture of the condylar neck. The fracture line starts above line A, and in more than half (the fracture distance) runs above line A. High condylar fracture.
3. Fracture of the condylar base. The fracture line runs behind the mandibular foramen and in more than half the distance below line A. Low condylar fracture.
4. Line A. A perpendicular line through the sigmoid notch tangential to the ascending ramus (Figure 7.6.1).

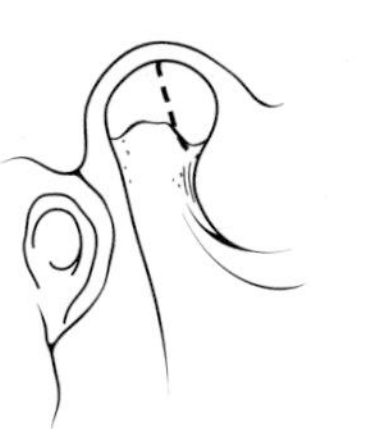

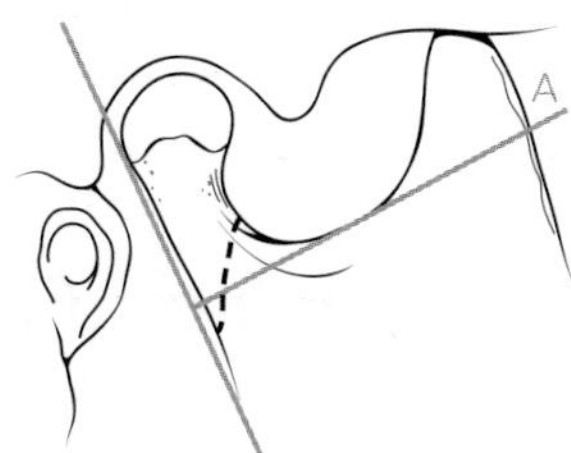

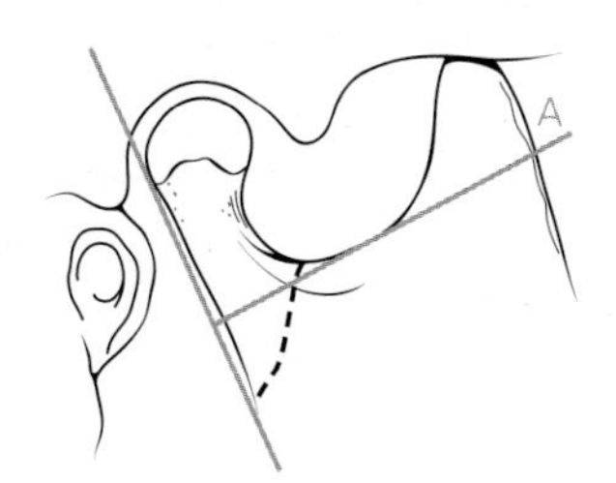

7.6.1 Classification of condylar fractures (modified with permission from Loukota RA, Eckelt U, De Bont L, Rasse M. *British Journal of Oral and Maxillofacial Surgery* 2005; **43**: 72).

INVESTIGATIONS AND IMAGING

A good history and clinical examination will be required as for all trauma patients. Condylar fractures may well be discovered in the 'secondary survey', as in Advanced Trauma Life Support (ATLS) protocols.

Clinical signs include pain, limited mouth opening, deviation on opening, lateral or anterior open bites, chin or external auditory meatus lacerations.

The mechanism of injury, associated injuries and the clinical findings will direct the imaging required. Imaging in two planes is the normal investigation, usually an orthopantomogram (OPG) and reverse Townes. With the advent of spiral computed tomography (CT) scanning some surgeons may have a CT as an initial investigation. A CT may well be helpful with bilateral fractures, gross medial displacement and impacted fractures where a contralateral open bite is present due to the 'crushing' of the condylar head.

TREATMENT OPTIONS AND OUTCOMES

Treatment options include the following:

- no treatment;
- closed reduction (management);
- open reduction;
- endoscopically assisted;
- free plating and grafting.

The most common clinical scenario is the management of the unilateral condylar fracture, with or without another mandibular fracture. Debate over this has been intense over the last decade with two consensus conferences and a recent prospective randomized multicentre study. In 1993, only 9 per cent of the surgeons questioned would consider open reduction and internal fixation (ORIF). While opinion is still divided, more evidence supports open reduction in defined clinical circumstances.

Patient-specific variables also impact on treatment decisions; age, ability to cooperate, other facial fractures and comorbidity all influence the management decision (Table 7.6.1).

Surgical variables include experience, fracture location (and imaging) and available instruments, e.g. endoscopic.

Table 7.6.1 Ideal outcomes of condylar fracture treatment.

Outcome
Pain free mouth opening >40 mm
Pain free lateral excursions >6 mm
Stable and pain free occlusion
Normal facial and jaw symmetry

No treatment

No treatment is considered when no occlusal discrepancy or functional impairment exists.

Closed reduction (management)

This is a blanket term, which implies no open intervention (Table 7.6.2). In common practice, it would involve the placement of arch bars, splints, intermaxillary fixation (IMF) screws or Rapid IMF™. All of these allow the placement of elastic intermaxillary traction/fixation.

Table 7.6.2 Indications for closed management.

Indications
Condylar neck fractures in children <15 years
Very high condylar neck fractures without dislocation
Intracapsular fractures

The precise post-operative course can vary from 2 weeks to three months using guiding elastics, with most surgeons using elastics for 2–4 weeks. It is now well accepted that there is no place for wire IMF.

Closed management was the previous treatment of choice for both displaced and nondisplaced fractures. Many surgeons had concerns about damage to the facial nerve with open reduction and it was not clear that reduced fractures gave better results. Complications of closed management can include painful or limited opening, deviation on opening, malocclusion and loss of posterior facial height. Outcome studies performed by Ellis *et al.* in 2000 confirm malocclusion, occlusal canting and loss of posterior facial height in patients treated with closed management compared to open reduction. The facial asymmetry was notable at 6 weeks.

Open reduction

Open reduction is not a new concept, having been proposed in certain defined circumstances by Zide and Kent in 1983. The impact of technology (Table 7.6.3) and the increased understanding of both the biomechanical and functional

Table 7.6.3 Impact of technology.

New technologies	
Plates	
Imaging	
Instruments	Endoscope
	90° screwdriver

advantages of plating supported by good randomized studies have encouraged surgeons to re-evaluate open reduction, and for others to explore endoscopically assisted reduction.

The principles of open management are similar for all fractures and include accurate reduction, stable internal fixation, preservation of blood supply and early active mobilization.

With open reduction of condylar fractures, the main specific concerns are facial nerve weakness/paralysis and scarring.

Much work has been carried out on evaluating open reduction (Table 7.6.4) and various surgical approaches have been described, including submandibular, retromandibular with transparotid access, pre-auricular, coronal and rhytidectomy. If mid-facial access is required, then a coronal approach may well be helpful; however, for the majority of cases a retromandibular incision tangential to the posterior border of the mandible with transparotid dissection will allow safe exposure of the fracture.

Table 7.6.4 Indications for open reduction.

Indications
Fracture dislocation angulation of >30°
Need to establish posterior facial height loss of >5 mm
Failed closed management
Displacement into middle cranial fossa or external auditory meatus
Bilateral condylar fractures with associated pan facial fractures
Medical contraindication to intermaxillary fixation, e.g. epilepsy

Materials used for fixation include, wires, K wire, screws and plates. The most common method of fixation is 2.0-mm titanium semi-rigid plates, although Asprino *et al.*'s biomechanical evaluation included one or two 2-mm plates with 4-, 6- or 8-mm screws (Figures 7.6.5–7). The most favourable mechanical behaviour was with two-plate fixation, although increasing screw length improved stability when only one plate was used.

A 70 per cent success rate has been reported by Davis with free grafting alone or in conjunction with a ramus osteotomy in cases when adequate reduction and fixation could not be obtained.

MANAGEMENT OF ISOLATED UNILATERAL CONDYLAR FRACTURE

Informed consent must be obtained including discussion of likely complications, including scarring and facial nerve damage.

Under endotracheal general anaesthesia, the patient is prepped and draped, allowing access to the oral cavity for downward distraction of the ipsilateral angle to aid reduction. An intravenous dose of antibiotic is given at induction. Ideally, two assistants are required for retraction and mandibular manipulation.

The retromandibular incision is marked 1 cm distal to the posterior border of the ramus, approximately 2 cm in length (Figure 7.6.2).

Wide dissection in the superficial layer above the parotid fascia is carried out to facilitate retraction. The parotid fascia is divided with blunt dissection under direct vision and the facial nerve branches are retracted out of the operative field. Once the masseter muscle is exposed, the surgeon uses a finger to palpate the underlying fracture and a vertical incision is made down to bone. Subperiosteal stripping exposes the fracture, although the condylar fracture can be 'trapped' in the muscle and requires careful freeing.

With retraction in a superior/inferior direction and use of a thin-bladed retractor behind the posterior border, the mandible can be displaced downwards and backwards with occlusal pressure, which increases the space and aids fracture reduction. Once fracture reduction has been achieved, adequate fixation is required. Some surgeons use intra-operative IMF, others will handhold the occlusion while it is fixed.

Options for plate fixation include one 2-mm DCP plate or two 2-mm plates placed as far apart as possible. Newer shaped plates may offer some ease of application. It is important to insert at least two screws (6–8 mm) in the distal aspect of the proximal fracture and placing the superior screw without the mandible in occlusion then rereducing the fracture and placing the second screw, prior to fixation of the distal fragment, can facilitate this. A fracture gap can open at this point and a two hole spaced plate with the space over the fracture is useful to close this gap by placing the superior screw and then securing manual reduction of occlusion with inferior traction on the distal screw holes of both plates to close the fracture gap prior to placing the final three screws (Figure 7.6.3).

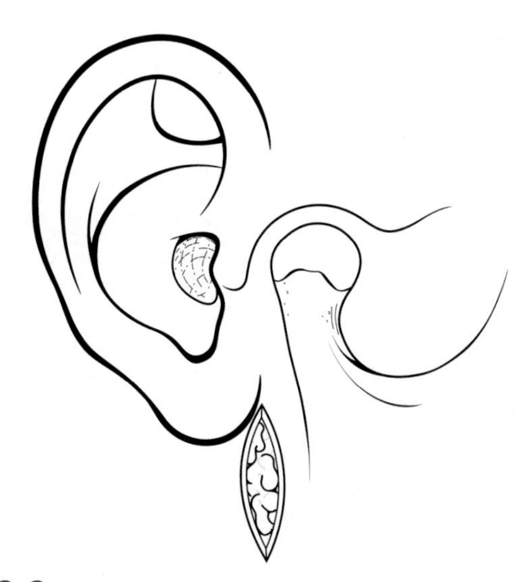

7.6.2 Retromandibular incision.

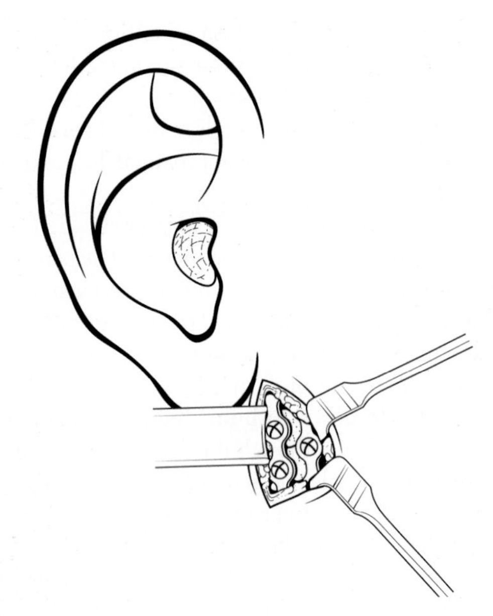

7.6.3 Fracture exposed and reduced.

The wound is closed in layers with attention to closing the masseter muscle and the parotid fascia/SMAS prior to skin closure with nonresorbable sutures.

In 2002, using this technique, 42 patients were reported by Devlin. A further 30 have since been treated with no patients having permanent facial weakness, five patients having transient facial weakness with a mean recovery of four months, two sialocoeles which settled with time, a wound infection and a plate failure, which did not impact on the clinical result.

Endoscopically assisted reduction of condylar fractures

While open reduction became more accepted, groups of surgeons have looked at using newer technology and applying this within maxillofacial surgery. Endoscopically assisted reduction is a good example, as it reduces the risk to the facial nerve and minimizes scarring. Work undertaken on the development of this technique confirms that there is a long and steep learning curve and that laterally displaced fractures are much easier than medially displaced fractures, and like all endoscopic procedures the surgeon must be able to convert to an open procedure to complete the surgery if needed.

With this development, plating companies have designed and produced special instruments to facilitate endoscopically assisted reduction; however, most institutions have the basic light sources, monitor banks and camera attachments.

The endoscopic approach uses an intraoral approach or a submandibular approach along with a transbuccal access for some fixation (Figure 7.6.4).

Using the intraoral approach, a ramus incision similar to one for a mandibular osteotomy is made and the masseter muscle stripped to create the optical cavity. A 4-mm 30° endoscope with an adapted retractor provides direct vision and this is aided by a Freer elevator with built in suction. Under vision and with special instruments the fracture is manipulated and reduced, this may require extensive dissection at the posterior border or the sigmoid notch, occasionally downward traction may be needed, this can be digital occlusal pressure or a wire at the angle. The transbuccal approach can be used to place screws using an adaptable plate holder or a 90° screwdriver can be used though this can be

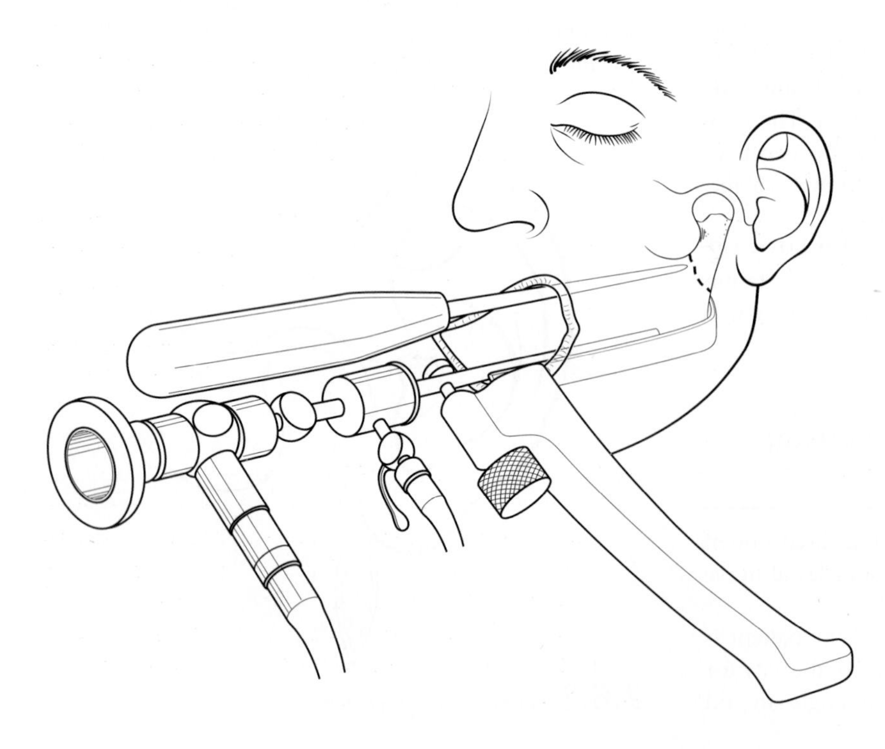

7.6.4 Endoscopic principle.

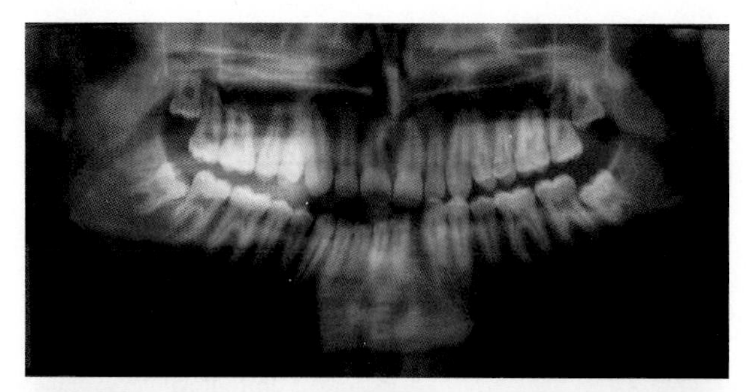

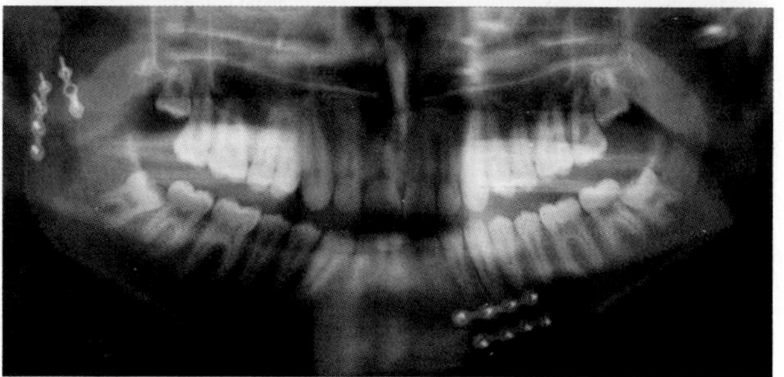

7.6.5 Combined pre- and post-operative orthopantomograms.

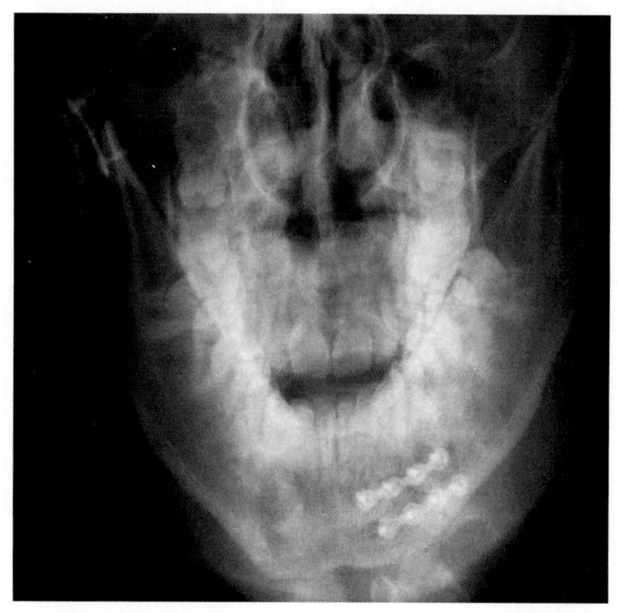

7.6.7 Post-operative posterioanterior mandible radiograph.

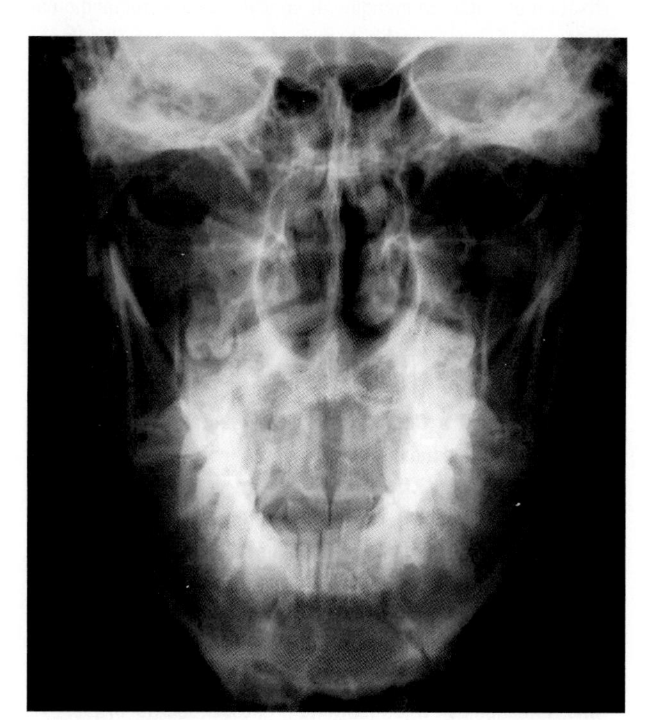

7.6.6 Pre-operative posterioanterior mandible radiograph.

difficult in a tight, soft tissue envelope, occasionally a second transbuccal stab may be needed to use a threaded fracture manipulator – 'the screw on a stick'. This can be used to place the initial screw in the proximal fragment.

In 2006, Muller *et al.* reported results of 150 fractures, where treatment times were down to 70 minutes, and 91 per cent obtaining primary plate fixation. Unfortunately, 9 per cent were aborted with either open or closed management initiated and fewer than 2 per cent having plate fracture or transient facial nerve weakness.

Further refinement of this technique will be required, as challenges exist with difficulty in reducing medially displaced fractures, a limited surgical cavity compared to other endoscopic procedures, e.g. brow lift and the need for special training and instruments.

PAEDIATRIC FRACTURES

Children with condylar fractures are a very different group. Children exhibit a regenerative capacity that adults do not and will regenerate condylar form and function, while adults compensate at an occlusal level with loss of posterior facial height.

In 2005, Dodson reviewed paediatric condyle–ramus fractures and reported good outcomes; however, increasing age was associated with poorer outcomes. These younger patients often require long-term follow up as they can in rare circumstances present in later years with developmental abnormalities including asymmetry, hypoplasia or ankylosis.

PAN-FACIAL FRACTURES

One of the clear indications for open reduction of condylar fractures is an associated mid-facial fracture. The correction of vertical height aids the correction of the mid-facial deformity, and should be carried out when the mandibular fractures are reduced, perhaps before definitive mid-face correction.

BILATERAL FRACTURES

When associated with a symphyseal fracture, this can lead to mandibular widening and great care must be taken to ensure accurate reduction at the symphysis or a post-operative malocclusion will be evident, in spite of anatomical condylar fracture reductions.

If two fractures are present, it is ideal to fix both; however, at least one needs to be fixed to regain height.

POST-OPERATIVE MANAGEMENT

Good post-operative care with elastic traction for closed management and jaw exercises and clear post-operative instructions for open or endoscopic treated fractures are needed.

COMPLICATIONS

Complications include the following:

- malocclusion;
- condylar necrosis, with associated open bite;
- wound infection (rare <1 per cent);
- hypertrophic scarring;
- facial nerve weakness, transient or permanent;
- sialocoele.

Top tips

- Treat the patient and the occlusion, not the radiograph.
- Ensure you have adequate assistance.
- Start with easier, low, laterally displaced fractures when starting open reductions.
- Do not attempt a high medially placed fracture as your first.
- Give clear post-operative instructions.
- Consider endoscopic approaches only when you master open surgery.

FURTHER READING

Asprino L, Consani S, de Moraes M. A comparative biomechanical evaluation of mandibular condyle fracture plating techniques. *Journal of Oral and Maxillofacial Surgery* 2006; **64**: 452–6.

Assael LA. Open versus closed reduction of adult mandibular condyle fractures: An alternative interpretation of the evidence. *Journal of Oral and Maxillofacial Surgery* 2003; **61**: 1333–9.

Baker AW, McMahon J, Moos KF. Current consensus on the management of fractures of the mandibular condyle. *International Journal of Oral and Maxillofacial Surgery* 1998; **27**: 258–66.

Brandt MT, Haug RH. Open versus closed reduction of adult mandibular condyle fractures: A review of the literature regarding the evolution of current thoughts on management. *Journal of Oral and Maxillofacial Surgery* 2003; **61**: 1324–32.

Davis BR, Powell JE, Morrison AD. Free grafting of mandibular condyle fractures: Clinical outcomes in 10 consecutive patients. *International Journal of Oral and Maxillofacial Surgery* 2005; **34**: 871–6.

Devlin MF, Hislop WS, Carton ATM. Open reduction and internal fixation of fractured mandibular condyles by a retromandibular approach: Surgical morbidity and informed consent. *British Journal of Oral and Maxillofacial Surgery* 2002; **40**: 23–5.

Dodson TB. Condyle and ramus–condyle unit fractures in growing patients: Management and outcomes. *Oral and Maxillofacial Surgery Clinics of North America* 2005; **17**: 447–53.

Eckelt U, Schneider M Erasmus F *et al.* Open versus closed treatment of fractures of the mandibular condylar process – a prospective randomized multicentre study. *Journal of Cranio-Maxillofacial Surgery 2006;* **34**: 306–14.

Ellis E, Simon P, Throckmorton GS. Occlusal results after open or closed treatment of fractures of the mandibular condylar process. *Journal of Oral and Maxillofacial Surgery* 2004; **58**: 260–64.

Loukota RA, Eckelt U, De Bont L, Rasse M. Subclassification of fractures of the condylar process of the mandible. *British Journal of Oral and Maxillofacial Surgery* 2005; **43**: 72–3.

Muller RV, Czerwinski M, Lee C, Kellman RM. Condylar fracture repair: Use of the endoscope to advance traditional treatment philosophy. *Facial and Plastic Surgery Clinics of North America* 2006; **14**: 1–9.

Zachariades N, Mezitis M, Mourouzis C *et al.* Fractures of the mandibular condyle: A review of 466 cases. Literature review and reflections on treatment and proposals. *Journal of Cranio-Maxillofacial Surgery* 2006; **34**: 421–32.

7.7

Middle third fractures

JOE MCMANNERS, JEREMY MCMAHON, IAN HOLLAND

DIAGNOSIS

The essential basic history, examination and directed special tests are the same as for any injured patient (see Chapter 7.1). Particular care in clinical examination should be sufficient to make most diagnoses of middle third fractures (see below under Classification).

Special tests

Plain radiography has a limited place in the diagnosis and treatment planning, as illustrated (Figure 7.7.1). Computed tomography scanning has enabled greatly improved visualization of the nature of the mid-face injury, which is usually much more complex than has previously been realized (Figure 7.7.2 and 7.7.3). Having said that, all that is revealed by a scan does not necessarily need internal fixation. Dental models from impressions taken once the patient is stabilized may be very helpful in diagnosing and restoring the occlusion at operation. Other imaging modalities may be necessary when indicated, e.g. contrast arteriography.

CLASSIFICATION

Mid-face fractures are often classified as central mid-face and lateral mid-face or zygomatico-orbital fractures.

Central mid-face fractures

- Low level, just above the tooth-bearing maxilla and alveolar process: Le Fort I (Figure 7.7.4 (a–d)).
- Mid-face, involving the inferior orbital margins and nasal complex (pyramidal): Le Fort II (Figure 7.7.5 (a–d)).
- High level, involving the arch of the zygoma, lateral, floor and medial orbit and root of the nose/frontal sinus: Le Fort III (Figure 7.7.6 (a–d)).

Naso-orbital ethmoidal injuries

Naso-orbital ethmoidal (NOE) injuries are central mid-face fractures forming an integral part of the higher level injuries: Le Fort II and III fractures. NOE fracture management may be particularly complex and is dealt with in Chapter 7.9.

USING EXAMINATION WITH CLASSIFICATION

Examination identifies and differentiates between these levels. This may be difficult and academic as 'imperfect' fracture lines often mean asymmetry, as well as impossible subclassifications (for example, is there a unilateral Le Fort III or a Le Fort I associated with a same side zygomatico-orbital complex fracture?).

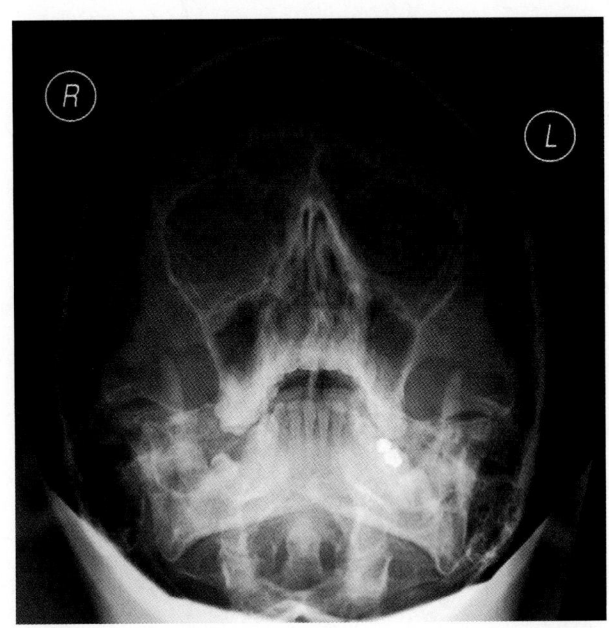

7.7.1 OM view of injury (not showing any obvious fracture).

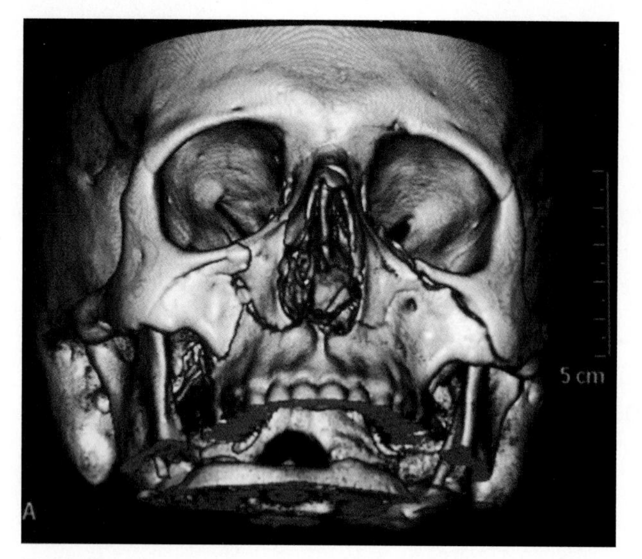

7.7.2 3D CT showing Le Fort II and I fractures.

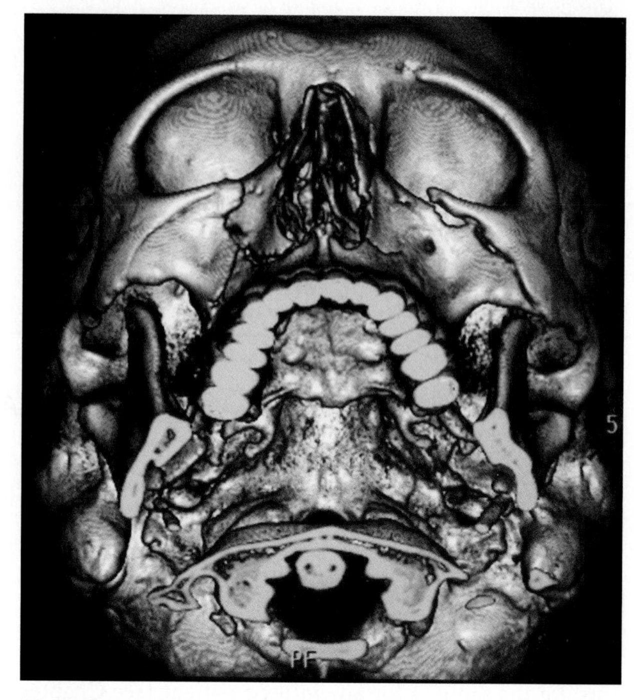

7.7.3 3D CT showing Le Fort II and I fractures.

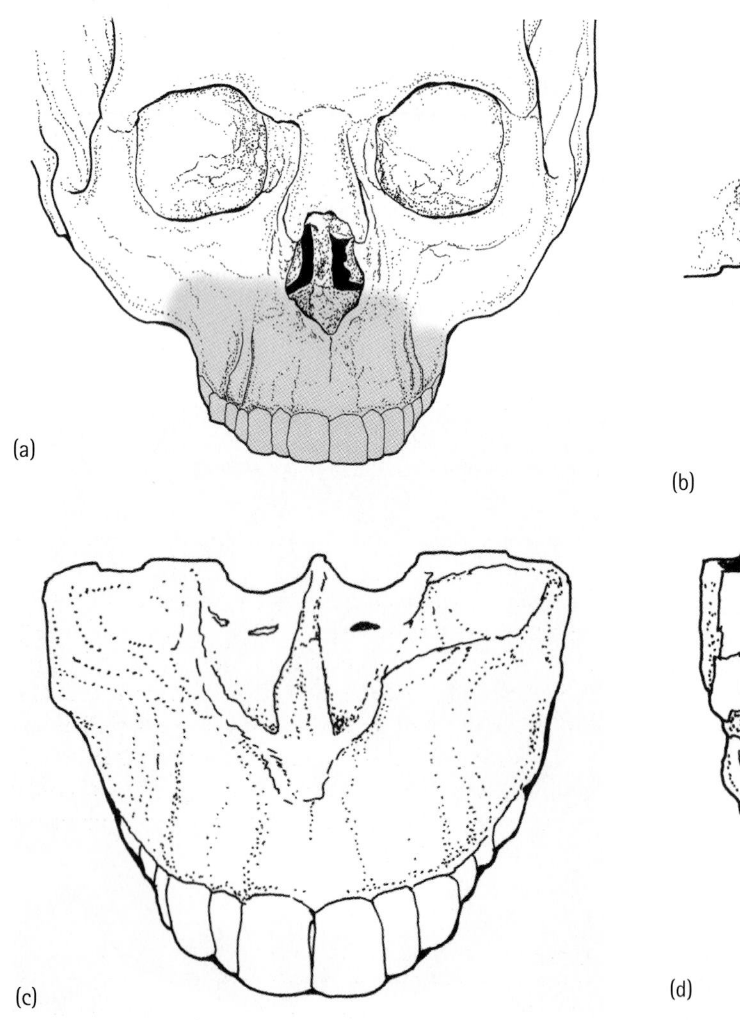

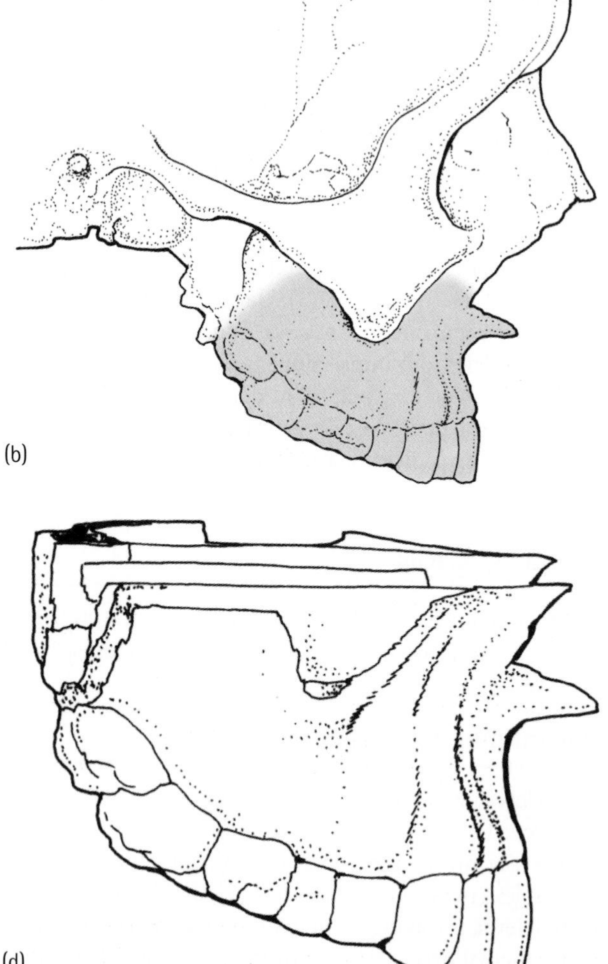

7.7.4 (a–d) Le Fort I

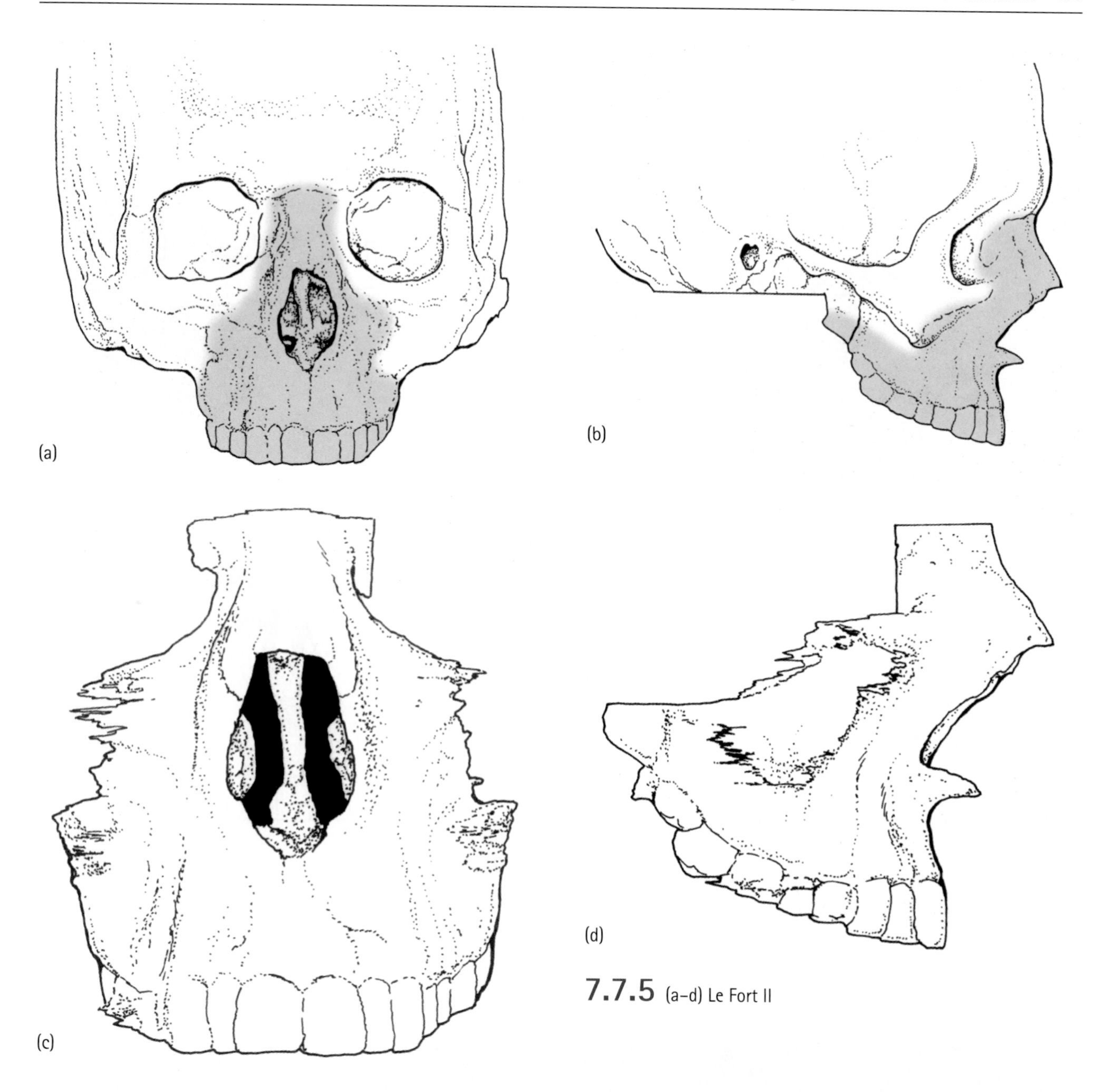

7.7.5 (a–d) Le Fort II

Look in particular for bruising, lacerations and loss of facial contour around the orbits and mid-face. This may be difficult to see because of swelling (balloon facies) disguising the underlying facial contour. Gentle palpation may be helpful around the orbits. Bilateral 'panda eyes' (indicating fractures within the orbit or base of skull), nasal deformities and lengthening of the face (the maxilla is often driven down and back) may also be seen.

Le Fort I

An isolated fracture may cause minimal facial deformity (Figures 7.7.7 and 7.7.8). Most higher level fractures will have a Le Fort I component (see below under Treatment). There may be lengthening of the face associated with the maxilla being driven down and back. Oral examination may reveal mobility of the whole maxillary dentition: dento-alveolar fractures may lead to more localized areas of mobility, split palate can give a traumatic central diastema and palpation of the zygomatic buttress may reveal irregularities from the fractures. An impacted, immobile maxillary fracture may exhibit a dull note when tapping the teeth ('cracked cup sign').

Le Fort II

Isolated fractures are rare and these injuries are often associated with other maxillary fractures and fractures of

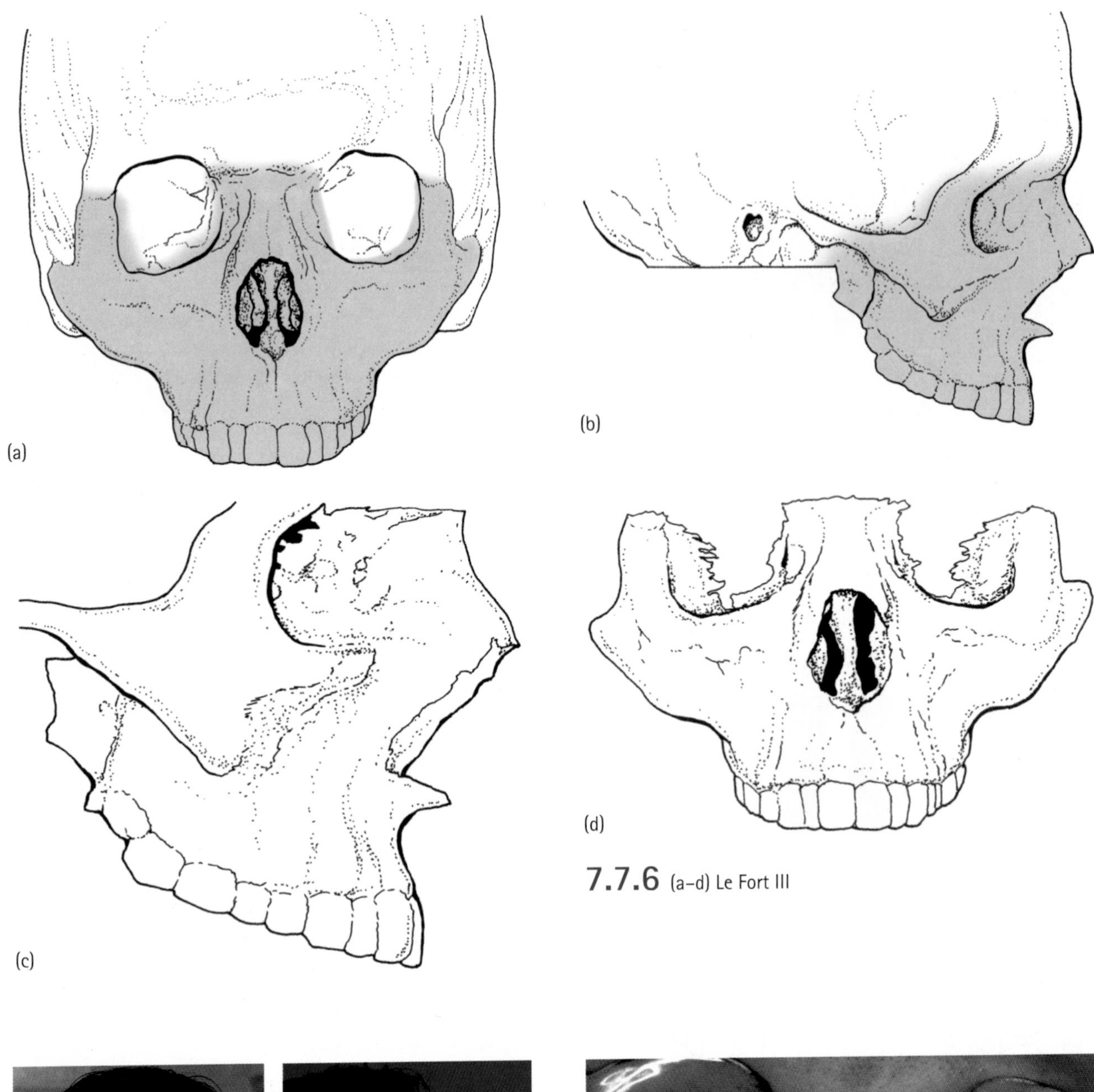

7.7.6 (a–d) Le Fort III

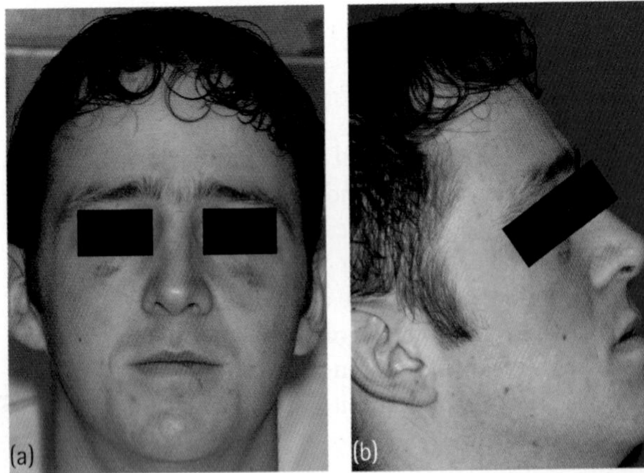

7.7.7 (a, b) AP and lateral views showing no significant clinical NOE injury or maxillary deformity

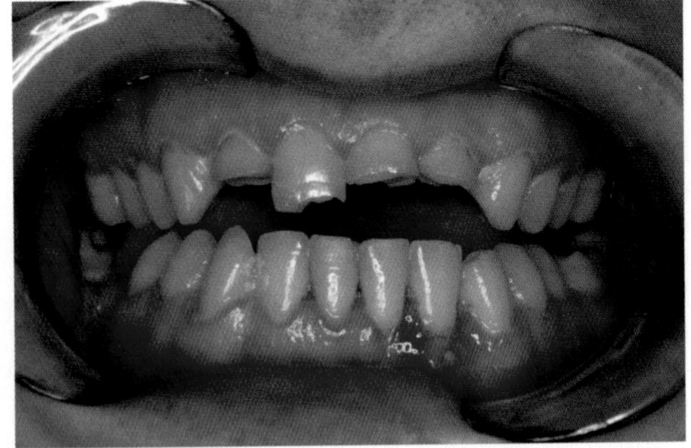

7.7.8 Anterior open bite deformity

the surrounding structures. The illustrated case does not have a significant NOE component; however, this should be assessed over time if there is significant swelling, as any functional problem or deformity may be disguised. Issues, such as medial canthal ligament attachment (tested using the draw sign – palpation of the tensed ligament), orbital involvement, e.g. a palpable step in the orbital rim or eye movement problems giving double vision, frontal sinus fracture (usually confirmed and assessed using imaging) and nasal disruption, should be addressed.

Le Fort III

Le Fort III fractures present a similar picture with even more chance of significant involvement of the surrounding structures. The main concern is of cranial involvement and scanning is mandatory. The higher level fractures both have the capability for increasing the width of the facial skeleton, as well as anteroposterior and height issues. This dimension is easily overlooked in planning the treatment of the grossly swollen face.

The authors' hope it is clear that the more complex higher level injuries will need assessment and treatment of the surrounding structures.

As well as the frontal sinus and base of skull already mentioned, the assessment of the NOE complex, the orbit and the zygomatic orbital complex need to be looked at in detail.

OTHER FACTORS

High or low velocity impact

High or low velocity impact will determine the likelihood of significant other injuries and the possibility of bone loss and the need for grafting.

Extremes of age

Older patients often have very thin bone, particularly when edentulous. This may have particular relevance when determining what kind of fixation to use and whether more simple 'closed' methods should be contemplated. Young patients may not have fully formed sinuses and exhibit unusual patterns of injury. The child's maxilla will be full of developing teeth, again posing potential problems for the use of internal fixation.

SURGICAL ANATOMY

Gruss and Mackinnon made an important conceptual advance in the mid-1980s describing the vertical supportive pillars of the mid-face: anteromedially the paired frontonasal maxillary pillars, laterally the zygomaticomaxillary pillars and posteriorly the pterygoid processes. In individuals with fully developed sinuses, these pillars are relatively weak in the mid-face. Unfortunately, for those repairing mid-face fractures, the most robust of these supportive pillars, the pterygoid plates (in fact, muscular processes) are inaccessible for direct operative repair. Subsequently, horizontal facial buttresses have been added: superiorly, the frontal bar of the upper facial subunit, inferiorly, the maxillary alveolus and palatal processes, with a contribution from the horizontal process of the palatine bone. The middle horizontal buttress is composed of the zygomatic arches, body of the zygomatic bones and the infraorbital rim. These transversely orientated supportive elements link the zygomaticomaxillary processes and nasomaxillary processes.

There are many issues with regard to the facial soft tissues and the effects of trauma, as well as wide undermining to access fractures. A feature of severe mid-face trauma is an appearance that suggests premature ageing when patients are reviewed later. This may be related to the changes within the soft tissue facial drape as a consequence of severe contusion. However, where wide access is employed, the entire superficial muscular aponeurotic system (SMAS) retaining adhesions and septa are detached. Soft tissue resuspension must therefore be part of any successful operative strategy.

PLANNING TREATMENT

The condition of the patient and their other injuries will be considered first. The authors work in a unit that delays treatment until brain swelling has had time to settle (usually 7–10 days). Only interventions that are absolutely necessary (for example, laparotomy, limb fracture stabilization and mandible fracture open reduction and internal fixation (ORIF)) are carried out earlier.

Operative planning for the facial injuries is facilitated with elective scans, involvement of other specialties (for example, neurosurgery, ophthalmology, otorhinolaryngology and maxillofacial technicians), use of dental casts and even photographs of the patients face prior to the trauma.

The management of the airway, if not already dealt with by tracheostomy, is a major issue. There are other methods of securing the airway, e.g. submental intubation; however, these issues need specialist planning. More simple fractures may be dealt with by nasal intubation. An experienced anaesthetist is needed when significant nasal disruption is present. In this type of case a change of tube to an oral intubation may be necessary once the maxilla is fixed internally, in order to deal with the nose.

Often mid-face fractures are present with multiple other facial and skull injuries. The definitive intervention is best planned meticulously, as several specialties may be involved. Sequencing of the various parts of the reduction and fixation are very important when dealing with multiple fracture levels (see a suggested sequence in Figures 7.7.9–7.7.15).

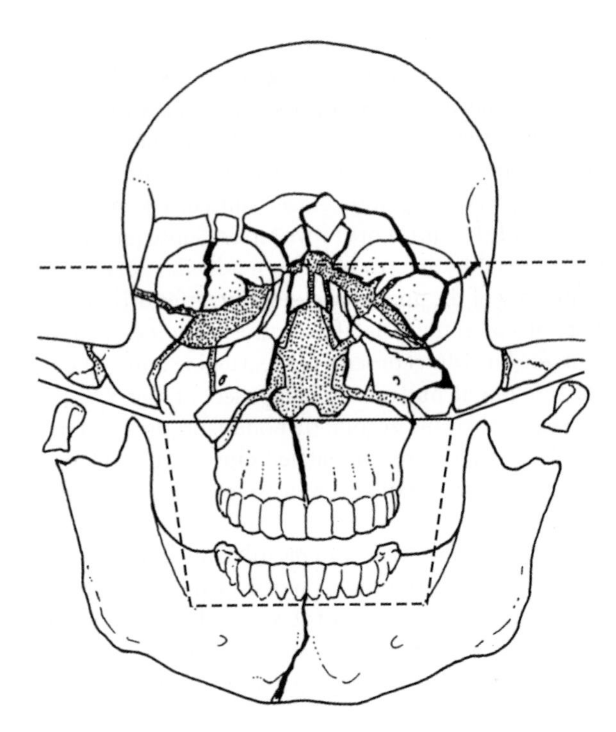

7.7.9 A useful way of looking at pan facial fractures is to divide them into two facial halves separated by a fracture at the Le Fort I level.

The upper facial half can be divided into an upper unit (comprising the frontal bone and a maxillofacial unit). The lower facial half is subdivided into an occlusal unit and a lower basal unit.

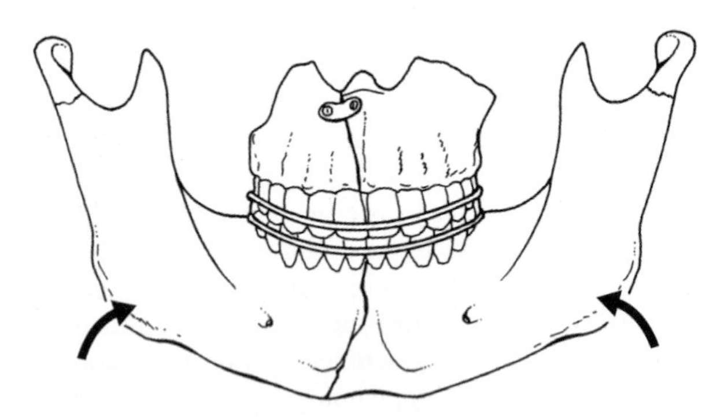

7.7.10 We suggest establishing facial width at the occlusal level first in order to deal with the sagittal element of maxilla and mandible factures.

The gross manipulation of the facial skeleton using the Rowe's disimpaction forceps needs to be completed before any fixation is applied. If the neurosurgeons are involved with anterior fossa repair, the reduction may be done under direct vision to minimise disruption.

When starting this part of the reduction, pressure at the gonial angles will reduce the splay until the anterior mandibular fracture begins to open. This is the moment to stop any further pressure on the reduction and apply the plates.

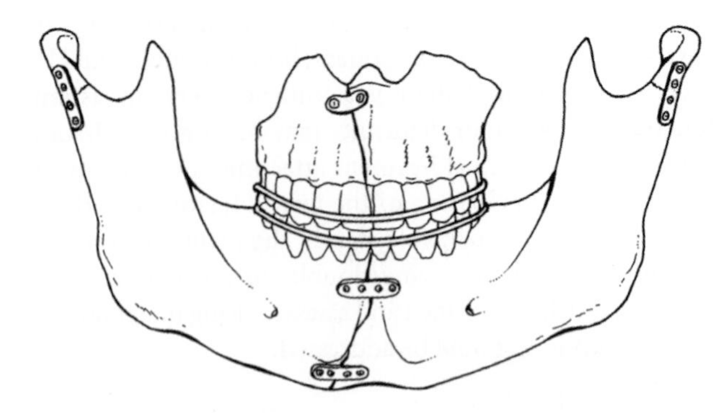

7.7.11 This is a good point to fix the condyles in order to finalise width issues and help with establishing posterior height (do not forget that the condyle may be accessible from the bicoronal flap approach).

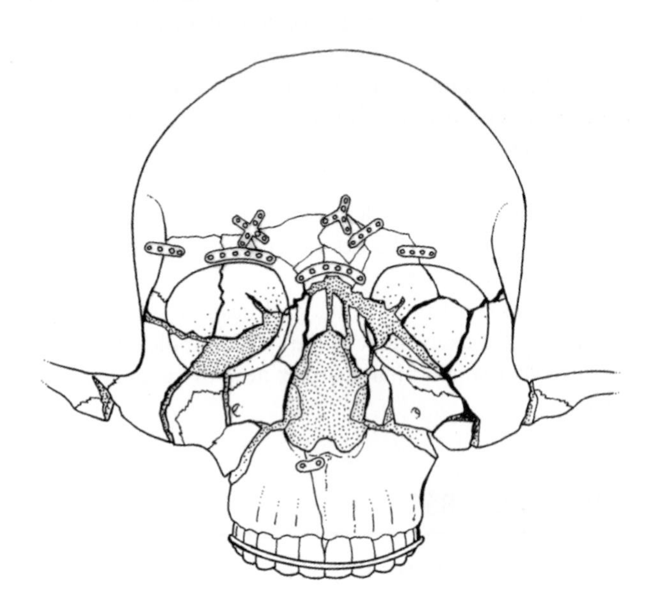

7.7.12 Next in our suggested sequence is the reassembly of the craniofacial/upper facial subunit.

The frontal sinus/base of skull repair/reconstruction including any dural repair (possibly needing local pericranial or galeofronteal flaps) will need to be finalised now.

TREATMENT

Conservative treatment

Conservative treatment is recommended when the dental occlusion is not disturbed and there is an acceptable facial contour with no other functional problems. There is more scope for this sort of treatment plan with an edentulous maxilla.

Open reduction and internal fixation

Open reduction and internal fixation is the treatment of choice for most displaced fractures. The sequence illustrated is of a minimally displaced Le Fort II fracture on the right with more

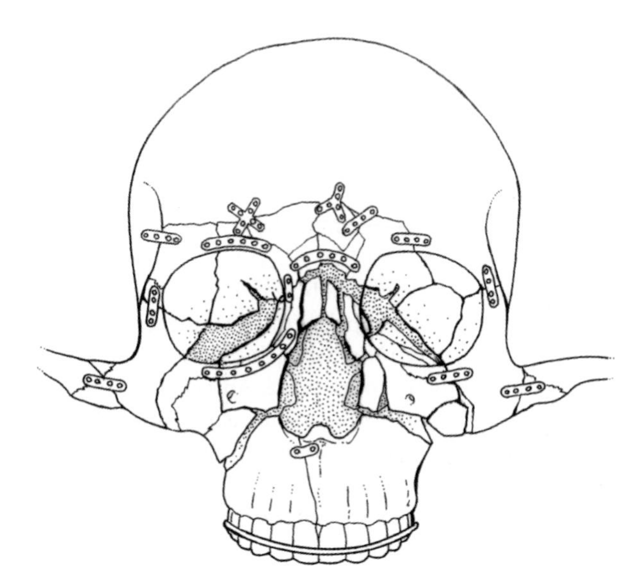

7.7.13 The mid face repair should begin at the area of least displacement so as to give the best chance of getting the correct AP projection and width in this region. The arch of the zygoma is straight, not curved.

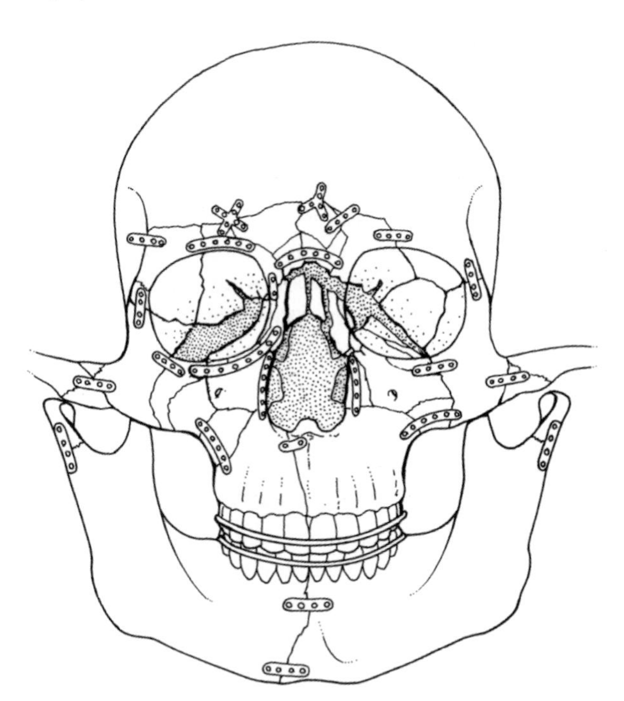

7.7.14 Finally the piriform fossa and zygomatic buttress plating is performed. The area of thin bone in between the buttresses can be severely comminuted. Occasionally in the high velocity injuries the buttress areas are missing too. Grafting may then be necessary.

displacement on the left. Examination of the face shows no obvious NOE injury with a reasonable nasal contour and no disruption of the medial canthi. A step defect was palpable at the left infraorbital margin and there was no clinical evidence of orbital floor or wall problems. There is a Le Fort I component to the fracture that gives a much more pronounced

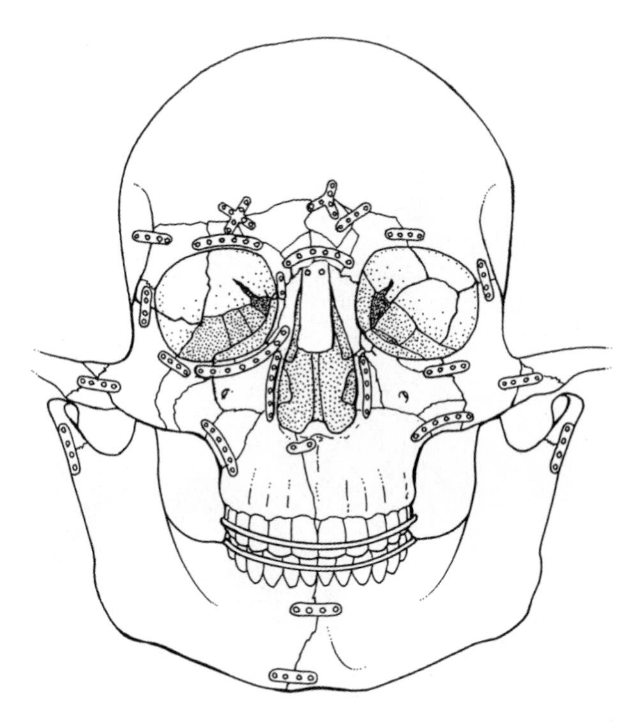

7.7.15 The last issue is to address any bone grafting issues within the orbit or onlayed on the nose. Soft tissue aspects such as soft tissue drape and suspension can be considered now. Any canthopexy issues can be finalised.

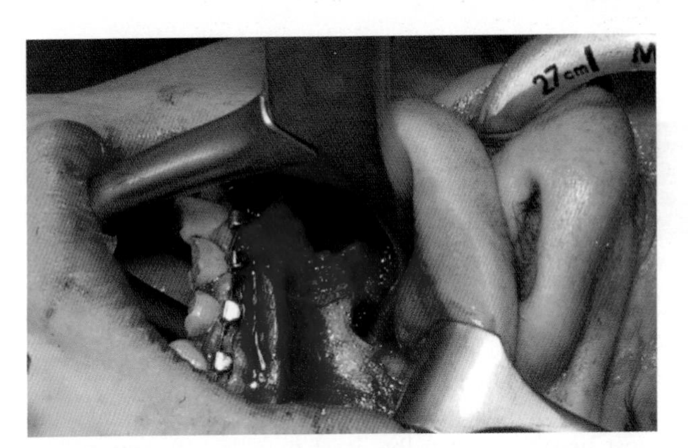

7.7.16 Application of the left Rowe's disimpaction forceps

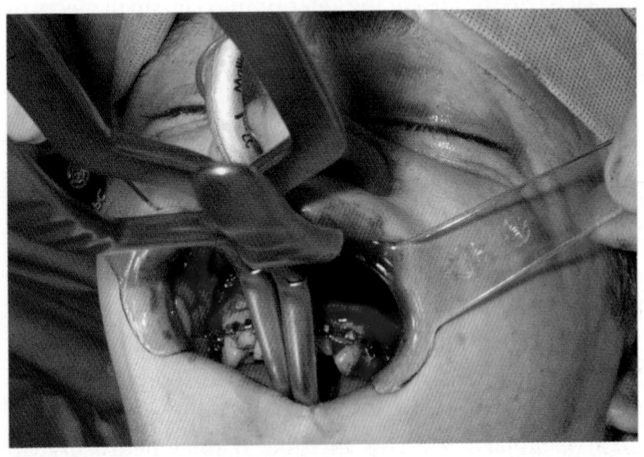

7.7.17 Application of both Rowe's disimpaction forceps

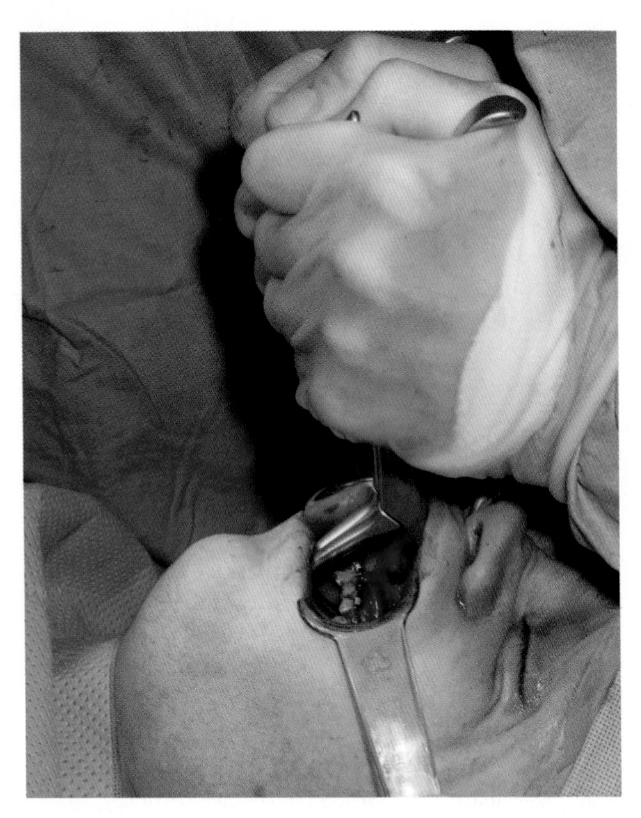

7.7.18 Mobilising the fractures using a careful rotatory movement

occlusal discrepancy of anterior open bite. CT scanning helps to delineate the injuries in great detail compared with plain radiographs (Figures 7.7.1–7.7.3).

Access

ORAL

The incision is placed high up in the buccal sulcus and is the most usual access to low level maxillary fractures. The dissection proceeds subperiosteally and care needs to be taken to keep in the correct plane when pieces of bone are displaced. In the area of the anterior maxilla, small pieces of comminuted bone may be best left attached to the periosteum so as to retain their viability.

FACIAL

These incisions would be as for access to the NOE complex (Chapter 7.8), orbital complex (Chapter 7.9) and zygomatic orbital complex (Chapter 7.10).

SCALP

For high level mid-face fractures, the bicoronal incision is used to gain access to the lateral and medial orbit, as well as the frontonasal region as for isolated injuries in the NOE area (Chapter 7.9). This incision enables neurosurgical access to the skull at the same time, if required.

Reduction

Direct reduction of the fractures relies on visualization of the mid-face fractures using the access described. The Rowe's disimpaction forceps are placed under the dissected nasal mucosa. The other prong of the forceps (which is usually padded with a silicone tube) is placed against the palatal mucosa (Figures 7.7.16–7.7.18).

The maxilla is typically mobile and displaced inferiorly and posteriorly. Occasionally, the maxilla is impacted superiorly and posteriorly, when it can be quite solidly impacted and difficult to mobilize. Anterior and inferior movement may require considerable manipulation in order to re-establish the correct anteroposterior and vertical dimensions and the intercuspation of the occlusion. This manipulation may restart or worsen the leakage of cerebrospinal fluid. There is a balance needed in manipulating the displaced maxilla so as to adequately reduce the fracture while minimizing further injury to the cranial base structures or orbital contents.

Sequencing mid-face fracture reduction when these fractures are part of pan-facial injuries may involve complex three-dimensional issues for the restoration of function and re-establishing facial contours. Typically, the major mobilization of the maxilla is performed early on in the operation as any fixation applied elsewhere would be disrupted by this. There are real issues with the correct orientation of the maxilla in high velocity injuries with bone loss and damage to neighbouring structures. In major craniofacial injuries, dealt with in collaboration with neurosurgeons, the mobilization of the maxilla is often performed only when the anterior cranial floor fractures are directly visualized following craniotomy and suitable brain retraction, so as to make sure further damage to the brain and dura does not occur.

Fixation

The majority of mid-face injuries are fixed internally using low profile titanium plates and screws (typically, 1.7 and 1.3 mm). They are usually placed in the areas of thickest bone which is most easily accessible, at the piriform aperture and the buttress of the zygoma in low level fractures. At higher levels, the orbital rims and glabellar region offer the best bone for plate application.

The use of arch bars and temporary intermaxillary fixation (IMF) may be very helpful in maintaining the correct reduction during application of the plates. The correct positioning of the fractured maxilla is guided by the anatomic position of the fractured bones, as well as the intercuspation of the dentition. The dental occlusion may not be easily attained if there is a pre-existing abnormal bite and/or missing teeth. Impressions and study models taken preoperatively with fabrication of an occlusal splint help attain the correct dental bite at operation and may be very helpful.

A source of error in positioning of the maxilla is distraction of the mandibular condyles when achieving the final position of the maxilla prior to plating. These issues are exactly the same as the problems facing the surgeon in correct positioning of the maxilla in mid-face osteotomy surgery. The solution is to make sure the mandible is passive when applying IMF or hand holding the occlusion prior to plating.

Return to function

There are real advantages in having arch bars in position for minor post-operative occlusal problems when treating maxillary fractures. Elastic IMF may be sufficient to finalise any small discrepancy. Jaw opening and lateral excursion exercises are helpful in regaining functional movements.

OTHER TREATMENT METHODS USED OCCASIONALLY

Closed reduction and fixation using intermaxillary fixation

Only contemplated in minimally displaced fractures in order to optimize the occlusion. Issues to do with the restoration of correct facial height, anterioposterior displacement or lateral facial splay cannot be addressed.

Closed reduction and external fixation

Again, there are limitations with this treatment, however the issues associated with facial height and anteroposterio position may be addressed to an extent. We would use this technique in the very rare situation of needing to stabilize the maxilla when packing the nose for a maxillary fracture complicated with a torrential mid-face haemorrhage.

The maxilla can be attached to an arch bar or cast splint by a projecting bar. Alternatively, projecting bars can be adapted from two bone pins placed directly into the premaxilla through small stab incisions, on either side at the alar base/nasal sill region, providing there is no comminution here. The projecting bars are connected to supraorbital pins or a halo frame.

Top tips

- Fractures of the mid-face are easily missed by inexperienced clinicians (often they are hidden beneath soft tissue swelling). All components, including the orbital and eye, nasal and eyelid attachment, and dental aspects are routinely underestimated.
- Computed tomography scanning is the imaging of choice. Scans often reveal extensive fractures unappreciated by clinical examination. These may not need active treatment, but it is useful to know of their presence.
- Work up for these injuries may involve other specialties. Surgical intervention is often delayed until associated head injury and facial swelling have resolved. This time should be utilized to develop a comprehensive surgical treatment plan.
- Having waited for the brain swelling to settle down, an operation if needed should not be delayed, despite any obtunded conscious level. Patients often make delayed recovery of brain function. Secondary correction is never as easy as primary anatomic repositioning of the basic mid-face structure. The planned intervention should be performed without further compromise to the damaged brain.
- The development of low profile (0.7 mm) and miniplate (0.3 mm) fixation systems has revolutionized our ability to reduce and fix these complex fractures.
- Despite apparent anatomic reduction at operation, post-operative elastic intermaxillary fixation using elastics is often required.

FURTHER READING

Gruss JS, Mackinnon SE. Complex maxillary fractures; role of buttress reconstruction and immediate bone grafts. *Plastic and Reconstructive Surgery* 1986; **78**: 9–22.

Manson PM, Clark N, Robertson B *et al.* Subunit priciples in midfacial fractures: The importance of sagittal buttresses, soft tissue reductions, and sequencing treatment of segmental fractures. *Plastic and Reconstructive Surgery* 1999; **103**: 1287–306.

McMahon JD, Koppel DA, Devlin M, Moos KF. Maxillary and panfacial fractures. In: Ward Booth P, Eppley BL, Schmelzeisen R (eds). *Maxillofacial trauma and esthetic facial reconstruction.* London: Churchill Livingstone, 2003: 237–61.

Moss C J, Mendelson B C, Taylor GI. Surgical anatomy of the ligamentous adhesions in the temple and periorbital regions. *Plastic and Reconstructive Surgery* 2000; **105**: 1475–90.

7.8

Orbital trauma

MICHAEL WILLIAMS

INTRODUCTION

Orbital trauma is common, the orbit being involved in approximately 40 per cent of all blunt facial injuries. Injuries can be subdivided into those occurring when the outer orbital frame is involved in other fractures (the most common being zygomatic complex, maxilla and nasoethmoidal fractures) and those in which the outer orbital frame is otherwise intact. This second group are often described as 'blow-out fractures', but it is probably more accurate to describe them as isolated wall or floor fractures.

Accurate assessment combined with meticulous attention to detail during the planning and operative procedure are essential to prevent or minimize poor aesthetic and, more importantly, functional outcomes.

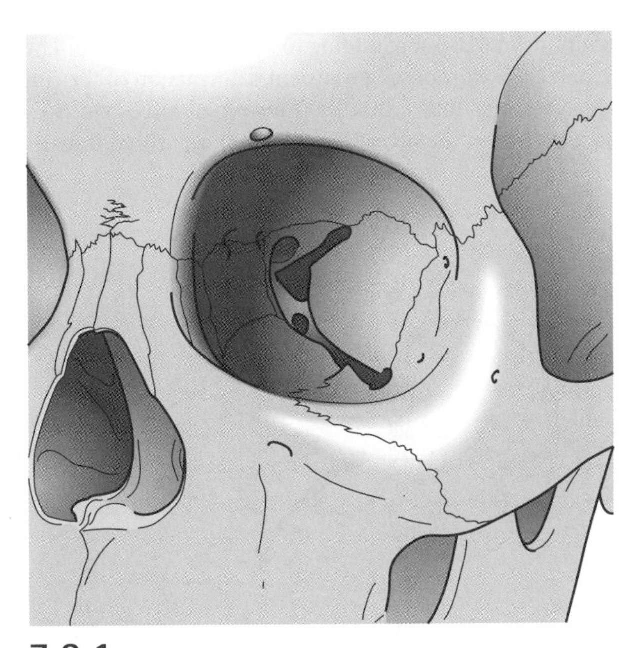

7.8.1 Orbital bones, frontal view.

ANATOMY

The orbit is comprised of an orbital frame or rim within which the walls can be conveniently described as floor, medial wall, roof and lateral wall (Figure 7.8.1). The orbital frame is strong and forms part of the mid-facial buttressing system. However, the walls, particularly the floor and medial wall, are extremely thin accounting for the frequency of fractures in these areas. The lateral wall and roof are stronger and, as a result, fractures of these walls are generally rare. It is important to note that the medial walls lie parallel to each other, and the lateral wall lies approximately 45° to the medial wall. The floor is concave upwards in the third, but then becomes convex upwards in the posterior two-thirds (post-bulbar bulge blending into the key area medially).

Although there are four walls at the orbital rim, as progress is made posteriorly, the medial wall and floor blend together and the orbit at this point becomes a three-walled pyramidal structure. This blending of the medial and lateral wall forms an important posteromedial bulge which has also been coined the 'key area'. It is an important area to replicate in orbital reconstruction to minimize post-operative enophthalmos. The anterior and posterior ethmoidal arteries pass through the medial wall and are important surgical landmarks. Passing through the floor is the inferior orbital fissure containing no structures of surgical importance.

At the orbital apex, the medially located optic canal passes through dense bone of the sphenoid transmitting the optic nerve and central artery of the retina; lateral to this lies the superior orbital fissure through which pass branches of the ophthalmic division of the trigeminal nerve together with the third, fourth and sixth cranial nerves. The 'superior orbital fissure syndrome' comprises total ophthalmoplegia, upper lid ptosis and anaesthesia in the distribution of the ophthalmic division of trigeminal nerve, 'orbital apex syndrome' includes these signs, together with blindness.

Within the orbit sits the globe supported by Lockwood's suspensory ligament and moved by the extraocular muscles, it is enclosed in periorbital fat whose loss can contribute to enophthalmos. Anterior to the globe, the upper and lower tarsal plates are attached to the medial and lateral walls by the medial and lateral palpebral ligaments. This tense fascial sheath constitutes the 'fifth wall' of the orbital pyramid thereby forming a closed box. It is important to recognize this, for if orbital pressure increases following trauma, release of this fascial band by way of a lateral canthotomy can be sight saving.

MECHANISM OF INJURY

Two theories have been proposed to explain the presence of isolated orbital wall fractures. In the first, an occluding force applied to the outer orbital rim leads to a transient increase in intraorbital pressure leading to a 'blow-out fracture'. The second theory proposes a transient deformation of the rim which remains intact, but the transmitted force leads to a fracture within the orbit (Figure 7.8.2), as orbital injuries rarely lead to significant ocular injury, this second theory is probably more likely.

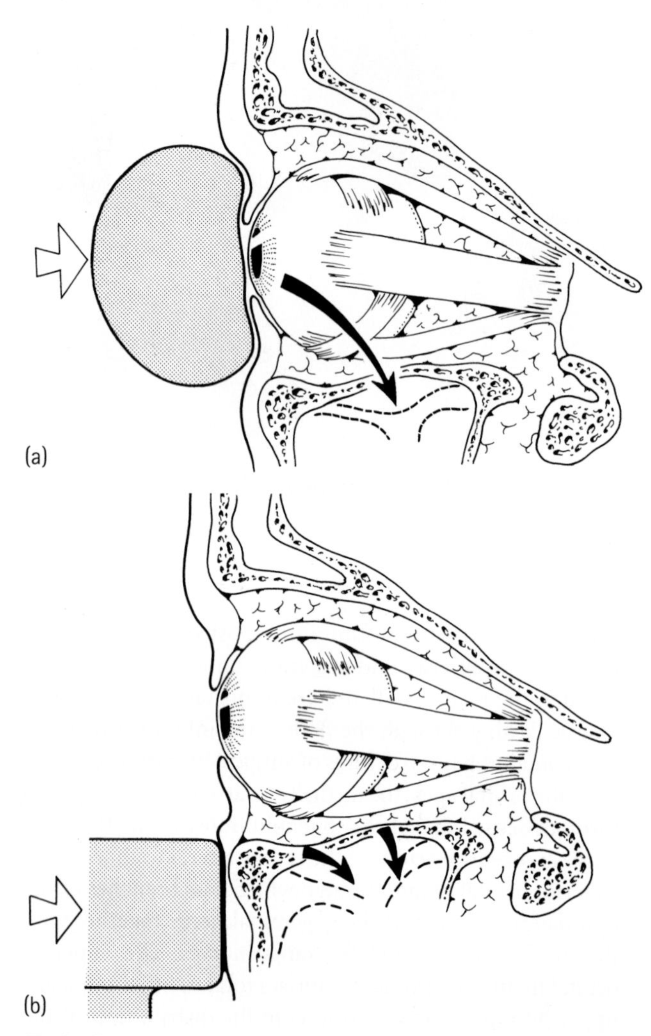

7.8.2 (a) and (b) Proposed mechanisms involved in blow-out fractures.

INITIAL ASSESSMENT

Following a full systemic and maxillofacial examination, the orbital injury should be carefully assessed. The mechanism of injury is important in particular to differentiate between blunt and penetrating trauma. Visual acuity must be assessed at an early stage and enquiries made regarding the presence of double vision and numbness around the orbit. Traumatic optic neuropathy is uncommon and presents a challenging management problem; surgical exploration is difficult and expertise may not be available locally. Furthermore, there is little evidence to support the use of megadose steroids.

Examination should include the periorbital soft tissues, especially the lid, cornea and anterior chamber of the eye, looking particularly for the presence of hyphema, corneal injury and iris injury. The presence of a subconjunctival haematoma without posterior limit indicates a likely breach in the orbital periosteum.

Examination proceeds with palpation of the outer orbital frame, following which eye movements are carefully assessed in the nine cardinal positions, carefully documenting the presence of diplopia in any of these positions. Red colour desaturation is an important sign which when combined with the swinging light test may indicate reduced optic nerve function.

INVESTIGATIONS

Radiology

Plain radiographs are of limited value in isolated orbital wall injuries, but the hanging drop sign may be noticed, and they are of value in assessing the outer orbital frame. However, the imaging modality of choice for orbital trauma is a fine cut spiral computed tomography (CT) which should include all four walls with coronal, sagittal and occasionally three-dimensional reformatting.

Orthoptic assessment

Orbital trauma should ideally be managed with ophthalmic surgeons and an important component is pre-operative orthoptic assessment. This will include clinical measurement of visual acuity and ocular motility, together with a cover test for near and distant vision. Any deviation is measured for consideration of prisms.

The Hess chart is a dissociation test allowing objective measuring and recording of ocular motility. The mobility of the injured eye being compared with the fellow uninjured eye.

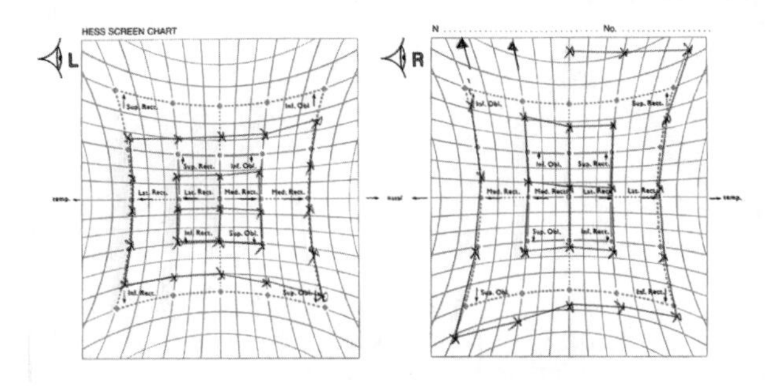

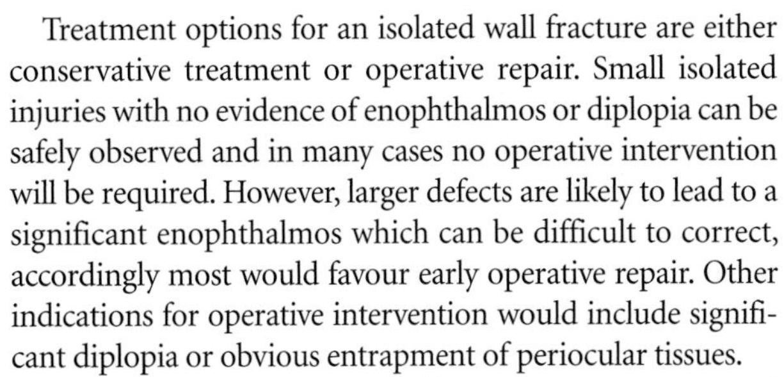

7.8.3 Hess chart indicating left orbital floor fracture. Note restricted movements in left chart but overcompensation in uninjured (right eye).

Restricted movement is observed in the injured eye and overcompensation seen in the normal eye (Herring's law) (Figure 7.8.3).

PAEDIATRIC INJURIES

Paediatric orbital fractures are less common due to underdevelopment of the associated paranasal sinuses. However, when they occur they often lead to a true trap door, greenstick fracture often trapping periorbital tissue. These are commonly missed injuries due to absence of other signs. It is imperative to operate and release the entrapped tissues as soon as possible, many emphasizing that this should be achieved within 5 days.

TREATMENT

For nonisolated orbital injuries, it is essential that the outer orbital frame is treated first, the orbital wall factures are then repaired in exactly the same way as for an isolated wall injury.

Treatment options for an isolated wall fracture are either conservative treatment or operative repair. Small isolated injuries with no evidence of enophthalmos or diplopia can be safely observed and in many cases no operative intervention will be required. However, larger defects are likely to lead to a significant enophthalmos which can be difficult to correct, accordingly most would favour early operative repair. Other indications for operative intervention would include significant diplopia or obvious entrapment of periocular tissues.

Following completion of all pre-operative tests and investigations, the surgeon should be able to formulate a clear treatment plan, including surgical approach, exposure and reconstruction of the involved walls. This should include the size and site of the defect and choice of reconstructive material.

OPERATIVE PROCEDURE

Positioning

The patient is placed supine on the operating table with a slight degree of head-up tilt with modest hypotension provided by the anaesthetist. Both eyes should be exposed and protected and a forced duction test performed to assess any restriction in ocular motility (Figure 7.8.4). There should be due attention to corneal protection, and this may be provided either in the form of a corneal shield if a transconjunctival incision is utilized or a temporary tarsorophy if a lower eyelid incision is used.

Exposure

The orbit can be exposed through a variety of incisions depending on which walls are fractured and the amount of exposure required. The floor can be approached by either a lower eyelid incision or a transconjunctival incision with or

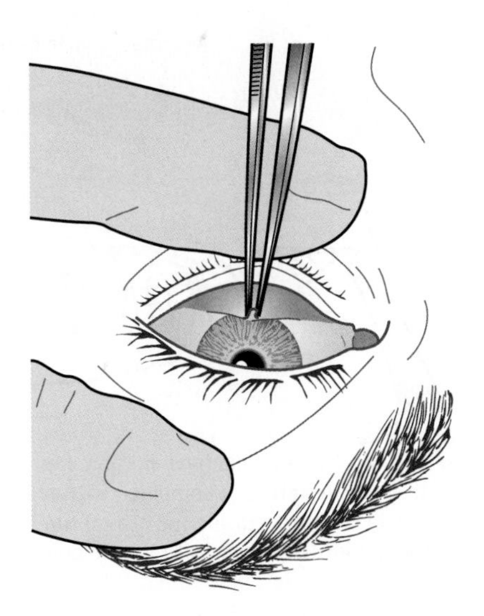

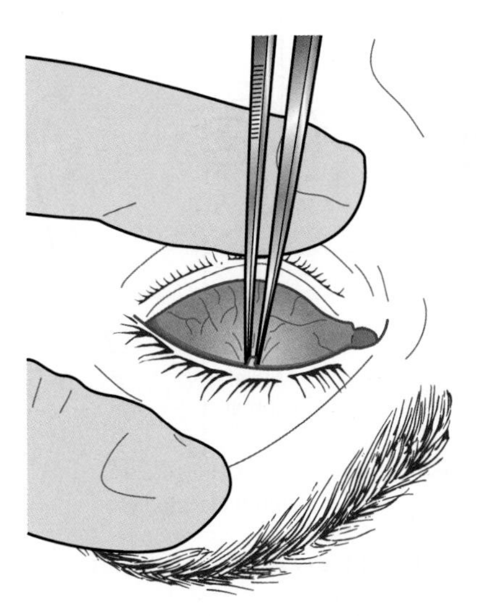

7.8.4 Forced duction test which should be performed pre-operatively and on completion of repair to exclude entrapment.

without a lateral canthotomy. There are three lower eyelid incisions: the subciliary (or blepharoplasty) incision, the midtarsal incision and the infraorbital incision (Figure 7.8.5). With regard to complications, the infraorbital incision has a very low incidence of ectropion, but an increased incidence of poor scarring. The subciliary or blepharoplasty incision has a very low incidence of scarring, but an increased incidence of ectropion, although this can be reduced by not suturing the wound and leaving a cuff of orbicularis occuli attached to the lid margin. The midtarsal incision combines the advantages of both these procedures, having very acceptable scarring together with a low incidence of ectropion, and is the author's preferred lower lid incision. The incision is carried through skin followed by careful sharp dissection through orbicularis oculi to reach the tarsal plate. Meticulous haemostasis with bipolar forceps is essential and further aided by pre-operative infiltration with lidocaine and epinephrine. Using careful retraction with a Desmare retractor, a clear plane is revealed between orbicularis oculi and tarsal plate which is followed by sharp dissection on to the anterior face of the orbital rim (Figure 7.8.6)

The transconjunctival incision can be made pre- or post-septally, the pre-septal approach is more complicated with few advantages and the post-septal approach is generally preferred. With the lower lid retracted anteriorly with a Desmare retractor, a malleable retractor can be placed directly behind the orbital rim, thus placing the tissues under tension (Figure 7.8.7). The conjunctival incision is then made, preferably with a needle point diathermy (Colorado micro needle®), following which the retractors are repositioned inside the wound allowing further dissection, again to the anterior face of the orbital rim.

Whichever incision has been used, the periosteum on the anterior aspect of the orbital rim is now incised. It is important to keep the dissection on the anterior surface of the orbital rim since this minimizes herniation of periorbital fat.

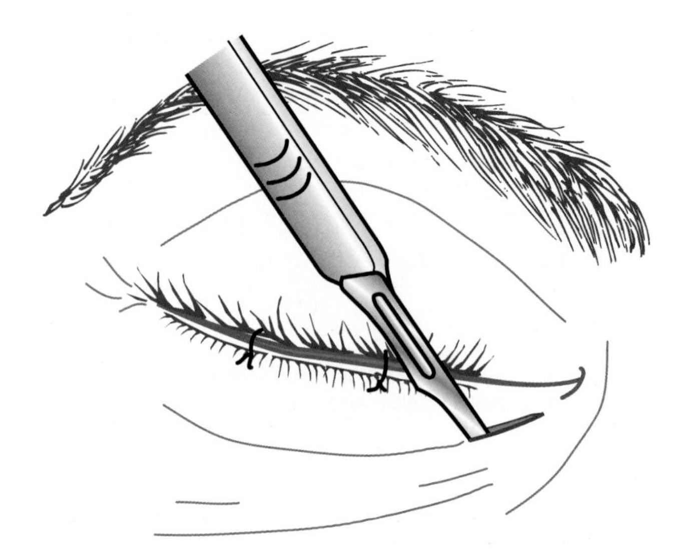

7.8.6 Retraction of wound edge revealing plane between orbicularis occuli and the tarsal plate.

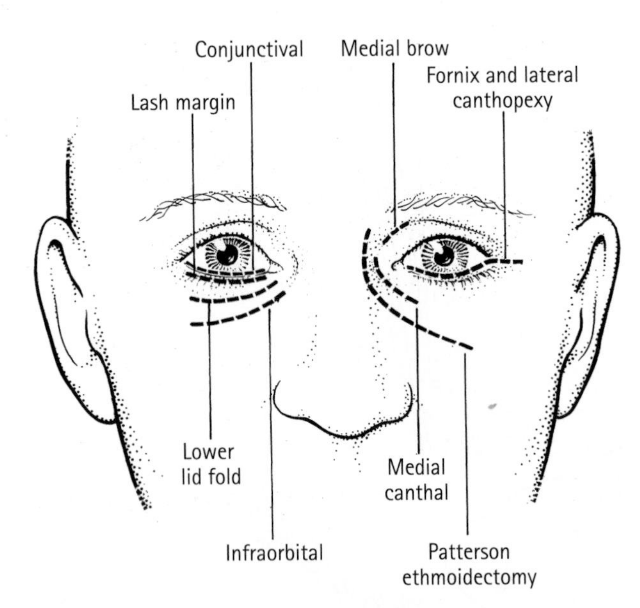

7.8.5 Surgical approaches to the orbital floor and walls.

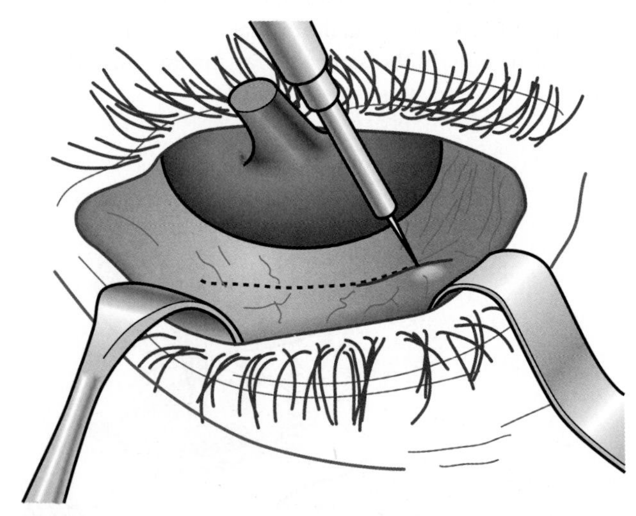

7.8.7 Transconjunctival incision. Retraction of lower eyelid with Desmare retractor combined with tension applied with blunt malleable retractor inside the orbital rim to place tissues under tension prior to division with needle point diathermy.

Greater exposure of the orbital floor can be gained by combining the transconjunctival incision with a lateral canthotomy. For this procedure, a small skin incision passes through the fornix between the upper and lower eyelids following which the lower limb of the lateral canthus can be divided (Figure 7.8.8). If this incision is utilized, it is generally more convenient to perform the lateral skin incision and canthotomy prior to dividing the conjunctiva.

Following incision of the inferior orbital rim periosteum, the periosteum is easily elevated over the rim and dissection proceeds in a downward direction before passing posteriorly until the anterior margin of the floor defect is identified, dissection should be careful and precise to avoid enlarging the defect. At this point, it is important to 'outflank' the defect and since the lateral wall is rarely fractured it seems more convenient to follow this as the next step. The inferior orbital fissure is then identified, which can be safely coagulated between bipolar forceps and then divided to give much improved access.

The presence of a significant medial wall fracture (often in combination with a floor fracture) requires a further incision to gain proper access. The established approach to the medial wall is via a coronal flap. The incision extends from a pre-auricular incision passing coronally across the scalp to be completed by a pre-auricular incision on the contralateral side. The so-called stealth variant zigzags the incision across the scalp to allow disguising of the scar by hair growth, although in the author's experience a wavy line incision is easier to raise and avoids hair loss at points of the zigzags (Figure 7.8.9).

The incision is ideally made with a ceramic blade passing through skin and the aponeurosis with careful vascular control provided with Raney clips. The flap can be rapidly mobilized in the subgaleal plane to a point just above the frontozygomatic suture, at which point the periosteum is incised and the incision carried laterally through the outer layer of the deep temporal fascia to the root of the zygomatic arch. By this means, the facial nerve is protected and temporal hollowing is minimized. By continuing dissection in a subperiosteal plane, the supraorbital notch is identified. If the supraorbital nerve is lying in a foramen, then the lower margin of this can be osteotomized to allow the supraorbital nerves to be freed. The periorbital rim periosteum is dissected and carried down the medial aspect. Flap mobility can be improved by incising the periosteum on the undersurface of the flap in the midline. By proceeding posteriorly generous exposure of the medial wall is obtained

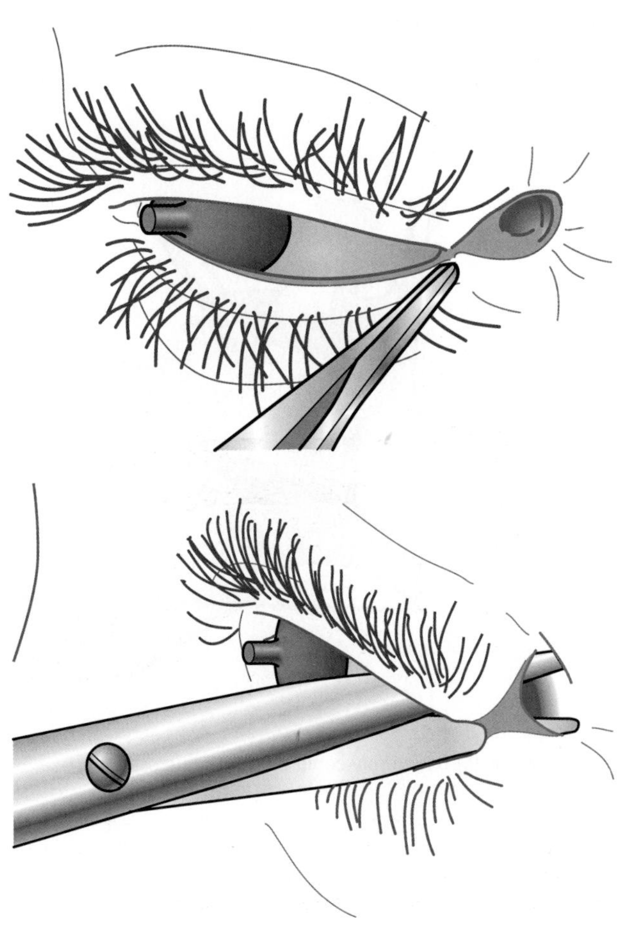

7.8.8 Lateral canthotomy, following skin incision the lower canthal band is identified and divided.

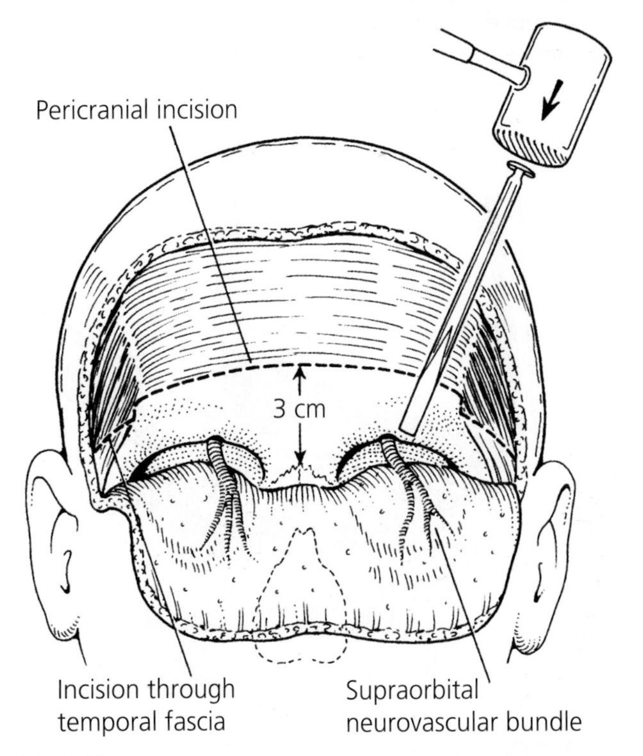

7.8.9 Coronal flap allows generous exposure of medial orbital wall.

(Figure 7.8.9). It is important to complete any lower eyelid incisions before raising a coronal flap, as it often leads to significant oedema in the lower eye lids.

The coronal flap can have significant morbidity including poor scarring, alopecia, injury to the temporal branch of the facial nerve and numbness in the distribution of the supraorbital and supratrochlear nerves. More recently, many have found the transcuruncular incision, which is essentially a medial extension of the transconjunctival incision, gives adequate exposure to the medial wall without such morbidity.

Dissection posteriorly along the medial wall almost certainly will require ligation or diathermy of the anterior ethmoidal vessels.

The posterior limit of dissection should ideally be to the posterior margin of the defect, but in deep orbital trauma there is clearly a limit to how far dissection can proceed without endangering the optic nerve. It has been suggested that subperiosteal dissection should not proceed beyond 35 mm from the orbital rim, but this guideline should not be used in the presence of an orbital rim fracture. Other guidelines are the level of the posterior ethmoidal artery. More recently, stereotactic navigation has been suggested, but this is not widely available and a recent paper has reiterated the importance of anatomical knowledge in such dissection.

On completing the subperiosteal dissection, exposure of the defect can be improved by undertaking a marginal orbitotomy. For this procedure the segment of inferior orbital rim to be removed is marked and a low profile microplate adapted and temporarily fixed to bridge the proposed osteotomy (Figure 7.8.10). The plate is removed and the orbitotomy completed. Removal of this segment of infraorbital rim certainly improves access, but is not always essential. Furthermore, it is extremely difficult to undertake in the presence of an orbital rim fracture.

Reconstruction

Following complete exposure of the defect, the surgeon is now in a position to plan the reconstruction. There are essentially two choices either to use autologous bone or an alloplastic material.

Historically, the use of alloplastic materials was associated with complications, including infection and extrusion, and as a result, autologous bone became the preferred reconstructive material. Autologous bone can be conveniently harvested from the calvarium if a coronal flap has been raised. Other sites include the anterior wall of the ipsilateral maxillary sinus if intact, iliac crest or rib. However, there can be significant donor morbidity from bone graft harvest and this, combined with unpredictable resorption, have led to new interest in alloplastic materials. There is now a wide range of such materials which can be divided into resorbable and nonresorbable groups.

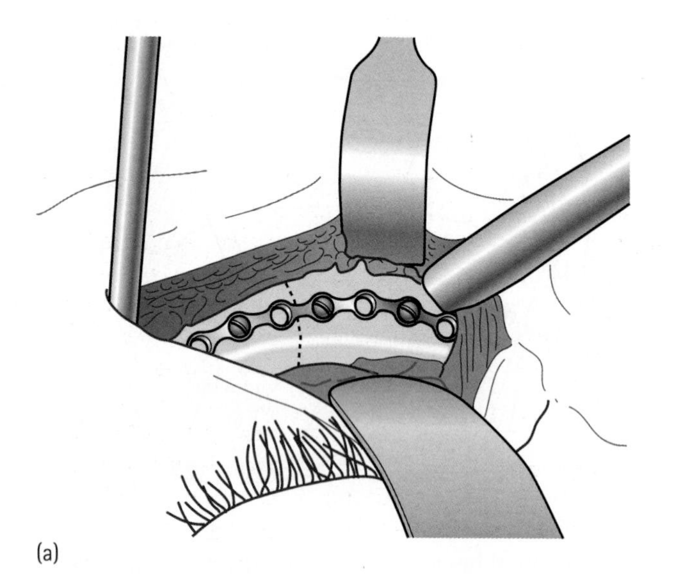

(a)

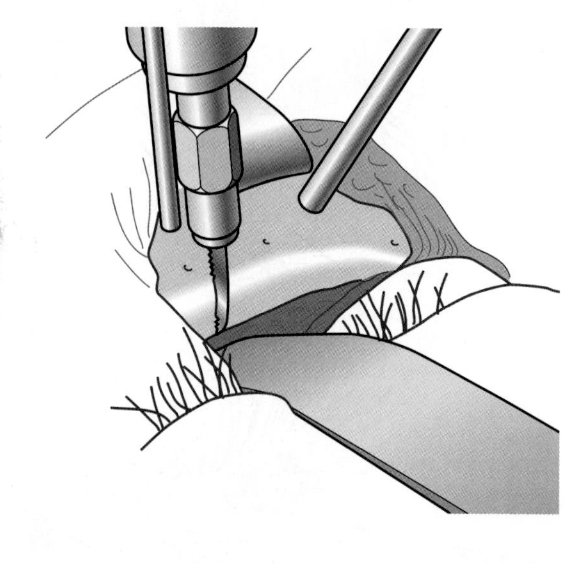

(b)

7.8.10 (a) Bridging plate adapted to the orbital rim over proposed osteotomy site. (b) Osteotomy completed with microsaw.

Resorbable membranes, such as PDS sheet and polylactic/glycolic acid, are thin and malleable, but are not suitable for large defects since they lack sufficient structural rigidity and have unpredictable resorption.

Nonresorbable materials include titanium mesh and polyethylene membranes (Medpore). Titanium mesh can be provided in simple plain sheet form which can be cut to shape, but most manufacturers are now providing preformed adaptable sheets allowing a very accurate three-dimensional reconstruction (Figure 7.8.11). They can be easily secured with titanium screws at the orbital rim and are generally very well tolerated with few complications.

Polyethylene sheet is very malleable, but does have some degree of memory. It has the advantage of providing a smooth surface against the orbital tissues which makes removal (if necessary) slightly easier than titanium mesh. However, fixation is less easy than with titanium mesh and can be achieved either with a titanium screw behind the orbital rim or with a PDS suture. More recently, polyethylene sheeting has been made over a titanium mesh framework, combining the advantages of both materials (Figure 7.8.12).

The chosen implant can be conveniently prepared by first making a malleable template to which the implant can be trimmed and adapted before insertion. There is great interest currently in producing sterile models of orbits to which alloplastic sheeting can be adapted, allowing accurate replication of orbital contour particularly in huge defects.

Following insertion of the implant, careful assessment is made with regard to correction of enophthalmos and the pupillary level and the forced duction test is repeated (Figure 7.8.3). Once the surgeon is happy with the reconstruction, the implant is fixed into position, ideally with titanium screws.

Wound closure can be made over a small vacuum drain and it is important to close the periosteum to allow proper

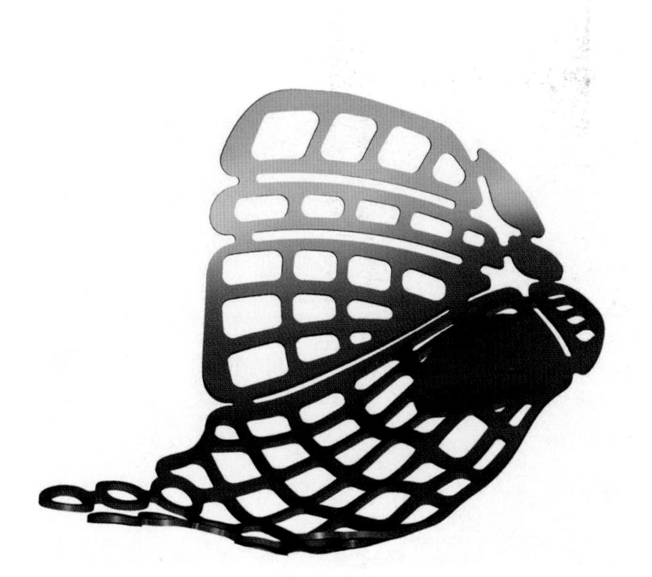

7.8.11 Preformed titanium mesh allowing accurate repair of complex orbital fractures. Example shown is a Synthes Ltd Matrix MIDFACE Performed Orbital Plate.

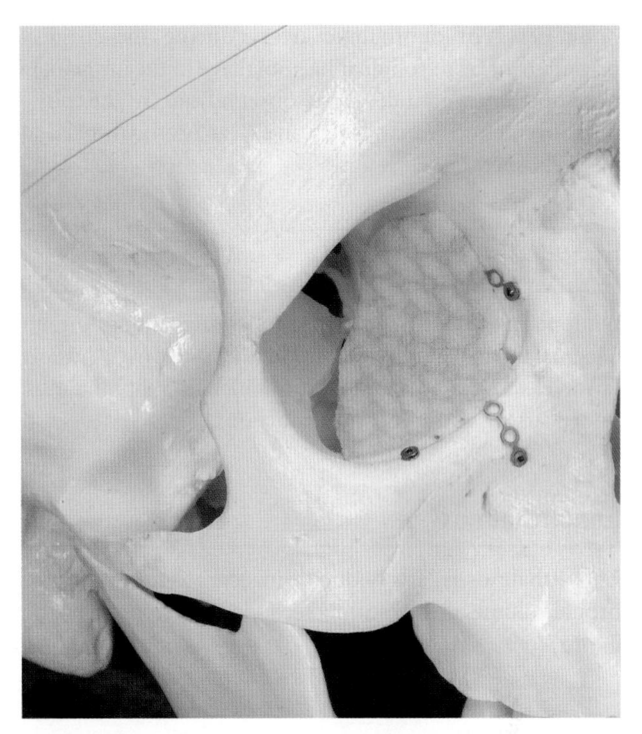

7.8.12 MEDPOR TITAN® OFW implant combines qualities of titanium mesh and high density polyethylene. Reproduced with permission from Porex Surgical Inc., Newnan, GA.

suspension of the malar fat pad, the muscle layer is not closed and the skin gently opposed with interrupted 6/0 nylon sutures. For transconjunctival incisions, following closure of the periosteum, there is debate as to whether the conjunctiva should be closed, with many preferring not to close the conjunctiva to reduce the risk of entropion. If a coronal flap is being utilized, it is important to carefully close the aponeurosis ideally using running 2/0 braided resorbable suture on a round-bodied needle. Following this, the skin can be conveniently closed with skin staples, but the pre-auricular incision should be carefully closed in layers with 6/0 nylon sutures to skin. Two large vacuum drains should also be used and it is advisable to apply a pressure dressing for the first 24 hours.

Post-operative care includes careful eye observations to include visual acuity, pupil reactions, ocular movements and most importantly increasing pain. The patient should be nursed with his head elevated to reduce periorbital swelling. He should be encouraged to mobilize his eyes as much as possible and avoid nose blowing.

COMPLICATIONS

Blindness

This is the most important complication of orbital surgery, the incidence being extremely low at approximately 1 in 1500. Visual impairment may follow either injury to the optic nerve or ophthalmic artery during the surgical procedure or by retrobulbar haemorrhage in the immediate post-operative period. Close observation in the post-operative period is mandatory and clear protocols need to be established.

Diplopia

Diplopia may be initially worse following surgery due to oedema or haematoma, but is likely to improve over the next few weeks. Long-term complications include enophthalmos, poor scarring and soft tissue distortion.

Enophthalmos

Enophthalmos is largely due to inaccurate restoration of orbital volume often requiring secondary correction (Figure 7.8.13).

Poor aesthetics

Poor scarring is more common with infraorbital incisions and rare with transconjunctival and blepharoplasty incisions. Malposition of the lateral canthus can occur and many suggest suturing the canthus with a nonresorbable suture to be hole drilled in the lateral rim of the orbit. Others have suggested dividing the lower rim of the canthus through the tarsal plate which can be more accurately sutured to the correct position.

Retrobulbar haematoma

A retrobulbar haematoma follows bleeding within the orbit and can either be within the cone of extraocular muscles or outside this cone. As bleeding continues, pressure increases within the orbit leading ultimately to pressure on the optic nerve head with the clinical signs of ophthalmoplegia, reducing visual acuity and pain leading to a fixed dilated pupil. This can occur either following the initial injury or following surgical correction. First aid measures include the use of steroids, mannitol and acetazolamide combined with a lateral canthotomy to give temporary control prior to formal surgical exploration and drainage.

More recently, the concept of a retrobulbar haemorrhage has been challenged and a better term may be 'orbital compartment syndrome', since in many cases the signs and symptoms are secondary to oedema, rather than true haematoma. It has been suggested that tonometry may provide some guidance on which cases require operative intervention and which can be safely observed. However, many would still recommend formal exploration in the presence of such signs.

Top tips

- Remember sight comes first. Visual acuity and full ophthalmic examination for all.
- Close working relationship with ophthalmic surgeons.
- Maintain high index of suspicion of orbital injury in all mid-third trauma.
- Assess the integrity of the orbital frame.
- Accurately record the size and location of the defect using high resolution axial scanning with coronal and sagittal reformatting.
- Children require urgent treatment.
- Plan access incisions with regard to size and location of defect, coexisting fractures and choice of repair material.
- Close observation in the post-operative period.

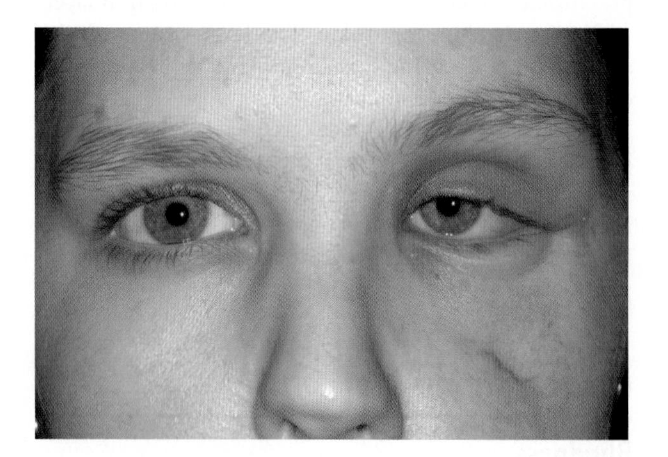

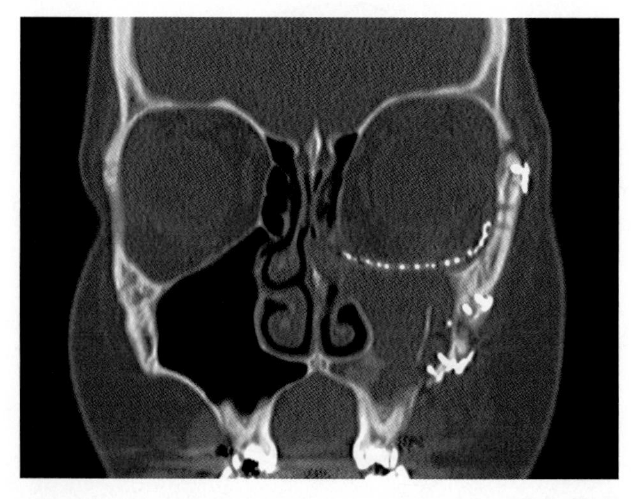

7.8.13 Enophthalmos clinical sequelae and imaging. The titanium mesh implant is malpositioned being too low on the medial wall (note the natural upward and medial slope of the uninjured right floor which has not been replicated). This has led to an expansion of orbital volume and enophthalmos as a consequence.

FURTHER READING

Bähr W, Bagambisa FB, Schlegel G, Schilli W. Comparison of transcutaneous incisions used for exposure of the infraorbital rim and orbital floor: A retrospective approach. *Plastic and Reconstructive Surgery* 1992; **90**: 583–91.

Ellis E 3rd, Tan Y. Assessment of internal orbital reconstruction for pure blow out fractures: Cranial bone grafts versus titanium mesh. *Journal of Oral and Maxillofacial Surgery* 2003; **61**: 442–53.

Evans BT, Webb AA. Post traumatic orbital reconstruction anatomical landmarks and the concept of the deep orbit. *British Journal of Oral and Maxillofacial Surgery* 2007; **45**: 183–9.

Kontio RK, Laine P, Salo A *et al.* Reconstruction of internal orbital wall fracture with iliac crest free bone graft clinical, computed tomography and magnetic resonance imaging follow up study. *Plastic and Reconstructive Surgery* 2006; **118**: 1365–74.

Kontio RK, Suuronen R, Salonen O *et al.* Effectiveness of operative treatment of internal orbital wall fractures with polydioxanone implant. *International Journal of Oral and Maxillofacial Surgery* 2001; **30**: 278–85.

Kwon JH, Moon JH, Kwon MS, Cho JH. The differences of blowout fracture of the inferior orbital wall between children and adults. *Archives of Otolaryngology – Head and Neck Surgery* 2005; **131**: 723–7.

Metzger MC, Schon R, Zizelmann C *et al.* Semiautomatic procedure for individual preforming of titanium meshes for orbital fractures. *Plastic and Reconstructive Surgery* 2007; **119**: 969–76.

Larian B, Wong B, Crumley RL *et al.* Facial trauma and ocular/orbital injury. *Journal of Cranio-Maxillofacial Trauma* 1999; **5**: 15–24.

Linberg JV. Orbital compartment syndromes following trauma. *Advances in Ophthalmic Plastic and Reconstructive Surgery* 1987; **6**: 51–62.

Steinsapir KD. Traumatic optic neuropathy. *Current Opinion in Ophthalmology* 1999; **10**: 340–2.

Sullivan WG, Kawamoto HK Jr. Periorbital marginotomies anatomy and applications. *Journal of Cranio-Maxillofacial Surgery* 1989; **17**: 206–209.

Tse R, Allen L, Matic D. The white eyed medial blow out fracture. *Plastic and Reconstructive Surgery* 2007; **119**: 277–86.

7.9

Craniofacial trauma, including management of frontal sinus and nasoethmoidal injuries

ROBERT P BENTLEY

BACKGROUND

Previously, patients sustaining craniofacial trauma were routinely treated separately by several disciplines independently achieving poor outcomes. However, it is now widely accepted that this group of patients are treated optimally by a multidisciplinary team approach in a neurosurgical centre with ready access to modern imaging technology and neurosurgical high dependency facilities. It has been this development, together with the realization that the first time is the best time to treat these injuries, that has led to the significant reduction in aesthetic and functional morbidity associated with such injuries over recent years.

CLASSIFICATION

While accepting the simple classifications of simple linear fractures of a given bone or fossa involved, a more useful working classification of fractures involving the frontobasilar region was suggested by Bernstein *et al.* who divided the injuries into central, lateral and complex groups. The central group includes fractures involving the central anterior skull base and cribriform region adjacent to the frontal, ethmoidal and sphenoidal sinuses (Figure 7.9.1). The lateral group include frontal bone fractures associated with the orbital roof, but lateral to the frontal sinus (Figure 7.9.2) and finally the complex group involving all areas often bilaterally (Figure 7.9.3, p. 514).

This classification helps relate the fracture pattern to involvement of adjacent structures and the possible functional sequelae. Thus, central injuries are far more likely to involve sinus-related problems, whereas lateral injuries are more often associated with orbital and globe issues. Second, the classification helps plan the craniotomy to gain sufficient access to perform a safe surgical repair.

CLINICAL ASSESSMENT

Due to the mode of injury, patients with craniofacial injuries will often present with associated head injury. In addition, 30 per cent of such patients will have another major life-threatening injury elsewhere in the body and up to 20 per cent will have an associated cervical spine injury. It is therefore imperative that the principles and management of advanced trauma life support (ATLS) are applied to this group of patients (Figure 7.9.4, p. 515).

Craniofacial assessment should include a full neurological examination paying particular attention to cranial nerve deficits. Ophthalmic assessment is mandatory and specialist help should be sought from an early stage even in the unconscious and intubated patient.

Any nasal or middle ear discharges should be tested for beta-2 transferrin to detect the presence of cerebrospinal fluid.

RADIOLOGICAL ASSESSMENT

The technical aspects have already been dealt with within the relevant section on radiological assessment of facial trauma, but suffice to say the role of high speed spiral computed tomography (CT) scanners and improved computer software has revolutionized the ability to produce high quality images quickly with the least embarrassment to the patient and permits accurate visualization of the fracture patterns in all three planes with three-dimensional reconstructions, aiding the surgeon to develop an operative plan.

INDICATIONS FOR COMBINED CRANIOFACIAL REPAIR

The indications for combined craniofacial repair include:

- central injuries, involving significant displacement of the anterior fossa floor and posterior wall of the frontal sinus;
- lateral injuries, involving the roof of the orbit leading to contour deformity, globe displacement or ocular motility disturbance;

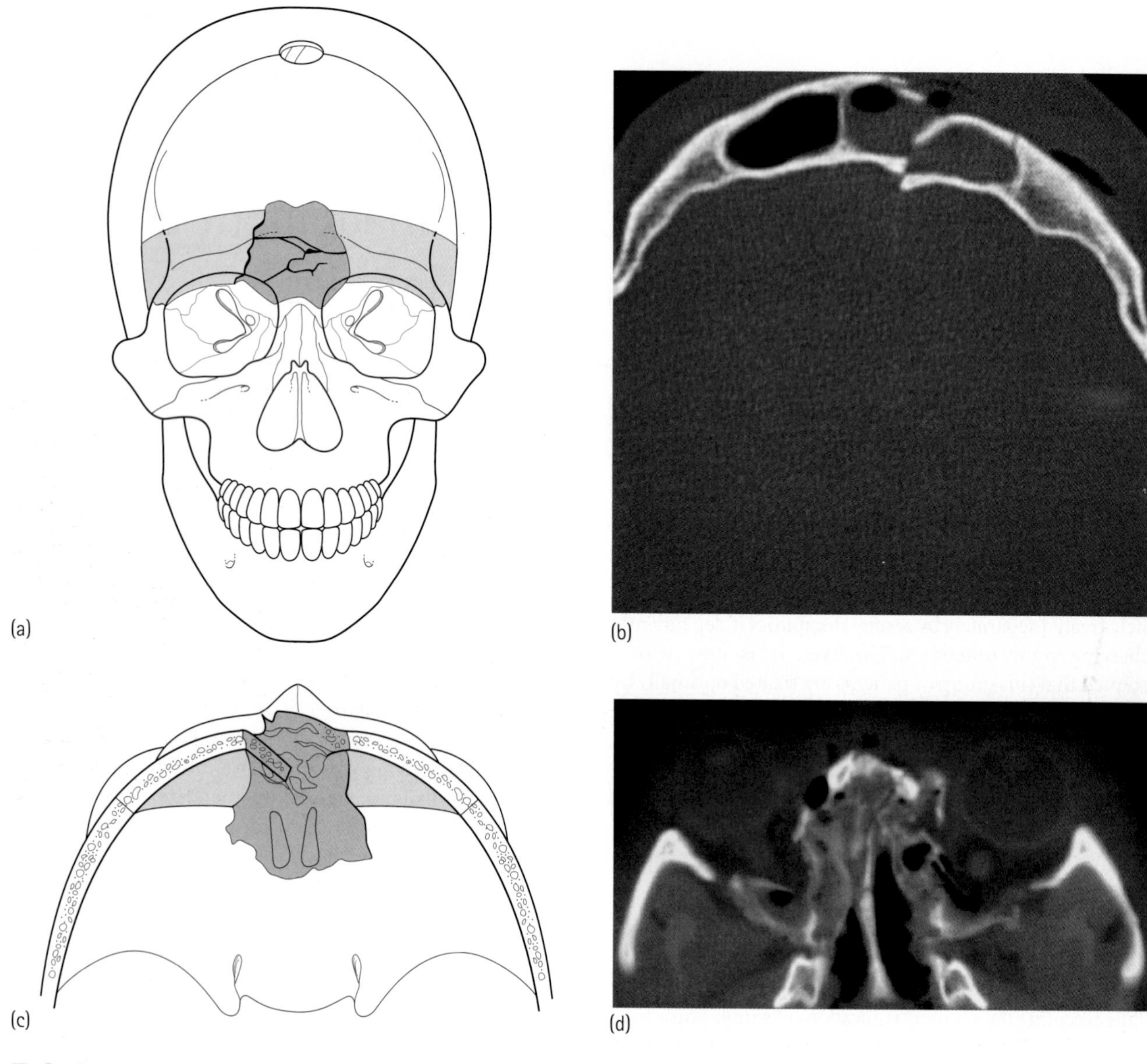

7.9.1 Central injuries.

- compound injuries with penetrating injuries or bone loss;
- growing fractures with dural lacerations, involving the orbit.

Surgical goals of a combined repair fall into two broad groups. First, to prevent the late sequelae of infection, cosmetic deformity and lastly functional deficits.

Principles underlying prevention of late infective sequelae

The principles underlying prevention of late infective sequelae include:

- accurate dural repair;
- achieving a functionally safe frontal sinus;
- repair of a deficient anterior skull base;
- the use of vascularized pericranial flaps to help seal off the dura from the nasal cavity.

Dural tears in communication with the nasal cavity and paranasal sinuses are common and place the patient at an increased risk of developing meningitis. There is no doubt that risk of infection is significantly increased by the presence of a cerebrospinal fluid (CSF) fistula. This may be reduced, but not abolished, by the use of antibiotics but may be reduced significantly by achieving a dural closure. The problem areas are not those cases where CSF leaks persist, but those that stop within a relatively short space of time and no formal repair is undertaken. Repair should be undertaken if the CSF leak has not stopped after 14 days.

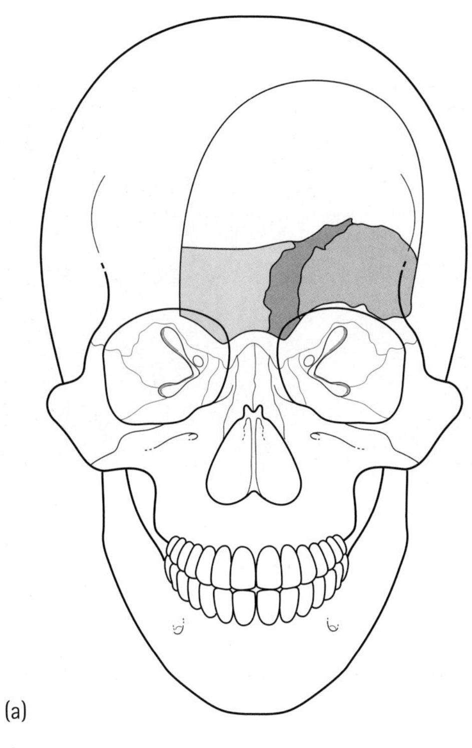

(a)

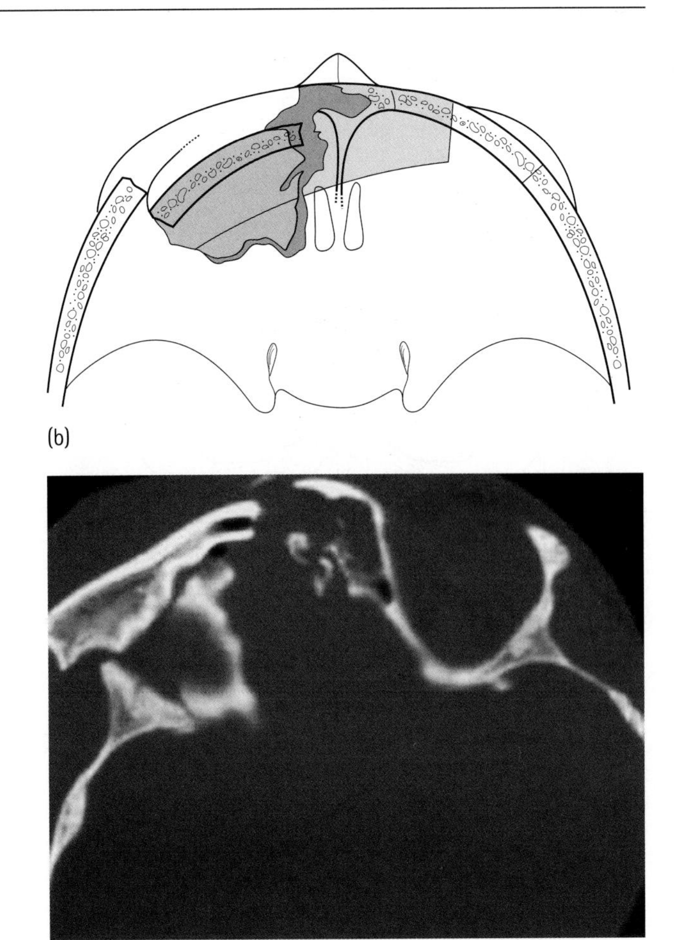

(b)

(c)

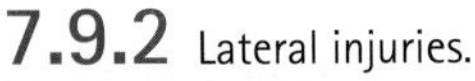

7.9.2 Lateral injuries.

Principles underlying prevention of post-traumatic cranio-orbital deformity

There is no doubt that the key to craniofacial repair is the accurate reassembly of the frontal bandeau which helps define a platform for facial height, width and projection, as well as allowing for accurate restoration of the convexity of the orbital roof, reducing the adverse effects on globe motility and minimizing the risks of altered orbital volume.

TIMING OF SURGERY

Surgery is usually directed towards life-saving neurosurgical compromise in the first instance based on GCS and CT findings supplemented with intracranial pressure monitoring where necessary. Assuming that these aspects have been addressed a time frame of 10–14 days has been shown not to adversely affect the patient's outcome.

SEQUENCING OF SURGICAL PROCEDURE

Anaesthesia

The choice of intubation may be normal oral intubation, but if injuries include pan-facial fractures requiring stabilization of the occlusion, then other options include nasal intubation, submental intubation with a possible tube switch to an oral tube at the end of the procedure to address the nasoethmoidal injuries. Tracheostomy may be required, especially if a prolonged period of post-operative ventilation is required due to a resolving head injury or thoracic injuries.

Position of the patient

Usually the patient would be placed supine in a head ring ensuring enough support to prevent excess head mobility, but allowing good access to the vertex and posterior scalp facilitating the coronal surgical approach and possible need to harvest calvarial grafts.

Adequate exposure

The abilty to restore normal form function and aesthetics can only come from the anatomical reduction of the facial skeleton and it is a prerequisite of this that all fracture sites should be exposed in a subperiosteal plane. Fortunately, previous experience has shown us that due to the abundant

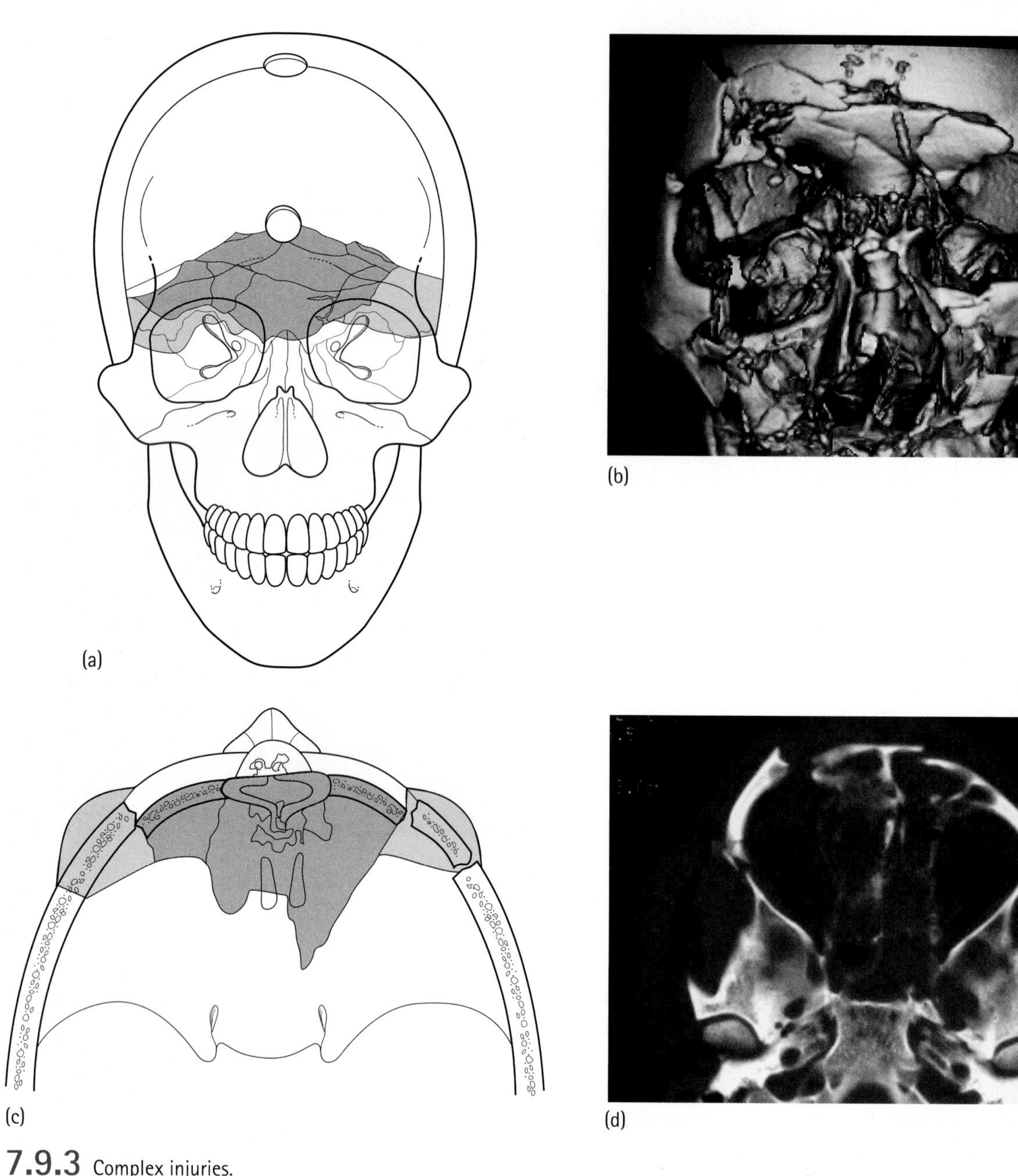

7.9.3 Complex injuries.

blood supply in the head and neck region, such a procedure is safe and does not lead to devitalization of the bone as long as it is firmly fixated and the soft tissues are accurately redraped.

Adequate exposure may be achieved by a coronal approach which may be modified depending on the fracture pattern to allow for various forms of pericranial graft to be used or extended to allow access further down to the mid-facial and condylar regions, respectively.

Consideration of the placement of the incision must take into account the hairline of the patient. The incision is best placed along the vertex of the scalp in a wave form so that the first curvature is directed posteriorly from the tragus ensuring the incisions amplitude is around 3 cm and it is important that the anterior aspect of the incision are kept within the hair line.

Pre-operative whole head shaving is not necessary, but parting of the hair with a comb helps positioning of the incision and this can be further aided by performing a 3-cm width shave with clippers and a hair razor. The hair may be treated liberally with chlorhexidine gluconate hand wash which acts as a good hair gel and allows the hair to be gathered into clumps and secured with elastic bands.

The whole site can be prepared with aqueous iodine after eye shields and simple eye ointment have been applied to each eye. Alternatively, temporary tarsorraphies may be performed with a 4/0 monofilament suture with an atraumatic needle utilizing 1-cm sections of paediatric silastic feeding tube to help prevent undue pressure on the delicate skin of the eyelids while maintaining protection. It is important to pass the needle through the grey line of the lids to ensure some of the tarsal plate is engaged helping prevent tearing of the eyelid skin (Figure 7.9.5).

Surgical drapes are secured to the posterior aspect of the proposed incision line with staples and a urology pouch secured in a similar fashion helps collect the extensive irrigation. The patient is positioned slightly head up taking care to remind the anaesthetist, as unexpected air emboli may infrequently complicate any cranial procedure with head up tilt on the table (Figure 7.9.6).

THE INCISION

The incision may be outlined using a pen and ink, preferably Bonney's blue, and the margins of the wound may be cross-hatched with a scalpel. A green needle may be used to tattoo marks using ink adjacent to the incision. The permanency of the marks may be improved by placing one's finger over the hub of the needle and passing the needle into the scalp tangentially twice ensuring good passage of ink into the tissues. Increased haemostasis may be achieved by injection of a 1 in 200 000 epinephrine (adrenaline) containing local anaesthetic solution into the subgaleal space which can be detected by distension of this space, which has the added benefit of defining the plane for subsequent dissection.

The initial incision is performed with a No. 10 blade to the level of the hair follicles in the mid part of the outlined flap for a distance of 5 cm (Figure 7.9.7). The incision is deepened using a needle point diathermy (Colorado micro needle®), set to minimize heat generation, but sufficient to help easy dissection down and through the galea to enter the subgaleal space. This procedure may be aided with gentle traction upwards and outwards with skin hooks inserted into the wound margins. This not only gives good access, but helps haemostasis. Having located the subgaleal layer, further dissection is achieved by placing McIndoe scissors with their tips up beneath the galea and opening the points widely. This action creates a pocket which may be held elevated by the skin hooks and clear of the underlying pericranium, so that extension of the incision along the galea can be achieved with the cutting diathermy without damaging the pericranium (Figure 7.9.8). As dissection progresses and the scalp flaps become more mobile, haemostasis is obtained with the use of bipolar forceps to accurately minimize the damage to the adjacent hair follicles. Rather than the use of Raney clips, this technique helps cut down on haemorrhage at the end of the procedure during wound closure and leads to a less hurried

7.9.4 Multiple injured patients with craniofacial injuries.

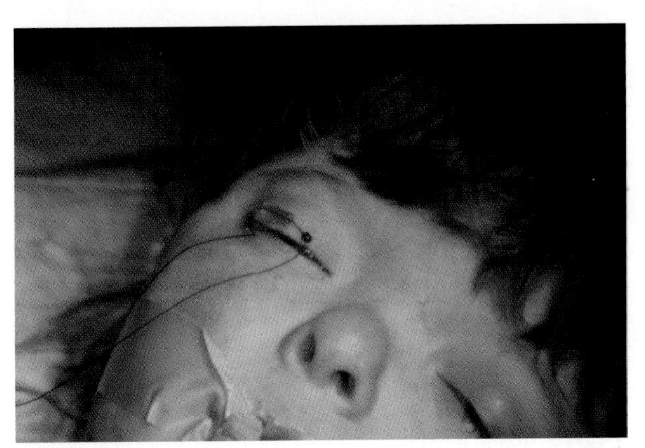

7.9.5 Temporary tarrsoraphies.

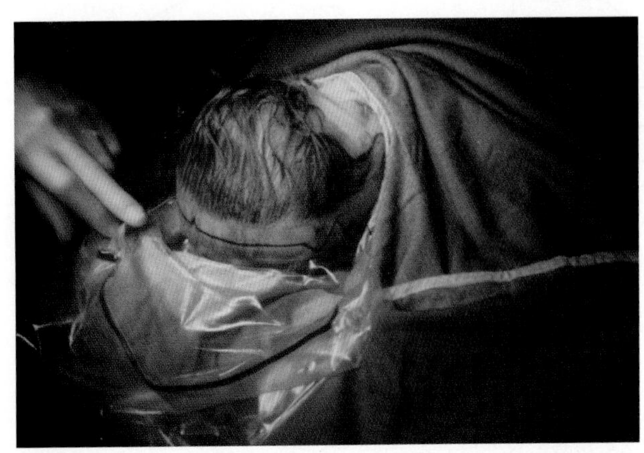

7.9.6 Patient preparation ,positioning and draping.

and accurate closure. Dissection progresses inferiorly into the preauricular region below the level of the superior temporal line keeping close to the underling temporal fascia. This latter point ensures that the dissection is beneath the level of the temporoparietal fascia which is a continuation of the galea beneath the level of the temporal line, and is important as the temporal branch of the facial nerve runs either on its deep surface or within it. Damage to this branch of the facial nerve results in weakness of the forehead and partial ptosis due to loss of innervation to the frontalis, corrugator, procerus and occasionally a portion of the orbicularis oculi.

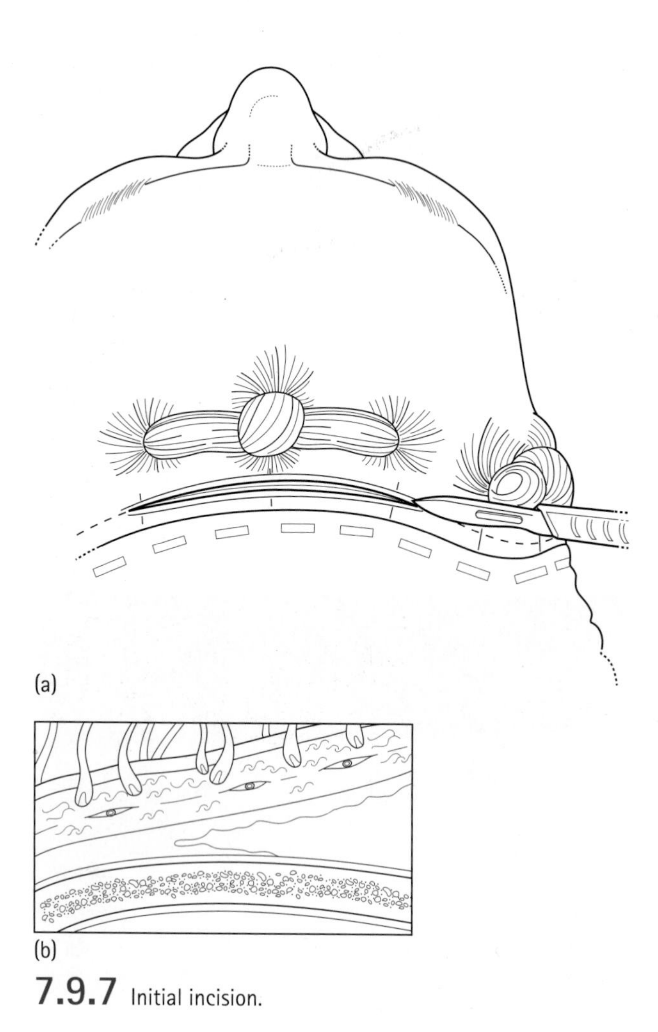

7.9.7 Initial incision.

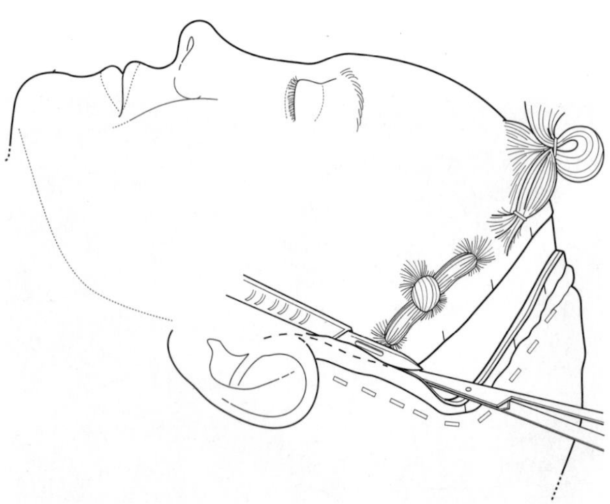

7.9.8 Development of coronal flap inferiorly.

Flap elevation may proceed easily in the subgaleal layer maintaining tension on the skin flap with skin hooks and Langenbeck retractors. Sharp pronged retractors should be avoided as they lead to damage to and bleeding from branches of the superficial temporal vessels on the surface of the coronal flap. Dissection proceeds using the sweeping action of a No. 10 blade or use of a ceramic monopolar diathermy blade, the latter having the advantage of reducing further blood loss. As the flap is freed, tension laterally has to be dealt with by incising the superficial layer of the superficial temporal fascia, paying due regard to the temporal branch of the facial nerve. As the flap is dissected inferiorly and anteriorly, an incision is made in the superficial temporal facia at an angulation of 45° from a point 2.5 cm above the superior aspect of the lateral orbital margin, to a point at the base of the zygomatic arch. This incision is best performed with a No. 15 blade midway along this line approximately 3–4 cm above the body of the zygoma. Having made the incision, the yellow colour of the superficial temporal fat pad is seen separating the superficial and deep layers of the temporal fascia. The incision is now extended superiorly to the temporal line and inferiorly to the zygomatic arch with dissecting scissors (Figure 7.9.9). The next stage to help reflect the flap further inferiorly is to decide at what level the pericranium should be incised. If an anteriorly based flap is required then the pericranium may be incised posteriorly using cutting diathermy just above the superior temporal line from a point marked from the superior aspect of the incised superficial temporal fascia. The extent of the posterior dissection of the flap should be enough to allow sufficient length of this flap to cover any base of skull defect without tension (Figure 7.9.10). Alternatively, if the viability of an anteriorly based flap is in question due to trauma, then two laterally based flaps may be raised with the blood supply coming from the lateral aspect (Figure 7.9.11). In either case, sharp subperiosteal dissection allows reflection of the flap inferiorly to the superior and lateral orbital margins. At this juncture, the surpraorbital neurovascular bundles will be encountered. In a proportion of cases, simple subperiosteal dissection will allow the bundle to be displaced inferiorly. If, however, there is a true foramen, the bundle may be freed by inserting the tip of a 5-mm fine osteotome into the foramen and hit inferiorly along already marked out triangular bone cuts. This usually delivers the inferior border of the foramen freeing the bundle (Figure 7.9.12).

Further subperiosteal dissection along the root of the nose may now proceed and may be aided by a vertical incision of the periostium on the undersurface of the flap, being careful not to attenuate the thickness of the skin flap unduly. This permits dissection along the medial orbital rim to the level of the medial canthal tendon. The tendon's attachments should not be unduly stripped of either its

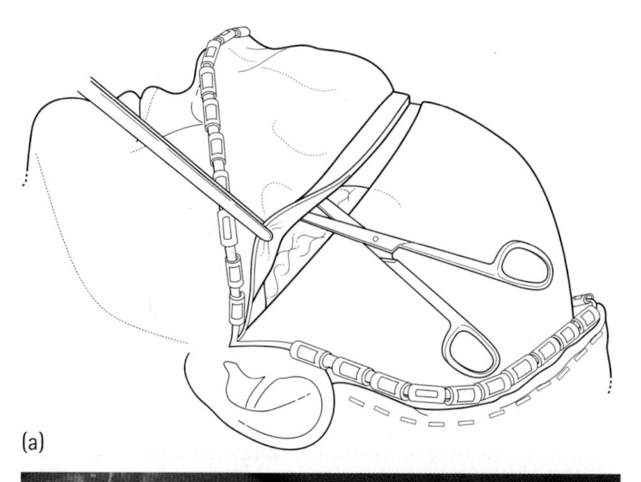

(a)

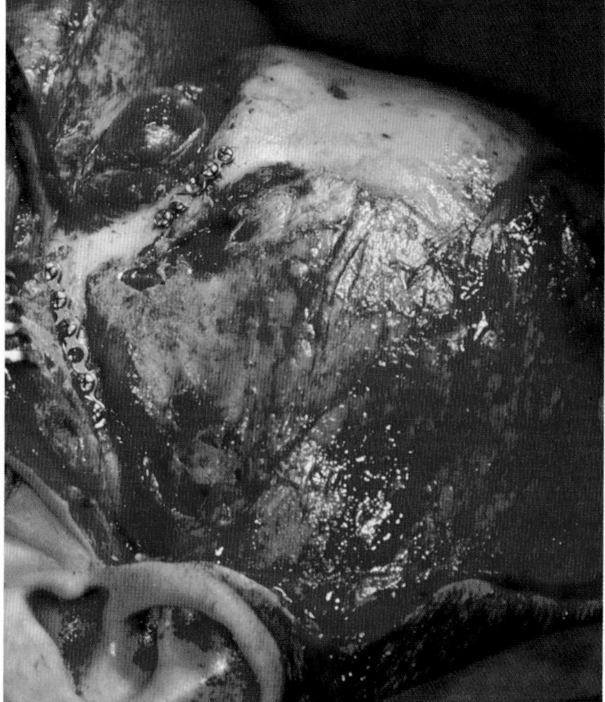

(b)

7.9.9 The incision of the superficial temporal fascia.

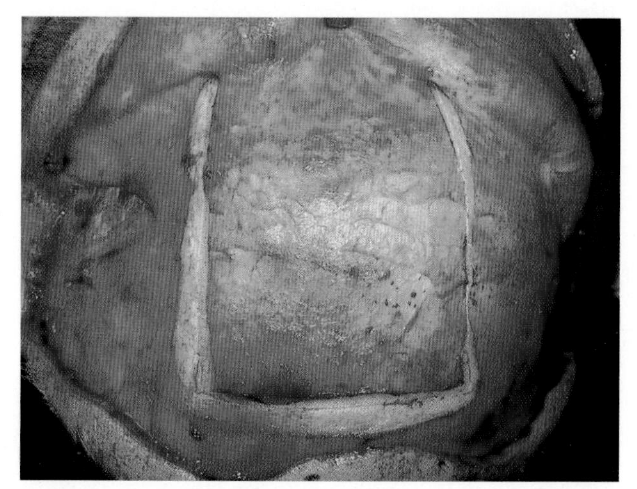

7.9.10 Anteriorly based pericranial flap.

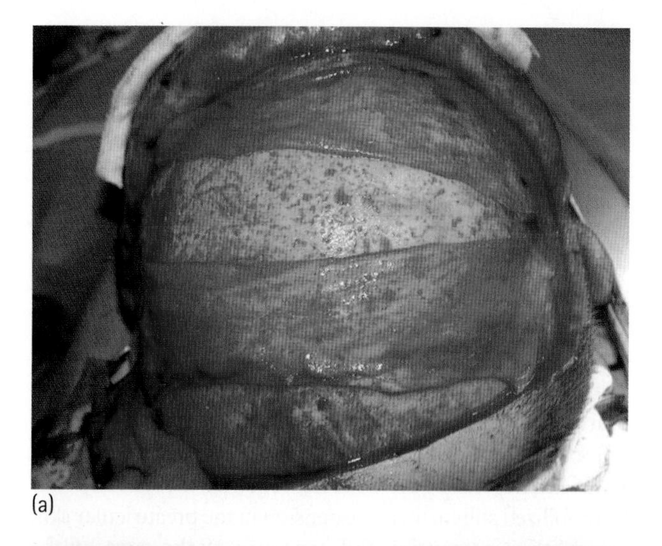

(a)

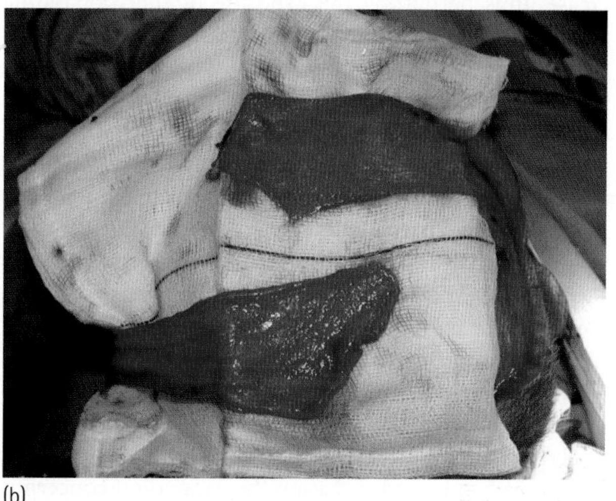

(b)

7.9.11 Laterally based pericranial flap.

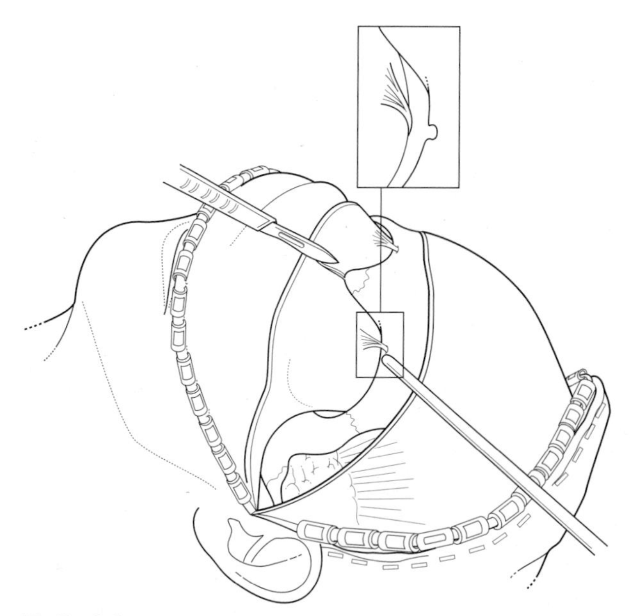

7.9.12 Release of supraorbital neurovascular bundle.

outer or inner insertions to the anterior and posterior lacrimal crests as this may lead to widening of the soft tissues across the nasal root and, in extreme cases, may induce telecanthus.

Laterally having now incised through the superficial temporal fascia and joined this superiorly with the reflected pericranium, the flap may be dissected more inferiorly by stripping of the lateral body of the zygoma and incising through the periosteum of the superior aspect of the zygomatic arch and posterior zygomatic body. Reflection of the flap exposes the body and arch of the zygoma leaving behind the superficial temporal fat pad intact. The temporal branch of the facial nerve is retracted in the flap beneath the reflected superficial temporal fascia.

Finally, depending on the access required, the skin flap may be mobilized still further by extension in the preauricular skin crease, thus permitting full exposure of the root of the zygomatic arch. Full subperiosteal orbital dissection is now possible mobilizing the attachment of the lateral canthal tendon and medially by identifying the anterior and posterior ethmoidal vessels. The ethmoidal vessels emerge at the level of the cribriform plate. The anterior and posterior vessels being 24 and 36 mm from the anterior lacrimal crest and the latter being 3–5 mm anterior to the optic foramen. Occasionally, very large facial lacerations may have to be incorporated into the line of the incision so as not to risk the vascularity of the flap. Lacerations by themselves, however, offer poor access and may compromise treatment by restricting the size of craniotomy that may be achieved, and for this reason, unless exceptionally large, extension of lacerations is to be avoided.

Having achieved retraction of the flap, the craniotomy must now be planned and again the paramount concern is adequate access to effect intracranial inspection and dural repair if necessary. This will depend on the site of injury and suggested craniotomies are shown for central, lateral and complex injuries as described by Burnstein. Burr holes should be placed to minimize subsequent aesthetic problems and also in a position that will allow a good low frontal craniotomy to deal with the frontal sinus, but also minimize the amount of brain retraction needed to explore the sub-basal region for dural repair and inspection of fractures of the orbital roof and anterior fossa floor. For this reason, burr holes may be placed laterally in the region of the pteryion after reflection of the temporalis muscle in this region. Not only does this permit good low access to the horizontal cut of the craniotomy, but may be covered with temporalis at the end of the procedure reducing visible defects in the bone. The craniotomy is raised using a combination of large burs with or without a cut out clutch to perforate the skull without damaging the dura. Depending on the size of the flap required, further bur holes are required superiorly and possibly adjacent to the midline to help mobilize the flap with a side cutting and end guarded craniotome, to avoid damage to the dura and if the midline has to be crossed, then the sagittal sinus. Finally, the bone flap is raised using blunt dissection from the underlying dura. Exposure should now permit easy tension-free retraction of the frontal lobes and allow inspection of the anterior and posterior walls of the frontal sinus, orbital roof and cribriform regions (Figure 7.9.13).

If there are sub-basal dural lacerations, retraction may already have been facilitated by loss of cerebrospinal fluid; alternatively, an osteotomy of the frontal bandeau may further aid access (Figure 7.9.14). A planned dural incision allows basal dural lacerations to be approached with minimal brain retraction, especially of the basal region, without damage to the olfactory tracts (Figure 7.9.15).

The next stage is to repair the frontal bandeau to restore frontal projection, width and height. This is closely linked to reductions in the temporal and zygomatic arch regions. Not only does reduction of these fractures form the basis for the accurate reposition of the mid-facial structures, but permits the size of defects of the orbital roof to be gauged and whether or not primary bone grafting is required.

If bone grafting is required, this is best performed now as use of any pericranial flap will preclude further bone work.

Bone grafts may be obtained by harvesting the inner table of the craniotomy segment. The cortices may be split initially using a fissure burr to define the plane between them, and the split is completed using a reciprocating saw and flexible

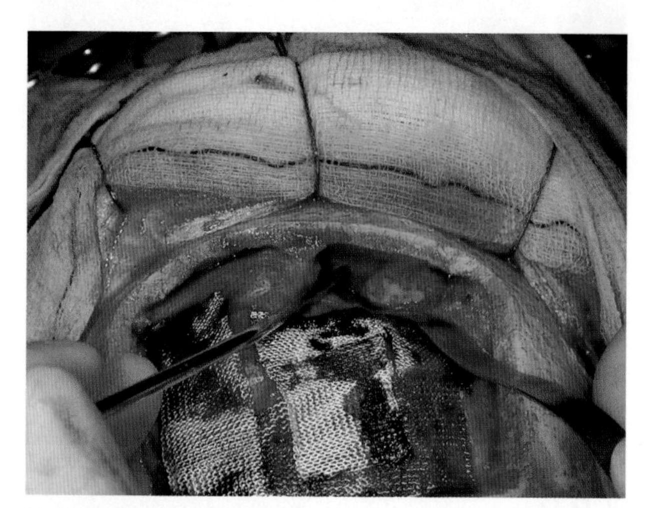

7.9.13 Retraction of frontal lobes.

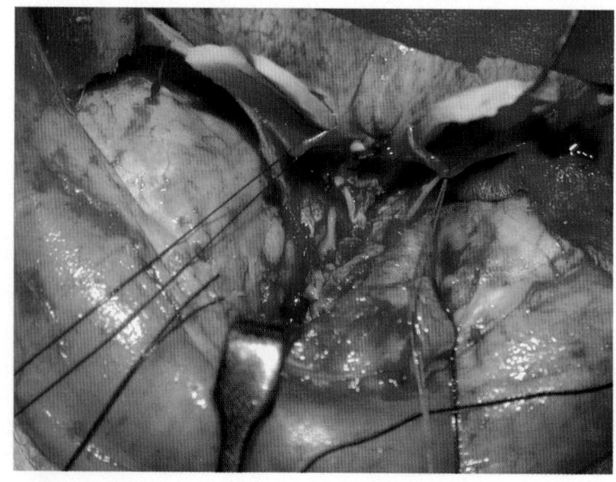

7.9.14 Temporary osteotomy of frontal bandeau.

osteotomes. The outer cortex may then be replaced over the donor site and the inner cortex used for grafting (Figure 7.9.16).

Outer cortical grafts may be obtained from the temporoparietal region overlying the the nondominant hemisphere. The size of the graft can be outlined with a fissure burr, used side on to cut through the outer cortex and the bone immediately outside the segment may be reduced in height using an acrylic burr. A slim osteotome can then be introduced into the diploic space and the graft harvested. Bleeding is arrested with a resorbable haemostatic agents which gives some bulk to the haematoma which can then be redraped with the periosteum to help minimize the subsequent depression (Figure 7.9.17).

The selection of osteosynthesis material requires maintenance of the reduced fractures and bone grafts in a stable position. Usually, titanium plates with a low profile utilizing screws 1–1.3 mm in diameter are used. This is sufficient as the scenario is not load-bearing other than to withstand the pulsation of the dura or in the case of the orbital roof the weight of the frontal lobes. Bone grafts must take into account the original anatomy of the defect and nowhere is this more important than in restoring the upward curving nature of the orbital roof, failure to realize this important point may result in vertical hypoglobus and potentially exophthalmos. Bone grafting within the orbital roof is important to separate the pulsation of the brain from the orbital contents which may result in very unsightly pulsation of the eye. Having restored the orbital roof, the anterior fossa floor and if necessary cranialization of the frontal sinus, then vascularized pericranial grafts may now be introduced. If an anterior flap is raised, this may be fed in beneath the frontal lobes and be secured with a few sutures and supplemented with fibrin glue to try and obtain a watertight seal and close off the nasopharynx from the anterior fossa. If damage to the pericranium anteriorly has necessitated a laterally based flap, then this may be introduced from the region of the lateral craniotomy cut and burr hole. Finally, the craniotomy segment may be repositioned taking care not to compress the pericranial graft and trying to position any subsequent space in the bone cuts to give the most cosmetically acceptable result.

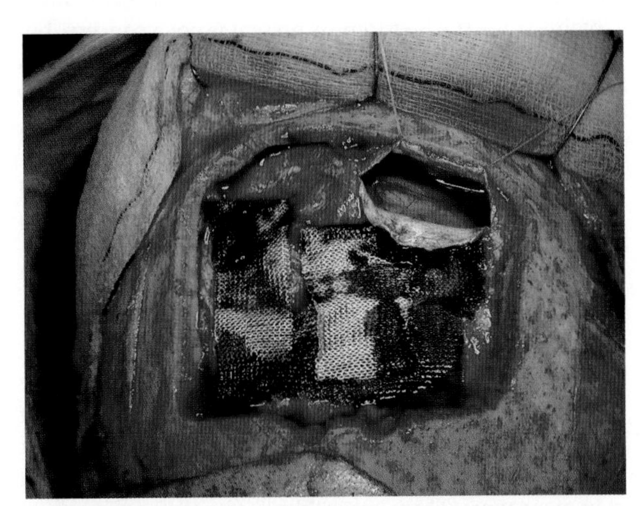

7.9.15 Intradural approach to basal region.

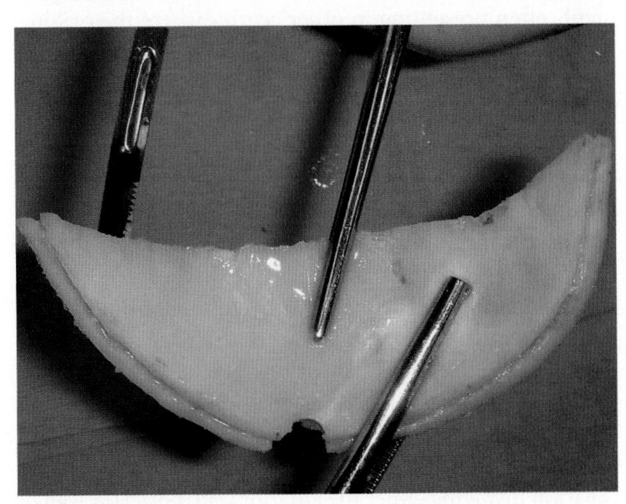

7.9.16 Craniotomy splitting with fine saw.

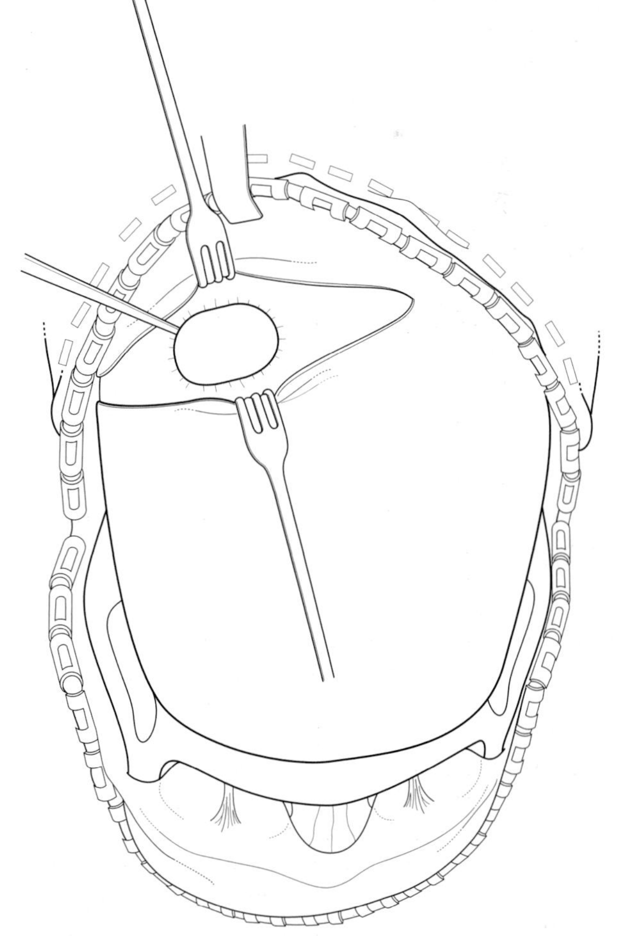

7.9.17 Harvesting outer table calvarial graft.

CLOSURE

A good closure will help achieve the correct soft tissue suspension over the anatomical hard tissue repair, failure to do so will result in gravity allowing the extensively mobilized tissue to move 'south'. This may be achieved in a number of ways. First, non-resorbable sutures are used to accurately attach the lateral canthal tendon and periorbita to fine drill holes positioned around the orbital aperture. This is combined with suspension sutures inserted into the periosteum overlying the zygomatic body and sutured to the temporal edge of the incised superior margin of the superficial temporal fascia. The temporalis must be replaced over the burr hole in the temporal region and any bone dust kept from the original access may be used in any residual bone defects. Finally, the inferior aspect of the incised superficial temporal fascia is attached to the temporal fascia at a slightly higher level, to help further support the soft tissue drape of the face (Figure 7.9.18). A drain is placed beneath the flap with the inferior aspect reaching into the side having undergone the most extensive dissection to avoid collection in this region. A system with variable ammonts of suction is ideal as leakage of CSF may require use of drains on gravity suction only. If CSF drainage is a real concern, then placement of a lumbar drain for a period of 5–7 days is favoured by some to allow time for the dural repair to establish itself. The scalp is closed with 2/0 resorbable suture, care being taken to use only the galea which allows for good soft tissue support and apposition of the wound margin.

In the region beneath the temporal line, more superficial sutures may be required and closure may be helped by removal of the staples placed initially to secure the drapes thus releasing tension from the posterior skin flap. Accurate positioning of the scalp is ensured by aligning the tattoo marks inserted at the beginning of the procedure. Skin closure is achieved very easily with staples ensuring that the wound margins are everted. A well-fitting head bandage is placed, making sure to cover the wound in the first instance with a non-adherent dressing and then absorbent swabs and finally cotton wool across the forehead and behind the ears before fitting a well-placed crepe bandage under tension. The cotton wool and avoidance of excessive tension in the dressing avoid pressure necrosis, particularly overlying the drain and forehead regions. The drain is secured only with tape to the head dressing allowing its removal when required without the need to disturb the head dressing thus helping to prevent further fluid accumulation which may lead to increased risk of infection and fibrosis.

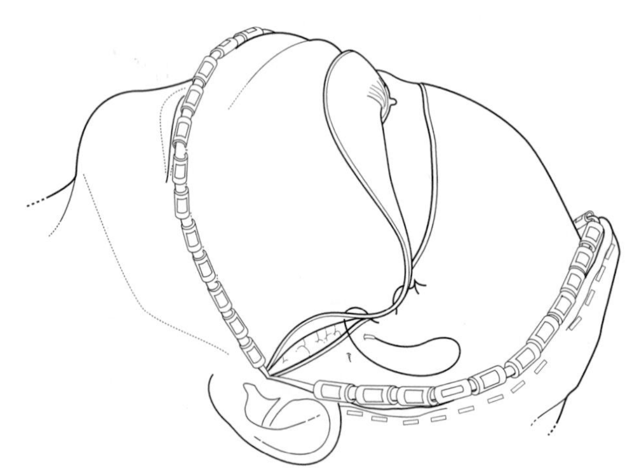

7.9.18 Temporal fascia closure.

POST-OPERATIVE CARE

The patient will be managed post-operatively in the neurosurgical high dependency unit. The decision to extubate at the end of the procedure will have been discussed previously with the anaesthetist, but occasionally due to intraoperative considerations, such as frontal lobe manipulation, CSF leakage and positioning of a spinal drain, blood loss and temperature control, a short period of maintained intubation may be advisable before extubation. Obviously if a tracheostomy is present is not a concern, but if the patient has had other forms of intubation, discussions over tube switching and acceptance of the tube post-surgery and in the weaning process will need to be decided upon. Antibiotics are usually continued for at least three post-operative doses and depending on the anterior fossa and dural repairs, as well as CSF leakage, these may be extended for several days.

MANAGEMENT OF THE FRONTAL SINUS

The treatment of the frontal sinus is controversial, not least of all as prospective studies in this area are few and most algorithms relate to the retrospective analysis of a unit's data over many years. There is a problem as studies certainly have shown complications many years after the original treatment, often presenting in other centres where the original treatment criteria is not known. It is safe to assume that one unit's complications may well be treated by another unit due to the time scales involved. Nonetheless, there has been a consensus about what one is hoping to achieve, namely a 'safe sinus' with the least intervention necessary. The frontal sinus is of variable size and is lined by respiratory epithelium that communicates via the frontonasal duct with the middle meatus of the nose. The duct is again in a variable structure, being well defined in some instances, but in more than 60 per cent of cases achieves its drainage via communication with the ethmoidal air cells (Figure 7.9.19).

Frontal sinus fractures occur in approximately 2–15 per cent of facial fractures and are far more associated with craniofacial fractures involving the skull base, but may occur in isolation involving either the anterior wall, posterior wall or floor with associated duct injuries (Figure 7.9.20). While

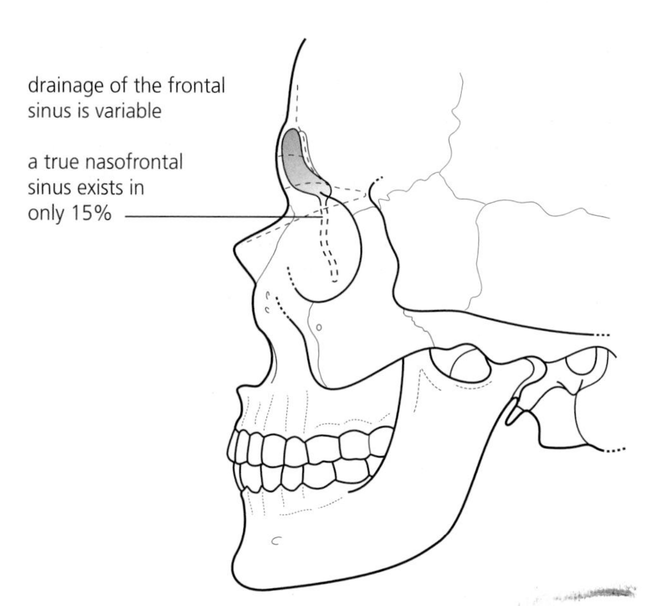

7.9.19 Anatomy of the frontal sinus and naso frontal duct. The frontal sinus is a pyramidal, air-filled cavity lying within the lamina of the frontal bone creating an anterior and posterior wall to the sinus. Drainage of the frontal sinus is variable. A true nasofrontal duct exists in only 15%.

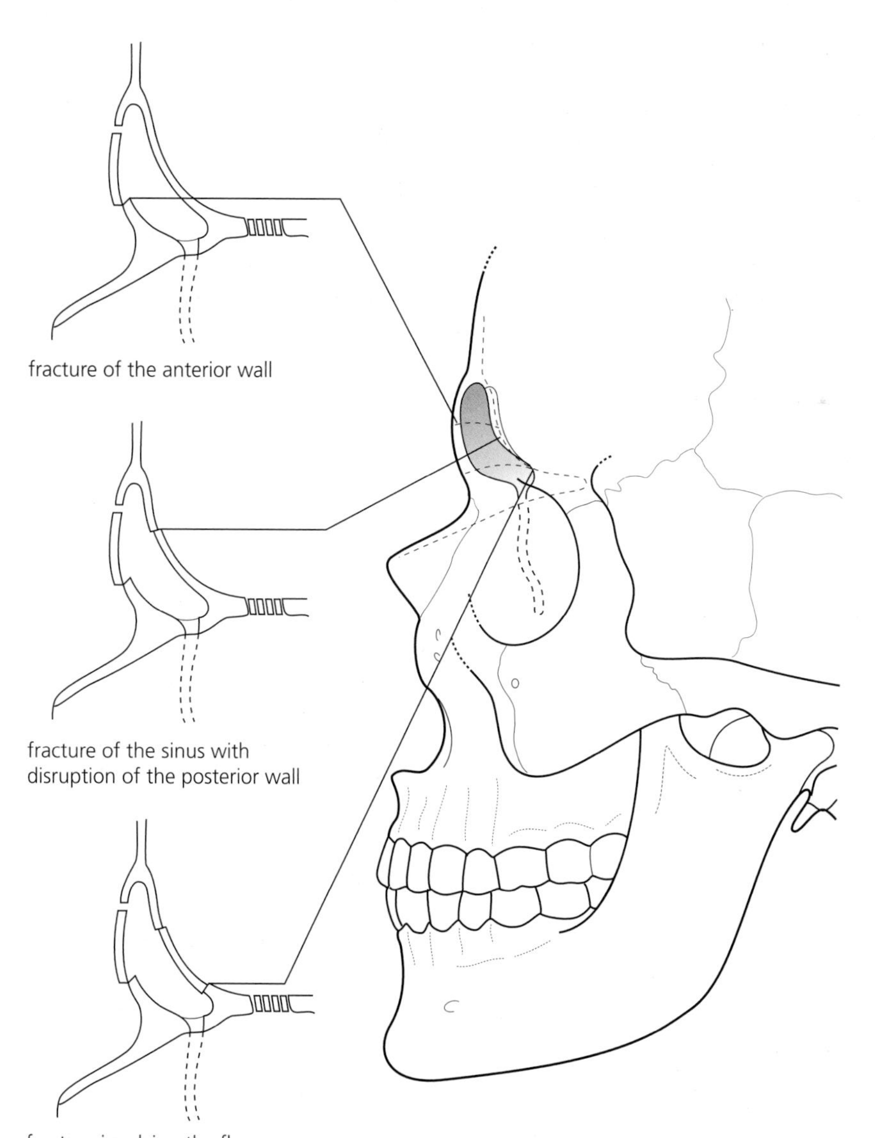

7.9.20 Classification of frontal sinus fractures.

there may be obvious cosmetic concerns with depression of the anterior wall of the frontal sinus, it is the functional problems including chronic sinusitis (up to 60 per cent), meningitis (6 per cent) and also mucopyocoele, osteomyelitis and cerebral abcess formation that drive the need for treatment.

Undisplaced anterior wall fractures may require no treatment; however, if displaced, access is achieved along the lines described previously as for craniofacial fractures only differing in the amount of exposure that is often necessary limiting exposure to between the superficial temporal lines, reducing the risk to the facial nerve. If the anterior wall is depressed, then it may be elevated without removal of the bone by placing 2-mm screws into the main fragments and elevated using forceps and subsequently fixated with low profile 1.3 mm or similar titanium systems (Figure 7.9.21). If fractures are more depressed, then the fragments will have to be temporarily removed and accurately laid out on a moist swab in the same orientation, to assist in their accurate reassembly and subsequent insertion. Any necrotic or damaged lining may then be removed carefully leaving all viable mucosa. The remaining mucosa will help seed subsequent re-epithelialization of the repaired sinus. If defects have occurred, then calvarial grafts may be harvested as previously described and fixated. If, after elevation of the bone fragments, they appear not to fit, it may be necessary to trim the bone margins to allow an accurate placement without overlap. This latter point results from the deformation of the bone segments during the fracture process.

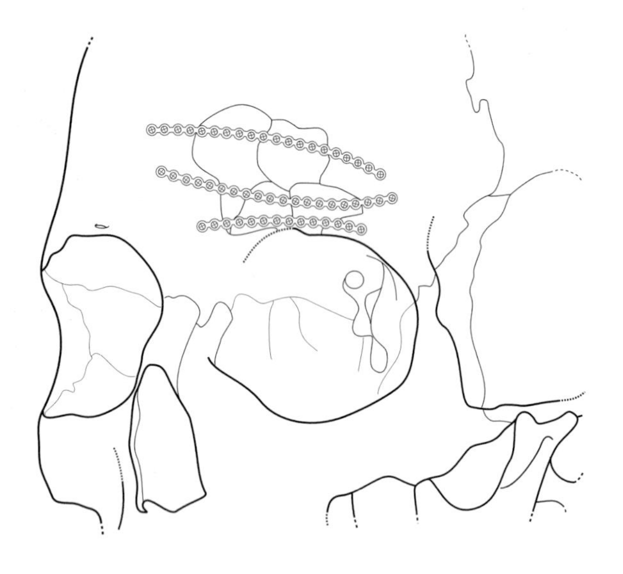

7.9.21 Reduction of anterior wall fracture of the frontal sinus.

Fractures of the frontal sinus floor may result in damage to the frontonasal duct which may subsequently lead to obstruction with mucocoele formation. Stenting of the ducts has been shown to be associated with long-term stenosis, the author prefers, therefore, to seal off the frontonasal duct in such circumstances. The procedure involves the temporary removal of the anterior sinus wall, but in this instance all the mucosal lining is removed meticulously and the surface of the bone drilled over to try and assure removal of all crypts of mucosa. The mucosa of the nasofrontal duct is mobilized and inverted through the infundibulum. Oxidized cellulose is then placed across and the defect is then filled with autogenous bone. The volume required may be large and, in some instances, iliac crest grafts may have to be utilized rather than morcelized calvarial grafts. Abdominal fat is to be avoided due to the variable levels of resorption and potential subsequent mucocoele formation. The anterior wall may then be replaced and fixated as previously described (Figure 7.9.22).

Isolated fractures of the posterior wall if displaced by more than 5 mm have been shown to be associated with dural lacerations and such fractures associated with a CSF leak should undergo cranialization. The technique utilizes the same exposure as before, but in this case following the low craniotomy, the posterior wall of the frontal sinus is removed, allowing all the frontal mucosa to be removed. The duct mucosa is inverted, as previously described, and covered with oxidized cellulose and this time a disc of cortical bone is placed over the duct orifice, and bone dust and milled bone obtained from the posterior wall is packed above it (Figure

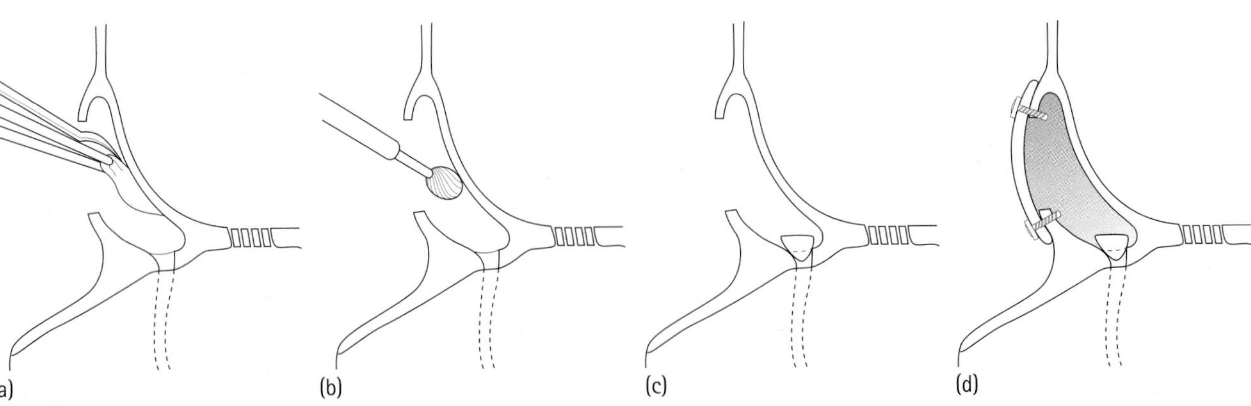

7.9.22 Frontal sinus obliteration.

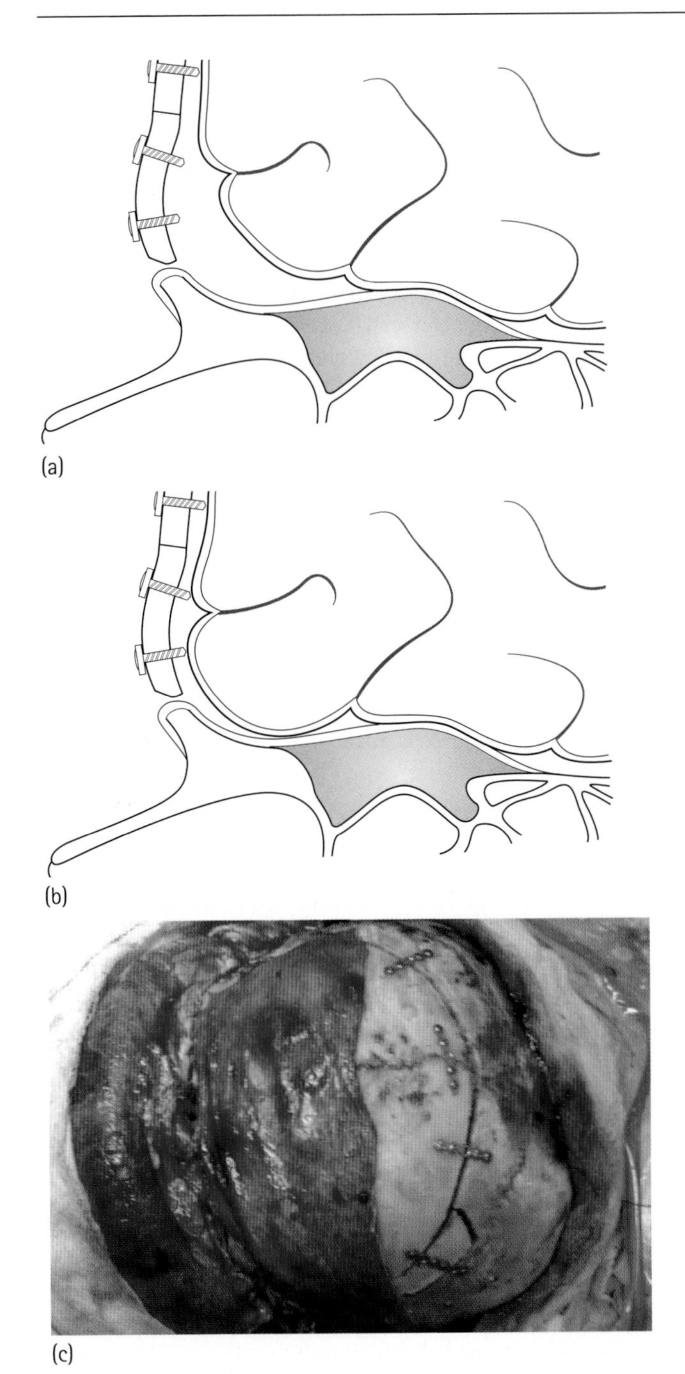

7.9.23 Frontal sinus cranilisation.

7.9.23). A vascularized pericranial flap is then placed across the infundibulum and bone grafts, so as to be supported beneath the frontal lobes with its vascularized surface against the bone graft. Any dural tears will have been repaired by this time, but if the tears are sub-basal then an intradural repair may be performed with the periocranium being introduced through the dural incision to lie under the frontal lobe (Figure 7.9.23), before the flap is secured with fibrin glue to achieve a watertight seal. The risk of a CSF leak may be further reduced by suturing the incised dural margin to the pericranial flap, but care has to be taken not to damage the vascularity of the graft. Closure is performed as described earlier in this section.

Recently, several authors have advocated the endoscopic repair of frontal sinus fractures and, while this is in the early stages, there is some promise in this minimally invasive technique in specific situations. The reader is referred to the relevant articles cited in the bibliography for a review of the technique.

Complications

INFECTION

This may be immediate in the form of meningitis, brain abscess or subdural emphyema, often related to failure to debride and gain adequate closure. Treatment involves antibiotic treatment with broad spectrum cephalosporins and metronidazole, together with possible reoperation and removal of infected craniotomy segments to allow the infection to settle and delay reconstruction to a later date. Late infection may be associated with the presence of a mucocoele due to an obstructed frontal sinus or CSF fistula that will need to be addressed. Mococoele formation may complicate 10 per cent of unrelated cases and require removal of the frontal sinus and formal cranialization to remove all the respiratory epithelium (Figure 7.9.24).

CEREBROSPINAL FLUID FISTULAS

Fistulas are relatively rare in closed injuries affecting only 2 per cent, which rises to 9 per cent in open or penetrating head injuries. Suggested investigations involve fine cut coronal CT or T_2-weighted magnetic resonance imaging (MRI) with contrast.

Cisternograms are more invasive and finally the use of fluorescein intrathecally combined with nasal endoscopy has been shown to be of benefit in defects which are difficult to identify.

NASOETHMOIDAL FRACTURES

Background

Nasoethmoidal fractures present several difficulties related not only to restoring the aesthetics of this region, but also the functional consequences related to the close proximity to the skull base and frontal sinus, the orbital contents, and walls and lacrimal apparatus. The force applied is well withstood by the stout bone of the orbital aperture, including the bone of the frontonasal buttress, but if anterior force overcomes this initial resistance then the pneumatized ethmoidal air cells and weak medial walls of the orbit offer little structural support and may become grossly disrupted in comparison to the greater resistance given by the anterior skull base and orbital apex, designed physiologically to help protect the brain and soft tissues of the orbital apex. The key to dealing with fractures in this region is understanding the relationship of the medial canthal tendon and its attachment to the so-called central fragment of the nasomaxillary

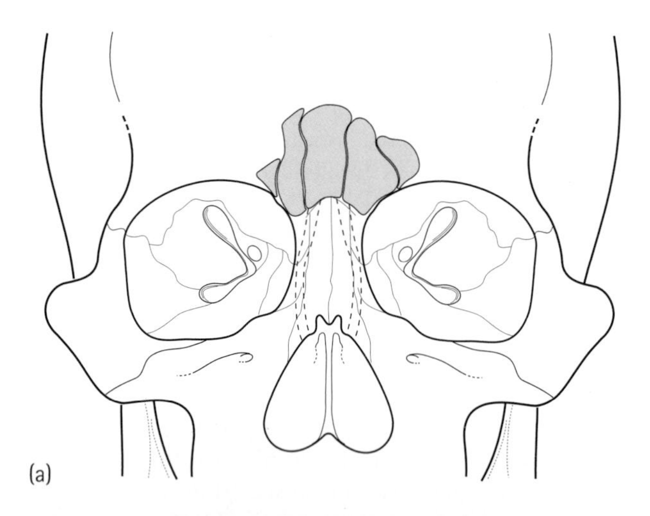

(a)

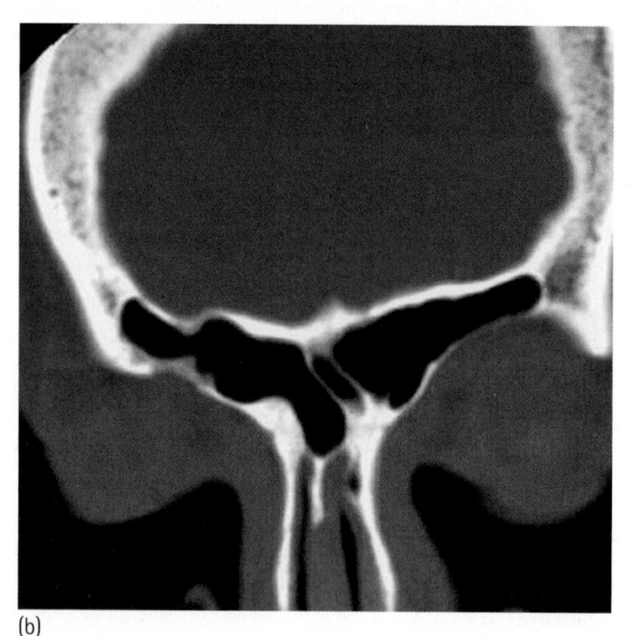

(b)

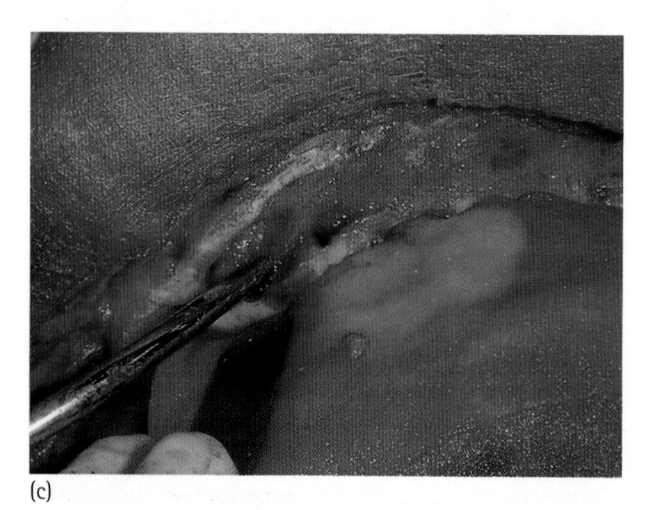

(c)

7.9.24 Aetiology of mucocoel formation. The risk of infection is linked to communication between the nasal cavity and dural tears via the frontal sinus. The aetiology of a mucocele appears to be related to obstruction of the nasofrontal duct in a diseased or injured frontal sinus.

complex and lacrimal bones. The medial canthal tendon attaches to the medial orbit by superficial and deep limbs attached to the anterior and posterior lacrimal crests, respectively. It is the medial extension of the upper and lower tarsi meeting, where the preseptal muscles divide into deep and superficial heads. This point is marked by the puntae of the upper and lower canuliculi within the lid margins. From this point, the canaliculi extend behind the medial canthal tendon into the lacrimal sac. The anterior horizontal segment of the tendon is attached firmly to the anterior lacrimal crest and is stronger than the posterior limb which is attached to the posterior lacrimal crest and serves to hold the eyelids against the globe in a posterior fashion. It is this medial and posterior relationship that has to be reconfigured in injuries involving the medial canthal tendon if the palpebral shape is to remain unaltered and the tarsal plates are to be supported in close apposition to the surface of the globe, and avoid epipora.

Nasoethmoidal fractures come as a spectrum ranging from simple dislocation to those which involve a pattern involving the medial wall of the orbit, frontal sinus, skull base, ethmoidal air cells, orbital rim and nasal bones. This means, therefore, that depending on the severity, other injuries associated with the frontonasal duct, lacrimal apparatus and medial canthal tendon must be addressed and the aims of treatment must not only address the reduction of the fractures, but deal with these functional and aesthetic issues. A classification of these injuries has been described by Markowitz, depending on the relative displacement of the medial canthal tendon, as types 1 to 3 (Figure 7.9.25).

Sequencing of nasoethmoidal fractures

Sequencing follows the following pattern:

- exposure;
- reduction and stabilization of the frontal bandeau and anterior fossa floor;
- restoration of the frontonasal angle;
- reconstruction of the outer orbital frame;
- repair of the medial orbital wall;
- reduction and fixation of midfacial buttresses;
- restoration of the medial canthal tendon;
- repair of the lacrimal system;
- closure;
- nasal plaster and septal splints.

Exposure

Apart from simple undisplaced rim fractures, the approach of choice is the coronal flap modified to reach the nasal bridge by incising the periosteum over the nasal bridge, as previously described, care being taken to identify the lacrimal apparatus and medial canthal tendon. In addition, the approaches previously described within the orbital fracture section may be used to achieve adequate exposure.

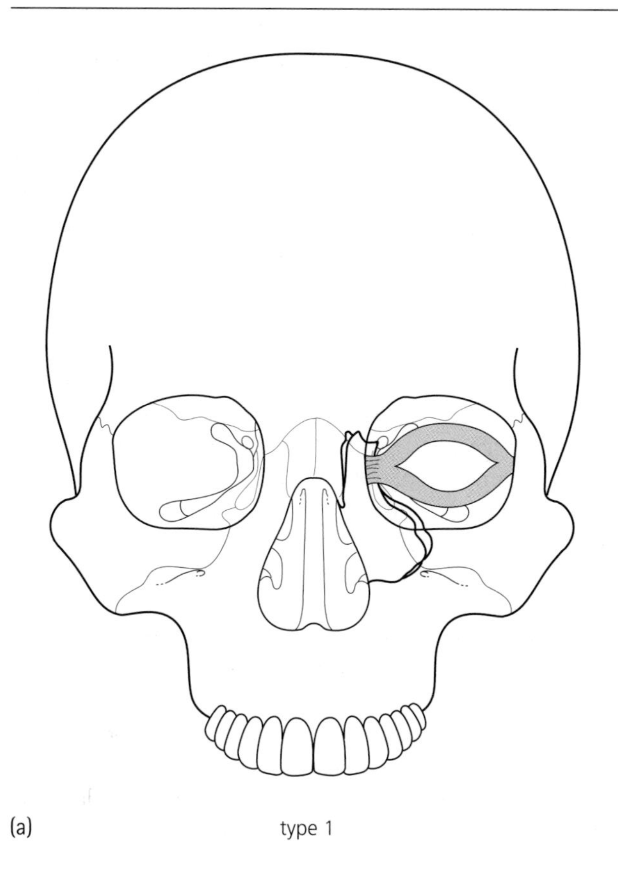

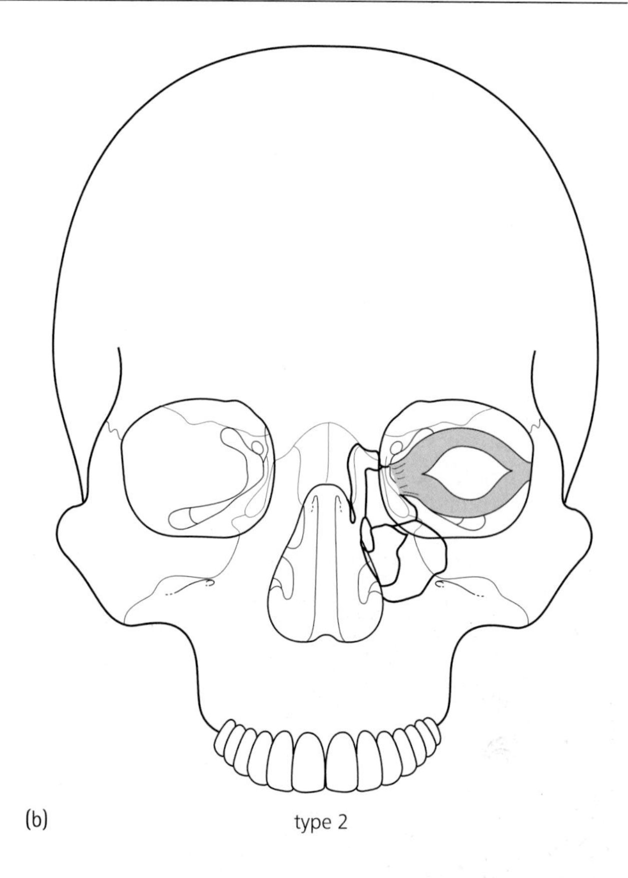

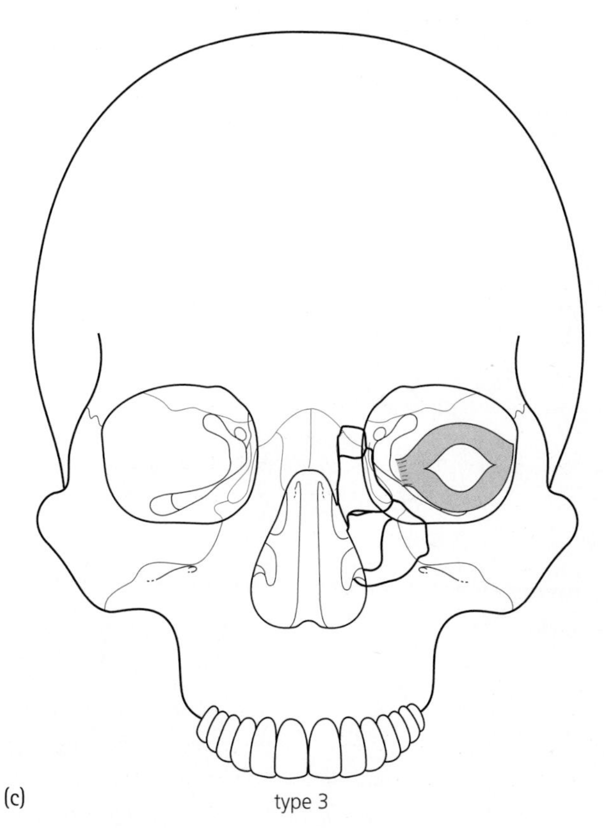

7.9.25 Classification of nasoethmodal fractures.

Assuming the frontal bandeau is intact or has been repaired, the frontal nasal angle must be restored by reduction of the fracture and fixation with low profile 1–1.3-mm plates and screws and, if necessary, primary bone grafting using split calvarium. It is important to ensure that the angle obtained is correct as significant shortening and posterior displacement can occur. This may mean slim osteotomes and spreaders being introduced to mobilize the fragments if impacted and especially if the fracture is more of a monobloc-type fracture than the more comminuted variety.

The lateral and inferior orbital wall may be approached via the coronal flap or adjuvant subciliary incisions so as to permit accurate alignment of the orbital margin taking care to use separate plates from above and below for fractures of the medial orbital rim, thus reducing excessive stripping of the anterior medial canthal tendon ligament which may lead to iatrogenic telecanthus and widening of the soft tissues across the bridge of the nose.

The alignment of the midfacial buttresses in the perialar and zygomatic regions via an intraoral approach will help further with orientating the position of the maxilla and establish facial height, width and projection and aid accurate alignment of the nasoethmoidal complex (Figure 7.9.26).

Having stabilized the outer orbital and facial frames and frontonasal angle, the medial orbital wall defects may be repaired with adaptive conical-shaped titanium plates which can be placed from the subciliary approach and visualized from above beneath the coronal flap. It is easy for different surgical planes to be developed via both approaches and to aid plate insertion, a polydioxanone sheet passed from below into the medial orbital region can easily be seen from above defining the subperiosteal layer, acting as a soft tissue retractor. The plates may be secured along the orbital rim, but if plates have already been placed, then two or three screws placed into the inferior lateral aspect of the orbit in the sounder bone found here will suffice.

The medial canthal ligament in type 1 injuries will have already been stabilized by reduction of the fractures.

In type 2 and 3 injuries, however, there is usually the need to identify the ligament with the aid of a canthopexy wire. Specialized wires are available (Synthes, Welwyn Garden City, UK). A stainless steel needle is passed externally through the medial caruncular region emerging interiorly through the inner surface of the down-turned coronal flap through the identified medial canthal tendon. This latter point may be identified by grasping the area behind the lacrimal apparatus with toothed forceps and sequentially observing the effects on the medial canthal tendon. It must be remembered that the angulation of the medial canthal region and the adaption of the eyelids depend on good support of the eyelids by a medial canthal tendon that is inserted superiorly and posteriorly. The best way to ensure this is to use a curved plate from the frontal region which may act as a point of support for the canthal insertion. In such cases, the tendon wire is passed through the lower hole of a suitable low profile plate. A passage for the needle is then made by drilling across the ethmoidal region behind the lacrimal apparatus to the contralateral side aiming slightly posteriorly. The use of a green needle will facilitate the passage of the wire's needle across the tract created. The curved plate may be so positioned and secured on the frontal bone to give support for the tendon insertion helping to restore the medial canthal angle, supporting the tarsal plates and addressing any telecanthus by tightening the wire to a superiorly placed screw (Figure 7.9.27).

The lacrimal sac and duct must be closely inspected for damage. Many late obstructions of the system result from inadequate reduction of the fractures and blockages in the intrabony part of the lacrimal system. Accurate fixation of the fractures will help this point. However, lacerations of the medial aspect of the lower eyelid carry significant risk of damage to the inferior canaliculus. If there is clear laceration in this region then identification of the severed ends may be cannulated with ophthalmic silastic stents, but it must be remembered that epiphora will not result if one of the canaliculi are present and functioning and if this is

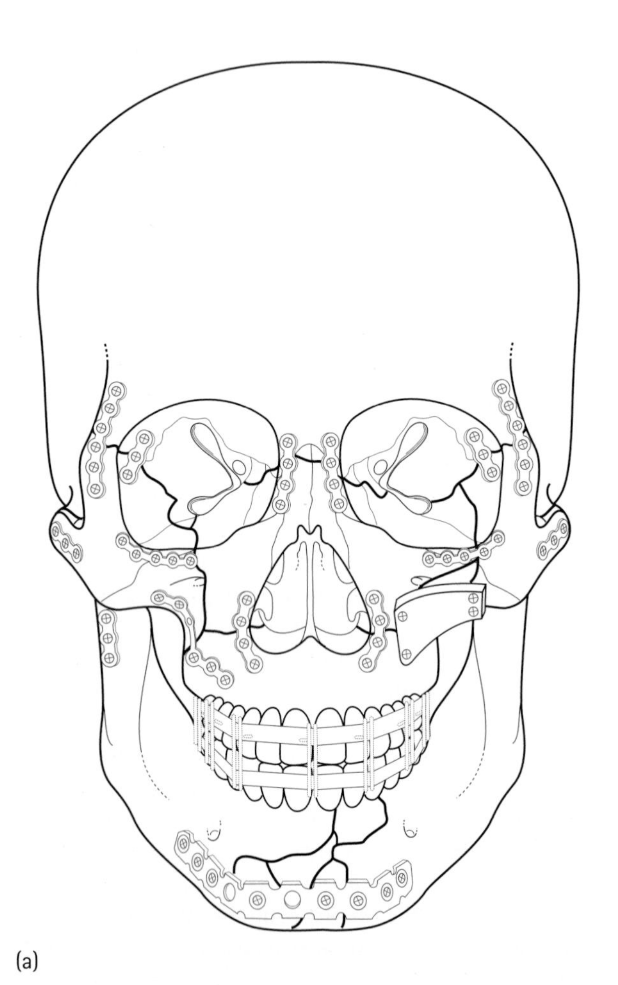

(a)

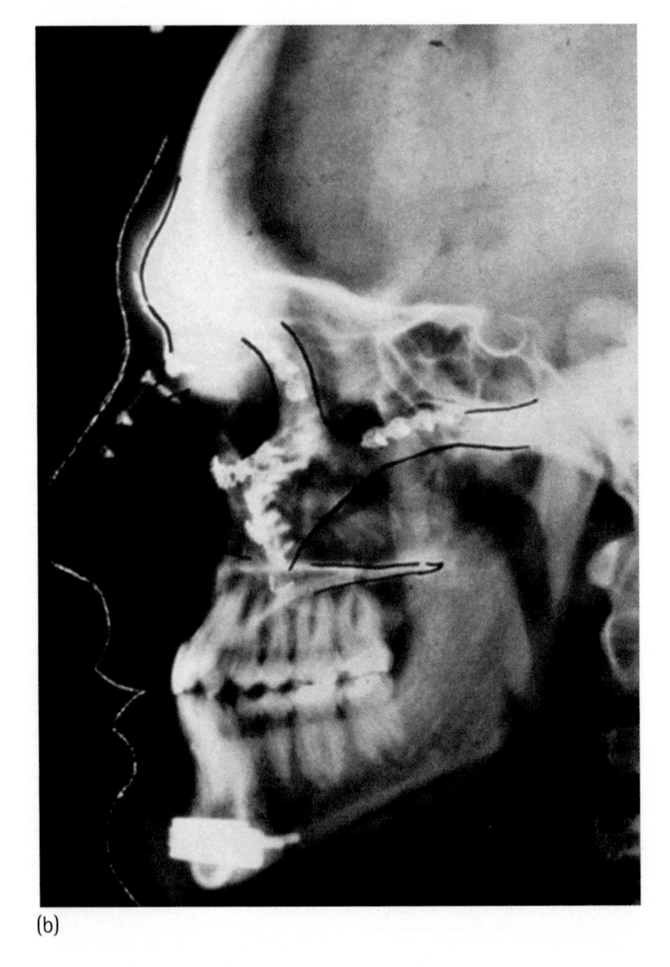

(b)

7.9.26 Reduction and alignment of midfacial buttresses.

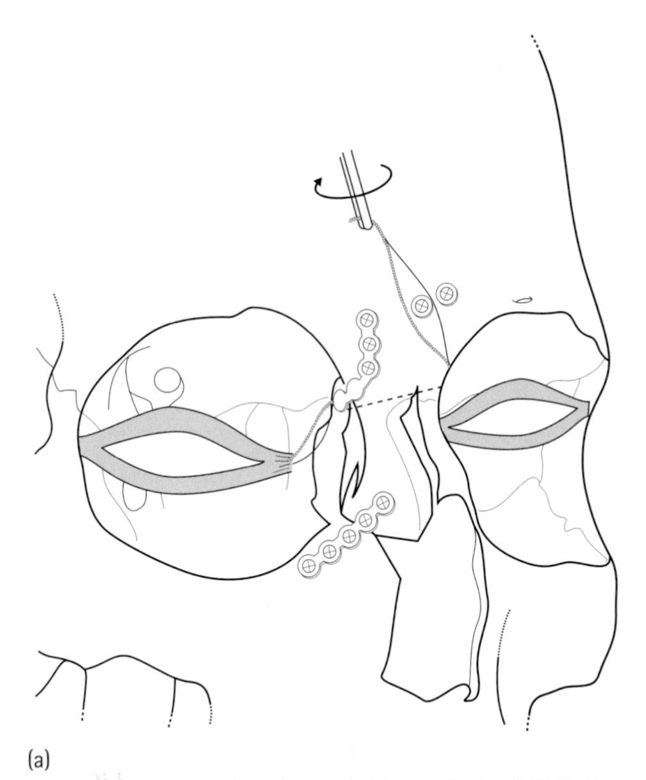

(a)

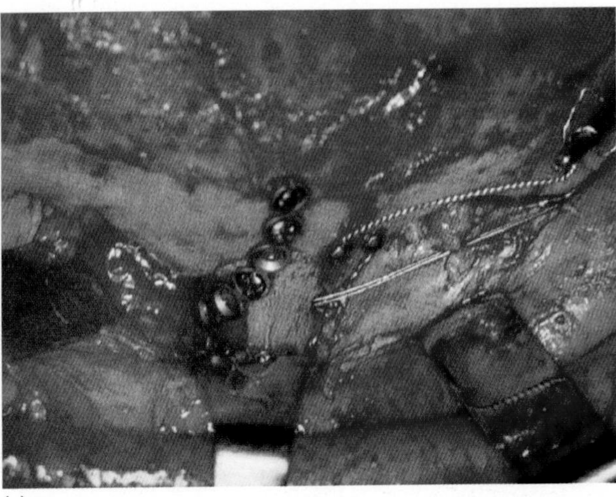

(b)

7.9.27 Alignment of medial canthal tendon using tendon wire and medial orbital plate.

not easily achieved then such procedures are best left as injudicious attempts at passing catheters may cause damage to the remaining canaliculus. It may be that further dacrocystorhinostomy may be necessary even in those cases where the duct has been repaired, as stenosis may occur even in stents left in place for six months.

Complications

Aesthetic blunting and vertical discrepancies of the medial canthal tendon are best dealt with through a combination of osteotomy and reattachment of the tendon if necessary; this latter point depends on the angle of the medial canthus. In general terms, trying to shorten the tendon without addressing the widening of the bone will not correct the defect.

Epiphora should be investigated by an ophthalmic surgeon, usually with a dacrocystogram and either the duct repaired or, more likely, a dacrocystorhinostomy. Cerebral sinus thrombosis (CST), fistulas, infection and mucocoele formation associated with frontal duct injuries and anterior fossa floor injuries are dealt with as described above. A final complication involves orbital volume changes to the associated medial wall defects.

Top tips

- Treat these injuries as part of a multidisciplinary team in specialized centres.
- Identify and treat appropriately associated life-threatening injuries.
- Outline a clear team plan for operation and sequencing on operation board.
- Avoidance of facial nerve injury by division of superficial temporalis fascia.
- Mobilization of supraorbital bundle with osteotomes.
- Preservation of pericranial flaps.
- Accurate soft tissue resuspension following coronal flap.
- Use of orbital plate to help give support for insertion of medial canthal tendon.

FURTHER READING

Becelli R, Renzi G, Mannino G *et al.* Posttraumatic obstruction of lacrimal pathways: A retrospective analysis of 58 consecutive naso-orbitoethmoid fractures. *Journal of Craniofacial Surgery* 2004; **15**: 29–33.

Bell RB, Dierks EJ, Brar P *et al.* A protocol for the management of frontal sinus fractures emphasizing sinus preservation. *Journal of Oral and Maxillofacial Surgery* 2007; **65**: 825–39.

Burstein F, Cohen S, Hudgins R, Boydston W. Frontal basilar trauma: Classification and treatment. *Plastic and Reconstructive Surgery* 1997; **99**: 1314–21, discussion 1322.

Donald PJ. Management of frontal sinus fractures. *Journal of Trauma* 2007; **62** (Suppl.): S91.

Ellis E 3rd. Sequencing treatment for naso-orbito-ethmoid fractures. *Journal of Oral and Maxillofacial Surgery* 1993; **51**: 543–58.

Markowitz BL, Manson PN, Sargent L *et al.* Management of the medial canthal tendon in nasoethmoid orbital fractures: The importance of the central fragment in classification and treatment. *Plastic and Reconstructive Surgery* 1991; **87**: 843–53.

Raveh J, Laedrach K, Vuillemin T, Zingg M. Management of combined frontonaso-orbital/skull base fractures and telecanthus in 355 cases. *Archives of Otolaryngology, Head and Neck Surgery* 1992; **118**: 605–14.

Shumrick KA. Endoscopic management of frontal sinus fractures. *Otolaryngology Clinics of North America* 2007; **40**: 329–36.

Strong EB, Pahlavan N, Saito D. Frontal sinus fractures: A 28-year retrospective review. *Otolaryngology – Head and Neck Surgery* 2006; **135**: 774–9.

Tiwari P, Higuera S, Thornton J, Hollier LH. The management of frontal sinus fractures. *Journal of Oral and Maxillofacial Surgery* 2005; **63**: 1354–60.

7.10

Zygomatic fractures

MICHAEL PERRY

Terminology can be confusing. 'zygoma', 'malar', 'cheek', 'zygomaticomaxillary', 'zygomaticomaxillary orbital', 'tripod' and 'tetrapod' are all terms used to describe essentially the same injury – a fracture of the zygomaticomaxillary orbital complex (Figure 7.10.1). Apart from isolated zygomatic arch fractures, nearly all other fractures involve part of the orbital floor and lateral orbital wall. Therefore, assessments of the orbit (and eye) are an integral part of management.

APPLIED ANATOMY

The cheek is predominantly formed by the zygomatic bone. This fuses with the frontal bone at the frontozygomatic (FZ) suture under the eyebrow, with the maxilla medially and with the temporal bone posteriorly and within the orbit. The body of the zygoma provides the aesthetic prominence of the cheek and together with the supraorbital ridge affords some protection to the eye. Superiorly, the body of the zygoma forms approximately the lateral two-thirds of the infraorbital rim, which is important for lower eyelid support. Consequently, any displacement in this area can affect eyelid function. Vertical displacement of the entire zygoma can lower the lateral canthus and lateral attachment of the globe with it (Whitnall's tubercle). This can result in diplopia, hypoglobus and an anti-mongoloid slant to the eye (Figure 7.10.2).

The facial skeleton is not a solid structure, but contains several 'cavities', notably the sinuses, orbits and nasal cavity. Around these, the bones condense to form a series of vertical struts known as 'buttresses'. The zygoma forms part of the lateral buttress. Horizontal buttresses also exist, but are much thinner. Consequently, the facial skeleton is very good at resisting vertically directed forces (biting/chewing), but is relatively weak at resisting horizontal forces (i.e. during most injuries). It has been suggested that sinuses have evolved to produce this survival advantage. Much like the chassis of a car, the face crumples, absorbing much of the kinetic energy during impact. The buttresses are a key element to facial repair and the support of any screws.

The temporalis muscle passes beneath the zygomatic arch to insert into the coronoid process of the mandible. Displaced fractures of the zygomatic arch can therefore impede mouth opening by interfering with this. The muscle is invested in the

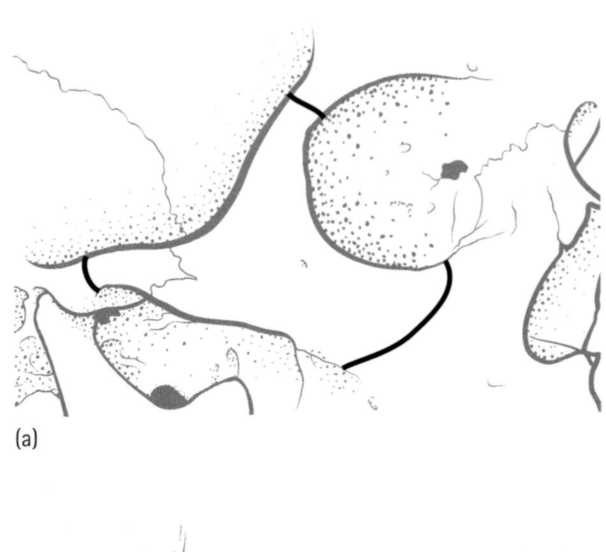

(a)

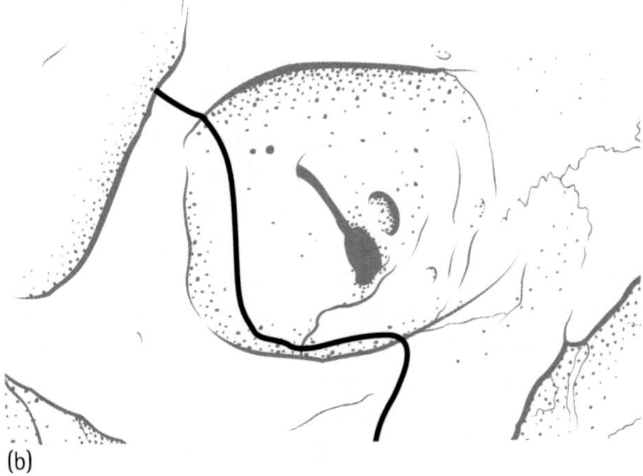

(b)

7.10.1 Fracture configuration.

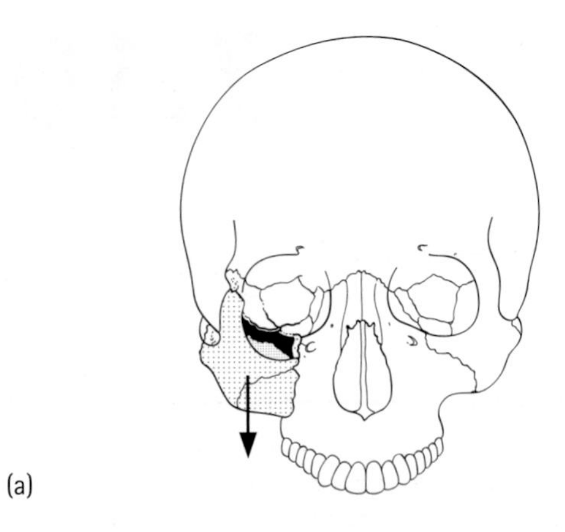

(a)

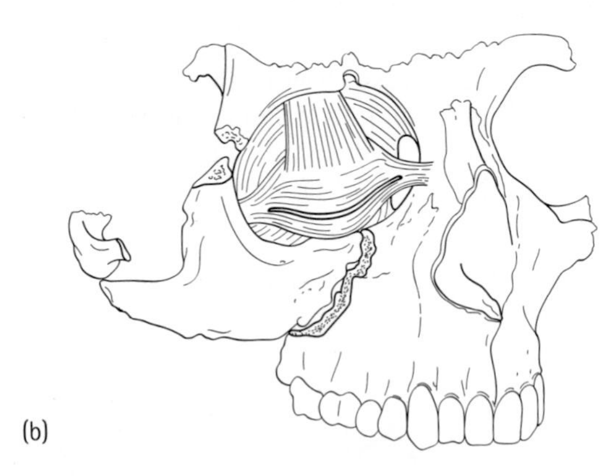

(b)

7.10.2 Downward displacement results in vertical ocular dystopia and an anti-mongoloid slant.

temporal fascia, which arises from the skull and passes down to insert into the zygomatic arch. This is an important surgical landmark (Gillies approach). The masseter muscle passes up from the mandible and attaches to the body of the zygoma and its arch. This may have a role in post-operative displacement of fractures which have not been internally (or externally) fixed. It is argued that fractures should be treated by open reduction and internal fixation (ORIF), as displacement may be caused by masseteric pull over the ensuing weeks. Just because the bone is accurately reduced immediately after surgery, it does not mean that it will stay there.

The zygoma and maxilla support many of the periorbital and perinasal muscles attached to the periosteum. In extensive repairs, degloving of much of these bones may be required. Resuspension of the soft tissues is important during wound closure to prevent sagging post-operatively. The infraorbital nerve supplies sensation to the majority of the cheek and the ipsilateral half of the nose and upper lip. This passes along the floor of the orbit and exits the infraorbital foramen approximately 1 cm below the infraorbital rim, approximately midway along its length. The infraorbital canal and foramen form a plane of weakness and fractures often pass nearby. The nerve is at risk during repair.

ASSESSMENT

A number of classifications exist. A practical one would be to consider fractures, as follows:

- isolated:
  - zygomatic arch
  - infraorbital rim
- minimally displaced;
- displaced fractured;
- comminuted fractured;
- associated with midface or complex orbital fractures.

With the exception of isolated arch fractures, all zygomatic fractures extend into the orbit. Following assessment of the head and neck (remember the ABCs (airways, breathing, circulation)), the eye therefore takes priority over any fractures. Check for ocular injury, diplopia and signs of entrapment. Clinical features of a fracture may include:

- pain;
- periorbital bruising and swelling;
- limitation of eye movements with diplopia;
- altered sensation of cheek/upper lip;
- restricted jaw movements;
- subconjunctival haemorrhage and chemosis;
- surgical emphysema;
- flattening of the malar prominence (often masked by swelling immediately after injury);
- palpable infraorbital step;
- anti-mongoloid slant;
- unilateral epistaxis (due to bleeding into the maxillary sinus);
- enophthalmos;
- exophthalmos;
- hypoglobus (vertical ocular dystopia);
- dysocclusion (premature contact on ipsilateral molar teeth, due to flexing of the upper dental arch).

RADIOGRAPHS AND OTHER USEFUL INVESTIGATIONS

Investigations include the following:

- Visual acuity.
- Force duction test under local anaesthetic (should detect entrapment of orbital soft tissues).
- Comprehensive orthoptic assessment (not just a Hess chart).
- Plain radiographs – occipitomental (OM), lateral face and submental vertex (SMV). Look carefully – sometimes the only clue is a fluid level in the antrum.
- Computed tomography (CT) scan, both axial and coronal. These are increasingly used in patient evaluation.

Indications include high energy injuries (is the orbital apex involved?), suspected orbital floor involvement, comminuted or severely displaced fractures, other midface fractures suspected, assessment of the arch.

- Ultrasound has been reported as useful for detecting fractures, but is not commonly used.
- Maxillary sinus endoscopy for orbital floor fractures (not commonly used).

FIRST AID MEASURES

These fractures do not require urgent intervention and can be assessed as an outpatient. In the interim, patients should be advised not to blow their nose, in order to avoid surgical emphysema. The concern here is not the air, but the associated contamination (mucus, etc.), which can pass into the orbit and soft tissues of the cheek through the fracture. This can result in orbital cellulitis, both a sight- and life-threatening condition if untreated. Patients may also be advised not to fly, although there is no good evidence base for how long in the literature; the author's advice is for 3 weeks. Some units may prescribe prophylactic antibiotics.

INDICATIONS FOR REDUCTION AND TIMING OF SURGERY

When there is clinical and radiological evidence of a displaced zygomatic fracture, indications include the following:

- facial deformity;
- loss of lower eyelid support;
- ocular dystopia;
- limitation of mandibular opening;
- sensory nerve deficit thought to be due to nerve compression.

Timing of treatment depends on the degree of swelling and the general condition of the patient (notably any head or ocular injuries). Surgery does not need to be carried out on an emergency basis, although on occasion it can be undertaken 'immediately' (i.e. within a few days). However, significant swelling may interfere with accurate clinical assessment, both as an indication for treatment (do not just look at the x-ray), and an on-table assessment (is this adequately reduced?). It also makes aesthetic incision placement particularly difficult. Furthermore, swelling may be exacerbated by surgical manipulation, so care should be taken if there is any proptosis. Surgery is therefore often carried out either immediately or about 5–10 days following injury. In the author's experience, acceptable results can still be obtained up to 5 weeks after injury, but all the fractures need to be openly reduced, callus ostotomized and accurate reduction becomes much more difficult. This may be necessary only in exceptional circumstances.

REDUCTION AND REPAIR

This depends on the fracture configuration and the degree of displacement. In determining treatment, consider the following:

- How displaced is the fracture? Accept if minimal, to avoid risks of surgery (especially in medically compromised and those on asprin/anticoagulants).
- Does the lateral buttress look comminuted on imaging? If so, some sort of fixation may be required to prevent collapse of the cheek. Do not use percutaneous hooks blindly – they may comminute this more.
- Is the zygomatic arch 'greensticked' or telescoped? The arch is important for cheek projection and may need to be reduced and aligned fully to maintain this. If telescoped, access to it for fixation may be required.
- Is the infraorbital rim comminuted? If so, it may need repair.
- Does the orbital floor also need exploration and/or repair (see Chapter 7.8)?
- Is the frontozygomatic suture 'greensticked' or displaced? If displaced, this may need open reduction and repair.

If none of the above apply, a closed reduction may suffice. Case selection is very important both pre-operatively and 'on the table', to identify those patients which are unlikely to relapse post-operatively due to lack of any fixation. Closed reduction techniques include the following:

- temporal approach (Gillies) (Figure 7.10.3);
- percutaneous or 'malar' hook (sometimes referred to as 'Poswillo') (Figure 7.10.4);
- eyebrow approach – zygomatic elevator;
- Carroll–Girard screw (now more of historical importance);
- intraoral approaches (upper buccal sulcus) (Figure 7.10.5, p. 534).

All of these involve making an incision somewhere on the patient and could therefore technically be argued as open techniques.

More recently, there has been a general move towards open reduction and internal fixation (ORIF), that is to place at least one plate (usually either a 'buttress' plate or one across the frontozygomatic suture). This is based on the concerns regarding masseteric and other forces acting on an unsupported reduction over the ensuing weeks. A buttress plate can be placed transorally and a frontozygomatic plate via a small upper blepharoplasty incision (Figure 7.10.6, p. 535). In both cases, scarring is virtually invisible. However, this is still a matter of personal preference for each surgeon and closed techniques still have an important role to play in management. Exposure to the infraorbital rim should be avoided if at all possible. These scars may be more noticeable, contraction can distort the lower eyelid, there is a risk of injury to the infraorbital nerve and the fixation is the weakest of all the fracture sites. It may be necessary,

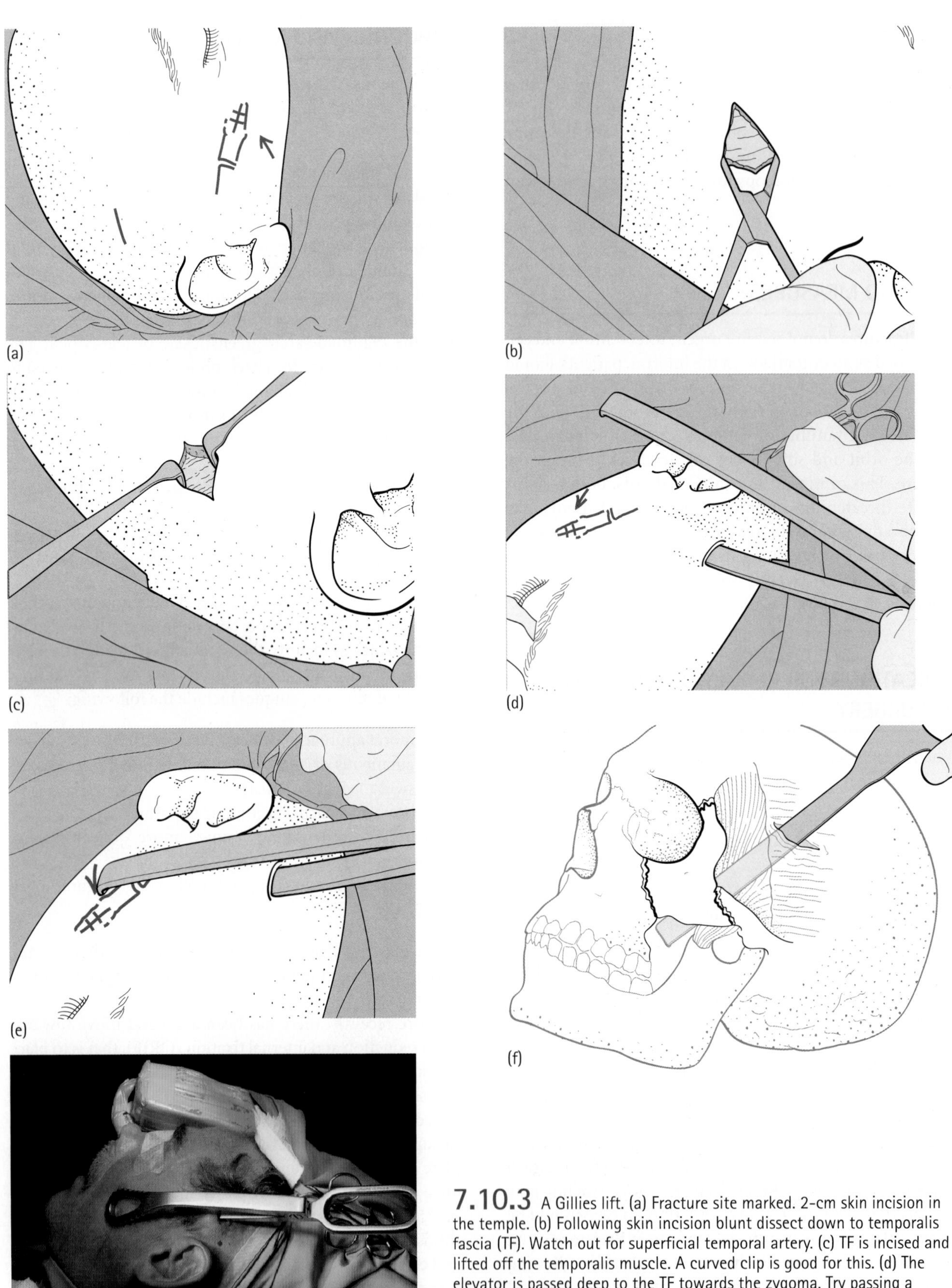

7.10.3 A Gillies lift. (a) Fracture site marked. 2-cm skin incision in the temple. (b) Following skin incision blunt dissect down to temporalis fascia (TF). Watch out for superficial temporal artery. (c) TF is incised and lifted off the temporalis muscle. A curved clip is good for this. (d) The elevator is passed deep to the TF towards the zygoma. Try passing a Howarth's periosteal elevator before – it helps open up the correct plane. (e) Make sure the elevator is under the bone before lifting (do not use the skull as a fulcrum). Schematic/operative view immediately prior to lift. (f) Surgical anatomy of lift.

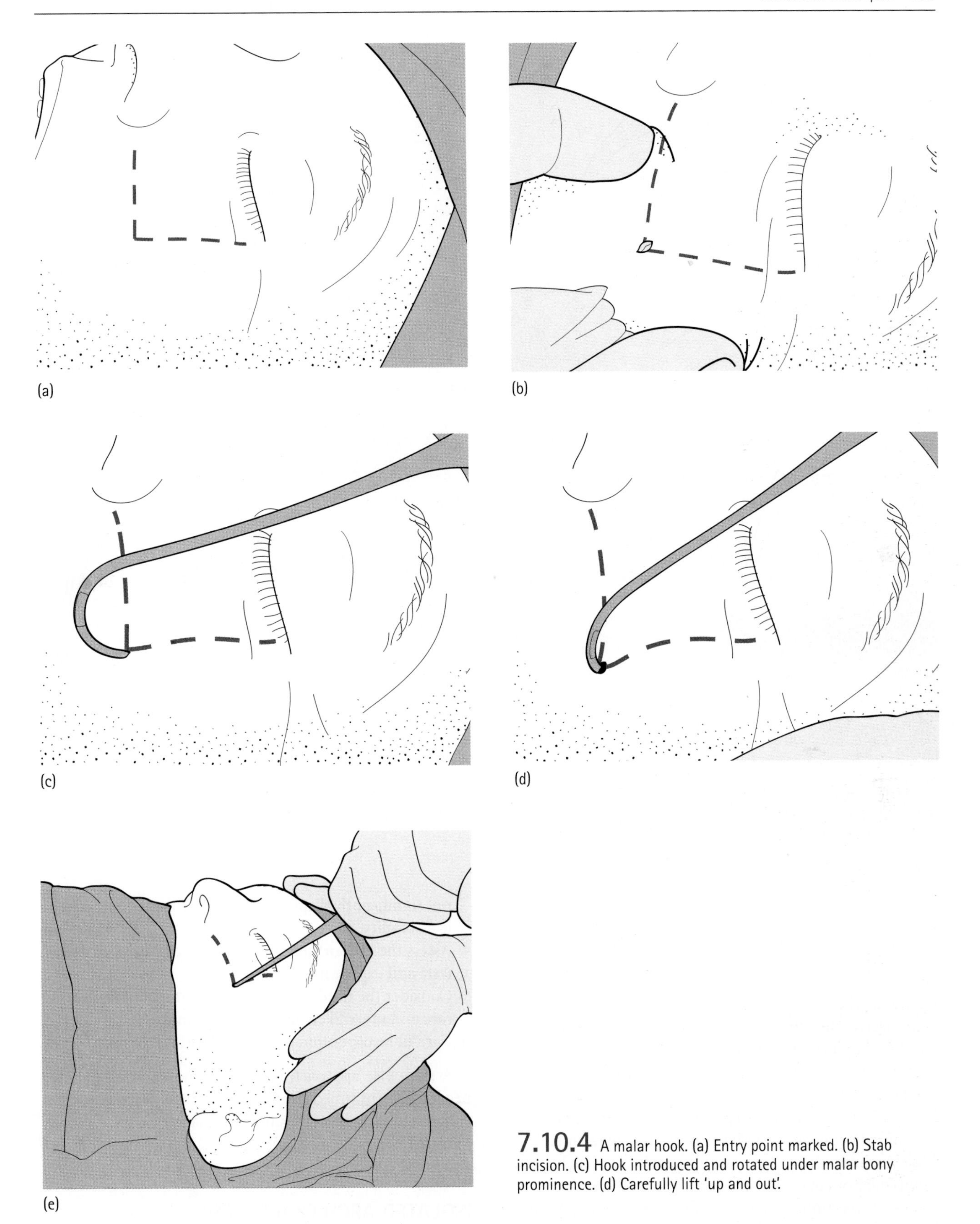

7.10.4 A malar hook. (a) Entry point marked. (b) Stab incision. (c) Hook introduced and rotated under malar bony prominence. (d) Carefully lift 'up and out'.

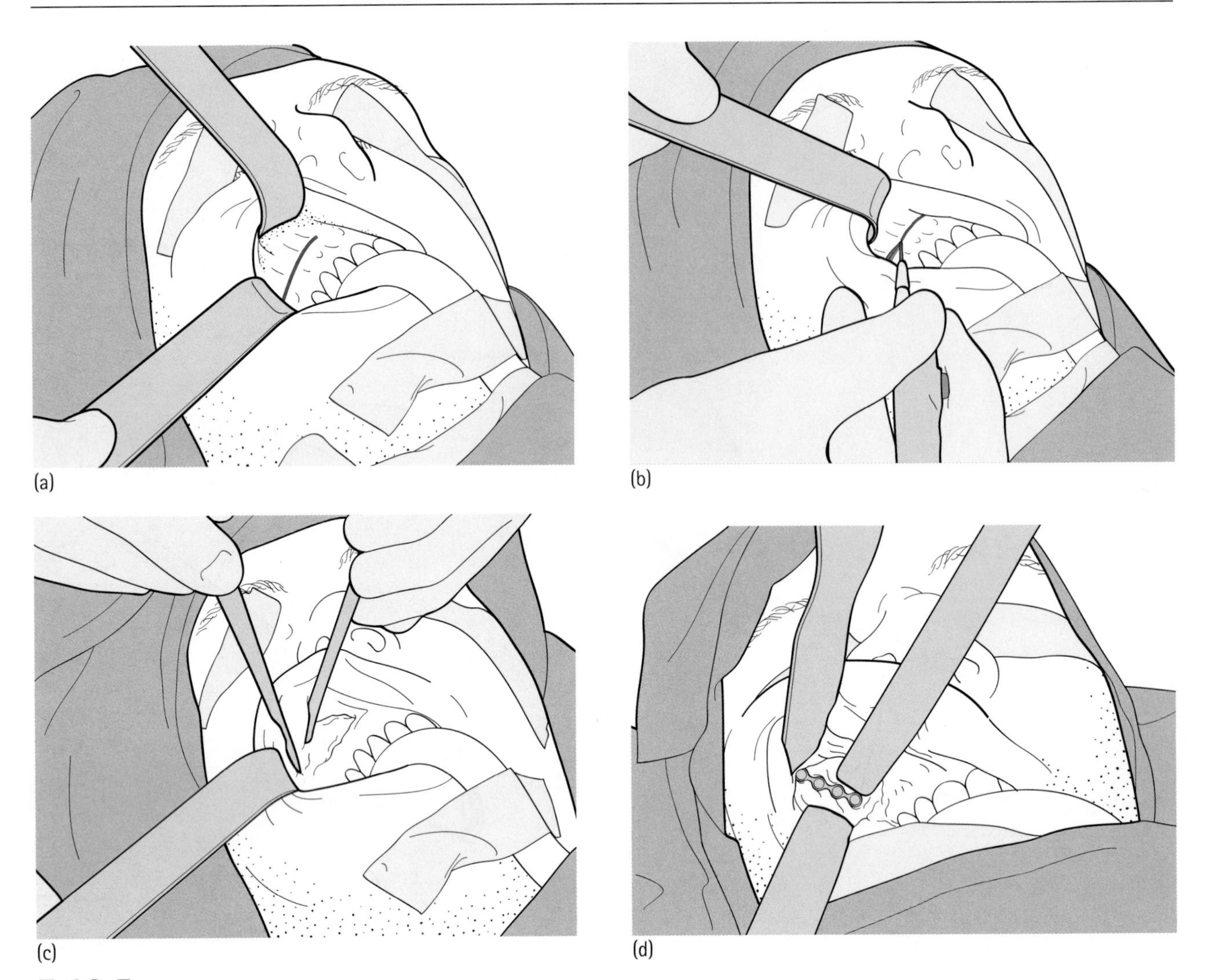

7.10.5 A buttress plate. (a) Mucosa marked allowing cuff to close. (b) Incision with knife or cutting diathermy (care with metal retractors). (c) Subperiosteal dissection to expose fractures. (d) Following fracture reduction (Gillies, hook or via incision) ORIF with four-hole plate (usually).

however, to access the orbit and/or repair multiple rim fragments.

Sequencing is a matter of choice. This author's approach is generally to:

1. Address the FZ suture first, if it is significantly displaced. The purpose of the fixation is to re-establish the vertical height of the fracture, and hopefully the correct height of the lateral canthal/Whitnall's attachments.
2. If necessary, reduce and repair the arch. This is only required occasionally and in significantly telescoped arches, but it does necessitate a posterior approach (pre-auricular or cutaneous incision). The arch is key to cheek projection. Careful assessment is necessary, even if not telescoped it may be bowed laterally and needs at least digital reduction.
3. Reduce and repair the lateral buttress. This is undertaken via an intraoral approach. In many cases, this may be the only procedure required, if (1) and (2) are not significantly displaced. This plate provides mechanical stability.
4. Assess the infraorbital rim/orbital floor (force duction test) and expose if necessary.
5. Consider the need for bone grafting the buttress. This is rare and more likely in high energy injuries.
6. Careful resuspension of the cheek prior to closure.

A step-wise approach is therefore needed and patients need to give informed consent appropriately. In many cases, either a closed approach or 'buttress' plate will suffice, usually the latter.

ISOLATED ARCH FRACTURES

These can often be reduced via a Gillies approach or transorally. They are usually stable, but occasionally can fall back down. If so, they may need support. Alternatives include the following:

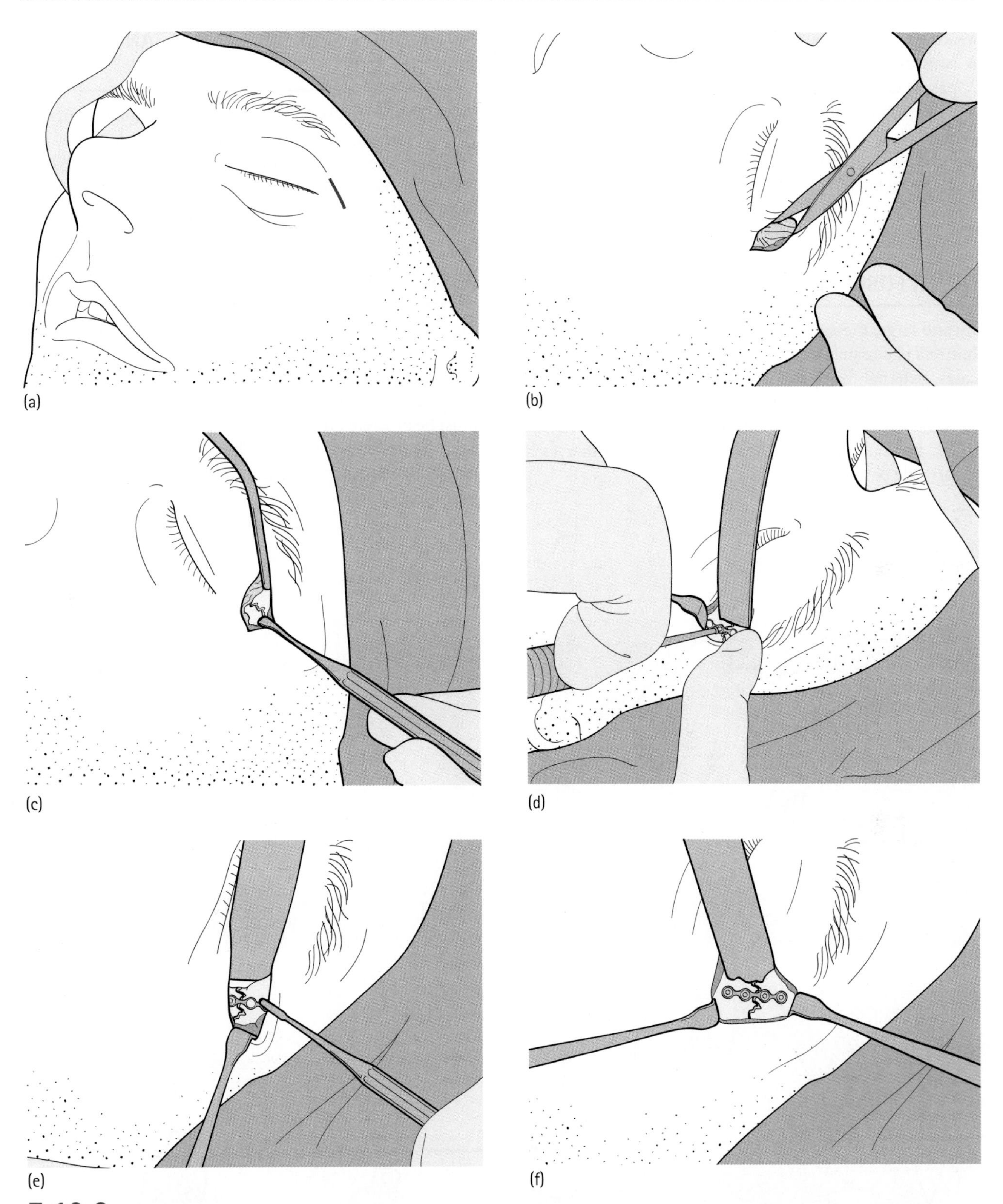

7.10.6 An FZ plate, via upper blepharoplasty incision. (a) Site of incision marked in upper eyelid. (b) Following skin incision, dissect down to perisoteum. (c) Incise periosteum and elevate to expose fracture. (d) Some fractures are easily elevated and plated. If very displaced, screw plate to lower half of fracture first. (e) Use a small hooked instrument or wire to lift and reduce the fracture by applying force through an unused upper hole (do not damage the plate). Drill and screw the other hole. (f) Place second screw. If correctly reduced this will accurately restore the vertical height.

- accept this and deal with any problems secondarily;
- suturing an external splint along the arch (suture is passed deep to the arch and tied over the splint);
- balloon inflation deep to the arch (a foley catheter will suffice);
- ORIF via a pre-auricular, or overlying incision (beware the facial nerve).

OTHER FORM OF FIXATION

By and large, these are rare, since reduction and a simple buttress plate can be undertaken relatively quickly in many cases. External fixation (Figure 7.10.7), like the mandible, may have a small role to play. Alternatively the zygoma can be 'kebabed' using a trans-antral K-wire. This is certainly quick, but is a blind procedure with risks to both eyes if incorrectly performed.

ANTIBIOTICS, STEROIDS AND TETANUS PROPHYLAXIS

Protocols may vary between different units. Antibiotics may be given to prevent sinusitis. Penicillin (or a cephalosporin) and metronidazole is one option, but many exist. Some surgeons prescribe steroids (dexamethasone/methylprednisolone) to reduce post-operative orbital swelling.

POST-OPERATIVE CARE

The main concerns here are to ensure that the fracture stays in the correct position, and serious complications such as loss of sight and severe infections do not develop. As patients wake up, they may be initially agitated and the repaired site must be protected from inadvertent injury. Various ways of achieving this are possible, but having the site clearly marked and an alert recovery/ward nurse go a long way to

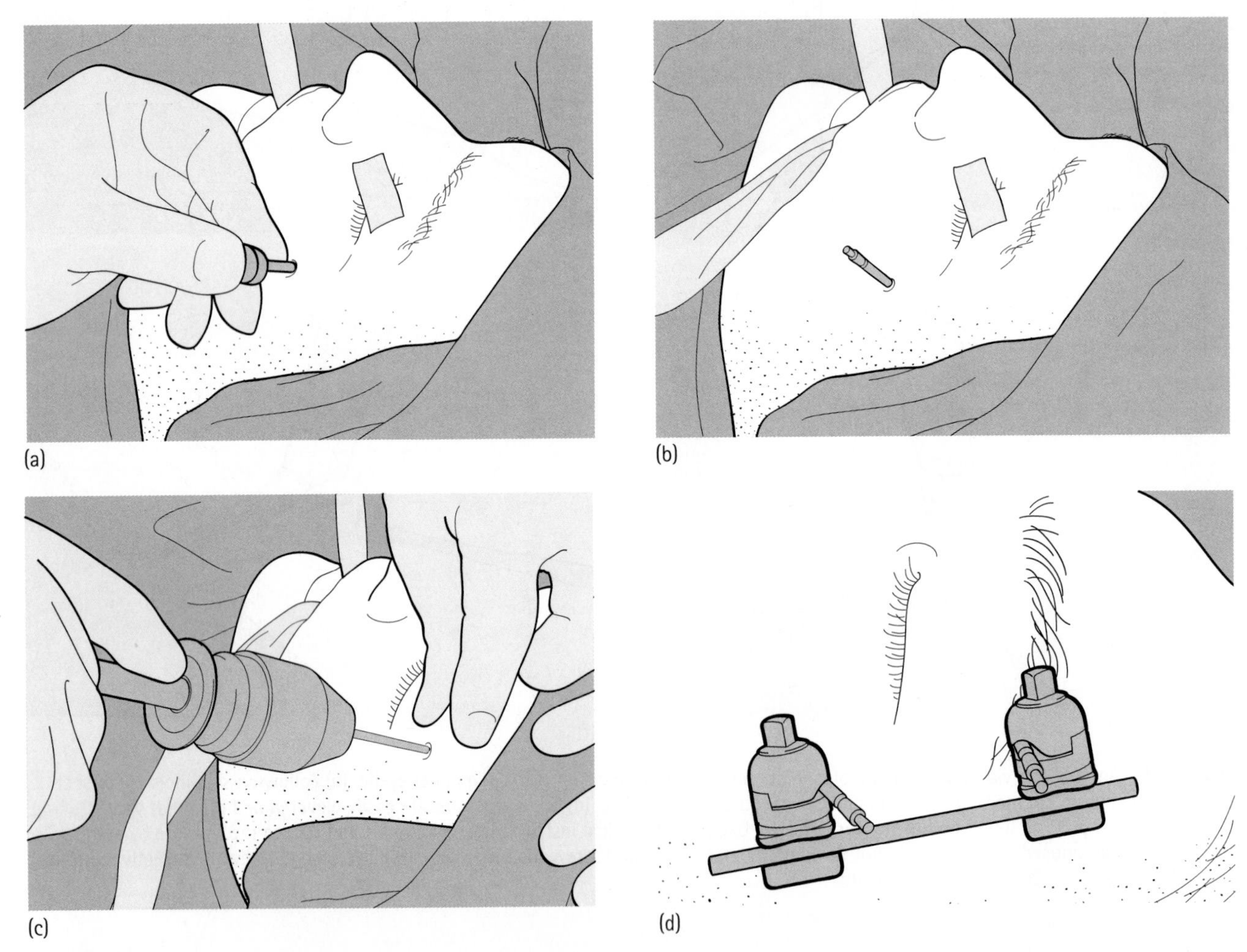

7.10.7 External fixation (see Chapter 7.5 for sequence). (a) Stab incision and trochar over cheek. (b) Following drilling, pin screwed into bone. (c) Procedure repeated for frontal pin. (d) Final assembly. Leave some space between joints and skin for hygiene and swelling.

achieving this. Swelling and bleeding behind the globe can occur, which unrecognized can result in loss of vision. Careful observation of the eye is therefore important, at least until the patient is awake. Various regimes exist. Antibiotics and steroids may be continued for a variable time and patients should be advised not to blow their nose.

RETROBULBAR HAEMORRHAGE/ORBITAL COMPARTMENT SYNDROME

Proptosis following injury or repair needs to be evaluated quickly and carefully (see Chapter 7.8, p. 501). The concern here is loss of sight following retinal/optic ischaemia. For this reason, the eye is put under careful observation, usually until the next day, although they can probably be stopped when the patient is fully awake. Progressive pain, deteriorating vision, proptosis and ophthalmoplegia are the main signs to check. Traditionally, acute proptosis is considered to be a retrobulbar haemorrhage (RBH), although in the author's experience (and as published) RBH is rarely the cause. Once the orbit/zygoma has been reduced, the orbit becomes a closed space and swelling is contained, resulting in an orbital compartment syndrome (OCS). For this reason, steroids are variably prescribed post-operatively. The key to urgency of treatment is the visual acuity, if the vision is normal, decompression is not required. Rarely do such cases need to be returned to theatre, but if they do it should be remembered that an OCS may not release blood, in which case if the proptosis is that severe, decompression will be required. Intravenous acetazolamide, mannitol, steroids and a lateral canthotomy buy time while theatre preparations are being made. If in doubt, globe tension should be measured by a 'tonopen' or other suitable device.

Top tips

- If the eyelids are swollen, gently pressing on them (not the globe) for a few minutes reduces this sufficiently to assess visual acuity.
- Numbness of the cheek and upper lip is an important sign that should generate a high index of suspicion for orbital or cheek bone fracture.
- Remember the nasolacrimal duct during infraorbital/eyelid access.
- Isolated arch or simple fractures which are incomplete at the frontozygomatic suture are those most suitable for closed reduction.
- Arch fractures with associated coronoid fractures are at risk of ankylosis.
- Correct alignment of the sphenozygomatic suture (lateral orbital wall) is a good on-table indication that the fracture is correctly reduced.
- A force duction test should be performed at the end of any reduction. As the fractures realign, orbital soft tissues may become trapped.
- Beware late enophthalmos – follow up patients closely.
- Place sticky tape over the repaired site. Do not draw on the patient – they may try and rub it off!
- Not all vision-threatening proptoses are due to retrobulbar haemorrhage.

PART 8

TEMPOROMANDIBULAR JOINT

8.1

Temporomandibular joint arthroscopy

JOSEPH MCCAIN, KING KIM

INTRODUCTION

Arthroscopy of the human temporomandibular joint (TMJ) was first introduced by Ohnishi in 1975. The current diagnostic and operative techniques are presented in this chapter. Meticulous attention to detail is required to successfully perform the procedure. Any alteration or compromise of the step by step surgical sequence will alter the ability to complete the planned procedure and will compromise the outcome. Operations are performed in the superior joint space, unless disc perforations exist which allows entry into the inferior joint space.

PATHOLOGY

The TMJ is a synovial joint subject to similar pathology as with other synovial joints. A basic difference, however, exists in that fibrocartilage rather than hyaline cartilage lines the articular surface. Osteoarthritis is the end point of the natural history of the disease. This may develop primarily or as a result of the traumatically dislocated interposing articular disc. Important structural anatomy of the TMJ can be seen in Figure 8.1.1.

The displaced disc causes pain and mechanical locking of the mandible. Synovial adhesions often accompany the herniation of the disc into the anterior recess. Central perforations of the disc occur in primary osteoarthritis. Perforation of the posterior ligament occurs in chronic dislocated discs secondary to micro- or macrotrauma. A conservative surgical cascade is advocated to manage the disease process. Evidence-based research has shown that restoration of normal anatomy or removal of the diseased perforated disc is not always needed to obtain a return to relatively pain-free function.

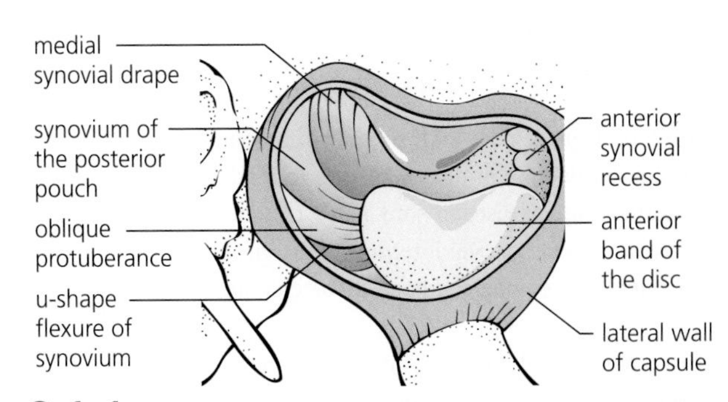

8.1.1 Anatomy of the temporomandibular joint as it relates to arthroscopy.

INDICATIONS

Although there are exceptions, patients who undergo initial consultation for TMJ internal derangement should undergo conservative nonsurgical therapy prior to any type of surgical intervention. This essentially includes teaching the patient about limiting eccentric jaw movements, eliminating any pathologic habits, having the patient undergo Boering therapy which educates the patient as to the nature of their problem, and instructing them to take a softer diet and to habitually perform nonclenching techniques. In addition, these patients should begin a regimen of oral anti-inflammatory medications to decrease any acutely inflamed process, and wearing a soft orthotic device to either eliminate a bruxing habit or to soften the load placed on the temporomandibular joints during bruxism. The chronic bruxer can also benefit from an oral muscle relaxant to minimize the load. The exceptions to this will include, of course, those patients who present for initial consultation who have already undergone orthotic therapy with little or no positive results.

After two to four months of conservative therapy, the patient is re-evaluated for their condition. Sometimes the problem will be resolved with these measures and no additional treatment is warranted. However, there are many who are refractory to this conservative approach and who desperately wish for a resolution to their problem. This is where a discussion with the patient about minimally invasive TMJ surgery is indicated.

The patient is made aware that arthroscopic TMJ surgery may not alleviate the patient's symptoms and that open joint surgery is a potential approach for the future. Additionally, the patient is made aware of the possibility of seventh nerve deficits secondary to extraoral punctures, malocclusion following surgery, possible scar formation from the punctures, as well as the possibility for pain, bleeding, swelling and post-operative infection.

The next step is making a decision on the type of arthroscopic procedure the patient will receive. This obviously must be ascertained based on the diagnosis made. For example, a patient with a clicking joint, intermittent pain and 35-mm maximum interincisal opening (MIO), with a Wilkes' stage II may benefit from a lysis of adhesions with lavage of the superior joint space to relieve the symptomsc (see Table 8.1.1). However, a patient who is in extreme pain with an anteriorly dislocated disc, which is nonreducing on magnetic resonance imaging (MRI), an MIO of 20 mm, with a preliminary Wilkes' stage IV, may benefit from a surgical arthroscopy procedure consisting of anteriorly releasing the disc with posterior repositioning, and fixating the disc to the condylar head arthroscopically.

PERIOPERATIVE CONSIDERATIONS

When the patient is ready for surgery, it is important to wrap the patient's head prior to entering the operating room to keep hair out of the operative field. When the head is wrapped securely, it allows the procedure to be clean and less cumbersome. In addition, the possibility of infection is minimized.

The procedures for TMJ arthroscopoy are best performed under general anaesthesia via nasal intubation. It is crucial that the assistant is able to manipulate the mandible and close the jaw into occlusion without the endotracheal tube getting in the way. If, however, the surgeon and patient elect to undertake a procedure, such as arthroscopic arthrocentesis, in an office setting under local anaesthesia and light sedation, the patient must be able to follow commands of moving the jaw open and closed and into excursions during the procedure. A diagram of patient positioning in the operating room setting can be seen in Figure 8.1.2 and the arthroscopic set up can be seen in Figure 8.1.3.

Perioperative medication considerations are crucial to attaining good results with TMJ arthroscopy. The use of prophylactic antibiotics to prevent post-operative infection is controversial. The orthopaedic literature surrounding arthroscopy is scant with good prospective studies, since the incidence for infection following arthroscopic procedures is so low. The American Academy of Orthopedic Surgeons has not elicited an advisory statement regarding the issue. However, literature does exist essentially stating that antibiotic prophylaxis for arthroscopic procedures is not indicated for healthy patients. It is the opinion of these authors that antibiotic usage is indicated for those prone to infec-

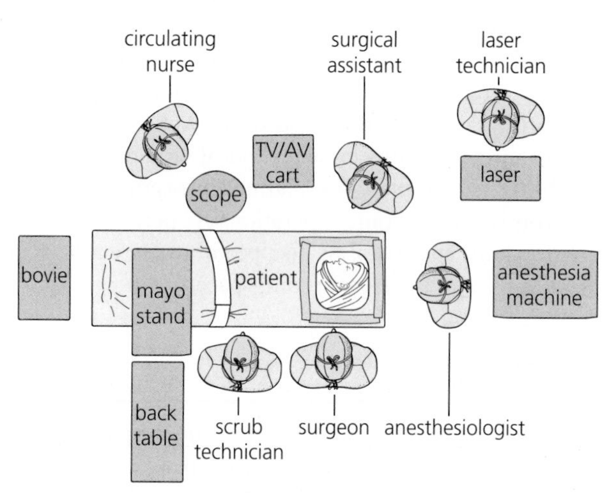

8.1.2 Patient positioning in the operating room.

Table 8.1.1 Clinical and radiologic criteria for Wilkes' staging of temporomandibular joint internal derangement.

Stage	Clinical findings	Radiological findings
I	No significant mechanical symptoms, no pain or limitation of motion	Slight forward displacement and good anatomic contour of disc
II	First few episodes of pain, occasional joint tenderness and related temporal headaches, increase in intensity of clicking, joint sounds later in opening movement, beginning transient subluxations or joint locking	Slight forward displacement and beginning anatomic deformity of disc, slight thickening of posterior edge of disc
III	Multiple episodes of pain, joint tenderness, temporal headaches, locking, closed locks, restriction of motion, difficulty (pain) with function	Anterior displacement with significant anatomic deformity/prolapse of disc, moderate to marked thickening of posterior edge of disc, no hard-tissue changes
IV	Characterized by chronicity with variable and episodic pain, headaches, variable restriction of motion and undulating course	Increase in severity over intermediate stage, early to moderate degenerative remodelling hard-tissue changes
V	Crepitus on examination, scraping, grating, grinding symptoms, variable and episodic pain, chronic restriction of motion, difficulty with function	Gross anatomic deformity of disc and hard tissue, essentially degenerative arthritic changes, osteophytic deformity, subcortical cystic formation

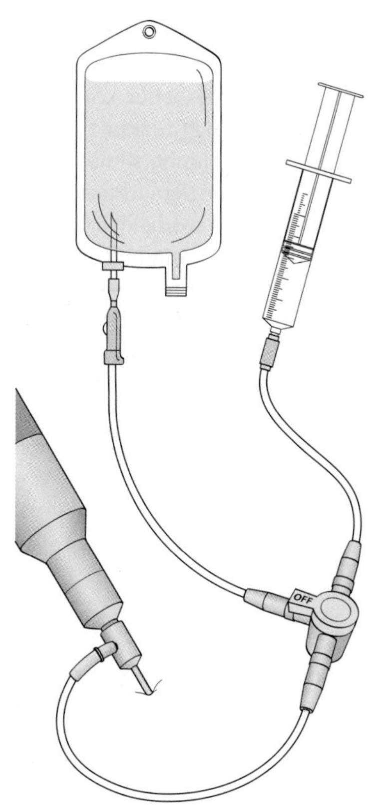

8.1.3 Temporomandibular joint arthroscopic set up.

tion. These include patients with diabetes, compromised immunity or skin disorders. When antibiotics are indicated, 1-g cefazolin i.v. 1 hour before the procedure provides good coverage to prophylactically manage these patients. Intravenous administration of corticosteroids prior to the procedure is an important consideration to prevent post-operative oedema. Many times after TMJ arthroscopic procedures, it is vital to initiate mandibular motion and opening to prevent arthrofibrosis, haemarthrosis and train the muscles of mastication to stretch. Oedema interferes with this ability to achieve the goal of improved mandibular functioning. Because of this, it is advisable to administer post-operative dosing regimens of corticosteroids in a tapered fashion.

As discussed earlier, the importance of instructing the patient to move the mandible post-operatively cannot be overemphasized. Patients are given these directions for jaw hinge exercises the day of or the day following surgery. These exercises are classified as stages I and II. Stage I exercises consist of taking the tongue, rolling it as far back on the palate as possible and opening as wide as possible without disengaging the tongue. The second of these exercises is to move the jaw in lateral and protrusive excursions as far as possible. Both sets of exercises are to be performed for 20 repetitions, four times a day. Stage II exercises involve the prybar, painting of teeth and rubber tubing. The prybar involves placing the thumb on the upper incisors, the middle finger on the lower incisors and gently prying open as far as possible. Painting of the teeth involves taking the tip of the tongue and starting at the buccal surface of the most posterior molar, painting all of the teeth from right to left and back again. Lastly, a piece of rubber tubing is placed between the canines on one side and moving into lateral excursions, while lightly biting on the rubber tubing. Each of these exercises is performed for 20 repetitions, four times per day.

Most patients are instructed to follow stage II exercise, but stage I exercises are indicated for patients under certain circumstances. For example, patients who undergo semi-rigid discopexy repair with the suture technique to treat anterior disc dislocation could very easily relapse back into the anterior position if translation is initiated too early. The same is true for those patients who receive posterior retrodiscal scarification procedures to treat slightly dislocated discs. Also, in those patients treated for condylar subluxation who undergo posterior retrodiscal release need to undergo opening exercises in reverse after surgery. This is to say that they need to prevent translating their condyles to allow the disc to settle into the correct position. In all three of these instances, the patient is only gradually worked into full function due to the instability of the disc position and potential for relapse.

SURGICAL CASCADE

Regardless of the pathology, the recommended surgical cascade is as follows:

1 arthroscopic arthrocentesis;
2 lysis and lavage with debridement;
3 discopexy;
4 contracture for mandibular dislocation.

A diagrammatic view of the relevant TMJ anatomy as it relates to puncture can be seen in Figures 8.1.4 and 8.1.5.

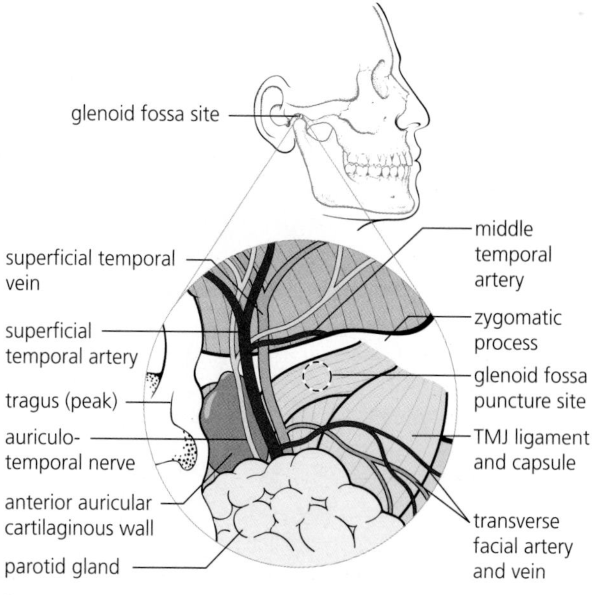

8.1.4 Anatomy relevant to single puncture technique.

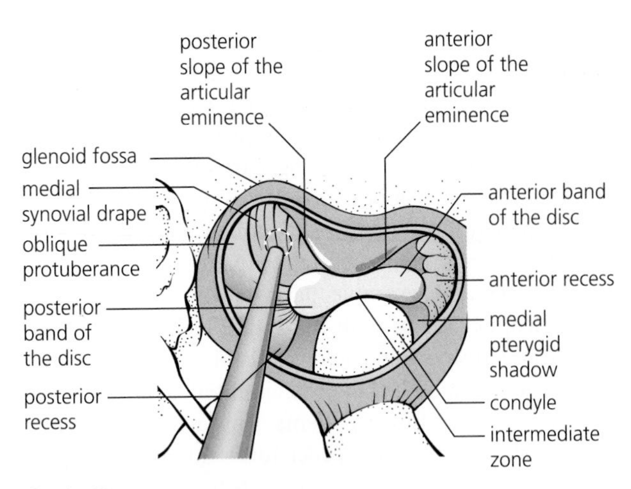

8.1.5 Anatomy and puncture location.

Arthroscopic arthrocentesis

This procedure essentially involves the single puncture technique, which can be seen in Figure 8.1.6.

The thumb is used to palpate the maximum concavity of the glenoid fossa at the junction between the periosteum and synovial capsule. The bony landmark is the maximum concavity of the inferior aspect of the zygomatic and temporal bones. To facilitate precision of the technique, this puncture should be performed with a sharp trocar. Throughout the puncture into the superior joint space, the trocar and cannula are advanced deeper into tissues utilizing a twisting and rotational motion to prevent injury to the facial nerve and to provide better control of the sharp instrument. After puncturing the skin, the trocar is used to scrape off soft tissue attachments subperiosteally at the maximum concavity of the glenoid fossa. The trocar and cannula are then redirected medially to enter the superior joint space. A depth of 20–25 mm indicates a safe puncture – any more and the risk of perforating through the medial synovial drape increases. It is important that the scope enters the joint as close to superolateral as possible for best visualization. Once inside the joint, the lavage of the joint ensues, and an irrigating needle is placed for outflow. The 22-gauge irrigating needle can be inserted 5 mm anterior and 5 mm inferior to the first puncture. It is important to insufflate with 2–3 cc of fluid prior to placing the irrigating needle to prevent collapse of the joint space (Figures 8.1.7–8.1.9).

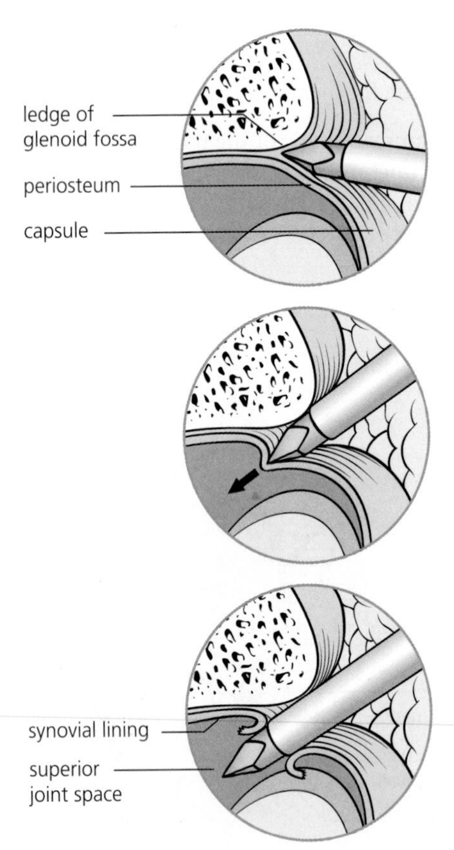

8.1.6 Single puncture technique.

Lysis and lavage with debridement

This procedure involves the double puncture technique. The fossa portal is created as described by the single puncture technique. Once the arthrosopic cannula with arthroscope

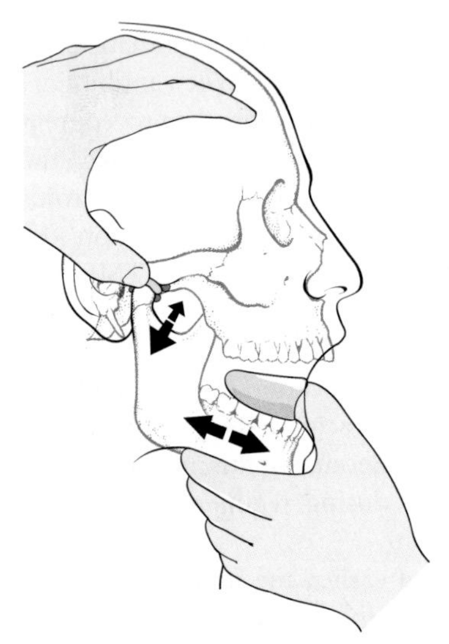

8.1.7 Operator and assistant collaborating to locate correct puncture location.

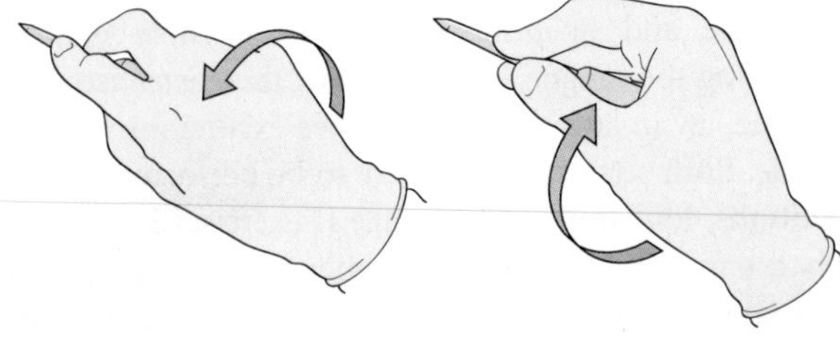

8.1.8 Rotational hand movement for puncturing superior joint space.

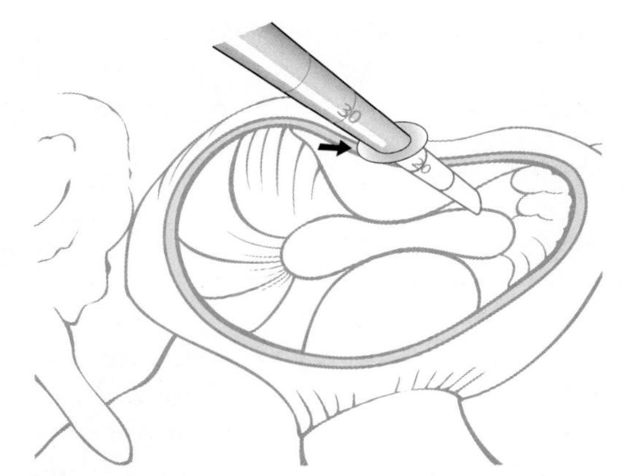

8.1.9 Diagrammatic representation of depth of puncture.

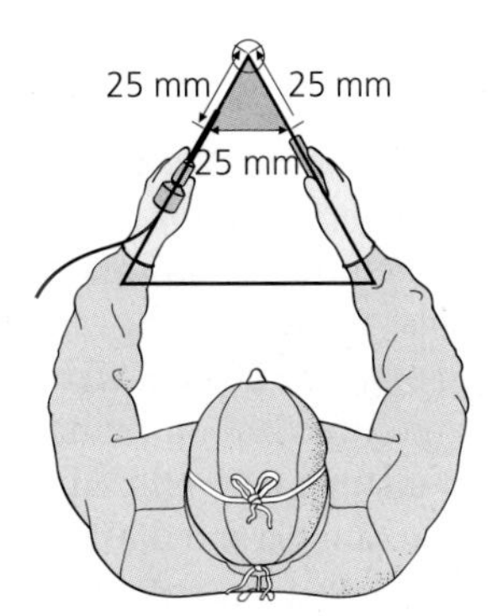

8.1.11 Triangulation concept.

is inserted, the articular eminence portal is then created by triangulation. To perform this technique, the most superior, anterior and lateral aspect of the articular eminence is targeted (Figures 8.1.10–8.1.14). The lavage needle is removed, and a 2/0 trocar and cannula is introduced into the superior joint space. The second cannula inserted is known as the working cannula. The working cannula is used to accommodate instrumentation, such as holmium lasers, shavers, graspers, straight probes, hook probes, as well as certain medicaments if they are needed. The size of the working cannula can be increased as needed.

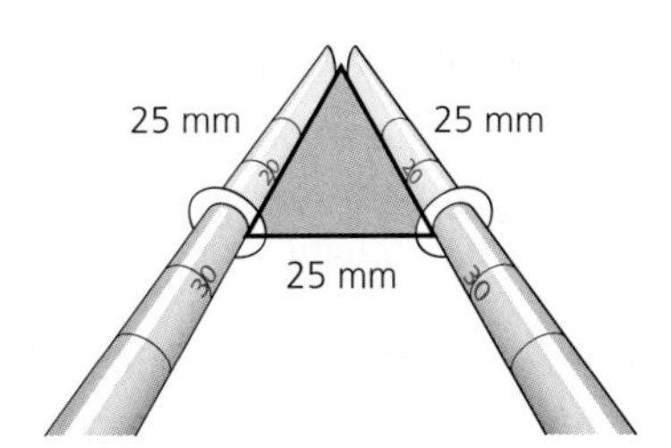

8.1.12 Triangulaton concept magnified.

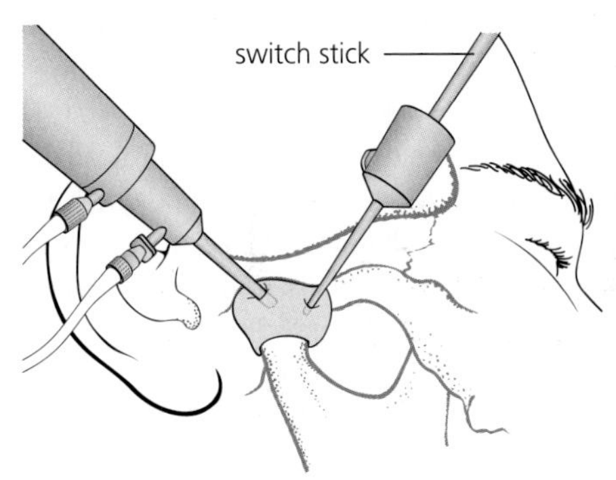

8.1.13 Triangulation on patient.

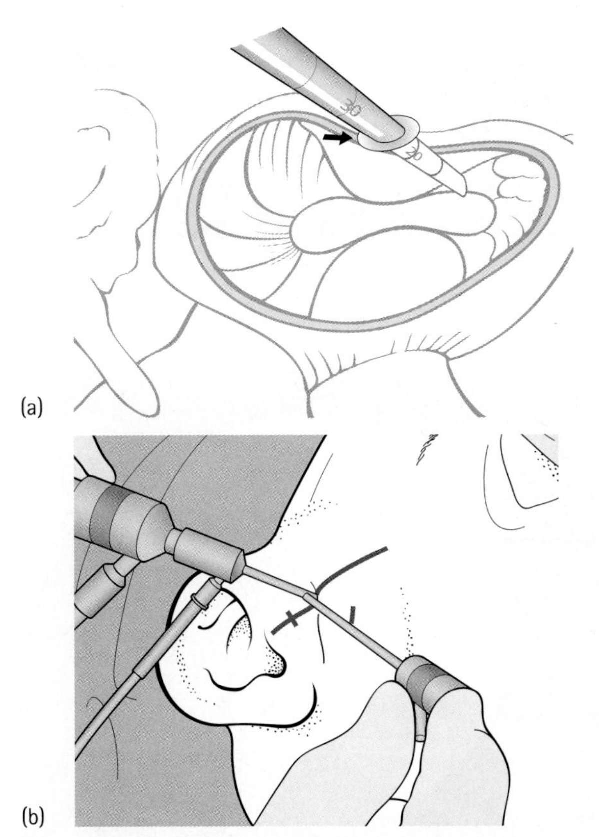

8.1.10 (a) Measuring second puncture point; (b) measuring the second puncture point.

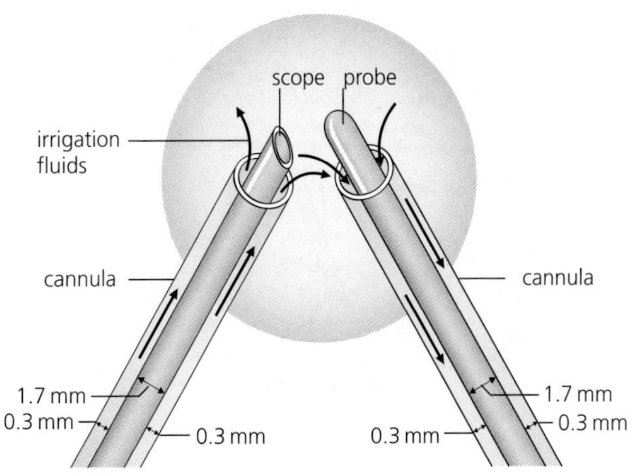

8.1.14 Instrumentation through both cannulas.

Discopexy

This procedure, which is the most complex, involves three or four punctures into the superior joint space. For rigid discopexy, three punctures are utilized. In addition to the arthroscopic cannula and the working cannula as previously described, the third puncture involves creation of the fixation portal for insertion of the fixation cannula. For semi-rigid discopexy, four punctures are utilized: the arthroscopic cannula, the working cannula and the fixation portal, which accommodates two needles: one anterior and one posterior.

For either rigid or semi-rigid discopexy, an anterior release must be performed prior to fixation. The anterior release is best performed through the working cannula with a holmium laser. The disc–synovial crease is delineated and scored with a hook probe, and the laser is used to cut along the scored area, making sure to detach the superior head of the lateral pterygoid from the discal tissues. After adequate release is performed, the straight probe is utilized to reduce the disc posteriorly, while the mandible is in the forward position. The retrodiscal tissues at this time can be ablated with bipolar cautery or the holmium laser, as needed, as a means to scar the tissues and keep the disc reduced.

For the rigid discopexy procedure, the fixation portal is created while a straight probe in the working cannula reduces the disc posteriorly. The trocar and cannula targets the posterior lateral disc attachment. A 22-gauge needle is used to sound the area predicted for puncture. While the mandible is in the forward position, the fixation portal is created 20 mm inferior to the fossa portal.

Rigid fixation of the disc to the condylar head can now be performed through the fixation cannula which is approximately 3.0–3.5 mm in diameter. Fixation is performed with either resorbable screws or nails, and can be performed with one, two or three points depending on the amount of access that is available. Post-operative rehabilitation consists of immediate functioning with stage II exercises, as disc position is secure. The correct position of the three cannulas can be seen in Figure 8.1.15, while the technique is demonstrated in Figures 8.1.16–8.1.18.

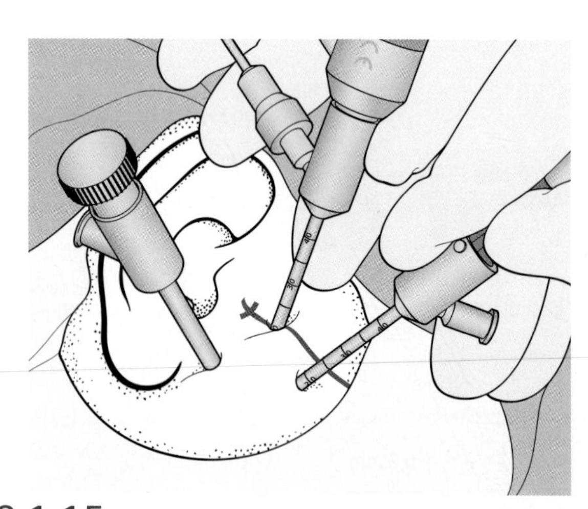

8.1.15 View of arthroscopic, working and fixation cannulas.

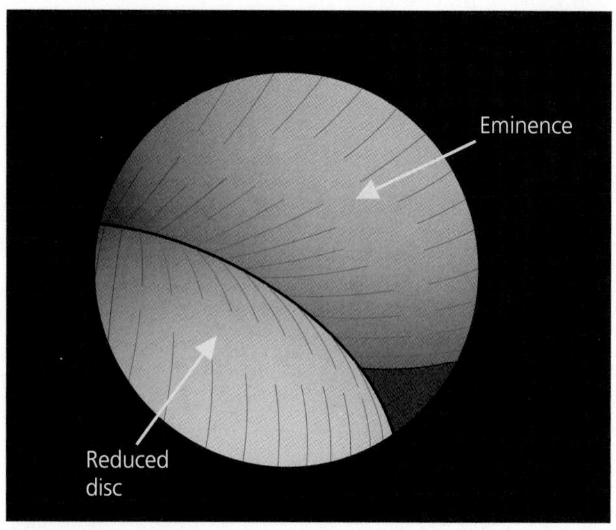

8.1.16 Arthroscopic view of disc in reduction.

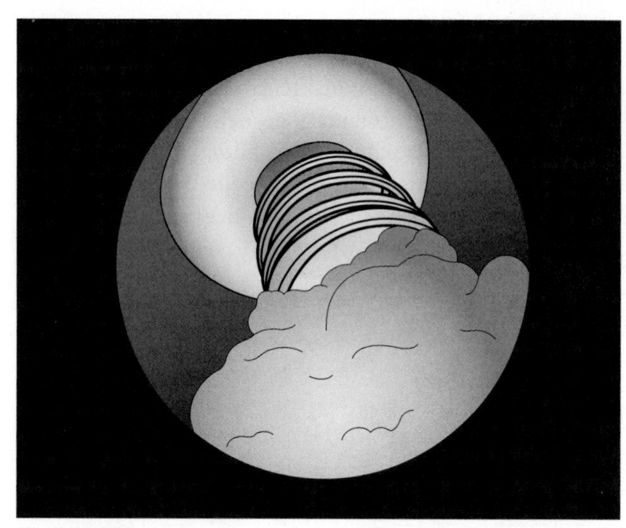

8.1.17 Arthroscopic view of rigid fixation technique.

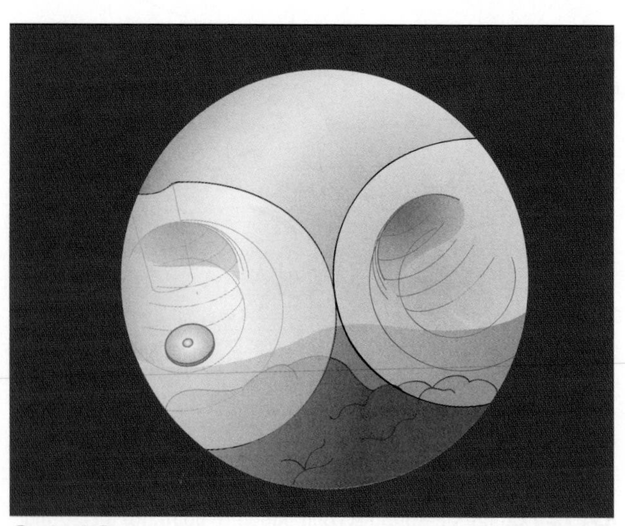

8.1.18 Arthroscopic view of resorbable screw fixation in place.

For semi-rigid fixation, or suture discopexy, the fixation portal is created the same way as in the rigid fixation technique. The anterior release can be seen sequentially in Figure 8.1.19a–c. Through the fixation cannula, a vector is aimed at the posterolateral attachment. A straight meniscus mender is then punctured under the reduction cannula to the condylar head, then superiorly through the posterior lateral portion of the disc. A second meniscus mender is then punctured through the skin and is used to catch the suture (Figure 8.1.20). A 0/PDS suture is then passed anteriorly and a snare is used to catch it posteriorly (Figure 8.1.21). The location of the suture when it is pulled through the skin is parallel and inferior to the apex of the tragal cartilage. A small skin incision is made after the suture is passed through, and a surgeon's knot is tied to the capsule and disc (Figures 8.1.22–8.1.25). Post-operative rehabilitation for these patients is slow and initially requires only a limited amount of jaw mobility, gradually increasing to stage II exercises and beyond.

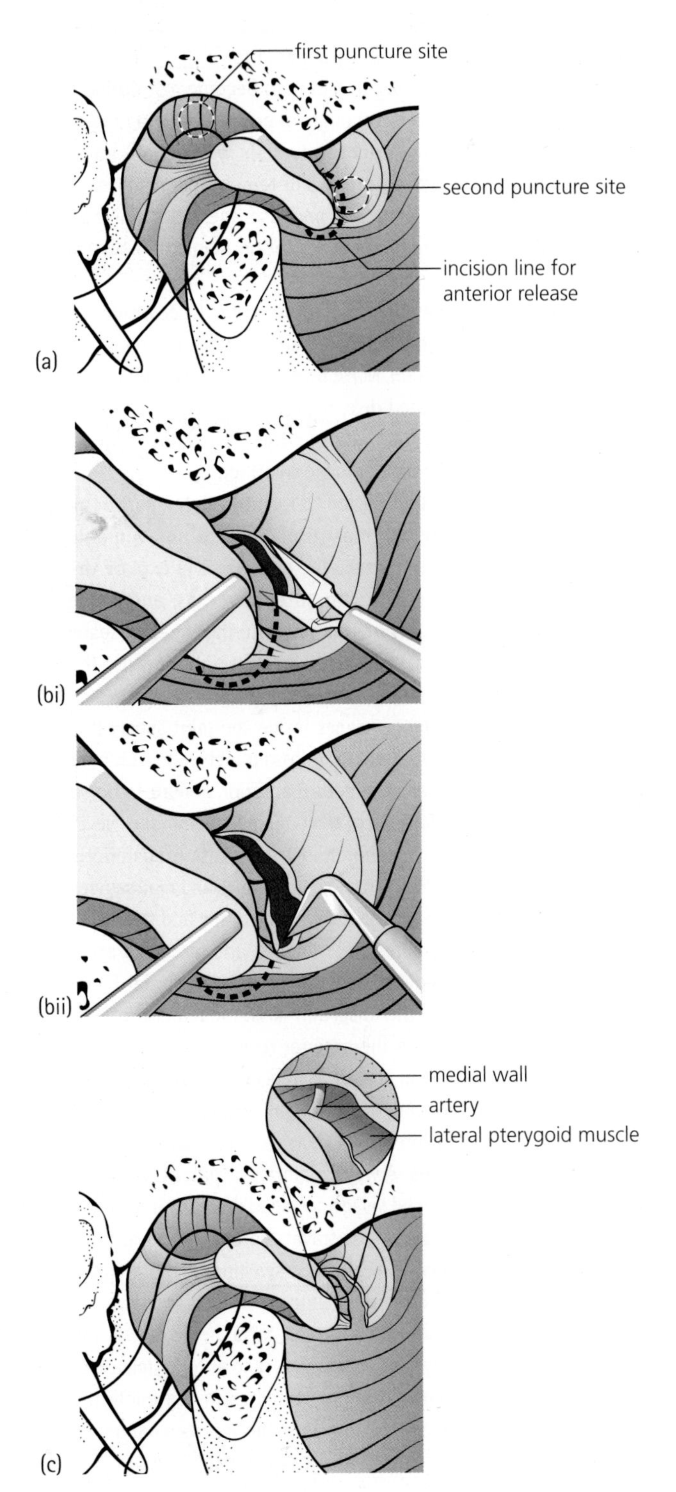

8.1.19 (a) Outlined location of anterior release; (b) performing anterior release; (c) anterior release completed with associate anatomical structures.

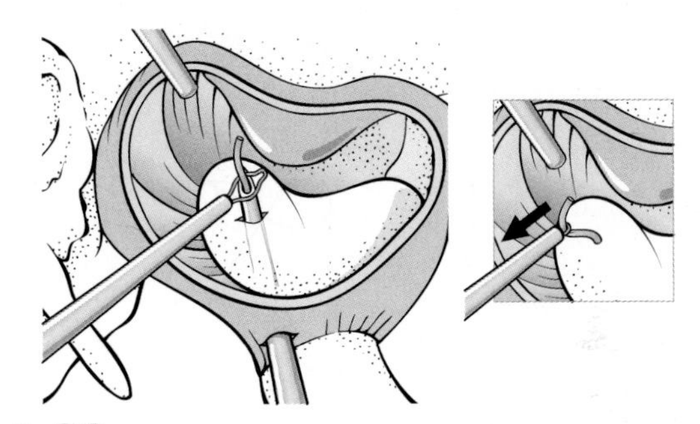

8.1.20 Suture discopexy.

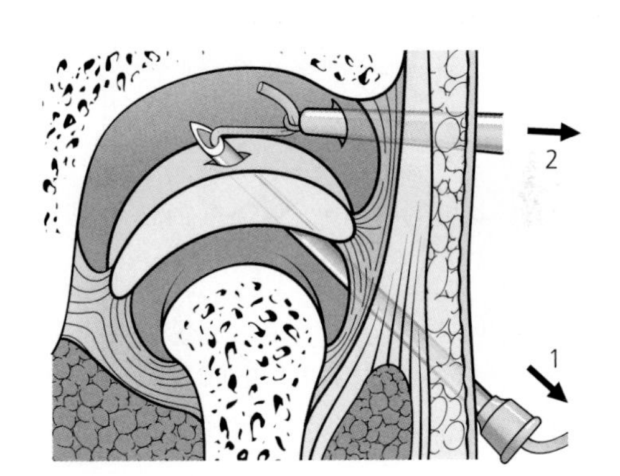

8.1.21 Suture discopexy.

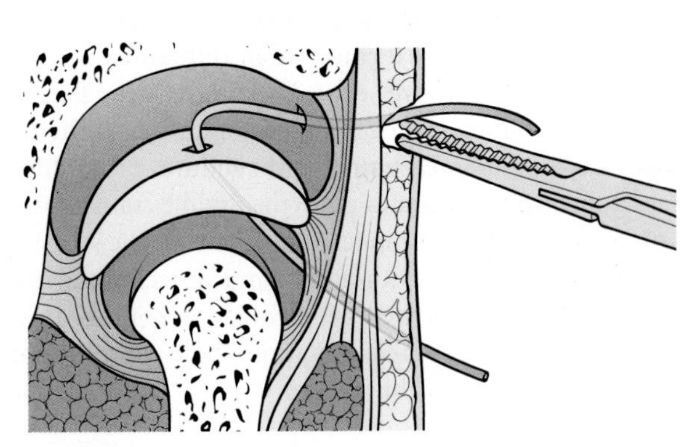

8.1.22 Suture discopexy.

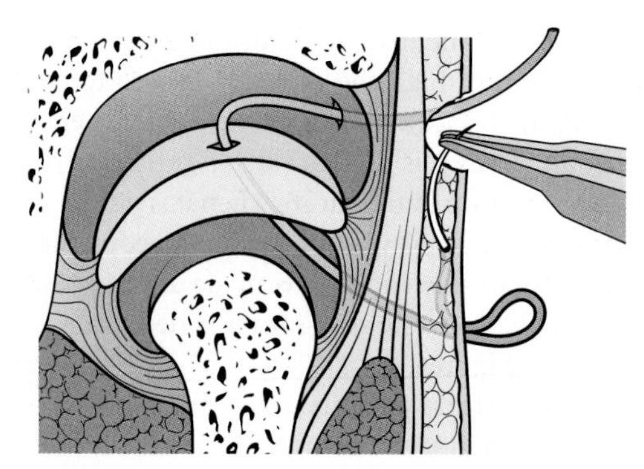

8.1.23 Suture discopexy.

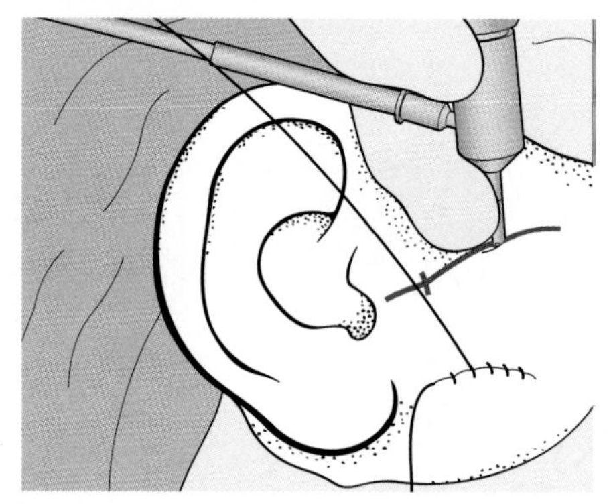

8.1.24 Suture discopexy.

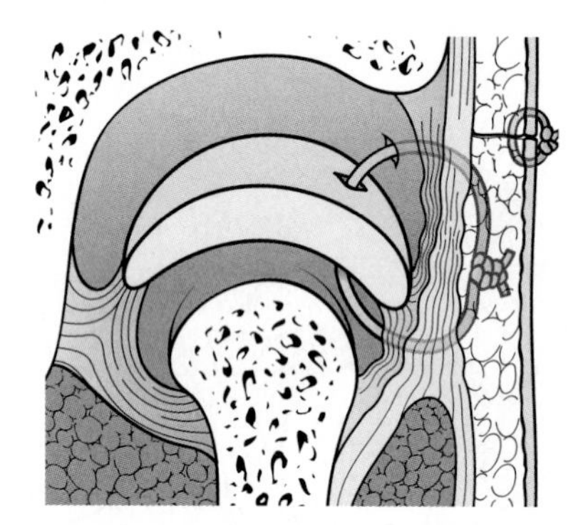

8.1.25 Suture discopexy.

COMPLICATIONS

Overall, TMJ arthroscopy is a safe procedure. It is minimally invasive and can be performed in an outpatient setting. Complications do, however, exist. These include facial nerve trauma, arthrofibrosis, infection, perforation into the ear canal or tympanic membrane, and subdural or epidural haematoma from perforation into the middle cranial fossa. Management of these complications is outside the scope of this chapter, however, with good surgical technique and attention to detail, as well as adequate and procedure-selective post-operative rehabilitation, these complication rates can be reduced to almost zero.

Top tips

- Patient positioning is paramount. If you start behind, you will become flustered for the entire procedure. Make sure the patient's head is turned and flat on the table, which will facilitate an easier puncture. Each step of arthroscopy is dependent on the successful completion of the previous one. It is impossible to perform advanced procedures if this principle is not strictly adhered to.
- Always use landmarks. It is easy to become lost during a puncture. If you feel as though no progress is being made, then back away, orient yourself with the known landmarks (zygomatic process of temporal bone, glenoid fossa and condylar head) and use these to make an accurate puncture. Use the vectoring measuring system for all multiple punctures.
- Make sure you gather all the information. Once inside the joint, a thorough diagnostic arthroscopy is crucial to treating the condition. Make note of everything that comes into view (perforated disc, hyperemic retrodiscal tissues, amount of dislocation, etc.) and use this knowledge to come up with the best possible treatment.
- Do not rush. The temptation to rush through a part or all of this procedure will most likely lead to unfavourable results. Make sure you take the extra time to explore the entire posterior pouch, the anterior recess, and if the second or third punctures are not entering the joint space in a timely fashion, be patient and do it right. It is not the job of the practitioner to make the patient worse.
- Be aware of all danger zones inside the joint space. It is important to keep the depth of fossa puncture to 25 mm or less and the vector of puncture anterior. Failure to do so may result in perforation of the tympanic membrane. Never move the operative cannula instrumentation posteriorly unless under direct arthroscopic control. Blind manoeuvres risk perforation of the medial synovial drape and the risk of injury to the tympanic membrane and or perforation through the glenoid fossa into the middle cranial fossa. Always visualize the insertion and movement of the operative cannula in the anterior recess arthroscopically. Blind manoeuvres may lead to a laceration of the middle meningeal artery and/or the lingual nerve.
- Make sure you prevent extravasation. Avoid careless multiple punctures. Always maintain a patent irrigation system. Lack of a good lavage needle to drain the insufflated joint space will result in extravasation of irrigating fluid, which can be seen clinically as a swelling of the affected side of the face. Extravasation into extracapsular tissues can lead to trismus, pain, malocclusion, facial nerve paresis and increased recovery time. In addition, if an anterior release of the disc is performed, the fluid could extravasate into the pterygoid space and further into the lateral pharyngeal space, leading to a very difficult airway situation.

FURTHER READING

Bert J, Giannini D, Nace L. Antibiotic prophylaxis for arthroscopy of the knee: Is it necessary? *Arthroscopy* 2007; **23**: 4–6.

Kurzweil PR. Antibiotic prophylaxis for arthroscopic surgery. *Arthroscopy* 2006; **22**: 452–4.

Ohnishi M. Arthroscopy of the temporomandibular joint. *Journal of the Stomatological Society of Japan* 1975; **42**: 207.

Smolka W, Iizuka T. Arthroscopic lysis and lavage in different stages of internal derangement of the temporomandibular joint: Correlation of preoperative staging to arthroscopic findings and treatment outcome. *Journal of Oral and Maxillofacial Surgery* 2005; **63**: 471–8.

Wilkes CH. Internal derangements of the temporomandibular joint: Pathological variations. *Archives of Otolaryngology – Head and Neck Surgery* 1989; **115**: 469–77.

8.2

Surgery to the temporomandibular joint

GEORGE DIMITROULIS

INTRODUCTION

Arthrotomy refers to the direct surgical exposure of a joint. A temporomandibular joint (TMJ) arthrotomy is technically one of the more difficult surgical dissections in the maxillofacial region. While the close proximity of the facial nerve is the main reason for the difficult surgical access, other important anatomical structures, such as the terminal branches of the external carotid artery and accompanying rich plexus of veins also add to the complexity of the dissection. With the middle cranial fossa above, and the middle ear behind the TMJ, there is little room for surgical error, as both these cavities are only a few millimetres away from the joint itself.

INDICATIONS FOR TMJ ARTHROTOMY

Surgery to the TMJ is undertaken for a wide range of joint disorders. Indications for surgical intervention are divided into relative and absolute.

Absolute indications

TMJ surgery has a definite and undisputed role in the management of uncommon joint disorders such as:

- dislocation, i.e. recurrent or chronic;
- ankylosis, e.g. fibro-osseous joint fusion;
- neoplasia, e.g. osteochondroma of the condyle;
- developmental disorders, e.g. condylar hyperplasia.

Relative indications

Unfortunately, the role of TMJ surgery in the management of common disorders, such as traumatic injuries, internal derangement and osteoarthrosis, is less clear and often ill defined. These may further be divided into the following.

GENERAL INDICATIONS

TMJ surgery for common conditions should only be considered under the following conditions:

- Where the joint disorder remains refractory to nonsurgical therapy, for example, occlusal splints, medication and physiotherapy.
- Where the TMJ is the source of the pain and dysfunction, hence pain is localized to the TMJ:
  - pain on functional loading of the TMJ;
  - pain on movement of the TMJ;
  - mechanical interferences within the TMJ.

Note: The more localized the symptoms are to the TMJ, the more likely surgery will have a favourable outcome.

SPECIFIC INDICATIONS

Clinical features which are refractory to nonsurgical treatment and TMJ arthrocentesis or arthroscopy, i.e.

- chronic severe limited mouth opening resulting from joint pathology;
- gross mechanical interferences, such as painful clicks;
- advanced degenerative joint disease with intolerable symptoms of pain and joint dysfunction;
- confirmation of severe joint disease on magnetic resonance imaging (MRI).

PRE-OPERATIVE PREPARATION

Anaesthesia

TMJ arthrotomy is performed under general anaesthesia using a nasoendotracheal tube to permit manipulation of the mandible that will help identify the position of the articular disc and mandibular condyle during the surgery.

Position of the patient

The head is turned to the opposite side of the surgery so that the ear is 60° to the perpendicular. The head is rested on a head ring covered by a waterproof drape to help stabilize it.

Preparation of the surgical site

The hair is shaved in front of the ear to the level of the superior tip of the pinna. Three inch (9–10 cm) wide waterproof tape ('sleke tape') is placed horizontally above the ear and another length of tape is placed vertically behind the ear to cover the hair (Figure 8.2.1). A marking pen is used to outline the proposed incision line. The surgical site, including the adjacent ear and ear canal, is liberally prepped with antiseptic solution. A sterile ear pledget with vaseline is inserted to protect the ear canal. A turban head drape is wrapped around the head which covers the anaesthetic tube exiting the nose (Figure 8.2.2). Marcaine (0.5 per cent) with 1:200 000 epinephrine is infiltrated into the subcutaneous tissues along the incision line and into the joint proper.

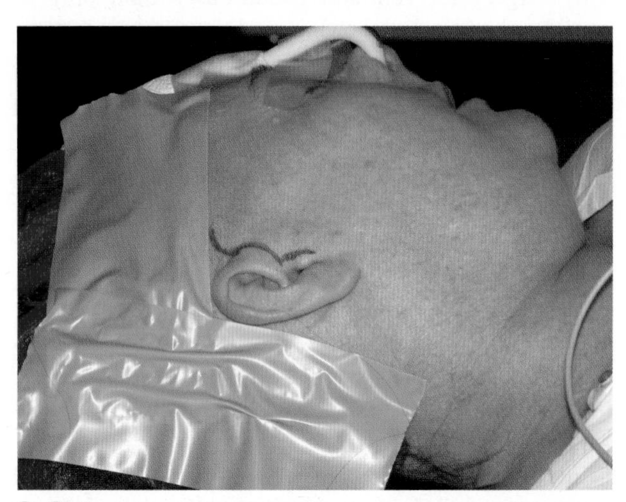

8.2.1 Sleek tape used to keep hair away from surgical site.

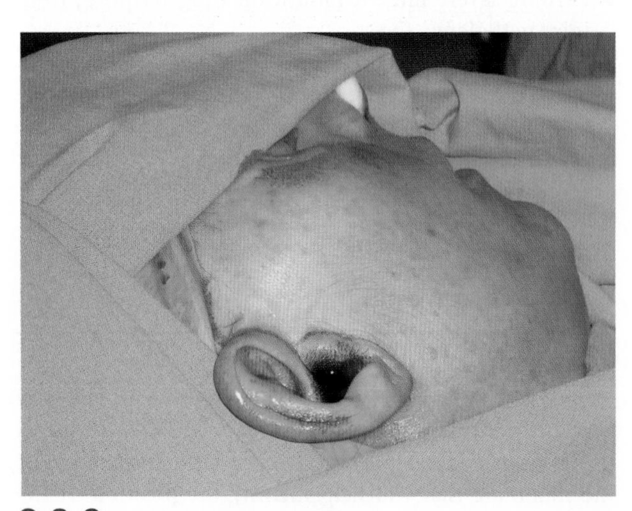

8.2.2 Draping of surgical site.

OPERATION

While there have been numerous surgical approaches to the TMJ described in the literature, the preauricular incision with a small temporal extension is the most common surgical approach. It allows direct surgical access to the joint and provides excellent access for most TMJ surgical procedures.

Incision

A 5–6-cm curvilinear preauricular incision, peaked posteriorly at the level of the tragus (Figures 8.2.3 and 8.2.4), is made through the skin and subcutaneous tissues to the level of the temporalis fascia. The preauricular incision runs around the insertion of the pinna, extending down to the lower border of the insertion of the ear lobe to the preauricular skin. Superiorly, a small temporal extension of the incision is made in a forward arc about 45° relative to the zygomatic arch and also deepened to the temporalis fascia.

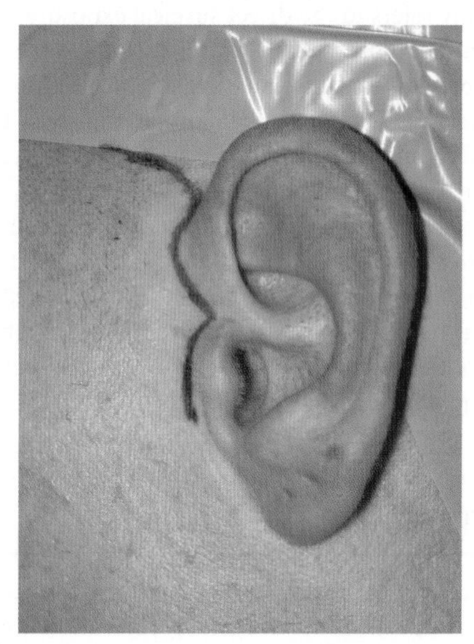

8.2.3 Preauricular incision with temporal extension.

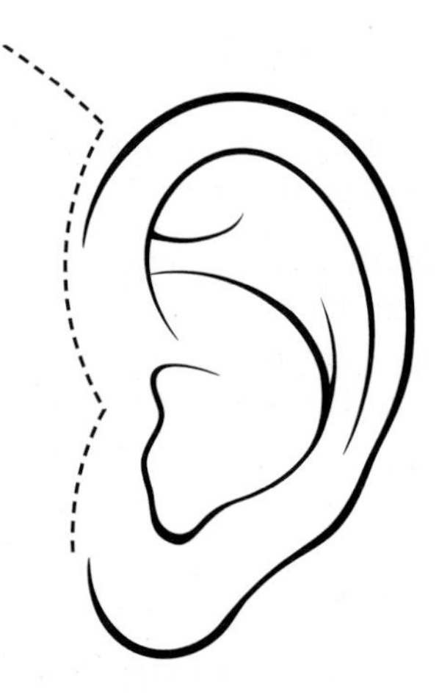

8.2.4 Diagram of preauricular incision.

Skin flap developed

Superiorly, the flap is extended anteriorly by blunt dissection with a periosteal elevator.

Inferiorly, the flap is developed in a relatively avascular plane parallel to the external auditory (tragal) cartilage which runs anteromedially (Figures 8.2.5 and 8.2.6).

Temporalis fascia

Once the temporalis fascia is exposed, it is then incised in the vertical direction (Figures 8.2.7 and 8.2.8). A flap is developed forwards by blunt dissection with periosteal elevator exposing the root of the zygomatic arch. At this stage, the surgical assistant should manipulate the mandible so that the surgeon can palpate and identify the position of the moving condyle.

Exposing the lateral joint capsule

Be prepared to diathermy a large vein which often runs just above the arch and deep to the fascia. A large periosteal elevator is used to expose the lateral part of the root of the zygomatic arch as far forwards as the articular eminence. From the pocket created over the root of the zygomatic arch, the capsule of the joint (Figures 8.2.9 and 8.2.10) is identified inferiorly by sharp and blunt dissection. A small triangular flap is then lifted and progressively rotated forwards by blunt dissection over the capsule and lateral margin of the glenoid fossa. This layer is relatively avascular, except inferiorly where branches of the superficial temporal vessels will be encountered. Access may be extended anteriorly and inferiorly depending on the surgery to follow. At this point, more Marcaine 0.5 per cent with 1:200 000 epinephrine (adrenaline) is injected through the capsule.

Entry through the joint capsule

With the condyle distracted inferiorly, pointed scissors are used to bluntly enter the superior joint space and it is opened to reveal the superior surface of the articular disc.

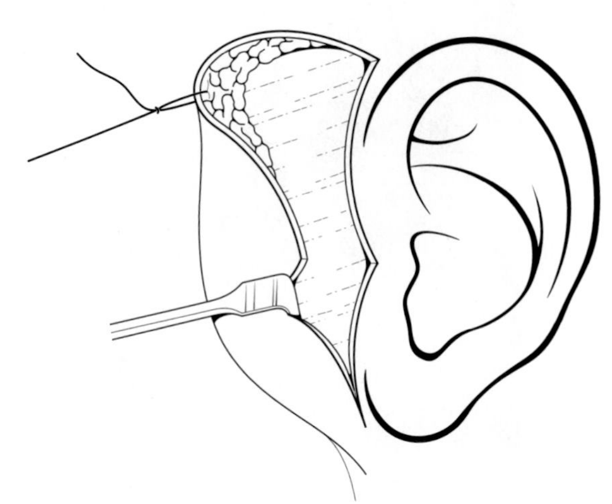

8.2.5 Raising full thickness skin flap.

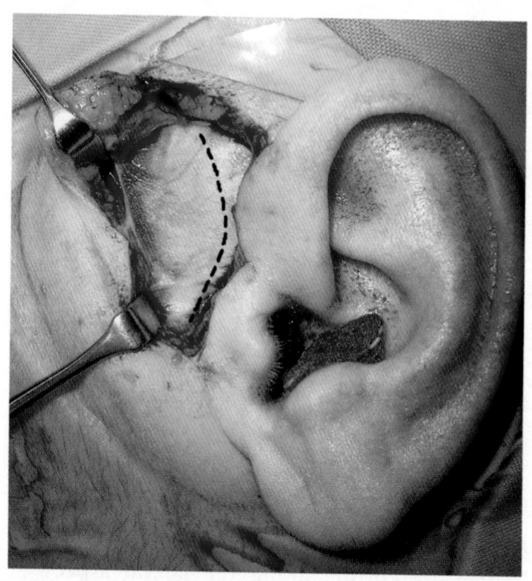

8.2.7 Curvilinear vertical incision of temporalis fascia.

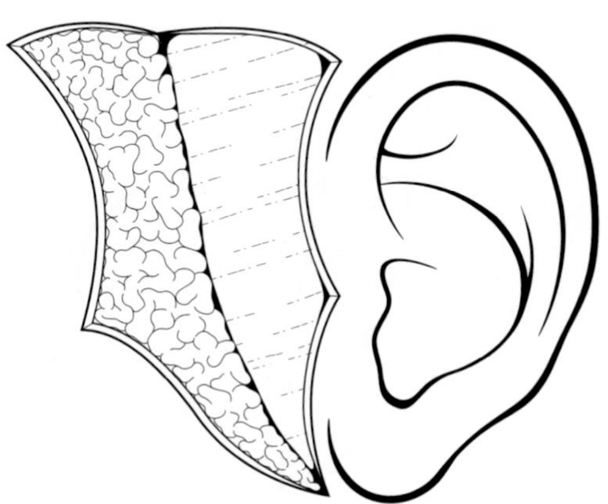

8.2.6 Temporalis fascia exposed.

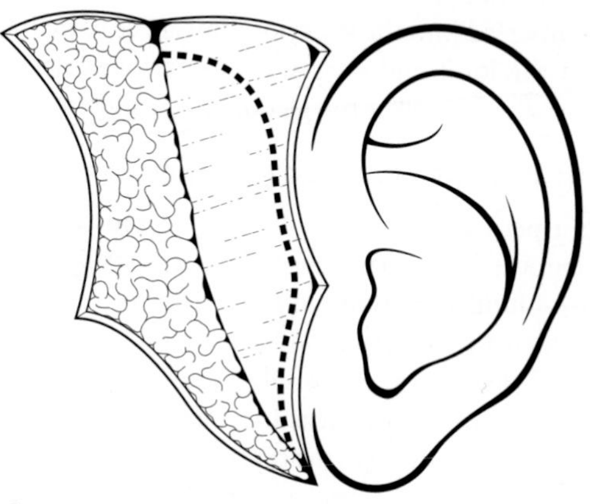

8.2.8 Incision of temporalis fascia.

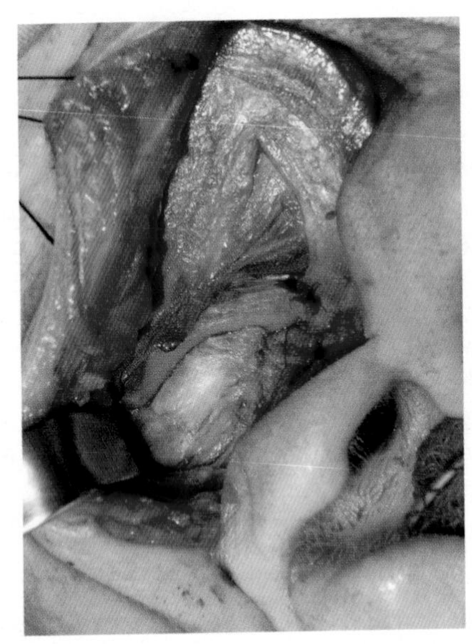

8.2.9 Exposure of lateral capsule.

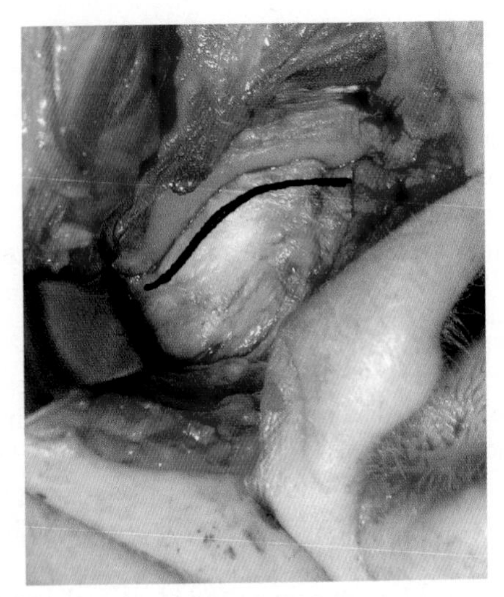

8.2.11 Incision into superior joint space.

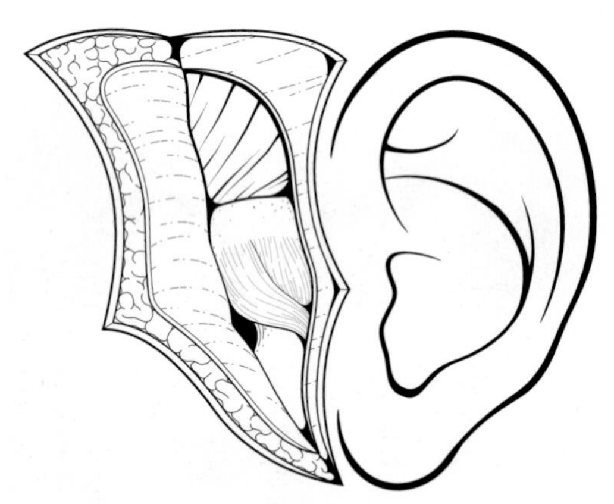

8.2.10 Exposed lateral joint capsule.

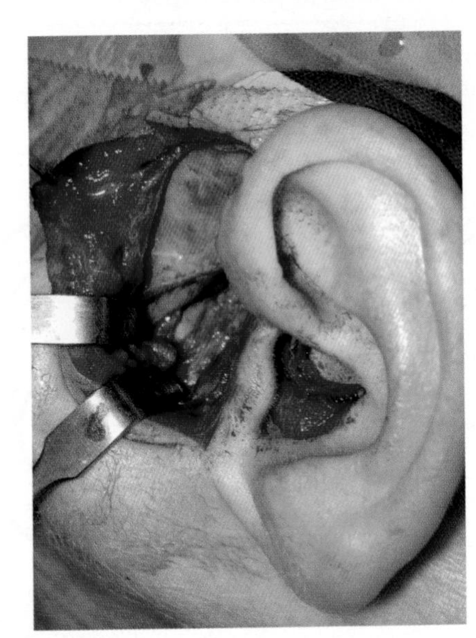

8.2.12 Exposure of superior joint space.

EXPOSURE OF SUPERIOR JOINT SPACE

With a small blade, the opening is extended anteriorly and posteriorly by cutting along the lateral aspect of the eminence and fossa (Figure 8.2.11). The capsule is reflected laterally to reveal the superior joint space (Figures 8.2.12–8.2.14). A broad spoon-shaped instrument, such as a Seldin, is then inserted into the superior joint space to help further distract the joint and expose the superior surface of the articular disc, as well as the glenoid fossa and eminence.

EXPOSURE OF THE ARTICULAR EMINENCE

Using a periosteal elevator, the periosteum covering the lateral aspect of the articular eminence is stripped off with forward blunt dissection along the root of the zygomatic arch. Once the anterior and posterior slopes are fully exposed, a small sharp periosteal elevator is directed medially below the greatest convexity of the articular eminence. The medial dissection through the capsule will expose the inferior aspect of the articular eminence which makes up the anterior boundary of the glenoid fossa (Figure 8.2.15).

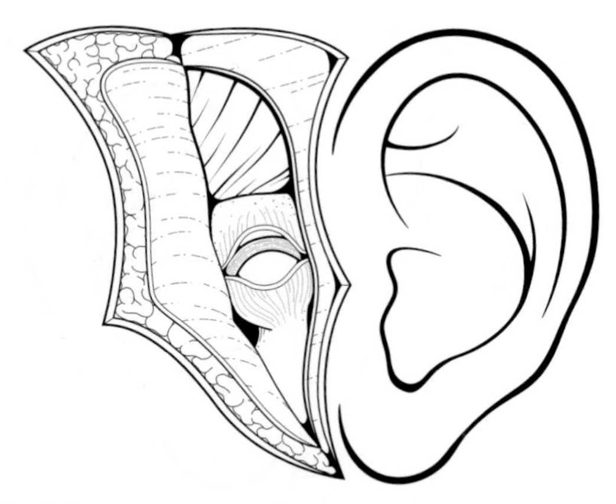

8.2.13 Diagram showing exposure of articular disc.

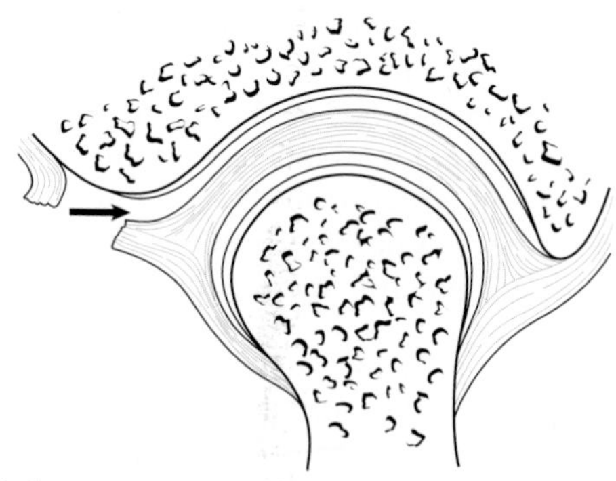

8.2.14 Coronal view of surgical approach to superior joint space.

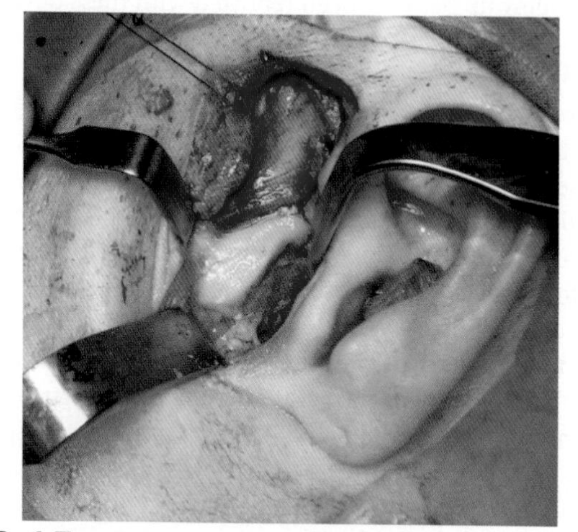

8.2.15 Surgical exposure of articular eminence.

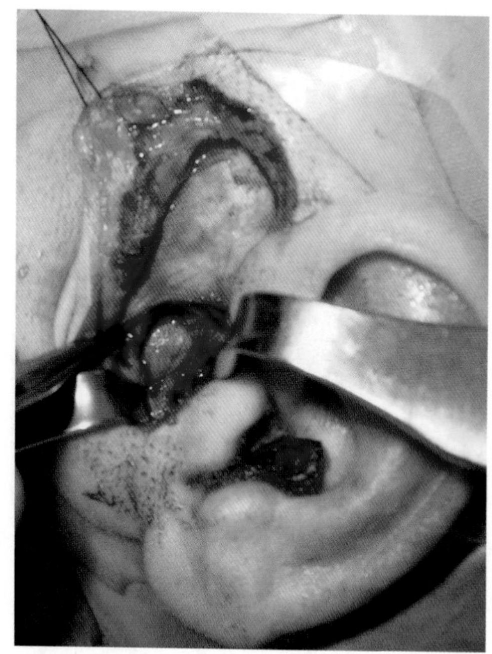

8.2.16 Exposure of condylar head.

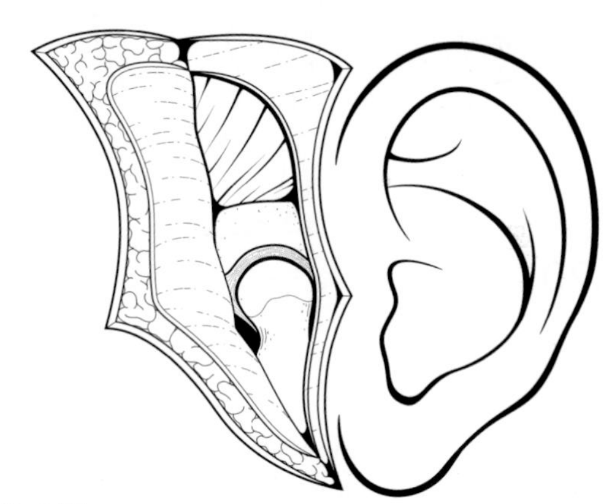

8.2.17 Diagram of exposed articular cartilage covering condylar head.

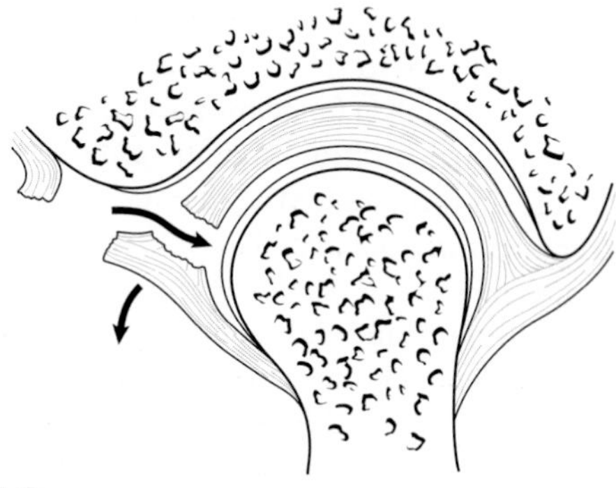

8.2.18 Coronal view of surgical approach to inferior joint space.

EXPOSURE OF THE INFERIOR JOINT SPACE

An incision is made along the lateral attachment of the disc to the condyle within the inferior recess of the capsule (Figures 8.2.16–8.2.18). Brisk haemorrhage may occur if posterior attachment of the disc is cut. A fine periosteal elevator is inserted into the inferior joint space to separate the disc from the condylar head and retract the disc superiorly to expose the articular surface of the condyle.

EXPOSURE OF THE CONDYLAR HEAD

To further expose the condylar head, a vertical relieving incision is made downwards behind the condyle. Special condylar retractors may then be inserted behind the condyle to fully expose and stabilize the condyle (Figures 8.2.19 and 8.2.20). Anteriorly, a small condylar retractor may be inserted below the attachment of the lateral pterygoid muscle to the fovea of the condyle.

SURGICAL PROCEDURES

Articular disc

The articular disc plays a central role in the complex mechanics of joint function. Any change in its physical

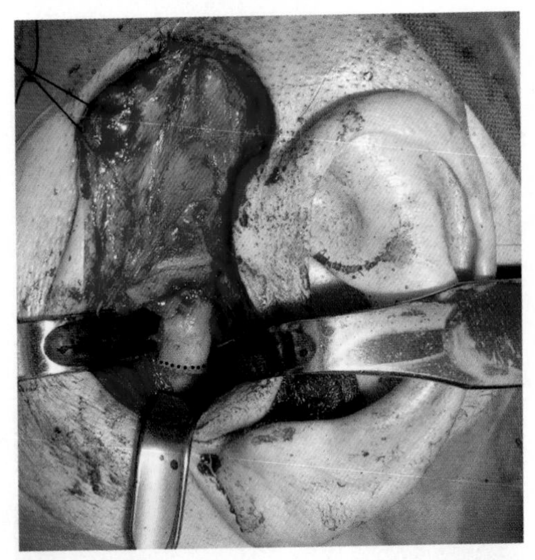

8.2.19 Dotted line showing osteotomy of condylar neck.

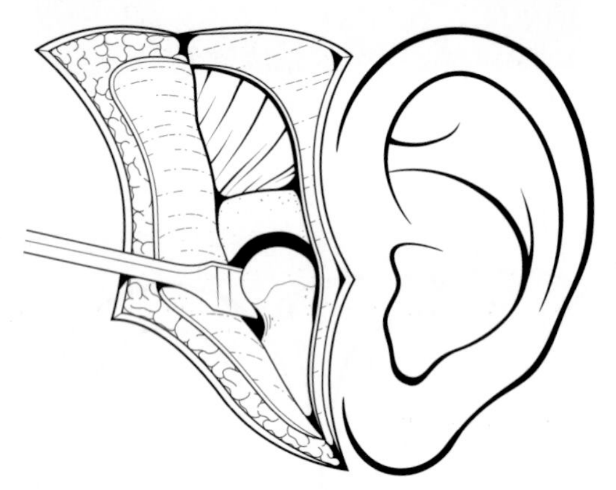

8.2.20 Exposure of condylar neck

structure, integrity or position may result in pain and joint dysfunction referred to as internal derangement.

Nevertheless, the two most common surgical procedures performed on the articular disc are disc repositioning and discectomy.

DISC REPOSITIONING

Upon exposing the superior joint space (Figure 8.2.14), a blunt instrument, such as a Howarth periosteal elevator or Seldin, is inserted to help free up the disc anteriorly and medially. The assistant then functions the mandible to determine the functional position and integrity of the disc (Figure 8.2.21). At this point, Marcaine (0.5 per cent) with 1:200 000 epinephrine (adrenaline) is injected into the posterior disc attachment and bilaminar tissues before the disc is freed up posteriorly and the vascular retrodiscal tissues are exposed. With minor anteromedial displacements, sufficient redundant tissue within the bilaminar zone can be surgically removed and the disc repositioned posteriorly and laterally. Multiple 5/0 interrupted mersylene sutures are placed to anchor the disc to the bilaminar tissues. In situations where the disc is severely displaced, the inferior joint capsule is also exposed (Figure 8.2.18). A blunt instrument is inserted into the inferior joint space to release the disc from the condylar head and mobilize it further. Redundant tissue lateral and posterior to the posterior band of the meniscus is excised using fine scissors, leaving a rim of vascularized tissue 2 mm from the avascular posterior band of the meniscus.

Buried horizontal mattress sutures (5/0 mersylene) are used to fix the disc to the remaining retrodiscal tissues in its new position (Figure 8.2.22). Various anchoring devices attached to the condylar head have also been reported as more stable fixation points for the disc, although no long-term follow up has ever been reported with these devices.

DISCECTOMY

In cases where the disc is found to be unsalvageable, it is completely excised. Both upper and lower joint spaces are exposed (Figures 8.2.14 and 8.2.18) and a vascular clamp is placed across the retrodiscal tissues (Figure 8.2.23). As the assistant distracts the mandible (and condyle) downwards and forwards, the posterolateral part of the disc is first excised with fine pointed scissors. The remaining anteromedial part of the disc is then clamped with Allis tissue forceps to help retract it laterally and posteriorly to facilitate excision of the remaining part of the disc (Figures 8.2.24 and 8.2.25). Infiltration with local anaesthesia and judicious diathermy of bleeding points will help reduce bleeding in the resultant joint cavity.

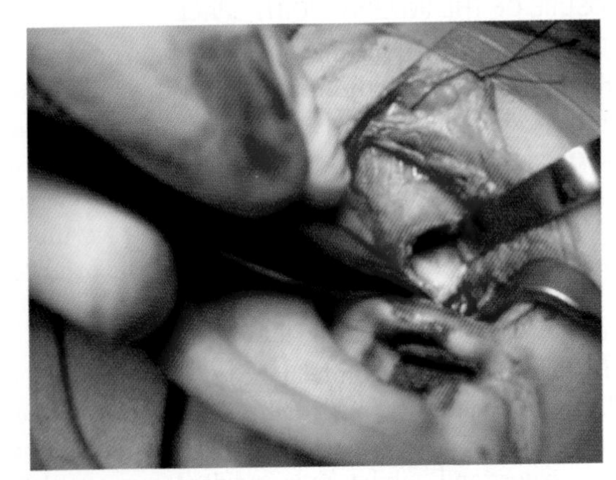

8.2.21 Surgical view of articular disc.

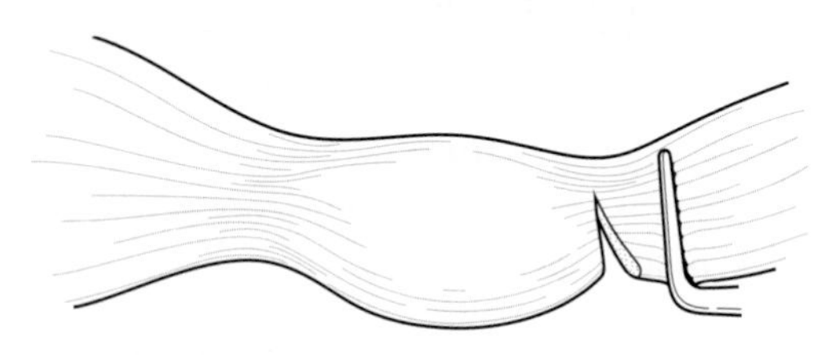

8.2.22 Partial excision of articular disc.

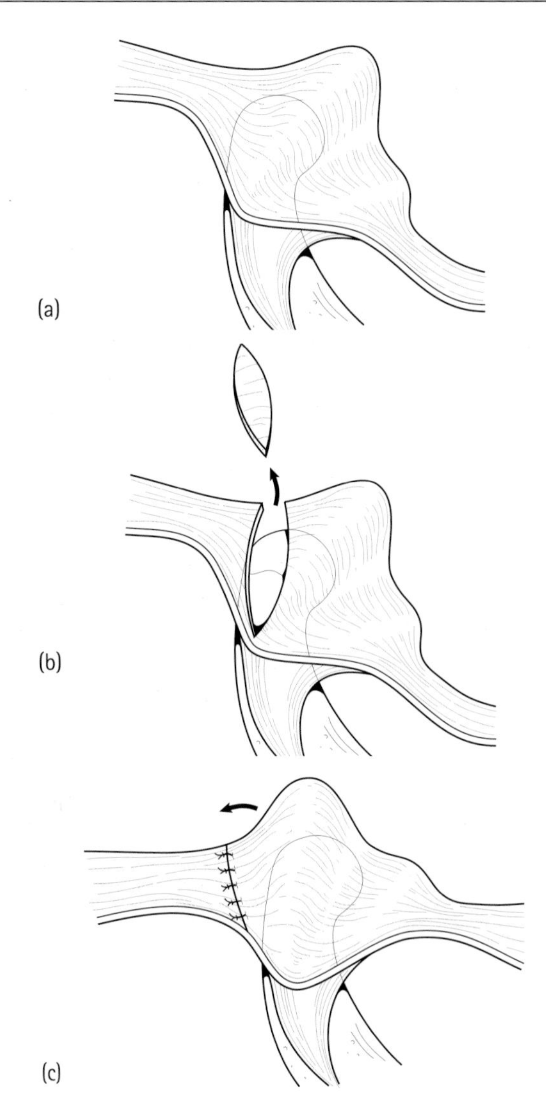

8.2.23 Excision of retrodiscal tissues (a) and (b) and posterior repositioning of disc (c).

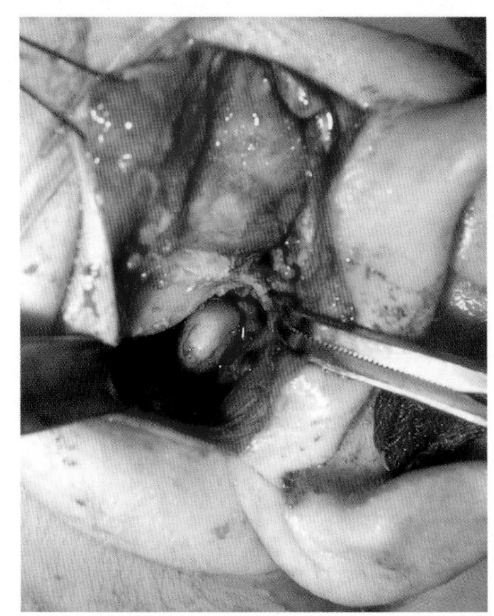

8.2.24 Exposed condylar head following discectomy.

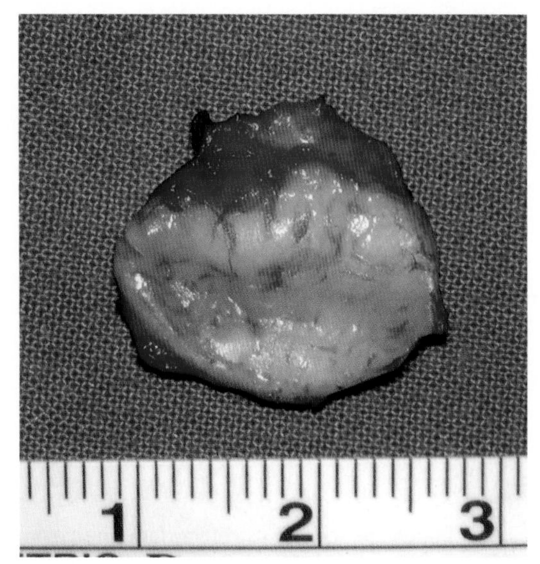

8.2.25 Disc specimen.

Many surgeons, however, leave the space empty following discectomy with good long-term results, while most other surgeons prefer to use pedicled temporalis muscle flaps.

Articular eminence

The articular eminence is often surgically remodelled in cases of recurrent dislocation. It may also be surgically altered to accommodate a fossa prosthesis during total joint replacement. Surgical procedures to the disc may also involve reduction of the articular eminence to facilitate the free movement of the operated disc. The articular eminence may either be surgically reduced (eminectomy) or augmented with osteotomies and/or grafts.

EMINECTOMY

The base of the eminence is identified by scoring the bone with a fine burr in a horizontal line joining the anterior and posterior slopes (Figure 8.2.26). The lateral part of the eminence is best removed with a fine curved chisel (Figure 8.2.27). The medial extension of the eminence is not as prominent as the lateral part and so a large round burr can be used to grind away the bony prominence (Figure 8.2.28) until the glenoid fossa is flush with the root of the zygomatic arch. Bone files are used to smooth the resultant surface.

EMINENCE AUGMENTATION

A number of augmentation procedures have been described to prevent the forward movement of the condyle in cases of recurrent dislocation. Unfortunately, the success of these techniques is limited, especially where the condylar head is small or atrophic and may slip medial to the augmented site.

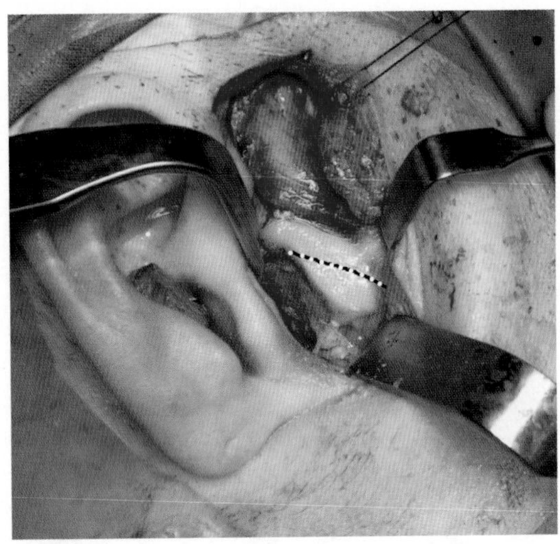

8.2.26 Dotted line showing osteotomy for eminectomy.

- Dautrey's osteotomy (Figure 8.2.29): This is where the zygomatic arch is divided just in front of the eminence and is then infractured. No fixation is used to hold the infractured arch which is held in position by friction alone.
- Onlay graft (Figure 8.2.30): Autogenous bone or allograft cartilage blocks are secured to the anterior slope of the eminence with miniplates and screws.
- Interpositional graft (Figure 8.2.31): A horizontal osteotomy is made along the base of the articular eminence. The inferior portion is downfractured and autogenous bone graft is placed as an interpositional graft which is secured with bone plates and screws.
- Alloplastic fixation: Metallic screws or plates are secured to the inferior surface of the eminence and left prominent to act as a physical barrier to the forward translation of the condyle.

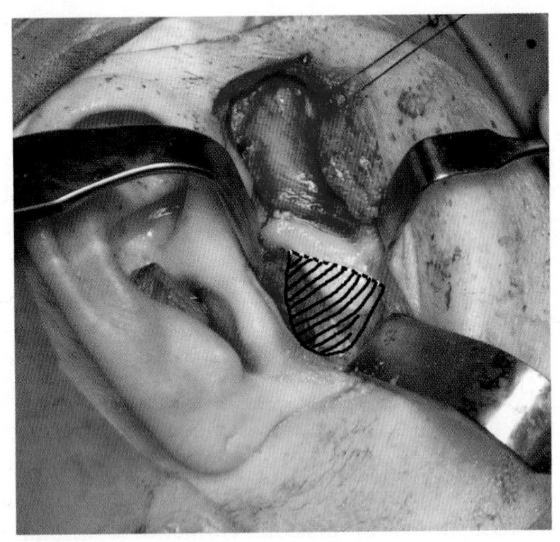

8.2.27 Shaded area showing bone removal required for eminence reduction.

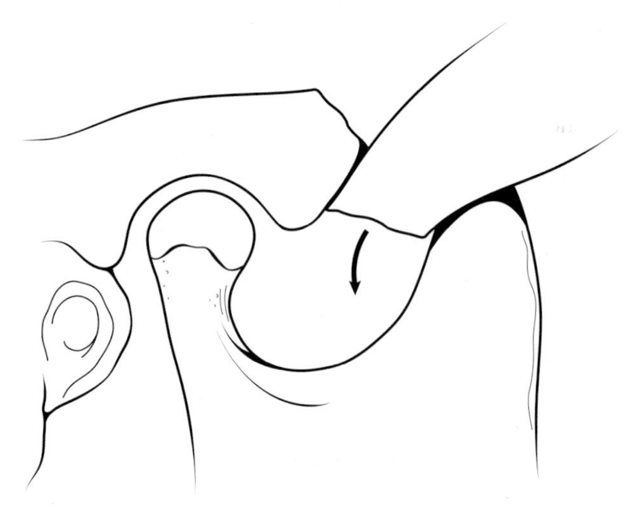

8.2.29 Downfracture of zygomatic arch to prevent forward translation of condyle.

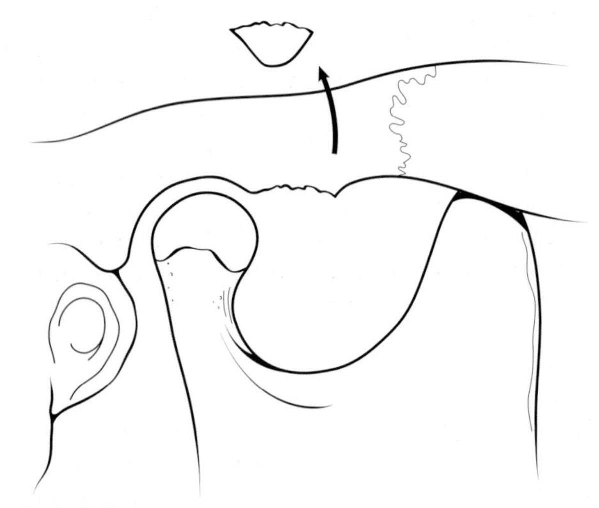

8.2.28 Eminectomy.

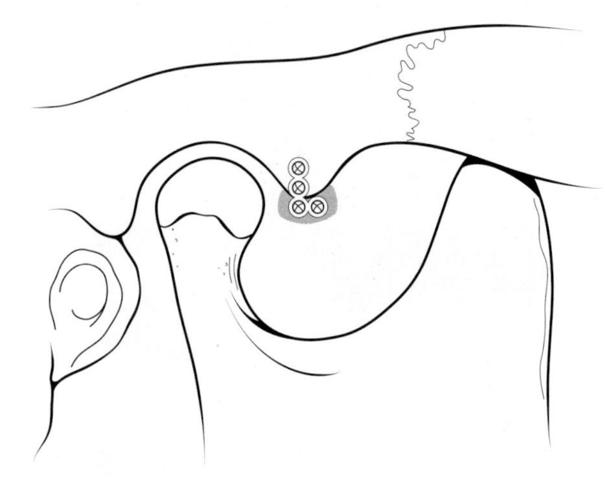

8.2.30 Augmentation of eminence with onlay grafts fixed with plate and screws.

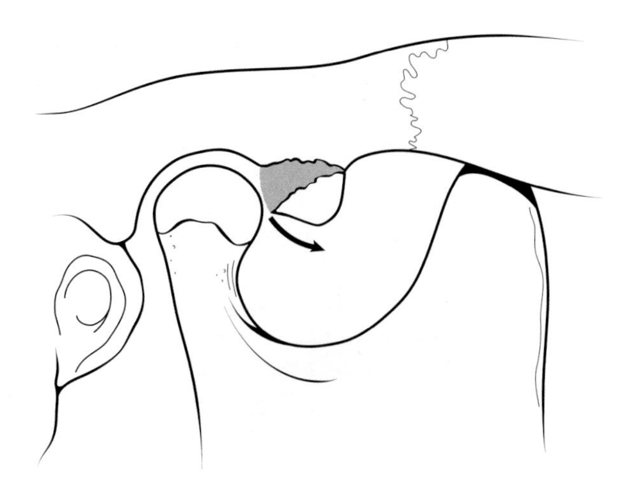

8.2.31 Augmentation of eminence by downfracture with interpositional grafting.

Condyle

The condyle is pivotal to the development, form and function of the mandible. Trauma, disease or developmental disorders which afflict the condyle will also have a significant impact on the mandible, in particular, the occlusion. Surgery to the condylar head may range from simple smoothing of irregularities in the fibrocartilagenous articular surface, and removal of osteophytes, to complete amputation of the condyle itself in cases of severe disease or tumours.

- Debridement: Upon entering the lower joint space (Figure 8.2.18), close inspection of the condylar head may reveal irregularities or defects within the fibrocartilagenous articular surface (Figure 8.2.24). With the condyle inferiorly distracted, a Moulte currette is used to gently shave the surface irregularities.
- Removal of osteophytes: These bony projections are often found on the lateral pole of the condyle and should be removed with chisels rather than powered handpieces so as to minimize surgical trauma to the condyle itself.
- High condylar shave: This technique is rarely used and it is now of historical interest. It was erroneously believed that a high condylar shave would create additional joint space. With the lateral pole of the condyle exposed, the top 5-mm layer is surgically removed with an osteotomy cut from the lateral aspect of the condylar head which is completed medially by chisel. The remaining surface is surgically smoothed with a bone file, ensuring there are no sharp margins around the circumference of the osteotomy site.
- Partial condylectomy: The lateral pole of the condyle may be excised (Figure 8.2.32) with the deep margin up to half the width of the condylar head. The aim is to preserve the medial pole of the condyle in order to maintain the height of the ascending mandibular ramus. A diagonal osteotomy is made from the posterior aspect of the condylar head (Figure 8.2.33) which is completed with chisels. Any sharp edges in the remaining defect are smoothly rounded with bone files.
- Total condylectomy: Blunt dissection is carried inferiorly to expose the neck of the condyle to the level of the sigmoid notch (Figures 8.2.19, 8.2.20 and 8.2.34). With two condylar retractors in place, the condylar process is stabilized as a reciprocating saw is used to section the condylar neck. A fine chisel is used to complete the osteotomy. The amputated condylar fragment is then held with bone holding forceps while the medial attachment of the articular disc is released with sharp scissors. Anteriorly, the thick attachment of the lateral pterygoid muscle is released with dissection scissors as a traction force is placed on the condylar fragment with the bone holding forceps. Once the condylar process is extracted (Figure 8.2.35) from its tissue bed, attention must be paid to the multiple bleeding sites. Total joint replacement with autogenous grafts or alloplastic prosthesis should always be considered at the same time as the condylectomy to prevent severe mandibular functional and structural deformity (see Chapter 8.4).
- Modified condylotomy: The surgical separation of the condyle from the mandible is used primarily for the management of internal derangement. The idea is that the resultant condylar sag will release the pressure within the joint space and allow the disc more room to move and therefore reduce the pain and clicking. While numerous approaches have been described, the most common is the transoral approach. A vertical incision is made through the mucosa from the external oblique ridge up along the ascending ramus to the tip of the coronoid process. A periosteal envelope is established and blunt dissection is carried posteriorly along the lateral surface of the ascending ramus until the posterior border of the mandibular ramus is reached. The mandibular sigmoid notch is identified superiorly and the angle of the mandible inferiorly. Sigmoid notch and posterior border retractors, preferably with fibreoptic lighting attached, are placed in the surgical space. A vertical osteotomy cut, similar to the vertical subsigmoid osteotomy, is then made with a 120° angled oscillating saw about 1–2 cm forwards from, and parallel to, the posterior border. The osteotomy cut is completed with osteotomes and the condylar fragment, together with the posterior border and the angle of mandible, is completely mobilized and separated from the rest of the mandible (Figures 8.2.36 and 8.2.37). The surgical wound is closed with dissolving sutures and the patient is placed in intermaxillary fixation for about 6 weeks, beginning with wire fixation for 2–3 weeks then followed by elastic fixation.

Gap arthroplasty

Gap arthroplasty is used for the management of TMJ ankylosis. Ankylosis release involves the removal of a block of bone: either the complete condyle (condylectomy) or full thickness section of condylar neck which is referred to as a gap arthroplasty. The gap must be as wide as possible.

A new joint space is created below the original joint space (Figure 8.2.39) and an interpositional graft is inserted within the new joint space to prevent bone union or reankylosis. Due to loss of ramus height, some post-operative occlusal derangement occurs and, if performed bilaterally, an open bite results.

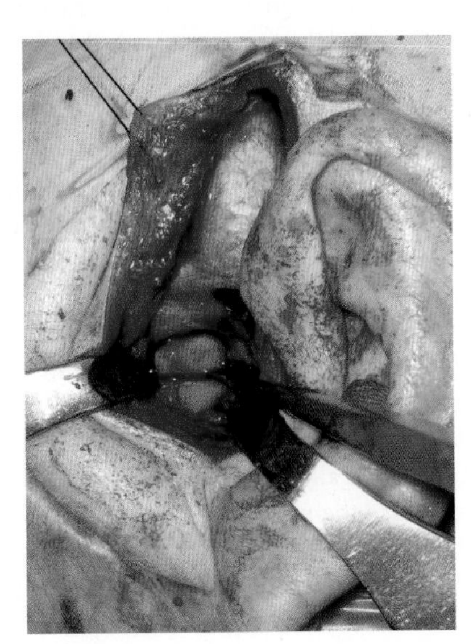

8.2.32 Osteotomy of condylar head.

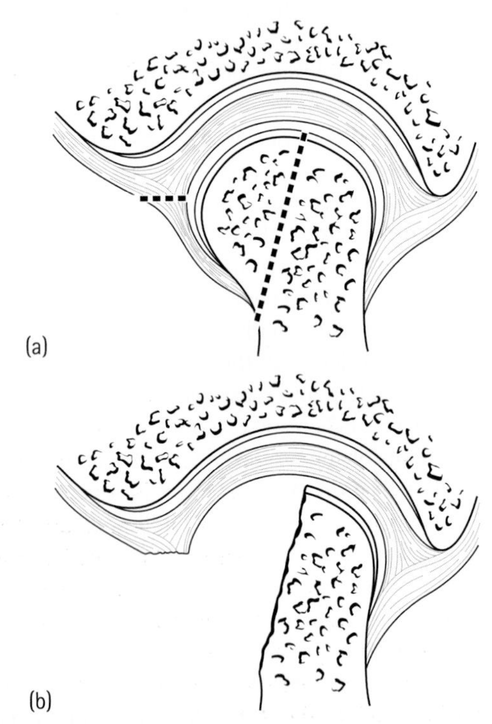

8.2.33 Sagittal ostectomy of lateral pole of condyle.

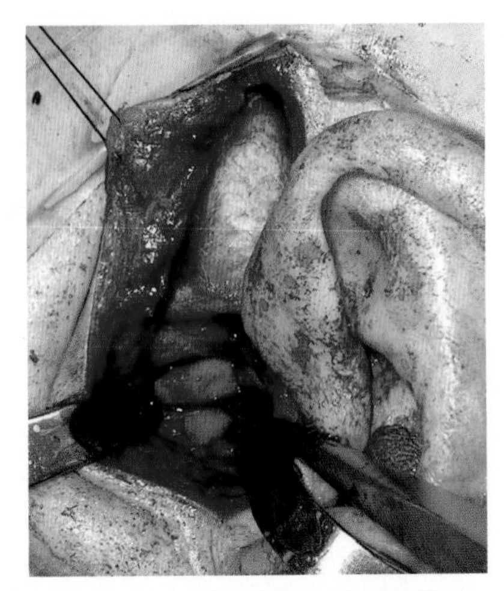

8.2.34 Osteotomy used for high condylectomy.

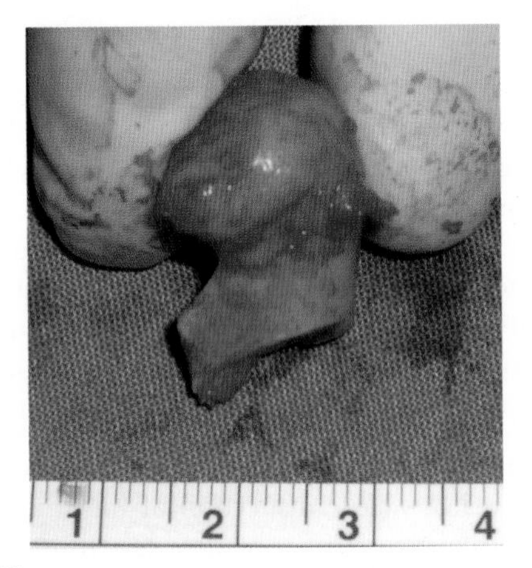

8.2.35 Surgical specimen of mandibular condyle.

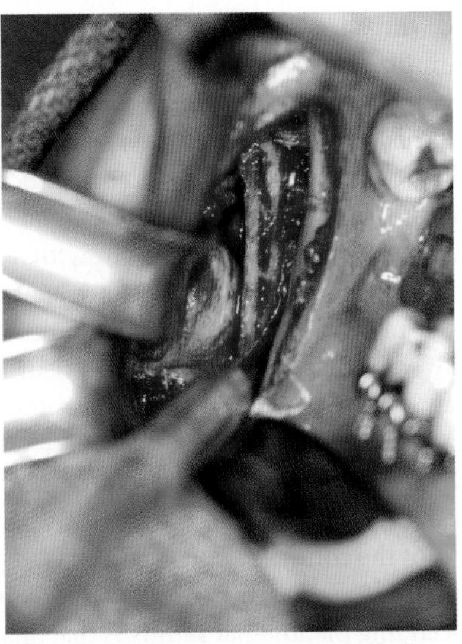

8.2.36 Intra-oral view of vertical subsigmoid osteotomy.

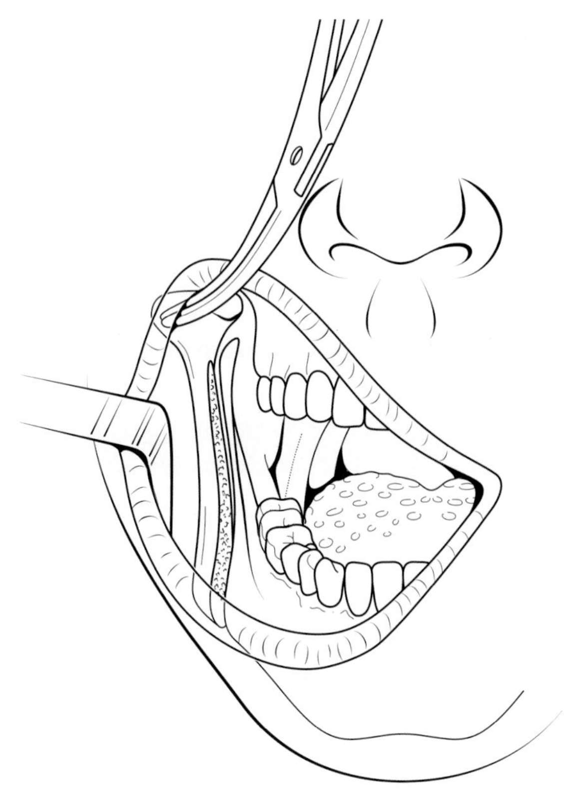

8.2.37 Diagram showing intra-oral approach to vertical subsigmoid osteotomy.

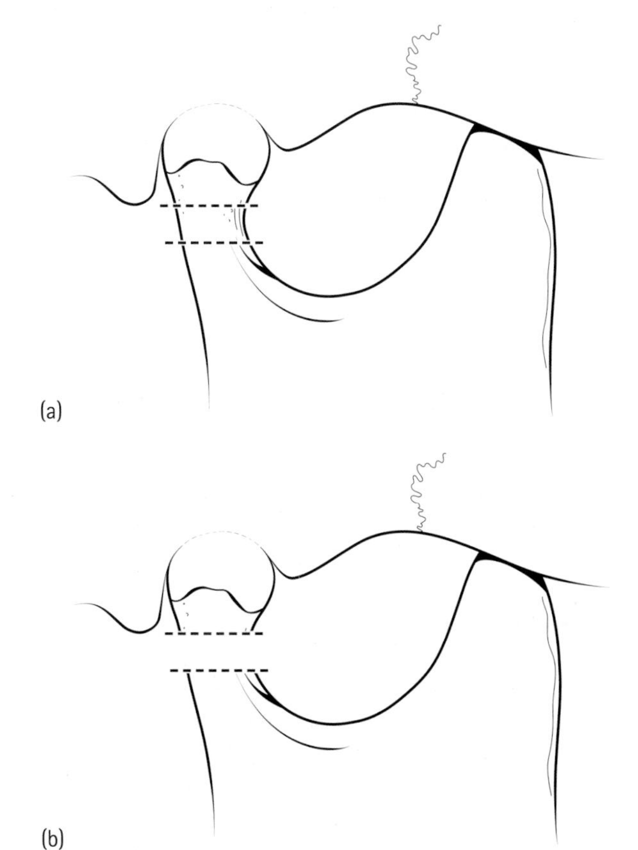

8.2.38 Ostectomy (a) and gap arthroplasty (b) for surgical release of TMJ ankylosis.

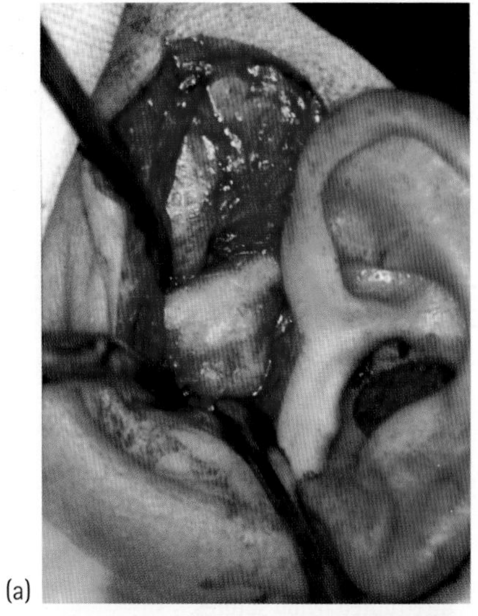

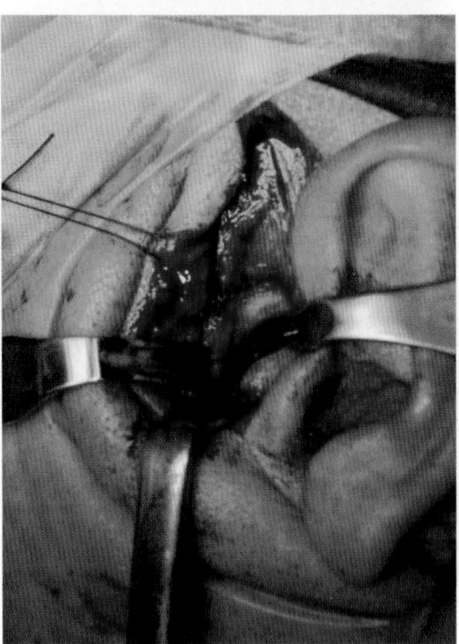

8.2.39 Bony ankylosis (a) following gap arthroplasty (b).

Closure

Careful attention to haemostasis is essential prior to closure. The surgical wound should be repaired in layers, i.e. capsule, temporalis fascia, subcutaneous tissues and skin. Resorbable 4/0 sutures, such as vickryl, are used for the deep layers and 5/0 nylon may be used for skin either as simple interrupted (Figure 8.2.40) or subcuticular sutures that are removed after 5 days. A mastoid-type pressure dressing (Figure 8.2.41) is applied for 24 hours. The ear must be padded with gauze or cotton before placing the dressing. Drains are rarely indicated.

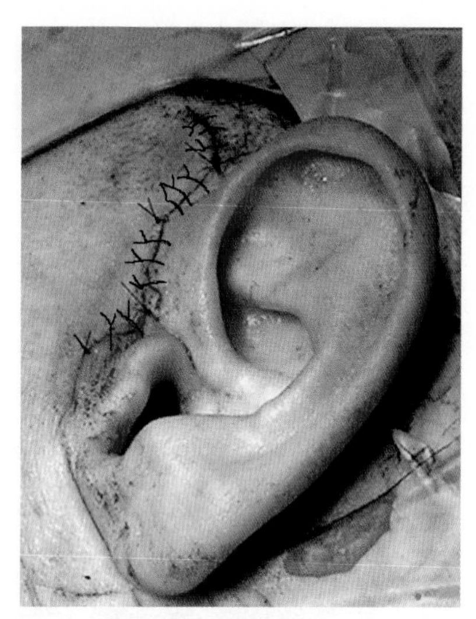

8.2.40 Interrupted nylon sutures.

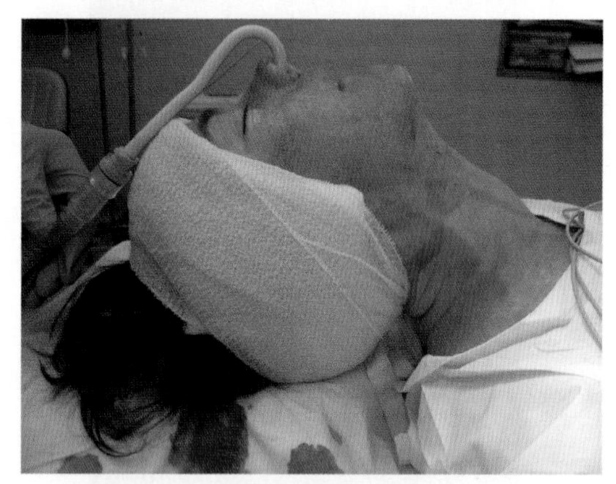

8.2.41 Barrel head bandage used as pressure dressing for 24 hrs following TMJ surgery.

COMPLICATIONS OF TMJ SURGERY (ARTHROTOMY)

1 Poor patient selection:
   - patient is an unreliable historian, i.e. secondary gain or compensation seeking;
   - patient has unrealistic expectations of surgical outcome;
   - psychiatric history;
   - significant medical history.
2 Inexperienced clinician:
   - poor diagnostic skills;
   - limited experience in TMJ surgery.
3 Poor surgical technique:
   - infection: haematoma, wound breakdown;
   - bleeding;
   - facial nerve paresis;
   - scarring;
   - deafness, middle ear surgically breached.
4 Malocclusion:
   - condylar resorption;
   - overzealous arthroplasty and disc surgery;
5 Limited mouth opening:
   - adhesions;
   - fibrosis;
   - ankylosis.
6 Persistent symptoms:
   - failure to continue supportive nonsurgical therapy;
   - poor patient compliance; cannot follow instructions;
   - misdiagnosis, chronic pain syndrome.

Top tips

- The operating table should be slightly inclined with the head elevated above the level of the heart to help reduce intraoperative bleeding.
- A condom-like rubber finger projection cut out of a urology drape is inserted in the mouth and taped to the lips to allow the surgical assistant to manipulate the mandible during surgery without unsterilizing the surgical field.
- The skin/fascia flap should be developed behind the superficial temporal vessels that will lie well protected in the anterior part of the flap.
- Staying beneath the temporal fascia will avoid the temporal branches of the facial nerve.
- Keeping a small periosteal elevator firmly on the bone, the soft tissues enveloping the condylar process can be bluntly dissected off the condyle as far inferiorly as the level of the mandibular notch.
- The role of disc repositioning surgery has diminished in the light of the success of less invasive procedures, such as TMJ arthroscopy and arthrocentesis.
- Bleeding is best controlled with a curved vascular clamp that is placed across the retrodiscal tissues immediately behind where the wedge excision of redundant tissue takes place (Figure 8.2.23).
- The author uses autogenous dermis-fat graft procured from the patient's lower abdomen to fill the resultant joint cavity following discectomy and gap arthroplasty.
- Aggressive debridement of articular cartilage must be avoided, as this will result in severe remodelling of the condyle.
- Where the lateral capsule has to be sacrificed, a flap from the deep layer of temporal fascia may be rotated down over the lateral side of the joint to form a pseudocapsule.
- Fixation should not be applied to the osteotomy site of the modified condylomtomy because the whole purpose is to allow the condyle to sag or drop slightly from its original position.
- Deliberately ignoring the original joint anatomy, a wide segment of ramus above the lingula is resected, leaving the ankylosed mass attached to the base of the skull (Figure 8.2.38).

FURTHER READING

Dimitroulis G. The role of surgery in the management of disorders of the temporomandibular joint: a critical review of the literature; Part 2. *International Journal of Oral and Maxillofacial Surgery* 2005; **34**: 231–73.

Dolwick MF, Dimitroulis G. Is there a role for temporomandibular joint surgery ? *British Journal of Oral and Maxillofacial Surgery* 1994; **32**: 307–13.

Dolwick MF, Sanders B. *TMJ internal derangement and arthrosis – Surgical atlas.* St Louis: CV Mosby, 1985.

Quinn PD. *Color atlas of temporomandibular joint surgery.* St Louis: CV Mosby, 1998.

8.3

Treatment of temporomandibular joint ankylosis

ANDREW J SIDEBOTTOM, ROBERT HENSHER

INTRODUCTION

Although the term 'ankylosis' suggests a crookedness (and the disease may produce deranged development when it affects young patients), ankylosis of a joint is commonly regarded as fusion across it, such that movement is either not possible or is greatly restricted. With regard to the temporomandibular joint (TMJ), the disorder is usually classified as intracapsular or extracapsular according to where the restriction occurs. A particular type of extracapsular ankylosis occurs when fusion takes place between the mandibular coronoid process and the adjacent zygomatic arch or maxilla.

The aetiology is usually due to trauma and/or infection, although it can be the endpoint of degenerative disease, bone or other malignancy or agenesis of the joint. In the Western world, the usual cause of ankylosis is post-traumatic following intracapsular condylar fractures. These may result in ossification of fragments of bone causing fusion between the mandible and the glenoid fossa.

MANAGEMENT

This may be broadly divided according to the age of the patient affected.

Infancy

It is unusual to see ankylotic disease in the first few months of life. Agenesis, infection and birth trauma all may lead to fixity of the TMJ, as may overgrowth of the mandibular coronoid process. The aims of treatment in this age group are to restore movement and function, leaving reconstruction to later in life.

Childhood

Up to the age of 15 years, ankylosis may be caused by trauma or infection (for example, from the middle ear or mastoid). As facial development is incomplete, the restriction may also affect growth from the condylar growth centre leading to a deranged occlusion and marked facial asymmetry, with occlusal cant upwards and centreline discrepancy towards the affected side as maxillary growth is also impaired. Additionally, there will be loss of vertical ramus height with associated undergrowth of the maxilla.

Treatment is aimed at first restoring function and movement of the TMJ with a bony replacement of the condylar head. This is usually achieved with a costochondral graft.

Subsequent correction of the occlusal and cosmetic deformity proceeds in the late teens with bimaxillary surgery or in the early teens with the assistance of distraction osteogenesis of the mandible. Both techniques should level the occlusal cant and in the growth phase, this may be achieved by levelling the mandible and holding back mandibular dentoalveolar growth permitting maxillary dentoalveolar growth to correct the cant. This requires close orthodontic co-operation.

Adults

Ankylosis in this age group (where dentofacial development is complete) is usually the result of trauma and treatment is aimed at restoration of satisfactory movement and function. Rare occlusal discrepancies are dealt with by standard orthognathic surgery, although an anterior open bite and other mandibular malpositions may be corrected during bilateral joint replacement surgery.

INVESTIGATIONS

Routine clinical assessment should be supplemented with adequate imaging of the degree of ankylosis. This is best achieved with computed tomography (CT) scanning, preferably with three-dimensional reformatting. Vascular assessment of the infratemporal fossa may require magnetic resonance angiography to determine the extent of involvement of the great vessels. The ankylotic process may extend widely and it is important to determine the extent and risks of the procedure pre-operatively to prepare adequately and obtain informed consent from the patient. In addition, patients with ankylosing spondylitis may need respiratory and spinal assessment.

ANAESTHESIA

These patients require specialist anaesthetic services with capability to provide fibreoptic intubation as their mouth opening is so restricted. If this is not possible, then pre-operative tracheostomy may be required either in the standard open fashion or by a percutaneous dilatational technique. Weight loss and dietary compromise may also be an issue, which may require pre-operative enteral feeding to supplement oral intake. Hypotensive anaesthesia aids the dissection, particularly of the deep tissues, and an anti-trendelenberg table (30° head up) will also reduce venous filling.

SURGERY IN THE ADULT

The aim of treatment is to restore adequate movement of the TMJ. Extra-articular ankylosis, such as that due to fusion of the coronoid process, may require simple intraoral coronoidectomy, possibly with trimming of bone from the upper point of fixity – the zygomatic arch or maxilla.

Prosthetic replacement of the TMJ is now the gold standard for restoration of function of the TMJ following ankylosis surgery. It provides a good 'gap' of greater than 1 cm and good function in the immediate post-operative period with the additional use of a Therabite® device as patient-provided passive motion. It reduces the risks associated with the harvest of a costochondral graft and reduces hospital stay, with a predictable long-term outcome.

SURGERY IN THE CHILD

The aim of treatment in the child is not only to regain mobility and function, but also to permit ongoing growth. For this reason, prosthetic joint replacements are usually contraindicated in the child and a costochondral graft is preferred, although Wolford has suggested the use of alloplastic replacement prior to cessation of growth, this area is controversial. A costochondral graft permits the possibility of ongoing growth, although this is unpredictable. In addition, they are more likely to reankylose and the patients and parents should be warned of these possibilities. Should the graft fail later in life (post-puberty) it should be converted to a prosthesis.

RESECTION OF THE ANKYLOTIC TISSUE

Preparation of the patient involves shaving the temporal region to provide a clean field for wound closure without the intervention of hairs. The patient is placed in a stable head ring (Ruben's pillow) with the nasal tube secured in the midline over the patient's forehead. Skin preparation should be carried out including a pre-operative rinse with chlorhexidene to cleanse the mouth. Draping should cover the mouth separately, as during the procedure the occlusion will need to be secured. The anaesthetic tube may be most safely secured using a clear adhesive dressing (such as OpSite®), although this should be left clear of the mouth. Two of these can be used in a bilateral case with the mouth free in the middle. The face is left clear of the other drapes to permit visualization for 'twitching' of the facial nerve during the procedure (Figure 8.3.1). The ear canal is cleansed and covered with OpSite.

Upper and lower arch bars are placed at this stage if access permits, or following restoration of opening with the face covered with a separate towel. All instruments used in this stage of the procedure should be kept separate to maintain asepsis of the facial operation site. Gowns and gloves are changed, the incision sites are marked and injected with local anaesthetic containing epinephrine (adrenaline) to reduce oozing. Five minutes should be allowed to permit action.

Upper approach

The joint is approached, in the manner described elsewhere, towards the capsule. The capsule of the joint is opened via an inverted L incision along the back border of the condyle and at the level of the disc. Bipolar diathermy should control any haemorrhage during this dissection. The anterior and posterior borders of the condylar neck are exposed in the subperiosteal plane and the condylar neck exposed with the

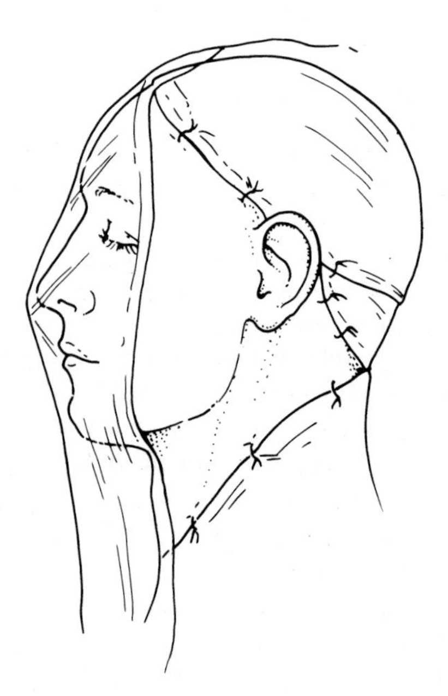

8.3.1 Draping of the patient prior to joint replacement surgery.

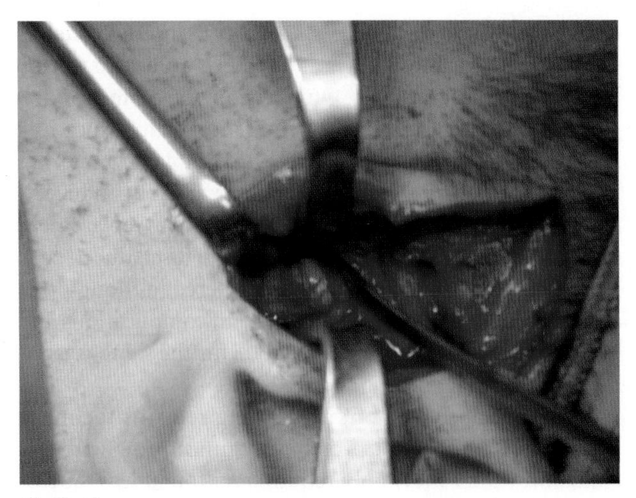

8.3.2 Exposure of the condyle of the mandible.

aid of Dautrey or similar retractors (Figure 8.3.2). This permits the lifting of the periosteum from the posterior surface of the condylar neck as the maxillary artery lies a few millimetres deep to this area (with the mandibular division of the trigeminal nerve emerging from the foramen ovale just deep to this).

Lower dissection

There are various approaches to the ramus of the mandible. The submandibular approach, whilst safe, stretches the tissues somewhat and makes the upper dissection of the condylar neck difficult to achieve. The Kent modification of this approach described in the first edition of this book reduces the stretching, while providing excellent access to the ramus. It does increase the risk to the marginal mandibular division of the facial nerve, but allows easier access to the external carotid artery in cases of vascular catastrophe. The authors prefer a retromandibular transparotid access described in Chapter 8.4. Whilst this carries risk of damage to the marginal mandibular branch, the authors have not seen this in primary cases as any branches traversing the wound can be seen and retracted if blunt dissection is used through the parotid. It provides a rapid access and permits access to the external carotid and retromandibular vein if required.

The retromandibular approach is described in Chapter 7.6, p. 487. On reaching the periosteum of the posterior border of the ramus, it is incised and subperiosteal dissection is continued to expose the lateral and posterior surfaces of the ramus up to the sigmoid notch and to join the superior dissection. A sigmoid notch retractor is useful in the notch and a swan neck retractor around the posterior border of the ramus permits exposure of the condylar neck from below while maintaining the closely related vessels away from the surgical field.

It is often easier to complete the condylectomy from below as the periosteum on the medial surface of the condylar neck is easier to retract without stretching the temporal branch of the facial nerve from above. The initial cut is marked by postage stamping in a 45° angle from the sigmoid notch posteroinferiorly to the posterior border of the ramus. This should be completed on the lateral cortex, but the inner cortex should be left somewhat intact to permit final separation of the condylectomy by insertion of a broad periosteal elevator (such as a Howarth) to prevent inadvertent drilling or osteotome placement through the medial periosteum into the maxillary or masseteric vessels. In any case, as much of the medial tissues as possible are held away subperiosteally by retraction. The lower portion of the resection is now complete and removal of the ankylotic mass can proceed, mostly from above.

Removal of the ankylotic mass

This stage of the procedure is different in every patient and only general guidelines can be given. The ankylotic mass can extend a long way along the base of the skull and therefore resection may be compromised by cranial nerves emerging from the skull base, the maxillary, middle meningeal and ultimately internal jugular and carotid vessels. It is for this reason that pre-operative vascular imaging may be useful and the assistance of a vascular or skull base surgeon may be required.

The upper limit of the ankylosis may be defined by a fine line in the bone exaggerated by either pulling down on the ramus prior to making the condylar cuts or by using a Juniper distractor across the joint. This may facilitate one plane of the upper dissection. Once the lower (condylectomy) cut is made, then the periosteum should not be transgressed. Although the condylectomy cut may generate some mobility, do not be tempted to pull on the fragment as this may avulse some deeper structure and haemorrhage control down a deep dark hole can prove troublesome! Proceed to carefully dissect around the mass anteriorly and posteriorly with the aid of bipolar diathermy to maintain a clear operative field. Carefully remove as much as possible of the mass until ready to fashion a new glenoid fossa. This may be a piecemeal process if the mass does not seem to want to come out whole. Cronoidectomy may also be required (Figure 8.3.3) via the lower approach under direct vision. Alternatively this may be simpler from above. Smooth all the remaining bone surfaces prior to accepting the final defect and proceeding to either the joint replacement (in an adult) or a costochondral graft (in a child). Ensure adequate haemostasis and satisfactory mandibular movement prior to proceeding. Recently the use of abdominal free fat packed around the prosthesis has been suggested to reduce the risk of re-ankylosis. If used this should be harvested just prior to placement to keep the fat fresh and improve the chances of revascularization and should be placed just prior to wound closure.

The mouth can now be thoroughly examined and any dental or periodontal condition dealt with. If the occlusion has been deranged by the disease process, once mobility has been

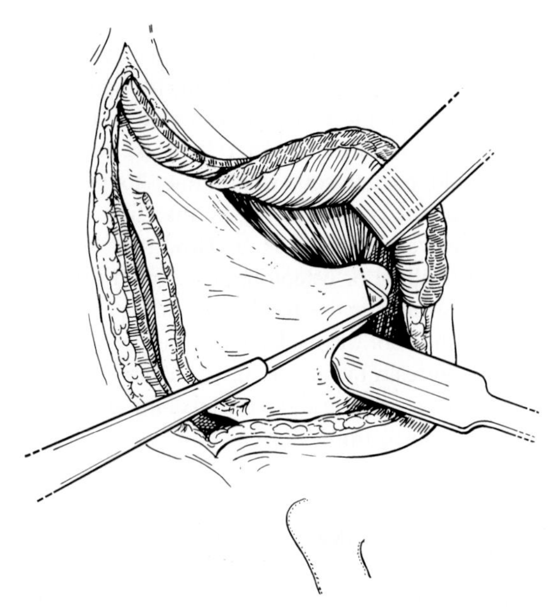

8.3.3 Coronoidectomy can be carried out under direct vision from below.

assured, the teeth can be placed in the desired occlusion and held with temporary intermaxillary wire fixation. In edentulous patients, Gunning splints may be used. If there has been maxillary undergrowth in a child then an intermediate wafer, providing space for levelling the occlusal plane with ongoing alveolar growth, may also be used. Gown and gloves are again changed, ensuring that the instruments used in the mouth do not contaminate the facial operative field.

At this stage in the procedure, the method of reconstruction varies between the child (costochondral graft) and the adult (prosthetic joint replacement).

COSTOCHONDRAL GRAFTING

This provides the main alternative to total joint replacement in the adult, but is a second option in the authors' opinion due to the risk of reankylosis. One of the prerequisites to management in the adult is to achieve an adequate gap between the bone surfaces. On occasion, the costochondral graft may be preferred due to either local factors such as a heavily irradiated bed, allergy to implant materials (although titanium-only prostheses can now be produced), lack of surgical expertise to perform prosthetic replacement or financial factors where a prosthesis is refused due to cost. Microvascular grafting may be considered, although this adds considerably to operative time and complications and has the same potential for reankylosis for the same reasons as costochondral grafting.

In the child, costochondral grafting remains the management of choice as a prosthesis cannot grow with the child and would inevitably require revision at least at cessation of growth. Costochondral grafts also permit ongoing growth, although this is unpredictable. For these reasons, we will only describe the technique for costochondral grafting in the child. The approach in the adult follows the same choices of access to the mandible as for resection of the ankylotic mass. In the child a lower cervical incision may be considered, as with growth this may rise towards the lower border of the mandible and if primarily too high, ultimately end as a scar on the face.

COSTOCHONDRAL GRAFT HARVEST

In the child, the contralateral rib usually provides the best curvature with the left rib being used for the right side and vice versa. The patient and anaesthetist should be warned of the possibility of pleural puncture and therefore the necessity for chest drainage post-operatively and difficulties with oxygenation intraoperatively.

In the female with breast development, the incision should be made directly below the breast skin fold. This leaves an almost invisible scar which in any case is cosmetically more acceptable. In the male, the approach should be lower and aimed at the sixth or seventh rib. The incision should follow the line of the ribs (Figure 8.3.4),

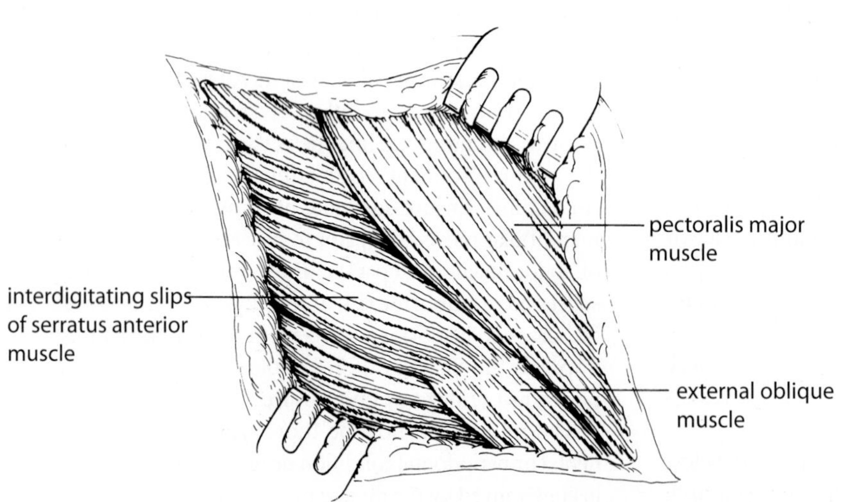

8.3.4 Exposure of the superficial chest wall muscles.

unless guided by the inframammary fold, and dissection is continued to the rib periosteum. Meticulous haemostasis permits better visibility and at this stage the periosteal envelope should be preserved. Carry the dissection under the periosteum commencing at the maximum curvature of the rib and developing the plane inferiorly, ensuring the preservation of the neurovascular bundle which lies on the inferior surface of the rib. Raise the periosteum superiorly (Figure 8.3.5) until continuity with the lower dissection is achieved. It may then be possible to insert a Doyen retractor initially to retract and subsequently elevate the periosteum.

The incision through the periosteum should now be continued towards the costochondral junction. About 1 cm from this junction, make the incision diverge in a 'Y' fashion, continuing on to the cartilage side to bring the incision edges back together and to complete a diamond shape. The cartilage may then be incised, with the remaining periosteum helping to maintain continuity with the rib and thus the costochondral junction. Finally, the length of rib required should be determined. The inner dissection is continued with a curved rib raspatory (Figure 8.3.6) and the lateral rib cut completed with a curved rib cutter (Figure 8.3.7). The rib is harvested and placed in saline-soaked gauze. The wound is closed in layers with deep resorbable sutures to the periosteum to aid rib regeneration. Vacuum suction drainage can be placed above this layer and the skin is closed with interrupted monofilament.

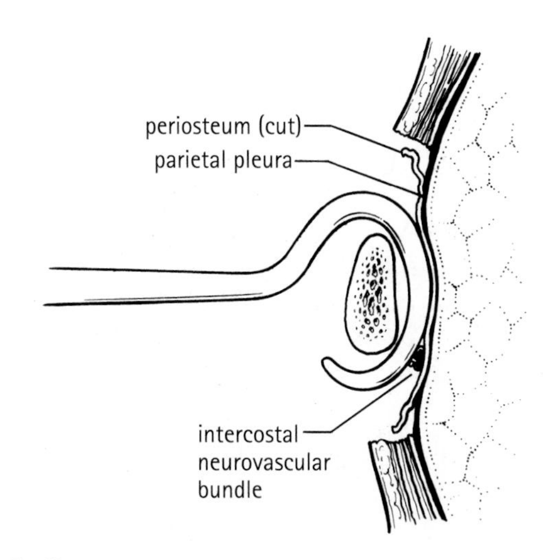

8.3.6 The inner dissection is continued using a curved rib raspatory taking care to preserve the pleura.

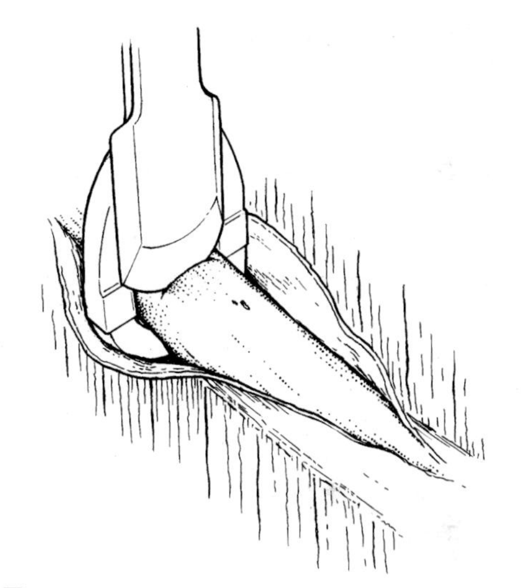

8.3.7 The lateral rib cut is completed with a rib cutter.

RECONSTRUCTION

The rib is trimmed and a temporalis interposition graft placed prior to rib fixation with the cartilage portion in the glenoid fossa (Figure 8.3.8). The rib is held with either cortical screws or plates to the lateral border of the ramus in the desired position (Figure 8.3.9). The lateral aspect of the mandible may be preprepared to enable direct fixation of the rib to cancellous bone, permitting a more accurate fit. The wound is closed in layers over suction drainage with deep resorbable and interrupted monofilamaent to the skin.

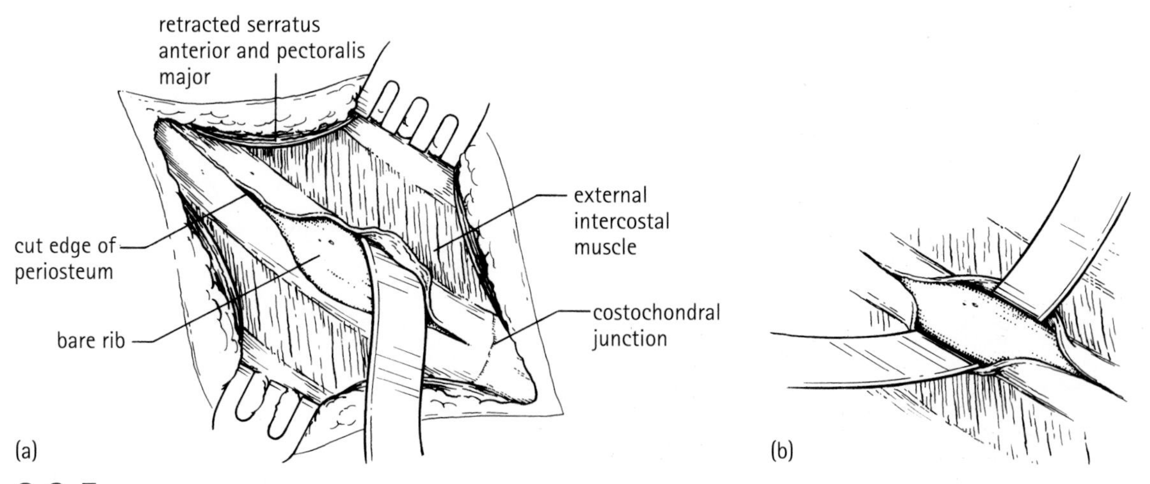

8.3.5 Subperiosteal dissection of the rib towards the costochondral junction with retraction of the pleura on the deep surface.

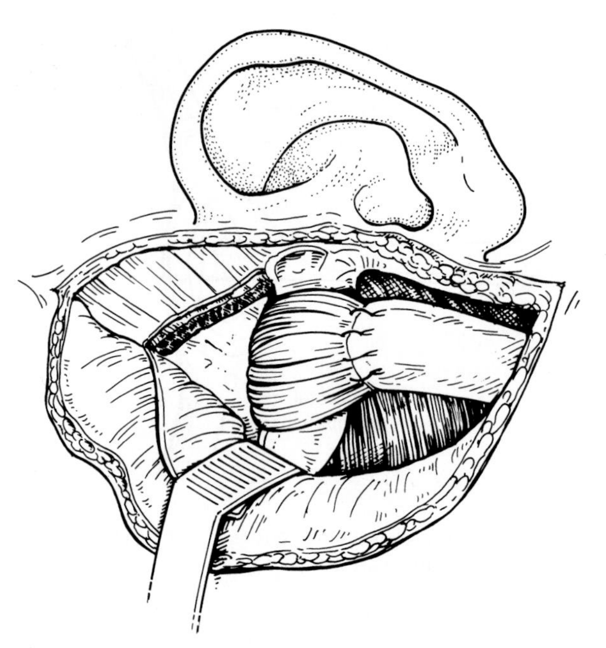

8.3.8 The costochondral graft in situe with temporalis interposition.

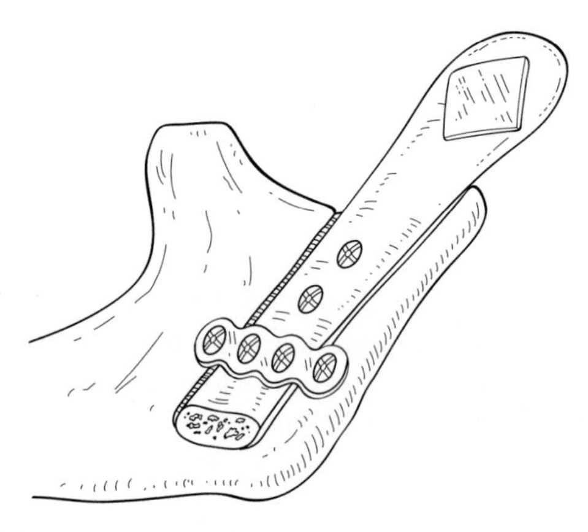

8.3.9 The costochondral graft is secured to the mandible with miniplate and or cortical screws.

Top tips

- Ankylosis of the TMJ is an uncommon problem in the Western world and should only be dealt with by a surgeon with experience in this area. The surgeon should have experience of the various approaches and methods of reconstruction and access to a neurosurgeon.
- Rapid access to the joint is facilitated by the pretemporal fascial dissection approach.
- Always group and save these patients as blood loss can be sudden and catastrophic.
- Ensure adequate mobilization post-operatively by use of the Therabite device.

8.4

Total prosthetic replacement of the temporomandibular joint

ANDREW J SIDEBOTTOM, ROBERT HENSHER

PROSTHESES IN COMMON USE

Total replacement of the temporomandibular joint (TMJ) has been an option since the nineteenth century, but the recent prosthetic choices arose following the development of the Christensen prosthesis in 1963. Initially, these were individually made prostheses of cobalt–chromium alloy fossa and ramus component with an acrylic condylar cap. Subsequently, this prosthesis was standardized and remained one of the prostheses of choice until the conversion of the condylar cap to an all cobalt–chromium condylar component in 1997, to give a metal-on-metal prosthesis. This latter is one of three currently available on the UK market and is used as either a stock or custom-made prosthesis. The stock prosthesis has three choices of condylar prosthesis length and 32 choices per side of fossa component (see Figure 8.4.1–8.4.3). The best fit of fossa component is used via the use of trial fossae. Clearly, this requires a large selection of alternative prostheses and surgical experience to guide in this choice. Even the best fit may require fossa modification and may have some mobility after screw fixation. Some surgeons carry out just hemi-arthoplasty with the fossa component as an alternative to discectomy and interposition graft. The longer term outcomes of this procedure have been questioned as a significant number require subsequent conversion to total joint replacement and the authors have abandoned this technique although others still find it a successful alternative.

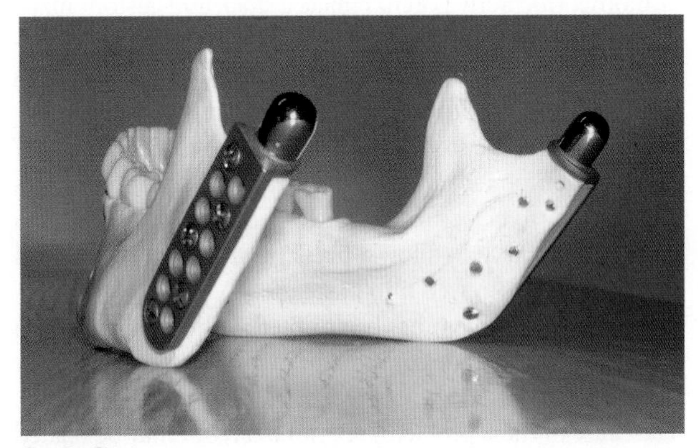

8.4.2 Fit of the Christensen condylar component to the mandible.

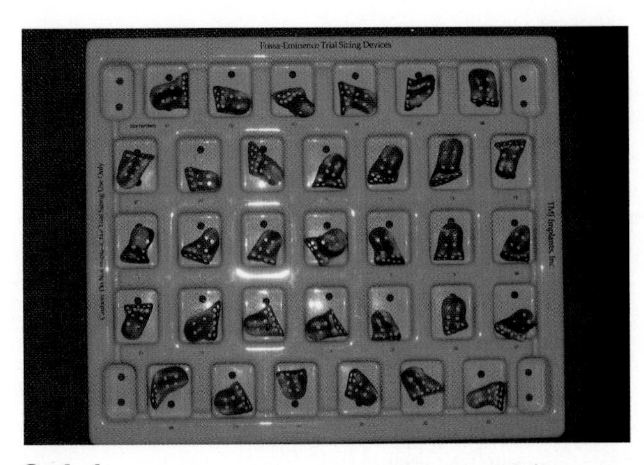

8.4.1 Selection of fossa components of the Christensen system.

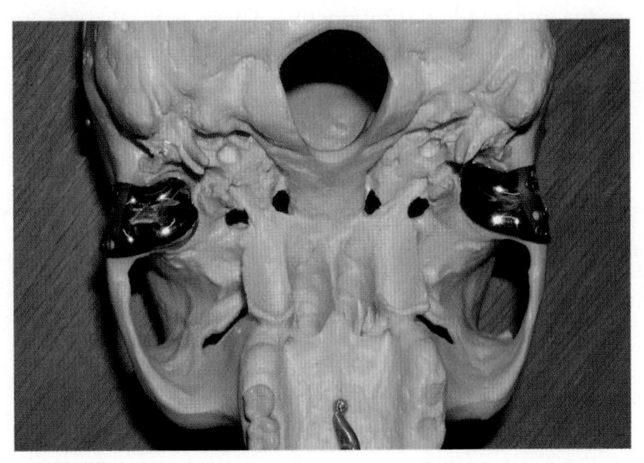

8.4.3 Fit of the Christensen fossa component to the base of the skull.

During the 1970s, the Kent prosthesis (VK I) came into and went out of vogue due to the reaction of the proplast component (which was on the fitting surface of the prosthesis) of this prosthesis to the surrounding tissues, causing destructive osteolysis and making revision of these prostheses extremely difficult. The adjusted VK II prosthesis, although successful, was withdrawn due to the litigation associated with its predecessor.

Techmedica developed a titanium ramus prosthesis with a cobalt–chromium condylar head and a titanium-based high molecular weight polyethylene fossa in 1989. This company was taken over and the prosthesis is now made by TMJ Concepts (Ventura, CA, USA). This is a custom-made prosthesis and is currently the authors' first choice of prosthesis. It requires a Protomed 3-D CT scan to create a CAD-CAM model on which the surgical cuts are determined and the prosthesis is subsequently made (the technique of construction can be seen from the case series illustrated). In patients with nickel, cobalt or chromium allergy, an all titanium condylar component can be constructed although the wear characteristics of a hardened titanium surface are less certain than cobalt chromium alloy. The prosthetic fit is superior with a custom-made prosthesis compared with a stock prosthesis and therefore less mobility in theory should lead to better success rates based on simple orthopaedic principles.

Biomet (formerly Lorenz) make a stock and custom made prosthesis with similar components to the Concepts system. The main difference is that the fossa component is all high molecular weight polyethylene without the titanium mesh fitting surface. The stock prosthesis has five choices of size of condylar component and three fossa sizes. The fossa requires eminectomy to be performed with specially designed burs to flatten the surface to allow a press fit of the prosthesis and permit it to be screwed into place.

Recently, a problem has been noted with metal-on-metal prostheses with a glide component in both orthopaedic knee implants and latterly with the Christensen metal-on-metal. The cause of these problems are not clear, but may be related to implant allergy at the time of placement or its development during implant wear. Around 10 per cent of the general population are nickel allergic with less than 1 per cent allergic to the other alloy components. There may also be an immune-mediated response to wear debris. Approximately 10 per cent of metal-on-metal TMJ prostheses in a UK series have failed and been found to have a giant cell foreign body reaction surrounding them. For this reason, the authors suggest all patients are at least patch tested for allergy to nickel, cobalt, chromium and molybdenum individually and if necessary proceeding to subdermal implantation of a prosthetic sample in the forearm skin prior to recommending a cobalt–chromium alloy-based prosthesis.

CHOICE OF PROSTHESIS

Prosthetic choice depends on indications, presumed benefits, personal preference and cost. While there are good long-term outcome studies for both the Christensen and Concepts prosthesis (90 per cent or more long-term survival), these studies should be taken in the light of studies involving orthopaedic implants. The long-term Christensen studies utilized the acrylic condylar head, which has now been discontinued due to excessive wear leading to anterior open bite formation after 15–20 years. These studies cannot be correlated with the newer metal-on-metal Christensen introduced in the late 1990s. Likewise, although the outcomes for the custom-made Concepts prosthesis are even more impressive, they only extend to 17 years. The outcomes for total knee replacement are similar at 15 years, but deteriorate from 20 years due to wear and it remains to be seen whether this will also be the case for the metal on high molecular weight polyethylene TMJ prostheses (Concepts and Lorenz). Patients should be warned of the possibility of long-term failure and for this reason prosthetic replacement should only be considered as a last resort and should only be used by high volume surgeons aware of the complications of insertion in order to give the best possible outcomes. Revision surgery carries more significant risk of morbidity, particularly related to the facial nerve, and certainly should only be contemplated by an experienced surgeon. TMJ replacement is not for the occasional surgeon.

INDICATIONS AND CONTRAINDICATIONS

The indications and contraindications for total replacement of the TMJ have recently been published by a UK consensus study group and can be seen in Tables 8.4.1, 8.4.2 and 8.4.3. These guidelines have now been accepted by NICE. The indications for surgery are more stringent than for an orthopaedic total joint replacement (Table 8.4.1). It is essential, prior to consideration of prosthetic replacement, that an appropriate trial of conservative management (including arthroscopy if possible) has been attempted and failed. Diagnosis of condylar disease should be made with the aid of CT or magnetic resonance (MR) scan as a

Table 8.4.1 Indications for total prosthetic replacement of the temporomandibular joint.

Disease processes (involving condylar bone loss)
Degenerative joint disease/osteoarthrosis
Inflammatory joint disease (rheumatoid, ankylosing spondylitis, psoriatic)
Ankylosis
Post-traumatic condylar loss/damage
Post-surgical condylar loss (including neoplastic ablation)
Previous prosthetic reconstruction
Previous costochondral graft
Major congenital deformity
Multiple previous procedures

Table 8.4.2 Clinical indicators for total prosthetic replacement of the temporomandibular joint.

A combination of the following:
Dietary score of <5/10 (liquid scores 0, full diet scores 10)
Restricted mouth opening (<35 mm)
Occlusal collapse/anterior open bite/retrusion
Excessive condylar resorption and loss of vertical ramus height
Pain score >5 out of 10 on visual analogue (in combination with any of the above)
Quality of life issues other than above

Table 8.4.3 Contraindications to total prosthetic replacement of the temporomandibular joint.

Contraindications
Ongoing local infective process
Severe immune compromise
Severe ASA 3 disease processes (relative)

minimum (not just plain radiographs). CT scan is preferable as it shows the bony anatomy in more detail and is required using a Protomed protocol (three-dimensional) if a custom-made prosthesis is to be constructed.

The clinical indicators (Table 8.4.2) give an idea of the severity of disability of the patient (similar to walking distance for total hip replacement) and also permit assessment of outcome following the procedure. Contraindications are rare (Table 8.4.3), but include severe local infective process or radiation reaction or associated severe immune compromise. These are relative, however, as most rheumatoid patients are on disease-modifying drugs, and with appropriate short-term adjustment of medication, prosthetic replacement can be safely carried out with minimal added risk.

Dental status should be checked pre-operatively and any teeth restored with compromised teeth being removed. Post-operative dental infection risks prosthetic biofilm infection with the required removal of the prosthesis. Revision surgery carries a significant increase in morbidity in addition to the cost of around US$10 000 (£6300) per prosthesis. Any post-operative dental infection should be dealt with aggressively, preferably with extraction. Prophylactic antibiotics are recommended according to the American Association of Orthopedics guidelines for invasive dental procedures for the two years following prosthetic insertion.

SURGICAL TECHNIQUE

Intravenous antibiotic prophylaxis (aimed at skin commensals) should be given on induction and planned for 24 hours intravenously with 5 days orally. Catheterization will aid in fluid monitoring, but may be removed at the end of the procedure.

The standard preauricular and retromandibular approaches to the TMJ are adopted. The patient is anaesthetized with a centreline tube extending over the vertex of the head. Arch bars are placed and the operating field around the mouth kept totally free from contaminating the operating field of the prosthetic replacement. The mouth is covered by the OpSite® free ends and local analgesic with epinephrine (adrenaline) infiltrated into the preauricular and retromandibular incision sites. The joint is exposed as described in Chapter 8.3 from below and above. The required condylectomy is carried out from below and the soft tissues of the capsule, disc and periosteum dissected gently with copious diathermy to maintain a blood-free field, while trying not to extend the dissection too far medially where the maxillary, middle meningeal and masseteric vessels and the mandibular division of the trigeminal lie within a few millimetres. It is essential that all disc and capsular tissue is removed to provide sufficient space for the prosthesis. Residual disc tissue, in particular, may interfere with prosthetic function and the disc can be removed most safely with the aid of diathermy and subsequent scissor freeing from the lateral pterygoid, which tends to ooze if just cut.

Once the fossa is completely cleared, the prosthetic fossa is tried in place. The fossa is irrigated with gentamicin-containing saline and the fit of the prosthesis checked and if necessary the bony fossa adjusted if there is any movement. The different types of prosthesis require slightly different techniques at this stage and will not be further described. The following will be a description of the technique of placement of a custom-made prosthesis.

The fit of the fossa is confirmed. The patient is placed in intermaxillary fixation to the desired occlusion and then all gowns and gloves are changed and the instruments for the intraoral procedure kept totally separate. The fossa is again trialled to ensure that adequate condyle and coronoid have been removed to enable free fitting of the fossa and rotation of the condylar component on mouth opening. There should be at least a 5 mm gap between the prosthetic fossa margin and the condylar stump. The cavity is again irrigated with gentamicin solution and the fossa fitted and secured, usually with three to four screws into the zygomatic arch.

The lower incision is now entered and the fit of the condylar component checked. It may be necessary to smooth down the lateral border of the mandible according to the pre-operative planning on the CT model. This has usually been necessary at the mandibular gonial angle, due to eversion of the bone tissues in this area at the lower attachment of the masseter. Once the fit to the lateral border has been confirmed, the fit into the fossa component is confirmed. This should match that seen on the prosthesis on the model (see Figure 8.4.4). Usually it lies about one-half to two-thirds of the way into the fossa. If the head lies too superficial to this, it suggests that insufficient condylar neck has been removed and this can be confirmed by direct vision and usually the prosthesis will move in the superoinferior plane. If necessary, more of the condylar neck

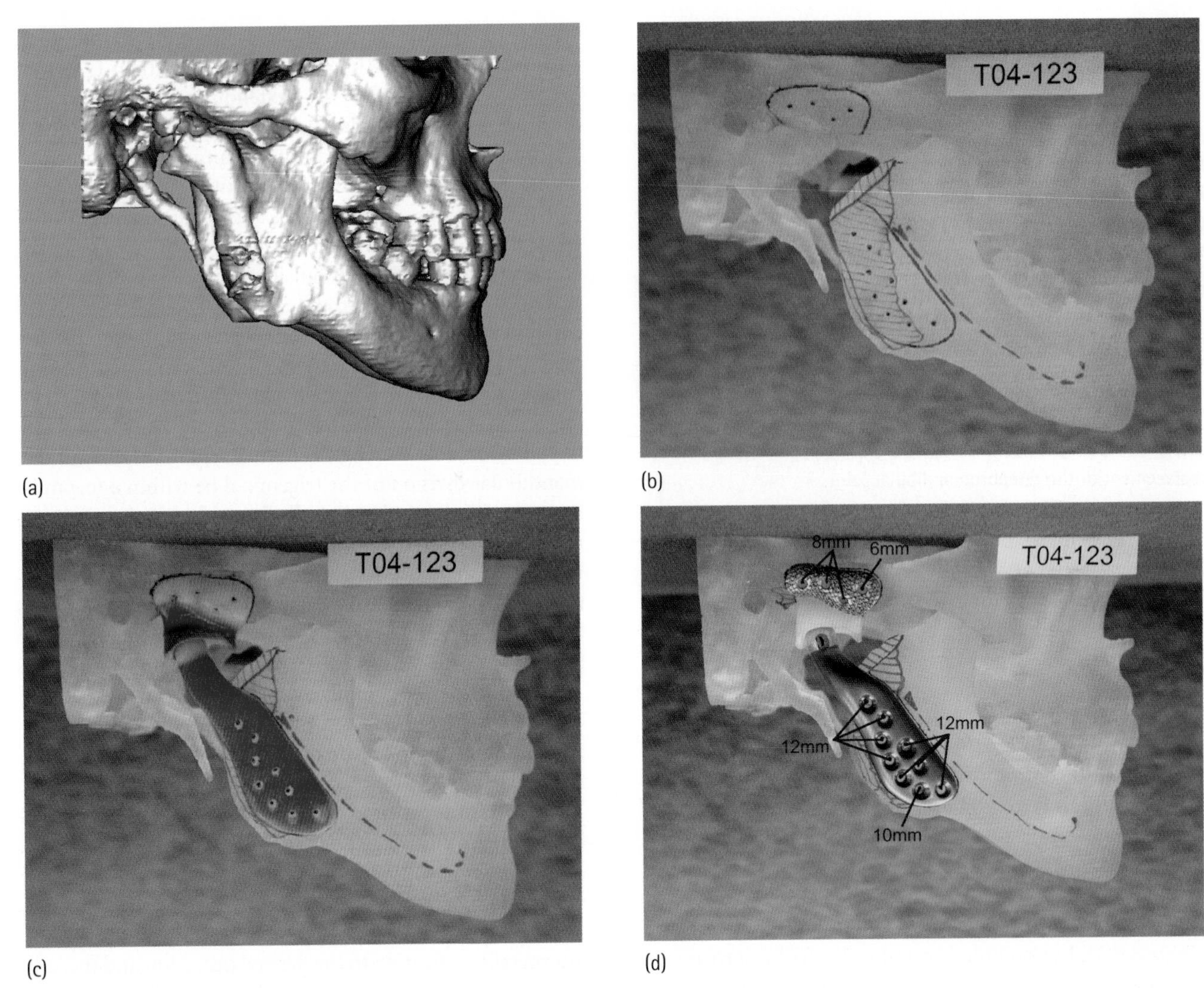

8.4.4 (a) Three dimensional CT pre-total prosthetic replacement of the temporomandibular joint; (b) model post-surgical adaptation; (c) model with waxed implant; (d) model with fine implant.

can be removed with extreme care not to damage the *in situ* fossa prosthesis. If necessary, this should be removed prior to further bone removal.

Once the fit of the condylar prosthesis is confirmed, this is secured initially with three screws to the length marked on the diagrams supplied by the company. The IMF is removed and the occlusion is checked. If this is not correct the prosthesis requires adjustment. Once the position and occlusion are correct the remaining screws should be inserted using copious irrigation. At least six screws should be used with the most important being the most proximal to the condylar stump. Movement of the prosthesis should now be checked in function. If there is dislocation then light IMF elastics will be required post-operatively for 1 week until the vertical stability is re-established. This can occur following previous coronoidectomy or with closure of anterior open bites, where the vertical pull of the temporalis has been reduced. Once the occlusion is satisfactory again, gown and gloves contaminated intraorally are changed. The fit and movement of the condyle within the fossa are checked and the wound is irrigated with gentamicin solution. If all is satisfactory, the wounds can then be closed.

The authors prefer a single 12-suction drain introduced through the upper wound extending over the prosthesis into the lower wound subperiosteally as this covers all the areas of potential wound leakage. This is secured behind the ear with black silk and is usually removed on the first post-operative day. At this stage the abdominal fat graft is placed if desired (see Chapter 8.3 Treatment of temporomandibular joint ankylosis). The upper wound is closed with continuous resorbable sutures (vicryl or PDS) to the temporalis fascia and periosteum to cover the joint, but ensuring that the drain is not inadvertently held too tightly into the wound. The subcutaneous tissues are then closed with interrupted vicryl to bring the wound edges together, and the skin is brought together with 6/0 monofilament. The lower wound is closed with continuous vicryl to the parotid fascia and subcutaneous tissues. This avoids involving the branches of the facial nerve in the closure. Monofilament is used to close the skin.

If there has been no dislocation intraoperatively, then the arch bars can be removed and the patient recovered. Antibiotics should be continued intravenously for 24 hours, then for 5 days orally. The authors prefer the patient to have low-dose non-steroidal anti-inflammatory drugs (NSAIDs) for 6 weeks as there is some evidence of a reduction in heterotopic bone formation in orthopaedics and this may reduce the likelihood of reankylosis. In any case, they provide good analgesic properties suitable to this form of surgery. Therabite passive mobilization should be commenced on the first post-operative day and continue for at least six months along the minimum recommended protocol of 7 seconds opening seven times, at least seven times a day, initially aiming to improve opening by 1–2 mm/day. The opening at the start of the day will have declined compared with the night before, so the measurements should be taken at the same time every day. Most primary joint replacement patients should achieve opening of above 30 mm within 6 weeks and the pain scores diminish rapidly towards zero.

Post-operative stay is between 48–72 hours in most instances. The patients should be advised according to the American Society of Orthopaedics guidelines to have prophylactic antibiotics prior to invasive dental surgery for two years following prosthetic insertion. The authors have had one prosthetic failure secondary to a dental infection occurring within 1 week of surgery, so pre-operative dental status should be ensured. Drains are removed at 24–48 hours and sutures are removed at 5–7 days.

All patient details should be entered into a database for long-term assessment of outcome and for comparison of outcomes of prostheses within a national/international database when available. The companies monitor failures as a requirement for the US Food and Drug Administration.

COMPLICATIONS

These may be divided into peri-operative and post-operative.

Haemorrhage

Peri-operative complications include haemorrhage. This can occur from the retromandibular vein behind the ramus, the superficial temporal vessels, the masseteric vessels deep to the sigmoid notch/condylar periosteum, the pterygoid venous plexus or occasionally deeper vessels medial to the condyle, such as the middle meningeal and even the internal jugular, which can be in close proximity either with a large ankylotic mass or following contracture due to previous surgeries. It is often difficult to control haemorrhage through the 1×1 cm wound that is the defect following condylectomy, hence the best method of control of haemorrhage is prevention by a careful technique. Blood should have been grouped and saved as transfusion is occasionally required. Usually, the haemorrhage can be temporarily controlled by pressure. The former sites are definitively controlled in the usual manner of ligation or diathermy, paying attention to the position of the facial nerve branches. Occasionally, more proximal ligation of the external carotid or jugular may be required and these can be accessed by a suitable extension of the retromandibular wound. Drainage of the wound will show any late reopening of vessels due to the hypotensive anaesthesia being reversed and the blood pressure should be permitted to rise before wound closure.

Dislocation

Dislocation of the prosthesis is rare and usually associated with previous coronoidectomy reducing vertical stability of the joint. Occasionally, closure of an open bite will cause a similar effect. If this occurs intraoperatively, then the arch bars should be left *in situ* and light IMF elastic used to control inadvertent wide opening for 1 week. By the end of 1 week, sufficient vertical stability has been regained. Post-operative dislocation may also be due to joint malpositioning. The patient should be returned to theatre to check the occlusion. If this is stable following relocation, which often occurs with inferiorly directed light pressure, then a means of obtaining IMF should be achieved and the patient placed in light elastics for 1 week. The wounds should only be opened as a last resort as this will markedly increase the risk of infection. If the prosthesis is malpositioned, then immediate revision may be the only option.

Facial nerve injury

Facial nerve palsies are common post-operatively, particularly in the temporal branch and especially following revision surgery. They are usually temporary due to stretching of the tissues to gain adequate access for placement of the prosthesis. Permanent palsies can be dealt with by brow lift and other cosmetic procedures.

Infection

Infection of any prosthesis is often staphylococcal and occasionally *Acinetobacter*-related and appropriate prophylactic antibiotics should be used. The authors recommend prophylaxis following invasive procedures causing bacteraemia similar to those for bacterial endocarditis prevention for two years post-operatively according to the American Association of Orthopedic Surgeons guidelines. Infection may present with obvious signs of redness and drainage of pus from the wounds. Prosthetic removal is almost inevitable and should be followed by a period of occlusal stabilization with a gentamicin-containing acrylic spacer.

Biofilm formation, whereby colonies of bacteria are covered by an almost impermeable polysaccharide membrane, may present more insidiously with ongoing pain and restriction, but with no other clinical or haematological signs of infection. Antibiotics cannot penetrate the biofilm and prosthetic removal, as above, is indicated.

Allergy

Allergy to the prosthetic material has recently been reported. Prevention by appropriate allergy testing pre-operatively may reduce this phenomenon, although there is a suggestion that patients with failing prosthetic hip replacements develop allergy. While most orthopedic patients are not tested for metal allergy, these findings cannot be confirmed; however, approximately 10 per cent of the population are allergic to one or more component of cobalt–chromium alloy (usually nickel), while 20 per cent of those with a functioning prosthetic hip are allergic, as are 60 per cent with a failing prosthesis. Other factors may be involved, however. Where allergy is suspected, the ongoing swelling may lead to traction facial nerve palsy and the prosthesis requires removal and ultimate revision to an all-titanium prosthesis.

Long-term complications are rare and the majority of patients gain significant improvements (80–90 per cent) in pain scores, dietary scores and mouth opening, which persist for more than ten years.

Prosthetic replacement has a growing place in the management of disorders of the TMJ, but should be confined at present to a few high volume operators to adequately assess outcomes.

POST-OPERATIVE CARE

The patient is transferred back to the ward for routine post-operative monitoring. If a chest drain was necessary this should be removed if possible the day post-operatively and a check chest radiograph should be obtained in all cases to exclude pneumothorax or haemothorax. Wound drains are removed on day one post-operatively and antibiotics can be discontinued after 24 hours.

The joint should be gently mobilised, bearing in mind that the bony surfaces will not be united for up to 8 weeks post-operatively, but also that the ankylotic process will have been induced by the bony resections.

Long term review for reankylosis or growth disturbance is necessary until adulthood when an assessment should be made regarding whether revision to a total alloplastic joint should be performed.

Complications

Early complications include pneumothorax and haemothorax and should be excluded by clinical examination of the chest and radiography. If present they should be managed appropriately with a chest drain if required.

Wound haemorrhage should be controlled locally with pressure and diathermy or ligation of the vessel. It is not unknown for the ankylotic mass to have encapsulated the maxillary or other vessels and control of these may be necessary via the neck. Exposure of the external carotid artery and ligation of the terminal maxillary branch should be within the competences of any TMJ replacement surgeon.

Long term only about one third of the costochondral grafts provide a satisfactory outcome. The remainder either re-ankylose, collapse and fail to grow or overgrow producing a condylar hyperplasia type picture. These require revision according to the age of the patient but preferably with an alloplastic joint replacement at cessation of growth.

PART 9

CLEFT LIP AND PALATE

9.1

Primary closure of unilateral cleft lip

CHRIS PENFOLD

PRINCIPLES

There is still controversy about the best way to repair a cleft lip. There is general agreement about the importance of muscle reconstruction and the fact that surgical scarring can be detrimental to facial growth. Opinion differs, however, on how best to achieve the former and avoid the latter.

In the past, attempts at restoration of nasal form and function were usually delayed until the age of 12 years to reduce the risk of growth impairment. Recognition of the importance of nasal breathing and the intimate relationship between form, function and growth of the nose and lip has encouraged an earlier radical approach to nasal repair which is now often attempted at the time of primary lip repair.

Traditional methods of lip repair focused on achieving balanced length and proportion of lip skin and vermillion and the production of a symmetrical 'cupid's bow' by the transposition of skin flaps. Various flaps involving rotation, advancement and triangular designs have been used in the repair of unilateral cleft lip. The most popular is the rotation advancement technique first described by Millard in 1976 (Figure 9.1.1). Numerous modifications of Millard's original design have since been proposed including measures to lengthen the columella and reduce scarring across the columella base. Delaire has described a design that respects the anatomical boundaries between the lip and nasal skin and avoids crossing aesthetically sensitive areas, such as the columella base and alar rim (Figure 9.1.2). Although this incision in itself has little facility to lengthen the lip, the incorporation of wavy lines and small triangular flaps above the vermillion allow some degree of lengthening. Delaire emphasizes the important contribution that the restoration of labiomaxillary muscle function makes towards achieving satisfactory lip length and aesthetics and considers this to be as important as geometric arrangement of skin flaps.

The author's technique of primary repair of the unilateral cleft lip is based on the principles described by Delaire and incorporates some modifications described by Talmant. The method of repair recognizes the major role played by abnor-

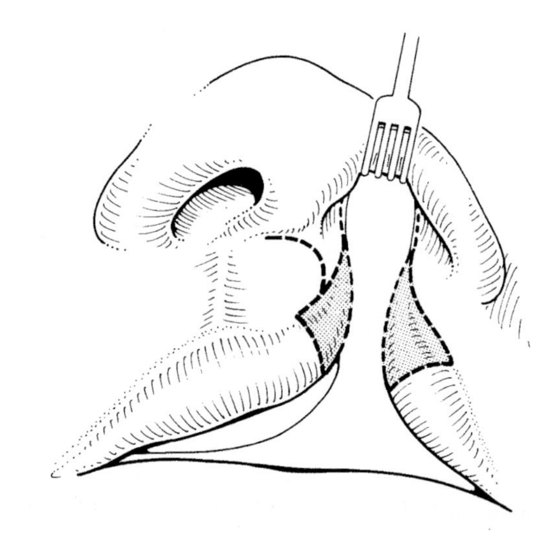

9.1.1 Outline for Millard incision.

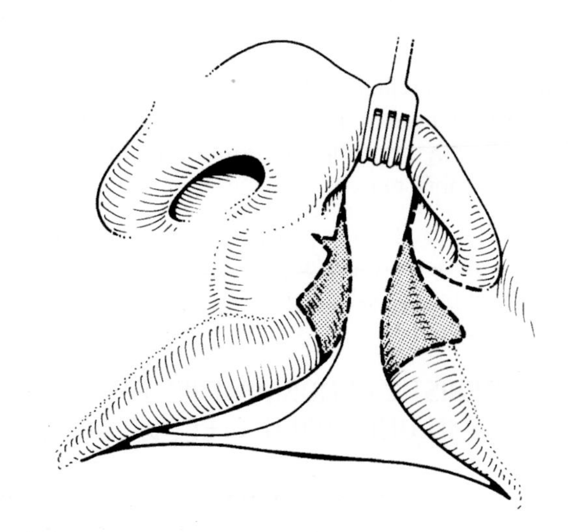

9.1.2 Outline for incision (based on Delaire).

mal muscle anatomy in defining the nature of the cleft deformity, in particular the effect that abnormal muscle function has on the growth and development of the nasal septum and the premaxilla. An understanding of normal facial muscle anatomy, as well as cleft muscle pathology, is therefore fundamental to achieving optimal outcomes in cleft lip repair.

NORMAL MUSCLE ANATOMY

There are a series of three interconnected muscle rings extending from the infraorbital rim and nose down to the chin and these rings form part of the fascial envelope in continuity with the SMAS (Figure 9.1.3). Although there is some controversy as to the exact nature of the inferior origin and insertion of the transverse nasalis muscle, some general observations from the perspective of cleft lip repair are apparent:

- The convergence of the upper and lower rings towards the anterior nasal spine (ANS) and nasal septum.
- The transverse nasalis muscle intermingles with the levator labii superioris and levator labii superioris aleque nasi as it turns around the lateral border of the ala cartilage to form a modiolus that fans out to insert into the nasal sill. It influences the shape and position of the ala cartilage and the height of the nasal sill. It then continues medially and mingles with the incisivus or myrtiformis muscle, which arises from the incisive fossa to insert into the ANS and nasal septum. The effect of this association is to prevent the nasalis muscle from lifting the nasal sill as it turns around the base of the nasal ala.
- The significance of the almost vertical orientation of the external or superficial part of the orbicularis oris and its connections with the muscles of the upper ring and with the lower ring through the modiolus. A major component of this muscle runs obliquely from the modiolus to the nasal septum.
- The four components of the medium septal system (MSS):
  - cartilagenous nasal septum;
  - Latham's ligament (which unites the septum to the premaxilla);
  - the medium cellular septum (which extends from the median frenum to the septal cartilage and unites the dermis with the median suture of the premaxilla);
  - the nasolabial muscles.

The MSS transmits to the premaxilla traction forces from both the anterior growth of the nasal septum and the movement of the nasolabial muscles.

CHARACTERISTIC ABNORMALITIES OF THE LIP AND NOSE IN UNILATERAL CLEFT LIP AND PALATE

In the unilateral cleft lip and palate, the upper and middle muscle rings are incomplete. All the muscle groups on the cleft side, which normally insert on to the ANS, septum and anterior surface of the premaxilla, become bunched up at the border of the cleft. The abnormal muscle function produces characteristic nasal and mucocutaneous abnormalities which have to be addressed at the time of primary lip repair.

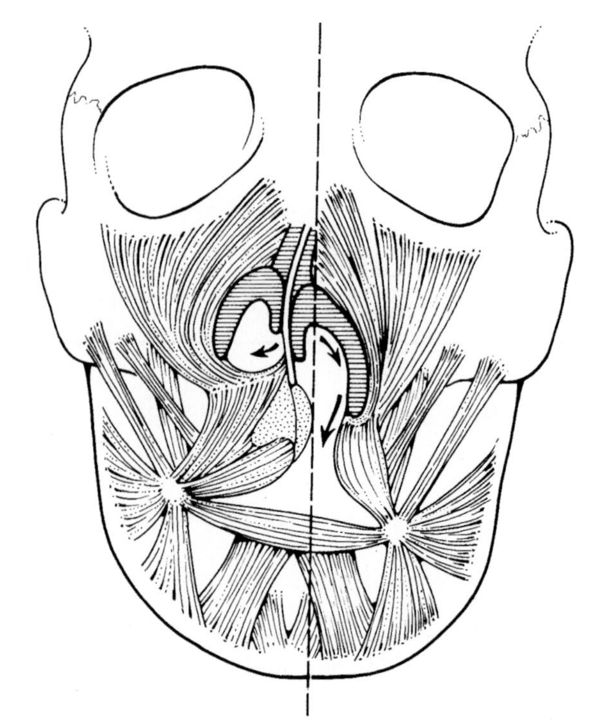

9.1.3 Nasolabial musculature in cleft lip.

Nasal abnormalities

The anterior nasal septum and columella are deviated to the cleft side.

The alar cartilage is deformed, but is not hypoplastic. Its lateral crus is pulled laterally and lengthened at the expense of the medial crus thereby flattening the dome on the cleft side. Its inferior border is also rotated posteriorly forming a web inside the nostril.

Mucocutaneous abnormalities

A detailed analysis of the skin around the cleft lip deformity shows that it is both retracted and displaced (Figure 9.1.4). The skin of the nasal floor is thin and hairless, and quite different from lip skin. It is pulled down into the upper part of the lip. On the lateral side of the cleft, the boundary between lip and nasal skin is represented by a perpendicular line extending from the mucocutaneous junction to point F at the base of the nasal ala (Figure 9.1.5). On the medial side, the boundary between lip and nasal skin is represented by the line 1–2 (Figure 9.1.5).

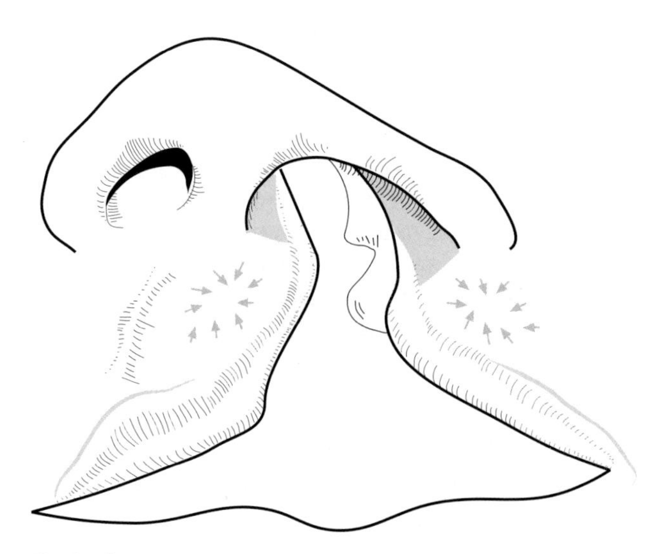

9.1.4 Skin abnormalities in unilateral cleft lip.

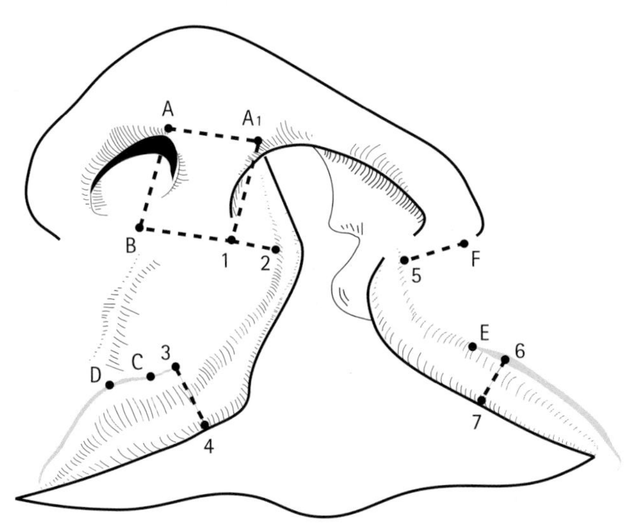

9.1.5 Identification of landmarks and skin markings for incision design (see text).

PRIMARY REPAIR OF UNILATERAL CLEFT LIP

Timing of surgery

Unilateral cleft lip repair is normally carried out between four and five months of age.

Pre-operative preparation

A single dose of a broad spectrum antibiotic, such as amoxycillin and clavulinic acid, is administered at the time of anaesthetic induction. The eyelids are closed with an adhesive protector.

Positioning

The patient is positioned on a paediatric surgical table with support under the shoulder to allow a degree of neck extension. The anaesthetic tube exits from the midline of the mouth in a caudal direction. This allows the surgeon to operate from a sitting position at the head of the table.

Skin preparation and markings

The skin of the face and oral mucosa is cleaned with an iodine-based antiseptic preparation.

The iodine skin preparation colours the skin and facilitates identification of the white roll.

The skin markings denoted by letters are identified by anatomical features from which the numerical markings are extrapolated. They can be considered in four groups:

I. Columella and noncleft side lip/nose junction – A, A1, B, 1 and 2;
II. Cupid's bow – C, D, 3 and 4;
III. Cleft side white roll – E, 6 and 7;
IV. Cleft side lip/nose boundary – F and 5;
A. Superior internal angle of the noncleft nostril;
A1. Superior internal angle of the cleft nostril;
B. Base of the columella on the noncleft side;
C. Base of the cupid's bow (in some clefts the bow is shallow and has to be approximated once the peak has been identified);
D. Peak of the cupid's bow on the noncleft side;
E. Point on the mucocutaneous junction on the cleft side where the white roll has completely faded;
F. Lateral and inferior pole of the alar base on the cleft side;
(1) Point at the base of the columella on the cleft side, which is established by extending a line from B parallel to A–A1, so that the lengths A–1 = A–B. It is important to spend some time establishing the points A, A1 and B so that the resulting rectangle A, A1 B, 1 outlines a symmetrical columella and so that B1 represents the junction of the columella with the philtrum. The use of a gentle traction to the roof of the nostrils with skin hooks helps in the identification of these landmarks.
(2) Point on the mucocutaneous junction established by extension of the line B1 (this marks the boundary between lip and nasal skin on the medial side of the cleft);
(3) Point on the mucocutaneous junction which establishes the peak of the cupid's bow on the noncleft side, so that C–3 is slightly less (by 0.5–1 mm) than C–D (this allows for some distension of the skin after muscle repair).
(4) Point on the junction between the dry and moist mucosa of the lip determined from a perpendicular line extended from the mucocutaneous junction;
(5) Point on the mucocutaneous junction determined by a perpendicular line that extends from the mucocutaneous

junction to F (this line represents the junction between nasal skin and labial skin);
(6) Point where the white roll begins to fade (usually 2–3 mm lateral to 'E').
(7) Point on the junction between the dry and moist mucosa of the lip determined from a perpendicular line extended from the white roll at '6'.

Incisions

Respect for the boundaries between nasal and lip skin in the design of skin incisions avoids transposition of nasal skin on to the lip. It is also important to note that incisions do not cross aesthetic boundaries, such as the columella base. Although the Delaire approach to cleft lip repair emphasizes the role of muscle function in determining the length of the repaired cleft lip, it is still necessary to establish balance between the lateral and medial lip heights and to create a symmetrical cupid's bow at the time of surgery. Before the incisions are made, it is advisable to check the relationship between length 2–3 on the medial side and length 5–6 on the lateral side of the cleft. It is usual for length 2–3 to be slightly shorter by no more than 1–2 mm than 5–6. The incorporation of a wavy line into the incision on both the medial and lateral incisions together with a small triangular flap will restore vertical balance and help establish a symmetrical cupid's bow at the end of the repair.

Incisions are now made using the 'numbered' landmarks as follows (Figure 9.1.6).

MEDIAL SIDE

Starting on the medial side an incision is made through skin only which begins in the floor of the nose at its junction with the nasal septum and runs parallel to the mucocutaneous junction (keeping on the skin side) to point 2. The incision is then continued to point 1 and then back along the skin side of the mucocutaneous junction to point 3. A double curve is incorporated into the incision as shown in Figure 9.1.6. The incision continues perpendicularly across the vermillion to point 4 and then along the junction between the dry and moist mucosa joining the line of the first incision as it enters the floor of the nose. The skin and mucosa outlined by these incisions is then discarded. Finally, a 2–3 mm long incision is made parallel and just above the white roll extending to a point directly above point C (the trough of cupid's bow). This is designed to accept a triangular flap from the lateral element. The marginal skin and mucosa is then undermined for 2–3 mm.

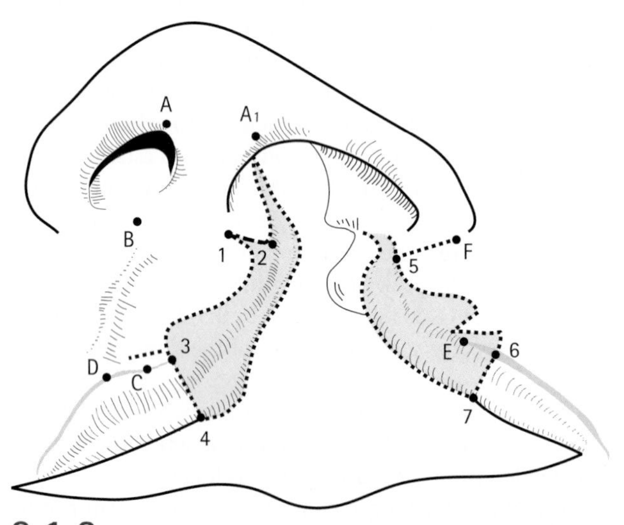

9.1.6 Incision design.

LATERAL SIDE

The incision through the skin starts posteriorly at the junction of the vestibular skin and oral mucosa at the pyriform rim (Figure 9.1.6). It runs parallel to the mucocutaneous junction (keeping on the skin side) and includes points 5, E and 6. A small curve incorporating a triangular flap is included at the inferior end of the incision. An incision is then made extending superiorly from point 7 along the junction between the dry and moist mucosa. This incision is continued into the labial sulcus up to the alveolus (Figure 9.1.6). A full thickness incision is then made through the skin and muscle from F to 5. This incision demarcates the nasal skin from the lip skin. The skin and mucosa outlined by these incisions is then elevated as a lateral vermillion flap, taking care to preserve the small pedicle at the base of the labial sulcus. This lateral vermillion flap is carefully conserved and extended towards the fornix of the labial sulcus as a modified Muir flap. This flap is available to fill in a defect created by a releasing incision made along the pyriform rim just anterior to the inferior turbinate (see below under Subperiosteal undermining).

Nasal cartilage undermining

A pair of curved tenotomy scissors is inserted between the skin and muscle through incision F–5 and, using a combination of blunt and sharp dissection, the nasal vestibular skin is freed from the ala cartilage up to and including the dome (Figure 9.1.7).

The same scissors are then inserted through incision 1–2 up between the medial crura of the ala cartilages up to the apex of the alar dome on each side (Figure 9.1.8). The scissors are then passed between the medial crura of the ala cartilages and the anterior border of the nasal septum. They are passed up between the skin and medial crura to the apex of the domes of the ala cartilage on both sides. No attempt is made to free the lateral crura of the ala cartilages from the overlying skin. Only the vestibular skin component is freed from the lateral crus on the cleft side.

The lower border of the nasal septum is then approached at its junction with the anterior nasal spine. The tenotomy scissors are used to dissect the perichondrium off the anterior border of the septum. The mucoperichondrium is then undermined from the cleft side of the cartilagenous septum using the scissors together with a Freer elevator. The

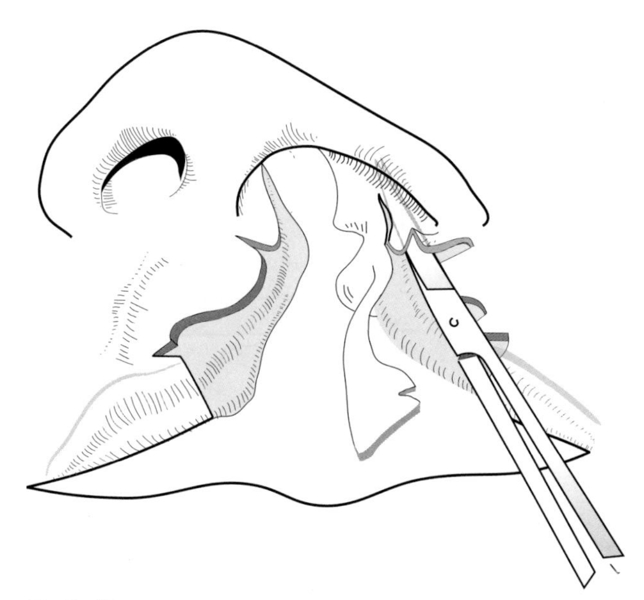

9.1.7 Dissection of lateral crus of ala cartilage.

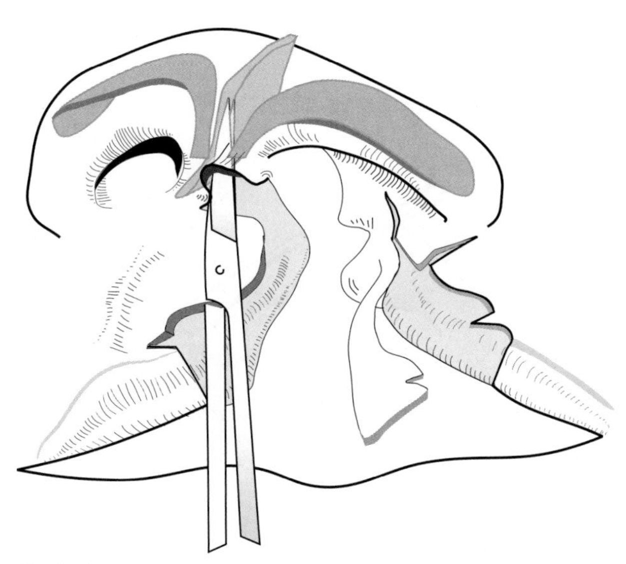

9.1.8 Dissection of medial crus of ala cartilage and septum.

nasal septum is deflected and usually curled towards the cleft and great care is needed to free the perichondrium from the anterior edge of the curled up septum. The undermining is continued up to the vomer superiorly and anteriorly past the junction of the septum and the upper lateral cartilage to join with the pocket previously formed by undermining the vestibular mucosa from the ala cartilage. An envelope of freed perichondrium and mucosa is thus created extending medially from the base of the septum to the lateral pole of the ala cartilage.

The perichondrium on the noncleft side of the septum is then elevated for a distance of 5 mm posteriorly, allowing the curled up anterior part of the septum to be straightened. No attempt is made to reorientate the main part of the cartilagenous septum (this will be achieved functionally following reattachment of the nasolabial muscles).

Subperiosteal undermining

An access incision is made laterally in the labial sulcus through which a small periosteal elevator is used to elevate the periosteum over the anterior maxilla. The undermining extends around the pyriform fossa and nasal bones, up to the infraorbital foramen, and up to the maxillary–zygomatic suture (Figure 9.1.9). The periosteum is then carefully incised to facilitate stretching of the fascial envelope medially. An incision just anterior to the inferior turbinate is then made extending from the base of the Muir flap superiorly along the pyriform rim to facilitate correct positioning of the alar base on the cleft side (Figure 9.1.10a). Occasionally in narrow clefts, positioning of the alar base can be achieved without the need for this relieving incision.

Muscle dissection

Identify the transverse nasalis muscle as it curls around the alar base on the cleft side. It lies above the incision (F–5) that demarcates the nasal skin from the lip skin. Its identification is confirmed by gentle traction with toothed forceps (Figure 9.1.11). The oblique or external fibres of orbicularis are identified lying more superficially and inferior to the nasalis muscle just below the incision line F–5. Finally, the horizontal or internal fibres of orbicularis are freed from the underlying glandular layer and vermillion for a few millimetres.

The vestibular access incision is closed first with 5/0 vicryl suture together with the vestibular mucosa at the cleft margins. The inferior one-third of the marginal mucosa near the vermillion is left open at this stage. The skin of the nasal floor is then repaired with 5/0 vicryl starting posteriorly to within a few millimetres of the nasal sill. The

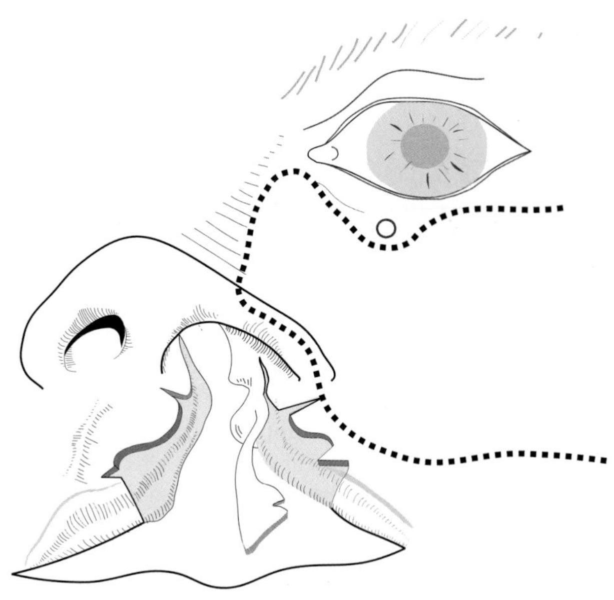

9.1.9 Subperiosteal undermining.

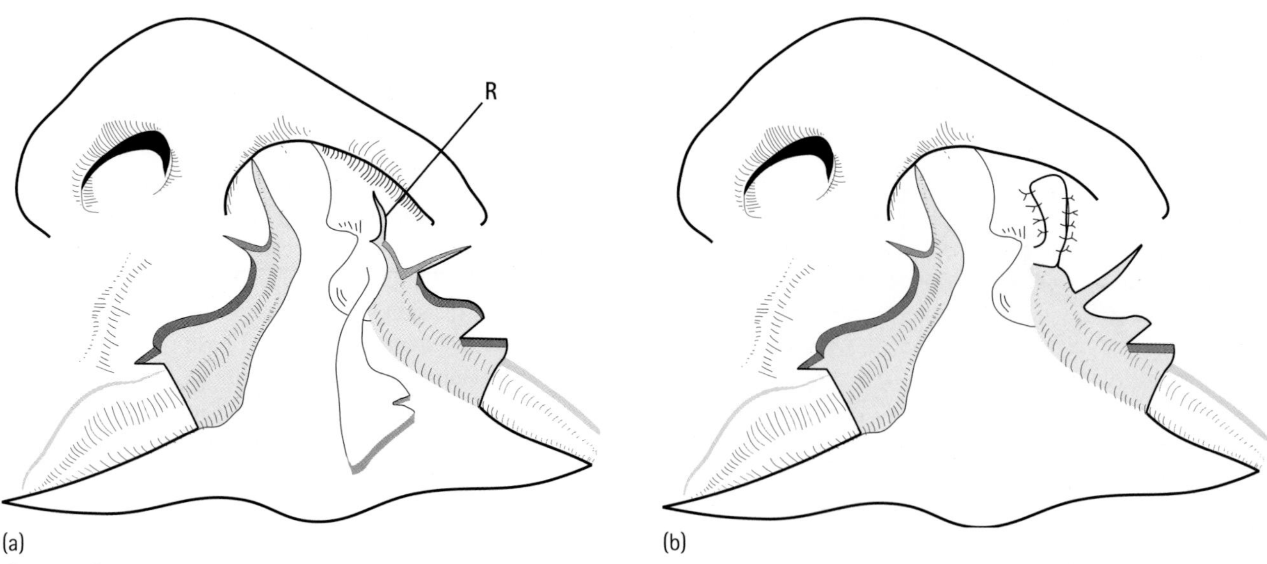

9.1.10 (a) Releasing incision; (b) defect from releasing incision filled with modified Muir (vermillion) flap.

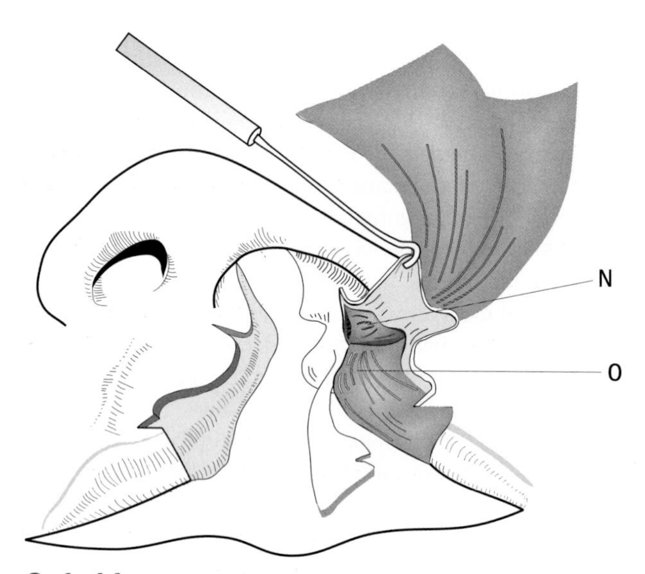

9.1.11 Identification of transverse nasalis muscle (N) and oblique fibres of orbicularis muscle (O).

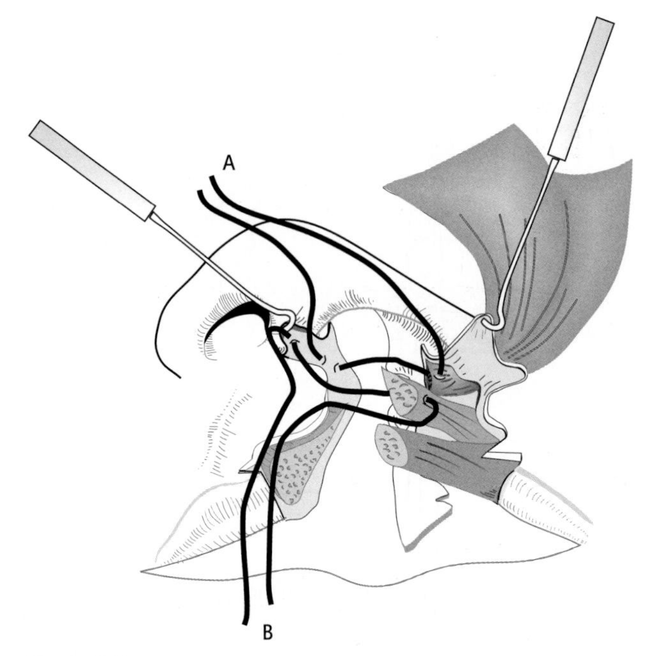

9.1.12 Muscle repair, sutures.

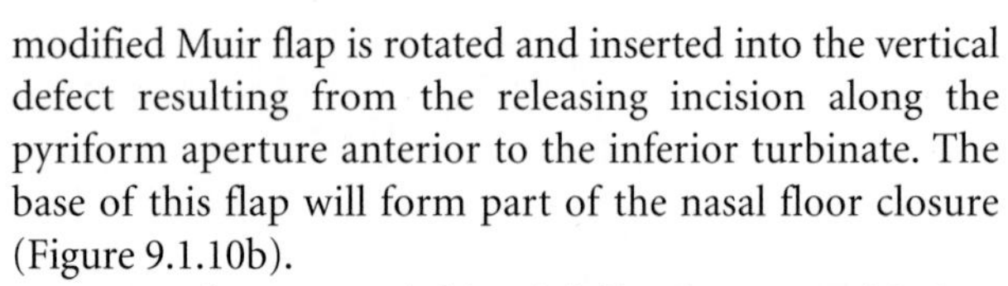

modified Muir flap is rotated and inserted into the vertical defect resulting from the releasing incision along the pyriform aperture anterior to the inferior turbinate. The base of this flap will form part of the nasal floor closure (Figure 9.1.10b).

A 4/0 prolene suture (ethicon) ('A' in Figure 9.1.12) is then inserted into the nasalis muscle and periosteum just lateral and inferior to the ANS. This will result in displacement of the muscle in a medial and slightly inferior direction. The suture is left free and not tied at this stage. A second suture is placed in the same muscle, but this time also including the dermis of the alar base, then across into the periosteum lateral and slightly superior to the first muscle suture. A suture (B) is then inserted through the oblique head of the orbicularis muscle and the perichondrium of the anterior nasal septum and soft tissue around the ANS. This suture will cross and be superficial to the sutures attached to the nasalis muscle. The sutures are then tied starting with the first nasalis muscle suture (A) and ending with suture B. After completion of the muscle sutures, it is important to ensure that the cleft-sided ala base is symmetrical with the noncleft side and is in the correct anteroposterior, horizontal and vertical plane. The horizontal or internal fibres of the orbicularis are then repaired with 5/0 vicryl taking care to align the muscle edges correctly at the vermillion.

Skin closure is achieved with interrupted 7/0 vicryl rapide suture (ethicon). The first suture is placed through the white roll. It is important to align this suture carefully. The medial element will rotate down to allow insertion of the small triangular flap situated just above the white roll. This should produce a symmetrical cupid's bow. Continue suturing the skin with 7/0 vicryl rapide ethicon from inferior to superior completing the procedure with closure of the anterior nasal floor and sill.

The nasal web is obliterated with a 4/0 PDS suture (ethicon) passed from inside the nostril and back through the same hole in the nasal skin. Another 4/0 PDS suture (ethicon) is passed medially and superiorly from inside the cleft side nostril just below the apex of the ala dome. It passes through a similar point on the medial aspect of the non cleft ala dome and then out into the non cleft side nostril. The suture is passed back in the opposite direction to exit in the cleft side nostril as shown in Figure 9.1.13. This suture helps support the ala dome. Cotton mittens or socks are placed over the baby's hands instead of arm restraints. Polyfax (Pilva Pharma Ltd) ointment is applied to the wound.

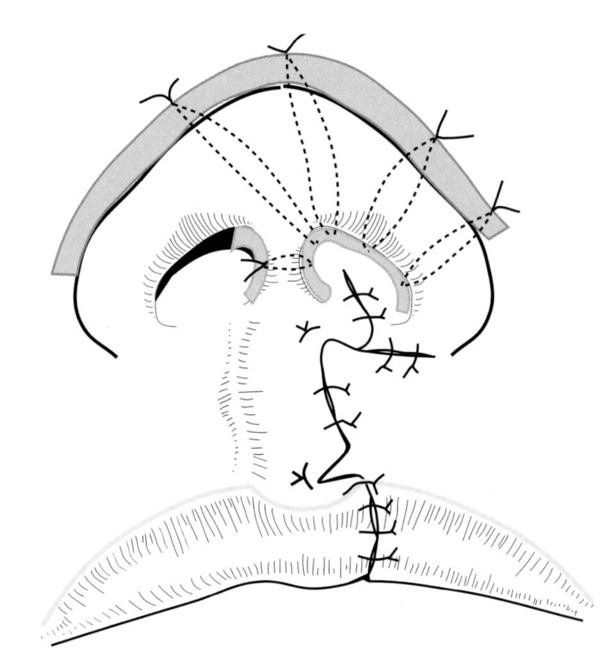

9.1.13 Skin repair and nasal splint.

POST-OPERATIVE CARE

The baby is returned to the ward and encouraged to start oral feeding. After 2 days, after which time feeding is usually re-established, the baby is discharged from the ward. The wound is kept lubricated with an antibiotic ointment for 7 days after which the nasal splint is removed.

Top tips

- Careful identification of anatomical landmarks and respect for anatomical boundaries between the nose and lip.
- Wide subperiosteal undermining of the anterior maxilla.
- Identification of the anterior border of the septum, subperichondrial undermining of the nasal septum and release of ala cartilage from the vestibular skin.
- Identification and dissection of the nasalis and orbicularis muscle.
- Reconstruction of the upper and middle muscle rings with fixation of the nasalis muscle to the periosteum, just below the ANS, and fixation of the oblique part of orbicularis to the ANS and septum.
- Correct alignment of the ala base, anterior septum and columella.
- Careful reconstruction of the horizontal fibres of orbicularis.

FURTHER READING

Brusati R, Mannucci N, Mommaerts MY. The Delaire philosophy of cleft lip and palate repair. In: Ward Booth P, Schendel SA, Hausamen JE (eds). *Maxillofacial surgery*, vol. 2. London: Chuchill Livingstone, 2007: 1027–47.

Delaire J. [Primary cheilorhinoplasty for congenital unilateral labiomaxillary fissure. Trial schematization of a technic]. *Revue de Stomatologie et de Chirurgie Maxillo-Faciale* 1975; **76**: 193–215 (in French).

Delaire J. General considerations regarding primary physiological surgical treatment of labiomaxillopalatine clefts. *Oral and Maxillofacial Surgery Clinics of North America* 2000; **12**: 361–78.

Delaire J. Theoretical principles and technique of functional closure of the lip and nasal aperture. *Journal of Maxillofacial Surgery* 1978; **6**: 109–16.

Delaire J. Traitement chirugicaux et orthopediques des becs de lievre et divisions palatines. *Revue d'Orthopédie Dento-Faciale* 1971; **5**: 104–40.

Markus AF, Delaire J. Functional primary closure of cleft lip. *British Journal of Oral Maxillofacial Surgery* 1993; **31**: 281–91.

McComb H. Anatomy of the unilateral and bilateral cleft lip nose. In: Bardach J, Morris HL (eds). *Multidisciplinary management of cleft lip and palate.* Philadelphia: WB Saunders, 1990: 144–9.

Millard DR. *Cleft craft. The evolution of its surgery.* Boston: Little Brown, 1976.

Mohler L. Unilateral cleft lip repair. *Plastic and Reconstructive Surgery* 1987; **80**: 511.

Muir J. Repair of the cleft alveolus. *British Journal Plastic Surgery* 1966; **19**: 30–36.

Randall P, Whitaker L, LaRossa D. Cleft lip repair: The importance of muscle repositioning. *Plastic and Reconstructive Surgery* 1974; **54**: 316–23.

Schendel SA. Unilateral cleft lip repair – State of the art. *Cleft Palate-Craniofacial Journal* 2005; **37**: 335–41.

Talmant JC. Nasal malformation associated with unilateral cleft lip. Accurate diagnosis and management. *Scandinavian Journal of Plastic Reconstructive Hand Surgery* 1993; **27**: 183–91.

Tennison CW. The repair of the unilateral cleft lip by the stensil method. *Plastic Reconstructive Surgery* 1952; **9**: 115.

9.2

Primary closure of bilateral cleft lip

KRISHNA SHAMA RAO

ANATOMY

- The prolabium located centrally is devoid of muscle and consists of skin, vermillion and oral mucosa.
- There is no definitive line of demarcation between the columella and prolabium.
- The premaxilla, containing the tooth buds for future permanent incisors, may be situated centrally or asymmetrically to the right or left, anteriorly, superiorly or inferiorly or a combination thereof.
- Sometimes permanent lateral incisors are missing/ hypoplastic.
- On the lateral segments, the lip vermillion is turned upwards to join the alar base. This is because both the extrinsic muscle (levator alaque nasi, levator labii superioris, nasalis), as well as the intrinsic upper lip muscles (orbicularis marginalis and peripheralis) are oriented upwards and inserted into the alar base and maxilla along the pyriform ring.
- The lower lateral cartilages are pulled laterally, resulting in a flattened appearance of the nose.
- The septum and premaxilla are attached to the vomer as a thin stalk.

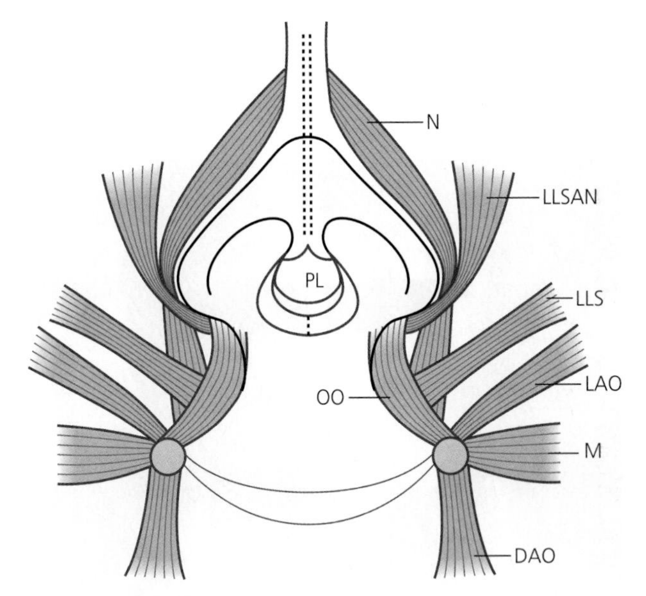

PL – prolabium. N – nasalis.
LLSAN – levator labi superiosis aleque nasi.
LLS – levator labi superiosis. LAO – levator anguli oris.
M – modiolus. DAO – depressor anguli oris. OO – orbicularis oris

9.2.1 Anatomy.

CLINICAL EVALUATION/RECORD KEEPING

- Photographs, both extra- and intraoral;
- study models;
- orthopantomogram after five years of age;
- check premaxilla for mobility and fracture.

TIMING OF SURGERY

- The ideal age for lip repair is three months.
- In less-informed societies, patients may present at any age.
- Protocols for primary repair of bilateral cleft lip presenting at any age is as follows:
    - three months to two years: lip repair;
    - two to seven years: palatoplasty first and then lip repair;
    - seven years to adulthood: palatoplasty first and then lip repair with alveolar bone grafting.

When the patient presents for surgery after the age of seven years, the premaxilla may be severely displaced and may occasionally require surgical repositioning.

HOW TO HANDLE THE PREMAXILLA

- In minimally displaced premaxilla in the newborn or when the child presents early (at less than three months of age), strapping of prolabium with dynaplast or elastics is helpful.

- In the more displaced premaxilla, nasoalveolar moulding with specially developed plates with nasal prongs to guide premaxillla and lateral segments into position can be fitted. It requires repeated visits to the clinic to adjust the plates.

Lip adhesion

This is a surgical procedure which allows mobilization of the nasal layer and closure of the lateral segment margins with the prolabium without mobilization and anastomosis of the orbicularis oris muscle. This allows repositioning of the premaxilla and definitive repair at the second stage some three months after the lip adhesion.

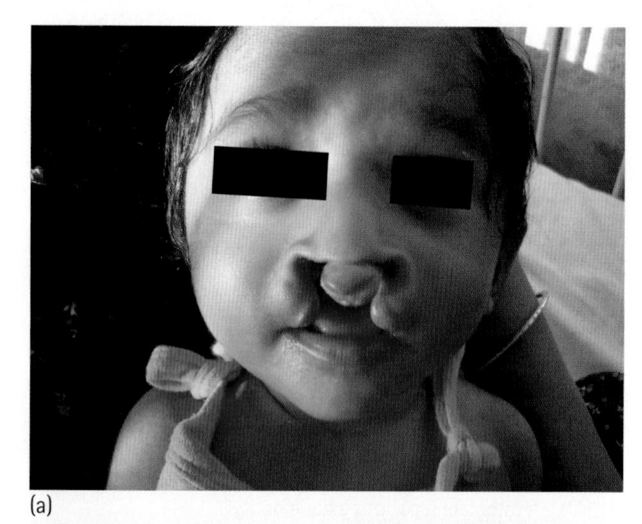

(a)

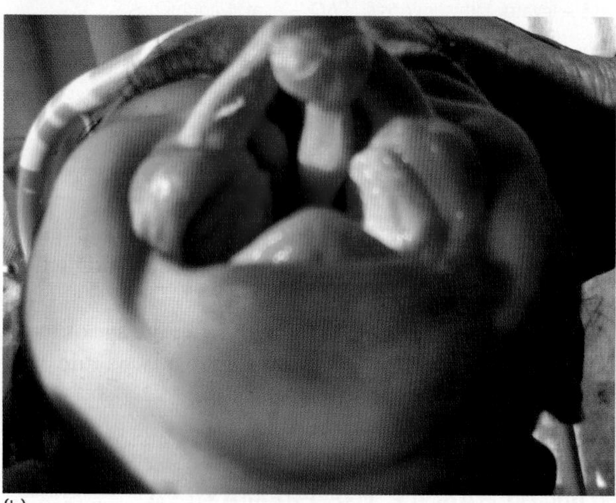

(b)

9.2.2 (a) Premaxilla at the tip of the nose, absence of columella and deficient prolabial tissue; (b) protruded premaxilla and deviated nasal septum.

Premaxillary osteotomy

INDICATION

Premaxillary osteotomy is indicated in the following conditions:

- patient aged about seven years;
- premaxilla more than 1 cm protruded and/or deviated;
- when other conservative techniques are not appropriate.

Primary premaxillary osteotomy is performed using longitudinal mucosal incision, use of cutting instruments to perform a predetermined oblique ostectomy, separation of the nasal septum from the vomer and retropositioning the premaxilla and stabilization with resorbable bone plates. After three months, primary repair of lip can be undertaken.

Pre-operative assessment is shown in Figures 9.2.6 and 9.2.7.

DEFINITIVE PRIMARY REPAIR OF BILATERAL CLEFT LIP

Anaesthesia

Patients are given general anaesthesia, using an oral endotracheal, reinforced tube.

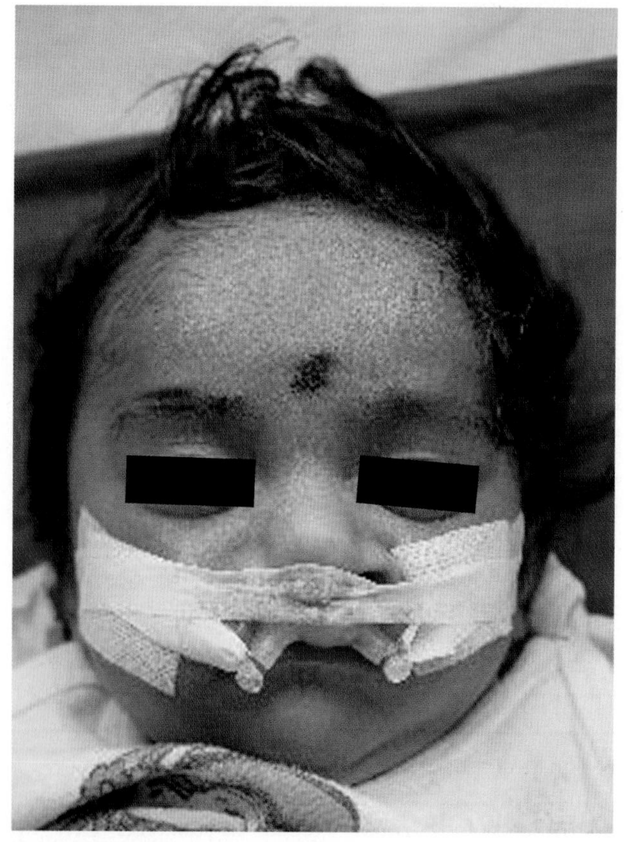

9.2.3 Appliance during first stage of alveolar moulding.

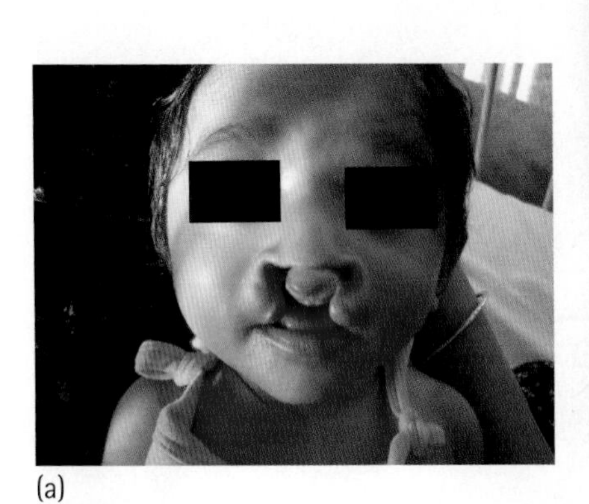
(a)

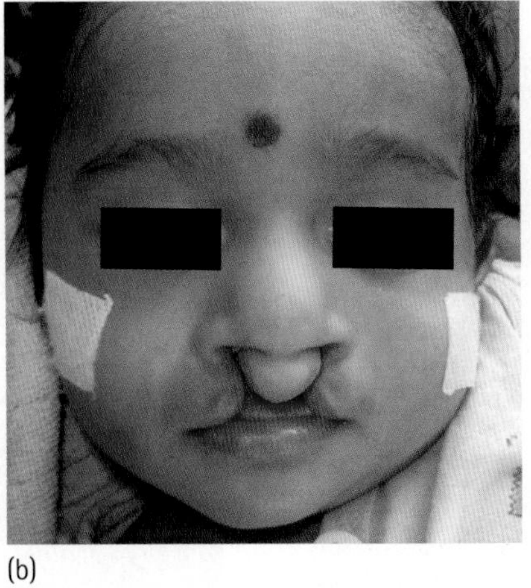
(b)

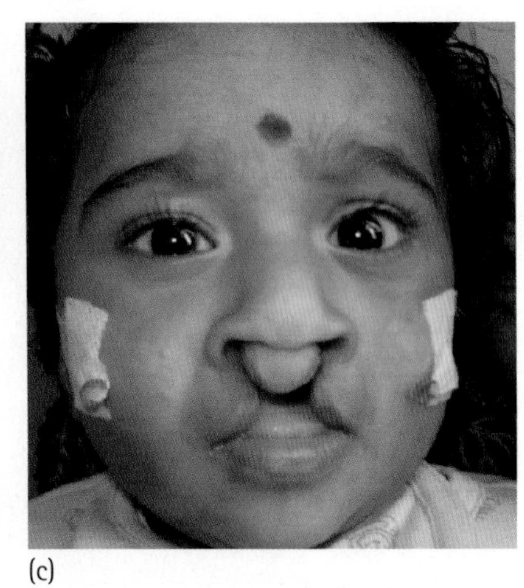
(c)

9.2.4 Treatment progression.

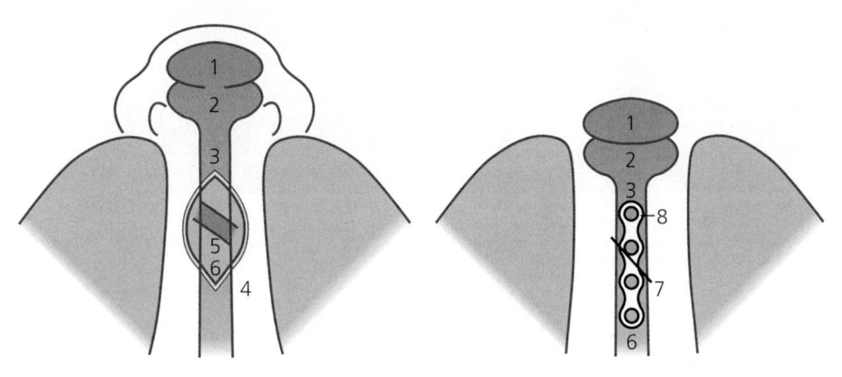

1 – prolabium. 2 – premaxilla. 3 – vomerine stalk. 4 – vomerine mucosa.
5 – osteotomy site. 6 – vomer exposed. 7 – osteotomy site after reduction.
8 – resorbable bone plates.

9.2.5 Premaxillary osteotomy.

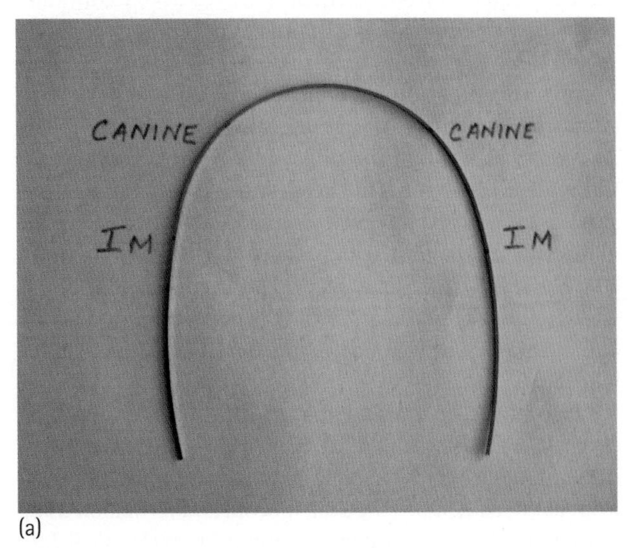

(a)

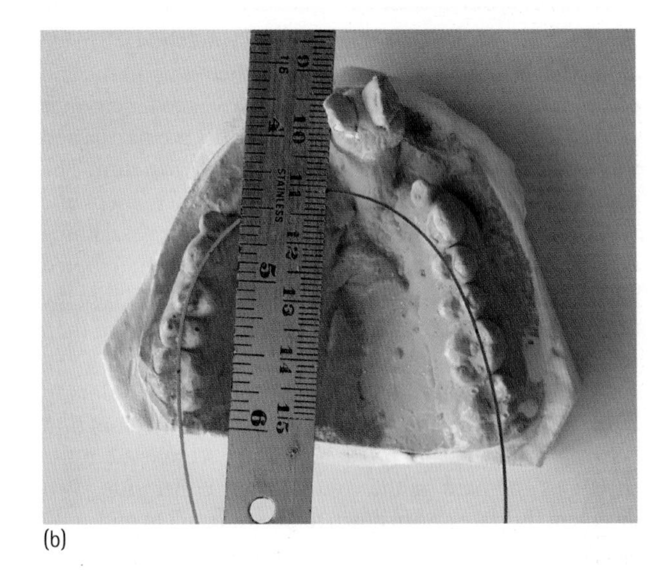
(b)

9.2.6 a,b Model analysis.

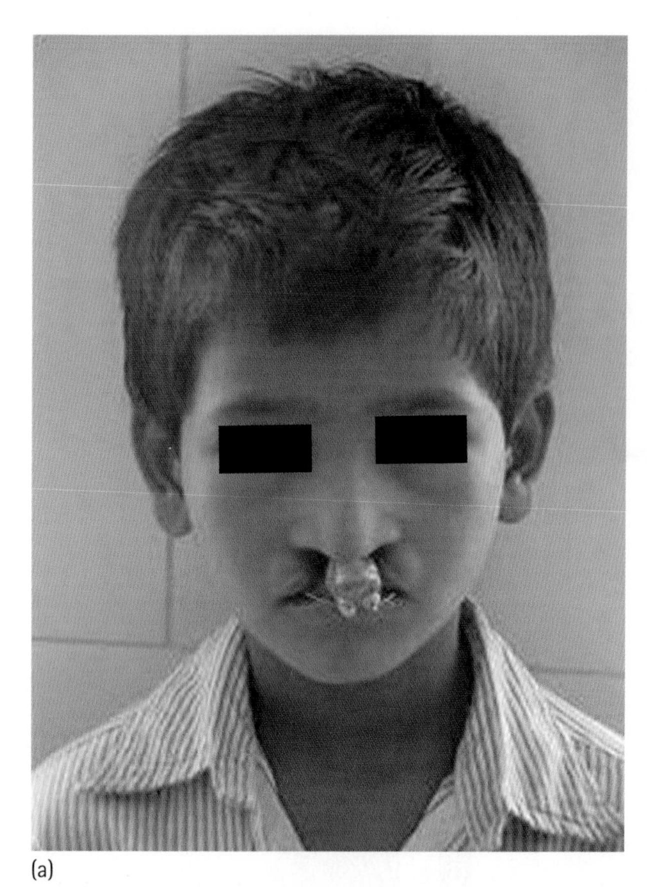

(a)

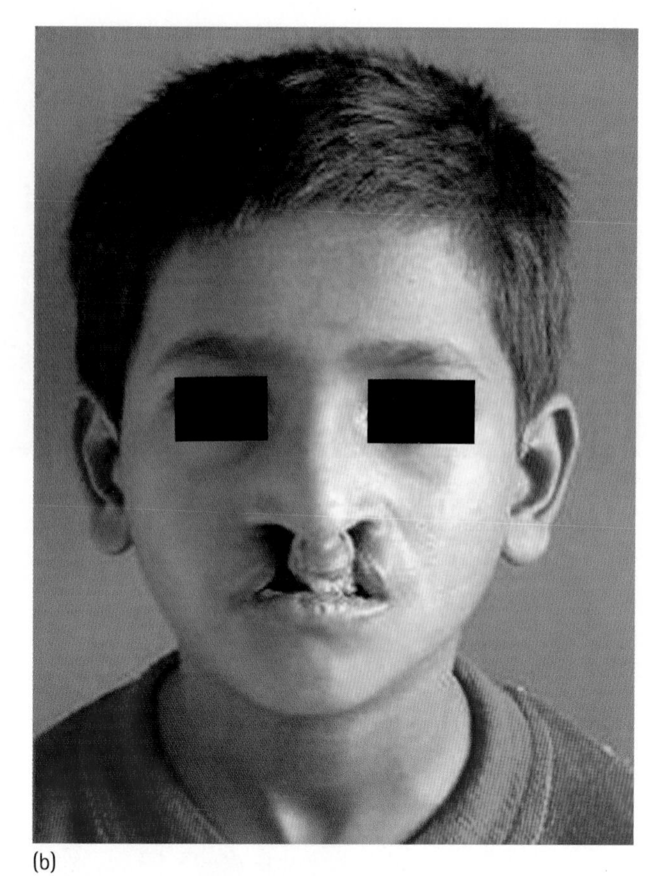

(b)

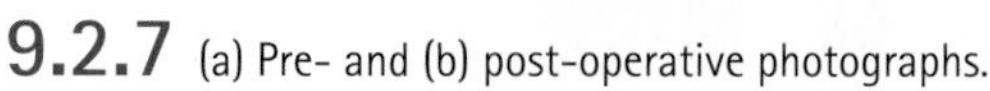

9.2.7 (a) Pre- and (b) post-operative photographs.

POSITION

Patients are positioned with the neck extended and a mouth gag applied.

PROCEDURE

After the mouth gag is applied, marginal incisions are made along the medial aspects of the palatal shelves up to the end of the hard palate. On the premaxilla, a Y-shaped incision is made with the two short limbs encircling the premaxilla and the long limb along the vomerine mucoperiosteum. The nasal layers are elevated using Mitchell's trimmer or a plastic instrument. A single layer mucosal closure of the nasal lining is achieved from the lip to the hard palate using interrupted resorbable vicryl 4/0 sutures with the knots inverted into the nasal cavity. The mouth gag and neck extension are then removed.

Next, lip marking should be planned, the key points to mark on the prolabium being: the apparent junction between columella and prolabium. Mark A1 and A2 at the corner of the base of the columella on either side. Two divergent lines are drawn down to the white roll to end at B1 and B2 as shown (Figure 9.2.8), B1 and B2 being slightly wider than A1, A2. Point C is the midpoint between B1, B2 and it is the lowest point of the cupid's bow. On the cleft side's right and left points, D1 and D2 are marked to represent the commissure of the lips. Points E1 and E2 are marked at the spot where the white roll just begins to fade. Thus, D1 to E1 is equal to D2 to E2. At E1 and E2, a perpendicular line is drawn towards the free margin of the lip. Points F1 and F2 are marked such that E1–F1 is equal to E2–F2 is equal to B1–C is equal to B2–C. F1–E1 continues along the white roll into the internal aspect of the nostril on either side. The incision is made using a No. 15 blade starting from A1 to B1 and then again on the other side from A2 up to B2. The two are joined together across C. The incision goes through the skin and incorporates a little of the underlying tissue. On the cleft sides, that is the lateral sides, incisions are started at E1 and continued along the white roll into the nostril and extended laterally to the point F1. At E1, the incision is also taken perpendicular to the white roll to the free margin of the mucosa and a mucosal flap is elevated on right side. A similar flap is elevated on the left side.

Once the incisions are completed, the orbcularis oris muscle is dissected free from its abnormal attachments on either side of the base of the ala and maxilla. The muscle is freed from its attachments to the skin, mucosa and vermillion using a No. 15 blade up to a distance of about 5 mm (Figure 9.2.9). Superiorly, where the abnormal insertion of the muscle into

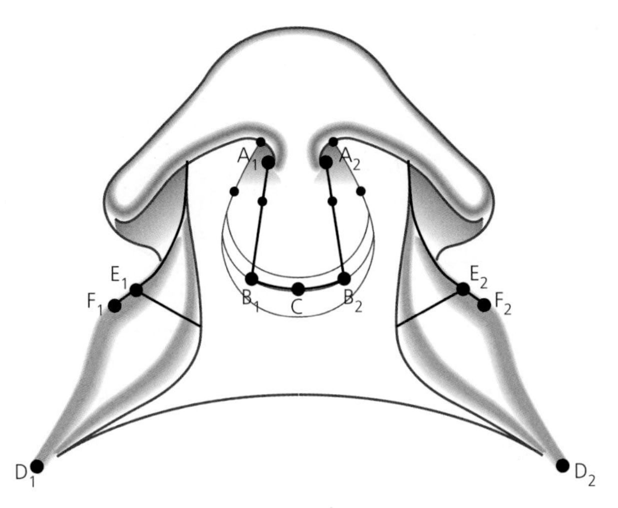

$A_1 A_2$ – junction of columella with prolabium.
$B_1 B_2$ – highest point of cupid's bow. C – lowest point of cupid's bow.
$D_1 D_2$ – commisure of lip. $E_1 E_2$ – white roll fades.
$F_1 F_2$ – back cut along white roll such that $E_1 F_1 = E_2 F_2 = B_1 C = B_2 C$.

9.2.8 Anatomic points for lip marking.

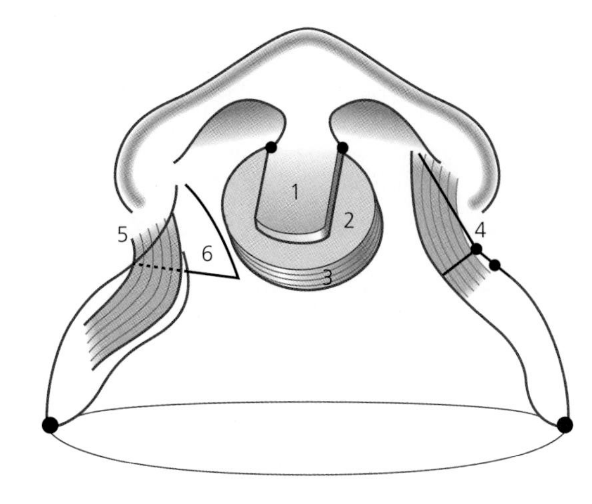

1 – prolabial skin flap. 2 – excess skin and mucosa. 3 – premaxilla.
4 – unoperated side showing orbicularis oris muscle bundle under intact skin/mucosa. 5 – exposed orbicularis oris muscle.
6 – mucosa elevated.

9.2.9 Muscle dissection.

the ala is seen, the muscle is freed using a combination of sharp and blunt dissection in order to free the entire corpus of orbicularis oris muscle along with the bundles of the nasalis and the other associated muscles. In order to mobilize the lip completely, the muscles are also freed from the underlying maxillary bone in a subperiosteal manner. The orbicularis and nasalis muscles are freed as far as the base of the alar margin and a sulcular incision is made into the depth of the sulcus from the free margin of the lip up to the premolar area. The subperiosteal dissection is carried out in order to elevate the entire lip complex along with its underlying and associated muscles away from the maxillary wall. The tissues are freed along the pyriform margin and also extended into the lateral aspects of the ala of the nose on either side. The incision along the white roll towards the nostril is carried on until it reaches the inferior aspect of the inferior turbinate mucosa. The mucosal flaps are raised to coincide with the nasal layer of the anterior aspect of the palatal mucosa. On the prolabial side, the incision B1–A1 is carried further backwards along the nasal mucosa over the vomer bone, such that the nasal flaps can be elevated on either side. This helps in having a continuous nasal lining from the palate forwards into the lip. As soon as the mobilization is complete, it will be seen that the lateral segments of the lip now assume a very comfortable horizontal position and they can be brought together with minimal or no tension at all. The excess lip mucosa which is medial to points E1 and E2 is used to form the sulcus of the future upper lip.

MOBILIZATION OF NASAL CARTILAGES

Blunt dissection of the lateral crura of the lower lateral cartilages on either side using a curved blunt-tipped tenotomy scissors. The scissors are placed through the lateral incision and blunt dissection is proceeded along the superior and inferior and the outer and inner aspects of the lower lateral cartilage up to the dome (intermediate crura). The medial crura of the lower lateral cartilage is approached from the prolabial side and also freed on all aspects. This mobilizes the lower cartilage completely and allows it to attain its natural form during closure of the lip.

CLOSURE

Closure is performed in three layers (Figure 9.2.10). First, the nasal layer is closed in continuity with the closure of the premaxillary nasal mucosa which was performed earlier. Once the nasal layer closure is complete, the mucosa on the inner aspect of the upper lip on either side is sutured to the prolabial mucosa in order to form the sulcus of the oral cavity. Closure is obtained using 4/0 vicryl sutures (5/8 of a circle cutting needle).

The next layer of the closure is the muscle. The nasalis is identified on either side by pulling it medially and seeing the inwards movements of lower lateral cartilage and the base of ala on either side. The orbicularis oris proper muscles are also identified and three sutures are placed using 4/0 vicryl in order to bring together the orbicularis and nasalis muscles comfortably in the midline over the prolabial mucosa. Along its length, skin hooks are positioned actively, giving a slight downward traction to the lip, in order to ensure that the entire nasalis and orbicularis muscles have been brought together.

SKIN CLOSURE

The prolabial skin is allowed to fall gently upon the closed orbicularis muscles, and the two lateral segments are then

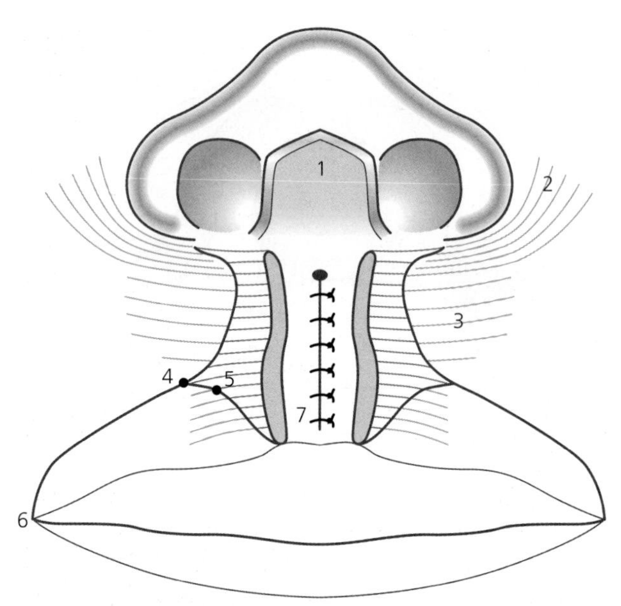

1 – elevated prolabium. 2 – nasalis muscle.
3 – orbicularis oris muscle. 4 – point F_1. 5 – point E_1.
6 – commisure point D.
7 – mucosa sutured with 4.0 vicryl

9.2.10 Closure.

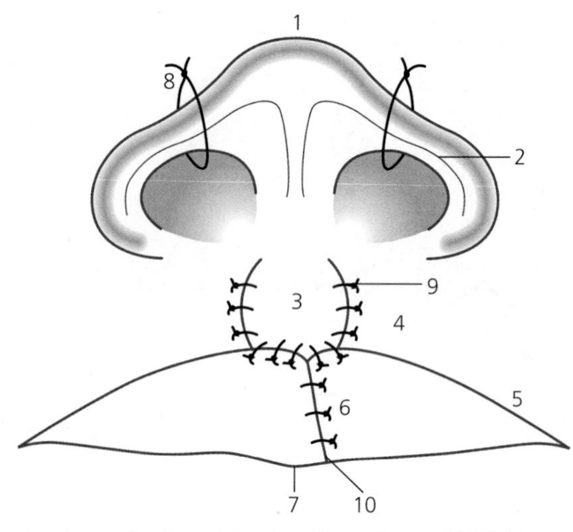

1 – dome. 2 – lower lateral cartilage. 3 – prolabial skin.
4 – lateral element skin. 5 – cupid's bow. 6 – vermillion.
7 – central tubercle. 8 – bolster stitch with 3.0 prolene.
9 – skin closure with 5.0 prolene.
10 – mucosal closure with 4.0 vicryl

9.2.11 Closure.

gently pulled across and held together with two skin hooks held in parallel along the long axis of the body of the patient (Figure 9.2.11). Any excess skin in the lateral segments resulting from the closure of the muscles can be incised in order to accommodate the prolabial skin in the midline and the wound is closed using 5/0 proline sutures. The vermillion and the oral mucosa are closed using 4/0 vicryl. Care is taken to achieve a central tubercle in the midline of the lip, thus giving the upper lip a pleasant and natural appearance. Bolster sutures are placed through the dome (intermediate crura) of the lower lateral cartilages in order to hold them up in a new position allowing the skin and the mucosa to adapt and heal in the new relaxed positions of the cartilages. The skin sutures and bolster sutures are removed after 7 days.

POST-OPERATIVE CARE

Steri strips are placed immediately after the suturing and they are removed after 2–3 days to inspect the wound and clean it. The wound is meticulously cleaned with normal saline and hydrogen peroxide and betadine and steri strips are replaced. On the 7th day, the sutures are removed under sedation, the wound is cleaned again and new steri strips are placed. The parents are advised to apply vitamin E cream to the wound post-operatively for a period of three months and massage the lip gently every day. Gentle massage of the lips is continued for at least three months.

RESULTS

The results of primary closure of bilateral cleft lip surgery are shown in Figures 9.2.12–9.2.15.

COMPLICATIONS

Intra-operative

FRACTURE OF THE PREMAXILLA

The premaxilla is continuous with the vomer along a very thin stalk and may sometimes be traumatized, especially if it is protruberant either prior to the surgery or during the procedure.

AVULSION OF THE PREMAXILLA

This is a rare, but unacceptable, iatrogenic complication.

Post-operative

EARLY

Infection

The wound may get infected, especially in chronically malnourished children in developing countries due to decreased immunity. Use of antibiotics and local wound management should salvage the surgical procedure.

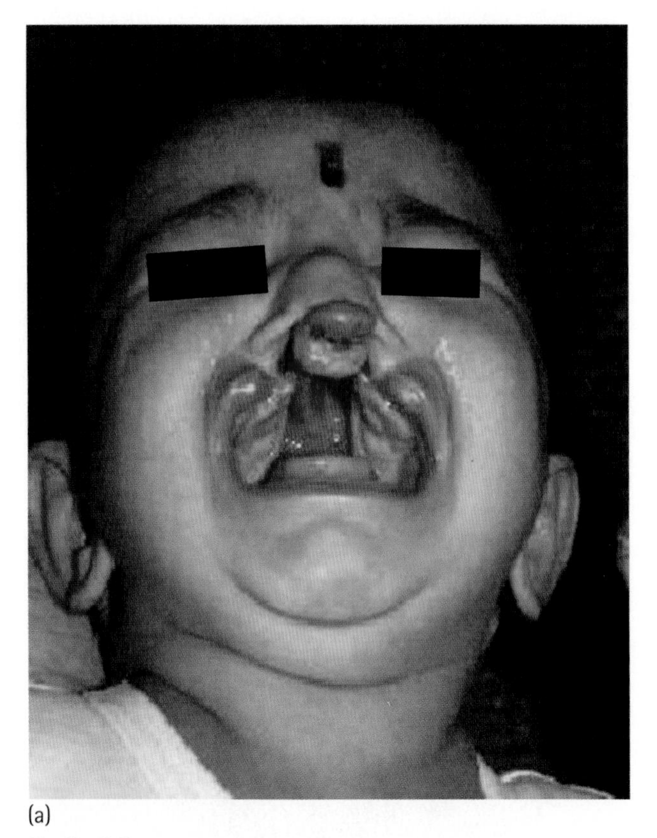

(a) (b)

9.2.12 Pre- and post-operative photographs.

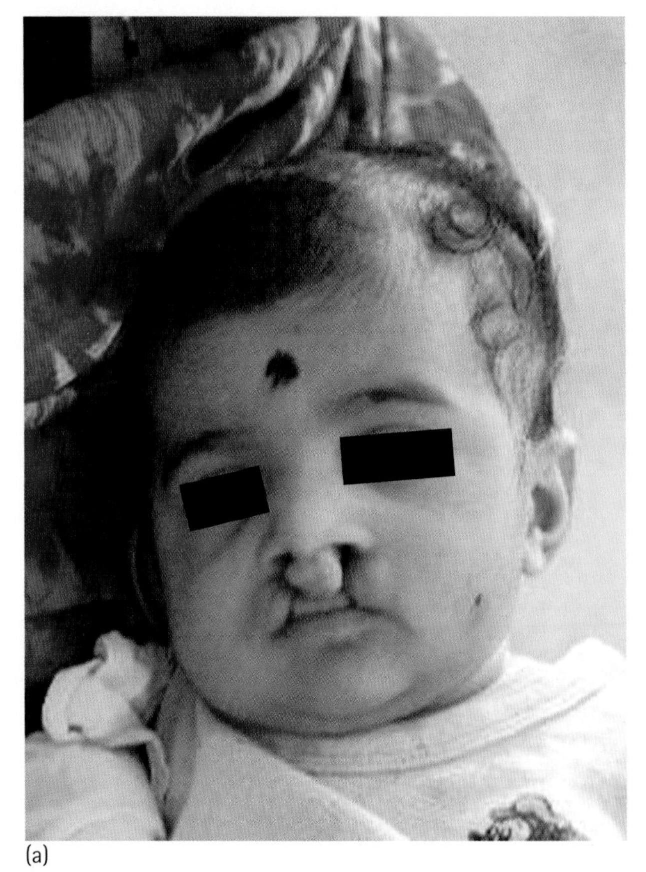

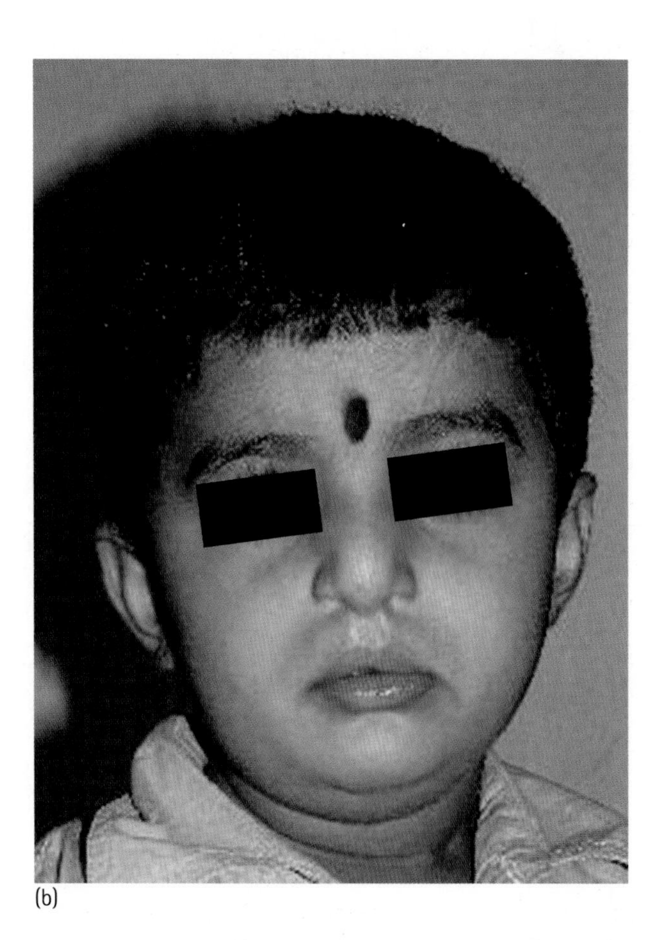

(a) (b)

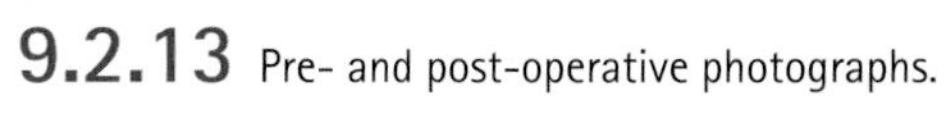

9.2.13 Pre- and post-operative photographs.

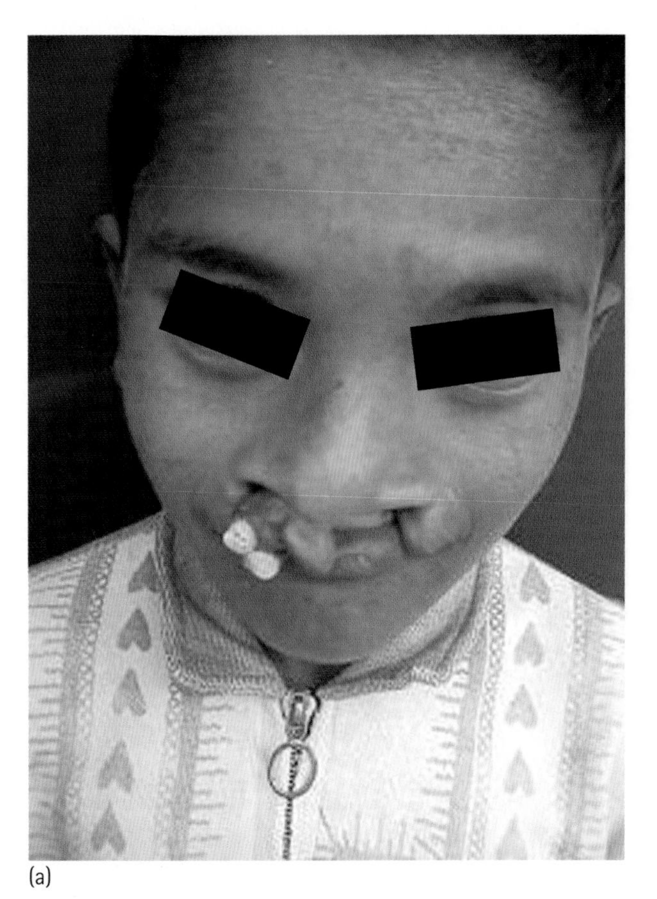

(a) (b)

9.2.14 Pre- and post-operative photographs.

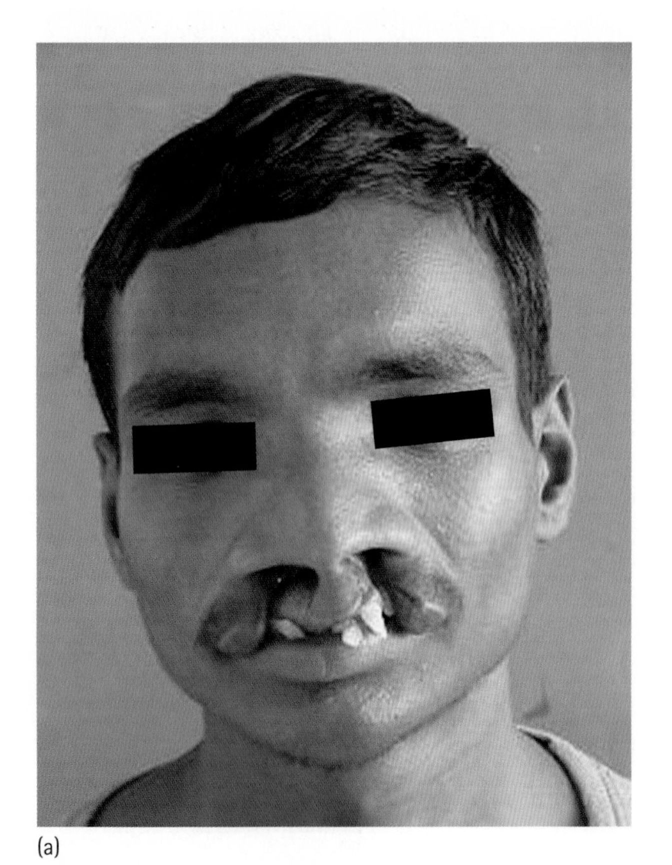

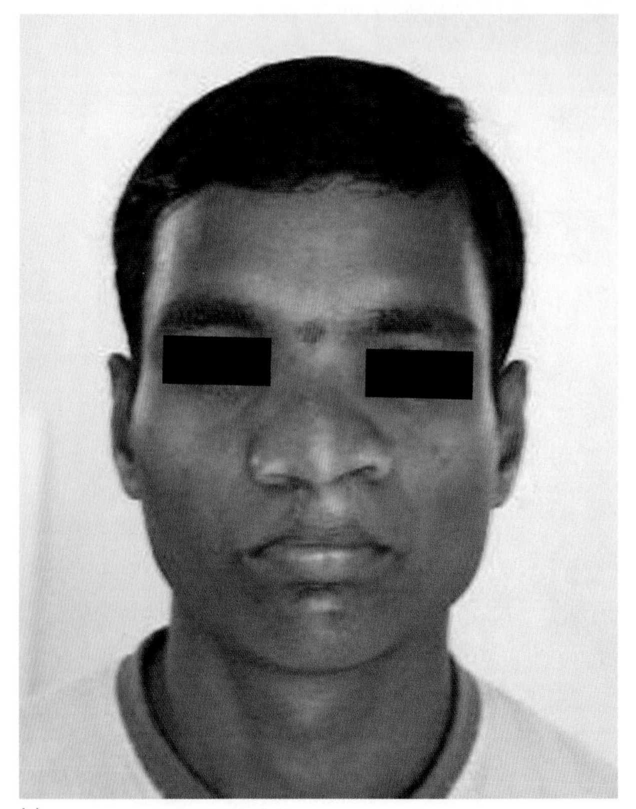

(a) (b)

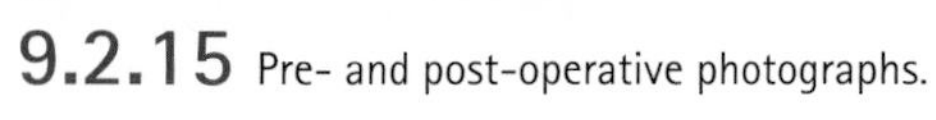

9.2.15 Pre- and post-operative photographs.

Dehisence of the wound

As a sequela to either wound infection or tension during closure, partial breakdown of the surgical repair may occur. Conservative management is followed by secondary correction after six months.

LATE

Oronasal fistula

Partial breakdown of the nasal layer may lead to small oronasal communications in the region of the premaxilla and lateral segments. Definitive repair of the fistula in two layers is taken up as a secondary procedure after six months.

Cupid's bow deformity

Mismatch of the white roll during suturing or wound contracture may lead to a deformed cupid's bone, which is corrected with Z-plasties or scar revision.

Whistling deformity

Generally, this is a severe deformity due to inadequate mobilization of nasalis and orbicularis oris muscles or dehiscence of these muscles due to closure with tension. Secondary repair is carried out in the form of a complete revision cheiloplasty.

Hypertrophic scar

Hypertrophic scar is a common sequel due to excessive tension in skin closure and is all the more apparent in pigmented skin (types IV–VI). Hypertrophic scars can be managed initially conservatively using vitamin E cream, massage, contratubex ointment, etc. Minimally hypertrophic scars can be resurfaced with erbium Yag lasers. Severely hypertrophic scars would need excision and resuturing in a tension-free environment.

Top tips

- The prolabium is devoid of muscle.
- The premaxilla may be situated centrally or asymmetrically in three dimensions.
- The ideal age of repair of the bilateral cleft lip is three months, but patients may present at any age in less-informed societies.
- There are several techniques to manage the premaxilla which include simple strapping (common), nasoalveolar moulding (common), lip adhesion (less common) and premaxillary osteotomy (occasionally).
- In the definitive repair of the bilateral cleft lip, it is important to first repair the nasal floor.
- Further important steps include careful marking of the incisions and meticulous mobilization of the muscles.
- The lip–nose complex is treated simultaneously and hence careful closed dissection and mobilization of the lower lateral cartilages are performed
- During mucosal closure, care is taken to achieve a good sulcus and, on the labial side of the alveolus, a gingivoalveolar periosteoplasty is achieved.
- Skin closure achieves symmetry of the lip and nose, and pleasing cupid's bow, philtral ridges and central tubercle.
- Potential complications though rare include intra-operative fracture or avulsion of premaxilla, post-operative infection or dehisence of the wound, and late problems such as oronasal fistula, whistling deformity, hypertrophic scars, etc.

FURTHER READING

Bardach J. *Salyer & Bardach's atlas of craniofacial and ceft surgery*, vol. II: Cleft lip and palate surgery. Philadelphia: Lippincott, 1999.

Bishara SE, Olin WH. Surgical repositioning of the premaxilla in complete bilateral cleft lip and palate. *Cleft Lip and Palate Journal* 1972; **42**: 139–43.

Cronin TD, Cronin ED, Roper P et al. Bilateral clefts. In: *Plastic surgery*, vol. 4. McCarthy J (ed.). Philadelphia: WB Saunders, 1990: 2653–722.

Delaire J, Precious D, Gordeef A. The advantage of wide sub-periosteal exposure in primary surgical correction of labial maxillary cleft. *Scandinavian Journal of Plastic Reconstructive Surgery, Hand Surgery*, 1988; **22**: 147–51.

Jackson IT, Yavuzer R, Kelly C, Bu-Ali H. The central lip flap and nasal mucosal rotation advancement: Important aspects of composite correction of the bilateral cleft lip nose deformity. *Journal of Craniofacial Surgery* 2005; **16**: 255–61.

Markus AF. Primary closure of cleft lip. In: *Operative maxillofacial surgery*, 1st edn. London: Chapman & Hall, 1998: 189–99.

Markus AF, Delaire J. Functional primary closure of cleft lip. *British Journal of Oral and Maxillofacial Surgery* 1993; **31**: 281–91.

Mulliken JB, Wu JK, Padwa BL. Repair of bilateral cleft lip: Review, revisions, and reflections. *Journal of Craniofacial Surgery* 2003; **14**: 609–20.

9.3

Primary repair of cleft palate

CHRISTOPH T HUPPA

INTRODUCTION

The first major step towards modern cleft palate surgery was made in 1862 by Bernhard von Langenbeck (1810–87) at the Charité in Berlin. He suggested closing the palate with two medially mobilized bipedicled mucoperiosteal flaps. In principle, this method is still in use today.

With the invention of local anaesthetic, surgical procedures could be refined as speed was no longer an issue. The first significant modification was introduced by F Ernst in 1925 who suggested suturing of the muscles, division of the palatine vessels and the formation of parapharyngeal pouches to reduce tension to the midline sutures.

Victor Veau from Paris refined the procedure in 1931 by dissecting the nasal mucosa, thus closing the soft palate in three layers. He furthermore developed a method using posteriorly based unipedicled flaps which helped to lengthen the velum according to the principle of a V–Y plasty. A similar procedure was developed by the British surgeons Thomas Pomfret Kilner (1890–1964) and WEM Wardill in the late 1920s and early 1930s. In 1959, this so-called 'push-back' procedure was modified by W Widmaier who suggested a supraperiosteal dissection of the flaps to reduce growth impediment of the maxilla. He introduced the use of a caudally based vomerine flap, first described by the British surgeon A Campbell in 1926, to close the hard palate.

In 1967, the German surgeon Otto Kriens from Hamburg published an article emphasizing the importance of an anatomically correct repair of the velar muscles which includes the detachment of the wrongly inserted musculature from the posterior aspect of the palatine bone. This concept of an intravelar veloplasty is still the basis of most modern techniques in primary and secondary cleft palate surgery.

In the 1950s, the ear, nose and throat (ENT) surgeon Wolfram Schweckendiek pioneered a method of a two-stage repair, previously described by Gillies and Fry in 1921, which included an early soft palate and a late hard palate repair to prevent maxillary growth disturbances which had been seen in many cases with the previous techniques. According to his protocol, he carried out the hard palate repair on a patient at the age of 12 years. Schweckendiek popularized this two-stage procedure in many cleft centres worldwide when he published excellent long-term results in 1978.

In 1976, Leonard T Furlow introduced a completely different method involving a double opposing Z-plasty to close and simultaneously lengthen the soft palate. This procedure had already been published in principle in 1966 by Karl Schuchardt. When Furlow presented some very encouraging results in 1986, the method gained popularity and is nowadays a very well-established procedure in many cleft centres around the world.

PRINCIPLES

The main target of the primary repair of the cleft palate is to reinstate the function of the soft plate. This is most important as the formation of certain speech sounds requires normal function of the velum. During the formation of, for example, explosives like [b], [p], [d] and [t], the nasal airway has to be sealed off by a craniodorsal movement of the soft palate. If this is not possible air escapes through the nose and the air pressure, which is necessary to form these sounds, cannot build up and speech sounds hypernasal. A nasal air escape can be noticed. This pathophysiological phenomenon is called velopharyngeal insufficiency (VPI) or velopharyngeal dysfunction (VPD). Therefore, it is paramount to repair the velar muscle layer in an anatomically correct position as pointed out by Otto Kriens in the 1960s.

A measure for VPI is the nasalance which is a quotient of nasal and oral acoustic energy. It can be measured by a nasometer (acoustic energy) or an aerophonoscope (air flow).

In order to lay the foundations for normal speech development, the repair of the soft palate should be carried out before onset of speech, i.e. in the first year of life.

A no less important aim of palate repair is to install the natural separation of the oral and nasal cavities and to establish two separate nasal cavities. This avoids nasal regurgitation of food, which can be socially very troublesome and prevents contact of food with the nasal mucosa.

On the other hand, an early intervention could lead to maxillary growth retardation and hypoplasia especially if the alveolar periosteum is detached during the procedure.

For this reason, some cleft surgeons advocate closure of the hard and soft palate in separate procedures. There is still some controversy about the question of whether a one- or two-stage palate repair is preferable. The two most common basic protocols are:

1. lip repair (uni- or bilateral) at the age of three to six months followed by a one-stage hard and soft palate repair at the age of six to 12 months;
2. lip repair (uni- or bilaterlal), in combination with soft palate repair followed by a hard palate repair at age 15 months to several years (in extreme cases, early teens).

In a two-stage procedure, early periosteal stripping of the hard palate can be avoided; however, it is still unclear if this gives a significant advantage for the midfacial growth. In fact some scientific studies suggest that differences in maxillary growth might not be significant. The disadvantage of persistent nasal regurgitation of food and fluids has to be taken into account.

Despite all the improvements in cleft palate surgery, in many cases speech and language therapy may still be needed to obtain a good result, but a significant proportion of patients can develop normal speech without any further therapy. Some patients may need further surgery for speech improvement later in life. Speech can still deteriorate during growth periods, such as the early teens, and special precaution has to be taken when planning maxillary advancement surgery.

Primary repairs in adulthood have been shown to be much less successful with regards to speech, but can still be helpful for the better functioning of dentures and to avoid nasal regurgitation of food.

ANATOMICAL CONSIDERATIONS

The physiological functioning of the soft palate is essentially due to an anatomically correct restoration and reorientation of the velar musculature which has to be detached from the posterior aspect of the palatine bone. Important muscles of the soft palate are:

- *Levator veli palatini* which originates from the petrous portion of the temporal bone, is attached to the medial wall of the Eustachian (auditory) tube and runs ventral to the tensor muscle into the velum to fuse with its counterpart on the opposite side. Its function is to lift the soft palate in a cranioposterior direction. This muscle is most important for the velopharyngeal seal and creates the velar 'knee' in a lateral videofluoroscopy. Functionally, it is most effective in a more posterior position.
- *Tensor veli palatini* which originates from the scaphoid fossa of the sphenoid bone and the lateral rim of the Eustachian tube, runs with a tendon through the sulcus of the pterygoidean hamulus and forms the palatal aponeurosis with the opposite side in the anterior third of the soft palate. Next to stretching the velum, its main function is to open the auditory tube.
- *Musculus uvulae* are a paramedian pair of muscles running from the posterior nasal spine to the tip of the uvula. Supports the levator bulge and thus helps with the oropharyngeal seal.
- *Palatopharyngeus muscle*, which forms the posterior pillar of the fauces (pharyngopalatine arch), originates with a wide base from the posterior and lateral pharyngeal wall and inserts with its posterior fasciculus at the posterior aspect of the hard palate and the anterior fasciculus into the soft palate. It can send the small salpingopharyngeus muscle to the Eustachian tube, but this muscle is not always present. Functionally, the palatopharyngeus elevates the pharynx and larynx, constricts the isthmus faucium while swallowing and depresses the soft palate opposing the action of the levator muscle.
- *Palatoglossus muscle* runs from the velar aponeurosis to the posterior superior parts of the tongue. It is another antagonist of the levator muscle and forms the anterior pillar of the fauces (palatoglossal arch).
- *Superior pharyngeal constrictor muscle* arises from the pterygoid hamulus of the sphenoid bone and the pterygomandibular raphe. The fibres run in a backward curve to unite in the median pharyngeal raphe with the opposite side. Its function is a constriction of the upper pharynx in collaboration with the levator veli palatini muscle while swallowing. If hyperplastic, this muscle is the anatomical substratum of the Passavant's ridge. Its significance for speech is doubtful.

PRE-OPERATIVE ASSESSMENT

Most children with cleft lip and palate are otherwise healthy and do not need any further pre-operative precautions. However, in some cases, especially where the cleft palate is part of a syndrome, attention has to be paid to other comorbidities involving especially the heart or kidneys. Therefore, it is important to have a paediatrician on the team to make sure these conditions are not missed.

Audiology and ENT assessment should be arranged prior to the palate repair as the insertion of grommets can be carried out simultaneously with the palate repair if indicated. As the palate repair can lead to significant haemorrhage, the clotting system should be assessed.

In case the cleft palate is part of a Pierre-Robin sequence, pre-operative sleep studies can be helpful. In these cases presurgical orthopaedic therapy with a modified Hotz plate can be useful to reposition the tongue in a more anterior position. The forward push of the tongue seems to stimulate mandibular growth.

As cleft surgery is in principle elective surgery, it should be carried out under optimal conditions. The procedure should be postponed whenever signs of common cold, respiratory tract infections or other acute medical conditions are seen. The parents need to be warned about this possibility in advance.

ANAESTHESIA

The surgery is undertaken under general anaesthetic which should be administered by an experienced paediatric anaesthetist. Due to their small body volume, infants are at much greater risk from hypothermia than adults. A temperature probe should be inserted and the infant has to be kept warm throughout the procedure. Monitoring during the entire surgery is most important.

For ventilation, an orotracheal tube is used and it should be fixed in the middle of the lower lip so it can be protected by the tongue spatula of the self-holding retractor (Dingman or similar). As paediatric endotracheal tubes do not have a cuff, it is paramount to prevent any gas leakage or fluid aspiration with a carefully placed throat pack.

To prevent a peri-operative wound infection, a single shot of an antibiotic (co-amoxiclav, combination of cephalosporin and metronidazole or similar) at induction is usually sufficient.

As the palate repair is physiologically stimulating for the infant, local anaesthetic with epinephrine (adrenaline) (2 per cent lidocaine with 1:80 000 epinephrine or similar) should be infiltrated into the soft and hard palate at the begining of the procedure to reduce the amount of general anaesthetics and to induce vasoconstriction in the surgical field.

Extubation is the most critical moment after palate repair and the infant has to be closely monitored during this process and during the first night afterwards. As the nasal airway resistance rises due to the surgery, the infants may experience airway problems and a nasal prong may have to be used. If this is at all necessary, it can be removed in most cases the next day as the infant adapts to the new situation and the post-operative oedema of the nasopalatal mucosa settles.

In children with Pierre-Robin sequence, however, it is sometimes necessary to keep the nasal airway for a while.

OPERATIVE PROCEDURE

There are a number of different surgical procedures available to close the cleft palate. The classical palate repair based on bilateral bipedicled von Langenbeck flaps, the Furlow repair and the two-stage Schweckendiek repair will be described in detail below.

Repair using bipedicled Langenbeck flaps (Langenbeck–Ernst–Veau–Kriens repair)

POSITIONING OF THE PATIENT AND LOCAL ANAESTHESIA

The patient rests in a supine position with a bulky gel pad or fluid bag underneath the shoulder. The neck has to be extended as much as possible to make sure the surgeon has good access to the palate and sits comfortably in the 12 o'clock position with the infant's head in his lap. The assistants sit at 9 and 3 o'clock (Figure 9.3.1). It is advisable to wear a head light.

The first step of any palate repair is the insertion of a self-holding retractor (Dingman or similar) which serves as a mouth gag, retracts the tongue and cheeks, and protects the orotracheal tube (Figure 9.3.2). Once the retractor is in its final position, sufficient ventilation has to be confirmed by the anaesthetist.

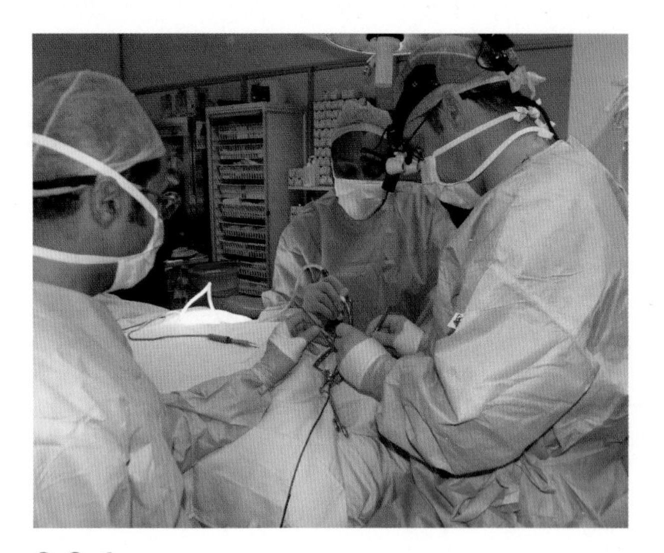

9.3.1 The surgeon's position at 12 o'clock with the infant's head in his lap.

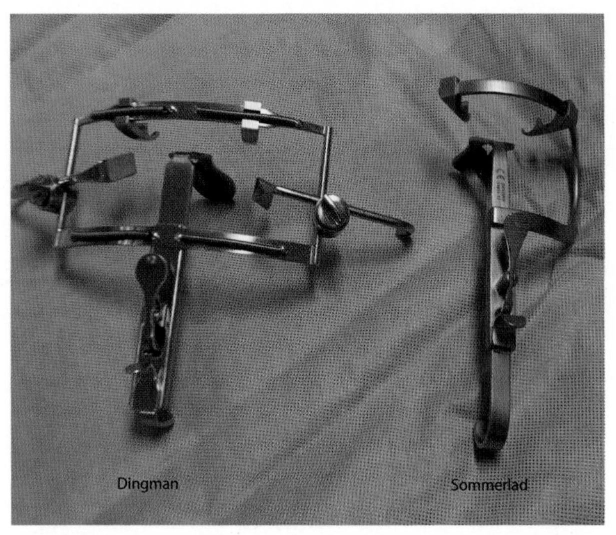

9.3.2 Different types of self-holding retractors.

The local anaesthetic is injected into the mucosa of the hard and soft palate. In order to give the adrenaline time to be effective, one should wait with the first incision until the bleeding in the injection channels stops.

MUCOSAL INCISIONS AND FORMATION OF BIPEDICLED LONGITUDINAL FLAPS

The procedure is started with the surgeon's right hand at the patient's left hand side. Using a size 15 blade, an incision is made along the borderline of the oral and nasal mucosa with excision of a little mucosal triangle at the medial aspect of the hemi-uvula (this creates a contact surface for the unification of both hemi-uvulae) (Figure 9.3.3). In the area of the hard palate, the incision goes right on to bone.

In wider clefts, lateral releasing incisions in the transition zone between alveolar and maxillary mucosa are necessary and should extend from the area above the space of Ernst posteriorly to the level of the anterior extension of the cleft (Figure 9.3.4). The incision is made right on to bone and an anterior pedicle should be preserved at this stage. The flap is now undermined subperiostealy with a curved sharp elevator and after thorough haemostasis the neurovascular bundle is luxated a few millimetres out of the palatine canal using a curved elevator anterior and posterior to the bundle. This step can be rather frightening for the inexperienced surgeon, but it is important because otherwise the flap cannot be mobilized towards the midline without tension. Care has to be taken in order not to damage the palatine artery.

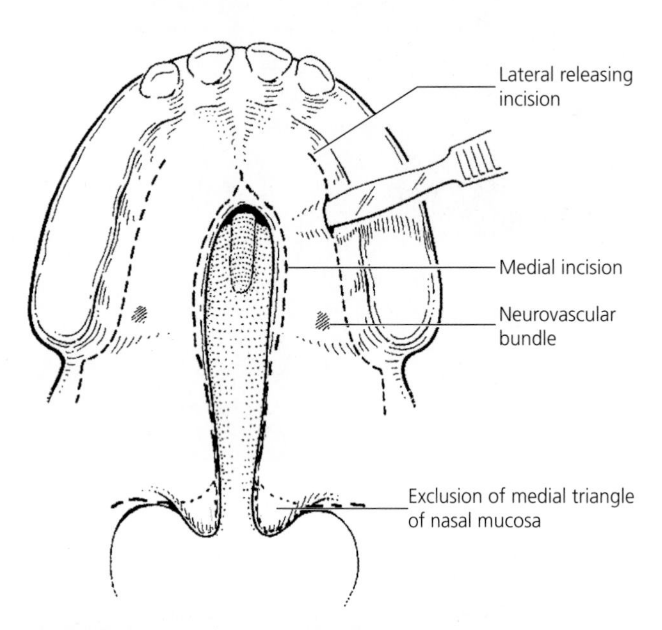

9.3.3 Incisions for formation of bipedicled longitudinal flaps.

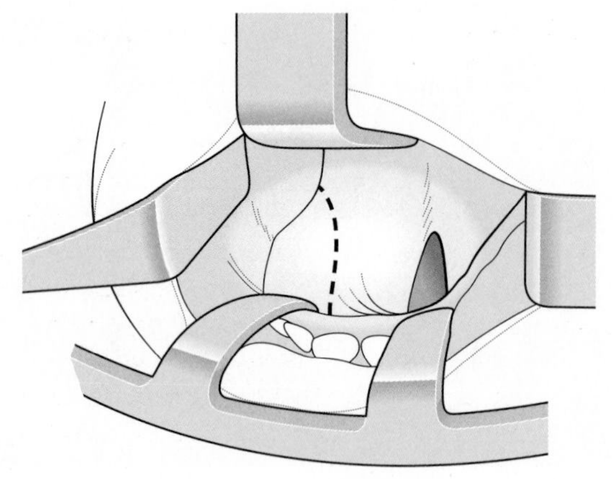

9.3.4 Marking for the left lateral releasing incision.

MUSCLE DISSECTION AND FORMATION OF A NASAL MUCOSAL LAYER

The muscle dissection and precise reconstruction is of paramount importance and should be carried out as carefully as possible. Loops with a magnification factor of 2.5–3.5 or a surgical microscope are most useful, but not indispensable.

The dissection begins with the detachment of the wrongly inserted musculature from the posterior aspect of the palatine bone. This is best undertaken with a sharp Freer's periosteal elevator and a Mitchell's trimmer. The nasal mucosa is detached from the nasal aspect of the palatal shelf with a fine sharp curved periosteal elevator to stretch it to the midline and thus make the closure with the opposite side possible.

The muscle is then lifted up with a skin hook and kept under tension to be dissected off the nasal mucosa laterally as far as the pterygoid plates. The dissection can be carried out with a pair of sharp pointed scissors or a size 15 blade.

It is important to keep the musculature attached to the oral mucosa because otherwise the blood supply to the mucosa can be compromised and oronasal fistulas are more likely to occur.

After analogous dissection on the patient's right side with the surgeon's left hand, an incision is made along the vomerine ridge with small release incision posteriorly at an angle of about 45° (Figure 9.3.5). The mucosa tends to bleed quite intensively due to its excellent blood supply.

Small vomerine flaps are formed and each of them is united with its adjacent counterfoil of nasal mucosa across the cleft using 5/0 monofilament resorbable sutures (Monocryl® or similar). The stitches should be inserted indirectly in order to place the knots towards the nasal cavity, so that two separate tubes of nasal mucosa are formed (Figure 9.3.6).

Next, the nasal mucosa of the velar area should be repaired from front to back in the same way using the same sutures.

MUSCLE REPAIR

The muscle repair is the most important step and should be carried out with slowly resorbing monofilament sutures (4/0 polydioxanone, i.e. PDS® or similar). Corresponding parts of the musculature are stitched together starting from the back to the front with three to four sutures. It is important to achieve a symmetrical result at this stage and the oral mucosa should align without tension after the

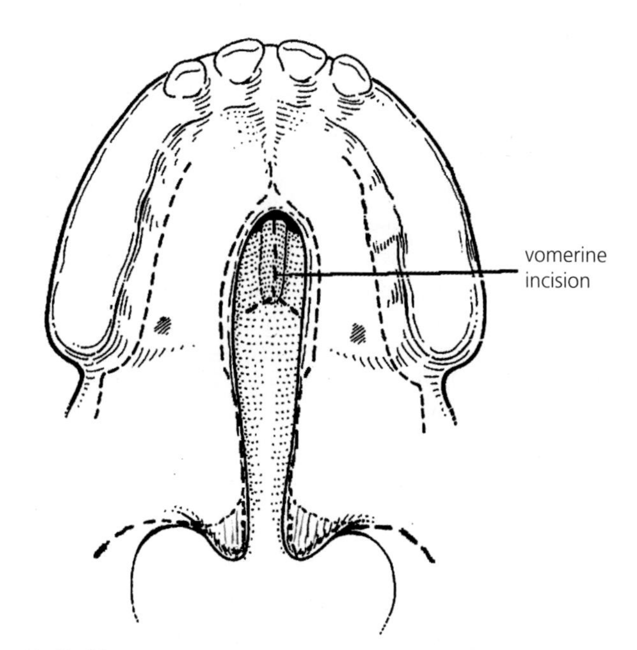

9.3.5 Incisions for the formation of bilateral vomerine flaps.

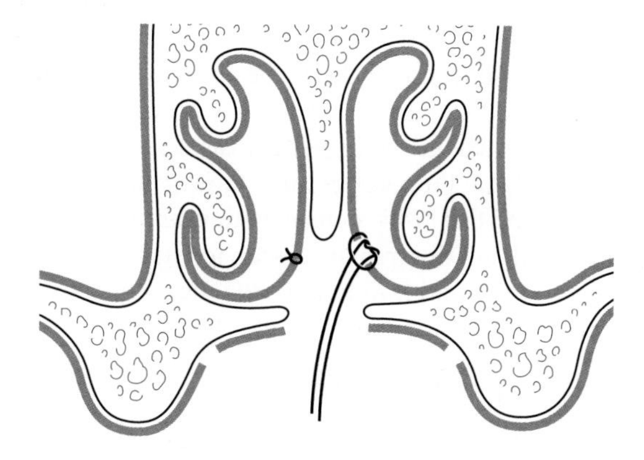

9.3.6 Cross-section of the anterior palate, reconstruction of two separate nasal tubes with vomerine flaps.

completion of the muscle repair. As a result of the repositioning of the muscle in a more natural posterior position, there should be a significant gap between the anterior aspect of the repaired muscle and the posterior ridge of the palatine bone.

REPAIR OF THE ORAL MUCOSA

The oral mucosa should be closed with 5/0 monofilament resorbable sutures. It is best to start the repair of the oral mucosa with two to three deep stitches which engage all layers (use 3/0 monofilament resorbable sutures) in the area of the hard/soft plate junction (Figure 9.3.7). They are placed and temporarily fixed with an arterial clip from back to front to be then tied one after the other from front to back. This is important to avoid a haematoma between the different layers which again reduces the risk of fistula formation. Furthermore, these stitches help to shape the typical palatal vault.

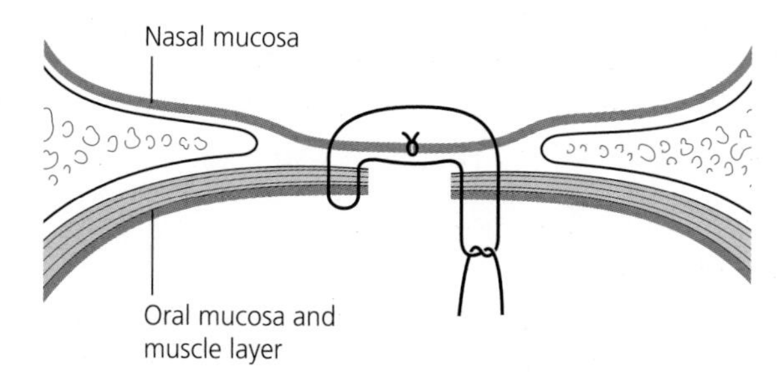

9.3.7 Cross-section of deep stitches at junction hard/soft palate to close down dead space and avoid haematoma formation

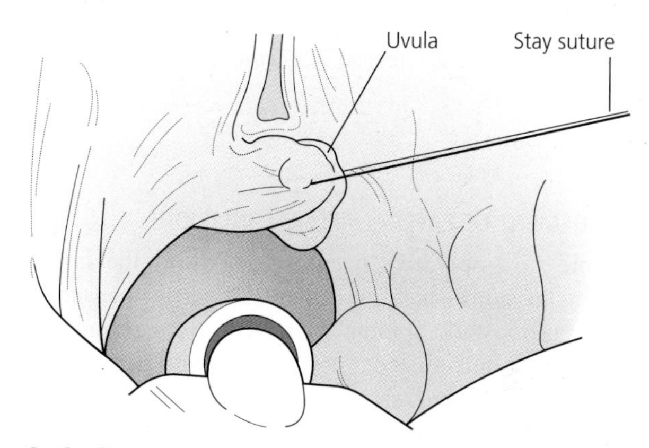

9.3.8 Tip of the reconstructed uvula fixed with a stay suture to access posterior aspect of the uvula for closure.

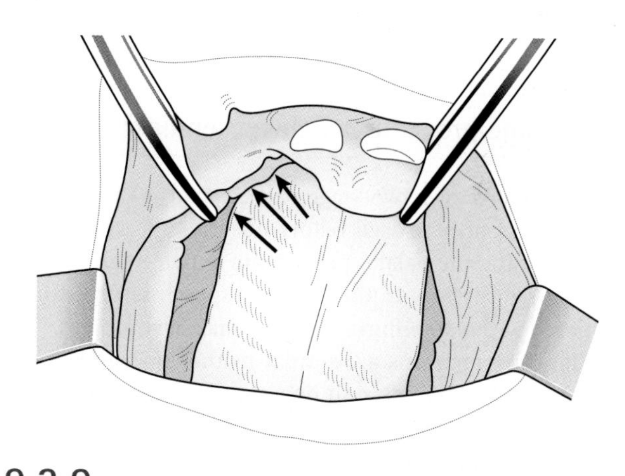

9.3.9 Wide alveolar cleft closed with the right detached anterior pedicle (arrows).

Next, the first 5/0 stitch is applied to the tip of the uvula. It should be used as a stay suture which can be attached to the retractor or clamped to the head towel (Figure 9.3.8). Following this, the stitches to the posterior aspect of the uvula can be put in easily. The stay suture is cut short and the oral mucosa can now be sewn without any tension from the back to the front using mattress stitches all along.

If the cleft is very wide, it is sometimes necessary to sacrifice one or even both of the anterior pedicles to close the anterior mucosa of the hard palate which would otherwise not be possible (Figure 9.3.9).

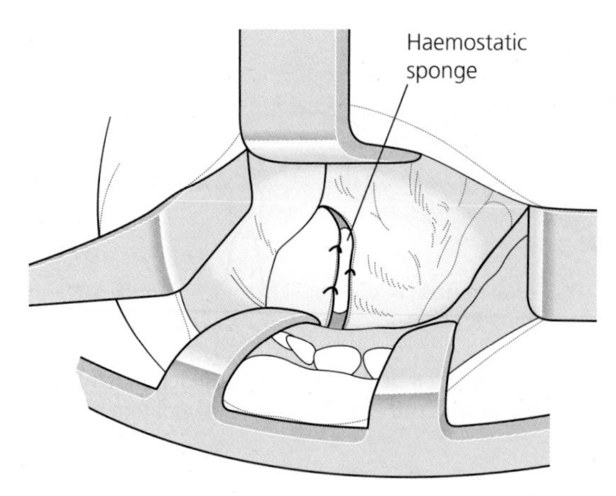

9.3.10 Left lateral releasing incision with haemostatic sponge *in situ.*

MANAGEMENT OF LATERAL RELEASE INCISIONS

To avoid post-operative haemorrhage from the lateral releasing incisions which remain at least partly open, some sort of haemostatic sponge (Surgicel®, Spongostan® or similar) can be introduced. They are fixed with two or three retaining stitches which should not be tied too tight in order to avoid tension at the primary closure site in the midline (Figure 9.3.10).

The releasing incisions will heal through free granulation and cannot be distinguished from the local mucosa with the naked eye after a few weeks.

Two-stage procedure (Schweckendiek)

The advantage of a two-stage palate repair is the fact that the velum can be closed before onset of speech without undermining the palatal periosteum which might lead to growth retardation. In theory, good speech results can be achieved without compromising on maxillary growth.

The velar incisions are similar to the von Langenbeck procedure, but the incision line at the border of oral and nasal mucosa stops in the area of the hard and soft palate junction to turn laterally at a right angle. Lateral to the pterygoid hamulus, a small back cut in the posterior direction is advisable.

The incorrectly inserted musculature has to be detached from the posterior aspect of the palatine bone (Freer, curved periosteal elevator) followed by a sharp dissection off the nasal mucosa with a blade or pointed pair of scissors (Figure 9.3.11).

The next step is the repair of the nasal mucosa with 5/0 monofilament resorbable (Monocryl or similar) interrupted sutures. As previously mentioned, the knots should be placed towards the nasal cavity. The muscle is now repaired as described for the one-stage procedure. The last step is the repair of the oral mucosa with 5/0 monofilament stitches in analogy to what was mentioned above.

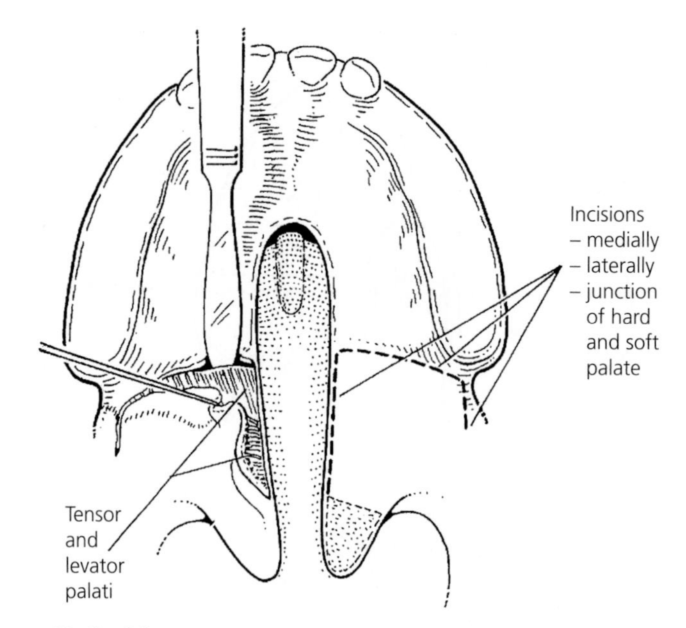

9.3.11 Incisions for stage one of two-stage procedure (isolated soft palate repair).

In wide cases an oral mucosa gap will remain at the hard and soft palate junction parallel to the posterior border of the palatine bone. It should not be closed with tight stitches as this would shorten the velum. In these cases, some resorbable haemostatic foam (Surgicel, Spongostane or similar) can be introduced and fixed with some retention sutures.

As a result of this repair, a scar forms in transverse direction. This could lead to a narrowing of the posterior hard palate due to scar contraction.

CLOSURE OF THE HARD PALATE

The closure of the remaining hard palate defect is carried out according to the particular protocol between 18 months and about 13 years of age. Nowadays, the tendency goes more towards early repair. Quite often, one will only find a relatively narrow but longitudinal defect as the gap tends to decrease with time. If the protocol involves a relatively late repair of the hard palate, a cover plate should be considered to reduce the inconvenience caused by the remaining oronasal communication.

The surgery is performed under general anaesthesia and follows the principles of a fistula repair. A two-layer closure is desirable. In order to create a nasal layer, the nasal mucosa has to be stretched and/or mucosa from the oral cavity has to be borrowed and turned over into the nasal floor. The remaining increased defect of the oral mucosa can then be closed with a rotation or sliding flap (similar to von Langenbeck flap) (Figure 9.3.12). It is important to design the oral mucosa flap as large as possible to avoid the reappearance of an oronasal fistula.

REPAIR WITH DOUBLE OPPOSING Z-PLASTY (FURLOW)

This technique follows a completely different approach to close the cleft palate. It uses an oral layer and a nasal layer

Z-plasty that oppose each other. Thus, a lengthening of the palate, as well as a reorientation of the muscles, can be achieved. The major disadvantage is that it produces an asymmetrical scar which is partly transversely orientated and could lead to some narrowing of the maxilla.

In a first step, a large Z-plasty is designed in the area of the velum with the end points of the lateral limbs lying in the area of the pterygoid hamuli, which can be palpated through the mucosa. The central limb lies parallel to the cleft (Figure 9.3.13).

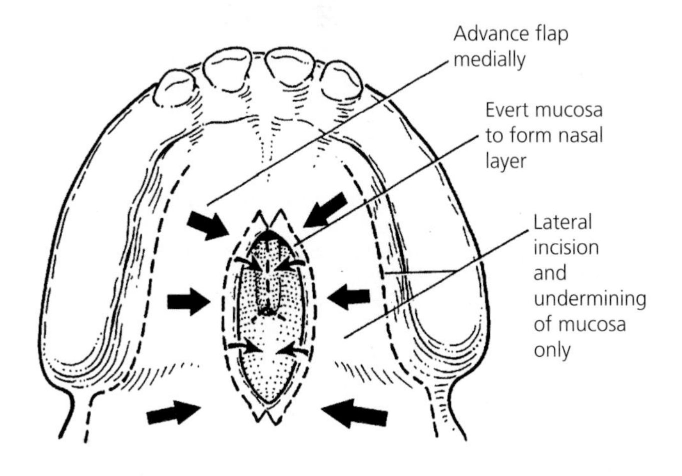

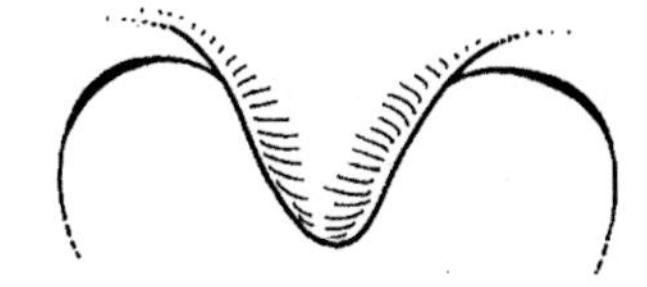

9.3.12 Incisions for second stage of two-stage procedure (hard palate repair).

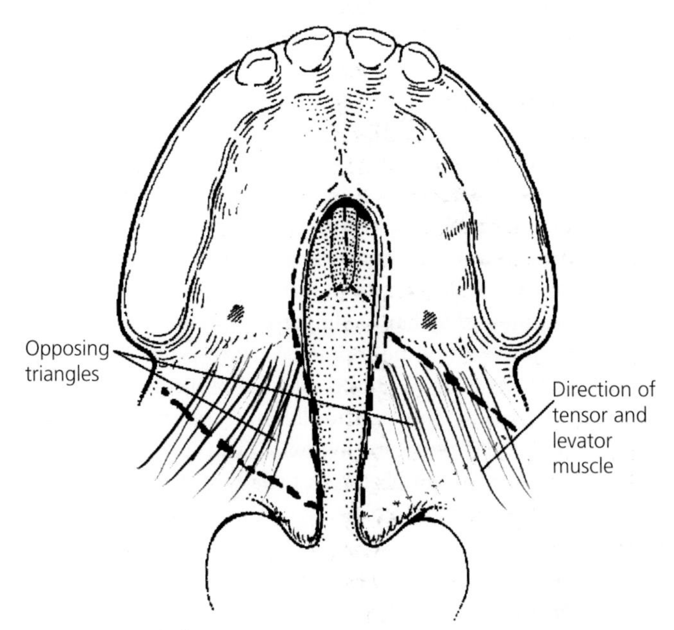

9.3.13 Incisions of oral mucosa for repair with double opposing Z-plasties (Furlow). Please note the sagittal direction of tensor/levator fibres.

The posteriorly based triangle has to be prepared as a myomucosal flap containing oral mucosa and tensor, as well as the levator veli palatini muscles. The muscles have to be detached from the posterior aspect of the palatine bone with a sharp Freer's elevator or Mitchell's trimmer and dissected off the nasal layer which stays intact at this stage. Nasal and oral mucosa have to be elevated from the bony shelves of the hard palate with a curved periosteal elevator, Mitchell's trimmer or Freer (Figure 9.3.14).

The opposite side in now dissected in the opposing way leaving the musculature attached to the nasal layer (Figure 9.3.15).

Next, the opposing nasal Z has to be designed with the end points of the lateral limbs situated just a few millimetres medial to the mouth of the Eustachian tube. As a result, a posteriorly based oral myomucosal flap opposes an anteriorly based oral mucosa flap (Figure 9.3.16).

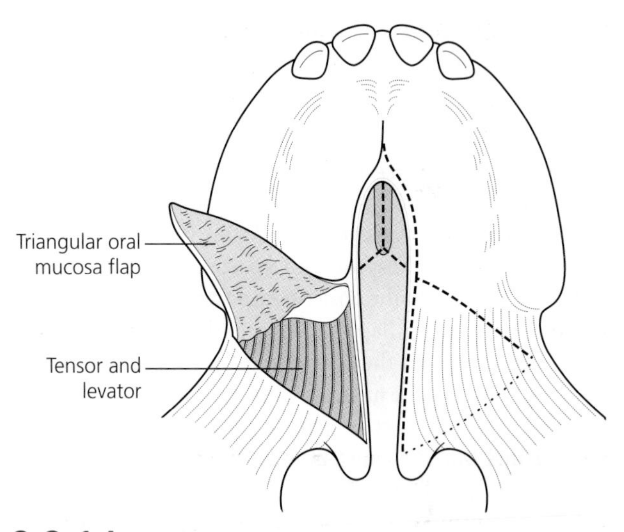

9.3.14 Dissection of anteriorly-based triangle of oral mucosa at the right hand side.

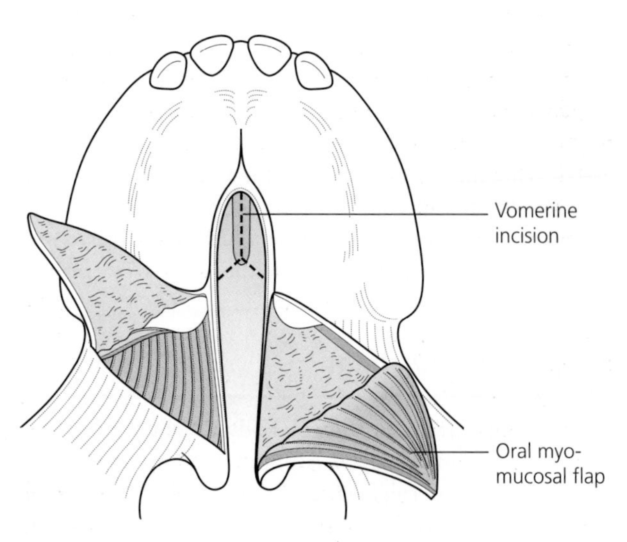

9.3.15 Dissection of posteriorly-based oral musculo-mucosal triangular flap at the left hand side.

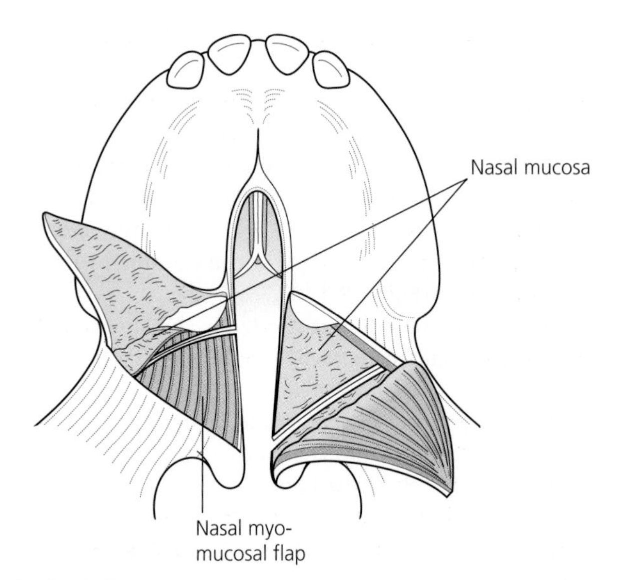

9.3.16 Dissection of anteriorly-based triangular nasal mucosa flap at the left and posteriorly-based triangular nasal musculo-mucosal flap at the right hand side.

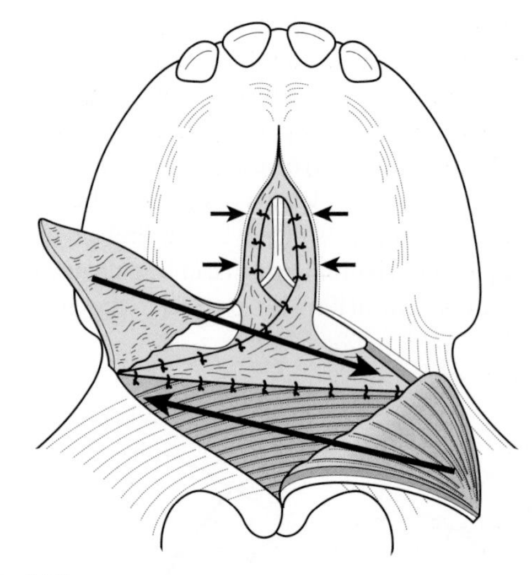

9.3.17 Situation after anterior nasal mucosa closure under formation of two separate nasal tubes and exchange of nasal triangular flaps just before exchange of oral triangular flaps in opposite direction (long arrows).

The nasal Z-plasty now has to be completed, creating a posteriorly based nasal myomucosal flap. As already performed on the opposite side, the muscle has to be detached from the posterior aspect of the palatine bone. Next, the Z-plasty flaps can be transposed, interposing the corresponding mucosa flap between the posterior aspect of the palatine bone and the myomucosal flap. A 4/0 monofilament stay suture is now placed through the base of the oral myomucosal flap engaging the tip of the nasal myomucosal flap and going back through the oral mucosa. This leads to an overlap of the musculature thus creating a muscle sling (Figure 9.3.17).

The nasal mucosa is now closed with a 5/0 monofilament resorbable suture and the stay suture can be tied (Figure 9.3.18).

The undermined mucosa of the hard palate can be closed in analogy to the above described procedure. A repair without tension, however, is not possible in very wide clefts as lateral releasing incisions are not provided.

The final result is a z-shaped scar with a transverse direction of the central limb is obtained. This procedure could be carried out in two stages, closing the soft palate first, leaving the hard palate open for a later repair.

Furthermore, it can be used as a modification in secondary palate surgery if lengthening of the velum as well as an intravelar veloplasty is required.

POST-OPERATIVE CARE

For post-operative pain control, body weight adjusted i.v. morphine administered by a pump as nurse-controlled analgesia (NCA) overnight is beneficial. Usually the morphine can be stopped after 24 hours and it should be replaced by regular paracetamol and ibuprofen for about 7 days. Under this regime, post-operative drinking and feeding is usually not a problem and should be encouraged immediately after the procedure. However, it is not unusual that infants refuse fluids and get on much better with purèed food as sucking can be more uncomfortable than feeding from a spoon.

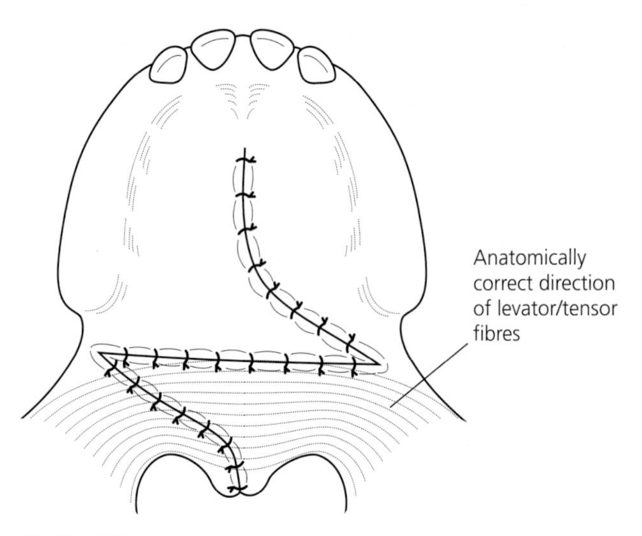

9.3.18 Situation after closure of oral mucosa. Please note the transverse direction of tensor/levator muscle fibres.

The infants should be monitored with pulse oximetry during at least the first 24 hours after the procedure, as post-operative swelling and a naturally increased nasal airway resistance could lead to hypoxia. The post-operative administration of antibiotics is usually not necessary in otherwise healthy children.

PROGNOSIS

Generally, speech and growth outcome after cleft palate repair have improved significantly over the last decades. The question of whether a single- or two-stage repair produces consistently better results has still to be answered. There is more agreement among cleft surgeons about the timing of the soft palate closure. An early repair before the onset of speech in the first year of life seems to lead to the best speech results. Nevertheless, a good proportion of children with cleft palate need speech and language therapy and should be regularly monitored for their speech outcome starting at the age of about two years. A minority of these children will need further surgery at a later stage to improve speech or to treat maxillary hypoplasia.

FURTHER READING

Furlow LT. Cleft palate repair by double opposing Z-plasty. *Plastic and Reconstructive Surgery* 1986; **78**: 724–38.

Gillies HD, Fry WK. A new principle in the surgical treatment of 'congenital cleft palate' and its mechanical counterpart. *British Medical Journal* 1921; **1**: 335–8.

Holland S, Gabbay JS, Heller JB *et al.* Delayed closure of the hard palate leads to speech problems and deleterious maxillary growth. *Plastic and Reconstructive Surgery* 2007; **119**: 1302–10.

Kilner TP. Cleft lip and palate repair techniques. *St Thomas Hospital Report* 1937; **2**: 127.

Kriens OB. An anatomical approach to veloplasty. *Plastic and Reconstructive Surgery* 1969; **43**: 29–41.

Kriens OB. Fundamental anatomic findings for an intravelar veloplasty. *Cleft Palate Journal* 1970; **7**: 27–36.

Mommaerts MY, Combes FA, Drake D. The Furlow Z-plasty in two-staged palatal repair modifications and complications. *British Journal of Oral and Maxillofacial Surgery* 2006; **44**: 94–9.

Ross RB. Treatment variables affecting facial growth in complete unilateral cleft lip and palate. *Cleft Palate Journal* 1987; **24**: 5–77.

Schweckendiek W, Doz P. Primary veloplasty: Long-term results without maxillary deformity. A twenty-five year report. *Cleft Palate Journal* 1978; **15**: 268–74.

Von Langenbeck B. Die Uranoplastik mittels Ablösung des mucösperiostalen Gaumenüberzugs. *Archiv für Klinische Chirurgie* 1862; **2**: 25.

Wardill WEM. Cleft palate. *British Journal of Surgery* 1928; **16**: 127–48.

Widmaier W. A new technique for closure of cleft palate. *Chirurgie* 1959; **30**: 274–8.

9.4

Secondary cleft surgery

JOHN F CACCAMESE JR

INTRODUCTION

Secondary cleft surgery can present a reconstructive challenge significantly greater than that of the initial deformity. The surgeon is frequently managing post-surgical deformities after having little or nothing to do with the primary procedure, as teams and protocols evolve over time. The cleft surgeon must be a student of the protocols and techniques of past years such that they are able to deal with the unique challenges of scarring and compromised blood supply manifest in these previously operated patients. Additionally, one must stay abreast of outcomes so that appropriate and effective secondary surgery can be offered to your patients with reasonable expectations.

EVALUATION AND CORRECTION OF SECONDARY CLEFT LIP DEFORMITIES

The appearance and function of the mended cleft lip are greatly impacted by the initial repair at infancy. The simultaneous reconstruction of functional nasal and labial muscles dictate the growth and development of the underlying facial skeleton, as well as the appearance of the lip. The aesthetic form of the lip is the result of both a carefully designed skin incision and the muscle repair at the initial surgery. Of the multiple skin incisions that have been used, the geometric triangular and quadrangular incisions violate the subunits of the upper lip, while the advancement rotation and its modifications more accurately replicate normal anatomic structures. Furthermore, disadvantages of the geometric repairs include the tendency to create a long lip which can be difficult to correct secondarily, and difficult to convert to a more anatomically appropriate skin incision if eventual revision is required.

As the habilitation of cleft lip and palate consists of a series of procedures whose timing is dependent on chronological and developmental milestones throughout life, the lip repair, which is often the first of many interventions, is critical to all procedures that follow it. It is also important to keep in mind that the staged reconstruction of these patients is a stepwise process, and that careful consideration must be given to each procedure and its downstream effects on subsequent procedures and growth, such that bridges are built and not burned.

While the construction of the labial and nasal muscular rings guides the eventual appearance and symmetry of the lip and nose, the individual's innate ability to heal and scarring tendencies also play a key role in the aesthetic appearance of the repair. Certain technical shortcomings in the repair can also lead to less than optimal results. The underlying skeletal platform must be considered when planning lip revision, as the presence or absence of a bony alveolar cleft or maxillary hypoplasia also greatly impacts the appearance of the nasolabial structures as the child grows. Regardless of attempted soft tissue correction and camouflaging techniques, facial harmony can only be accomplished when these hard tissue problems have been addressed. Therefore, it is recommended that depending on the age of the child and the degree of skeletal dysplasia, major soft tissue revisions be deferred until bone grafting or LeFort osteotomy has been accomplished when possible.

When trying to determine whether a minor revision or a complete takedown of the lip is required, an understanding of the initial deformity and the goals of primary surgery are important. Understanding the secondary deformity, and its global functional and aesthetic shortcomings, are also crucial. Lesser procedures, transpositions and simple scar revisions can be used to address minor height mismatches of the white roll, vermillion notching or vermillion fullness, when the muscle is otherwise noted to be functional and united across the cleft. If applied inappropriately, however, these 'minor' procedures might only serve to amplify defects, increase scarring or leave the patient well short of a complete correction. A complete takedown of the lip should be considered if there are significant issues with lip height or symmetry, nasal symmetry, substantial vermillion/white roll mismatches or a dehiscent orbicularis oris. Finally, when there is significant damage and scarring to the cleft adjacent tissue, especially in the case of the bilateral cleft lip, one may have to recruit nearby tissue to reconstitute the philtral complex and reconstruct the muscular ring.

Reopening the lip may also be advantageous in that it provides an excellent opportunity and additional access to address residual nasal and septal deformities or turbinate issues. While nasal revision is often simply an extension of lip revision surgery, it will be covered in detail separately in Chapter 9.6.

Note on sutures: Unless otherwise specified, the author uses 3/0 or 4/0 chromic gut or polyglactin on tapered needles for mucosal closure, 4/0 polyglactin for muscle approximation, 5/0 or 6/0 polyglactin or poliglecaprone on cosmetic cutting needles for deep dermal facial sutures, and 5/0 or 6/0 nylon on cosmetic cutting needles for skin. Suture selection depends somewhat on the age and size of the patient.

CUTANEOUS LIP PROBLEMS

Long upper lip

The long upper lip is infrequently seen with the predominance of advancement rotation repairs performed today. Excessive lip length was primarily a problem of the triangular and quadrangular repairs, but can be encountered as a result of overzealous rotation in an advancement rotation. The long lip can be a difficult problem to correct, frequently requiring the horizontal excision of tissue at the supravermillion level or in the subalar region. The scars left by these revisions, though reasonably well camouflaged by the white roll and the alar crease, respectively, are less than optimal in appearance.

REDUCTION OF LIP HEIGHT

Subalar excisions or supravermillion excisions can be used to adjust the height of a lip when excessive lip length is encountered. Either form of excision can be combined with philtral modifications as needed, and both generally require the removal of both skin and muscle. Both the subalar and the supravermillion excisions can be designed symmetrically or asymmetrically to address specific length issues (Figure 9.4.1).

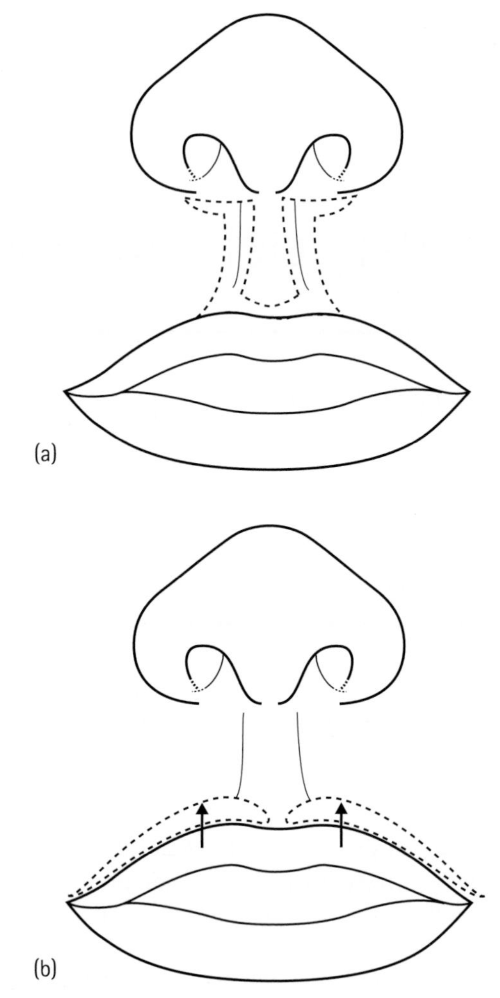

9.4.1 Reduction of lip height.

Tight upper lip

The tight upper lip can stem from overly aggressive soft tissue excision at the time of primary or secondary repair, or be the result of a protuberant premaxilla. The appearance of tissue deficiency can be further accentuated by maxillary hypoplasia, or a full lower lip. Further lip revision that includes soft tissue excision might only serve to enhance the problem unless distant tissue is recruited in the form of an Abbé flap. This pedicled crosslip flap, based on the labial artery, will add width and appropriate bulk, while decreasing the width differential between the upper and lower lip. The Abbé flap may also be of value when the prolabial tissue has been severely damaged by scar.

RECRUITMENT OF DISTANT TISSUE

When the philtral region has been destroyed by scar or when there is a significant full thickness tissue deficiency, a pedicled Abbé flap or lip switch flap is designed based on the labial arterial pedicle of the lower lip (Figure 9.4.2). The flap, as well as the inset defect, can be customized based on the recipient site requirements for height and aesthetics.

- The upper lip incision can be designed to allow downward rotation of the lateral lip elements (Y-shaped, Figure 9.4.2a–c), or it can involve a full thickness excision (Figure 9.4.2d–g) of damaged/scarred tissue.
- A full thickness shield, W- or rectangular shaped flap is designed in the lower lip, including skin, vermillion and mucosa.
- One side of the flap remains pedicled at the vermillion, based on the labial artery.

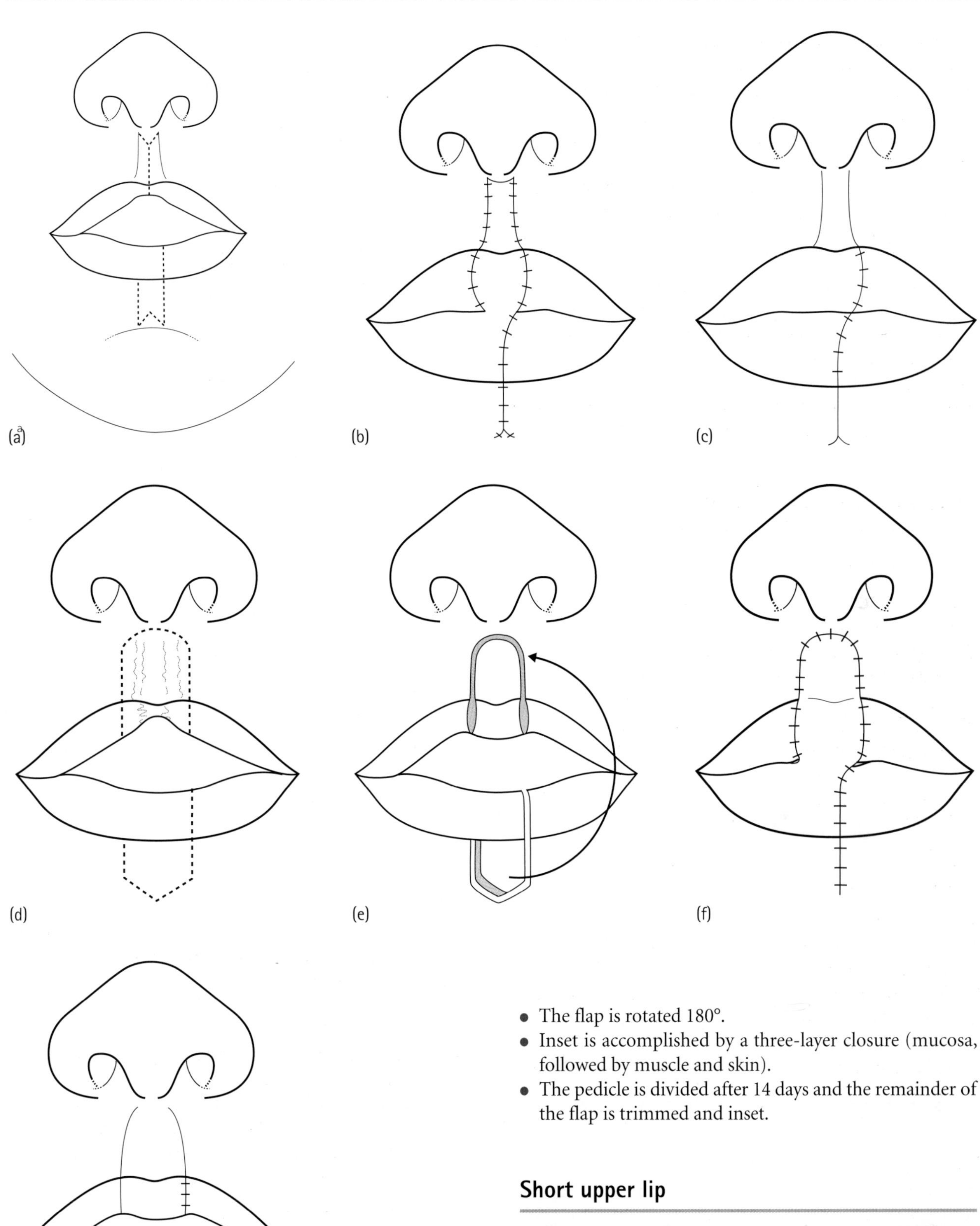

9.4.2 Recruitment of distant tissue.

- The flap is rotated 180°.
- Inset is accomplished by a three-layer closure (mucosa, followed by muscle and skin).
- The pedicle is divided after 14 days and the remainder of the flap is trimmed and inset.

Short upper lip

The short upper lip may be the result of several different shortcomings in the primary lip repair. Most commonly, it is the result of an under-rotated, improperly/incompletely repaired, or dehiscent muscle and this will require a rerepair of the lip. In this case, the original repair scar can be used to access the nasal and labial muscles for an exacting functional repair. If conversion to an advancement rotation from a geometric repair is feasible, it should be considered, as this places the cutaneous scars in a more natural position. Vertical scar contracture might also play a role in the short lip. When the muscle is found to be intact and is dynamically symmetric, and the height discrepancy or contracture involves only one aspect of the lip, such as the vermillion or the vermillion–cutaneous junction, this can sometimes be corrected with a more limited cutaneous or musculo-cutaneous revision.

MINOR NOTCHING OF THE VERMILLION

- *Vermilion Z-plasty.* Vermilion muscle flaps are created at the site of the notch and transposed to fill the vermilion defect. Once the flaps are raised, they can be transposed with skin hooks and the incisions then more specifically extended or trimmed to fill the given defect.
- *Vermillion V–Y-plasty.* A V-shaped musculomucosal incision is created approaching the vermillion notch with the apex of the V pointing towards the maxillary vestibule. The incision is then closed as a Y, advancing the leading edge of the incision into the notch (Figure 9.4.3).

ASYMMETRIES AND/OR WHITE ROLL MISALIGNMENT

- *Wavy line excision.* A wavy line excision of an unaesthetic scar can be used to create symmetry of cupid's bow when it is peaked, and there is otherwise no notch of the lip (Figure 9.4.4). This is based on Pfeiffer's wavy line lip closure, where the wavy line helps to lengthen the skin of the lip along the philtral column.
- *Diamond excision.* Similar to the wavy line, a diamond-shaped excision can be used to eliminate white roll misalignment and cupid's bow asymmetry, based on its geometry and ability to lengthen (Figure 9.4.5).
- *Z-plasty.* When the defect simply involves a white roll misalignment, a simple Z-plasty can be performed (Figure 9.4.6).
- *Complete revision.* The cleft deformity is recreated and a complete muscular reconstruction and cutaneous revision is accomplished. Anatomic points are marked as they would be for a primary lip repair.
- *Unilateral cleft.* The skin is marked similar to that of a primary repair, and for this, the author favours Delaire's markings with a functional muscular repair (Figure 9.4.7):
  - A, superior internal angle of the non-cleft nostril;
  - A′, superior internal angle of the cleft nostril;
  - B, the base of the noncleft columella;
  - C, the depth of cupid's bow;
  - D, the noncleft peak of cupid's bow;
  - E, the end of the white roll on the cleft side;
  - 1, point marks base of the columella on the cleft side (A–A′–1–B should form a parallelogram);
  - 2, point from B–1 extended to the best skin adjacent to the scar (separates nasal skin from lip skin);
  - 3, point should equal D–C (or slightly less, as white roll permits);
  - 4, point at the wet–dry line that equals the distance from D–C, when measured from the frenum;
  - 5, point at the junction of alar base and lip;
  - 6, point on the cleft side skin adjacent to the scar, where a line from 5–6 separates nasal skin from lip skin;
  - 7, point marks the best/thickest white roll on the cleft side;
  - 8, point at the wet–dry line perpendicular to line drawn from 7, coincides with widest portion of dry vermillion.

Additional length in the repair can be obtained through the use of a wavy line as the incision approaches the mucocutaneous junction or by creating a small triangular flap from the noncleft side to be inserted above the white roll. This should enable 1–3 to equal B–D in length.

Careful attention is given to dissecting out and reconstructing the transverse nasalis and the orbicularis oris muscles. Wide subperiosteal undermining of the anterior maxilla, zygoma and nasal bones should be utilized as needed to facilitate advancement.

- *Bilateral cleft.* The skin is marked similar to that of a primary repair, and for this, the author favours a

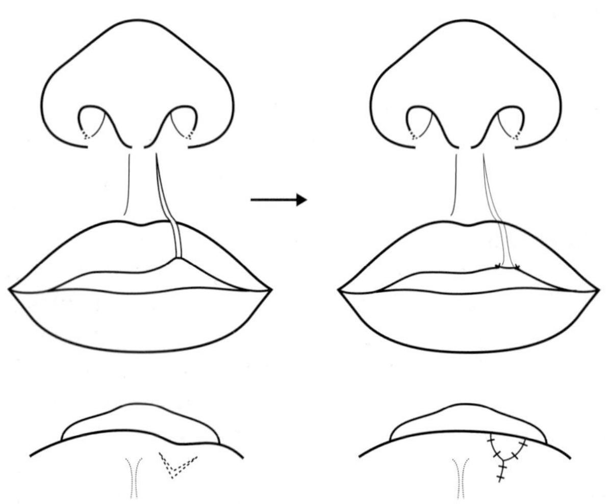

9.4.3 Vermilion V–Y plasty.

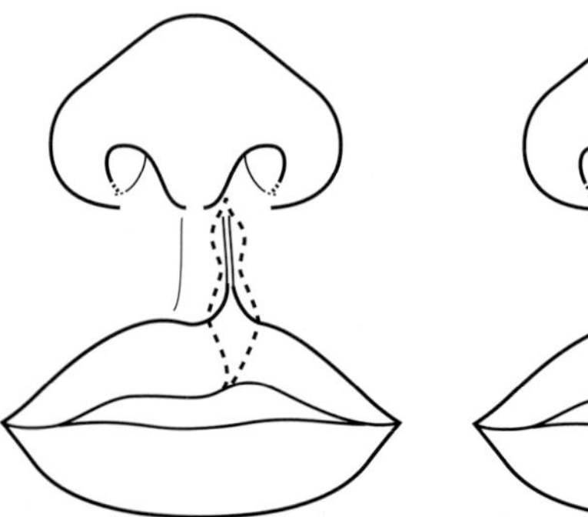
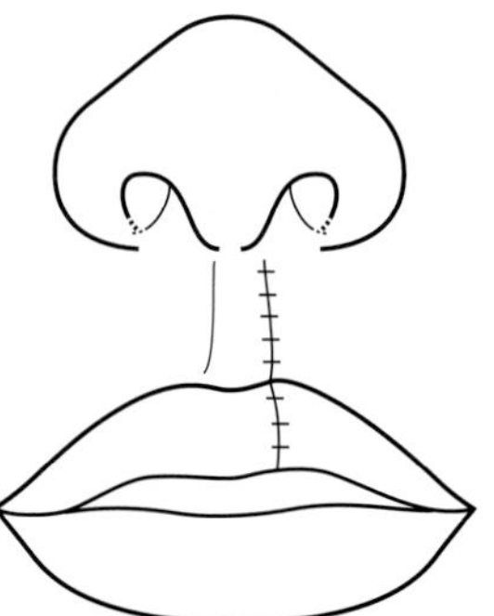

9.4.4 Wavy line excision.

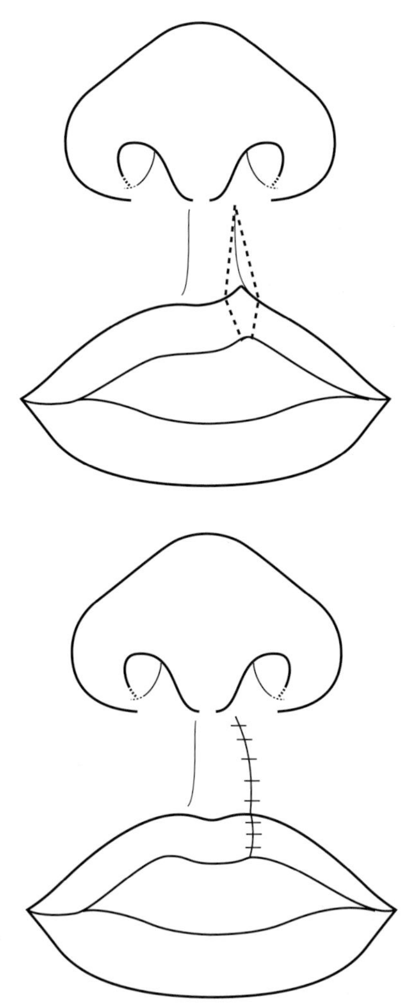

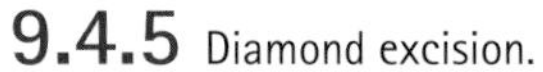

9.4.5 Diamond excision.

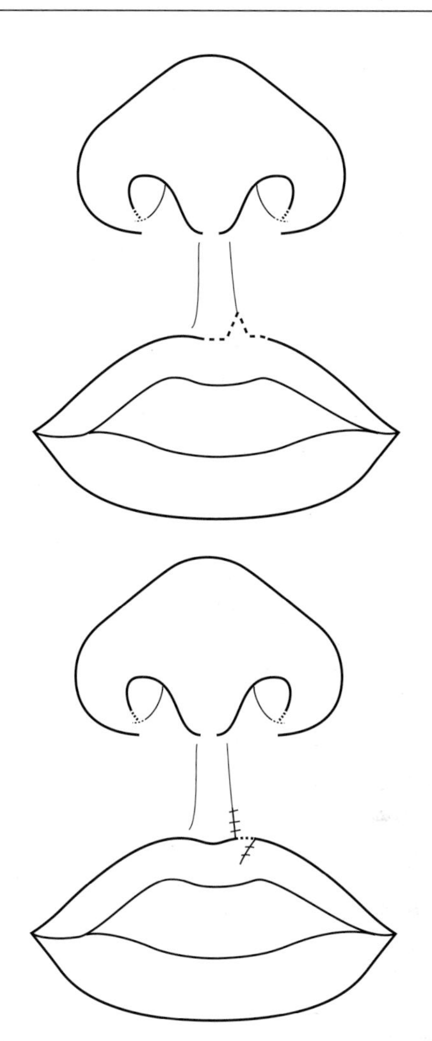

9.4.6 Z-plasty.

modification of Millard's skin markings with functional muscular repair (Figure 9.4.8):

- A, the junction of the alar base and lip;
- B, line from A–B delineates the nasal skin from the lip skin;
- C, the extent of the back cut (C–D) superior to and including the best/thickest white roll (D); also lateral contribution to the peak of cupid's bow;
- D, point marks the best/thickest white roll; also the lateral contribution to the depth of cupid's bow;
- E, marks the greatest width of the wet–dry line, perpendicular from line D (these turndown flaps, C–D–E, form the lateral lip that will be used to reconstruct the central vermillion);
- 1, point marks the superior internal angle of the nostril;
- 2, the base of the columella;
- 3, the depth of cupid's bow;
- 4, point marks the medial contribution to the peak of cupid's bow (3–4 is slightly concave).

The muscular reconstruction, like the vermillion, is accomplished via the lateral nasolabial elements. Again, wide subperiosteal undermining should be utilized to facilitate this process.

PROBLEMS OF THE PHILTRUM

Obliteration of the philtral dimple and cupid's bow asymmetries are occasionally seen following primary lip repair. A flat cupid's bow is sometimes the result of a triangular repair. The philtral dimple can often be preserved in unilateral clefts with minimal cutaneous undermining of the noncleft side at the time of initial repair. A natural dimple is difficult to restore secondarily. Additionally, widening of the scar in the philtral column position can occur as a result of early wound tension, poor suturing or wound breakdown at the initial repair. This can often be treated with simple excision and augmented with other surface treatments, such as CO_2 laser or dermabrasion.

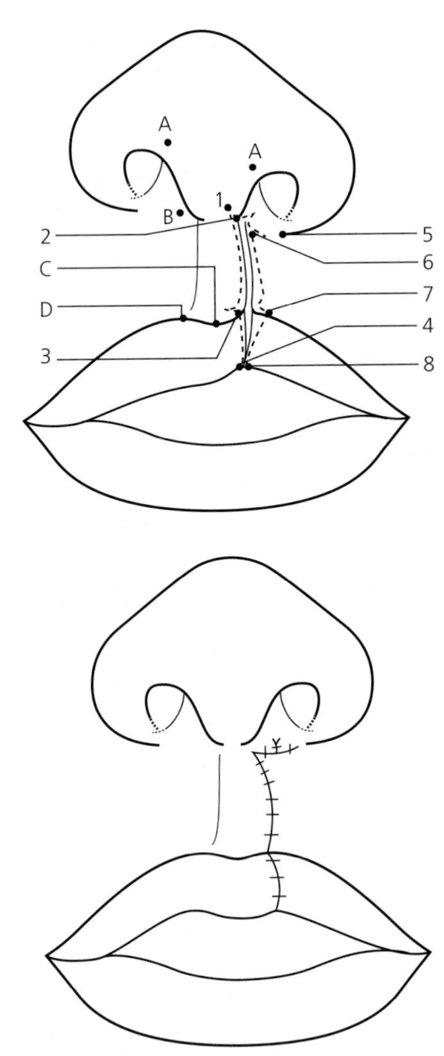

9.4.7 Unilateral cleft.

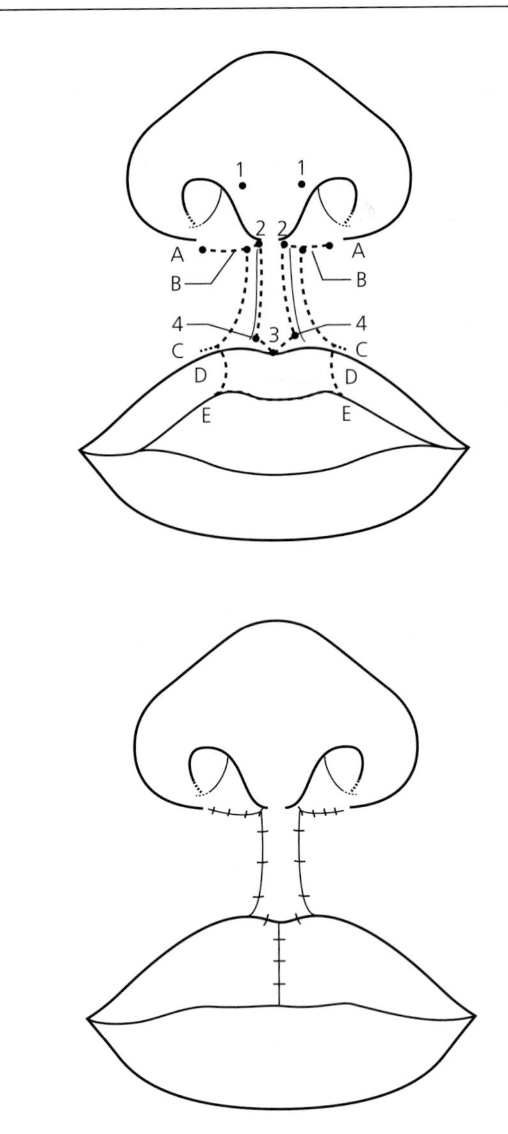

9.4.8 Bilateral cleft.

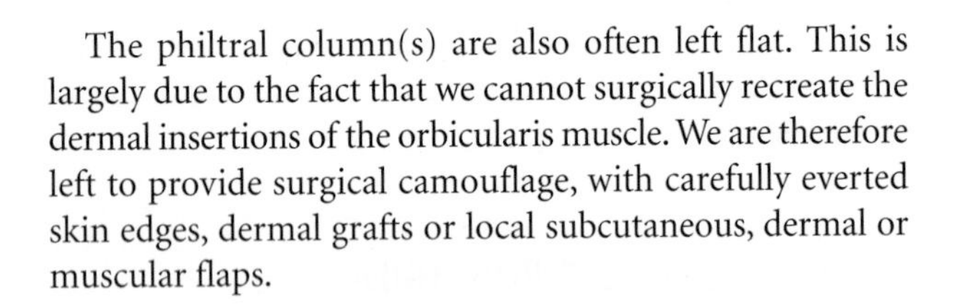

The philtral column(s) are also often left flat. This is largely due to the fact that we cannot surgically recreate the dermal insertions of the orbicularis muscle. We are therefore left to provide surgical camouflage, with carefully everted skin edges, dermal grafts or local subcutaneous, dermal or muscular flaps.

CUTANEOUS DEFECTS

Isolated unaesthetic cutaneous lip scarring can be managed similar to other facial scars, by excision, dermabrasion, etc. One must keep in mind the orientation of the philtral column and other local lip structures. For example, the horizontal orientation of a running W-plasty might not suit this area as well as a wavy line excision to recreate the philtral column. One must also be mindful that the skin of the nose and the skin of the lip are of different quality, much as the skin of the white and red lip. If the skin of the nose has bled down on to the skin of the upper lip or conversely, the skin of the vermillion has bled into the cutaneous lip, this must be addressed in the revision.

SECONDARY CLEFT PALATE SURGERY

Speech and facial growth are the primary outcome measures of cleft palate surgery. Both are highly dependent on the type and the timing of the initial repair. Despite appropriate interventions at the correct time, maxillary hypoplasia, velopharyngeal dysfunction (VPD), and oronasal fistulas can occur. In order to identify patients in need of revision surgery, they should be followed and evaluated by an interdisciplinary team that will provide interval palatal evaluations, dental care, orthodontic care, hearing evaluations and speech evaluations. For the purposes of this chapter, the discussion will be limited to VPD and oronasal fistulas.

ORONASAL FISTULAS

Oronasal fistulas have been reported with a wide range of occurrence. They are frequently left intentionally at the alveolus, to be repaired at the time of secondary bone grafting. They can, however, occur anywhere on the palate and frequently occur in the middle of the hard palate or at the hard palate–soft palate junction. The failure rate of fistula repair increases with each unsuccessful attempt at revision. Many techniques have been described, including the application of local flaps (palatal rerepair), tongue flaps, pedicled flaps, free tissue transfer and augmentation with the acellular dermis.

Midpalatal and junctional fistula repair

The palatal rerepair, raising the original hard palatal flaps and if necessary performing a functional revision of the soft palate, is most useful in most circumstances (Figure 9.4.9). For large fistulas, acellular dermis can be useful as an additional layer and might facilitate healing in the eventuality of dehiscence.

(a) Incisions are made in the mucosa around the fistula and it is turned in toward the nasal side to allow creation of a nasal layer (wound edges everted and sutures tied to the nasal side).
(b) A two-flap or von Langenbeck palatoplasty is performed on the remaining hard palate mucosa, scoring or release is performed laterally and around the neurovascular bundle as needed.
(c) Acellular dermis can be interposed and secured between the oral and nasal flaps, as needed.
(d) The flaps are sutured in the midline.

Velopharyngeal dysfunction

Continuous perceptual speech evaluation is the primary tool for evaluating VPD. The longitudinal evaluation of speech intelligibility can begin shortly after palate repair. Early identification and correction of VPD is critical to avoid the development of compensatory misarticulations. Characteristics of VPD include hypernasal resonance, nasal escape, nasal turbulence and inadequate intraoral air pressure. In addition to perceptual speech evaluation, video-

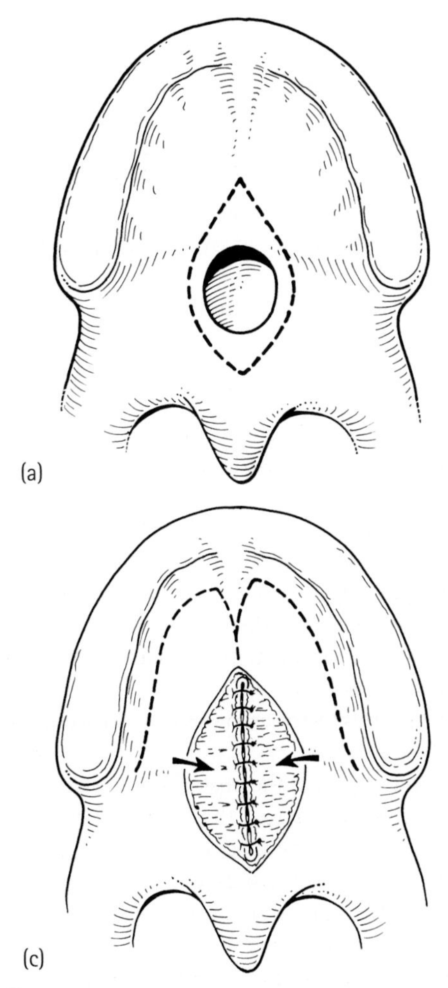

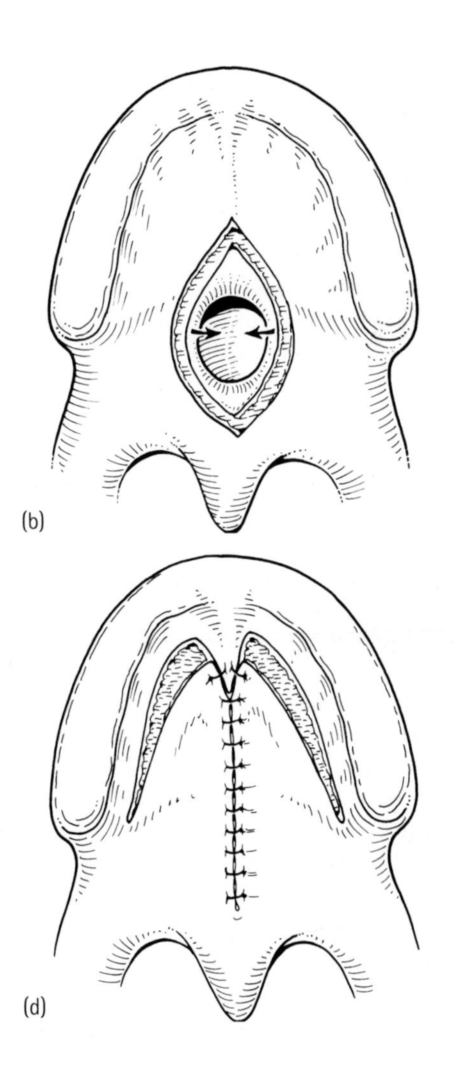

9.4.9 Midpalatal and junctional fistula repair.

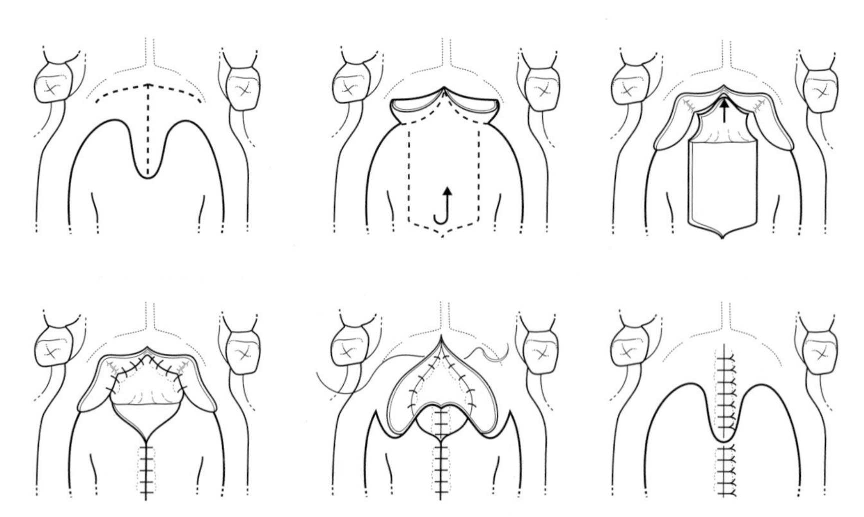

9.4.10 Superiorly base pharyngeal flap.

fluoroscopy, nasal endoscopy and nasometry might be useful in identifying the size and nature of the velopharyngeal defect.

Surgical treatment largely consists of three modalities: revision palatoplasty, superiorly based pharyngeal flap and sphincter pharyngoplasty.

REVISION PALATOPLASTY

Revision palatoplasty, in an effort to avoid the morbidity of pharyngoplasty, is an effort to restore functional continuity to the palatal muscles and length to the palate, especially in patients who have had little to no dissection of the velar muscles. In this group, the velar muscle bundles are seen to be oriented sagitally, instead of transversely. Techniques described for this purpose include intravelar veloplasty with retropositioning of the muscle sling or Furlow palatoplasty. Both achieve retropositioning of the velar sling and have demonstrated efficacy in limited cohorts. These revision procedures are felt to be more physiologic than pharyngoplasty and are best utilized for those who demonstrate small anteroposterior gaps as viewed by nasoendoscopy or videofluoroscopy. Should VPD persist following six to 12 months of additional speech therapy, pharyngoplasty is still an option.

SUPERIORLY BASED PHARYNGEAL FLAP AND SPHINCTER PHARYNGOPLASTY

Both the pharyngeal flap and the sphincter pharyngoplasty have demonstrated value in the management of VPD, but more so than the selection of the procedure, the VP gap size and closure pattern are likely to influence the clinical outcome of the operation, regardless of which procedure is performed. Despite multiple attempts in the literature to delineate the best operation for specific VP defects, recent randomized controlled comparisons of sphincter pharyngoplasty and pharyngeal flap for VPD demonstrated no difference in long-term speech outcomes. Therefore, one must consider specific patient issues and the potential morbidities of the operation when selecting a VPD technique.

SUPERIORLY BASED PHARYNGEAL FLAP

- The palate is divided in the midline a few millimeters from the hard palate through the uvula (Figure 9.4.10). Lateral incisions (nasal flaps) are made anteriorly and extended toward the pharyngeal walls.
- A superiorly based flap is elevated at the depth of the prevertebral fascia approximately two-thirds the width of the posterior pharyngeal wall, long enough to reach the anterior extent of the palatal incision without tension.
- The tip of the flap is inset into the apex of the palatal incision, the lateral aspect of the flap is sutured to the lateral edges of the soft palate flaps.
- The nasal flaps are closed over the raw surface of the pharyngeal flap.
- The palate is closed in the midline.

MODIFIED HYNES SPHINCTER PHARYNGOPLASTY

- The palate is retracted superiorly with an instrument or by a suction catheter passed through the nose and sewn to the palate.
- Vertical incisions are made along the anterior aspect of the posterior tonsillar pillars in a cephalocaudal direction.
- A similar incision is made on the posterior aspect of the tonsillar pillars, capturing the palatopharyngeus muscle in a superiorly based flap.
- The flaps are transected as low as possible to allow tension free apposition.
- The superior aspect of the posterior tonsillar incisions are joined transversely across the posterior pharynx at the depth of the prevertebral fascia.
- The pillar flaps are transposed and sutured end to end (Figure 9.4.11c) or in an overlapping fashion (Figure 9.4.11d) (to decrease the port size).
- The superior and inferior transverse incisions are closed.
- The tonsillar pillar defect is closed.

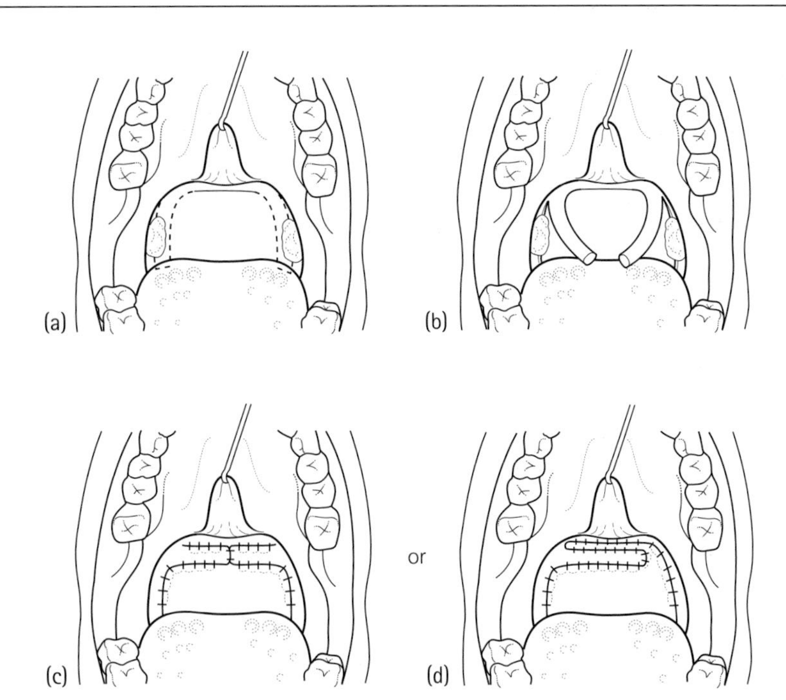

9.4.11 Modified Hynes sphincter pharyngoplasty.

Top tips

- Consider the totality of the lip/nose defect as this frequently leads to and is best served by total lip revision and muscular reconstruction.
- Consider revision palatal surgery for small to moderate velopharyngeal gaps when an intravelar veloplasty has not been previously performed, it is a more physiologic option than pharyngoplasty.
- The first opportunity to close a palatal fistula is the best one. Do not limit your results by performing less surgery than is required. Consider augmenting the closure with acellular dermis when appropriate.

FURTHER READING

Abyholm F, D'Antonio L, Davison-Ward SL *et al.* Pharyngeal flap and sphincterplasty for velopharyngeal insufficiency have equal outcome at 1 year postoperatively: Results of a randomized trial. *Cleft Palate Craniofacial Journal* 2005; **42**: 501–11.

Boorman JG, Shivaram Barathwaj V. Secondary palatal surgery and pharyngoplasty. In: Ward Booth P *et al.* (eds). *Maxillofacial surgery*, vol. II. St Louis: Churchill Livingstone Elsevier, 2007: 1102–19.

Brusati R, Mannucci N, Mommaerts MY. The Delaire philosophy of cleft lip and palate repair. In: Ward Booth P *et al.* (eds). *Maxillofacial surgery*, vol. II. St Louis: Churchill Livingstone Elsevier, 2007: 1027–47.

Eufinger H, Machtens E. Microsurgical tissue transfer for rehabilitation of the patient with cleft lip and palate. *Cleft Palate Craniofacial Journal* 2002; **39**: 560–7.

Hynes W. Observations on pharyngoplasty. *British Journal of Plastic Surgery* 1967; **20**: 244–56.

Kirschner RE, Cabiling DS, Slemp AE *et al.* Repair of oronasal fistulae with acellular dermal matrices. *Plastic and Reconstructive Surgery* 2006; **118**: 1431–40.

Markus AF, Delaire J. Functional primary closure of cleft lip. *British Journal of Oral and Maxillofacial Surgery* 1993; **31**: 281–91.

Markus AF, Delaire J, Smith WP. Facial balance in cleft lip and palate. I. Normal development and cleft palate. *British Journal of Oral and Maxillofacial Surgery* 1992; **30**: 287–95.

Markus AF, Delaire J, Smith WP. Facial balance in cleft lip and palate. II. Cleft lip and palate and secondary deformities. *British Journal of Oral and Maxillofacial Surgery* 1992; **30**: 296–304.

Millard DR. Personal approach to cleft lip. In: *Cleft craft: The evolution of its surgery*, vol. 1: The unilateral deformity. Boston: Little Brown, 1976: 165–88.

Millard DR. A radical rotation in single harelip. *American Journal of Surgery* 1958; **95**: 318–22.

Millard DR. Shaping and positioning the lip-switch flap in unilateral clefts. In: *Cleft craft: The evolution of its surgery*, vol. 1: The unilateral deformity. Boston: Little Brown, 1976, 593–628.

Noorchashm N, Dudas JR, Ford M *et al.* Conversion Furlow palatoplasty: Salvage of speech after straight-line palatoplasty and 'incomplete intravelar veloplasty'. *Annals of Plastic Surgery* 2006; **56**: 505–10.

Perkins JA, Lewis CW, Gruss JS *et al.* Furlow palatoplasty for management of velopharyngeal insufficiency: A prospective study of 148 consecutive patients. *Plastic and Reconstructive Surgery* 2005; **116**: 72–80, discussion 81–4.

Pfeifer G, Schmitz R, Herwerth-Lenck M, Gundlach KKH. Long term results following primary lifting of the nose and labioplasty according to the wave line procedure in unilateral complete clefts. In: Pfeifer G (ed.). *Craniofacial anomalies and clefts of the lip, alveolus and palate*. Fourth Hamburg International Symposium. New York: Thieme, 1991: 239–46.

Sommerlad BC, Mehendale FV, Birch MJ *et al.* Palate re-repair revisited. *Cleft Palate Craniofacial Journal* 2002; **39**: 295–307.

Talmant JC, Markus A, Precious DS, Mommaerts MY. Secondary cleft surgery. In: Ward Booth P *et al.* (eds). *Maxillofacial surgery*, vol. II. St Louis: Churchill Livingstone Elsevier, 2007: 1073–91.

Ysunza A, Pamplona C, Ramirez E *et al.* Velopharyngeal surgery: A prospective randomized study of pharyngeal flaps and sphincter pharyngoplasties. *Plastic and Reconstructive Surgery* 2002; **110**: 1401–7.

9.5

Alveolar bone grafting

TIM FLOOD

INTRODUCTION

There are many types of facial clefting disorders reported in the literature. The cleft lip and palate anomaly is the most common of these, being reported in approximately 1:700 live births. In 75 per cent of cleft lip and palate cases, the cleft runs through the alveolus.

Perhaps the most important development in the treatment of cleft lip and palate patients followed the work of Boyne and Sands and was the introduction of reconstruction of the alveolar cleft with bone, at a time when the growth of the maxilla is largely completed (secondary alveolar bone grafting). Attempts at alveolar bone grafting go back as far as 1901 when Von Eiselberg used a pedicled bone graft to fill the defect. However, in 1908, Lexter was the first to demonstrate the use of free bone grafts.

CLASSIFICATION

Alveolar bone grafting can be classified as follows:

- primary (0–3 years), often undertaken at the time of lip repair and now of historical significance only;
- early secondary (3–6 years), before the eruption of the permanent incisor teeth;
- secondary (6–13 years), before the eruption of the permanent canine teeth;
- late (after 13 years), after the eruption of the permanent canine teeth.

PRESENTATION AND TREATMENT AIMS

Functional and aesthetic problems are associated with cleft lip and palate. The severity of these will depend upon the type of cleft (unilateral or bilateral).

Common presenting problems:

- discharge and smell from the nose;
- oral food/fluids leaking from the nose;
- poor speech;
- inability to suck up a straw or blow up balloons;
- poor appearance of the incisor teeth, which traumatize the upper lip;
- missing or supernumerary teeth within the cleft area, which are often decayed;
- difficulty cleaning teeth in the cleft area;
- poor facial appearance.

The objectives of alveolar bone grafting are therefore aimed at addressing the above complaints as follows:

- complete closure of all oronasal fistulas with significant improvement in speech;
- restoration of the continuity of alveolar/dental arch with bone;
- providing stability to the premaxilla and dental arch;
- allowing normal eruption of the permanent teeth in the cleft area and providing sufficient bone for the placement of dental implants, where needed;
- allowing orthodontic alignment of the maxillary dentition.

Additional benefits can also be achieved with reconstruction of the nasal floor and piriform aperture, as follows:

- improvement of nasal symmetry;
- a functional nasal airway;
- support for the upper lip.

TIMING OF SURGERY

Primary bone grafting was adopted by many centres in the 1950s and early 1960s; however, reports emerged demonstrating a significant detrimental effect of this procedure on maxillary growth. Secondary bone grafting was advocated by Boyne and Sands. This approach was popularized by further work undertaken by Abyholm *et al.* Where possible, alveolar bone grafting should be undertaken between the ages of six and 13 years. Perhaps the ideal age is eight years following the peak in maxillary growth and before the unerupted canine tooth has started to erupt from bone into the cleft. This is usually before the canine root has developed two-thirds of its final length. Waiting until maximal transverse growth of the maxilla has been achieved may avoid the need for presurgical maxillary expansion or at least minimize the presurgical orthodontic treatment required. Timing of surgery is largely guided by dental age, although other factors such as psychological development, speech and social circumstances should be taken into account in a multidisciplinary and child-friendly setting. Where the permanent canine tooth has already erupted into the cleft area, this will significantly compromise the graft and consideration should be given to delaying the grafting procedure until the canine is fully erupted and can be aligned by presurgical orthodontic therapy to optimize the surgical outcome.

Late alveolar bone grafting is known to be less successful. This is due to a number of factors including poor hygiene and tobacco smoking. This patient group, however, should not be excluded from treatment and it is important that alveolar bone grafting is offered to older patients requesting facial reconstruction and dental rehabilitation. Careful and comprehensive treatment planning is essential and most patients will require presurgical orthodontic treatment. It is essential that alveolar bone grafting precedes facial osteotomy surgery and reconstructive rhinoplasty for optimal results.

PATIENT ASSESSMENT

Patients should be assessed within a multidisciplinary setting. A full history should focus on previous surgical episodes and complications related to these. Examination of the cleft area should note the presence of supplemental and supernumerary teeth and the presence of dental caries in the remaining dentition. Deciduous teeth which have erupted into the cleft will compromise the available soft tissue for flap reconstruction and should be removed prior to definitive surgery.

Photographic and radiographic records (panoramic, occlusal and periapical films) are essential for treatment and audit. Fully coned three-dimensional computed tomography (CT) scanning is becoming increasingly important as this gives full visualization of the cleft defect at a reasonable radiation dosage. When used post-operatively, it is possible to accurately assess the volume of successfully grafted bone and is a powerful audit tool.

Study models are obtained and, for the bilateral cleft cases, an interocclusal acrylic wafer is constructed to the predetermined agreed post-operative position of the premaxilla.

SURGICAL TECHNIQUE

Surgery is undertaken under general anaesthesia with nasal intubation in both unilateral and bilateral cases. Use of ilium is the author's preferred option for harvesting bone as this site reliably produces large volumes of donor bone and allows a second team to harvest bone simultaneously. Infiltration of the oral cavity with local anaesthetic solution with vasoconstrictor helps intraoperative haemostasis and dissection, and aids post-operative pain control. The mouth is irrigated with a chlorhexidine solution and prophylactic antibiotic therapy instituted and continued for 5 days. The primary objectives of the surgery are to close all oronasal fistulas and therefore the whole of the cleft area, including the hard palate, needs to be widely exposed. Scar tissue lying within the cleft alveolus and nasal floor area should be excised to create room for grafted bone.

Bone grafting

Through a small incision over the iliac crest, dissection is taken to the perichondrium of the crest. The cartilaginous cap is divided along its length with stop cuts at either ends and the cartilage cap retracted medially to expose the inner aspect of the ilium. A corticocancellous block is now harvested with additional cancellous bone (Figure 9.5.1). The cortical sheet is now separated from the cancellous block and the cancellous portion morcellated. The wound is closed primarily with insertion of an epidural catheter into the wound to provide post-operative analgesia with a local anaesthetic solution.

Unilateral clefts

Incisions for flaps are made starting in the buccal suclus posteriorly along the gingival margins from the upper first molar tooth to the cleft margin on the lesser segment (Figures 9.5.2 and 9.5.3).

A second flap is raised on the greater segment sufficient to expose the piriform aperture on the noncleft side.

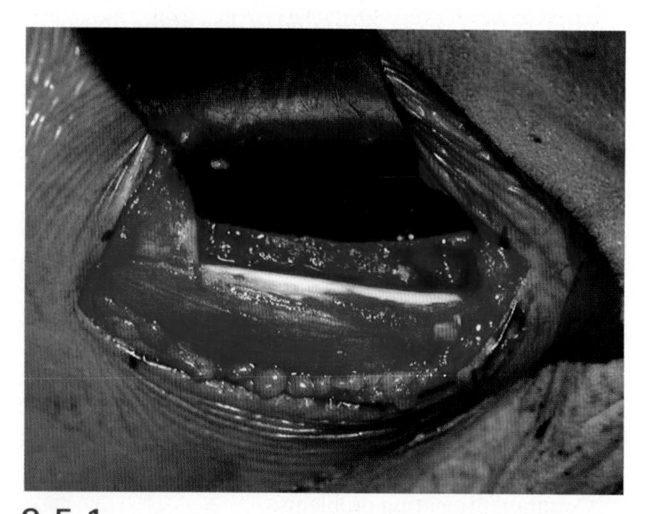

9.5.1 Cartilage splitting approach to ilium and volume of available bone.

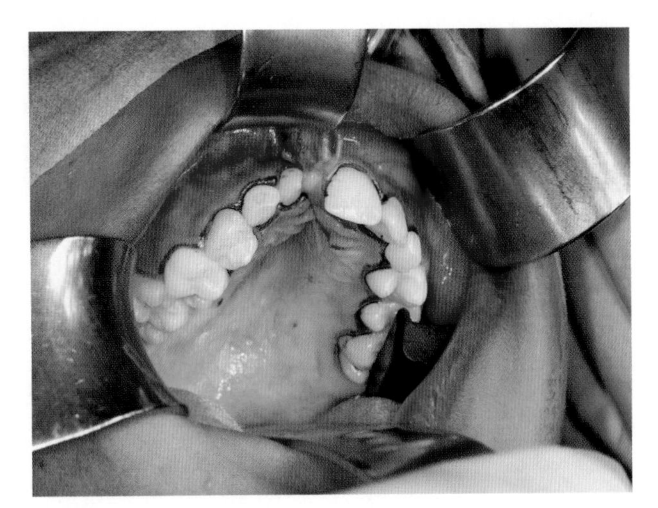

9.5.2 Planned incisions.

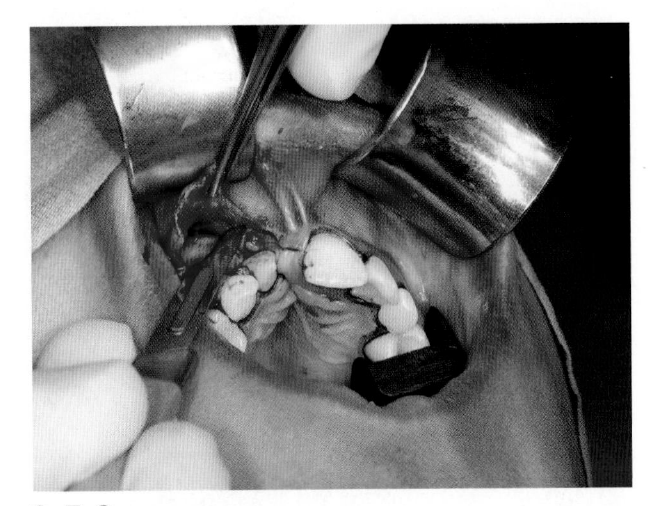

9.5.3 Dissection of labial mucoperiosteal flaps from the cleft area.

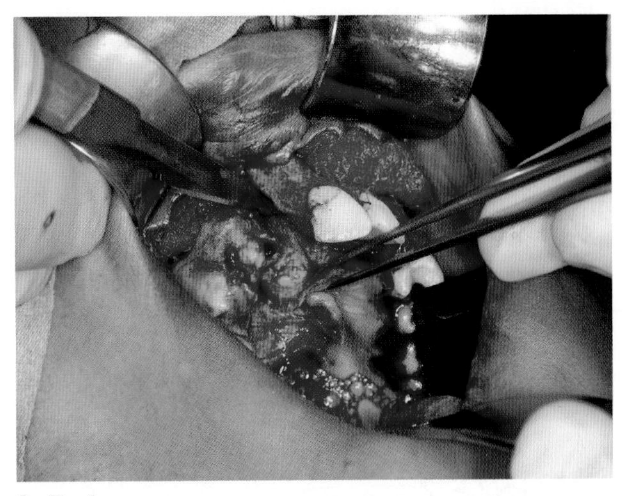

9.5.4 The horizontal incision into the cleft to separate the nasal layer from the palatal tissues with Veau flaps being elevated.

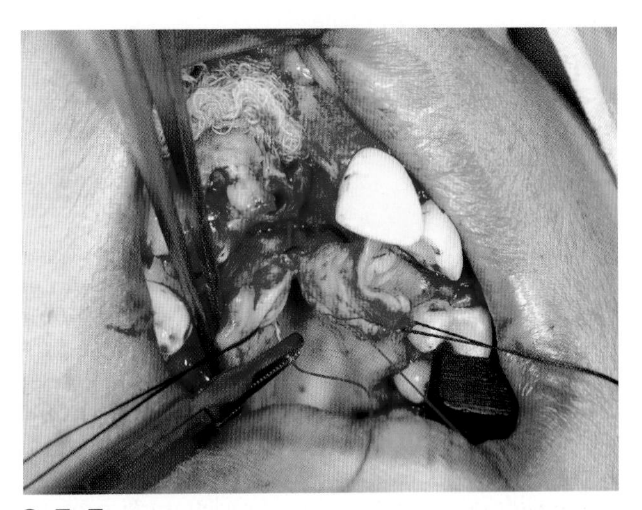

9.5.5 Approximation of the Veau flaps following wide exposure of the cleft area.

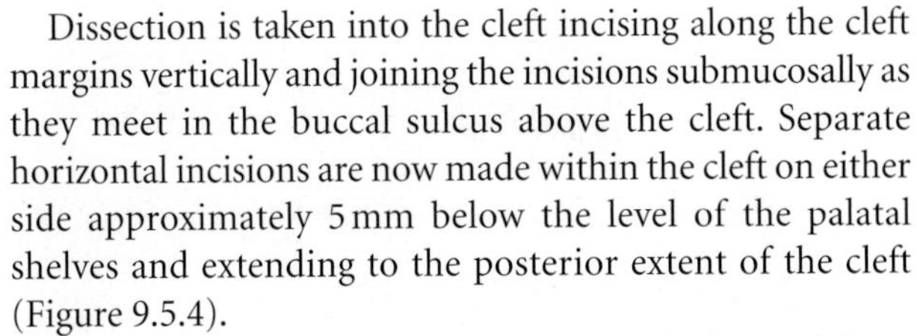

Dissection is taken into the cleft incising along the cleft margins vertically and joining the incisions submucosally as they meet in the buccal sulcus above the cleft. Separate horizontal incisions are now made within the cleft on either side approximately 5 mm below the level of the palatal shelves and extending to the posterior extent of the cleft (Figure 9.5.4).

Bilateral Veau palatal flaps are raised as far posteriorly as possible to fully expose the cleft in the hard palate. Where necessary, a backcut is made medial to the molar teeth should advancement be required. The cleft is now fully exposed.

The medial margins of the Veau flaps are trimmed and approximated with a continuous suture (Figure 9.5.5). Where the inferior turbinate has hypertrophied and is lying within the cleft alveolus, this is trimmed to above the level of the palatal shelves as described by Iino (Figures 9.5.6 and 9.5.7).

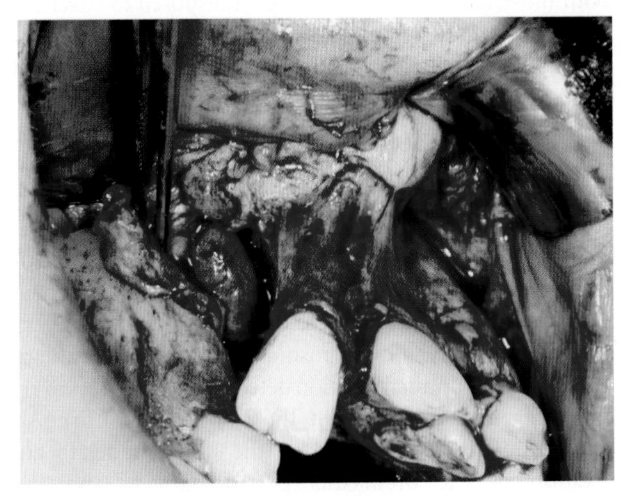

9.5.6 The hypertropy of the inferior turbinate lying within the alveolus area of the cleft.

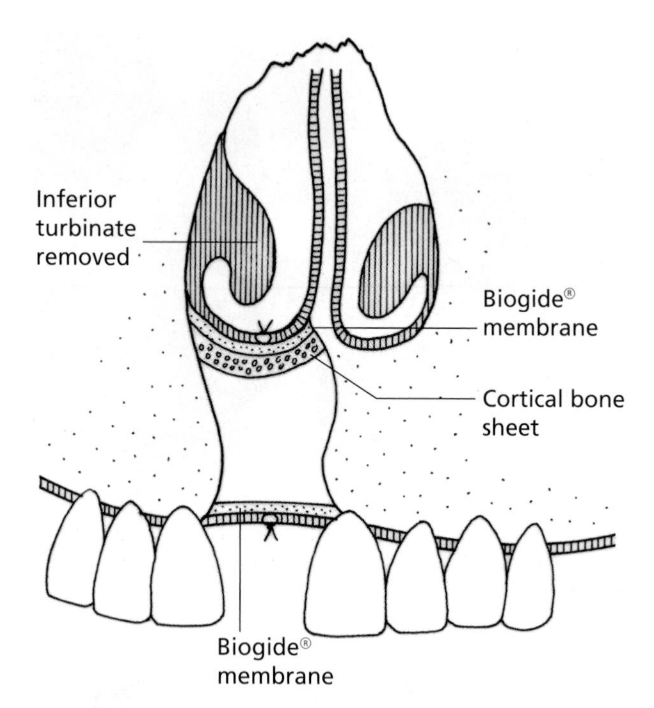

9.5.7 Inferior turbinectomy and reconstruction of the nasal floor with a Bio-Gide biomembrane overlying a thin sheet of cortical bone.

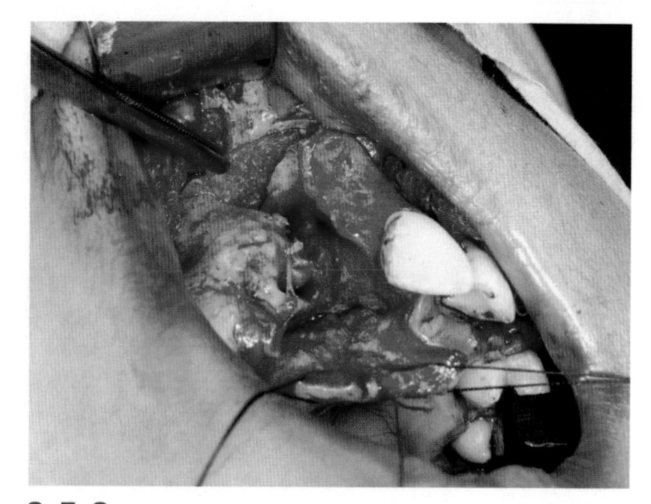

9.5.8 Formal reconstruction of the nasal floor at the level of the piriform aperture with a thin sheet of cortical bone.

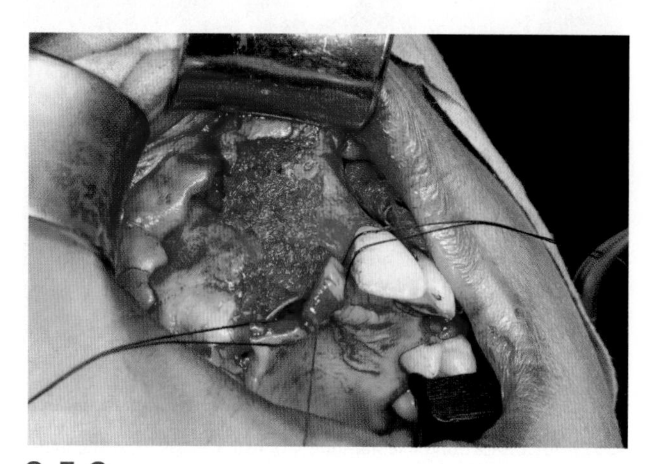

9.5.9 Reconstruction of the alveolus with cancellous bone chips. Note the Bio-Gide biomembrane on the palatal surface of the bone.

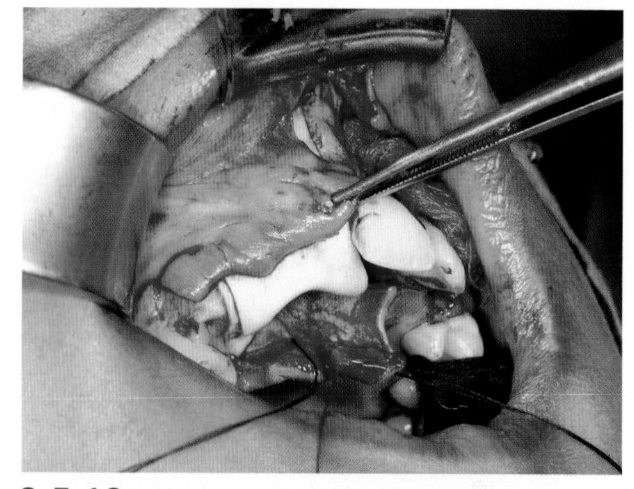

9.5.10 The graft covered with Bio-Gide and the mucoperiosteal release flap rotated to cover the graft without tension.

Following removal of any excess mucosa, the nasal layer is approximated closing the fistula along its length. A thin sheet of cortical bone is inserted at the level of the piriform aperture reconstructing the nasal floor (Figure 9.5.8). A biomembrane (Bio-Gide®; Geistlich Pharma, Wolhusen, Switzerland) is placed above the cortical sheet which acts as a barrier to ingress of infection and promotes guided tissue regeneration.

Bio-Gide is also placed on the cleft surface of the approximated Veau flaps (Figure 9.5.9) and the cancellous bone chips are packed tightly into the cleft defect.

The buccal surface of the grafted cleft is then also covered with Bio-Gide and the buccal flaps transposed to cover the graft and sutured without tension (Figure 9.5.10). Rotation of these flaps ensures a satisfactory sulcus depth in the cleft area.

Bilateral clefts

Full exposure of the bilateral cleft is required for closure of the nasal layer and to facilitate a reliable palatal flap repair. The surgical technique therefore includes premaxillary osteotomy which allows repositioning of the premaxillary segment to an optimal position determined pre-operatively following consultation with the cleft orthodontist. An acrylic wafer is constructed on the study model to aid fixation of the premaxilla post-operatively and the orthodontist is asked to band and place brackets on the maxillary teeth.

Buccal mucoperiosteal flaps are raised as before; however, special care is taken when performing the vertical incision on the premaxillary side of the cleft (Figure 9.5.11). The mucoperiosteum on the labial aspect of the premaxilla has to remain attached on a wide base to the premaxilla as this will form the vascular supply to the premaxillary segment.

Horizontal incisions into the cleft on either side are made at the level of the nasal floor and these are extended to the midline and join on the palatal aspect of the premaxilla and are designed in such a way as to leave a generous cuff of mucosa attached to the premaxilla. The posterior horizontal incisions inside the cleft are then extended as one incision in the midline over the caudal end of the hypertrophied vomerine/maxillary suture freeing up the whole of the nasal mucosal layer (Figure 9.5.12).

The vomerine/maxillary suture area is now osteotomized with either a small osteotome or drill. The premaxilla can now be reflected in a superior direction based on the labial pedicle and the nasal layer is closed along the length of the cleft (Figure 9.5.13).

Finally, bilateral Veau flaps are raised, as described previously, with backcuts if necessary to give additional length. These are trimmed medially and approximated. A cortical bone sheet, covered by Bio-Gide, is now placed on both sides of the cleft and a further sheet placed to bridge the palatal shelves to reconstruct the nasal floor. The premaxilla is repositioned in the planned post-operative position and the attached lingual cuff of mucosa sutured to the Veau flaps across the width of the anterior palate (Figure 9.5.14).

Bio-Gide is placed on the inside of the suture line and cancellous bone is packed into the cleft defect from both sides and covered with further Bio-Gide. Finally, the buccal mucoperiosteal release flaps are rotated and advanced to cover the grafted clefts and sutured into place (Figure 9.5.15). The acrylic wafer is now wired into place securely.

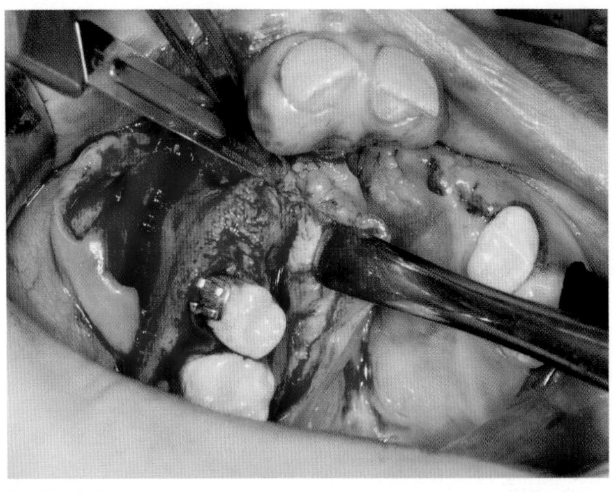

9.5.12 Division of nasal and palatal tissues and elevation of flaps. Note the generous cuff of mucosa on the palatal aspect of the premaxilla.

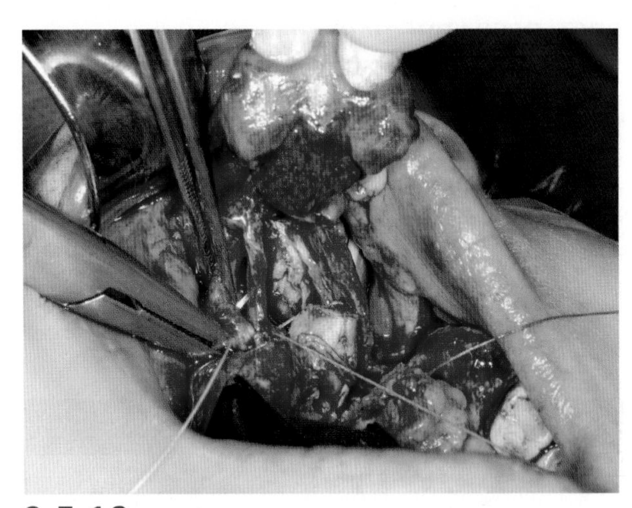

9.5.13 The osteotomized premaxilla is retracted anteriorly allowing excellent vision for accurate closure of the nasal layers.

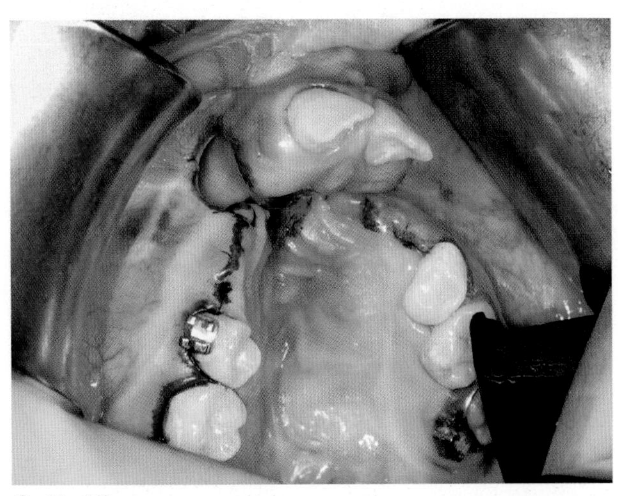

9.5.11 Incisions in a bilateral case.

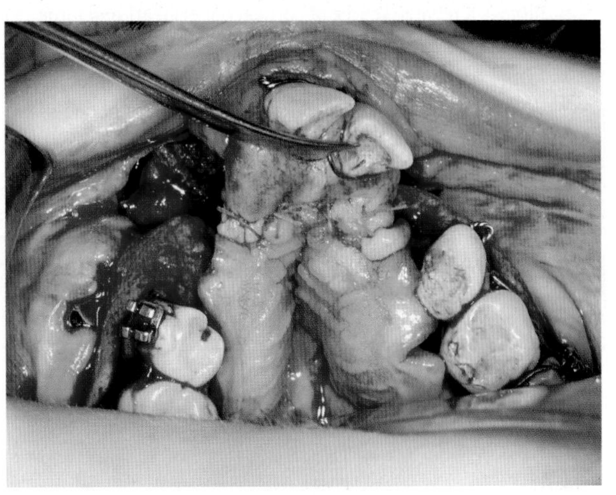

9.5.14 The premaxilla is repositioned and palatal tissues approximated prior to final placement of the cancellous graft.

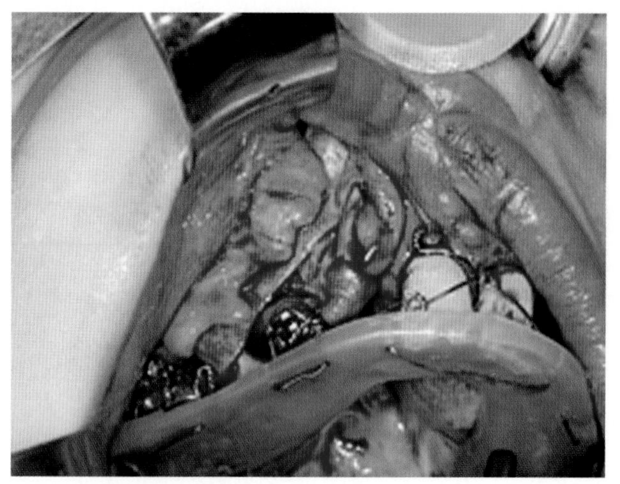

9.5.15 Rigid fixation of the premaxilla into a locating wafer prior to final closure over the Bio-Gide biomembrane covering the graft.

POST-OPERATIVE CARE

Antibiotics and a chlorhexidine mouthwash are continued for 1 week and the patient is placed on a liquidized diet and strict oral hygiene measures for 3 weeks. Ambulation is encouraged on the first post-operative day. Complications are rare with these procedures, although minor wound dehiscence is not uncommon. Infection of the graft is the most serious complication and where dehiscence occurs, it is wise to extend the prophyactic antibiotic cover.

Top tips

- Planning of treatment is best undertaken in a multidisciplinary team setting.
- Optimum age for alveolar bone grafting is between seven and nine years of age.
- Wide exposure of the cleft is essential for success.
- Ilium is a reliable source of cortical bone sheets and large volumes of cancellous bone.
- In the bilateral case, premaxillary osteotomy, combined with guided tissue regeneration, followed by a period of rigid fixation produces predictable results.
- Computed tomography is a powerful audit tool as bone volumes can be measured accurately.
- It is essential that alveolar bone grafting precedes facial osteotomy surgery and cleft rhinoplasty for optimal results.

FURTHER READING

Abyholm FE, Bergland O, Semb G. Secondary bone grafting of alveolar clefts. A surgical/orthodontic treatment enabling a non-prosthodontic rehabilitation in cleft lip and palate patients. *Scandinavian Journal of Plastic and Reconstructive Surgery* 1981; **15**: 127–140.

Arctander K, Klobenstvedt A, Aalokken TM *et al.* Computer tomography of alveolar bone grafts 20 years after repair of the unilateral cleft lip and palate. *Scandinavian Journal of Plastic and Reconstructive Surgery* 2005; **39**: 11–14.

Banks P. The surgical anatomy of secondary cleft lip and palate deformity and its significance in reconstruction. *British Journal of Oral Surgery* 1983; **21**: 78.

Boyne PJ, Sands NR. Secondary bone grafting of residual alveolar and palatal clefts. *Journal of Oral Surgery* 1972; **30**: 87–92.

Bureau S, Penko M, McFadden L. Speech outcome after closure of oronasal fistulas with bone grafts. *Journal of Oral and Maxillofacial Surgery* 2001; **59**: 1408–13.

Iino M, Kondoh T, Fukuda M *et al.* Partial inferior turbinectomy during secondary alveolar bone grafting. *International Journal Oral and Maxillofacial Surgery* 2002; **31**: 489–94.

Kazemi A, Stearns JW, Fonseca RJ. Secondary grafting in the alveolar cleft patient. *Oral and Maxillofacial Surgery Clinics of North America* 2002; **14**: 477–90.

Posnick J. The staging of cleft lip and palate reconstruction: Infancy through adolescence. In: Rose R, Ross A (eds). *Craniofacial and maxillofacial surgery in children and young adults.* Philadelphia: WB Saunders, 2000: 785–815.

Scott JK, Webb RM, Flood TR. Premaxillary osteotomy and guided tissue regeneration in secondary bone grafting in children with bilateral cleft lip and palate. *Cleft Palate Craniofacial Journal* 2007; **44**: 469–75.

9.6

Cleft rhinoplasty

ILANKO ILANKOVAN

It is natural for the harelip surgeon to be so pleased with the satisfactory lip repair, that his eyes will be temporarily out of focus while gazing upon the nose.

Gillies and Millard (1957)

Despite all the improvements in primary cleft surgery, cleft nasal deformity still remains a functional and aesthetic dilemma for both patients and surgeons.

There is inherent composite tissue abnormality or hypoplasia. The developmental problems therefore can be divided into the following three categories: the covering, the framework (bone and cartilage) and the lining. The questions are: What are the deformities and what is the optimal time for correction?

There is adequate information in the literature that early limited correction of the lower lateral cartilage provides no subsequent growth disturbance, allows better nasal growth and reduces the psychological trauma to the child. Developmentally, the explanation falls into two distinct factors which are responsible for the cleft nasal deformity. First, there is agenesis of tissue due to the lack of mesodermal and ectodermal quantity. Second, there is associated deformation as a result of mechanical stresses located within the cleft margins.

The deformities of the unilateral cleft nose are:

- Septum
  - perpendicular plate deviating to the cleft side;
  - quandranticular cartilage deviating cordally towards the noncleft side;
  - nasal spine deviating to the noncleft side.
- Dorsum
  - bony pyramid deviating to the noncleft side;
  - asymmetry of the nasal bone and flattened at the cleft side;
  - asymmetry of the upper lateral cartilage on the cleft side;
  - disturbed junction between the upper and lower lateral cartilages on the cleft side;
  - downward displacement of the lower lateral cartilage on the cleft side;
  - tendency for bifidity;
  - buckling of the lateral crura on the cleft side;
  - reduced height of the medial crura on the cleft side.
- Columella
  deviation at the top to the cleft side and at the base to the noncleft side.
- Alar base
  - lateral displacement resulting in a horizontal rotation of the nostril at the cleft side.

The deformities of the bilateral cleft nose are:

- Septum
  - no specific deviation;
  - disturbed caudoventral outgrowth.
- Dorsum
  - lack of projection and flattening of the osseo-cartilaginous vault;
  - disturbed junction between the upper and lower lateral cartilages.
- Tip
  - bifidity;
  - downward rotation of the alar cartilage;
  - buckling of the lateral crura on both sides.
- Columella
  - very short.
- Alar base
  - lateral displacement resulting in horizontal rotation of both nostrils.

Alveolar cleft, hypoplasia and retroposition of the maxilla compound the nasal deformity.

We divide our approach to cleft rhinoplasty into three stages. They are:

1. Rhinoplasty procedures at the time of primary cleft lip surgery.
2. Cleft rhinoplasty during the preschool years.
3. Definitive cleft rhinoplasty once growth has stopped.

Pre-operative assessment is the most important step. The family's and patient's impression of the deformity and their expectations should be discussed in detail. The aim is always improvement and not perfection.

RHINOPLASTY PROCEDURES AT THE TIME OF PRIMARY CLEFT LIP SURGERY

We describe two different approaches. One is based on McComb's technique where patients undergo presurgical orthopaedics and the other is based on Ahuja's technique, where no presurgical orthopaedics is carried out.

Unilateral

At the time of the lip repair, the skin of the nose on the cleft side is freed from the underlying bony and cartilaginous skeleton. Sharp pointed scissors are passed up through the incision in the upper buccal sulcus on the side of the cleft, extending the dissection over the cleft half of the nose. The same scissor is also used to free the dome of the alar cartilage and the medial crura. The dissection is carried out in this same plane up to the nasion.

Now the affected lower lateral cartilage should be able to be easily lifted upwards with the attached nasal lining.

The alar lift will be maintained by two mattress sutures (Figure 9.6.1). A straight needle with 3/0 nylon suture is started at the nasion, just cranial to the dissection boundary. The needle is passed through the intercrural angle into the nostril. A bolster is passed through the needle, then the needle is passed through the nasal lining and lateral crura and then passed subcutaneously to the exit point at the nasion. Here, another bolster is applied and the two ends of the suture are held in a clip and the needle is cut. A similar second suture is placed, if necessary, towards the lower third of the lateral crura (Figure 9.6.2). Alar lift is carried out to the desired contour, compared to the noncleft side and both sutures held in a clip until the primary lip repair is completed. The final knotting is completed once a desirable height is contoured. The mattress sutures are removed at 5–7 post-operative days.

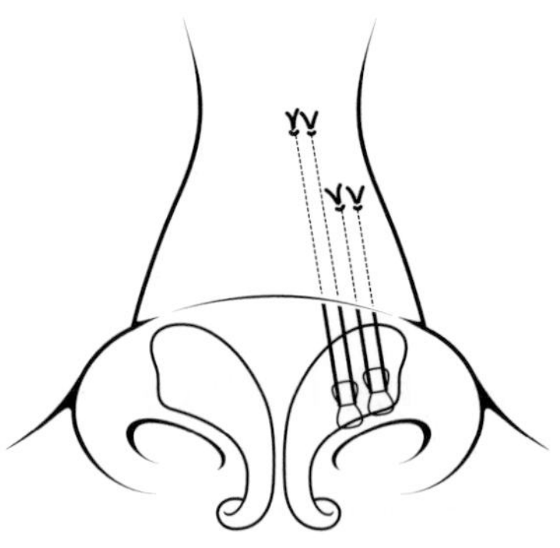

9.6.2 Second mattress suture placed towards the lower third of the lateral crura.

Bilateral

The procedures are carried out exactly the same as in the unilateral procedure, however, there is no landmark position to place the alar lift. The upper lateral cartilages should normally be at the same height as the lower lateral cartilage. Therefore, the aim of lifting should be to the height of the upper lateral cartilage and to reduce the nostril size equally (Figures 9.6.3 and 9.6.4).

This is based on Ahuja's 'limited open' approach, where elevation, medial rotation and suture fixation of the lateral crura, reconstruction of the nostril sill, alar base positioning and correction of the vestibular webbing is carried out along with lip repair.

The nasal tip and lower half of the dorsum were exposed and an inverted U incision on the cleft side and a marginal incision on the non cleft side (Figure 9.6.5).

The inverted U incision on the cleft side is joined with the buccal sulcus incision. The upper half of the medial crura, the dome and the lateral crura of both alar cartilages were dissected from the dorsal nasal skin. The base of the lateral crura on the cleft side is released from the pyriform margin.

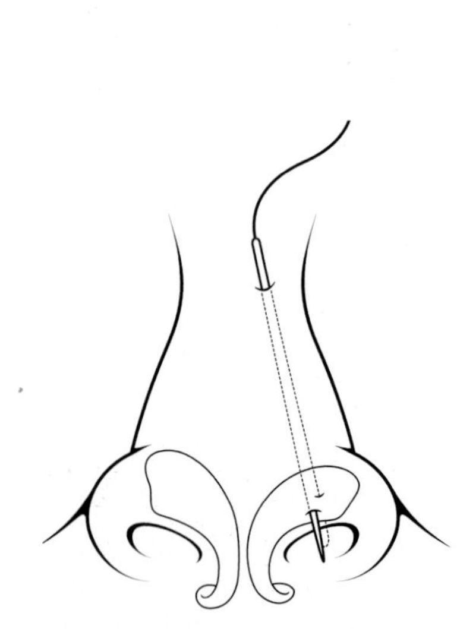

9.6.1 First mattress suture in a unilateral cleft placed via the intercrural angle.

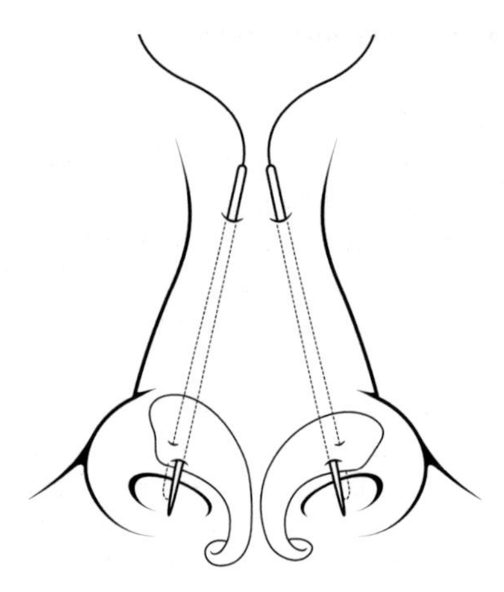

9.6.3 First mattress suture in bilateral cleft.

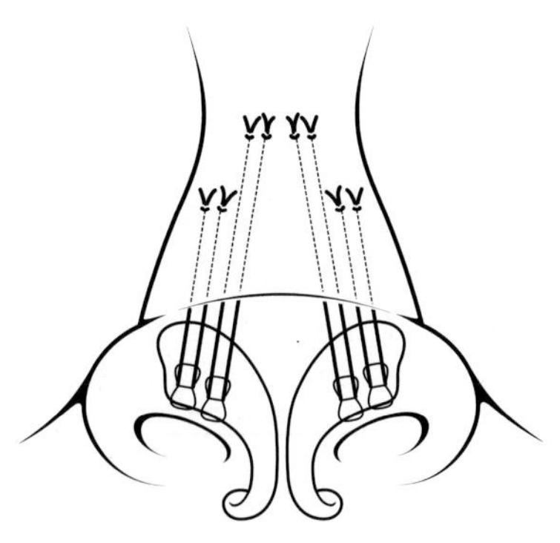

9.6.4 Second mattress suture in bilateral cleft.

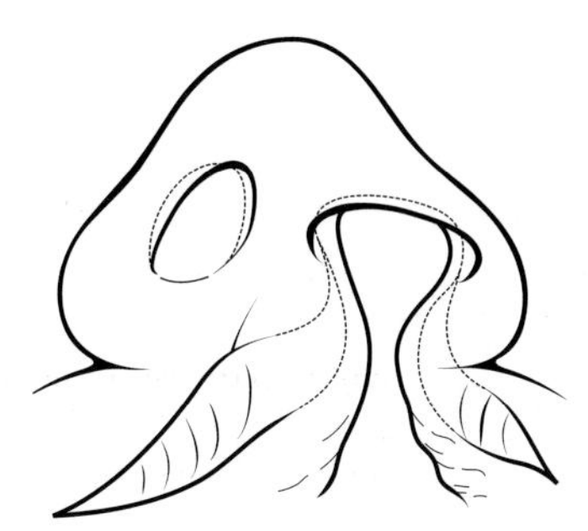

9.6.5 Inverted U incision on the cleft side and the marginal incision on the non cleft side.

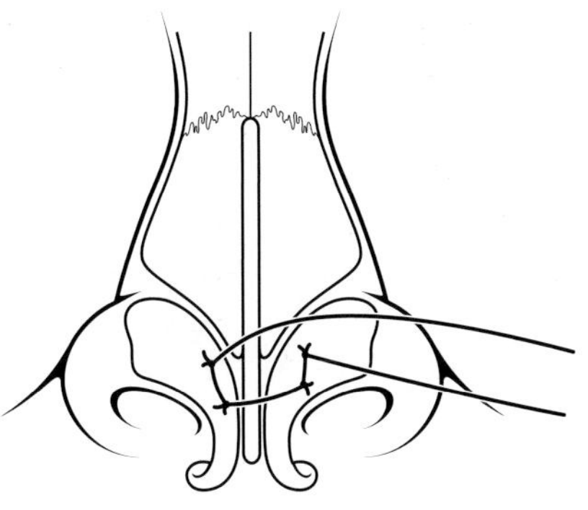

9.6.6 Horizontal mattress suture from the cleft side to the non cleft side.

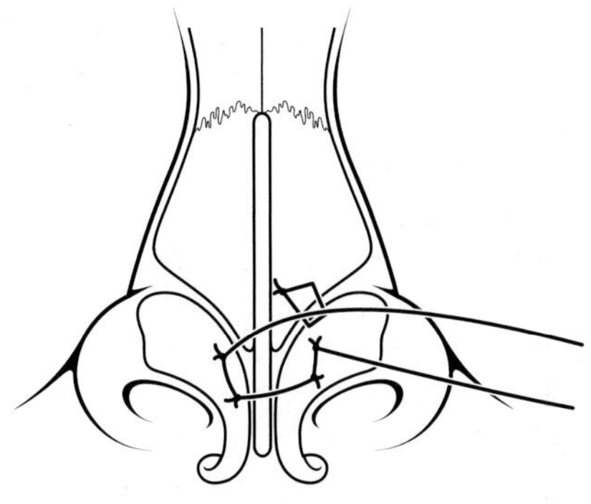

9.6.7 Second horizontal mattress suture from the lateral crura on the cleft side to the lower end of ipsilateral upper lateral cartilage.

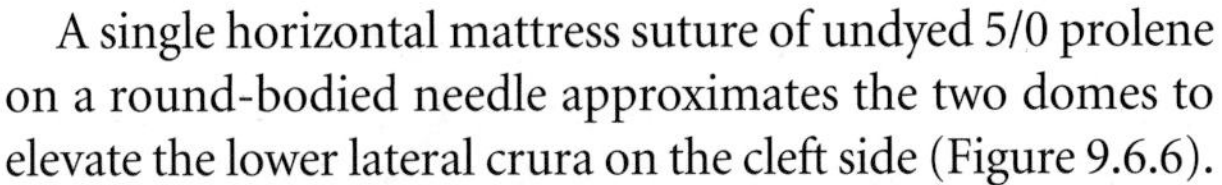

A single horizontal mattress suture of undyed 5/0 prolene on a round-bodied needle approximates the two domes to elevate the lower lateral crura on the cleft side (Figure 9.6.6).

A second suture of the same material is used to fix the lateral crura on the cleft side, to the lower end of the ipsilateral upper lateral cartilage (Figure 9.6.7). This mattress suture is placed in a differential manner on both ends, depending upon the adjustment required. On the cleft side from the lip repair, the part of the advanced mucosa is fed into the vestibular incision to compensate for the shortage of the lining that can lead to the vestibular web or fold.

The cleft lip is repaired in the usual way, together with reconstruction of the nostril sill and floor.

A suitable nasal splint is placed and maintained as long as possible (Figure 9.6.8). In Ahuja's technique, he recommended a vaseline gauze for 5–7 days. The authors prefer the former.

Bilateral inverted U incisions are used. Dissections of the upper half of the medial crura on both sides, as well as the dome and lateral crura from the overlying skin. The base of the lateral crura on both sides is dissected from the pyriform margins.

The desired alar height is checked in relation to the height of the upper lateral cartilage and the sutures placed accordingly. The advanced mucosa from both sides of the lip repair is fed into the vestibular incisions (Figure 9.6.9). The bilateral cleft is repaired in the usual way, together with reconstruction of the nasal sill and floor. Suitable nostril splints are placed and maintained as long as possible.

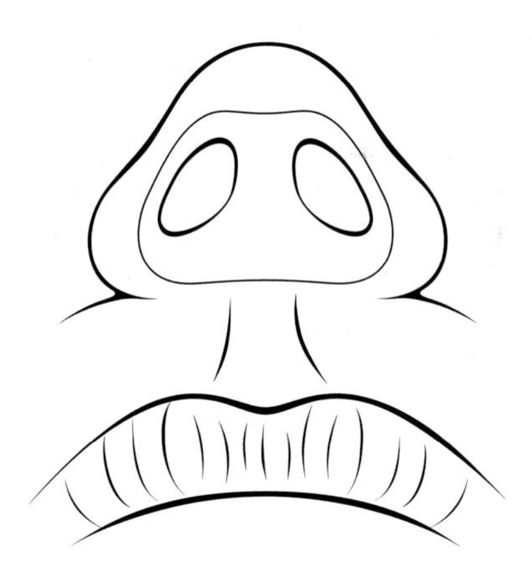

9.6.8 A silicone nasal implant *in situ*.

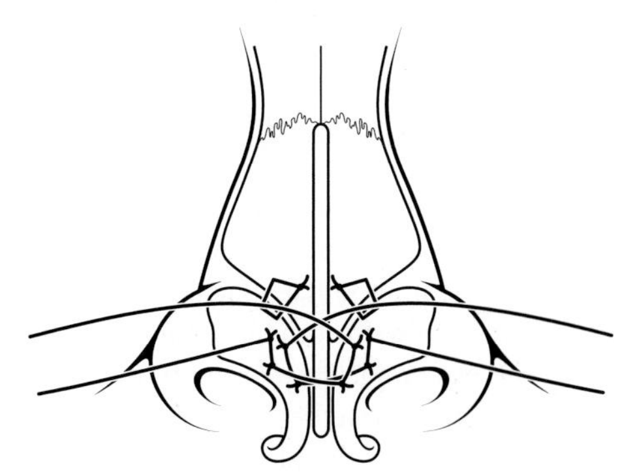

9.6.9 Two horizontal mattress sutures placed for bilateral clefts.

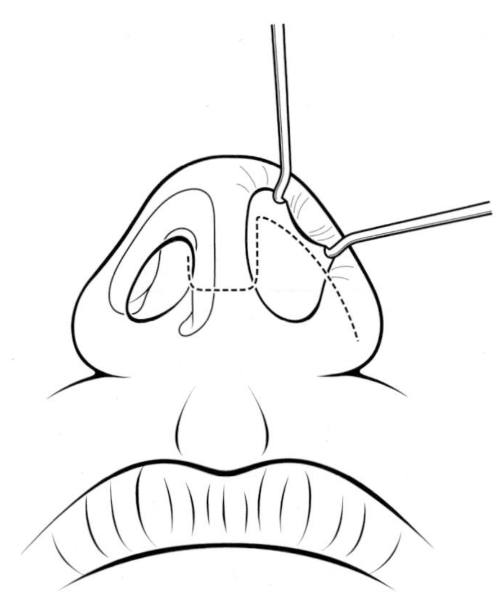

9.6.10 A mid columella transverse incision with bilateral infracartilaginous incision.

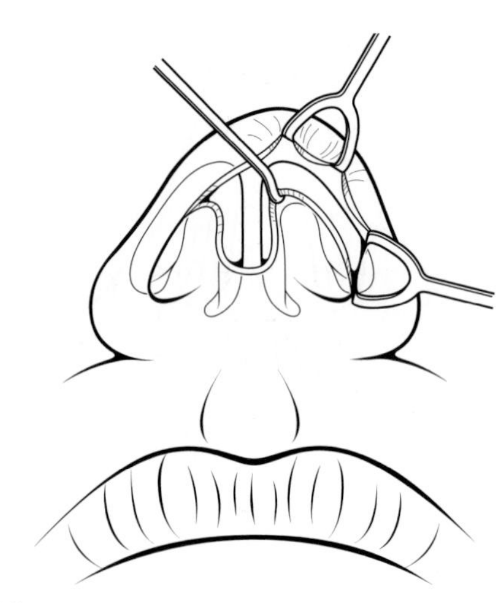

9.6.11 The required mobilisation on the cleft side is assessed by placing a skin hook.

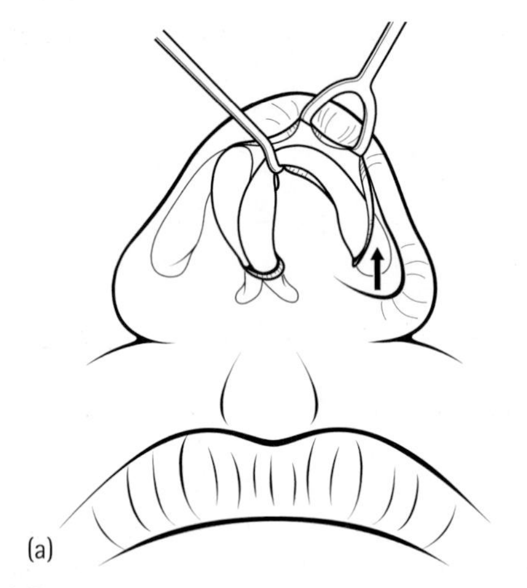

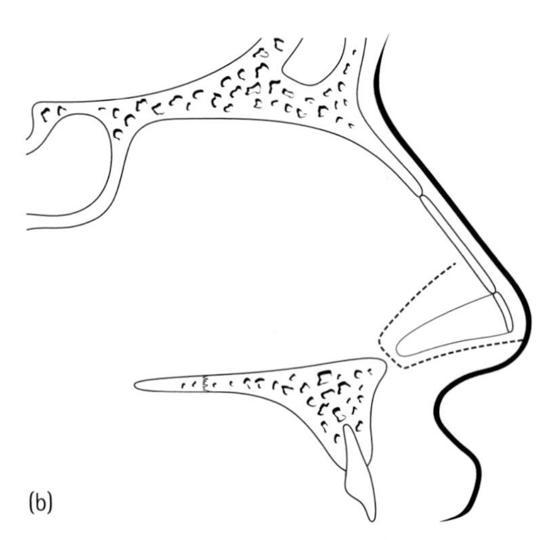

9.6.12 (a) Frontal view of lateral mucosa dissection towards the inferior turbinate. (b) Lateral view showing the inferior turbinate mucosal flap.

CLEFT RHINOPLASTY DURING THE PRESCHOOL YEARS

Unilateral

A mid-columella transverse incision is made across the columella. It is extended superiorly on the inner edge of the columella to the dome, continuing as an infracartilaginous incision down to the pyriform aperture. The lower lateral cartilage and upper lateral cartilages are exposed (Figure 9.6.10). The fibrous attachment of the lower lateral cartilage to the upper lateral cartilage and the rim of the maxilla are freed by sharp dissection. The interdomal attachment between both lower lateral crura are also freed. This should allow the lower lateral cartilage to be completely free and mobile, allowing it to be evaluated for mucosal tethering on the lateral end.

The deficiency of the cleft side mucosa is evaluated by placing a hook in the intermediate crura margin and advancing the freed lower lateral cartilage with attached mucosa to match the height of the noncleft side (Figure 9.6.11). If there is tethering of the lower lateral cartilage, re-evaluation of the previous release of the lower lateral cartilage from the upper lateral cartilage and the rim of the maxilla is made to ensure that only the mucosal attachment remains (Figure 9.6.12). If the mucosa is still tight and limits elevation of the lower lateral cartilage, an inferior turbinate mucosal flap is raised, which is attached to the lower lateral cartilage and the mucosa and this flap is completely elevated into the pyriform fossa.

After release of the lower lateral cartilage and correction of the mucosal deficiency, the chondromucosal unit is advanced into its correct position and held in two places; first, it is fixed to the apex of the medial crura, which is fixed to the opposite side medial crura on the noncleft side (Figure 9.6.13). Second, the lateral third of the lower lateral crura on the cleft side to the lower part of the upper lateral crura. No sutures are placed to the septal cartilage.

The skin is redraped and closed over with 6/0 prolene sutures. Additional support can be provided with alar transfixation sutures to the skin at the alar crease. The number can vary from one to three (Figure 9.6.14). The advantages are that it reconstitutes the alar crease, supports the nasal tip projection and prevents vestibular webbing.

A suitable nostril splint is applied and maintained as long as possible. The sutures are removed on the 7th post-operative day.

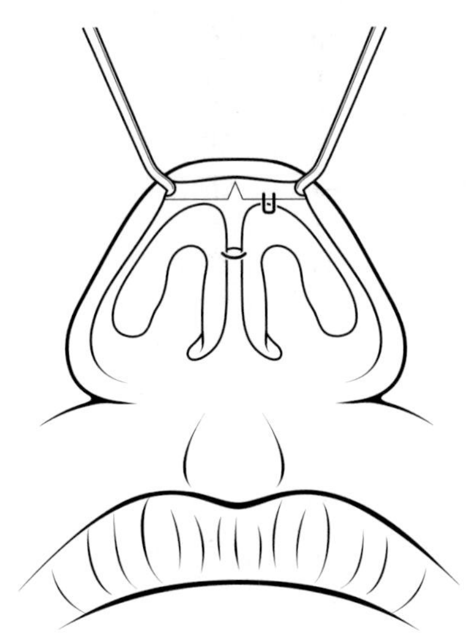

9.6.13 Two mattress sutures placed at the apex of the middle crura and the lateral crura to the upper lateral cartilage.

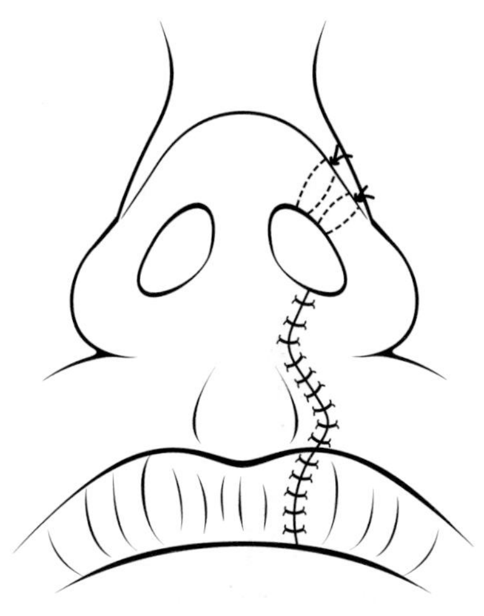

9.6.14 Alar transfixation sutures to the skin at the alar crease.

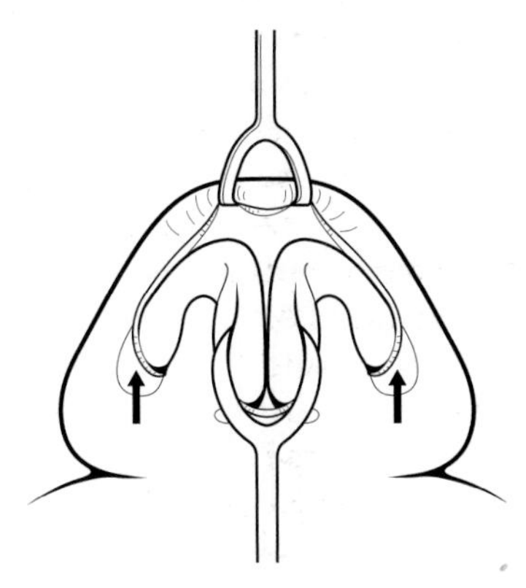

9.6.15 Mid columellar incision and bilateral infracartilaginous incision extending towards the inferior turbinate.

Bilateral

A mid-columellar transverse incision is made across the columella (Figure 9.6.15). Similar to the unilateral approach, here a bilateral approach is made along the columella and along the infracartilaginous area. The whole of the lower half of the nose is exposed after blunt and sharp dissection. Bilateral inferior turbinate flaps are raised to ensure that there is no mucosal tethering (Figure 9.6.16). The chondromucosal unit is advanced to an acceptable height and held by two sutures as before.

The skin is redraped and closed with 6/0 prolene sutures. Additional sutures can be provided with alar transfixion sutures bilaterally.

When redraping the columella skin, if there is a deficiency along the columella, a composite earlobe graft can be used in the defect. A word of caution here, however, if the bed vascularity is not adequate, the graft may not take.

DEFINITIVE CLEFT RHINOPLASTY ONCE GROWTH HAS STOPPED

Septal correction

The approach is two-fold. First is a dorsal approach once the nasal lobule is degloved via a columellar and infracartilaginous incision. The second is a hemi-transfixion incision as in any septoplasty procedure.

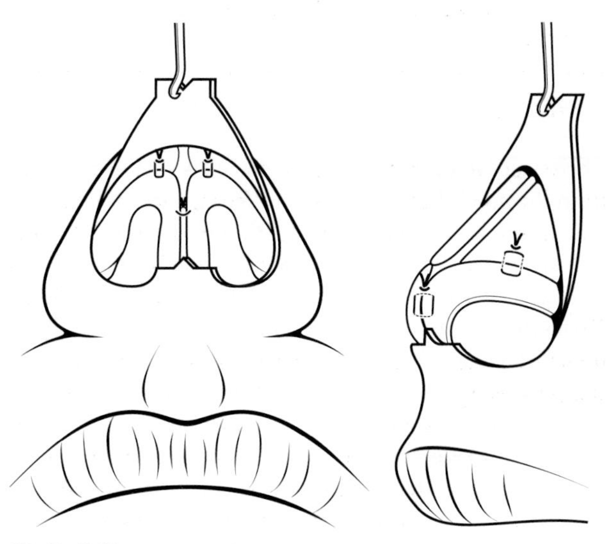

9.6.16 Bilateral inferior turbinate chondro-mucosal flaps and placement of three sutures as before.

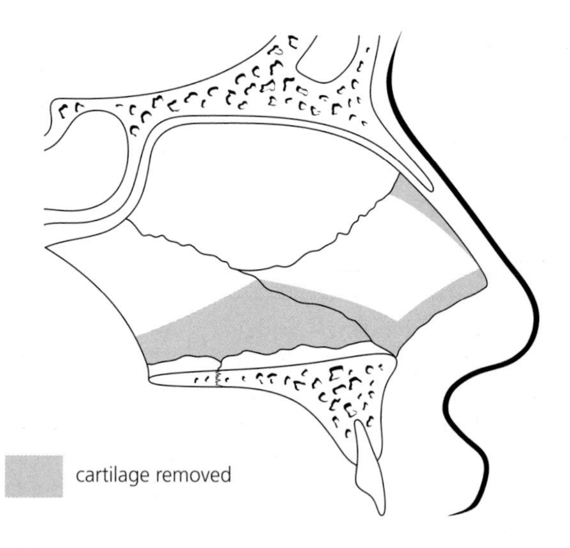

9.6.17 Areas marked where the septal cartilage is removed.

In the former, the medial crura and fibrous attachments are separated and a mucoperichondrial flap is raised to the base of the nasal floor from above.

The anterior nasal spine is inspected and if it is displaced, a 3-mm osteotome is used to mobilize it from the maxillary bone to the correct midline. Once the midline position is stabilized, it is held by the attached soft tissues by 4/0 PDS round-bodied suture.

The lower one-third of the septal cartilage is resected and a septal straightening is carried out in the usual way (Figure 9.6.17).

If the approach is carried out via a hemi-transfixion incision, a mucoperichondrial and mucoperiosteal dissection was carried out in order to expose both sides of the cartilaginous and bony part of the nasal septum. Then the lower third of the nasal cartilage together with vomarian bone, if required, is removed. This would aid in centralizing the nasal septum.

The cartilage which has been removed is used as a grafting material.

Lower lateral cartilage correction

The lower lateral cartilage from the cleft side is dissected from the nasal skin and the lining. Sharp curved dissecting scissors are very valuable towards this procedure.

The required amount of cephalic excision is carried out to create an alar crease (Figure 9.6.18). This is carried out bilaterally. Due to the cleft-side hypoplasia, the amount of cephalic excision would be less than the noncleft side.

The removed septal cartilage, or separately harvested conchal cartilage, is used to support the lower lateral cartilage in a tailor-made fashion (Figure 9.6.19). The septal cartilage can be trimmed to form an intercrural graft. Conchal cartilage can be used as an on-lay graft to the lateral crura or as an extension from an intercrural graft to the lower lateral cartilage contour.

The intercrural graft sits on the anterior nasal spine and is stabilized to the desired height with two or three 4/0 PDS round-bodied mattress sutures, holding the medial crura (Figure 9.6.20). In the past, the noncleft side lower left cartilage was dissected in its entirety and it was found that it was not necessary to do so unless there is gross secondary deformity. In spite of mobilization and stabilization, the dome height may not be equal. Next, an on-lay graft should be placed over the intermediate crura and sutured with 4/0 PDS sutures. It is preferable to place the knot on the dorsal surface.

If there is gross hypoplasia of the lower lateral cartilage, a conchal cartilage can be used as an intercrural graft and an onlay graft to provide support and height.

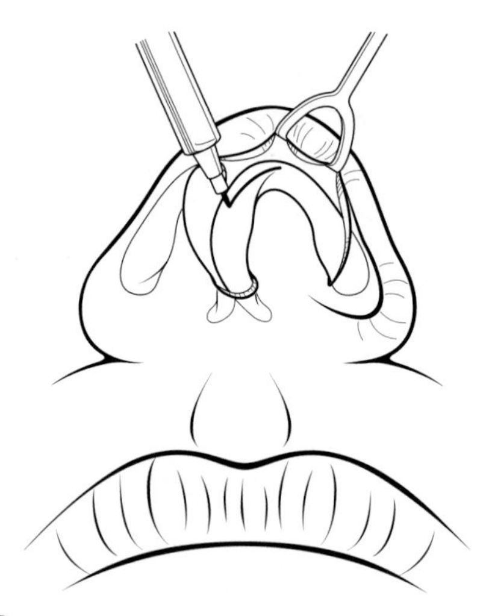

9.6.18 Selective cephalic excision.

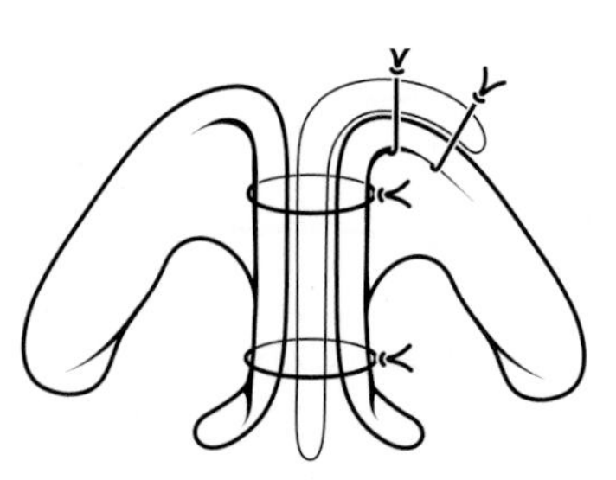

9.6.19 Intercrural graft with extension into the dome of the cleft side and stabilised with mattress sutures.

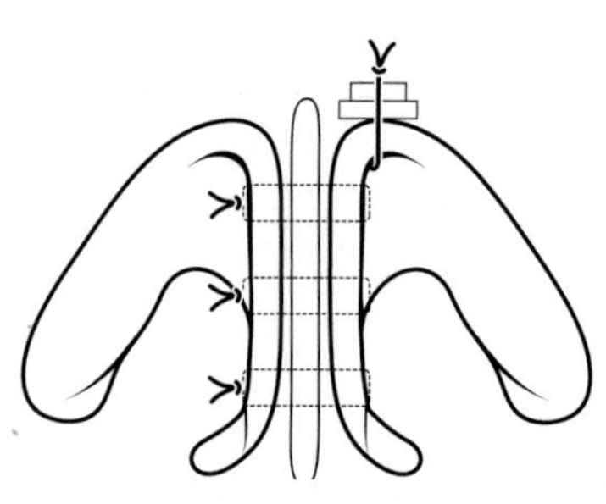

9.6.20 Intercrural graft stabilised with mattress sutures and onlay graft along the dome of the cleft site.

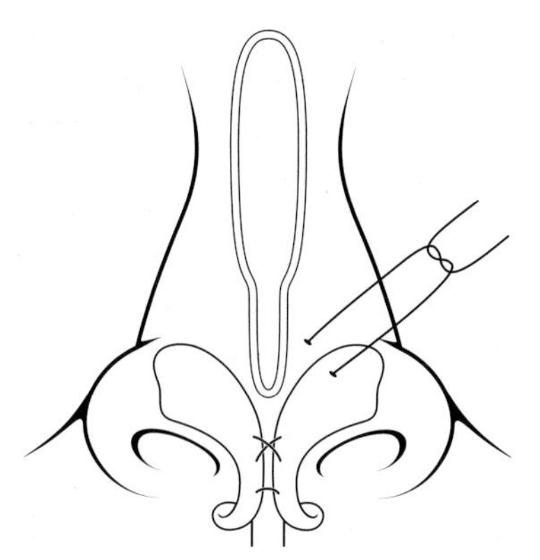

9.6.21 Horizontal mattress suture from the lateral crura to the ipsilateral upper lateral cartilage.

Once the symmetry of the nasal lobule is achieved, a horizontal mattress suture is placed from the lower end of the upper lateral cartilage to the upper end of the lower lateral cartilage, along the lateral third of the affected side (Figure 9.6.21).

Correction of lining deformity

If there is lining deficiency in spite of good mobilization of the fibrous attachment to the maxilla, a finger extension to the inferior surface of the inferior turbinate is obtained.

The benefit of mobilizing the nasal lining on its own is the freedom to overcome any webbing deformity and in turn provide a symmetrical nostril shape. The disadvantage, however, is introducing further scarring on the ventral surface of the lower lateral cartilage.

Hump reduction and medial and lateral osteotomy

This procedure is in the main not necessary. A midline osteotomy of the nasal bone is carried out using a 5-mm osteotome. Depending upon the size of the nose, between two and five stab incisions are made along the lateral end of the nose and the bridge. Transcutaneous osteotomies are made using a 2-mm osteotome. Infracture is carried out like any other rhinoplasty procedure. If there is gross hypoplasia of the nasal bone, the infracture would not provide the necessary height, in which case an on-lay calvarial or costal cartilage graft is required.

Redraping

The skin is redraped, examination is carried out for residual asymmetry and irregularity. Crushed cartilage is used to overcome these problems.

Suturing

The nasal lining is repaired with 5/0 vicryl suture and the columella skin with 6/0 prolene sutures.

Splinting and dressing

Support tape is applied to minimize any chance of haematoma, following which a suitable thermoplastic nasal splint is applied. These procedures are exactly similar to any standard rhinoplasty operation. The difference here is placement of a suitable nostril splint, which should remain for a period of three to six months. This is a social embarrassment to some patients, but it must be used at night, at the very least.

Bilateral

The main difference is the columella shortening, bifid blunt nasal lobule and broad nasal bridge. The columella incision is designed to maximize the columella skin height (various modifications are shown in the diagram) (Figure 9.6.22a–d). The dissection is carried out as before. Bilateral lower lateral cartilage mobilization is carried out, following which septal centralization is achieved. An intercrural graft is placed and stabilized with the medial crura to the desired height. On-lay conchal cartilage is placed and sutured as before (Figure 9.6.23).

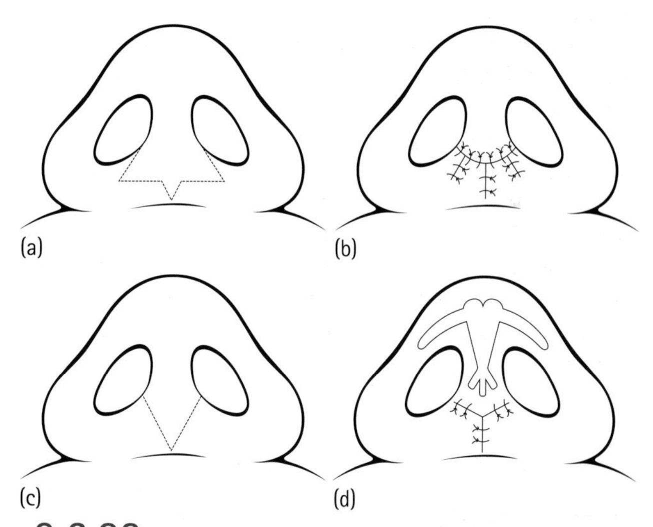

9.6.22 Various modifications of the columella incision designed to maximise the columella skin height.

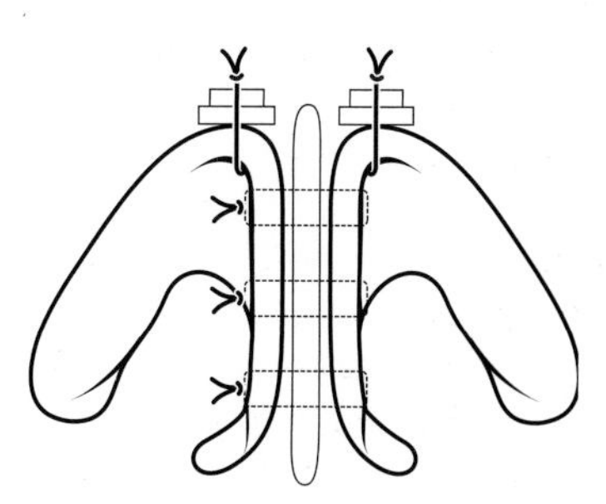

9.6.23 Intercrural graft held by mattress sutures. Onlay graft of the dome held by mattress sutures.

Hump reduction is a rare event in the bilateral cleft. However, if needed, medial and lateral osteotomy is carried out with infracture. A spreader graft has a role to play in providing stability to the nasal septum and the nasal bridge. An on-lay cartilaginous graft is placed if necessary and upper and lower lateral cartilages are sutured as before.

Nasal lining is extended to the inferior turbinate. The skin is repositioned and irregularities checked and corrected with crushed cartilage. The skin is repaired with 6/0 prolene and the lining repaired with 5/0 vicryl and the dressing is as before. Competency should be obtained in the standard aesthetic rhinoplasty prior to engaging in cleft rhinoplasty procedures.

FURTHER READING

Ahuja R. Primary rhinoplasty in unilateral cleft patients: The 'limited open' approach and other technical consideration. *Cleft Palate – Craniofacial Journal* 2006; **43**: 492–8.

Malek R. Nasal deformities and their treatment in secondary repair of cleft lip patients. A clinical study of 175 cases. *Scandinavian Journal of Plastic Reconstructive Surgery* 1974; **8**: 131–41.

McComb H. Primary correction of unilateral cleft lip. Nasal deformity: A 10 year review. Journal of Plastic Reconstructive Surgery 1985; **75**: 791–7.

PART 10

CRANIOFACIAL SURGERY

10.1

Segmental surgery of the jaws

PAUL JW STOELINGA

PRE-OPERATIVE ASSESSMENT

The need for segmental surgery, with the intention to align the dentoalveolar arches, has greatly been reduced, since it is now widely accepted that orthodontic treatment should be part of the treatment plan in patients with dentofacial deformities. Alignment of teeth and elimination of dentoalveolar compensation is usually achieved by orthodontic treatment alone, yet there still are indications for segmental surgery and they will be discussed for each separate osteotomy. In general, however, segmental osteotomies carried out in the dentate area require enough available space for these osteotomies to be performed safely without damage to the periodontal apparatus. This implies that when segmental surgery is contemplated, this aspect should be carefully considered in the treatment plan so that spaces are created in the dental arches.

This advice is particularly relevant for mandibular segmental surgery because the mandibular bone is usually more dense when compared to the maxilla and, therefore, less abundantly vascularized. In general, a diastema of 5 mm, allowing for approximately 2 mm of septal bone to be attached to the root of the tooth next to the osteotomy, is considered to be safe.

ANTERIOR MAXILLARY SEGMENTAL OSTEOTOMY

History

The first account of an anterior maxillary segmental osteotomy (AMSO) was probably from Cohn-Stock in 1921, but a single stage set-back osteotomy through a vestibular approach was first described by Wassmund in 1926. In 1962, Wunderer presented an important improvement of Wassmund's technique in that he recommended a predominantly palatal approach, which simplified the procedure. In 1980, Bell introduced the concept of the 'down-fracturing' in which the anterior segment is approached through a horizontal vestibular incision.

Principles and indication

The main consideration for the AMSO is to reposition and fix the fragment in the desired position without jeopardizing the vascular pedicle. The vascular pedicle is either predominantly buccally or palatally. Either way, care should be taken not to impair the blood supply by inadvertent cutting of the important vessels or by stretching or folding of the mucoperiosteal flap that contains the vascular pedicle.

The anterior fragment may be moved upwards, downwards, rotated and set back. An additional mid-line osteotomy allows for expansion or elimination of a central diastema. Most importantly, however, this allows for correct positioning of the canines by the rotation of both anterior fragments slightly by pulling the canines down. At present, this osteotomy is mainly carried out to correct an extremely reversed curve of Spee by intruding the anterior segment, i.e. in Class II division 2 anomalies. For this reason, the Wunderer approach is to be preferred.

Techniques

WUNDERER TECHNIQUE

Two vertical, vestibular incisions are made with a distal slant, to provide a maximum buccal, soft tissue pedicle (Figure 10.1.1). The mucoperiosteum is gently elevated cranioanteriorly to reach the nasal aperture. A periosteal elevator or small Langenbeck retractor is used to retract the mucoperiosteal flap, but care should be taken not to strip off the gingival attachments around the anterior teeth. With a short Lindemann burr, a bone cut is made from the nasal aperture slightly curved towards the alveolar crest (Figure 10.1.2). Care should be taken not to damage the periapical area of the canines. It is recommended that a 5 mm margin with regard to the apices of these teeth be left in order to avoid permanent neurovascular damage. The cut through the alveolar portion may be completed at this stage. Attention is then directed towards the palate and an anteriorly curved incision is made through the palatal mucosa (Figure 10.1.3). The mucoperiosteum is elevated posteriorly and the palatal cut is made connecting both alveolar cuts (Figure 10.1.4). At this stage, attention should be paid to the position of the nasal tube and cuff as they can easily be damaged during this procedure. After completion of the bone cuts, the anterior segment can be rotated upwards, thereby tearing the cartilaginous nasal septum from the nasal crest. A chisel may then be used to cut the nasal septum in a more controlled fashion once the fragment is beginning to rotate.

The fragment may be rotated all the way up, just pedicled to the vestibular mucoperiosteum (Figure 10.1.5). In this way, excellent access is obtained for trimming the bony interferences that exist when the fragment is to be set back or intruded. An acrylic burr is ideal to reduce the bony margins, particularly on the palatal side and the paranasal buccal bone plates. The nasal spine should be reduced, if necessary, for which a bone cutter may be used.

A mid-line osteotomy is often necessary. This allows for widening of the fragment and better positioning of the canines in the dental arch. A thin Lindemann burr is best used to start approximately 5 mm away from the palatal gingival margin and continue all the way through the segment towards the palatal cut. Separation is achieved by gently wiggling with an osteotome; this causes fracturing of the interdental septum and buccal plate (Figure 10.1.6). This way, the least possible damage is inflicted to the periodontal apparatus. If elimination of a central diastema is required, the interdental bone should be reduced from a palatal approach with a short Lindemann burr.

WASSMUND TECHNIQUE

The Wassmund approach also begins with two vertical vestibular incisions that may be curved anteriorly to expose the nasal aperture. The bone cuts are made as described

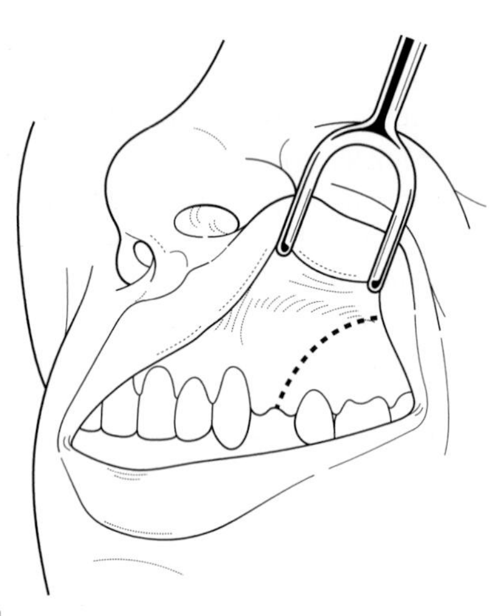

10.1.1 Incision is curved backwards to allow a broad, buccal pedicle.

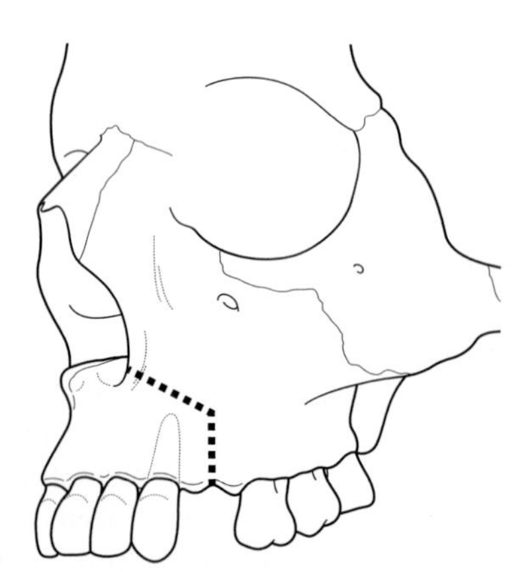

10.1.2 Curved bone cut running from the nasal aperture to the alveolar crest. A 5 mm margin is left with regard to the apex of the canine tooth.

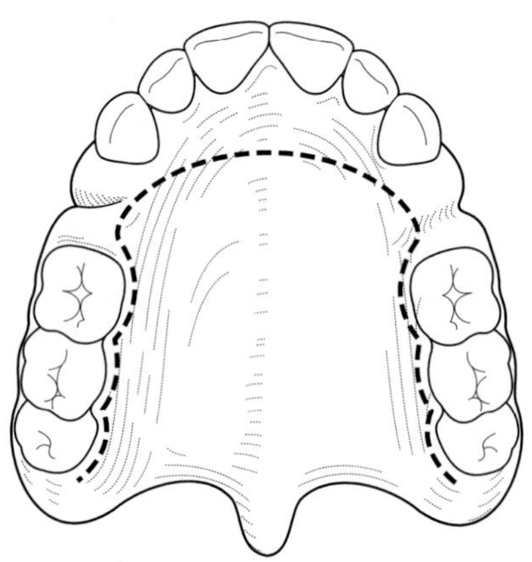

10.1.3 Anteriorly curved incision made in the palate. Posterior of the line of the supposed osteotomy, the cut may be made in the gingiva to allow reflection of the flap.

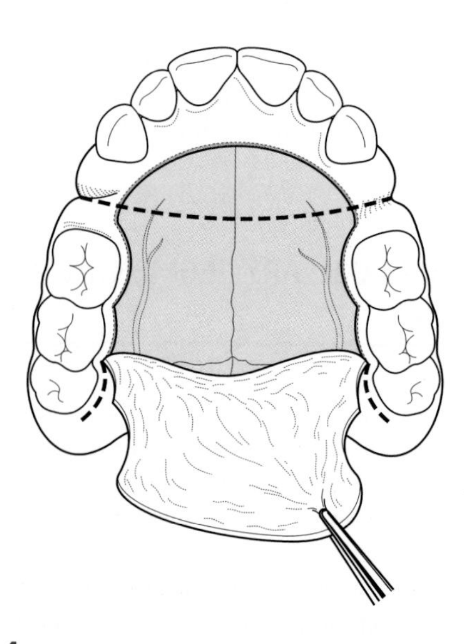

10.1.4 The palatal bone cut running straight over the palate connecting the two alveolar cuts.

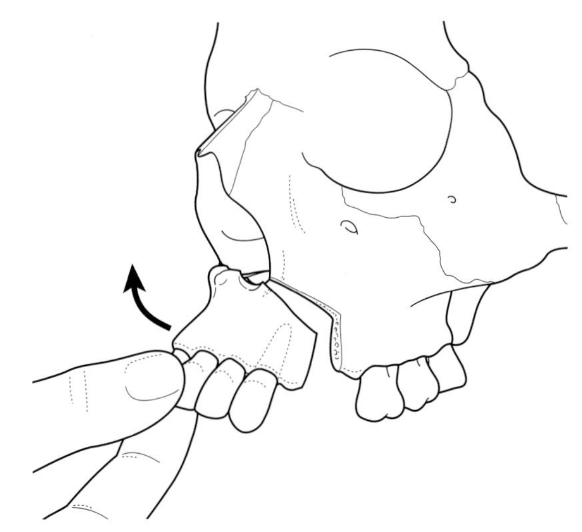

10.1.5 Anterior fragment rotated upwards still pedicled to buccal mucoperiosteum.

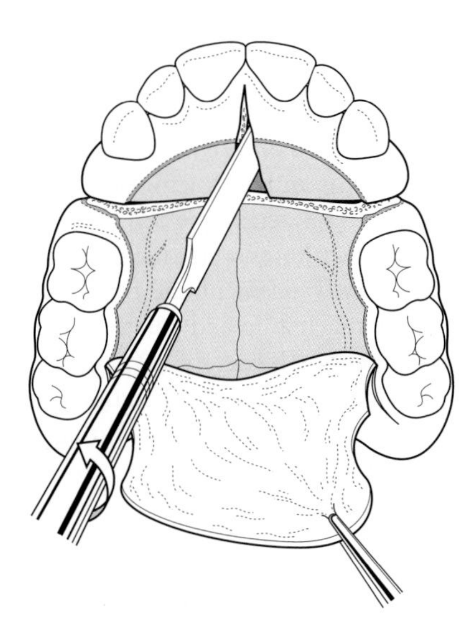

10.1.6 After a groove is made with a thin Lindemann burr, an osteotome is used to 'fracture' the buccal cortical plate by wiggling.

above. On the palatal side, bilateral marginal gingiva incisions are made from the lateral incisor to the second premolar, after which the palatal mucosa is elevated from the bone in a tunnelled fashion (Figure 10.1.7). The palatal bone cut is made through the buccal cuts with a long Lindemann burr. This procedure is essentially carried out blindly. The separation from the nasal septum is achieved through a small vertical mid-line incision in the buccal vestibule. The nasal spine is exposed and the septum cut from the nasal crest with a forked chisel.

It is the appropriate reduction of bone on the palatal side that makes this procedure a less attractive alternative. This, again, is to be carried out blindly with the obvious risk of taking away too much bone. Mid-line splitting, if necessary,

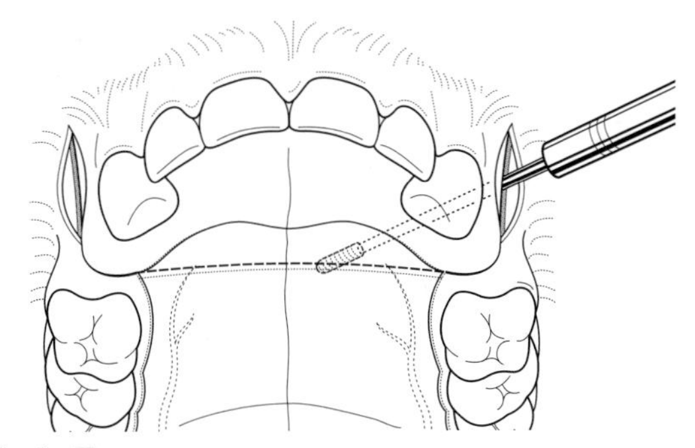

10.1.7 The palatal bone cut is made with a long Lindemann burr after the palatal mucosa, that is still attached to the anterior fragment, has been lifted.

should be done from the buccal side with a thin fissure burr and thin osteotome. For this reason, a small vertical incision is made over the nasal spine in the vestibule. The spine is exposed by limited subperiosteal dissection.

DOWN-FRACTURING TECHNIQUE

For the down-fracturing technique, a horizontal vestibular incision is made extending at least one tooth distal to the proposed osteotomy on both sides. The mucoperiosteum is reflected to expose the nasal aperture, while the alveolar crest at the side of the osteotomy is also carefully exposed. The bone cuts are made as in the Wassmund technique but the vertical cuts are used to gain access to the palatal bone. The palatal cut is completed with a thin tapered fissure burr or 4 mm osteotome. During this manoeuvre the palatal mucosa should not be damaged since this will be the sole vascular pedicle once the fragment is down-fractured. When the anterior fragment is down-fractured the bone can be trimmed to fit the new position.

FIXATION

If no posterior segmental osteotomies are carried out, fixation is relatively simple. A prefabricated acrylic splint, reinforced with a steel wire with which loops are made, is used to stabilize the fragments. The anterior fragment is manoeuvred into place, after which the splint is first fixed to the posterior teeth using pull wires, that are fed through the loops in the wafer (Figure 10.1.8). Once this is done, pull wires should be used to first pull the canines in the splint, and if necessary, followed by the central incisions. Since a tendency exists for the fragment to be slightly rotated upwards when pushed backwards, the canines tend to be in supraposition. This undesirable effect can be counteracted by a mid-line split and the use of canine pull wires. To secure the position of the anterior segment(s), two four-hole miniplates can be used to fix the fragment (Figure 10.1.9).

The acrylic splint may be removed in a few days if the patient still has orthodontic brackets. A rigid arch wire will then usually suffice to keep the teeth in the proper position. Intermaxillary fixation is never necessary and is not to be recommended. In case the anterior segmental osteotomy is

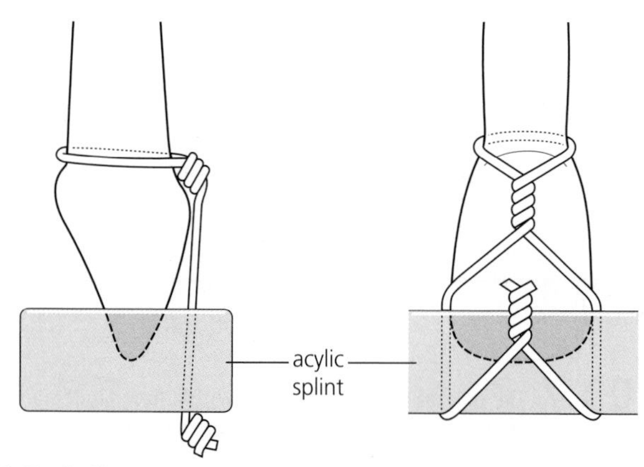

10.1.8 Acrylic splint secured to the posterior teeth first using pull wires. Pull wires are also used to fix the anterior fragment in the splint. These wires are twisted around the canines and then tightened to the splint.

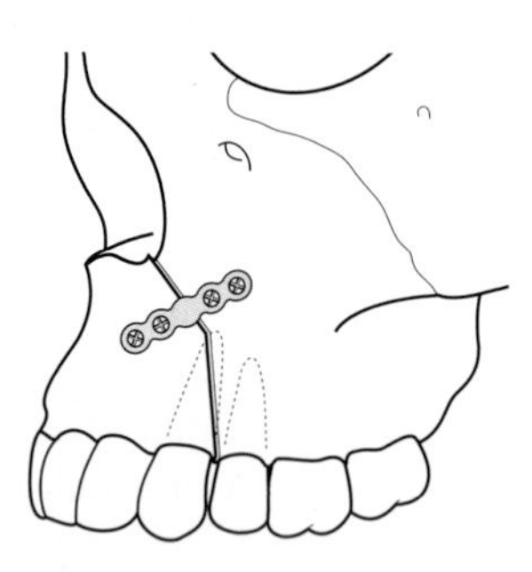

10.1.9 Four-hole microplate securing anterior fragment to the posterior maxilla, above the level of the apices.

combined with posterior segmental osteotomies, the posterior fragments should be stabilized first with an acrylic splint, temporary IMF and miniplates. Once secured, the anterior fragment can be treated as described above. The incisions are closed using 3/0 sutures.

Post-operative care

Apart from some swelling apparent for a few days, hardly any complications can be expected. However, when intrusion is the main purpose of the procedure and the palatal mucosa is left intact (Wassmund or down-fracturing technique), it is recommended that the colour of the buccal gingiva is carefully checked. A bone step at the site of the palatal osteotomy may cut off the blood supply and, thus, endanger the viability of the anterior segment.

POSTERIOR MAXILLARY SEGMENTAL OSTEOTOMY

History

The posterior maxillary segmental osteotomy (PMSO) was introduced in 1954 by Schuchardt as a two-staged procedure to correct anterior open bite. In 1960, Kufner described a one-stage modification. Several modifications of the PMSO have been described with either horizontal or vertical buccal incisions, a direct or transantral approach to the palate and varying degrees of exposure of the palatal bone before osteotomy. In 1972, West and Epker provided an extensive review, emphasizing the versatility of this procedure.

Principles and indications

As in the AMSO, special attention should be paid during the whole procedure to the buccal gingiva to maintain adequate blood supply to the fragment. Inadvertent tearing of the buccal or palatal mucoperiosteal flap may jeopardize the vitality of the segment.

Typical indications include anterior skeletal open bite treated by bilateral PMSOs with intrusion of the segments. Although at present this deformity is often treated by a one-piece Le Fort I tilting and intrusion osteotomy, the indication is still valid, particularly in patients with a steep SN–A angle, because tilting of the whole tooth-bearing maxilla tends to cause an obtuse nasolabial angle.

Extrusion, widening and narrowing of the posterior arch are also possible with this technique and vertical movements are often combined with transverse movements. One of the best applications is advancement and rotation of the lesser segment in unilateral cleft lip and palate (CLP) patients or the posterior segments in bilateral CLP patients. The PMSO allows for reconstruction of an uninterrupted arch form in many of these patients, simultaneously with grafting of the alveolopalatal cleft.

In general, elimination of edentulous spaces in the arch can be achieved by advancing the posterior segment.

Technique

A vertical incision is made in the buccal mucoperiosteum of the interdental area (Figure 10.1.10) and carried over to the palatal side. With the alveolus exposed by reflection of the mucoperiosteum, the bone cut is made with a fine tapering fissure burr (short Lindemann). Bucally, submucoperiosteal tunnelling is carried posteriorly towards the tuberosity. A flat, malleable retractor is placed under the buccal pedicle with care taken not to tear off the attached gingiva. The lateral, horizontal bone cut is made with a long Lindemann burr in an 'inside to outside fashion'. It is first placed into the antrum at the uppermost point of the vertical osteotomy, approximately 5 mm above the apices of the posterior teeth (Figure 10.1.11). This distance is considered to be safe with regard to the neurovascular regeneration of the pulp of the teeth involved. The cut can be completed almost to the tuberosity, the last millimeters finished with a 4 mm osteotome.

The palatal osteotomy can be performed with a fine tapering fissure burr or osteotome directly through the

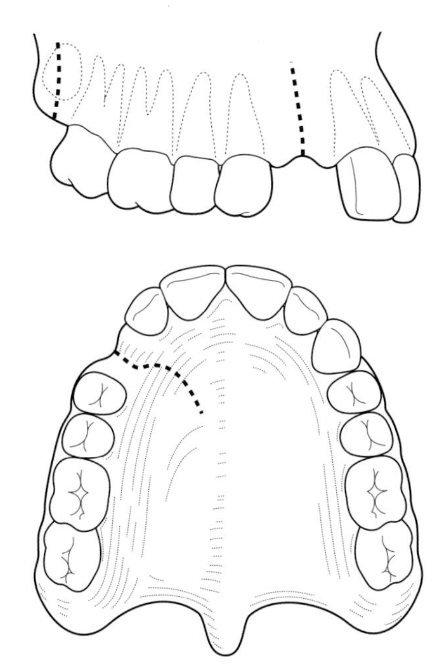

10.1.10 Position of buccal and palatinal incisions for posterior segmental osteotomy.

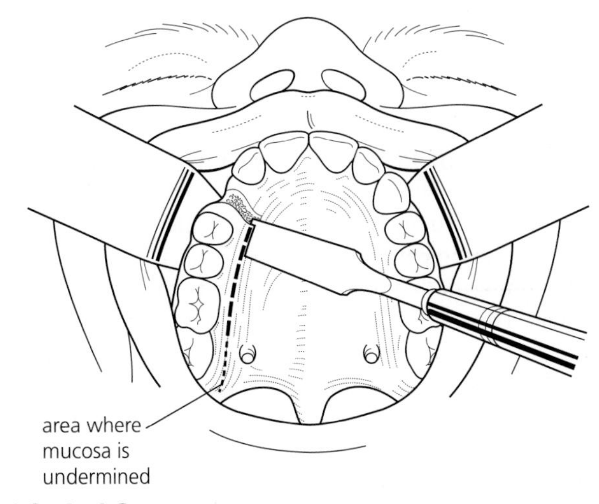

10.1.12 Palatal bone cut made at the junction of the alveolar process and the palate. The cut should be made lateral to the greater palatal foramen. The mucosa in the posterior palate can be left intact by guiding the osteotome under the mucosa and completing the bone cut in a tunnelled fashion.

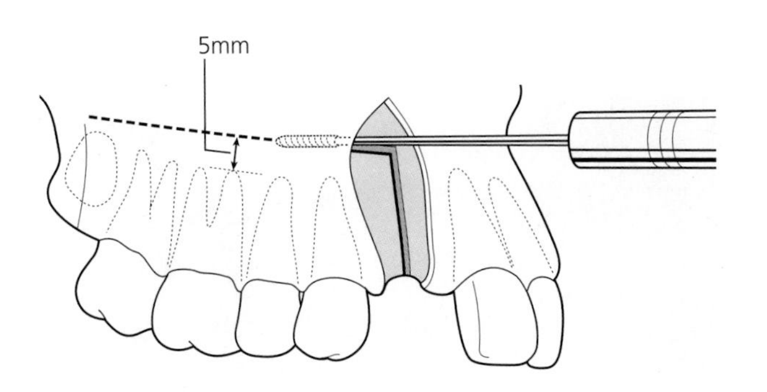

10.1.11 Bone cut made in a tunnelled fashion approximately 5 mm above the level of the apices.

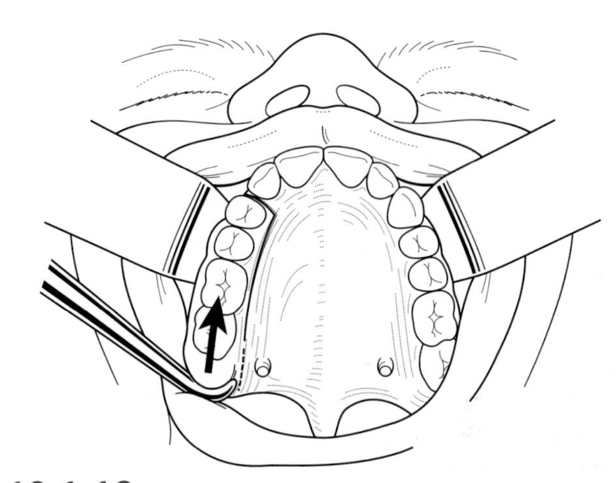

10.1.13 A curved osteotome is used in the tuberosity area to mobilize the segment and also to manoeuvre it forwards.

palatal mucoperiosteum, without direct exposure of the bone. The aim is to place the bone cut at the junction of the alveolus with the horizontal palatal process, above the root apices and lateral to the greater palatine artery. With a 4 mm osteotome angled at 45° to the vertical plane, a series of punctures into the antrum can be made, after which the cut is completed with a 10 mm wood-handled osteotome. This way the palatal mucoperiosteum still maintains a pedicle to the soft palate, which contributes to the blood supply to the segment (Figure 10.1.12). The final step is the posterior osteotomy through the tuberosity region which is the same as described for the Le Fort I osteotomy.

Mobilization is achieved by rotating the wood-handled osteotome in the palatal osteotomy and by forward mobilization with a curved osteotome in the tuberosity region (Figure 10.1.13).

FIXATION

The segment(s) are moved into the desired position and fixed with the aid of an acrylic, prefabricated splint and pull wires much the same as described for the AMSO. Once in position and fixed, a mini- or microplate can be used to provide additional stabilization (Figure 10.1.14). Due to the limited access, usually only one plate on each side can be placed. The acrylic splint should therefore be maintained for a period of 6 weeks, but IMF is not necessary. The incisions are closed with 3/0 sutures.

Post-operative care

The same considerations are applicable as for the Le Fort I osteotomy with regard to swelling and possible post-operative bleeding. There are no special aspects to be considered apart from occlusal factors.

Application of PMSO in cleft patients

The PMSO is extremely suitable for advancing and rotating the lesser fragment in unilateral CLP patients or for repositioning both posterior fragments in bilateral CLP patients. This can be done while the alveolopalatal cleft is simultaneously grafted. For this purpose, an incision is made around the cleft extended upwards (Figure 10.1.15). The soft tissue in the alveolopalatal cleft is mobilized and pushed upwards to form the nasal layer. The vertical incision is used to reflect the buccal mucoperiosteum, just as described for the PMSO. The palatal osteotomy is made lateral to the scar tissue that is usually present in the palatal cleft. After the tuberosity split, the fragment is mobilized as described before.

At this stage, the nasal layer is closed after appropriate trimming of the redundant scar tissue. The segment is then advanced and rotated or brought downwards as required, and fixed with the use of an acrylic splint and one four-hole miniplate (Figure 10.1.16). Once stabilized the narrowed alveolopalatal cleft is grafted with autogenous corticocancellous bone, and the palatal and buccal mucosa can be closed with 3/0 sutures because the advancement has approximated the soft tissues. This technique usually corrects the paranasal depression often seen in cleft palate patients and considerably improves the existing asymmetry of the alar base (Figure 10.1.17). Long-term follow-up studies have shown that the technique provides predictable and stable results.

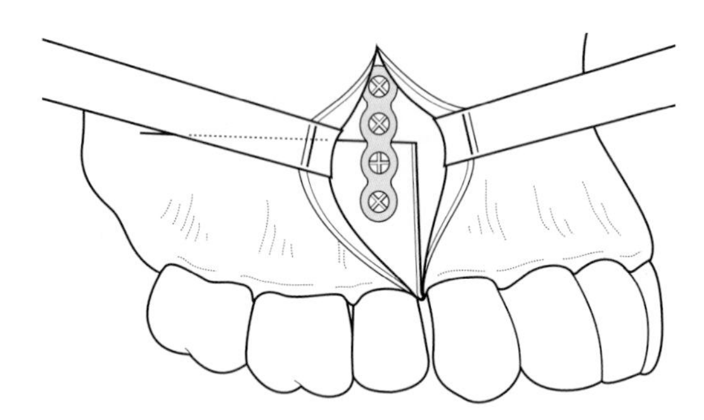

10.1.14 Mini- or microplate can be used to fix the posterior segment to the remaining maxilla.

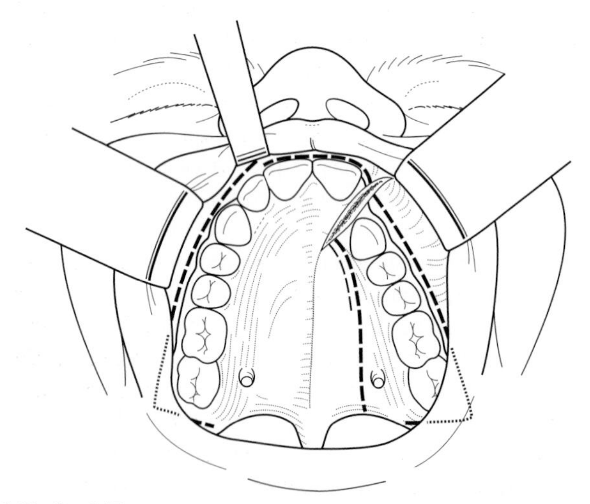

10.1.15 Segmental osteotomy of the lesser fragment in patients with unilateral cleft lip and palate. The major fragment can be mobilized using the Le Fort I technique.

ANTERIOR MANDIBULAR SUBAPICAL OSTEOTOMY

History

The first description of an anterior subapical mandibular osteotomy was by Hullihen in 1849. However, in 1942, Hofer made this procedure popular by recommending its use for dentoalveolar set-back as well as advancement. In 1959, Köle advocated this osteotomy to treat anterior skeletal open bite by interposition of a bone graft taken from the lower border of the mandibular symphysis.

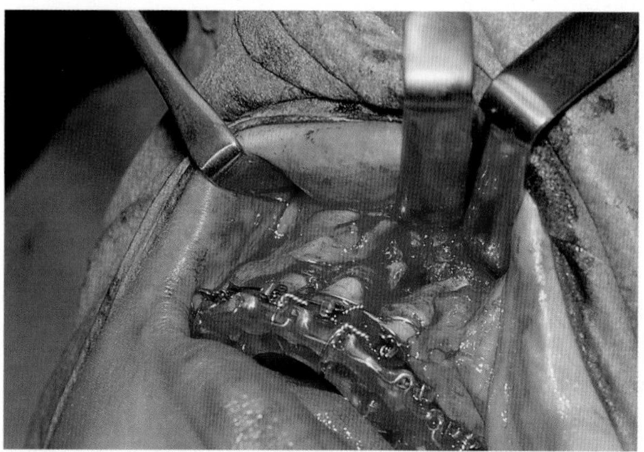

(a)

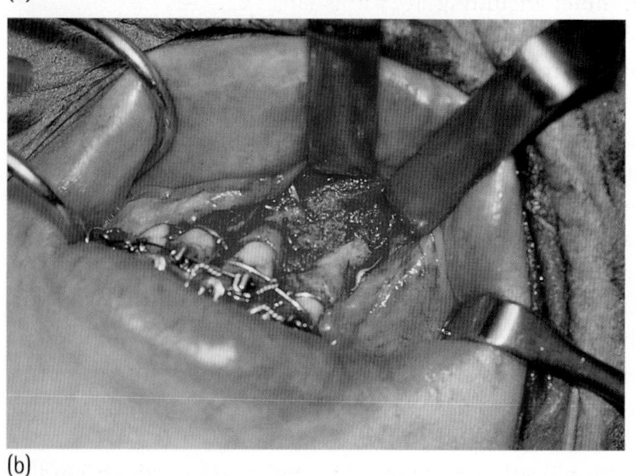

(b)

10.1.16 (a) Lesser fragment advanced and fixed in the splint with wires. (b) Alveolopalatal cleft is grafted with particulate autogenous bone.

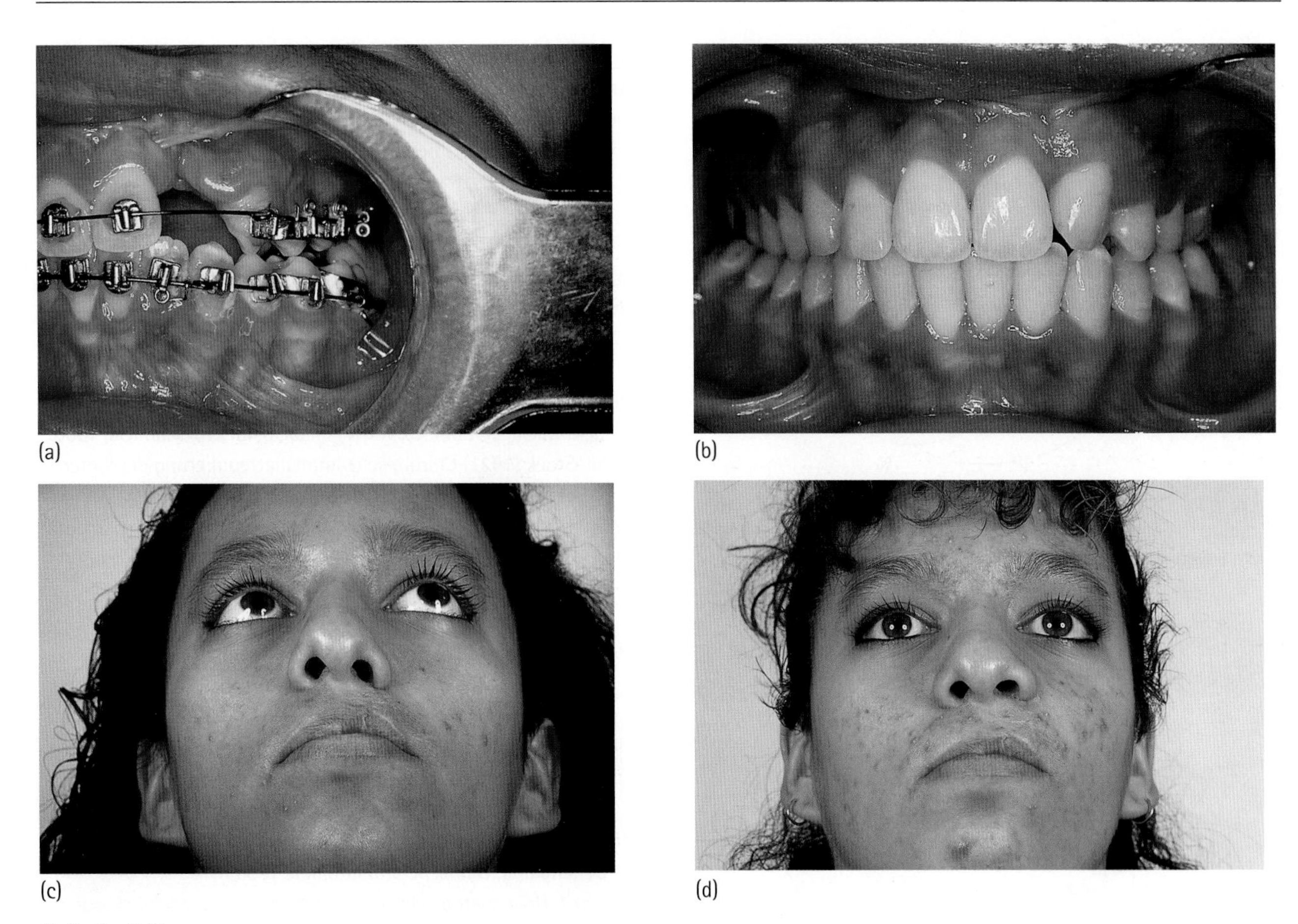

10.1.17 Pre-operative (a,c) and post-operative (b,d) situation in patient with left-sided unilateral complete cleft. Note elimination of edentulous space and alignment of segment. Symmetry of the alar base has been achieved by advancing the lesser fragment (c,d).

Principles and indications

The anterior subapical mandibular osteotomy is, at present, mainly used to level an extruded anterior dentoalveolar part. In principle, however, movements in all directions are possible, including forwards and backwards and even upwards if the gap is grafted. It is also possible to correct asymmetries.

Its vascularization is completely dependent on the lingual mucoperiosteum–muscle pedicle and therefore attention should be paid during the whole surgery not to tear this pedicle. This is particularly relevant when relatively large movements are planned.

Technique

Vertical incisions are made in the mucoperiosteum of the interdental area and these are joined up by a vestibular incision that is carried out into the buccal vestibule (Figure 10.1.18). After subperiosteal dissection, the whole buccal side of the chin is exposed and the flap pulled downwards with a chin retractor as described for the genioplasty.

Vertical bone cuts are made in the areas designated and they are connected by a horizontal bone cut. These bone cuts are made with a tapered fissure burr and, if possible, carried just through the lingual cortex. The horizontal bone cut should be at least 5 mm away from the apices of the roots of the anterior teeth. A 4 mm osteotome may be used to finish the osteotomy. If the segment is to be brought down, a strip of bone should be removed so as to allow the segment to fit the new position. A prefabricated acrylic splint helps to position the segment correctly in the desired position.

FIXATION

The anterior segment, once manoeuvred into place, is ideally fixed with miniplates. The four-hole plates are bent to fit the contour and placed in the corners of the box (Figure 10.1.19). If necessary, an additional plate may be placed in the middle of the horizontal bone cut. If orthodontic treatment is carried out, the wafer does not need to be fixed. Instead, a rigid orthodontic arch wire should be inserted which will be sufficient to maintain the position of the front teeth. In case no orthodontic treatment is planned, an arch bar or acrylic splint fixed to the teeth will be necessary to maintain the position.

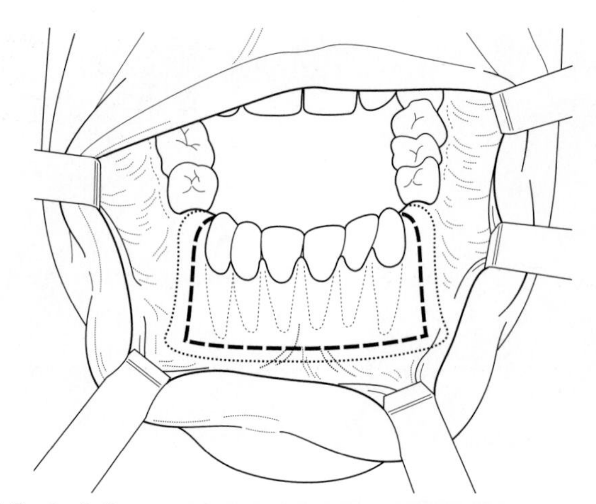

10.1.18 Incision in the interdental areas carried out in the vestibule to approach the anterior subapical area and bone cuts for the subapical anterior mandibular osteotomy.

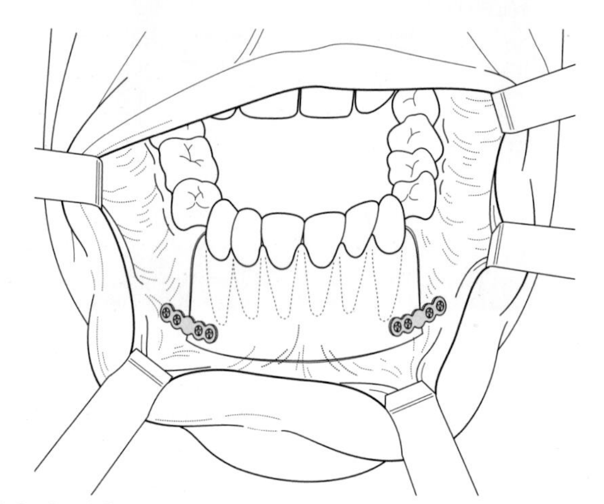

10.1.19 Fixation of the anterior segment with two four-hole miniplates.

KÖLE TECHNIQUE

In 1959, Köle recommended the use of this osteotomy to close an anterior open bite while the gap was grafted with bone taken from the lower border. This author advises strongly against this method because this will most likely change the contour of the chin in an unacceptable manner. Detachment of the periosteum and muscles and resection of the rounded inferior fragment will create a square 'fleshy chin' that is aesthetically not pleasing. If this technique is selected, the interpositional graft should be harvested from another location.

Post-operative care

This osteotomy does not usually create unforeseeable problems although, as in genioplasties, severe haemorrhage in the floor of the mouth may be encountered. This is due to damage to the vessels located in the genioglossal muscle. Ice packs and positioning of the patient in an upright position are supportive measures to be taken. Apart from occlusal factors, no other aspects need be considered.

FURTHER READING

Bell WH, Levy BM. Revascularisation and bone healing after posterior maxillary osteotomy. *Journal of Oral Surgery* 1971; **29**: 313–20.

Bell WH, Proffit WE, White RP (eds). *Surgical correction of dentofacial deformities.* vol 1. Philadelphia: WB Saunders, 1980.

Cohn-Stock (1921) Chirurgische immediatregulierung der Kiefer. *V Schr Zahnheilk* (cited by Wassmund, 1926).

Erbe M, Stoelinga PJW, Leenen RJ. Long-term results of segmental repositioning of the maxilla in cleft palate patients without previously grafted alveolo-palatal clefts. *Journal of Cranio-Maxillofacial Surgery* 1996; **24**: 109–17.

Hofer O. Die operative behandlung der alveoläre retraktiones unterkiefers und ihre anwendungsmöglichkeit für prognathie und mikrogenie. *Zahn-, Mund- u Kieferheilk*, 1942; **9**: 121–32.

Hullihen SP. Case of elongation of the underjaw and distortion of the face and neck, caused by burn, successfully treated. *American Journal of Dental Science*, 1849; **9**: 157.

Köle H. Formen des offenen Bisses und ihre chirurgische Behandlung. *Deutsche Stomatologie* 1959; **9**: 753.

Kufner J. Nove metody chirurgiekele leceni osteureneho skusu. *Cslka Stomat* 1960; **60**: 387.

Moloney FB, Stoelinga PJW, Tideman H. The posterior segmental maxillary osteotomy. Recent application. *Journal of Oral and Maxillofacial Surgery* 1984; **42**: 771–81.

Schuchardt K. Chirurgie für offenen Bisses. In: Bier A, Braun A, Kümmel H (eds), *Chirurgische Operationslehre*, 7. Leipzig: Aufl, band 2, 1954.

Stoelinga PJW, Van de Vyver HRM, Leenen *et al.* The prevention of relapse after maxillary osteotomies in cleft palate patients. *Journal of Cranio-Maxillofacial Surgery* 1987; **15**: 226–331.

Stoelinga PJW, Hinderks F. The concept of segmental repositioning of the alveolar arches and simultaneous grafting in CLP patients. *Journal of Craniomaxillofacial Surgery*, 1992; **21** (Suppl. I): 70.

Tideman H, Stoelinga PJW, Gallia L, Le Fort I. Advancement with segmental palatal osteotomies in patients with cleft palates. *Journal of Oral Surgery* 1980; **38**: 196–9.

Wassmund M. From: *Lehrbuch der Praktische Chirurgie des Mundes und der Kiefer* (1939) Joh Ambrosius Barth, Leipzig, **I**, 1926: p.277.

West RA, Epker BN. Posterior maxillary surgery: its place in the treatment of dentofacial deformities. *Journal of Oral Surgery* 1972; **30**: 562–3.

Wunderer S. Die prognathie operation mittels frontal gestiltem maxilla fragment. *Österreichische Zeitschrift für Stomatologie*, 1962; **59**: 98–102.

10.2

Orthognathic surgery of the mandible

PAUL A JOHNSON

INTRODUCTION

Orthognathic mandibular surgical techniques are used mainly to correct mandibular prognathism and retrognathia. In addition, lower facial asymmetries, anterior open bites and post-traumatic malocclusions can be rectified. They can be used alone as single jaw procedures or in combination with midface procedures as a bimaxillary procedure.

They are widely used for the correction of dentofacial deformities and indications include malocclusions causing masticatory difficulties, temporomandibular dysfunction, sleep apnoea and unaesthetic appearance with its attendant psychosocial effects.

Orthodontic preparation for surgery is usually required to align, decompensate and coordinate the dental arches. Ideally, treatment planning should be performed jointly between the surgeon and orthodontist to clearly identify treatment goals. Orthodontic preparation time varies but usually requires approximately one year of fixed appliance therapy. Post-surgical orthodontic detailing normally takes about six months.

The most frequently used mandibular techniques are the bilateral sagittal split osteotomy (BSSO) and the horizontal genioplasty. Other techniques, such as the vertical subsigmoid, inverted-L and C-osteotomies, although they still have some adherents, are infrequently indicated and relatively rarely performed.

THE BILATERAL SAGITTAL SPLIT OSTEOTOMY

The BSSO was first described in 1957 by Trauner and Obwegeser and subsequently modified by DalPont, Hunsuck and Epker amongst others.

Its main advantage is its versatility. Mandibular advancement, setback and rotation can all be achieved. An anterior open bite can be corrected by anticlockwise rotation. It is carried out by an intraoral approach avoiding external scarring. Direct fixation of the osteotomy sites by miniplate or bicortical screw osteosynthesis is easily achieved, thereby negating the need for post-operative intermaxillary fixation with its associated safety and patient comfort implications.

Major complications are rare. Excessive haemorrhage is uncommon, although the facial vessels are at risk when making the buccal bone cut unless adequately protected by a retractor. There is a risk of distraction of the condyle when advancement of the mandible is carried out with consequent incorrect occlusion which may only be recognized post-operatively, necessitating an early return to the operating theatre for revision. The most frequent complication and major risk of the BSSO, however, is damage to the inferior dental nerve. Reported incidences vary, but it is common in the immediate post-operative period. Permanent anaesthesia is rare, however, with recovery usually occurring over a period of weeks or months. Finally, unfavourable fracture at the osteotomy site can resulting in a 'bad split'. This is largely technique dependent. Ideally, lower third molars should be removed at least six months before surgery to minimize the risk of this occurring.

SURGICAL TECHNIQUE

Incision

The incision is made down the external oblique ridge down the lateral mandibular ridge and deepened down to bone using cutting diathermy (Figures 10.2.1 and 10.2.2). Subperiosteal dissection is carried out on the buccal surface of the mandible inferiorly to the antegonial notch. It is not necessary to raise the periosteum over the angle of the mandible. The lingual surface of the ramus of the mandible is then approached by elevating periosteum over the anterior surface of the ramus towards the coronoid process for approximately 2 cm above the occlusal plane. Retraction of mucosa is achieved using either a forked retractor or by clamping the anterior surface of the coronoid process using a curved Kochers clamp. The lingual surface of the ramus is now exposed by introducing a periosteal elevator above the level of the mandibular foramen and progressing inferiorly (Figure 10.2.3) Usually, the lingula can be easily identified and the periosteal elevator can be positioned immediately above the lingula and used as a retractor protecting the inferior dental nerve.

The bone cuts

The lingual cut is made using a Lindeman bur as far posteriorly as the lingula and deepened into cancellous bone (Figure 10.2.4). Care must be taken to ensure that it is sufficiently deep posteriorly. The Kocher and lingual retractor are then removed and a buccal channel retractor inserted.

The buccal bone cut is again carried out using a Lindeman bur and extends from the lower border of the mandible to the lateral mandibular ridge. It extends into cancellous bone. Care must be taken to ensure that the cut extends through the lower border of the mandible as far lingually as possible (Figure 10.2.5).

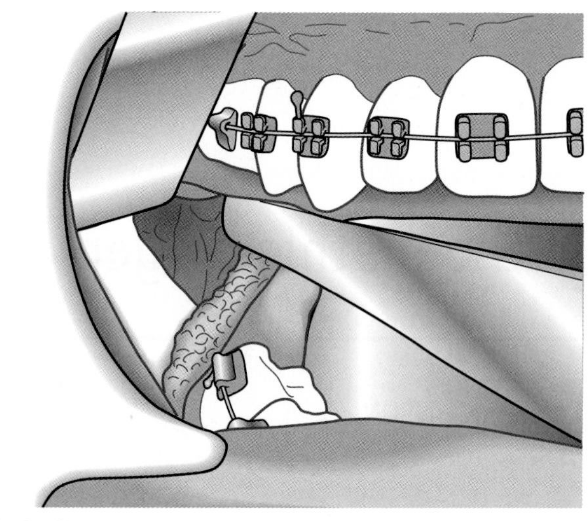

10.2.3 Periosteal elevator being used to expose the lingual aspect of the ramus.

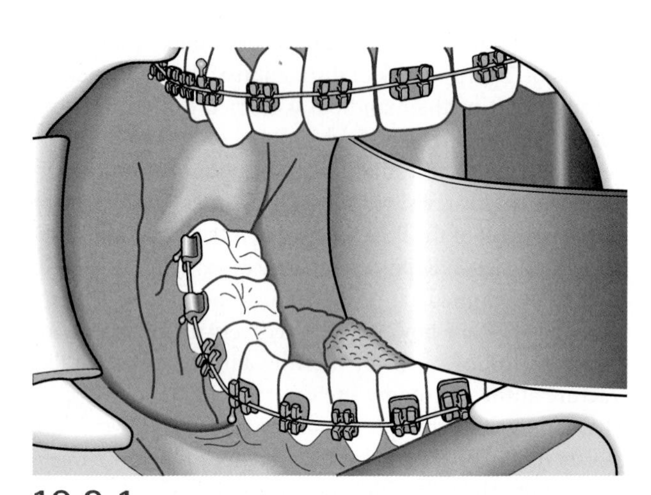

10.2.1 Incision line on the external oblique ridge.

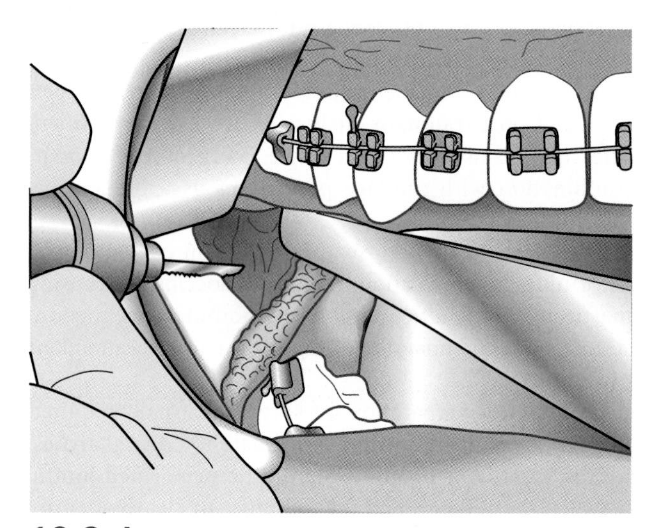

10.2.4 Lingual cut being made with a Lindeman bur.

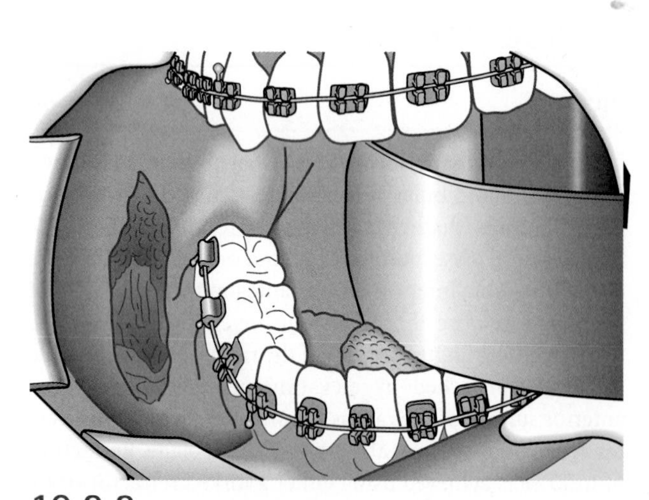

10.2.2 Incision will be extended down to bone.

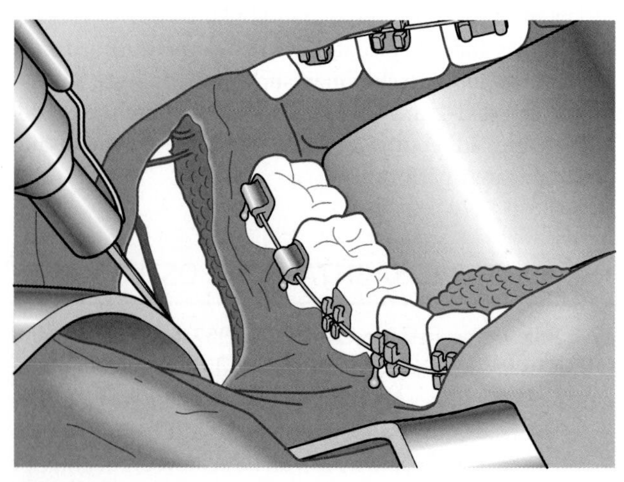

10.2.5 Buccal cut being extended down to the lower border of the mandible.

The Kocher and lingual retractor are then again inserted and the joining cut linking the lingual and buccal cuts is performed at the junction between the buccal cortical plate and cancellous bone (Figure 10.2.6).

The split

A controlled split is carried out.

This is commenced using a curved osteotome placed at the junction of the lingual and connecting cuts and tapped through posteriorly so that the superior end of the split line is initiated in a downwards direction from above the lingual (Figure 10.2.7).

An osteotome is then inserted at the junction of the buccal and connecting cuts and the buccal plate is gradually prised laterally (Figure 10.2.8). The same ostotome can be used to separate the buccal cortical plate from the cancellous bone. Once the lower border of the mandible can be seen the osteotomy line can be propagated posteriorly using an osteotome and Smith's spreader to join the lingual cut and complete the split.

The inferior dental nerve is usually easily identified during the split and can be protected (Figure 10.2.9). However, it can remain completely contained within the distal fragment in which case it is not visualized. If it crosses from the lingual to the buccal side it may be partly or completely within the bone of the proximal segment. In this circumstance, it must be carefully freed from the surrounding bone using a fine osteotome.

Fixation

After completion of the BSSO the patient is placed into intermaxillary fixation. Usually a prefabricated splint is used to locate the correct occlusion.

Fixation of the osteotomy sites can be achieved using either a single buccal miniplate or bicortical screws placed transbuccally (Figure 10.2.10). Control of the proximal fragment is crucial. The mandibular condyle must be seated in the glenoid fossa and not distracted downwards or forwards. This is largely a matter of feel. The proximal segment is pushed posteriorly and upwards using a curved osteotome (Figure 10.2.11).

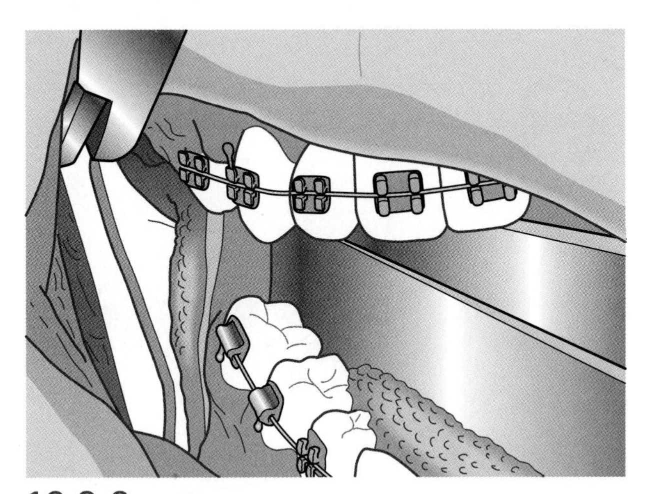

10.2.6 The cut joining the lingual and buccal cuts has been completed.

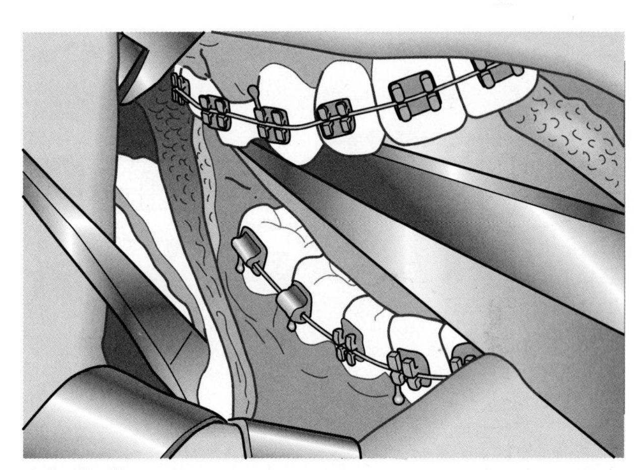

10.2.8 The buccal plate is being prized laterally with an osteotome.

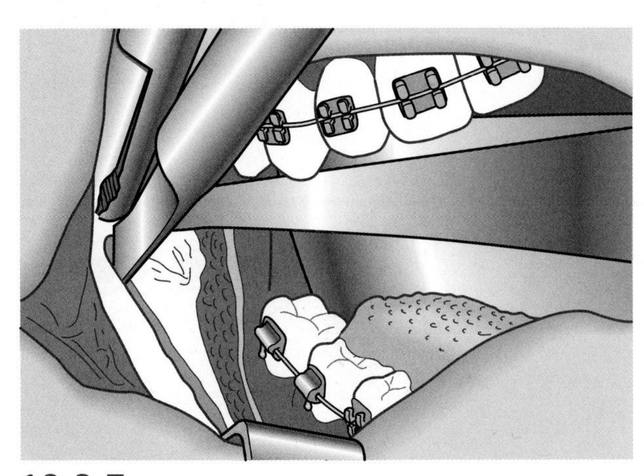

10.2.7 The lingual split is being developed using a curved osteotome.

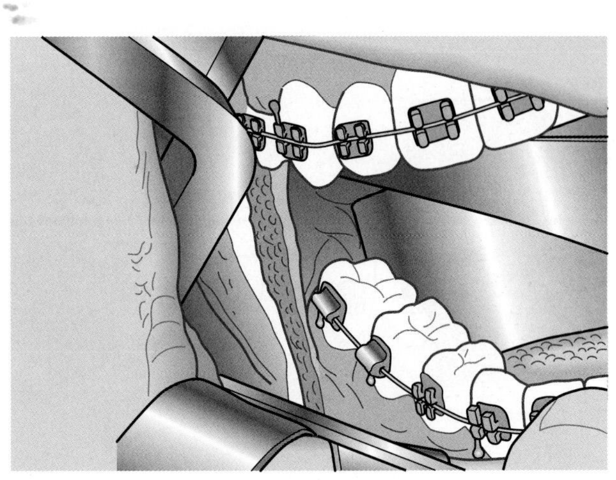

10.2.9 The inferior alveolar nerve has been identified and protected.

Completion of procedure

The intermaxillary fixation is released, the splint removed and occlusion checked (Figure 10.2.12). The intraoral incisions are sutured and the cheek incisions are Steri-stripped.

A NOTE ON FIXATION

The osteotomy sites can be fixed with either plates or bicortical screws (Figure 10.2.13). These can be either titanium or resorbable. In the event of a 'bad split', i.e. lingual (Figure 10.2.14) or buccal (Figure 10.2.15) cortical plate fracture, a combination can be used.

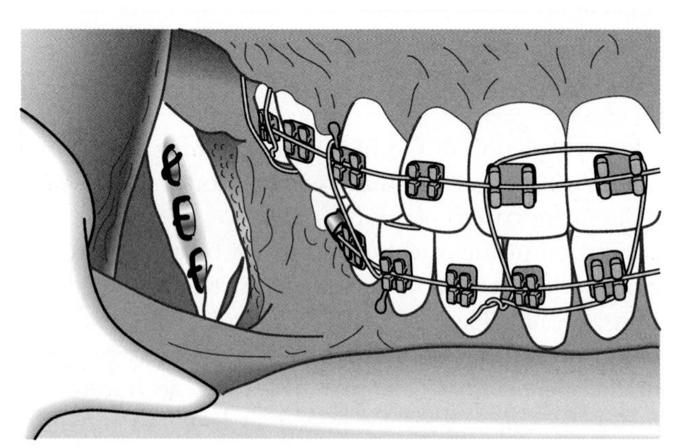

10.2.10 The osteotomy has been immobilised with three bicortical screws.

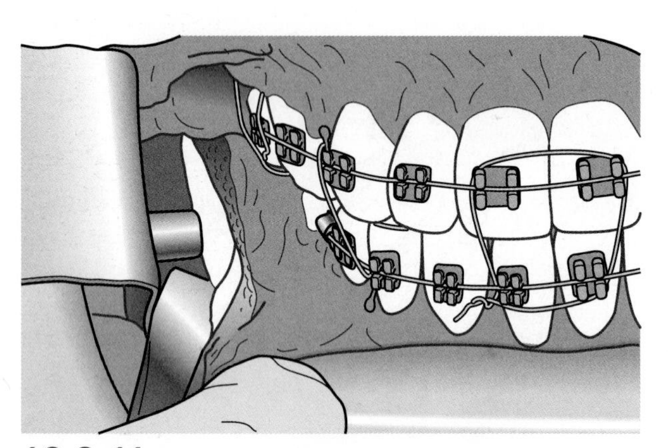

10.2.11 Whilst the transbuccal holes are being drilled, the proximal segment is pushed posteriorly with a curved osteotome.

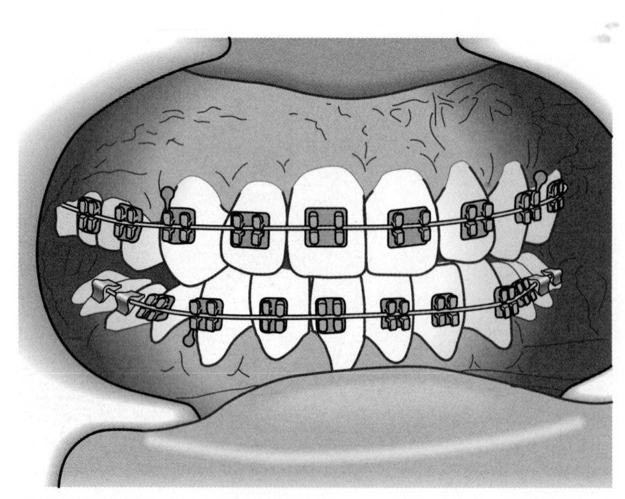

10.2.12 The intermaxillary fixation has been released in order to check the occlusion.

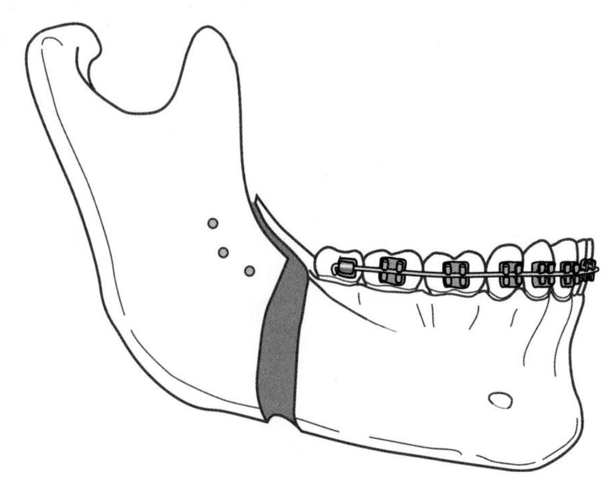

10.2.13 The ideal position of the holes when bicortical screws are used for immobilisation.

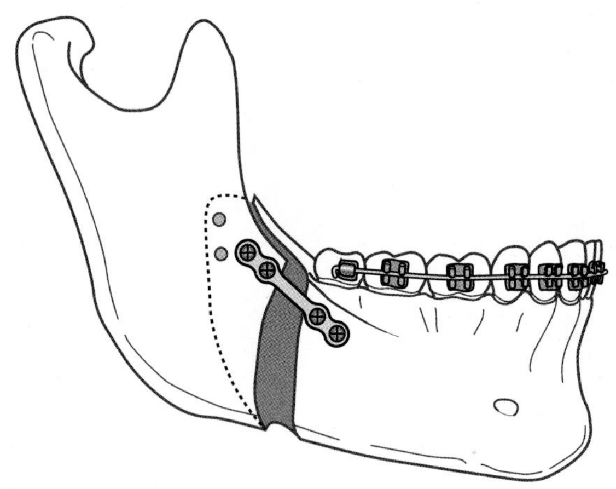

10.2.14 An additional bone plate is used when there has been a 'bad' lingual split.

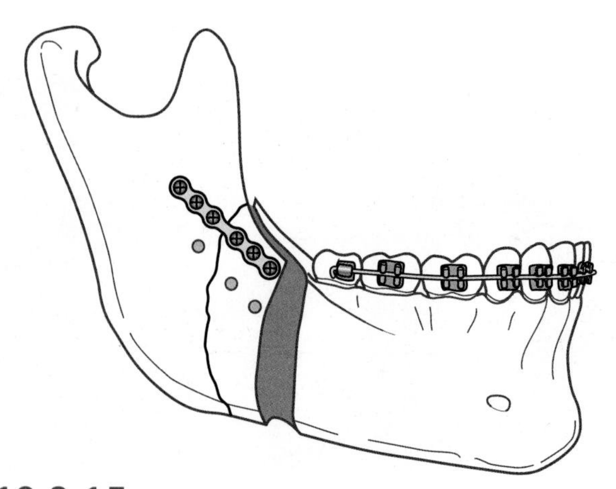

10.2.15 In this case an additional bone plate is being used to control a 'bad' buccal split.

GENIOPLASTY (HORIZONTAL SLIDING OSTEOTOMY)

This was first described in 1958 by Obwegeser. Horizontal osteotomy of the anterior mandible allows the chin to be repositioned in three dimensions. It can be advanced or set back to correct retro- or progenia. The lower face height can be either decreased or increased by excising bone or downgrafting the chin. Finally, rotational osteotomy can be performed to correct a lower facial asymmetry.

Surgical technique

If combined with a sagittal split osteotomy, the genioplasty is performed after the BSSO. It is easier if the patient is left in intermaxillary fixation while the genioplasty is carried out.

Incision

Using cutting diathermy an incision is made in the lower lip approximately 5 mm above the reflection of the lower labial sulcus and deepened to the anterior surface of the mandible (Figure 10.2.16). The mentalis muscles are transected in the process. Subperiosteal dissection is carried out towards the chin prominence. However, it is not necessary to deglove the chin. Extending laterally, the mental nerve is identified (Figure 10.2.17).

The bone cuts

A reference cut is first made in the line of the mandibular symphisis to mark the midline (Figure 10.2.18).

An Aufricht retractor is introduced into the lateral extent of the subperiosteal pocket on first one side and then the other below the mental foramen, while the horizontal osteotomy is performed. The mental nerve is directly visualized and protected. The osteotomy can be completed laterally using an osteotome (Figure 10.2.19). Having completed the bone cut on the first side, the saw is reversed and the cut extended on the contralateral side to complete the osteotomy (Figure 10.2.20).

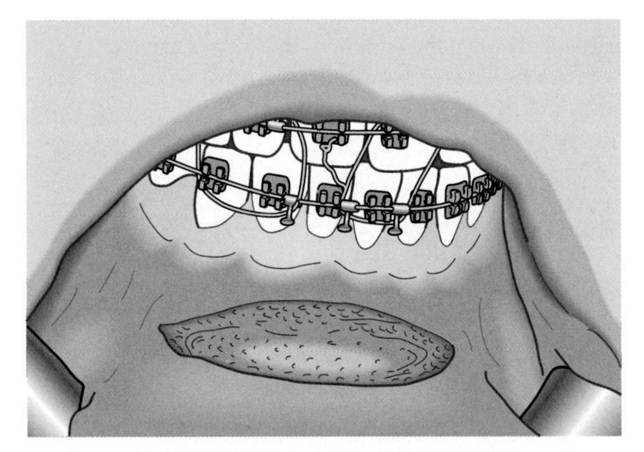

10.2.17 The mental nerves are identified laterally.

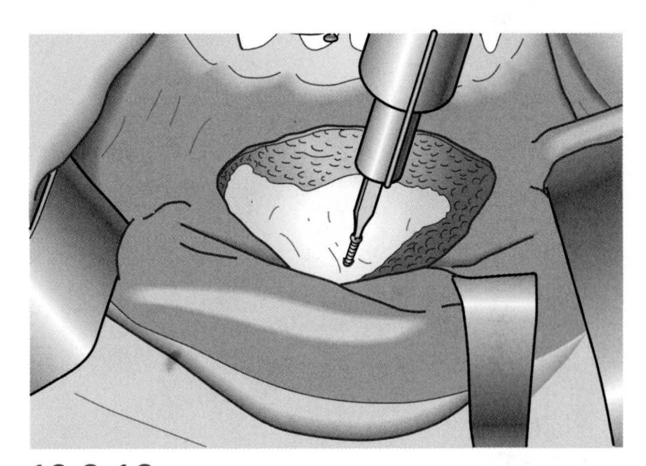

10.2.18 A small bone screw is used to mark the midline.

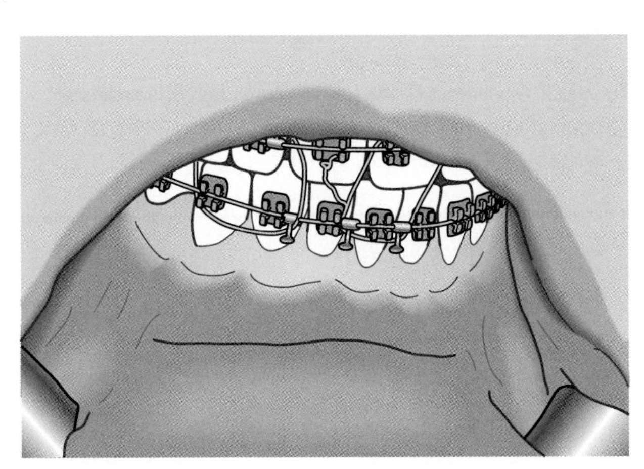

10.2.16 A sulcus incision is used to expose the anterior surface of the mandible.

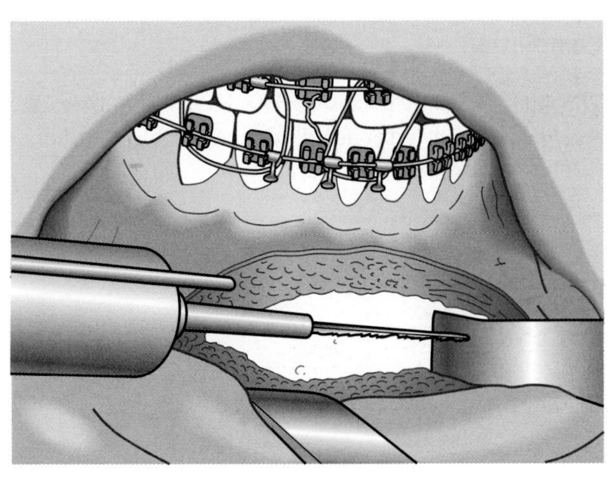

10.2.19 The horizontal osteotomy is being done with a reciprocating saw.

Fixation

The chin is mobilized into the planned position and fixed using either plates or screws. The author uses screws when possible (Figures 10.2.20 and 10.2.21). When the chin is advanced it is held in the planned position using a Kocher clamp. It is often easier to use plates to fix the osteotomy in this situation, particularly when the symphysis thickness is narrow.

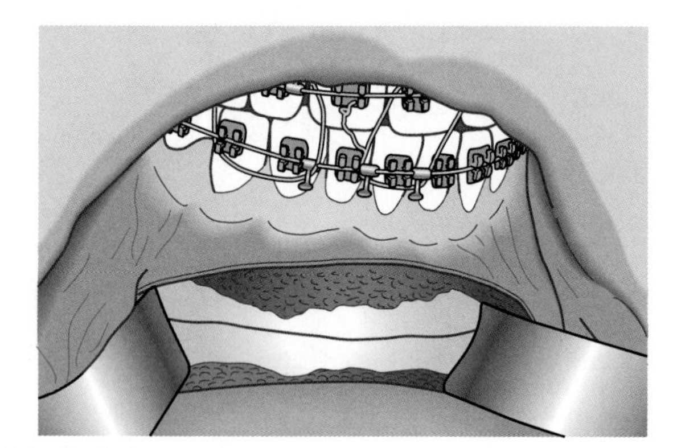

10.2.20 The horizontal cut has been completed.

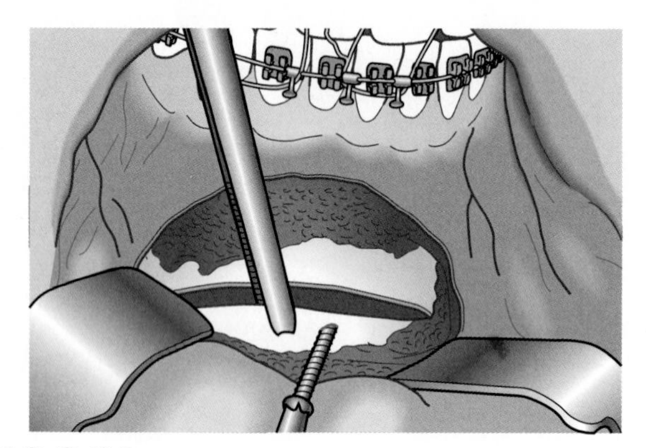

10.2.21 The mobilised segment is being held with a Kocher clamp whilst a screw is being inserted to immobilise the osteotomy.

Completion

The incision is then closed. The mentalis muscles are repaired. The mucosa is closed using resorbable, continuous sutures. A pressure dressing is applied.

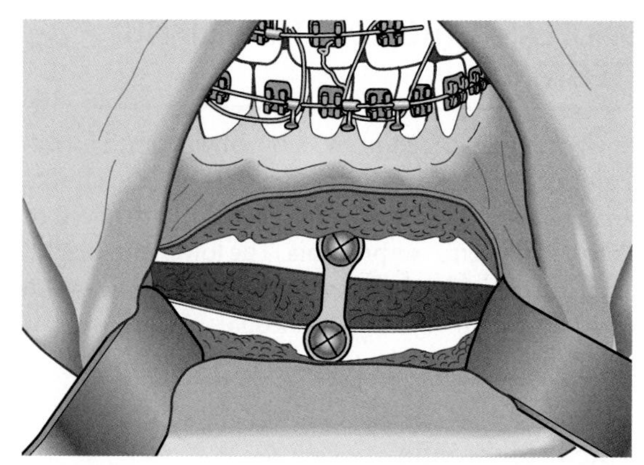

10.2.22 A bone plate may be used to immobilise the segment if there is not good bone contact.

Top Tips

- Ensure optimal operating conditions. Use a headlight and ask for hypotensive anaesthesia.
- Keep it simple. Avoid difficult and unusual procedures. The sagittal split osteotomy is uniquely versatile and, once mastered, is easy to perform and predictable. It is easily combined with a genioplasty.
- Perform a controlled split from anterior to posterior.
- Visualize the inferior dental nerve early and protect it.
- Use rigid fixation with either bicortical screws or a plate fixation.

FURTHER READING

Dal Pont G. Retromolar osteotomy for the correction of prognathism. *Journal of Oral Surgery* 1961: **19**: 42–7.

Epker BN. Modifications in the Sagittal osteotomy of the mandible. *Journal of Oral Surgery* 1977; **35**: 157–9.

Hunsuck EEA. A modified intraoral technique for correction of mandibular prognathism. *Journal of Oral Sugery* 1969; **26**: 249–52.

Obwegeser H. Die Kinnvergrosserung. *Oestereiche Zeitschrift fuer Stomatologie* 1958; **55**: 535.

Trauner R, Obwegeser H. The surgical correction of mandibular prognathism with consideration of genioplasty 1 and 11. *Oral Surgery* 1957; **10**: 677–89, 787–92.

10.3

Orthognathic surgery – maxilla (Le Fort I, II and III)

GEORGE OBEID

LE FORT I

Indications

- Correction of maxillary:
  - Hypoplasia and hyperplasia
  - Vertical excess and deficiency
  - Asymmetry
  - Transverse anomalies
  - Occlusal plane abnormalities
- Obstructive sleep apnea
- Access to the pharynx and base of skull for resection of tumours.

Planning fundamentals

POSITION OF THE UPPER INCISORS IN THE ALVEOLAR BONE

One of the cornerstones of planning for a maxillary osteotomy is to understand the position of the upper central incisors as they relate to the upper lip and the face. For this evaluation to be dependable, the central incisors must have the correct location and inclination inside the alveolar process. If at the time of evaluation the incisors are in an abnormal position, appropriate adjustments must be incorporated in the assessment.

VERTICAL POSITION OF MAXILLA

- Assess relationship between the upper central incisors to the upper lip. The incisor show is about 2–3 mm in repose; it is normal to show 1–2 mm above the gingivocervical margin when smiling. Since this measurement depends on a normal upper lip length, variation in the length and shape of the upper lip may have significant impact on this measurement. For instance, if the upper lip is abnormally short (males normal values 22 ± 2 mm, females 20 ± 2 mm) the upper incisors should not be moved to accommodate an abnormally short lip. Failure to take this into consideration may lead to imbalance of the facial structures.
- Assess facial thirds which are equal when measured from hairline to glabella, glabella to subnasale, and subnasale to soft tissue menton.

ANTERIOR POSTERIOR POSITION OF MAXILLA

- Clinical examination:
  - Observe the midpoint of the facial surface of the clinical crown of the central incisor as it relates to the forehead in profile, while smiling as described by Andrews. In a well balanced face, this point does not project beyond glabella. The relationship is universal and is consistent across age, gender and racial groups.

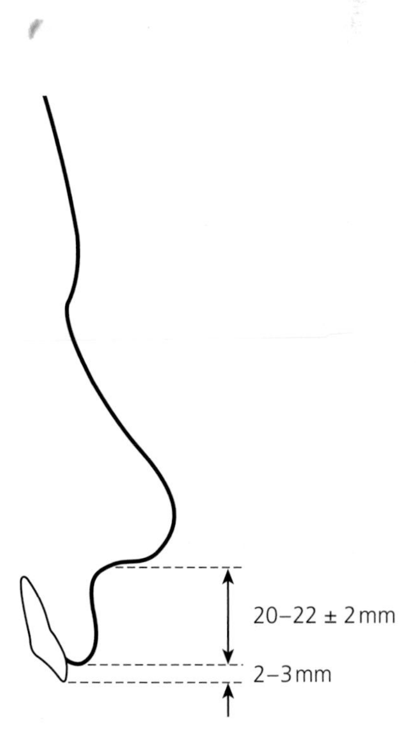

10.3.1 Upper lip length and incisor show.

- Cephalometric analysis:
  - SNA Sella-nasion-A point angle (82°). For this angle to be useful, the inclination of the SN to the Frankfort horizontal should be adjusted to about 7°.
  - Maxillary depth angle. NA – Frankfort horizontal (90°).

MIDLINE POSITION OF THE MAXILLA

The midline between the maxillary central incisors should relate to the lower central incisors, the philtrum, the chin, the nose and the forehead. Photographs, penciled in line and a string applied to the face all help determine if an asymmetry is present.

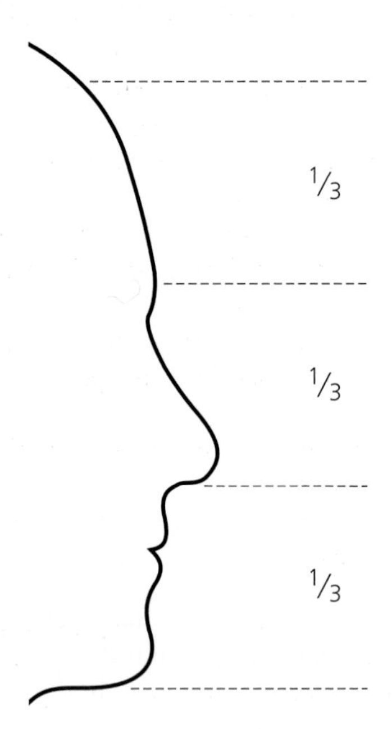

10.3.2 Facial thirds.

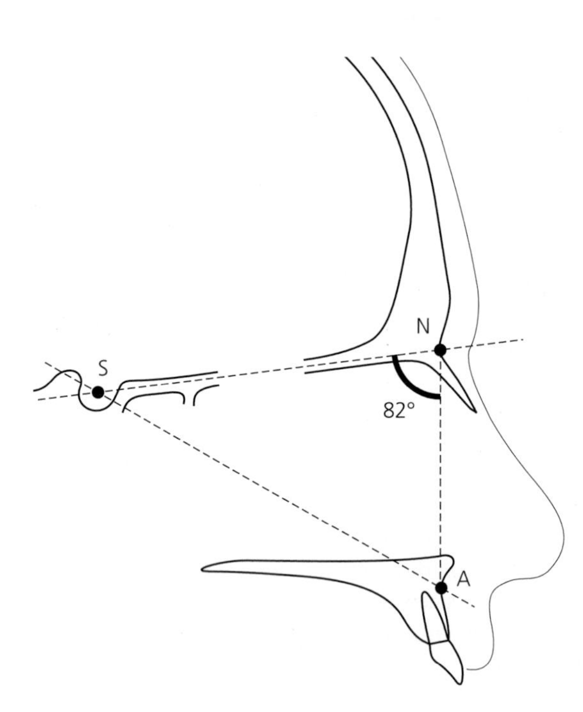

10.3.4 AP position of maxilla using SNA angle.

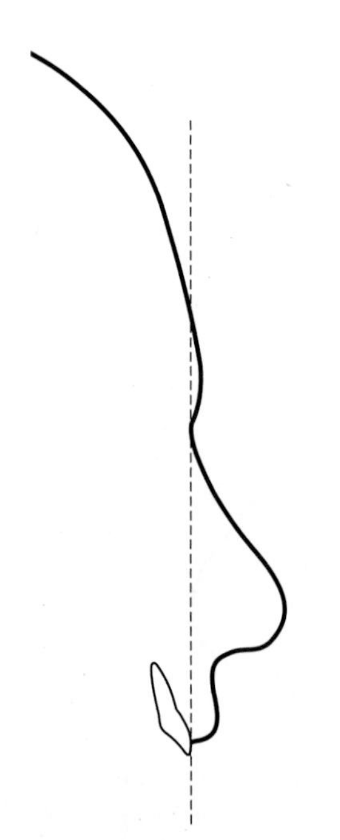

10.3.3 AP position of maxilla using relationship of upper central incisor to forehead.

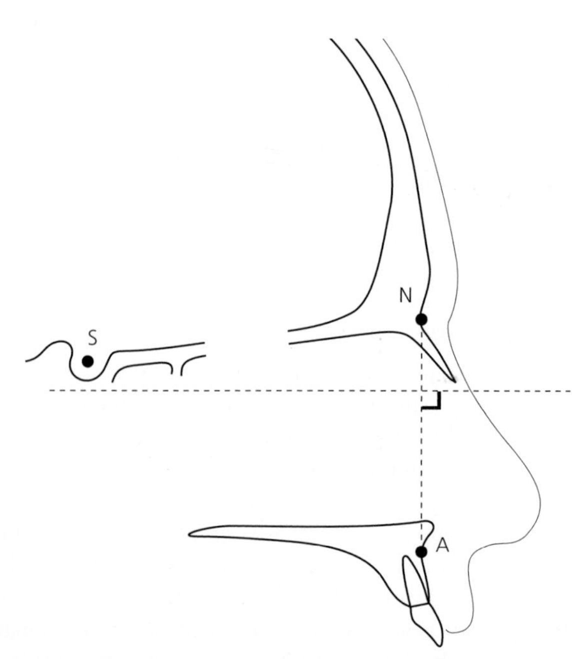

10.3.5 AP position of maxilla using facial angle.

MAXILLARY CANT

Measure the distance between the medial canthal ligament, to the incisive edge of the central and lateral incisors, and canine on one side and compare it to the other side.

OCCLUSAL PLANE INCLINATION

The inclination of the occlusal plane, about 8° from Frankfort horizontal, has an impact on the facial aesthetics and the need for double jaw surgery.

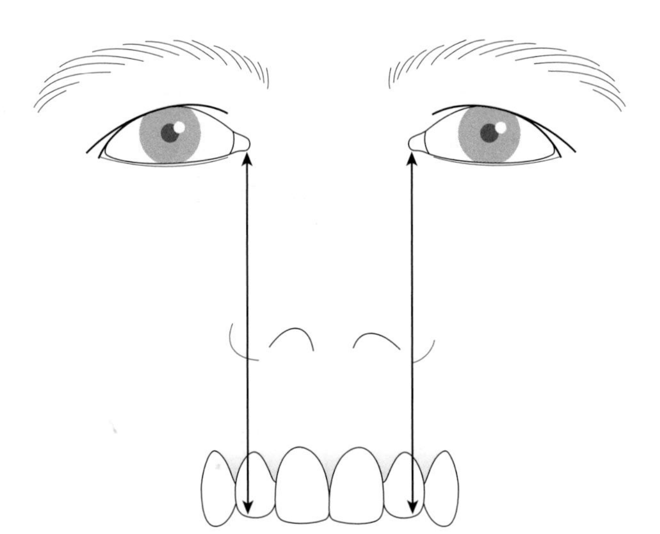

10.3.6 Assessment of maxillary cant.

Operation

- Anaesthesia is accomplished with a nasotracheal tube well secured to the forehead.
- About 10 mL of 0.5 per cent lidocaine with vasoconstrictor is injected in the buccal vestibule for haemostasis.
- Hypotensive anaesthesia, particularly at the time of down-fracture, reduces oozing and improves visibility.
- A non-threaded Kirschner wire is placed in the bridge of the nose to be used as an external reference marker. Distances from the wire to the central incisors are recorded.
- Place a circumvestibular incision, using a blade or electrocautery, in the buccal vestibule from molar to molar. The use of the electrocautery should be done with caution; orthodontic forces sometimes bring the apices of the teeth close to the surface of outside the bone, putting them at risk of thermal injury. Additionally, the use of electrocautery in the anterior region risks the formation of a wide scar band and possible shortening of the upper lip.
- Expose the piriform aperture, the infra-orbital nerves and the zygomatic buttresses.
- Expose the posterior maxilla by subperiosteal tunnelling to the junction of the maxillary tuberosity with pterygoid plates.
- Reflect mucoperiosteum of the floor of the nose, starting with a small Molt curette and then with an angled Freer elevator. Bothersome oozing can be minimized with the use of strips of ribbon gauze impregnated with a vasoconstrictor.
- It is preferable to perform the lateral bony osteotomy in the form of a step, instead of a straight line. The anterior limb of the step is kept horizontal. The step, 4–5 mm in length, is placed in the zygomatic buttress region. The step

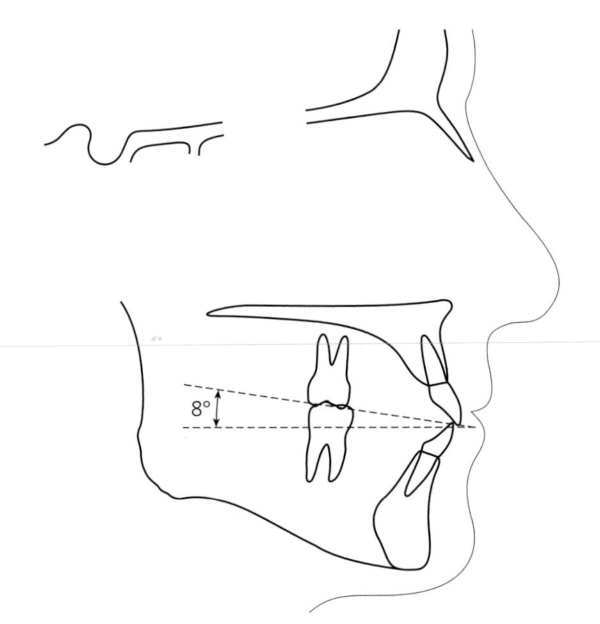

10.3.7 Assessment of inclination of occlusal plane.

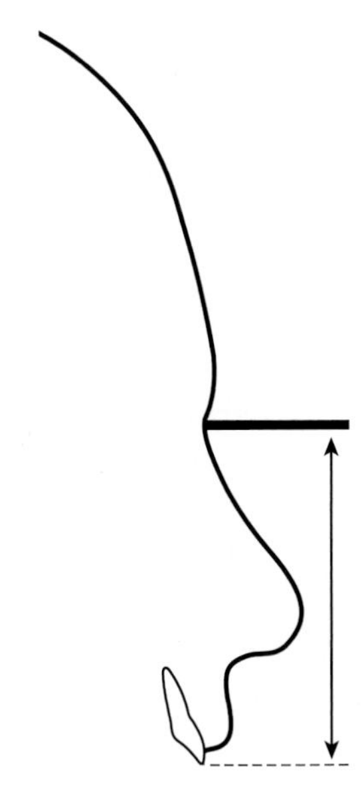

10.3.8 External reference marker.

reduces the risk of shortening the face as the maxilla is advanced horizontally forward rather than on a ramp. The step also offers an intraoperative verification of the bony movement, in addition to providing a suitable location for the placement of bone graft when needed. The osteotomy can be performed with burs or reciprocating saw. Visibility is improved by starting the osteotomy posteriorly and moving forward.

- Score the posterior wall of the maxillary antrum, without going through it, with a thin spatula osteotome introduced through the lateral osteotomy and directed in a downward direction.
- Separate the nasal septum with the double beaded osteotome directed downward and backward.
- Separate the maxilla from the pterygoid plates with a small curved osteotome placed at, or just behind, the tuberosity, as perpendicular as possible, and driven in a downward and medial direction. The operator's index finger is placed inside the mouth on the palatal side of the tuberosity to verify the position and direction of the osteotome.
- While protecting the nasal mucosa with a periosteal elevator, cut the lateral nasal wall with a thin spatula osteotome placed anteriorly in the nasal aperture and

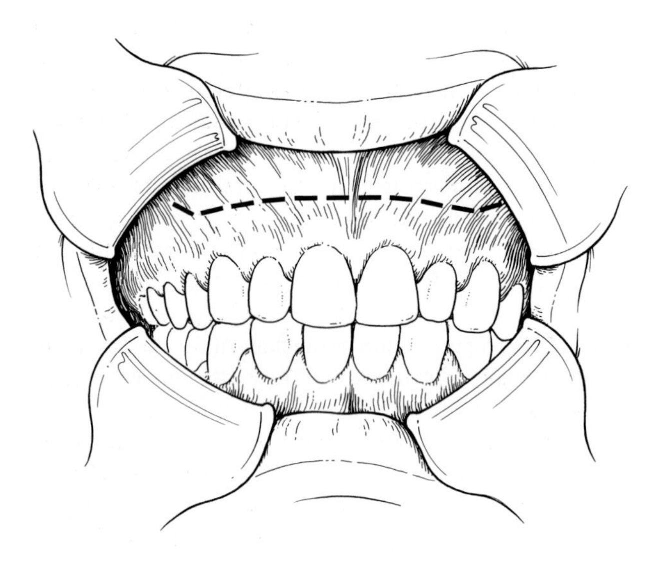

10.3.9 Soft tissue incision in buccal vestibule about 1 cm above the junction of mobile and fixed mucosa. The incision is curved slightly cranially in the posterior region.

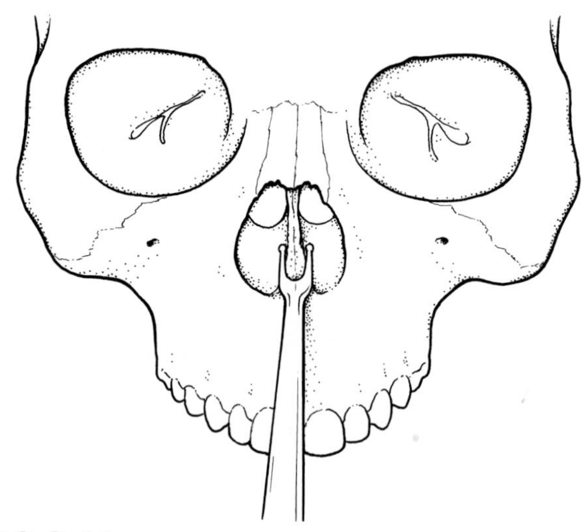

10.3.11 Septal osteotome is used to separate the nasal septum from the maxilla. Note the blunt end of this instrument which avoids tearing the nasal mucosa.

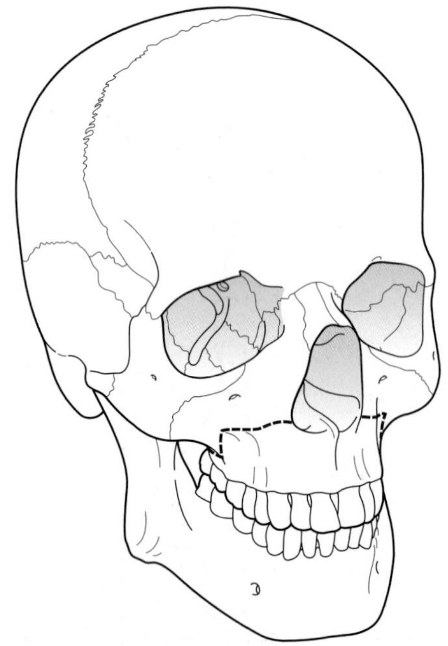

10.3.10 Outline of Le Fort 1 osteotomy.

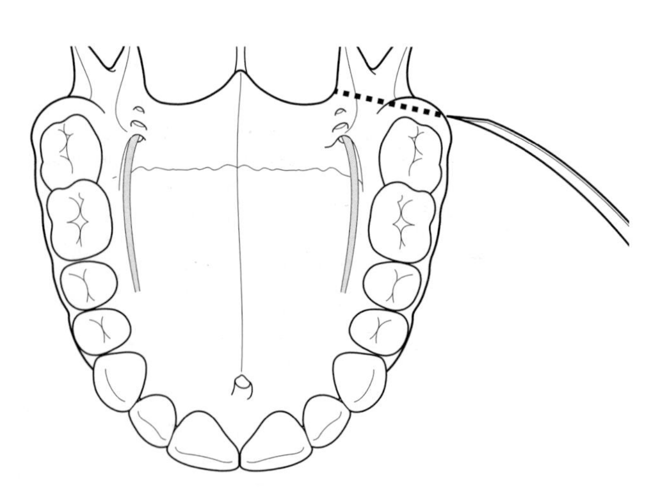

10.3.12 Place a slightly curved osteotome to cut through the tuberosity in a downward and medial direction.

directed in a posterior and downward direction to about 30 mm without reaching the descending palatine vessels. This step is repeated with increasingly thicker osteotomes, slowly wedging the maxilla down.

- Down-fracture the maxilla with light digital pressure, if resistance is encountered, repeat use of the osteotome. Down-fractured maxillas that have pterygoid plates attached to the tuberosity have markedly restricted movements. The descending palatine vessels can be safely coagulated.

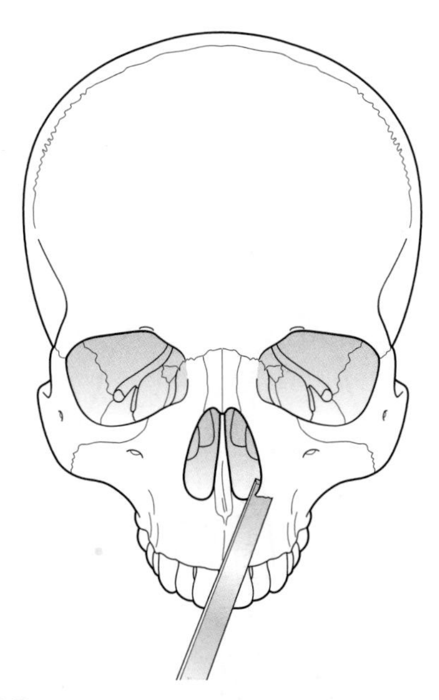

10.3.13 The lateral nasal wall is cut with an ostotome with a blunt end so as not to damage the nasal mucosa.

- Mobilize the maxilla with spreaders, Seldon elevators, curved osteotomes and Tessier mobilizers in addition to digital manipulation. Once the desired mobility is accomplished, the maxillary and mandibular teeth are wired together with or without a splint. With the maxilla and mandible attached together and the condyles properly seated in the glenoid fossa, the complex is passively closed to the desired vertical dimension using the external reference point.
- Reduce the nasal septum enough to prevent buckling. Deep bony structures are trimmed to allow free movements without interferences. To avoid excessive bone trimming, the lateral wall of the maxilla is reduced under direct vision, trimming only the bony spots that are preventing the planned movement.
- When 4–5 mm posterior maxillary expansion is needed, a midline split along the maxillary suture can be carried out. Once the maxilla is down-fractured, a slim spatula osteotome is hammered in the middle of the nasal spine towards the centre of the alveolar process. There is no need to use a bur or to reflect the gingival tissue over the buccal surface of the anterior teeth. With the maxilla supported with one hand, the osteotome is driven into the bone for about 1 cm. The step is repeated with a Smiley osteotome which is then slowly rotated to split the maxilla along the midline suture from the hard palate to between the central incisors. The two segments are then slowly stretched to reach the desired movement.
- Patients undergoing maxillary impaction may require the removal of the inferior turbinates to provide needed space and to reduce nasal airway obstruction. With the maxilla in the down-fracture position, the nasal mucosa is incised lengthwise on both sides and the inferior turbinates are

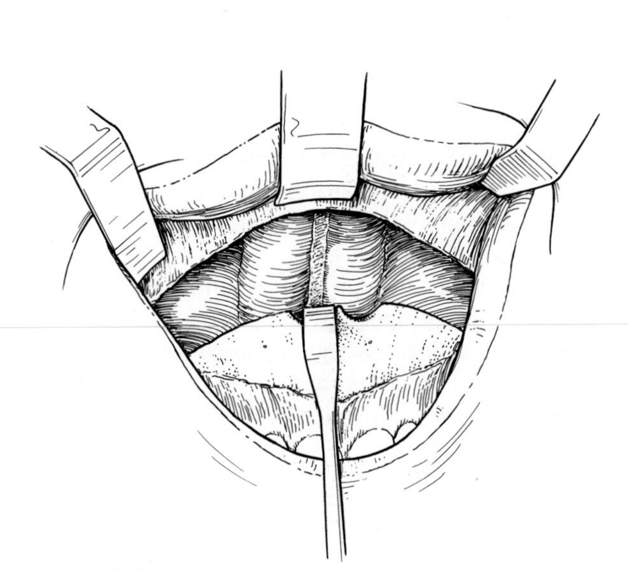

10.3.14 Down fractured maxilla.

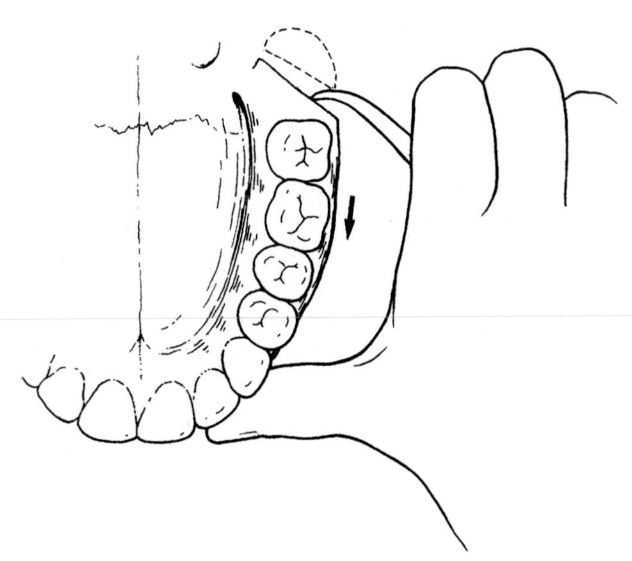

10.3.15 Curved instruments such as the Seldon elevator are used to mobilize the maxilla and move it forward.

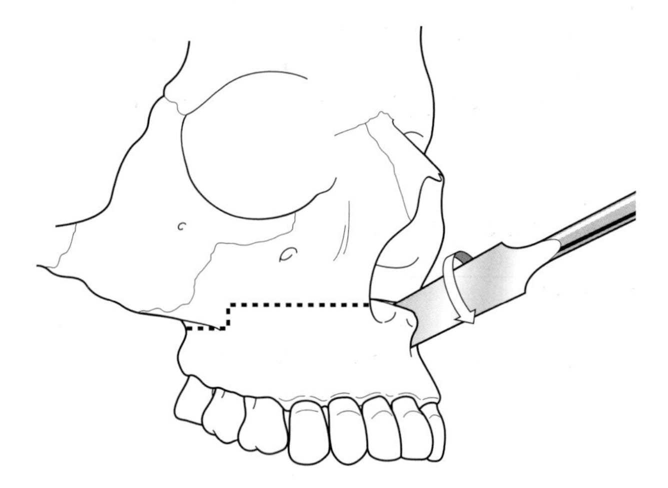

10.3.16 For small maxillary expansion, osteotomes are used for opening the midline sutures to expand the maxilla posteriorly.

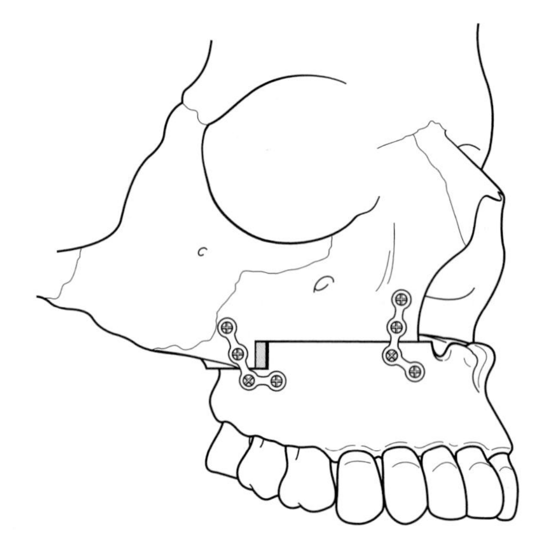

10.3.17 Two small plates, in the piriform rim and zygomatic buttress, are used to fix the maxilla.

resected with scissors and electrocautery. The nasal mucosa is then close with 4/0 chromic gut sutures.

- Fixation of the maxilla is ideally carried out with two plates and screws on each side, one in the piriform rim area and a second one in the malar buttress region. The maxilla, still attached to the mandible, is brought to its final position using the mandibular condyle as a guide. It is critical to have the condyle properly seated in the glenoid fossa. This step begins prior to surgery, by understanding the patient's specific occlusion and centric relation. If interim splints are used they must be accurate, otherwise a cant or side to side movements of the maxilla may occur. The anterior plates are placed first; constantly referring to the external reference point to avoid inadvertent shortening or lengthening the midface. Plate placement requires precision; any inaccuracies lead to malocclusion.
- Verify accuracy of the fixation. This can be done by manually maintaining the mandible in occlusion while the IMF wires are removed. Observing any shift of occlusion while the teeth are slowly released is helpful in recognizing an error in fixation. Malocclusion that is secondary to inaccurate plating needs to be addressed at this stage.
- Alar cinch suture is often needed to prevent alar flare that occurs as the result of the maxillary surgery. Evert the lip and grasp the fibrous tissue located immediately below the alar cartilage. Pass a 0 Vicryl or similar suture through the tissue and visualize the pulling effect on the alar region to assure proper placement of the suture. Repeat step on the opposite side. The suture is tied to the desired tension in the midline.

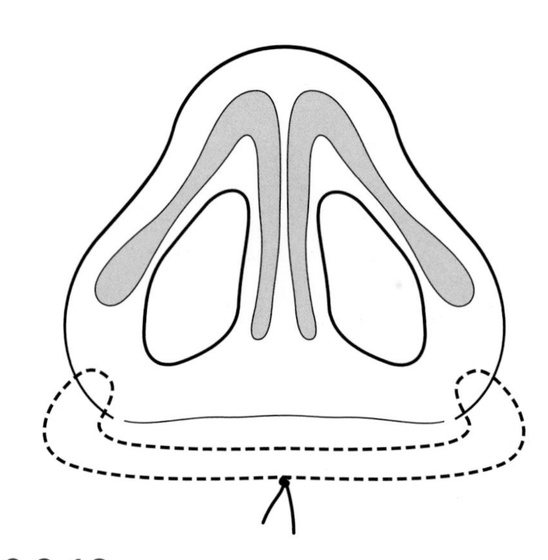

10.3.18 Alar cinch suture.

- V-Y closure of the anterior wound can affect the protrusion of the upper lip and preserve its length. The rest of the maxillary incision is closed with interrupted or running 3/0 vicryl suture.
- Light elastics may be applied between the maxillary and mandibular teeth

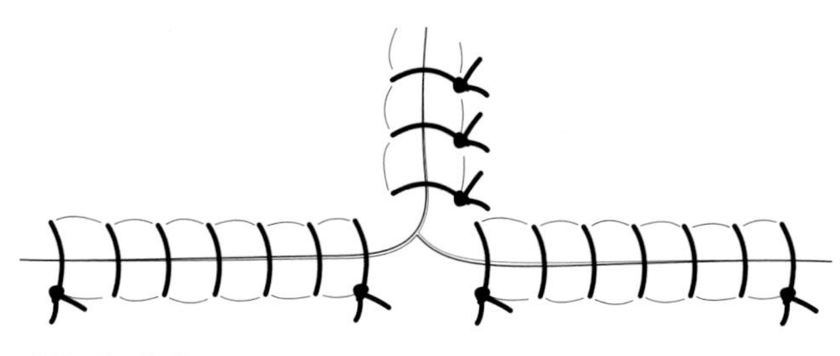

10.3.19 VY closure of soft tissue incision.

Post-operative care

- Obtain cephalometric radiographs to verify the planned movement and to monitor any future relapse.
- Check the occlusion; minor occlusal interdigitation problems are corrected with light elastics. More significant midline or anterior posterior (AP) discrepancies may require a return to the operating room for correction.
- Monitor for infection and wound dehiscence.
- Orthodontic tooth movement can be started as early as 4–6 weeks post-surgery.

OSTEOTOMIES ABOVE THE LE FORT I LEVEL

HIGH LE FORT I OSTEOTOMY

Principles

Also known as quadrangular Le Fort I. It is similar to the standard Le Fort I except that it extends higher on the anterior wall of the maxilla and the body of the zygoma.

Indication

Maxillary and zygomatic horizontal deficiencies in patients that have normal nasal projection. The principal movement is advancement with midline split when necessary.

Operation

- Identical to the Le Fort I approach except for the osteotomy on the lateral wall of the maxilla.
- Start bony cuts low at the lateral wall of the nose.
- Extend superiorly to just below the infraorbital rim.
- Continue laterally, below the infraorbital rim, skirting around the infra orbital foramen, to the zygomatic body.
- Turn downward into the zygomatic buttress.
- Continue horizontally backward to the pterygomaxillary fissure.
- Down-fracture maxilla with attention not to break the thin lateral maxillary wall.
- Fixation with miniplates and screws and bone graft as needed.

LE FORT II OSTEOTOMY

Indication

Adult patients with nasomaxillary hypoplasia to accomplish mostly advancement and some downward movements.

Operation

- Intraoral circumvestibular incision from molar to molar.
- Bilateral oblique paranasal skin incisions or coronal flap.
- Bony outline.
  - Horizontal line across the nasofrontal and nasomaxillary sutures.
  - Extend vertically downward through the lacrimal bone, keeping the canthal ligaments intact.
  - Continue posterior to the lacrimal apparatus to cross the medial aspect of the infraorbital rim.
  - Continue from the intraoral side, in a downward and lateral direction to finish in the pterygomaxillary fissure.

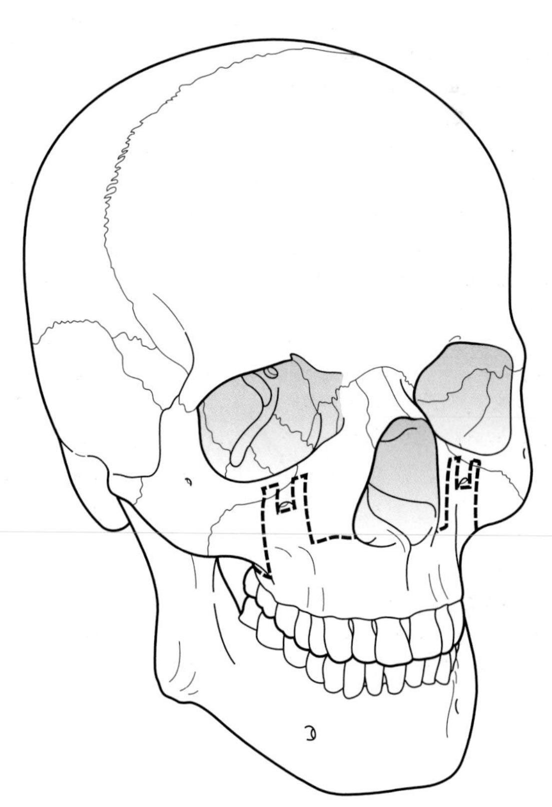

10.3.20 Outline of high Le Fort I osteotomy.

- Separate the nasal septum from the base of the skull with an osteotome starting at the level of the bridge of nose and sloping in a posterior and inferior direction. Pre- operative CT scan can help assess the midline structures and their proximity to the proposed septum osteotomy.

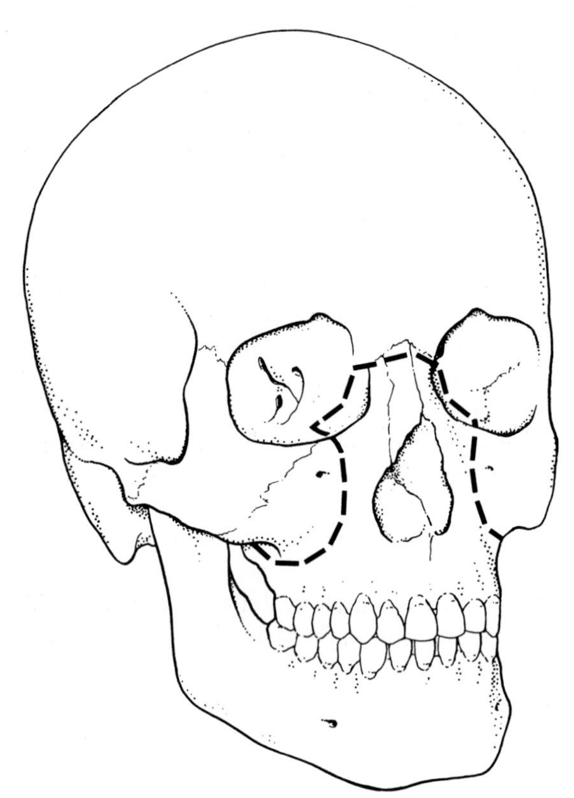

10.3.21 Outline of the Le Fort II ostetotomy.

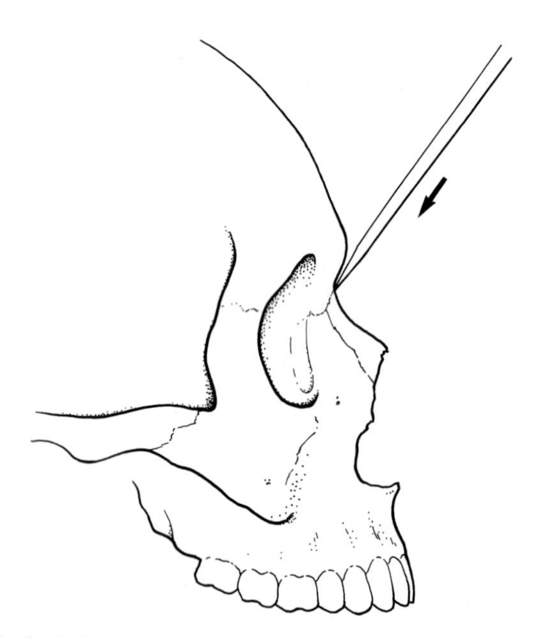

10.3.22 Direction of nasal septum cut the level of the nasal root.

- Mobilize with Rowe's disimpaction forceps and Tessier mobilizers.
- Fixation is with miniplates and screws with bone grafts placed primarily in the bridge of the nose and other areas as needed.

QUADRANGULAR LE FORT II OSTEOTOMY

Principles

Follows similar outline to the high Le Fort I osteotomy with the exception of including the infraorbital rims. The infraorbital nerve is overly manipulated in this osteotomy, increasing the risk of long-term injury.

Indication

Maxillary and zygomatic deficiencies in patients who have increased scleral show and normal nasal projection. The movements are mostly advancement. Often, aesthetic and functional movements needed at the tooth level differ from what is needed at the infraorbital rim level.

Operation

- The entire osteotomy can be accomplished from an intraoral circumvestibular incision; the orbital floor is cut with osteotomes introduced from either side of the osteomized infraorbital rims. If unfeasible, additional skin or transconjunctival access is performed.
- Fixation is with miniplates and bone graft as needed.

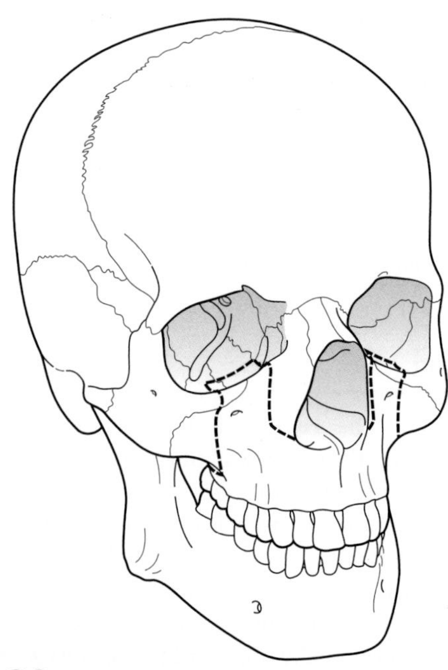

10.3.23 Outline of the Quadrangular Le Fort II osteotomy.

LE FORT III OSTEOTOMIES, TRANSCRANIAL FRONTOFACIAL OSTEOTOMIES, MONOBLOC OR SAGITTAL BIPARTITION

Indication

Correction of concurrent nasal, orbital, zygomatic and maxillary deficiencies in mostly syndromic or post-traumatic patients. Abnormalities in the shape of the forehead will affect the selection between a transcranial approach and a subcranial Le Fort III osteotomy.

Timing of surgery is selected on a case-by-case basis with early intervention often influenced by severe proptosis, sleep apnoea and need to improve the child's appearance around school age. It is important to take into account that early intervention will have a restrictive growth on the facial skeleton and even with overcorrection, repeat surgery, once the growth is completed, may be indicated.

Operation

- Tracheostomy may be indicated.
- Coronal flaps; additional access to the orbital floor may require lower cutaneous eyelid incision or a transconjunctival approach.
- The bony outline of the Le Fort III osteotomy runs bilaterally through:
  - The zygomatic arch, frontozygomatic suture and lateral orbital wall
  - Extends to the floor of the orbit and the infraorbital fissure
  - Continues behind the nasolacrimal apparatus onto the medial wall of the orbit to the bridge of the nose
  - The nasal septum is separated from the base of skull as described for Le Fort II osteotomy
  - The pterygoid plates are separated from the tuberosity with osteotome introduced either from the coronal flap approach or through a small intraoral incision in the tuberosity region.
  - Concurrent midfacial and supraorbital rim deficiencies require a transcranial approach whereby the supraorbital rims and the midface are advanced as a single unit 'monobloc'. The outline for this osteotomy differs from that of the Le Fort III procedure in that the superior cuts run across the anterior cranial fossa to include the entire orbital rim.
  - Patients with associated hypertelorism and palatal constriction can, in addition, have 'facial bipartition'. The face is divided in the central area down to the hard palate and a predetermined column of bone is removed. As the two halves are brought together, the hypertelorism, as well as the palatal constriction, are corrected and the face is advanced as a single unit.
  - Mobilize with spreaders, Rowe's disimpaction forceps and Tessier mobilizers, avoiding unplanned fractures that are common in the infraorbital rim and the palate.
  - Preserve medial canthal attachment whenever possible. Should there be need to detach it, appropriate canthopexy is carried out at the conclusion of surgery.
  - Mobilize the face to the planned position and temporarily wire together the maxillary and mandibular teeth.
  - Blocks of autogenous bone graft, calverial, rib or iliac crest are placed primarily in the areas of the zygomatic arch, lateral orbit wall and nasal bridge.
  - Use miniplates and screws to stabilize the osteotomy and the grafted bone. Concerns of migration of metal plates and restriction of growth make a strong case for the use of biodegradable plates and screws in children.
  - Decision to release the intermaxillary fixation depends on the stability of the osteotomy.
  - Dental arch discrepancies may require an additional Le Fort I osteotomy. Although this procedure can be performed concurrently with the midface advancement, it is preferable to do it separately at a later date.

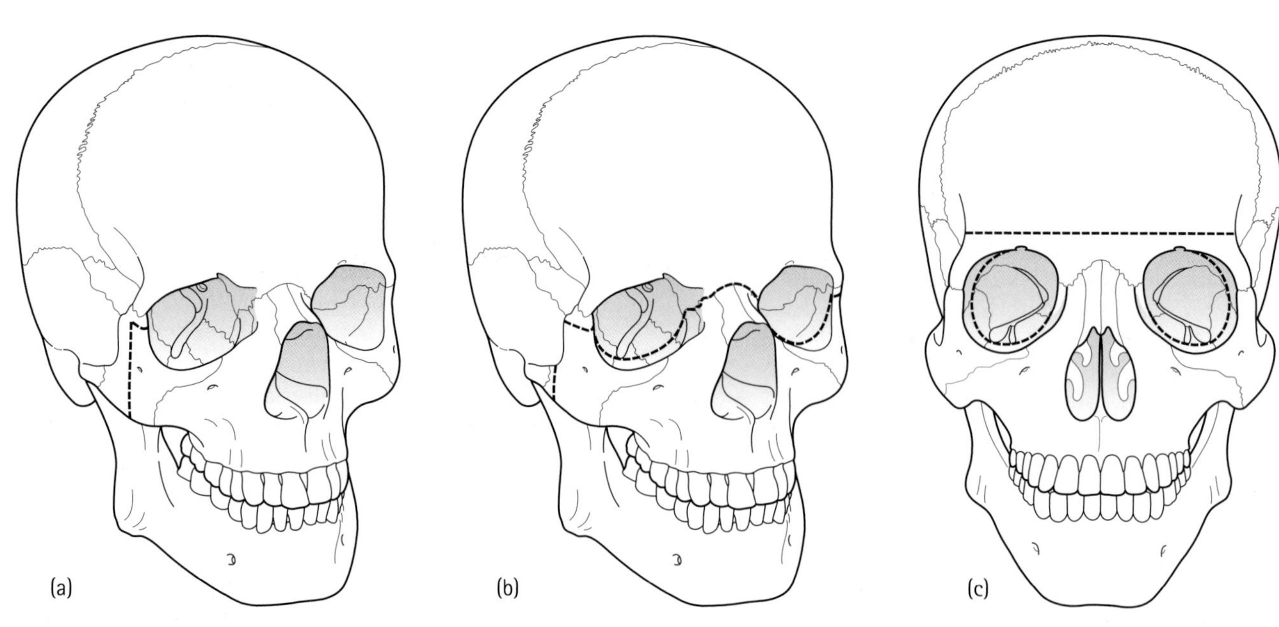

10.3.24 Various outlines of Le Fort III osteotomy.

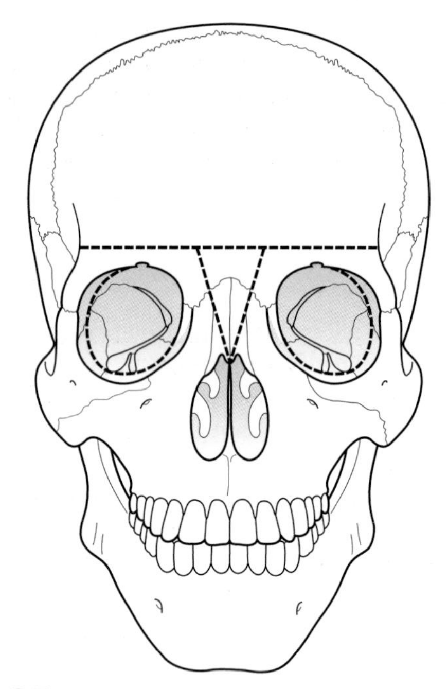

10.3.25 Outline of facial bipartition.

Top tips

- Meticulous planning entails placing the upper central incisors in an ideal vertical and AP position, in addition to having the occlusal plane leveled in the proper inclination.
- External reference point is essential in placing the maxilla in the desired position.
- Proper seating of the condyles in the fossa while fixing the maxilla.
- Eliminate any bony or septal cartilage interferences.
- Plate bending should be accurate; minor imperfections lead to malocclusion.

FURTHER READING

Frost DE. Orthognathic surgical techniques. In: Ward Booth P, Schendel SA, Hausamen JE (eds). *Maxillofacial surgery.* St. Louis, MO: Churchill Livingstone Elesevier, 2007: 1224–46.

Perciaccante VJ, Bays RA. Maxillary orthognathic surgery. In: Miloro M. (ed.). *Peterson's Principles of oral and maxillofacial surgery.* London: BC Decker, 2004: 1179–204.

Posnick JC, Muhling J. Surgical treatment of craniofacial dysostosis syndrome and single-suture craniosynostosis. In: Ward Booth P, Schendel SA, Hausamen JE (eds). *Maxillofacial surgery.* St. Louis, MO: Churchill Livingtstone, Elsevier, 2007: 876–900.

Schlosser JB, Preston CB, Lampasso J. The effect of computer aided anteroposterior maxillary incisor movement on ratings of facial attractiveness. *American Journal of Orthodontics and Dentofacial Orthopedics* 2005; **127**: 17–24.

Wolford LM, Fields RT Jr. Diagnosis and treatment planning for orthognathic surgery. In: Betts NJ, Turvey RA (eds). *Fonseca, oral and maxillofacial surgery, orthognathic surgery,* vol. 2. Philadelphia, PA: WB Saunders. 2000: 24–55.

10.4a

Mandibular distraction osteogenesis by intraoral and extraoral techniques

DAVID A WALKER

INTRODUCTION

Distraction osteogenesis (DO) is a powerful technique utilized to gradually lengthen the mandible significant distances. Distraction osteogenesis creates new bone without the need for bone grafting and donor site morbidly. The distraction technique requires proper understanding and application of the biologic principles of distraction osteogenesis that are age appropriate and anatomically sound. Distraction osteogenesis has a wide range of applications (Table 10.4a.1) and requires selection of an appropriate intraoral or extraoral distraction device.

Table 10.4a.1 Indications for mandibular distraction osteogenesis.

1. Severe mandibular retrognathia/micrognathia
2. Craniofacial syndromes: Hemifacial Micosomia, Treacher Collins syndrome, Nager syndrome, Pierre Robin sequence
3. Post-traumatic deficient mandibular growth and temporomandibular joint ankylosis
4. Severe mandibular asymmetry
5. Revision mandibular orthognathic surgery
6. Mandibular retrognathia with obstructive sleep apnoea
7. Mandibular retrognathia with temporomandibular joint disease or juvenile rheumatoid arthritis
8. Mandibular defects from tumour resection

PRE-OPERATIVE ASSESSMENT

A thorough history and clinical examination is appropriate with utilization of diagnostic imaging; including panoramic; posterior anterior, and lateral cephalometric radiographs. Computed tomography (CT) scans with three dimensional (3D) reconstructions of the mandible and temporomandibular joint are helpful. Dental study models mounted on a semi-adjustable articulator with prediction model surgery are of benefit. In selected instances stereo lithographic models may aid in treatment planning. Standardized 3D cephalometric prediction tracings are appropriate. All clinical and diagnostic tools are utilized to plan out the proper 3D distraction vector selection.

Distraction osteogenesis device selection is based on available bone stock, ease of application, distance of distraction osteogenesis and ability to adjust the distraction vector post device placement. It is the author's preference to utilize an intraoral device (Tables 10.4a.2 and 10.4a.3) although extraoral devices, in selected instances, have advantages. (Tables 10.4a.4 and 10.4a.5).

Table 10.4a.2 Advantages of intraoral distraction osteogenesis.

1. Allows bidirectional and tridirectional mandibular lengthening of 10–30 mm and avoids intermaxillary fixation
2. Avoids external skin scars of distraction, pin loosening or pin tract infection
3. Allows longer consolidation times with minimal to no skeletal relapse after extreme mandibular lengthening
4. Can be applied to neonates, infants, paediatric and adult patients
5. Avoids more invasive bone grafting procedures and potential donor site morbidity
6. Can be utilized for mandibular widening
7. Potential for less temporomandibular joint adverse affects in response to asymmetric lengthening
8. Decreased length of hospital stay and cost compared with bone grafting with less chance of blood transfusion

ANAESTHESIA CONSIDERATIONS

Standard pre-operative medical evaluation, diagnostic tests and anaesthesia consultation regarding the patient's airway are appropriate. Many of the patients undergoing mandibular lengthening by distraction osteogenesis have

Table 10.4a.3 Disadvantages of intraoral distraction osteogenesis.

1. Requires additional pre-operative work up and is technique sensitive
2. Requires patient compliance, increased post-operative care and monitoring
3. Requires second procedure for DO device removal

Table 10.4a.4 Advantages of extraoral distraction devices.

1. Applicable to small mandibles in infants and small children due to less available bone stock
2. Extraoral device results in less disruption to periosteum and blood supply
3. Able to distract greater distances than intraoral devices
4. Offers the potential for three dimensional vector adjustments after device placement. Adjustments can be made in the horizontal vertical and transverse planes

Table 10.4a.5 Disadvantages of extraoral distraction devices.

1. External skin scars
2. Distraction pin loosening
3. Pin tract infections
4. Psychosocial considerations
5. Inadequate consolidation time resulting in skeletal relapse
6. Temporary or permanent cranial nerve VII palsy

severe mandibular retrognathia with significantly compromised airways. Pre-operative polysomnography is a strong consideration in patients with suspected obstructive sleep apnoea. An awake fibreoptic nasoendotracheal intubation of the trachea may frequently be required. Distraction procedures for lengthening of the mandible are more commonly carried out under general anaesthesia although in selected cases sedation and local anaesthesia has been used.

OPERATIVE TECHNIQUE FOR INTRAORAL DISTRACTION DEVICE PLACEMENT

The patient is placed in a supine position with appropriate head support and is prepped and draped in the normal fashion for an oral and maxillofacial surgical procedure. The author prefers appropriate intravenous antibiotic prophylaxis. After establishing general anaesthesia, preferably by nasoendotracheal methods, local anaesthesia (typically 2 per cent lidocaine with 1/100 000 epinephrine or 0.5 per cent bupivacaine with 1/200 000 epinephrine) is infiltrated throughout the planned area of incisions. Care is taken to avoid toxic local anaesthetic dosages, particularly in infants and children. A bite block is placed on the contralateral side to open the mandible and bring the ramus forward. An incision is made over the external oblique ridge a distance of two to three centimeters. The length of incision is based on the length of osteotomy and degree of surgical access. A sharp dissection is carried out through buccinator muscle down to the external oblique ridge. The subperiosteal dissection is carried out exposing the anterior aspect of the ramus of the mandible to the level of the insertion of the temporalis muscle and a notched ramus retractor is used to retract tissues. The subperiosteal dissection is carried out down to the angle of the mandible and the antegonial notch region, stripping off the masseter muscle. The dissection is carried out anteriorly to an extent that is required for placement of the distraction device. Care is taken to identify the mental nerve, particularly in infants and children. A careful superior medial subperiosteal dissection is carried out at the body ramus junction in preparation for the osteotomy cut and to protect the lingual nerve.

The planned osteotomy is a linear osteotomy at the body ramus junction, distal to the second molar and is placed in an oblique angle (it is helpful to remove the third molar if present some three to six months predistraction). The superior and inferior aspect of the osteotomy is located and marked with a 701 burr. The lateral cortex osteotomy is completed with the 701 burr or reciprocating saw. Appropriate pre-operative diagnostic imaging will help to identify the position of the inferior alveolar neurovascular bundle. The inferior border osteotomy is made in a through and through fashion to the medial aspect of the mandible with a channel retractor in place to avoid the facial artery and vein. Care is taken to ensure that this cut does not encroach upon the inferior alveolar neurovascular bundle. The superior aspect of the osteotomy cut is not completed at this time.

Prior to placing the sterile distraction device (Figure 10.4a.1) it is important to open and close the device to ensure all components are functional and then the device is typically placed at the zero position. The intraoral distraction device is contoured with plate bending pliers to lie passively on the lateral aspect of the mandible. It is particularly important to ensure the correct distraction vector in three planes of space, which is more frequently parallel to the occlusal and sagittal planes rather than parallel to the inferior border of the mandible (Figures 10.4a.2a–e). It is helpful during this stage of the operation to have the mouth closed by a surgical assistant. Screw holes are drilled, one anteriorly and one posteriorly, and screws (preferably 2.0 mm) are utilized to secure the device. If access is difficult posteriorly, a 5 mm percutaneous stab incision can be utilized for introduction of a trocar through which drilling and screw placement can occur. It is advisable to place three to four screws per bony segment a minimum of 5 mm away from the edge of the osteotomy. The length of screws is dependent on the position of important structures such as the inferior alveolar neurovascular bundle, teeth

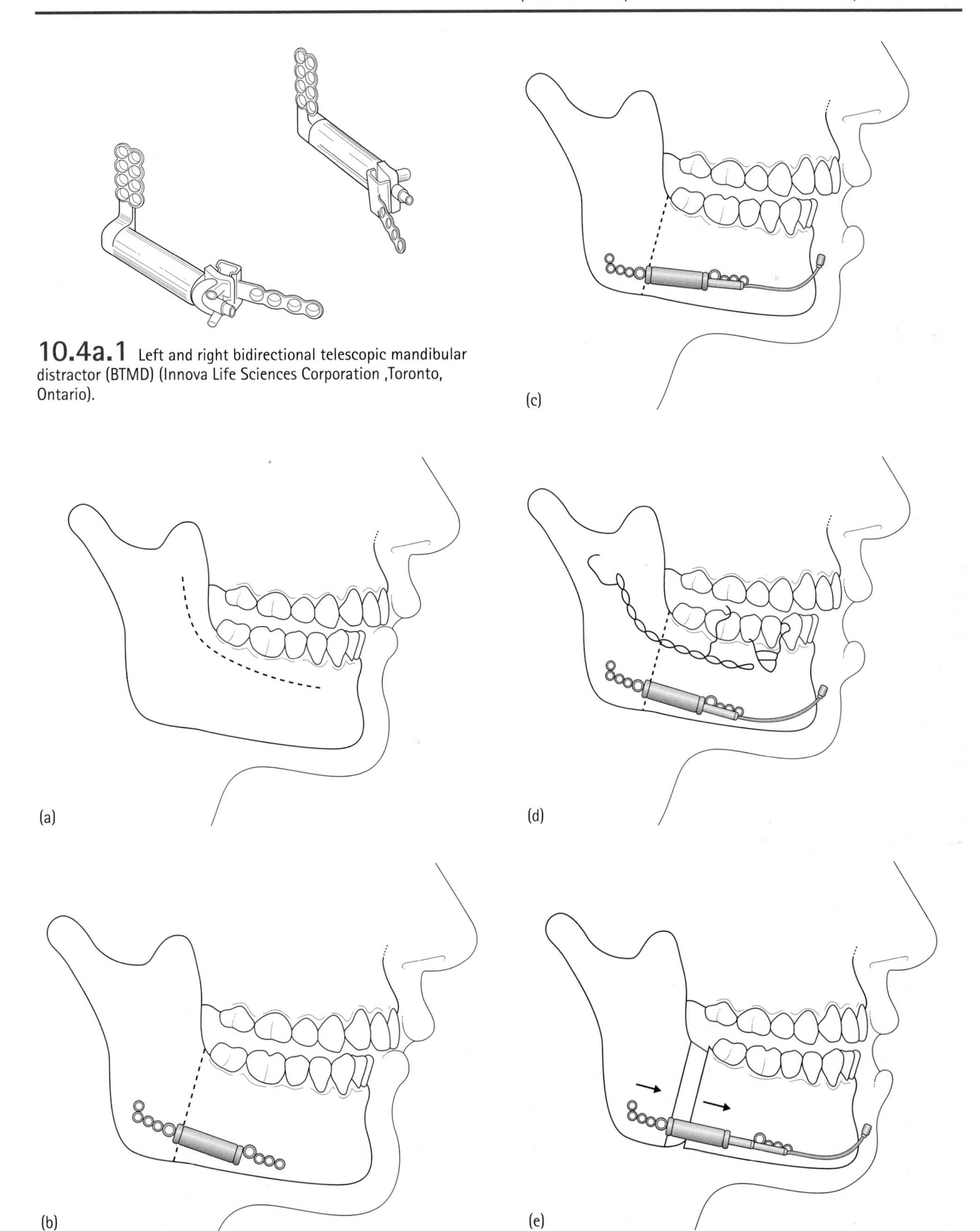

10.4a.1 Left and right bidirectional telescopic mandibular distractor (BTMD) (Innova Life Sciences Corporation ,Toronto, Ontario).

10.4a.2 (a) An incision is made through mucosa down through buccinator muscle over the external oblique ridge. The distance is 2–3 cm based on planned surgical access and distraction device size. (b) The BTMD is contoured and secured on the lateral aspect of the mandible after partial completion of the osteotomy at the body ramus junction. (c) The BTMD distracter has been secured with monocortical and bicortical screws and the osteotomy is completed. (d) The activation arm can be placed such as it emerges transmucosally or percutaneously depending on the size of the mandible and surgical access. (e) The distraction device is activated to ensure complete movement of both segments of the mandible and the inspection of the inferior alveolar neurovascular vascular bundle.

roots and developing tooth buds in infants and children. The DO device is typically secured with a combination of moncortical and bicortical screws.

After the distraction device is secured, and with adequate soft tissue retraction with a seldin retractor on the medial aspect of the mandible, the superior aspect of the body ramus osteotomy is now completed utilizing a 701 burr and reciprocating saw leaving a small area of bone around the lingual aspect of the inferior neurovascular bundle. Initially a wedging osteotome is tapped into place superiorly above the inferior alveolar nerve, and utilizing a torquing motion a fracture is created through the remaining portion of the mandible. At this stage it is important to open the distraction device and see that the bony segments move freely and also to inspect the inferior alveolar neurovascular bundle. If there is difficulty separating the bony segments the distraction device may be removed, the osteotomy completed and device re-applied.

Placement of the distraction activation arms is undertaken prior to closure. The activation arm can emerge trans-mucosally or percutaneously depending on the size of the mandible or surgical access. If it is elected to have the activation arm exit percutaneously, a small incision is made in the symphysis region of the mandible approximately to the level of the inferior border. It is important that there is no soft tissue drag on the exiting area of the activation arm. Copious irrigation is carried out and after haemostasis is achieved, the mucosa is closed with a combination of horizontal mattress sutures with 3/0 or 4/0 vicryl, and a running 4/0 chromic gut for water tight closure. Most cases require bilateral application of distraction devices. Occasionally unilateral distraction may be undertaken in younger patients.

OPERATIVE TECHNIQUE FOR EXTRAORAL DISTRACTION DEVICE PLACEMENT

The external distraction device can be placed through an external percutaneous submandibular approach or by a combination of intraoral and extraoral approaches.

Combined intraoral and extraoral approach

An intraoral approach as described previously is undertaken and the osteotomy is partially completed. Percutaneous incisions (1–1.5 cm) are placed in the submandibular area close to the planned area of pin placement. The pins are best placed approximately 6–8 mm away from the distraction osteotomy site and should be 4 mm apart depending on the distraction device (Figures 10.4a.3a–d). Pinhole sites will determine the initial vector of distraction and should be placed in locations based on pre-operative diagnostic studies. In a four-pin device the skin or soft tissue is pinched between the two pairs of pins to reduce the length of resulting scar. Fifty mm half pins are inserted through a trocar through the external incisions. The external distraction device is attached to the pins. The completion of the osteotomy is then accomplished in the superior border as described previously. The devices are opened to allow direct visualization of the distraction osteotomy site and then backed down to zero position.

Extraoral approach

The osteotomy and device placement can also be undertaken through a totally extraoral approach to the mandible, in which case a bolster underneath the shoulders and neck with the head extended somewhat improves access to the submandibular region The classic Risdon or submandibular approach is utilized with the skin incision being slightly higher, close to the inferior border. The skin and subcutaneous tissues are incised, the platysma muscle is divided with care being taken to ensure identification and preservation of the marginal mandibular branch of the facial nerve. A blunt dissection is carried out down the inferior border of the mandible and angle region. In order to provide adequate surgical access, the facial artery and vein frequently require dissection, clamping, transection and ligation. A subperiosteal dissection is carried out stripping off the masseter muscle and anteriorly to visualize areas of pin placement. Depending on the position of the incision the distraction pins can emerge through the incision or in separate percutaneous incisions. Osteotomy completion and pin placement are as described previously. Tissues are closed in layers, muscle periosteum and platysma 3/0 vicryl, subcutaneous tissue 4/0 vicryl and skin with 5/0 monofilament nylon. The device activation is similar as described for intraoral devices. The distraction device removal should be accomplished with the same criteria as established for intraoral devices with adequate osseous fill of the distraction gap visualized on radiographs, CT scan and/or ultrasound. The device removal is usually carried out under local anaesthesia after the appropriate time of bony consolidation. This may range from two months in very young children to five months in adult patients.

POST-OPERATIVE CARE

If the patient has significant airway compromise with obstructive sleep apnoea, patient admission to the ICU with endotracheal intubation overnight or until ready for extubation is a consideration. Alternatively, extubation could be achieved if the patient is awake and alert and able to protect their own airway. Requirements for discharge from hospital are adequate pain control and PO intake, and otherwise stable recovery from anaesthesia and surgery. A "minimal chew" soft diet is recommended for 6–8 weeks. In older children and adults, chlorhexidine 0.12 per cent mouthrinse is a consideration during distraction device activation. Use of post-operative oral antibiotics requires judgement and is based on patient wound healing and clinical progress. Skin sutures, if used, are usually removed

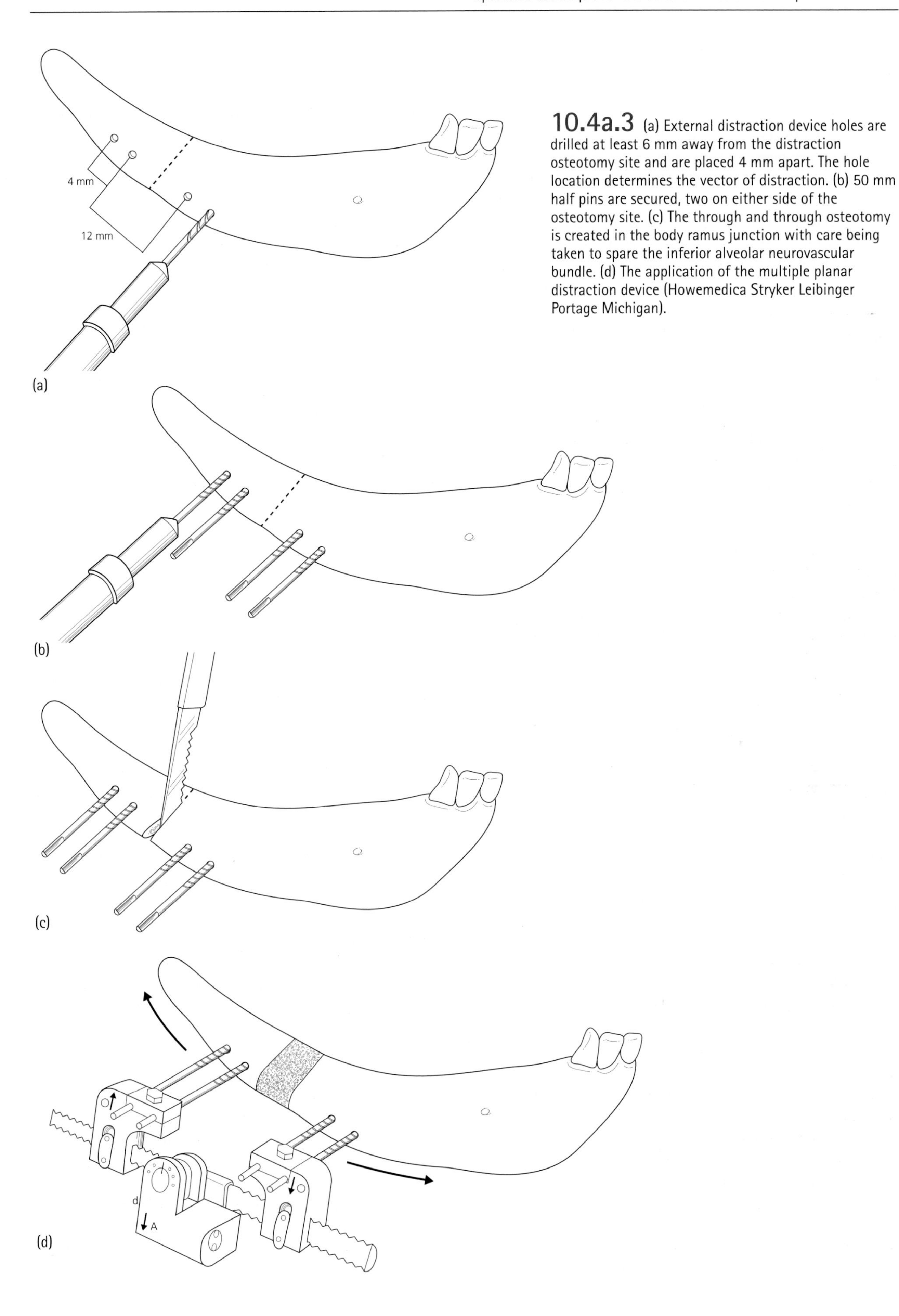

10.4a.3 (a) External distraction device holes are drilled at least 6 mm away from the distraction osteotomy site and are placed 4 mm apart. The hole location determines the vector of distraction. (b) 50 mm half pins are secured, two on either side of the osteotomy site. (c) The through and through osteotomy is created in the body ramus junction with care being taken to spare the inferior alveolar neurovascular bundle. (d) The application of the multiple planar distraction device (Howemedica Stryker Leibinger Portage Michigan).

seven to ten days post-operatively (or longer) depending on wound tension during distraction.

DISTRACTION DEVICE ACTIVATION

Activation of the distraction device is typically started on post-operative day 5, although earlier distraction may be commenced in younger patients. The distraction rate is typically 1 mm a day divided in two or three activations. It is important that responsible adults or patients activate the devices properly. In patients from the age of birth to two years a distraction rate of 1.5–2 mm a day may be appropriate based on rapid ability to create new bone and concern with premature bony consolidation. Monitoring of distraction with periodic radiographs and visual inspection is appropriate one to two times per week. Frequent assessment during distraction allows recognition of complications or aberrant distraction vectors and is necessary to determine the completion of distraction. Three dimensional vector adjustments can be made during distraction with selected multivector intraoral and extraoral DO devices (Figures 10.4a.4–10.4a.6). These are best done after approximately 10 mm of lengthening has occurred due to compression and stretching of the distraction regenerate. Vector alterations may be accomplished in sequential activations depending on the degree of distraction regenerate and the desired 3D changes.

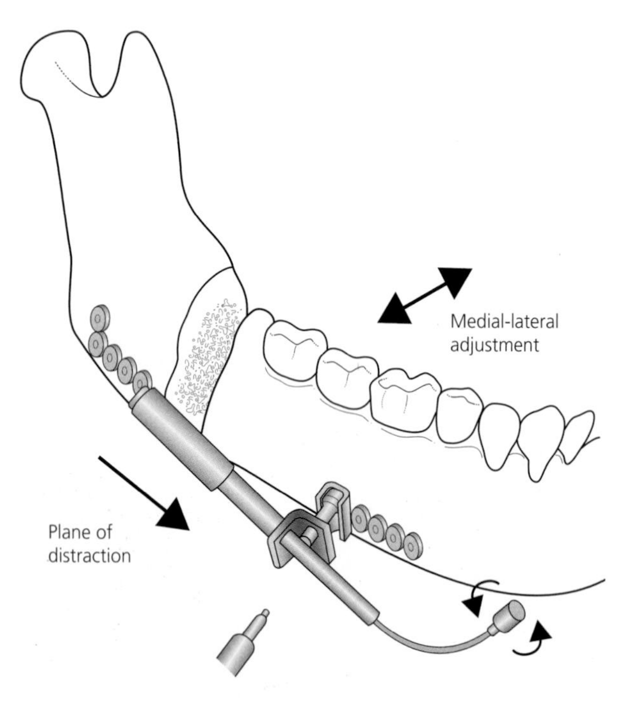

10.4a.4 Bidirectional telescopic mandibular distractor with opportunity to distract longitudinally and mediolaterally.

Activation arms are typically removed under local anaesthesia and conscious sedation after the completion of the distraction activation. Device retention is based on the radiographic appearance of adequate ossification of the distraction regenerate which can range from two to five months. Intraoral devices are better tolerated by the patient during the consolidation period. Intraoral or extraoral distraction device removal is accomplished under local anaesthesia with sedation as a separate procedure or under general anaesthesia particularly if a Le Fort I osteotomy and/or other surgical procedures are to be performed. Orthodontic intervention is frequently helpful in distraction cases to optimize occlusal outcomes.

COMPLICATIONS FROM DISTRACTION OSTEOGENESIS

Routine surgical problems can be addressed with appropriate post-surgical care including management of bleeding, haematoma, infection and wound dehiscence. Distraction device complications may include the following: loosening of the device secondary to inadequate stability which can result in fibrous union; failure of the device to activate due to device malfunction or premature bony consolidation; paraesthesia of the inferior alveolar, mental neurovascular bundle or lingual nerve which is usually temporary but on occasions can be permanent. Temporary cranial nerve VII palsy can occur with extraoral approaches but is rarely permanent. Skeletal relapse is uncommon if adequate distraction rates and consolidation times are utilized. Relapse may occur at the temporomandibular joint or the distraction osteotomy site.

SUMMARY

This chapter has focused on the surgical technique of osteotomy and distraction device placement by intraoral and extraoral approaches for mandibular lengthening by distraction osteogenesis. Distraction osteogenesis research and techniques are constantly evolving. This work is designed to supplement the reader's surgical knowledge of distraction osteogenesis, but it would be expected that a responsible practicing surgeon would attend appropriate continuing education courses and lectures and have reviewed textbooks and important articles to provide the knowledge base to appropriately apply distraction techniques. In order to successfully apply distraction techniques the practitioner should have a very good understanding of the biologic basis and principles of distraction as treatment modifications and adjustments are frequently required. Distraction osteogenesis is a powerful surgical technique and, when applied appropriately, distraction can be very rewarding to the patient and the practitioner.

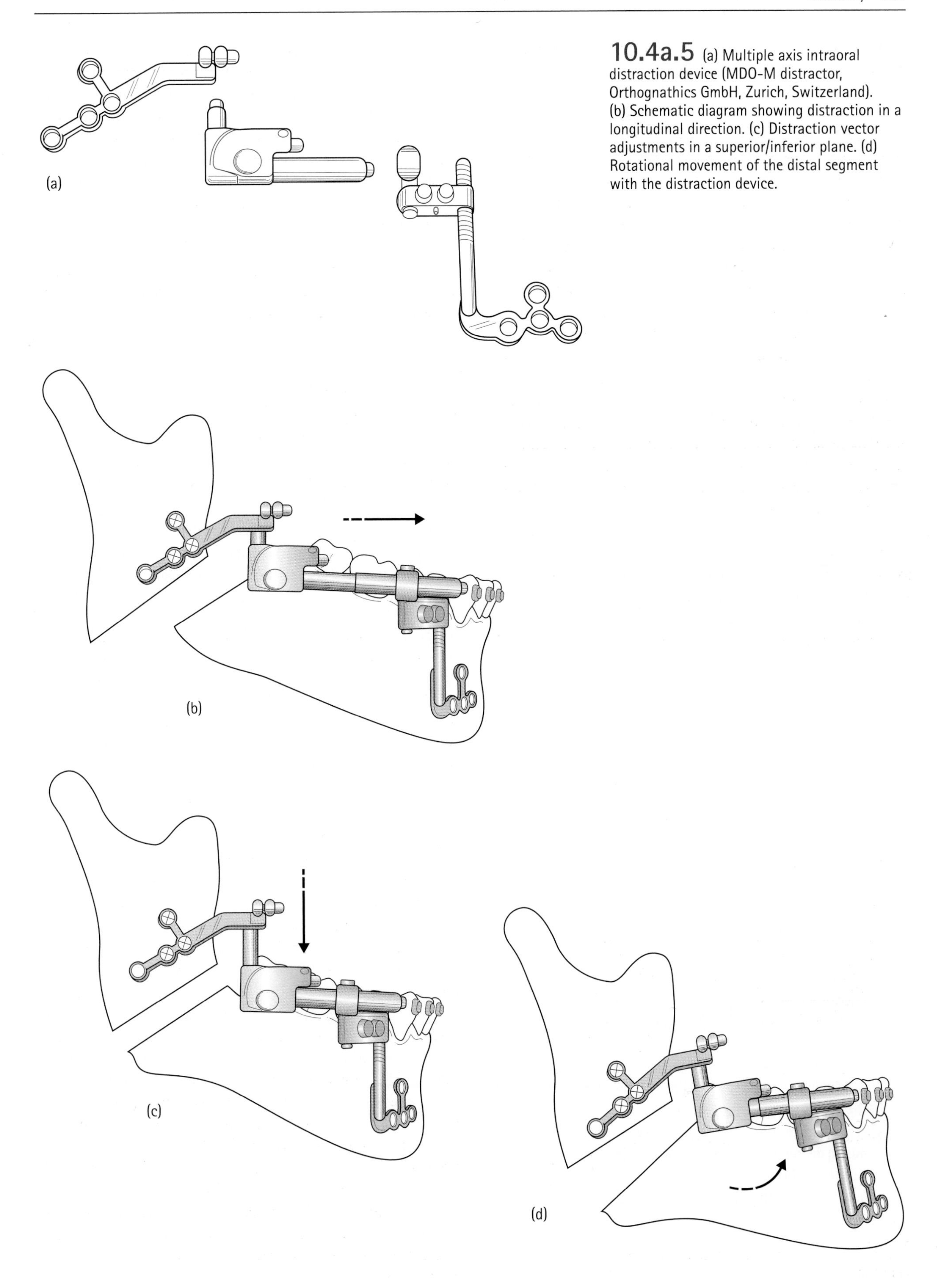

10.4a.5 (a) Multiple axis intraoral distraction device (MDO-M distractor, Orthognathics GmbH, Zurich, Switzerland). (b) Schematic diagram showing distraction in a longitudinal direction. (c) Distraction vector adjustments in a superior/inferior plane. (d) Rotational movement of the distal segment with the distraction device.

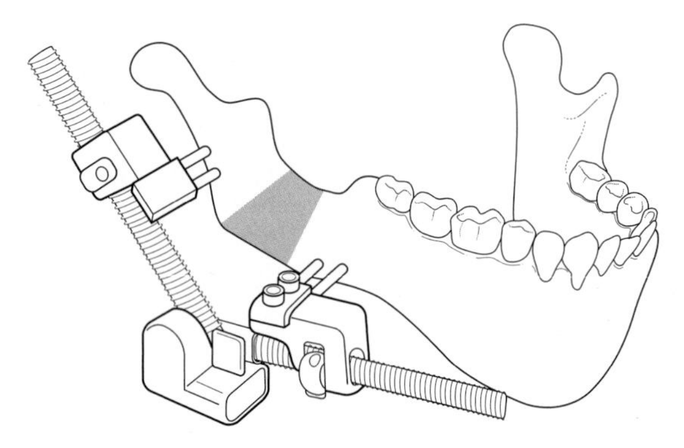

10.4a.6 Multi-Guide II external distraction device shown on the paediatric mandible. Device can activate longitudinally, mediolaterally and superiorly/inferiorly (Stryker Leibinger, Portage Michigan).

Top tips

- Distraction osteogenesis techniques require proper understanding and application of the biologic principles of distraction osteogenesis that are anatomically sound and age appropriate.
- Distraction osteogenesis device selection is based on available bone stock, ease of application, distance of distraction osteogenesis, and ability to adjust the distraction vector post device placement.
- When performing the lateral cortex, inferior border, and superior border osteotomies care is taken to ensure that these cuts do not encroach upon the inferior alveolar neurovascular bundle, facial artery and vein or the lingual nerve.
- When the platysma muscle is divided, care is taken to ensure identification and preservation of the marginal mandibular branch of the facial nerve.
- When securing the distraction device to the mandible, it is important to ensure the correct 3-D distraction vector.
- The length of the mono and bicortical distraction device screws is dependant on the position of the inferior alveolar neurovascular bundle, teeth roots and developing tooth buds in infants and children.
- After completion of the osteotomy cuts, a wedging osteotome is tapped into place superiorly above the inferior alveolar nerve, and utilizing a torquing a motion a fracture is created through the remaining portion of the mandible.
- Distraction rates can range from one to two mm per day, divided in two to three activations per day, depending on the age of the patient.
- Three dimensional vector adjustments can be made during distraction with selected multivector intraoral and extraoral DO devices and are best done after approximately 10 mm of lengthening has occurred.

FURTHER READING

Ilizarov GA. Transosseous osteosythesis: Theoretical and clinical aspects of the regeneration growth of tissues. Berlin, Germany: Springer-Verlag, 1992: 287–328.

McCarthy J, Grayson B, Williams J et al. Distraction of the mandible: the New York University experience. In: McCarthy J (ed.). Distraction of the craniofacial skeleton. New York, NY: Springer-Verlag, 1999: 80–203.

Samchukov M, Cope J, Cherkasin A. Biological basis of new bone formation under the influence of tension stress. In: Samchukov M, Cope J, Cherkasin A (eds). Craniofacial distraction osteogenesis. St. Louis, MO: Mosby, 2001: 21–36.

Triaca A, Minoretti R, Dimai W et al. Multiaxis intraoral distraction of the mandible. In: Samchukov M, Cope J, Cherkasin A (eds). Craniofacial distraction osteogenesis. St. Louis, MO: Mosby, 2001: 323–33.

Walker D. Buried bidirectional telescopic mandibular distraction. In Samchukov M, Cope J, Cherkasin A (eds). Craniofacial distraction osteogenesis. St. Louis, MO: Mosby, 2001: 313–22.

Walker DA. Management of severe mandibular retrognathia in the adult patient using distraction osteogenesis. Journal of Oral and Maxillofacial Surgery 2002; **60**: 1341–6.

Walker D. Mandibular lengthening by distraction osteogenesis. In: Bell W, Guerrero C (eds). Distraction osteogenesis of the facial skeleton. Hamilton, Ontario: BC Decker, 2007; 327–40.

10.4b

Maxillary distraction osteogenesis by intraoral and extraoral techniques

DAVID A WALKER

INTRODUCTION

Distraction osteogenesis (DO) of the maxilla is a technique utilized to gradually lengthen the maxilla (predominantly the cleft maxilla) extensive distances. Distraction osteogenesis creates new bone without the need for bone grafting and donor site morbidity. Maxillary distraction osteogenesis has many significant differences from mandibular distraction osteogenesis. Anatomically, the maxilla is comprised of thin-walled membranous bone and distraction vectors are predominantly in a tangential vector from the osteotomy site as opposed to a perpendicular vector from the osteotomy site in the mandible. It is important to have a sound understanding of the biologic principles of distraction osteogenesis and maxillary osteotomies when applying distraction techniques. There are a multitude of distraction devices including bone-borne, tooth-borne and intraoral and extra oral devices. The indications, advantages and disadvantages for maxillary distraction osteogenesis are listed in Tables 10.4b.1, 10.4b.2 and 10.4b.3.

PRE-OPERATIVE ASSESSMENT

A thorough history and clinical examination is appropriate with utilization of diagnostic imaging, including panoramic, posterior anterior and lateral cephalometric radiographs. Computed tomography (CT) scans with three-dimensional (3D) reconstructions of the maxilla are helpful. Dental study models mounted on a semi-adjustable articulator with prediction model surgery are of benefit. In selected instances, stereolithographic models may aid in treatment planning, osteotomy location and device contouring. Standardized 3D cephalometric prediction tracings are appropriate. In cleft maxilla patients, pre-operative speech assessment with nasopharyngeal airflow studies and/or fibreoptic nasopharygoscopy is important to identify borderline or frank velopharyngeal incompetence which may worsen with distraction. All clinical and diagnostic tools are utilized to plan out the proper 3D distraction vector selection and distance of distraction.

Maxillary distraction osteogenesis device selection is based on available bone stock, ease of application, distance of distraction osteogenesis and ability to adjust the distraction vector post device placement. Intraoral bone-borne devices have many advantages including good device

Table 10.4b.1 Indications for maxillary distraction osteogenesis.

Indications
Severe maxillary retrognathism
Cleft Maxilla
Post-traumatic maxillary deficiency
Revision orthognathic surgery
Craniofacial syndromes including Apert's and Crouzon's syndrome

Table 10.4b.2 Advantages of maxillary distraction osteogenesis.

Advantages
Greater distance of maxillary lengthening compared with conventional maxillary osteotomies
No bone grafting or donor site morbidity
Greater stability compared with conventional orthognathic surgery
Overcomes the soft tissue scarring and deficiencies (cleft patients)

Table 10.4b.3 Disadvantages of maxillary distraction osteogenesis.

Disadvantages
Requires two procedures; device placement osteotomy and device removal
Less occlusal control
Possible velopharyngeal incompetence with long distraction osteogenesis distances

stability and longer consolidation times, although extraoral devices with cranial stabilization, in selected instances, have advantages such as longer distraction distances and ability to adjust distraction vector, but typically have shorter consolidation times.

ANAESTHESIA CONSIDERATIONS

Cleft palate patients with previous pharyngeal flap surgery require extra care and attention for nasal endotracheal intubation which may best be performed through fibreoptic approaches. Some craniofacial syndromes have choanal atresia and pre-operative CT scans and anaesthesia consultation would be appropriate. An anaesthesia approach can be either from an oral or naso-endotracheal approach. Occasionally, patients with severe maxillary retrognathism with sleep apnoea have tracheostomy tubes which can be utilized for inhalational anaesthesia.

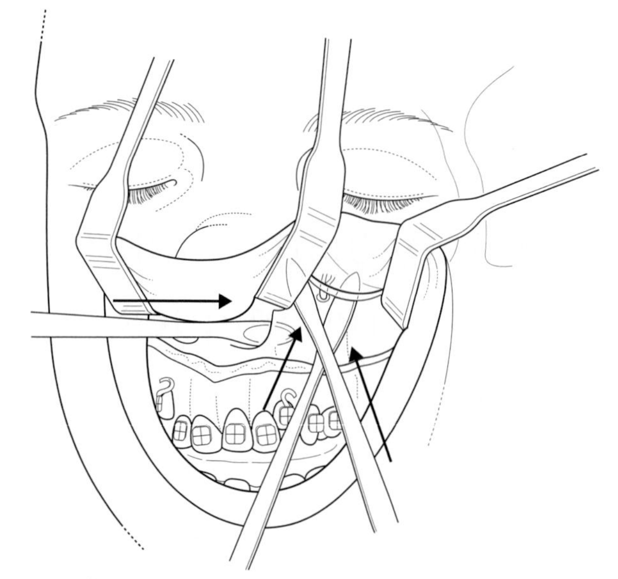

10.4b.1 The subperiosteal dissection is carried out exposing the piriform rim, the infraorbital nerve, the zygoma and a subperiosteal tunnel is carried out posteriorly back to the pterygomaxillary junction.

OPERATIVE TECHNIQUE

The operative technique is similar to the classic Le Fort I osteotomy with some important modifications. After establishing general anaesthesia and administering appropriate antibiotic prophylaxis, attention is directed to the maxillary vestibule where local anaesthetic 2 per cent lidocaine 1/100 000 epinephrine is infiltrated in the planned area of incision. Toxic dosages should be avoided, particularly in paediatric patients or those patients with cardiac anomalies. After allowing suitable time for haemostasis, a vestibular incision is made a minimum of 5 mm above the attached gingiva from zygoma to zygoma. It is desirable to leave significant labial attached gingiva pedicled to the maxilla. Adjustments in the incision location can be made in areas of cleft alveolus. The subperiosteal dissection is carried out exposing the piriform rim, the infraorbital nerve, the zygoma and a subperiosteal tunnel is carried out posteriorly back to the pterygomaxillary junction (Figure 10.4b.1).

Osteotomy location is based on the need for adequate bone above and below the osteotomy site for application of the bone-borne distraction devices. At this point, the level of the osteotomy is marked with a 701 tapered fissure bur or with a reciprocating saw. All bone cuts or osteotomies are made with adequate soft tissue retraction and copious saline irrigation. It is advisable at this time to contour and secure the left and right bone-borne distraction devices with two screws above and below the osteotomy site. It is important to have the vector of the distraction device close to the sagittal plane and not convergent. The distraction devices are now removed and stored in a safe sterile location. Typically, it is desirable to have approximately 5 mm of bone height above the apices of the dentition. The osteotomy location may have to be higher in younger patients where the developing canine teeth are unerupted. It is advantageous to have a step osteotomy in the zygoma region. The angle of the osteotomy will also control the vector of distraction and this can be adjusted to either inferiorly or superiorly depending on available bone stock (Figure 10.4b.2a,b). External maxillary devices utilize a tooth-borne component which allows greater flexibility of osteotomy location. A Frier elevator is used to strip the nasal mucosa from the inferior and lateral aspect of the lateral nasal wall to the posterior extent of the nasal wall. A periosteal retractor is placed along the lateral nasal wall to prevent tearing of the tissues. An osteotomy is made with the reciprocating saw from the zygoma to the piriform rim at the appropriate level. With the Langenback toe out retractor placed to the pterygomaxillary junction, the osteotomy is carried out posteriorly and inferiorly back to the pterygomaxillary junction (Figure 10.4b.3a).The osteotomy is performed on the contralateral side of the maxilla care being taken to ensure it is symmetric. Next the anterior nasal spine is dissected free and initial area of the attachment of the nasal septal cartilage to the maxilla is freed up. The nasal mucosa is stripped from the floor of the nasal cavity and the inferior aspect of septal cartilage. With adequate tissue retraction and a finger placed at the posterior nasal spine (oral side), the nasal septal osteotome is tapped with a mallet separating cartilaginous septum and vomer from the maxilla (Figure 10.4b.3b).With a periosteal elevator in place protecting lateral nasal mucosa, a spatula osteotome is gently tapped along the lateral nasal wall until a increase in resistance is felt, ensuring the descending palatine neurovascular bundle is not transected (Figure 10.4b.3c).

At this point, it is the author's preference to use the curved pterygoid osteotome to separate the maxilla from the pterygoid plates just prior to down-fracturing the maxilla. It is important to place the osteotome near the inferior aspect of the pterygomaxillary junction and angled inferiorly in

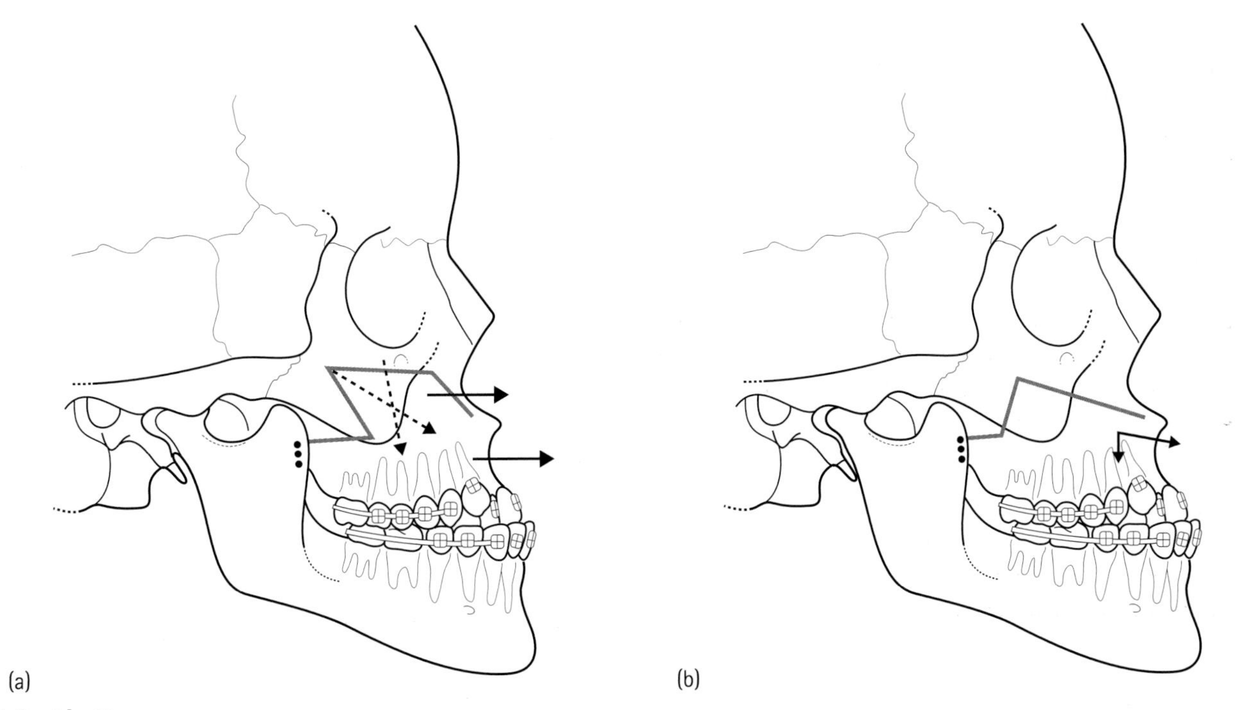

10.4b.2 (a) The angle of the osteotomy is in the horizontal plane with a step at the zygoma for bone borne distraction device. (b) The angle of the osteotomy will also control the vector, of distraction and this is placed in a superior to inferior position allowing vertical lengthening of the maxilla during distraction, depending on available bone stock.

order to avoid the internal maxillary artery (Figure 10.4b.3d). The operating surgeon controls the pterygoid osteotome and places a finger on the palatal aspect of the pterygomaxillary junction, while the surgical assistant strikes the osteotome with the mallet. Subsequently, the maxilla is digitally down-fractured with pressure on the anterior maxilla and midface. Extensive mobilization is not required, just enough to free up the maxilla (Figure 10.4b.3e). If difficulty is experienced in mobilizing the maxilla, recheck all osteotomy cuts, and if necessary the Rowe disimpaction forceps can be placed on the nasal floor below nasal mucosa and on the hard palate to free up the maxilla. Care is taken to avoid damage to the incisors.

It is advisable to remove the sinus mucosa from the inferior aspect of the maxillary sinus and to remove any bony irregularities along the Le Fort I cut that may impede distraction movement (Figure 10.b4.3f). Next, the bone-borne distraction devices can be placed and secured with 1.5–2.0 mm self-tapping screws of appropriate length. The devices should be activated a few millimetres to ensure maxillary movement then backed down to zero (Figures 10.4b.4.a,b and 10.4b.5a,b).When using external distractors, there is no bone-borne stabilization and if there is significant mobility of the maxilla a transosseous 3/0 gut suture can be placed in the piriform area. If there is concern with respect to alar base flaring an alar base suture with 2/0 vicryl can be placed. Copious saline irrigation is carried out, haemostasis is obtained and tissue are closed in a two layer fashion with 3/0 vicryl interrupted horizontal mattress sutures in the muscle periosteum layer. The mucosal incision is closed with 4/0 monofilament nylon horizontal mattress sutures for wound eversion then 4/0 chromic gut running suture for watertight closure. The incision may have considerable tension on it during long distraction distances. It is typical to have the device activation arm exit through the incision line or through a separate transmucosal stab incision depending on device position.

External maxillary distraction devices have a tooth-borne component which is usually placed by the orthodontist pre-operatively or intraoperatively and are attached to the external distraction framework connected to the halo frame (Figures 10.4b.6 and 10.4b.7a,b). Alternatively, bone plates can be attached to the maxilla and attached via stainless steel wire to the external vertical bar (Figure 10.4b.8). Placement of the halo frame should be based on bone quantity and quality measured on pre-operative CT scan. The halo frame should be parallel to Frankfort horizontal plane and should be sized to fit not more than approximately 2 cm from the patient's head and be placed far enough anterior to allow the maxillary distance of distraction. The screws should penetrate the scalp and calvarium into the outer cortex only. Three to four screws per side is desirable, 2–4 cm above the helix of the ear, avoiding the thin bone of the temporal fossa. The vertical component of the external system should be in the midline parallel to the facial plane and is attached to the orthodontic intraoral device (Figures 10.4b.7a,b and 10.4b.8).

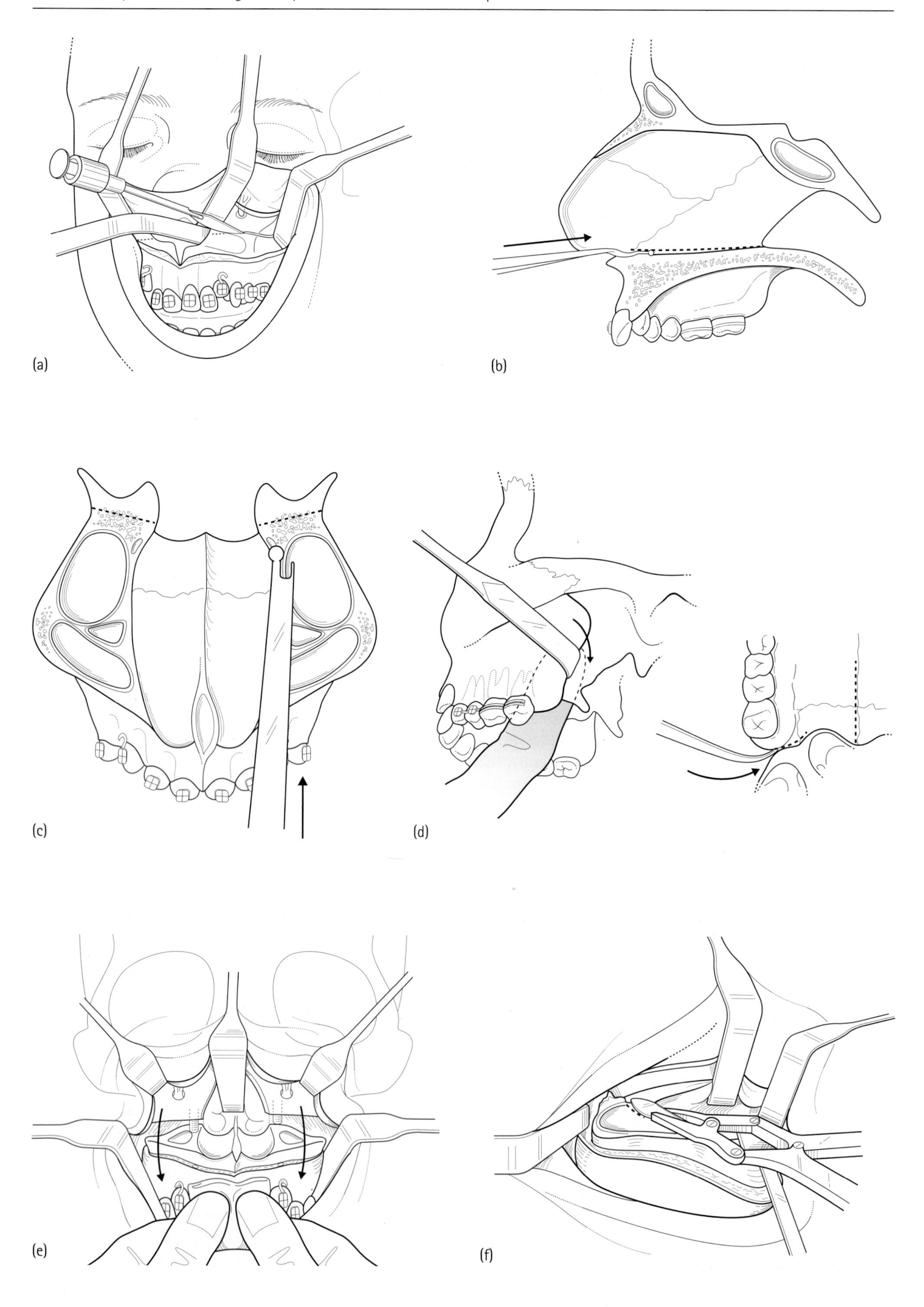
(a)
(b)
(c)
(d)
(e)
(f)

10.4b.3 (a) A periosteal retractor is placed along the lateral nasal wall to prevent tearing of the tissues. An osteotomy is made with the reciprocating saw from the zygoma to the piriform rim at the appropriate level. With the Langenback toe out retractor placed to the pterygomaxillary junction, the osteotomy is carried out posteriorly and inferiorly back to the pterygomaxillary junction. (b) With adequate tissue retraction and a finger placed at the posterior nasal spine (oral side), the nasal septal osteotome is tapped with a mallet separating cartilaginous septum and vomer from the maxilla. (c) With a periosteal elevator in place protecting lateral nasal mucosa, a spatula osteotome is gently tapped along the lateral nasal wall until a increase in resistance is felt ensuring the descending palatine neurovascular bundle is not transacted. (d) It is important to place the osteotome near the inferior aspect of the pterygomaxillary junction and angled inferiorly in order to avoid the internal maxillary artery and have a finger palpating the pterygomaxillary junction from the oral side. (e) The maxilla is digitally downfractured with pressure on the anterior maxilla and midface. Extensive mobilization is not required, just enough to free up the maxilla. (f) It is advisable to remove the sinus mucosa from the inferior aspect of the maxillary sinus and to remove any bony irregularities along the Le Fort I cut that may impede distraction movement.

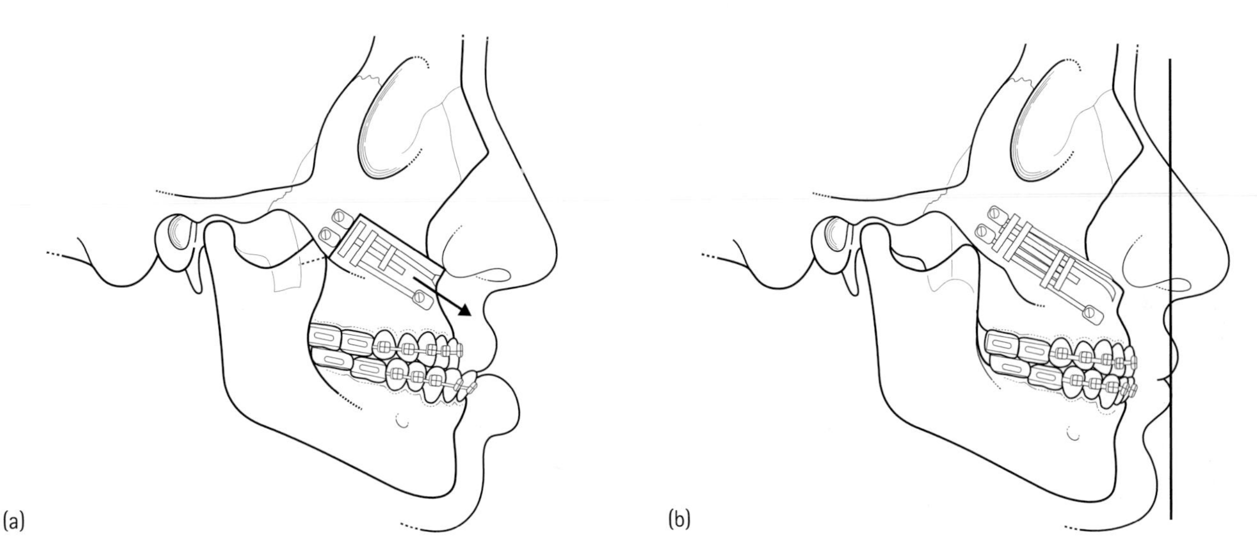

10.4b.4 (a,b) Bone-borne distractor after osteotomy and placement and after the completion of distraction (Dynaform, Stryker, Leibinger Inc, Kalamazoo, MI).

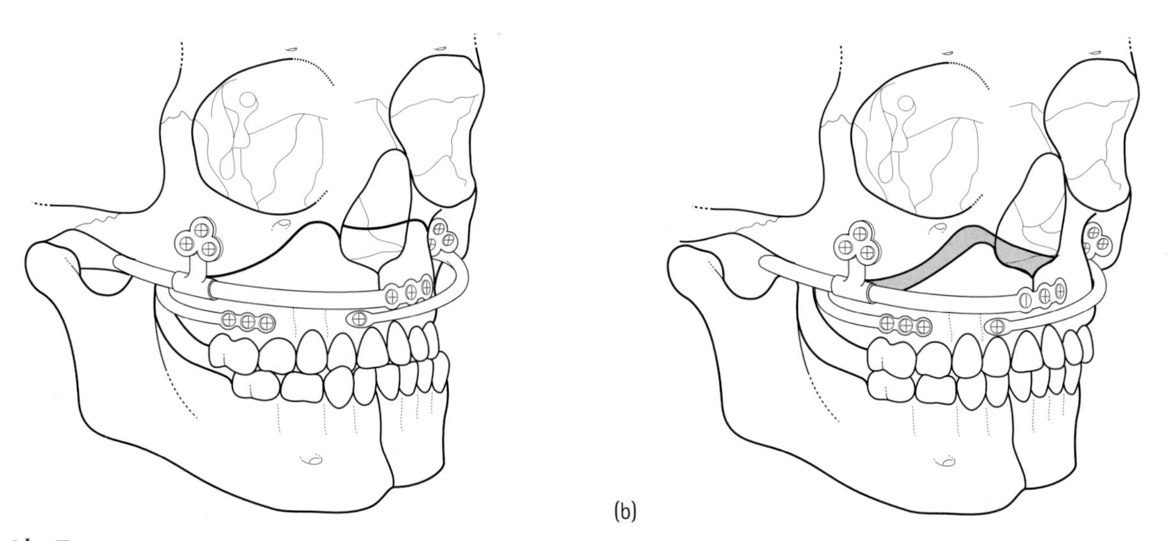

10.4b.5 (a,b) Bone-borne distractor in paediatric patient after osteotomy and placement and after the completion of distraction (Zurich Pediatric Maxillary Distractor, KLS Martin Jacksonville, FL).

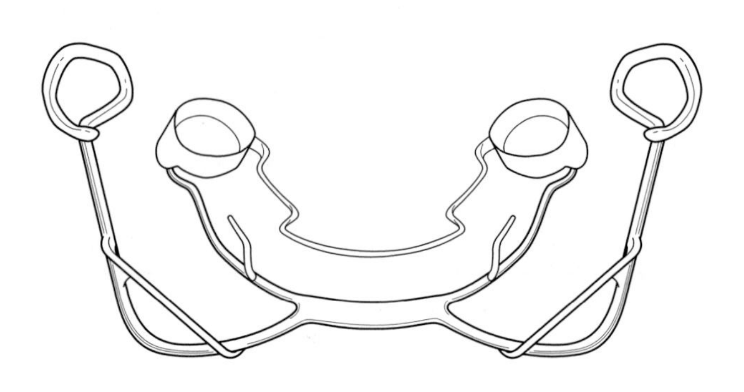

10.4b.6 Orthodontic device to be cemented on to molars with external arms to be connected to external distraction device.

POST-OPERATIVE CARE

If the patient has significant pre-operative airway compromise, patient admission to the ICU with endotracheal intubation overnight, or until ready for extubation, is a consideration. Alternatively, extubation could be achieved if the patient is awake and alert and able to protect their own airway. Periodic nasal clearing of significant blood clots with a Q tip and hydrogen peroxide may be appropriate. Topical or systemic sinus decongestants can be used depending on patient age and clinical need. Requirements for discharge from hospital are adequate pain control and p.o. intake, and otherwise stable recovery from anaesthesia and surgery. A 'minimal chew' soft diet is recommended for 6–8 weeks. In older children and adults, chlorhexidine 0.12 per cent mouth rinse is a consideration during distraction device activation. Use of post-operative oral antibiotics requires judgement and is based on patient wound healing and clinical progress. No specific care is required for halo screws.

DISTRACTION DEVICE ACTIVATION, REMOVAL

Activation of the distraction device is typically started on post-operative day 5–7, although earlier distraction may be commenced in younger patients. The distraction rate is typically 1 mm a day divided in two or three activations. It is important to have responsible adults or patients to activate the devices appropriately. Monitoring of distraction with periodic radiographs and visual inspection is appropriate 1–2 times per week. Frequent assessment during distraction allows recognition of complications or aberrant distraction vectors and is necessary to determine the completion of distraction. Three-dimensional vector adjustments can be made during distraction with selected extraoral DO devices. Vertical vector alterations may be accomplished in sequential activations depending on the degree of distraction regenerate and the desired 3D changes. If orthodontic appliances are in place class III and or vertical elastics may aid in occlusal correction.

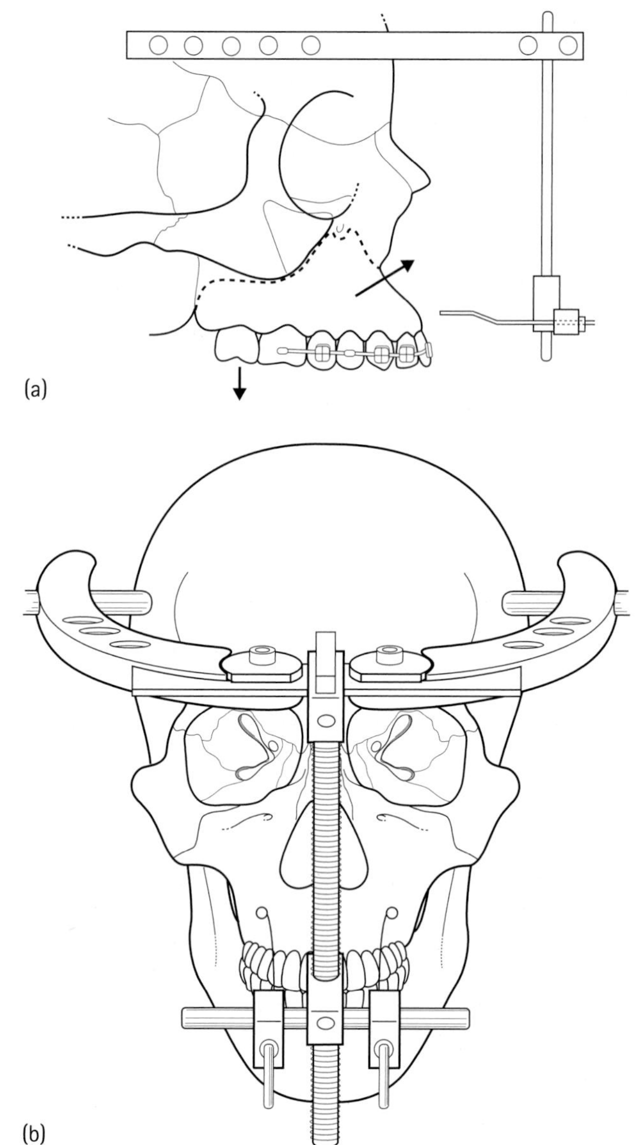

10.4b.7 (a,b) Rigid external distraction (RED) device with attachment to orthodontic devices (KLS Martin, Jacksonville, FL).

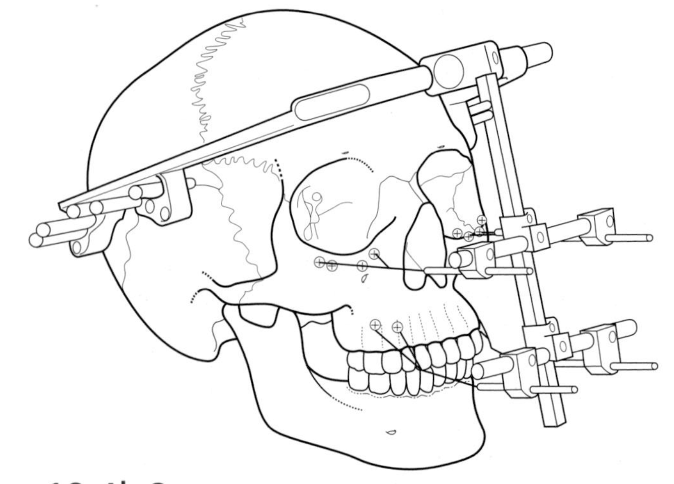

10.4b.8 Halo frame external distractor with bone plate attachments on the maxilla and midface (BLUE Device Multi-Vector Distraction, Biomet Microfixation, Jacksonville, FL).

Activation arms are typically removed under local anaesthesia and conscious sedation after the completion of the distraction activation. In devices with nonremovable activation arms, tissues are monitored periodically. Device removal is accomplished under local anaesthetic and sedation and is based on the radiographic appearance of adequate ossification of the distraction regenerate which can range from 6 weeks to five months. Intraoral devices are better tolerated by the patient during the consolidation period. If external devices are removed after shorter consolidation times, an orthodontic facemask appliance should be worn at night time for an additional two to three months to minimize relapse. Orthodontic intervention is frequently helpful in distraction cases to optimize occlusal outcomes.

COMPLICATIONS FROM MAXILLARY DISTRACTION OSTEOGENESIS

Routine surgical problems can be addressed with appropriate post-surgical care including management of bleeding, haematoma, infection and wound dehiscence. Distraction device complications may include the following: loosening of the device secondary to inadequate stability and failure of the device to activate (breakage, activation gear malfunction). Surgical intervention with replacement or restabilization of the DO device would be appropriate. Aberrant distraction vectors can produce occlusal problems which can be remedied with orthodontic treatment with elastic traction or on occasion with mandibular surgery. Premature bony consolidation is rare, but occasionally fibrous union can occur and may be treated with application of bone plate fixation and or autologous bone grafting. Paraesthesia of the infraorbital nerve is usually temporary but on occasion can be permanent. Skeletal relapse at the distraction osteotomy site is uncommon if adequate distraction rates and consolidation times are utilized. Velopharyngeal incompetence is documented in cleft maxillas after long distraction distances and may require a pharyngeal flap to correct speech problems. Intracranial pin migration with halo frame (particularly with craniofacial syndromes or previous cranial vault surgeries) has been reported.

Top tips

- Maxillary distraction techniques require proper understanding and application of the biologic principles of distraction osteogenesis that are anatomically sound and age appropriate.
- Anatomically, the maxilla is comprised of thin-walled membranous bone and distraction vectors are predominantly in a tangential vector from the osteotomy site as opposed to a perpendicular vector from the osteotomy site in the mandible.
- Maxillary distraction osteogenesis internal or external device selection is based on available bone stock, ease of application, distance of distraction osteogenesis, osteotomy location and ability to adjust the distraction vector post device placement.
- In cleft maxilla patients, pre-operative speech assessment with nasopharyngeal airflow studies and or fibreoptic nasopharygoscopy is important to identify borderline or frank velopharyngeal incompetence which may worsen with distraction.
- Cleft palate patients with previous pharyngeal flap surgery require extra care and attention for nasal endotracheal intubation which may best be done through fiberoptic approaches.
- Maxillary osteotomy location is based on the need for adequate bone above and below the osteotomy site for application of internal bone-borne distraction devices, and can be placed in a higher position with external DO devices
- When securing the internal distraction devices to the maxilla, it is important to ensure the correct 3D distraction device vector close to the sagittal plane and not convergent.
- The external distractor halo frame should be parallel to Frankfort horizontal plane and should be sized to fit and not be more than approximately 2 cm from the patient's head, and be placed far enough anterior to allow the maxillary distance of distraction
- When securing the halo frame with screws, avoid the thin bone of the temporal region and select CT scan-guided screw position in craniofacial syndromes or those patients with previous cranial surgery.
- Distraction rates can range from 1–2 mm per day, divided into two to three activations per day, depending on the age of the patient.
- Three-dimensional vector adjustments can be made during maxillary distraction with selected multivector extraoral DO devices.

FURTHER READING

Altuna G, Walker D, Freeman E. Surgically assisted rapid orthodontic lengthening of the maxilla in primates – a pilot study. *American Journal of Orthodontics* 1995; **107: 531–6.**

Bell WH. Le Fort I osteotomy for correction of maxillary deformities. *Journal of Oral Surgery* 1975; **33**: 412–26.

Bell WH, Fonseca RJ, Kennedy JW, Levy BM. Bone healing and revascularization after total maxillary osteotomy. *Journal of Oral Surgery* 1975; **33**: 253–60.

Bell W, Pinto L, Chu S *et al.* Simultaneous correction of three-dimensional maxillary deformity by the Le Fort I osteotomy and distraction osteogenesis technique. In: Bell W, Guerrero C (eds). *Distraction osteogenesis of the facial skeleton.* Hamilton, Ontario: BC Decker, 2007: 327–40.

Figueroa AA, Polley JW, Ko E. Distraction osteogenesis for treatment of severs cleft maxillary deficiency with the RED technique. In: Samchukov M, Cope J, Cherkasin A (eds).

Craniofacial distraction osteogenesis. St Louis, MO: Mosby, 2001: 85–93.

Guerrero C. (eds). *Distraction osteogenesis of the facial skeleton*. Hamilton, Ontario: BC Decker, 2007: 327–40.

Guyette TW, Polley JW, Figueroa AA, Smith BE. Changes in speech following maxillary distraction osteogenesis. *Cleft Palate Craniofacial Journal*, 2001; **38**: 199–205.

Polley JW, Figueroa AA. Rigid external distraction: its application in cleft maxillary deformities. *Plastic and Reconstructive Surgery* 1998; **102**: 1360–72.

Rachmiel A. Regenerate bone formation during maxillary and midface distraction. In: Samchukov M, Cope J, Cherkasin A (eds). *Craniofacial distraction osteogenesis*. St Louis, MO: Mosby, 2001: 477–84.

Samchukov M, Cope J, Cherkasin A. Biological basis of new bone formation under the influence of tension stress. In: Samchukov M, Cope J, Cherkasin A (eds). *Craniofacial distraction osteogenesis*. St Louis, MO: Mosby, 2001: 21–36.

10.5

Surgical management of craniosynostosis

GE GHALI, DAVID M MONTES

JUSTIFICATION

Craniosynostosis is the premature closure of one or more sutures resulting in a variety of cranial vault deformities. Successful management of craniosynostosis demands a multidisciplinary approach. Nonsyndromic craniosynostosis of one or more sutures is the most common craniofacial anomaly with the prevalence in the United States being 1 in 2500 births. Virchow's postulation of compensatory growth following premature suture closure has been confirmed and allows for prediction of skull form based on suture closure patterns. This results in stereotypical growth limited to one side of the vault when the attached sutures are perpendicular to the synostosis and growth which is bilateral when the compensatory attached sutures are parallel to the synostotic suture. Diagnosis is based on both clinical and radiographic evaluations. The clinical evaluation involves the palpation of the skull for any movement, ridging and absence or presence of the anterior and posterior fontanelles. Quantitative measurements of the superior orbital rims, relative to the most anterior aspect of the cornea, is also useful in treatment planning of superior orbital rim advancements. The radiographic evaluation of craniosynostosis is used to quantitatively define aberrant anatomy, plan surgical procedures and to provide a means to demonstrate to parents the difference between stenosed and nonstenosed sutures. Computed tomography provides the craniofacial team with a baseline record, a means of surgical planning and a modality to document surgical changes *in vivo*, thereby allowing longitudinal comparisons.

INDICATIONS

Functional considerations

INHIBITION OF BRAIN GROWTH

Although the neurodevelopmental morbidity of nonsyndromic craniosynostosis is not fully understood, children manifesting nonsyndromic synostosis exhibit significant speech, behavioural and cognitive abnormalities as compared with the general population.

INTRACRANIAL HYPERTENSION

Varying degrees of intracranial hypertension, decreased cerebral perfusion pressure and episodic respiratory obstruction are documented complications associated with complex craniosynostosis. Intracranial hypertension of greater than 15 mmHg develops in 13 per cent of single suture synostosis and 42 per cent of multiple suture synostosis patients. Multisuture stenosis is accompanied by hydrocephalus in 10 per cent of cases. Acute intracranial hypertension manifests as papilloedema, headache and nausea/vomiting; chronic signs are optic and cerebral atrophy.

NEUROMOTOR DEVELOPMENT

In a series of scaphocephalic patients, auditory short-term memory and language developmental impairment persisted following cranial vault corrective surgery. Neuromotor development improves with surgery. Functional studies suggest regional cerebral circulation improvement following corrective surgery for unilateral or simple craniosynostosis.

VISUAL/AUDITORY IMPAIRMENT

Glucose metabolism and brain function relative to visual development and spatial co-ordination significantly improve following corrective surgery for single-suture synostosis. Although posterior plagiocephaly comprises less than 3 per cent of all isolated synostosis cases, diagnosis is critical because of its relationship to significant hemifield visual asymmetry. The degree of visual field impairment does not correlate to the degree of deformation or the laterality of the defect.

Aesthetic and psychosocial considerations

Correction of the deformity provides a more normal contour to the naso-orbital region, supraorbital unit and cranial vault. Children who fail to undergo timely repair of craniosynostotic deformities often represent due to social hardships and parental concerns for their child's successful integration into society.

CLASSIFICATION AND CHARACTERISTICS

- Sagittal synostosis (Figure 10.5.1):
  - scaphocephaly;
  - transverse skull narrowing;
  - Anteroposterior skull elongation;
  - premature sagittal fusion;
  - represents 50 per cent of synostosis cases in the USA.
- Unilateral synostosis (Figure 10.5.2):
  - frontal plagiocephaly;
  - asymmetric skull shape;
  - forehead flattened and retropositioned on abnormal side;
  - premature unilateral coronal fusion;
  - differential diagnosis includes infant positioning, moulding;
  - congenital torticollis and lambdoid synostosis;
  - represents 20 per cent of synostosis cases in the USA.

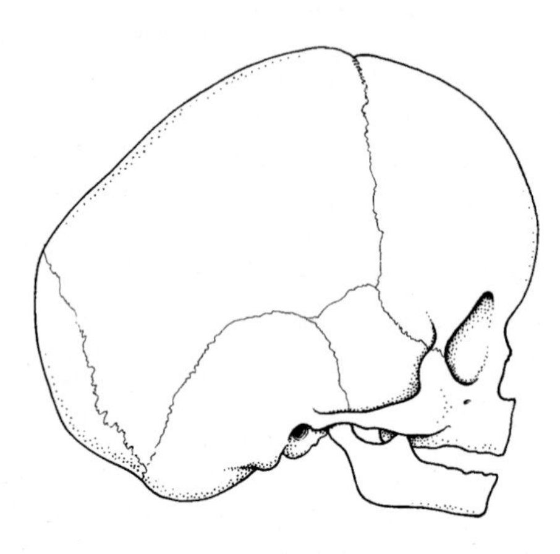

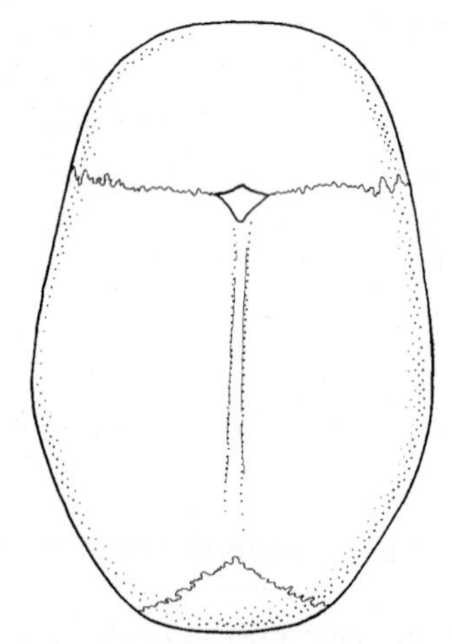

10.5.1 Sagittal synostosis in lateral and superior views.

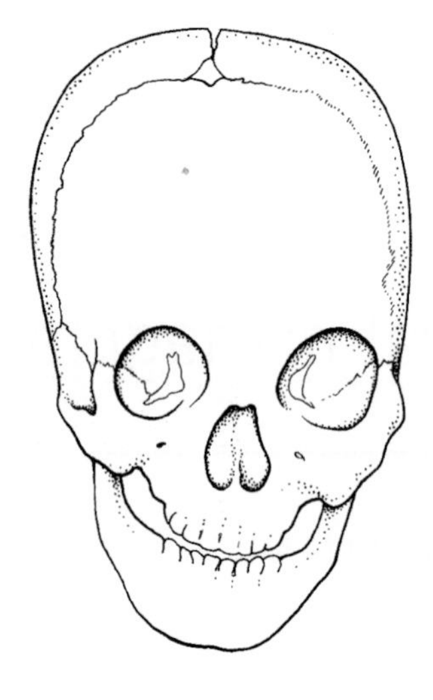

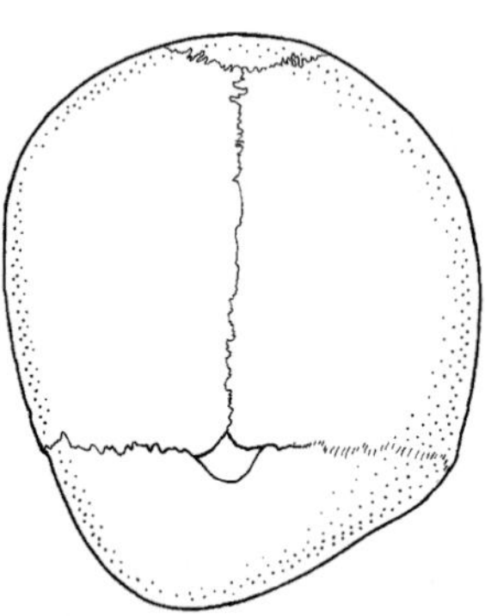

10.5.2 Left anterior plagiocephaly in frontal and superior views.

- Bilateral coronal synostosis (Figure 10.5.3):
  - brachycephaly;
  - sagittal skull shortening;
  - lower forehead;
  - recessed supraorbital bar;
  - excessive transverse dimension of forehead;
  - most common syndrome-associated;
  - premature bilateral coronal fusion;
  - represents 20 per cent of synostosis cases in the USA.
- Metopic craniosynostosis (Figure 10.5.4):
  - trigonocephaly;
  - triangular skull;
  - prominent midline keel;
  - relative hypotelorism;
  - premature metopic fusion;
  - represents 10 per cent of synostosis cases in the USA.

TIMING OF SURGERY

Brain volume in the normally developing child nearly triples in the first year of life growing from 350 to 950 g; at 24 months the brain reaches 1250 g with the adult brain weighing 1350 g. Rapid brain growth requires that the cranial vault achieves 80 per cent of the adult size by birth and readily expands until three years of age. A good indication of cranial

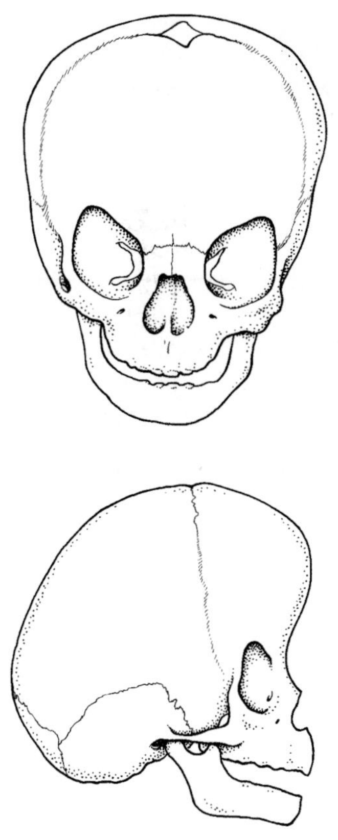

10.5.3 Bicoronal synostosis in frontal and superior views.

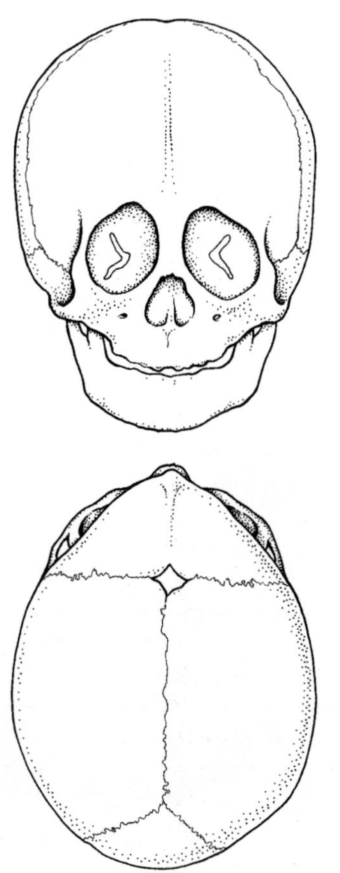

10.5.4 Metopic synostosis in frontal and superior views.

growth can be ascertained by skull circumference measurements. Low figure measurements for any age group may be a sign of craniosynostosis or microcephaly. The relationship between the anteroposterior length and bitemporal width provides additional insight. The normal length to width ratio is 3:2. A lower ratio suggests restricted growth as in craniosynostosis. In craniosynostosis, premature suture fusion is combined with continued brain growth. Precise timing remains controversial and individualized. We prefer surgical repair between four and eight months, while other centres have reported good results when treatment is completed between two-and-a-half and three years of age. Timely surgical intervention allows for rapid frontal lobe growth which supports the forehead and supraorbital ridge. Additionally, at this age the cranium is highly malleable and therefore easier to contour. Children over one year of age have thicker bone which is more difficult to modify. Although some patients may require multiple staged surgical procedures, early intervention may have a positive effect on facial growth and result in a lessening of the facial deformity as the child grows.

OPERATIVE TECHNIQUE

Pre-operative preparation

The pre-operative assessment should include a coagulation panel, complete blood count, and a basic metabolic panel. It is imperative that the child be cross matched for at least two units of packed red blood cells and fresh frozen plasma prior to surgery. The blood must be available in the operating theatre prior to incision. Central venous catheterization and large bore peripheral venous access greatly assists the anaesthesia team in the monitoring for and recognition of critical signs associated with significant blood loss and fluid shifts that may occur during the operation. In addition to routine electrocardiography, peripheral oxygen saturation and capnography monitoring; arterial line placement and precordial Doppler monitoring are useful adjuncts in patient monitoring. All fluids and blood products are warmed. It is critical that the operating theatre be kept warm during induction, patient preparation and draping to ensure the maintenance of normal body temperature.

Unilateral coronal synostosis

- The patient is positioned supine with head secured on a Mayfield headrest. Via a coronal incision, a subperiosteal anterior scalp flap is elevated along with the temporalis muscle bilaterally. Pre- or postauricular extensions may be utilized if needed (Figure 10.5.5a,b).
- Bilateral subperiosteal reflection extends to the periorbital and temporal regions anteriorly while maintaining the attachment of the medial canthal tendons. Posteriorly, the scalp flap is reflected midway between the coronal and

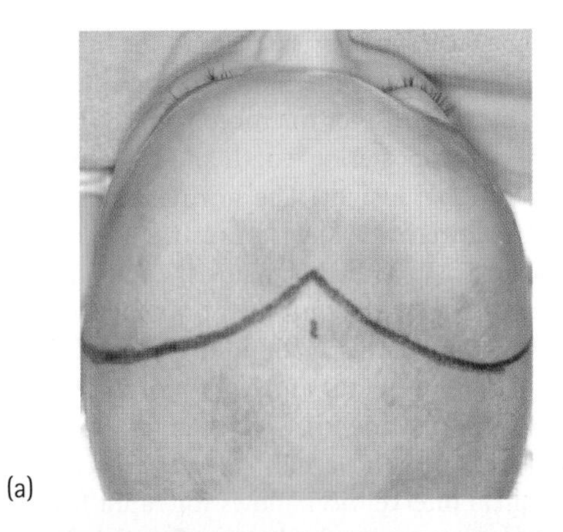

(a)

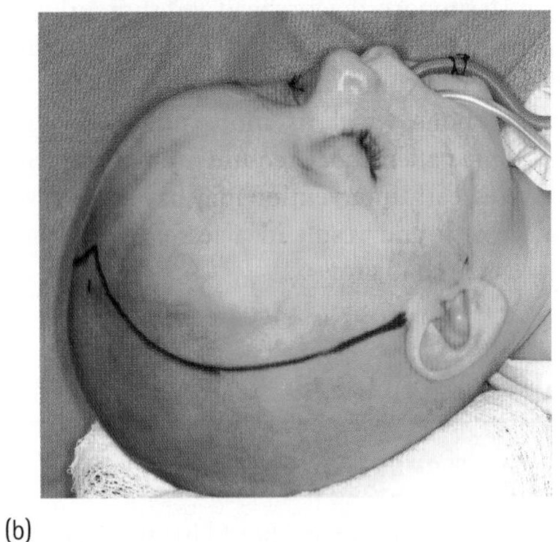

(b)

10.5.5 Superior (a) and lateral (b) views of coronal markings in preparation for plagiocephaly correction.

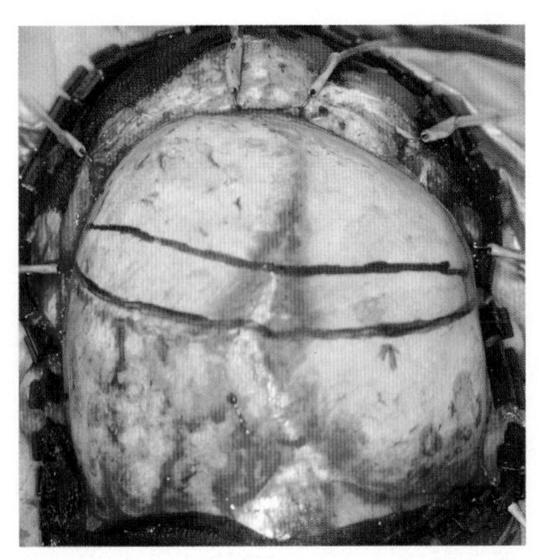

10.5.6 Superior view demonstrating extent of subperiosteal reflection, as well as degree of right-sided anterior plagiocephaly.

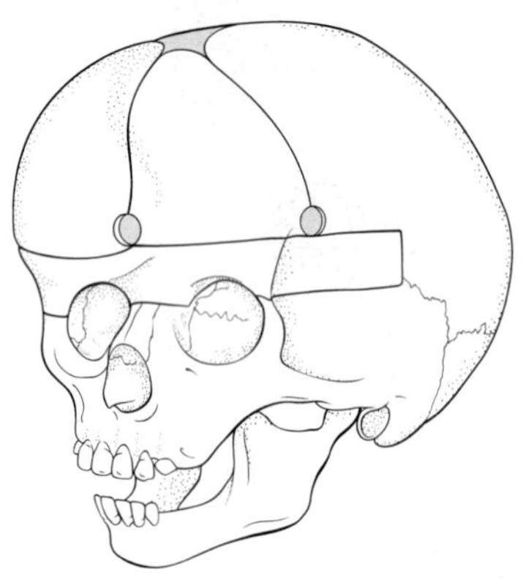

10.5.7 Bur holes in preparation for bifrontal craniotomy at the level of the supraorbital region.

lambdoid sutures (Figure 10.5.6). Markings for the bifrontal craniotomy and frontoorbital bar/bandeau are indicated (Figure 10.5.7).

- Bifrontal craniotomy using the Midas Rex drill developing a 1 cm bandeau (Figure 10.5.8).
- Retraction of the frontal and temporal lobes of the brain facilitates superior orbital and temporal osteotomies. Bilateral tongue-in-groove (tenon) extensions developed via a reciprocating saw to the level of pterion (Figure 10.5.9).
- Intracranial retraction of frontal lobes (Figure 10.5.10), as well as intraorbital retraction of the periorbita (Figure 10.5.11) is necessary to achieve the anterior skull base osteotomy. One may tailor the level of the lateral orbital rim osteotomy based on aesthetic needs.
- Removed bandeau is adjusted bilaterally via removal of wedges from the recessed side and scoring of the over-projected side (Figure 10.5.12a). Bandeau is recontoured by bending the recessed side and straightening the over-projected side (Figure 10.5.12b).
- Barrel-staving osteotomies are placed in the parietal and/or temporal bones as needed for reshaping (Figure 10.5.13).
- Resorbable plates and screws are utilized for stabilization of the bandeau and forehead (Figure 10.5.14a,b).

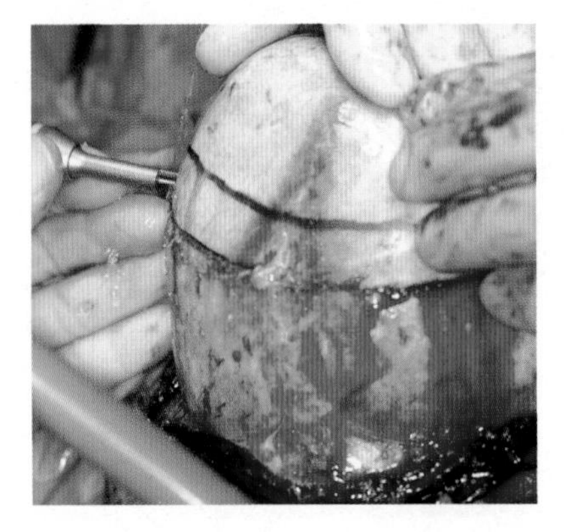

10.5.8 Neurosurgeon performs craniotomy using Midas Rex drill.

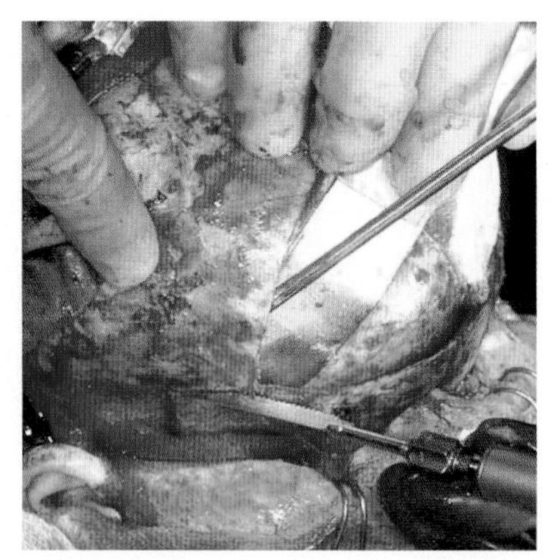

10.5.9 Reciprocating saw is utilized to perform bifrontal tenon extension osteotomies.

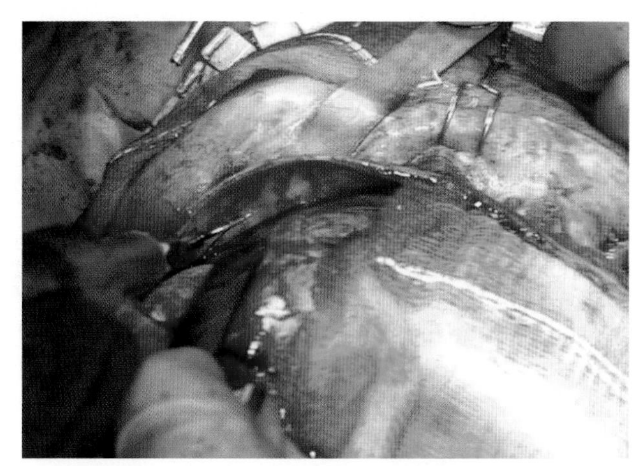

10.5.10 Intracranial retraction to expose anterior cranial base for osteotomy.

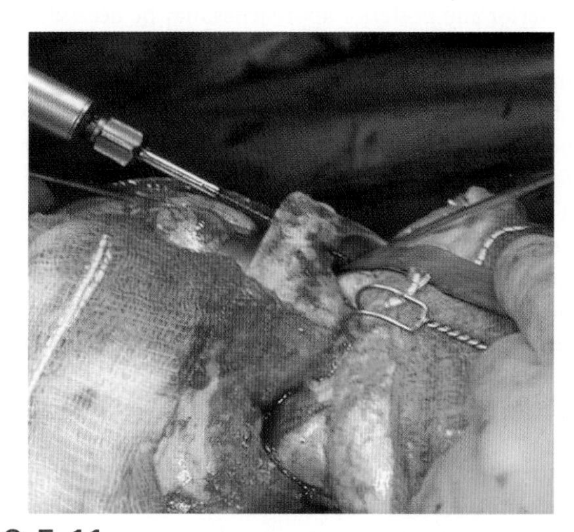

10.5.11 Combined intracranial and intraorbital retraction to complete the anterior cranial base osteotomy along the orbital roof.

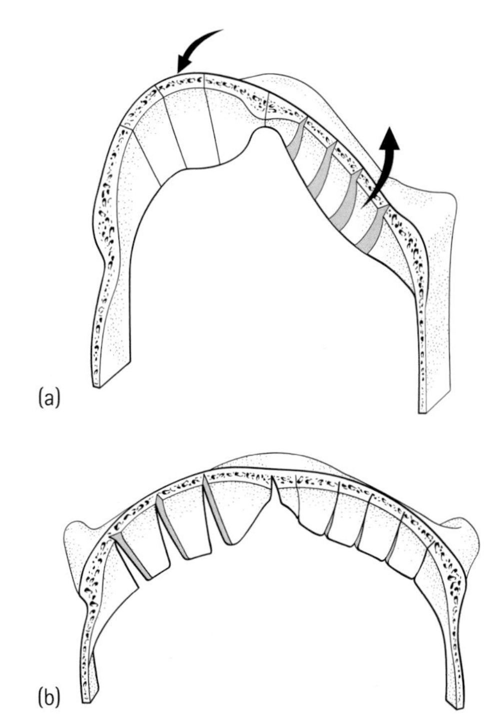

10.5.12 Removed bandeau prior to (a) and after (b) wedge and scoring osteotomies.

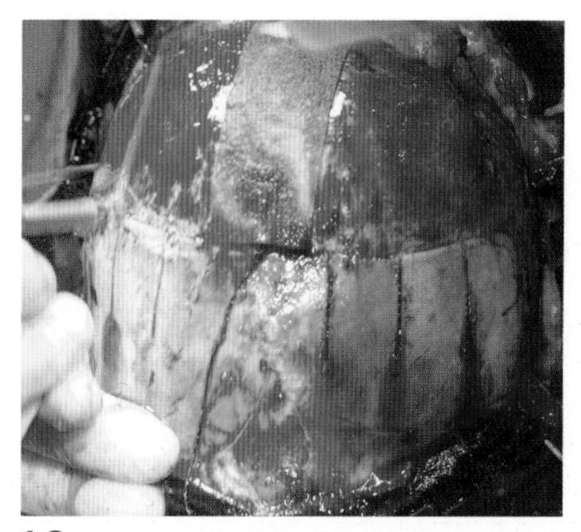

10.5.13 Barrel-staving osteotomies achieved via Midas Rex or reciprocating saw to impart plasticity to the bone.

Bilateral coronal synostosis

- Surgical positioning, approach and osteotomy design is similar to that previously described for plagiocephaly repair. Sites of osteotomies bilaterally as indicated (Figure 10.5.15).
- Following osteotomies, reshaping and fixation of the bandeau and forehead (Figure 10.5.16).

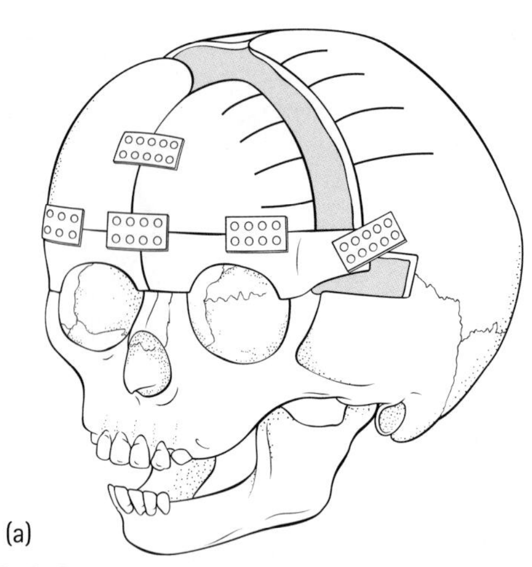

10.5.14 Oblique (a) and superior (b) views following resorbable plate fixation.

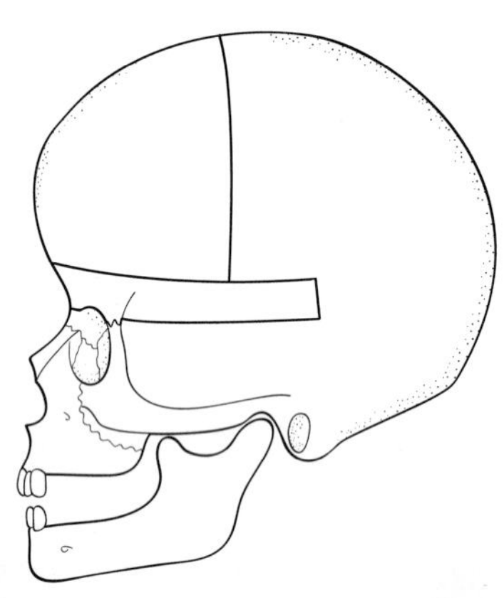

10.5.15 Lateral view of proposed osteotomy design for repair of bicoronal synostosis.

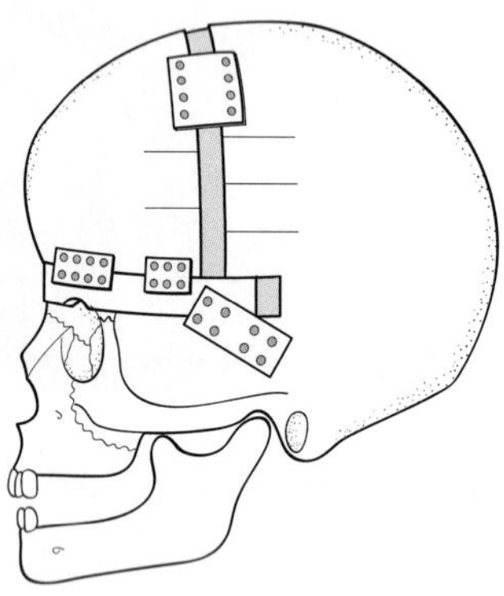

10.5.16 Lateral view after resorbable plate fixation.

Metopic synostosis

- Surgical positioning, approach and initial osteotomy design is similar to that previously described. Site of osteotomies of the anterior cranial vault and superior orbital rims from a frontal (Figure 10.5.17a) and lateral (Figure 10.5.17b) views.
- Superior view of bandeau prior to (Figure 10.5.18a) and after (Figure 10.5.18b) reshaping.
- The bandeau is sometimes vertically split at the midline and an autogenous cranial bone graft placed to correct true hypotelorism (Figures 10.5.19 and 10.5.20).
- Assessment of the gap between the bandeau and anterior cranial base assists in determining symmetric correction and bitemporal expansion (Figure 10.5.21).
- Barrel staving is often needed to widen the temporal region prior to final anterior cranial vault reshaping and fixation (Figure 10.5.22a,b).

Sagittal synostosis

- Premature closure of the anterior two-thirds of the sagittal suture requires formal total reshaping of the cranial vault, with or without superior orbital rim shaping. When the entire sagittal suture is fused, a combination of both anterior and posterior approaches may be necessary. For children over 12 months or children with the need for upper orbital reconstruction, we prefer the supine position at one operative setting, or rarely, in two stages with posterior reconstruction preceding anterior treatment by four to six months.
- The forehead is tilted posteriorly and the occiput is tilted anteriorly, thereby reducing the anterior–posterior dimension; resorbable fixation is used to secure the segments. Barrel-staving, as well as interchanging of the temporal segments, helps widen the transverse dimension (Figure 10.5.23).
- The patient must be prone when the posterior half of the sagittal suture is involved with protection of the airway and globes. Unless a significant concomitant supraorbital deformity exists, we prefer to treat full sagittal suture stenosis via total cranial vault reshaping at one operative setting with the patient in the prone position (Figure 10.5.24).

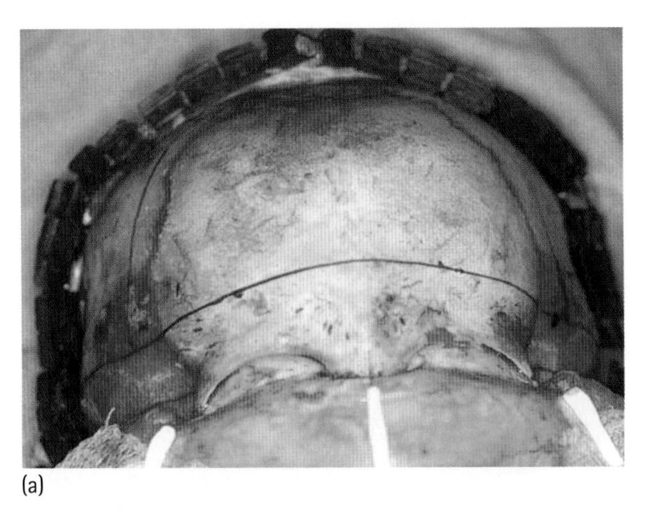

(a)

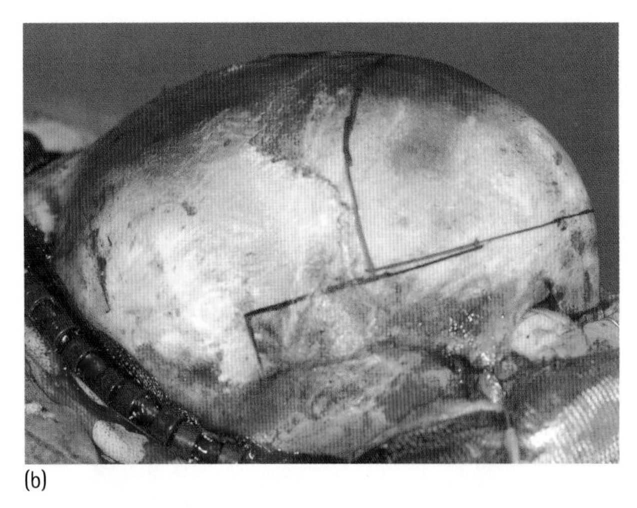

(b)

10.5.17 Proposed osteotomy markings from frontal (a) and lateral (b) views.

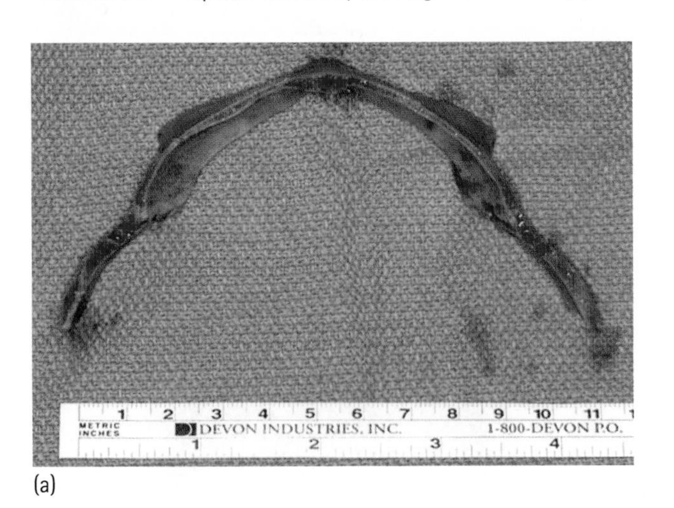

(a)

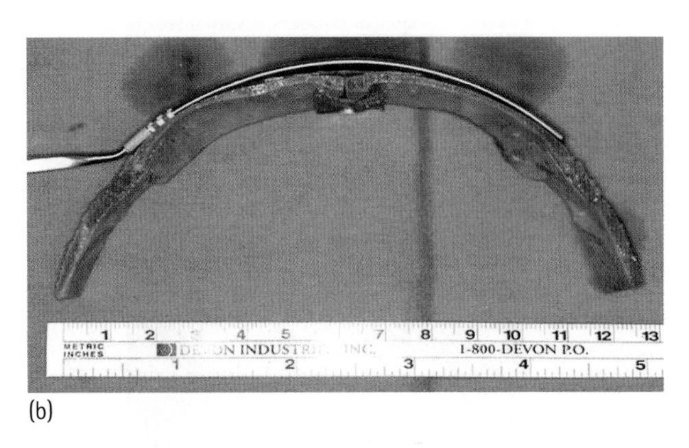

(b)

10.5.18 Bandeau before (a) and after (b) reshaping and resorbable plate fixation.

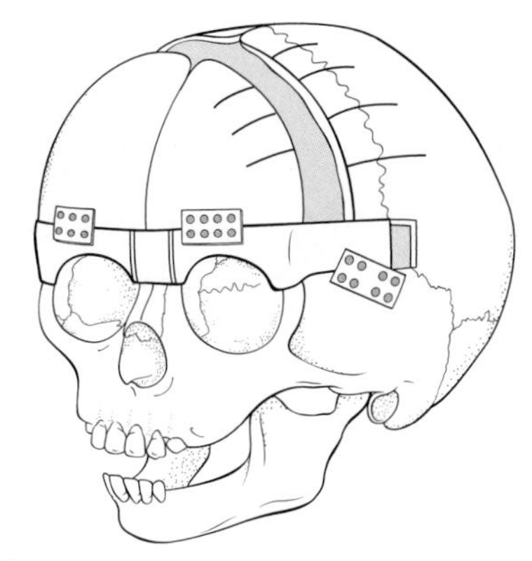

10.5.19 Fixation following metopic synostosis correction from an anterior view.

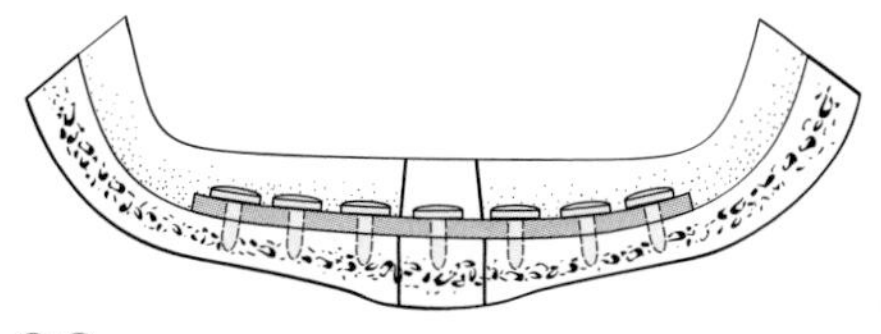

10.5.20 Internal resorbable plating of the bandeau at the midline with autogenous bone grafting.

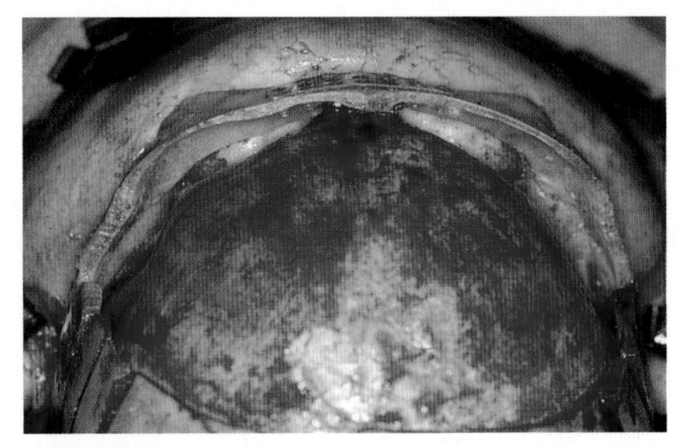

10.5.21 Superior view following fixation of bandeau but prior to placement of frontal segments.

- Intraoperative (Figure 10.5.25a) and schematic (Figure 10.5.25b) pre-operative superior views of the proposed osteotomy sites for total cranial vault reshaping without orbital osteotomies.
- Intraoperative (Figure 10.5.26a) and schematic (Figure 10.5.26b) superior views after total cranial vault reshaping to increase the biparietal width and reduce the frontal and occipital projection.
- Intraoperative left lateral view prior to reshaping (Figure 10.5.27a) and after reshaping and fixation (Figure 10.5.27b).

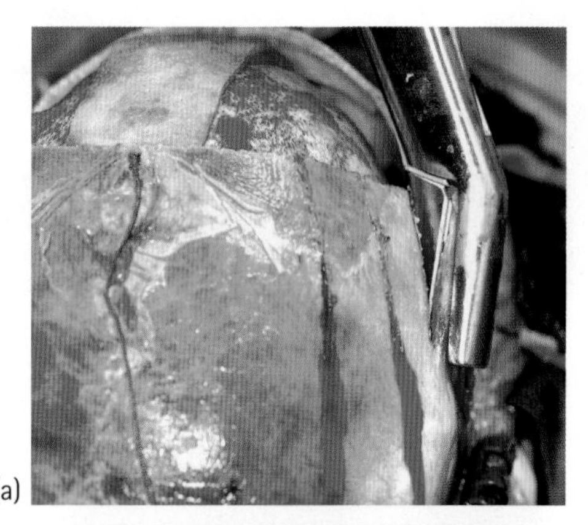

(a)

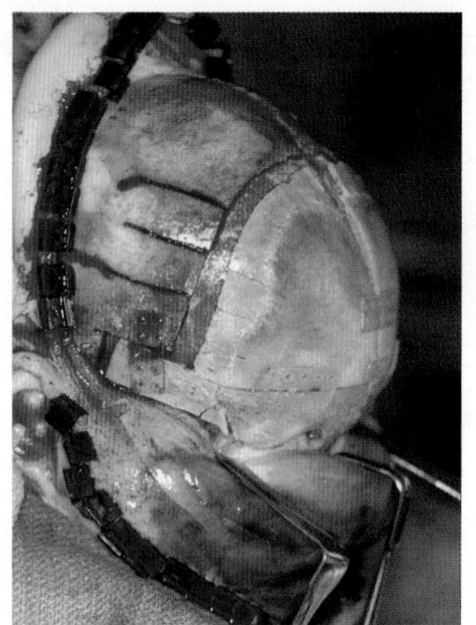

(b)

10.5.22 Barrel-staving bone cuts are manipulated via bone benders (a) and final fixation achieved via resorbable plates (b).

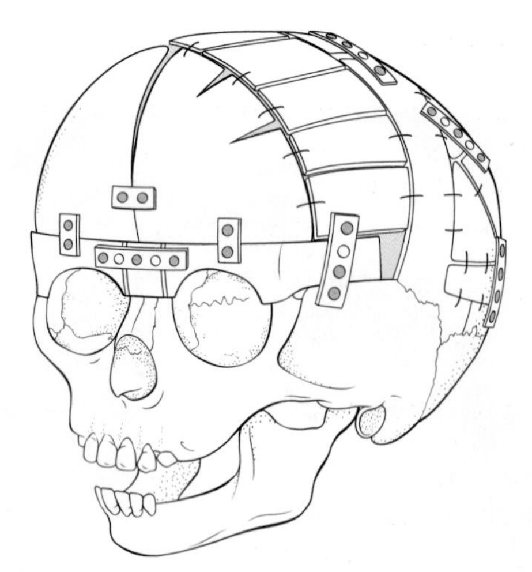

10.5.23 Total cranial vault reshaping and resorbable plate fixation to correct sagittal synostosis.

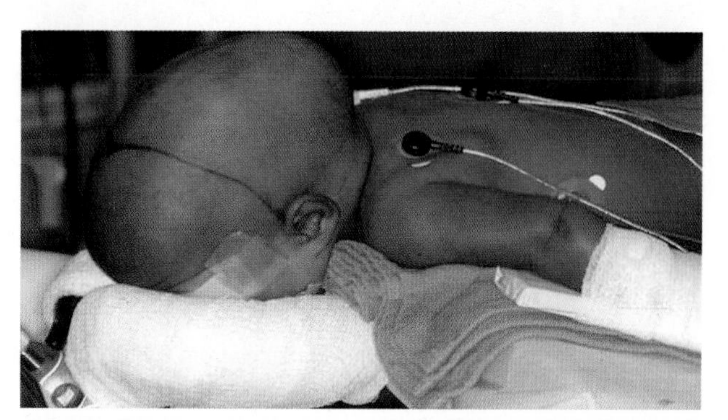

10.5.24 Prone positioning for total cranial vault reshaping.

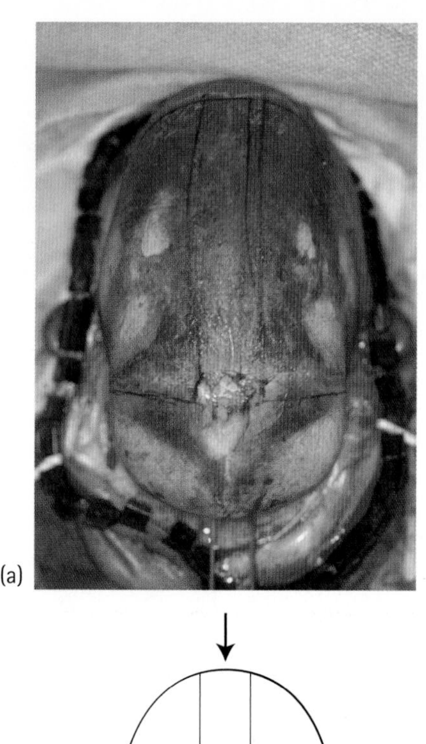

(a)

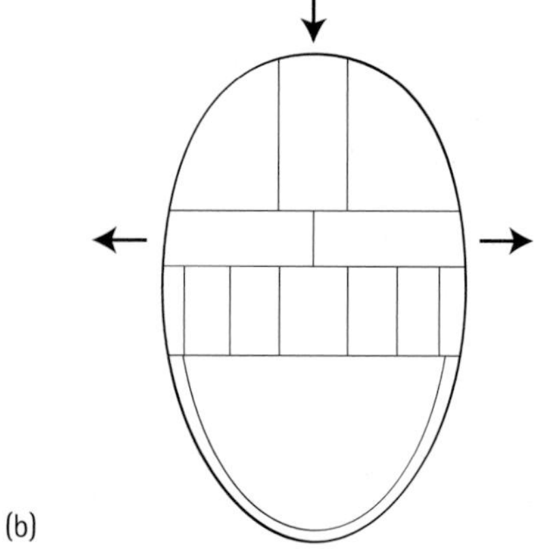

(b)

10.5.25 Superior intraoperative (a) and schematic (b) views prior to total cranial vault reshaping and fixation.

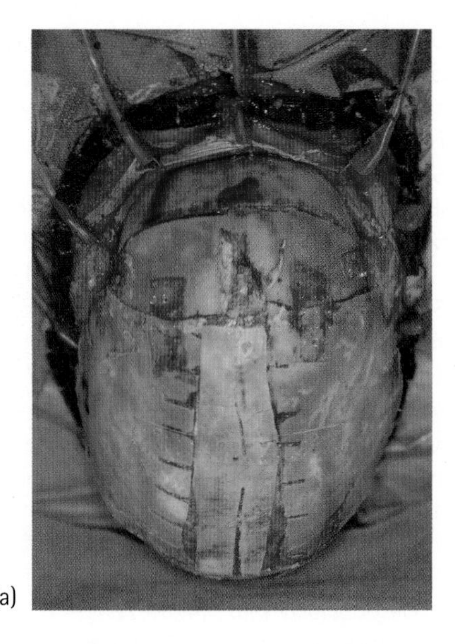

(a)

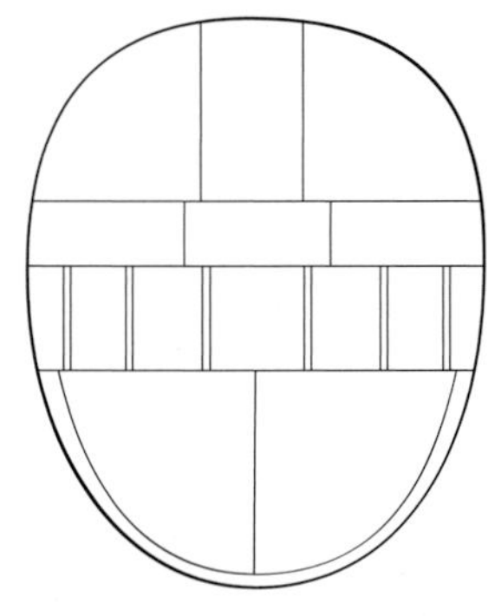

(b)

10.5.26 Superior intraoperative (a) and schematic (b) views following total cranial vault reshaping and fixation.

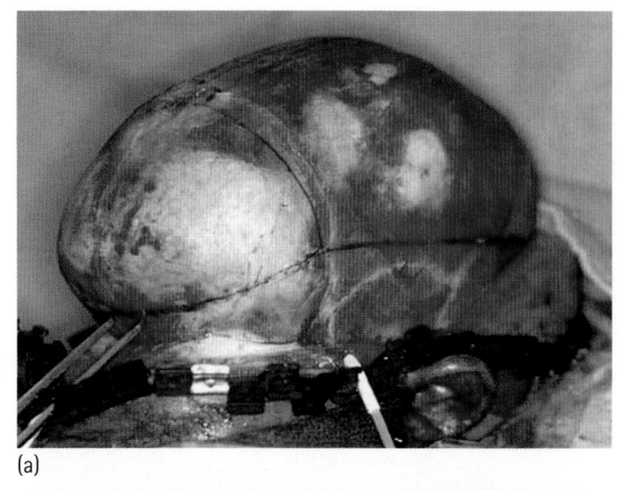

(a)

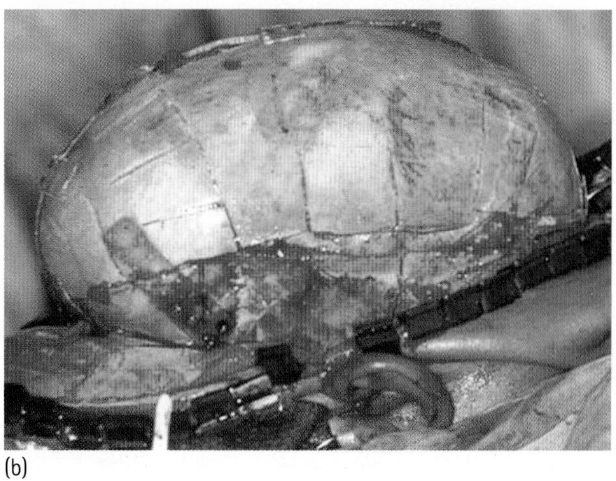

(b)

10.5.27 Lateral intraoperative views prior to (a) and following (b) total cranial vault reshaping.

COMPLICATIONS

Operative

- Excessive blood loss
- Subdural hematoma formation
- Cerebrospinal fluid loss
- Anaesthetic complications
- Periorbital injury
- Death.

Early post-operative

- Bleeding
- Haematoma
- Corneal abrasion
- Stitch abscess
- Cerebrospinal fluid leak
- Volume and electrolyte disturbances (SIADH and CSW syndromes)
- Infection/meningitis
- Loss of vision
- Airway obstruction
- Death.

Late post-operative

- Incisional alopecia
- Hypertrophic scarring
- Skull and orbital irregularities
- Diplopia, strabismus or canthal drift
- Sterile abscess secondary to plate hydrolysis.

Top tips

- Elevation of a coronal flap should be in the subperiosteal plane with inclusion of the temporalis muscles maintaining attachment to the flap.
- Development of a supraorbital bandeau with a minimum height of 1.5 cm.
- Liberal placement of barrel-staving osteotomies to facilitate intraoperative three-dimensional changes and post-operative moulding if necessary.
- Use of resorbable plate fixation thereby avoiding the need for plate and screw removal or migration.

FURTHER READING

Becker DB, Petersen JD, Kane AA *et al.* Speech, cognitive, and behavioral outcomes in nonsyndromic craniosynostosis. *Plastic and Reconstructive Surgery* 2005; **116**: 400–7.

Burrows AM, Mooney MP, Smith TD *et al.* Growth of the cranial vault in rabbits with congenital coronal suture synostosis. *Cleft Palate-Craniofacial Journal* 1995; **32**: 325–246.

David LR, Genecov DG, Camastra AA *et al.* Positron emission tomography studies confirm the need for early surgical intervention in patients with single-suture craniosynostosis. *Journal of Craniofacial Surgery* 1999; **10**: 38–42.

Ghali GE, Sinn DP. Nonsyndromic craniosynostosis. In: Miloro M, Ghali GE, Larsen PE, Waite PD (eds). *Peterson's Principles of oral and maxillofacial surgery*, 2nd edn. Hamilton, Ontario: BC Decker, 2004: 887–900.

Ghali GE, Sinn DP, Tantipasawasin S. Management of nonsyndromic craniosynostosis. In: Haug RH, Steinberg B (eds). *Atlas of the oral and maxillofacial surgery clinics of North America*. Philadelphia, PA: WB Saunders , 2002: 1–41.

Hayward R, Gonsalez S. How low can you go? Intracranial pressure, cerebral perfusion pressure and respiratory obstruction in children with complex craniosynostosis. *Journal of Neurosurgery* 2005; **102**: 16–22.

Marchac D, Renier D. Treatment of craniosyonostosis in infancy. *Clinics in Plastic Surgery* 1987; **14**: 61–72.

Ozgur BM, Aryan HE, Ibrahim D *et al.* Emotional and psychological impact of delayed craniosynostosis repair. *Child's Nervous System* 2006; **22**: 1619–23. 2006.

Siatkowski RM, Fortney AC, Nazir SA *et al.* Visual field defects in deformational posterior plagiocephaly. *Journal of AAPOS* 2005; **9**: 274–8.

Virtanen R, Korhonen T, Fagerholm J, Viljanto J. Neurocognitive sequelae of scaphocephaly. *Pediatrics* 1999; **103**: 791–5.

10.6

Hemifacial microsomia

JANICE S LEE

INTRODUCTION

Hemifacial microsomia is the second most common congenital anomaly of the craniofacial region. Abnormal development of the structures derived from the first and second branchial arches results in unilateral hypoplasia and asymmetry of the orbit, mandible, ear, cranial nerve VII and overlying soft tissue. Extracranial anomalies may occur. The characteristic finding of hemifacial microsomia, including bilateral involvement, is the asymmetry in craniofacial development.

Treatment is determined by the age of the patient (potential for growth) and the severity of the facial deformity affected by the mandibular type. The patient's psychosocial development should be considered in the timing of the surgical treatment. The timing of treatment remains controversial and influenced by the theories surrounding progressive or stable asymmetry.

Using the Pruzansky classification with the Kaban modification, most surgeons agree that the mandible type I and IIa may be treated with conventional orthognathic surgery or distraction osteogenesis. The mandible type IIb and III typically require construction of the missing or deficient glenoid fossa-condyle-ramus (GCR) unit using costochondral grafts. Construction of the affected ear often occurs between six and nine years of age when the child is of adequate size to harvest an adequate amount of costochondral cartilage. The soft tissue augmentation is typically carried out after skeletal construction. Augmentation can be achieved with microvascular free-tissue transfers, most commonly the scapular free flap, or fat injections as we have noted with excellent aesthetic results. This chapter will describe the comprehensive work-up and the craniofacial surgical skeletal treatment after growth is complete for the type IIb or III mandible in a patient who has completed pre-surgical orthodontic preparation.

EXAMINATION OF THE PATIENT

Many patients tend to posture the head toward the affected side or may have musculoskeletal restrictions. In such cases, the patient should be examined in resting and corrected position with the horizontal facial plane established (Figure 10.6.1). Skin markings may help establish the facial planes. The extent of the facial asymmetry should be documented and diagnostic photographs should be obtained.

Assessment should include:

- facial animation, smiling and facial nerve function;
- occlusal cant (a tongue blade may be helpful) and position of dental midlines;
- profile view from left and right (Figure 10.6.2);
- temporomandibular joint examination (deviation with opening, any symptoms and range of motion, although it is not often limited);
- masticatory muscles presence and function;
- degree of microtia;
- soft tissue deficiency;
- submental view (Figure 10.6.3);

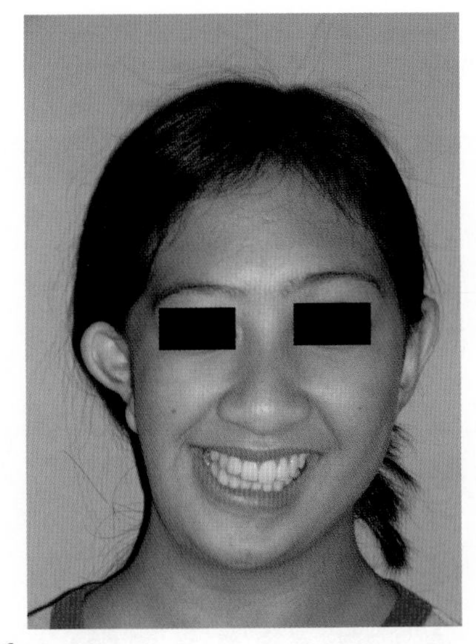

10.6.1 Pre-operative frontal smiling view with patient in corrected head position. The mandible and chin point are deviated to the right and there is an obvious maxillary and mandibular cant and rotation. The facial nerve is intact.

- intraoral examination, including the overjet and overbite relationship, the amount of oral opening, the presence of a lateral shift or centric relation-centric occlusion (CR-CO) discrepancy that is often seen in HFM patients, and the movement of the soft palate.

DIAGNOSTIC IMAGES

As well as the 2-dimensional radiographs, panorex, lateral and posterior-anterior (PA) cephalograms, 3-dimensional images such as a spiral or cone-beam CT with 3D reformatting prior to surgery helps to appreciate the skeletal deformity in all planes (Figures 10.6.4 and 10.6.5). The 3D images have demonstrated skull base asymmetry and the extreme rotation of the maxilla and mandible. The 3D CT allows for the fabrication of anatomical models that may be incorporated into the model surgery.

MODEL SURGERY

Advanced technology is allowing for surgical treatment planning using virtual surgery software. This chapter will describe the more conventional treatment planning method.

Ideally, two anatomical models are requested for each surgical patient. One anatomical model is marked at all the midline structures while the second model is used to compare the baseline asymmetry. Using the orbital rims for the horizontal facial plane or an arbitrary horizontal facial plane if there is orbital dystopia, the projected facial midline is established by bisecting the horizontal plane with a perpendicular line. The foramen magnum or sella in the skull base may provide a reasonable midline structure in the submental view of the skull. The mandible and maxilla are then disarticulated from the skull base. For an ideal aesthetic result, particularly in profile, the steep occlusal and mandibular planes need to be corrected, often with the

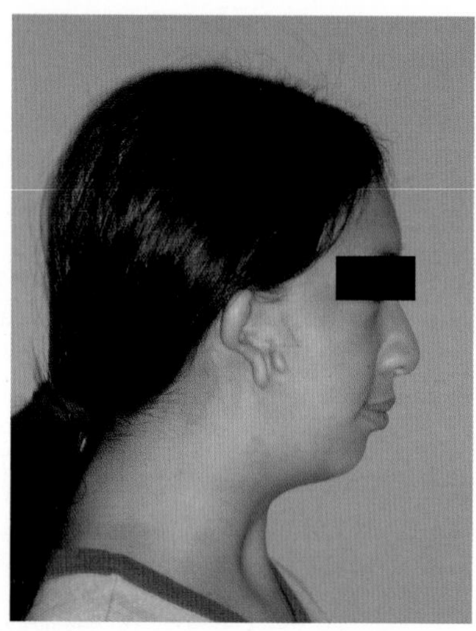

10.6.2 Pre-operative right lateral view demonstrating right microtia, retrognathia and short posterior face height.

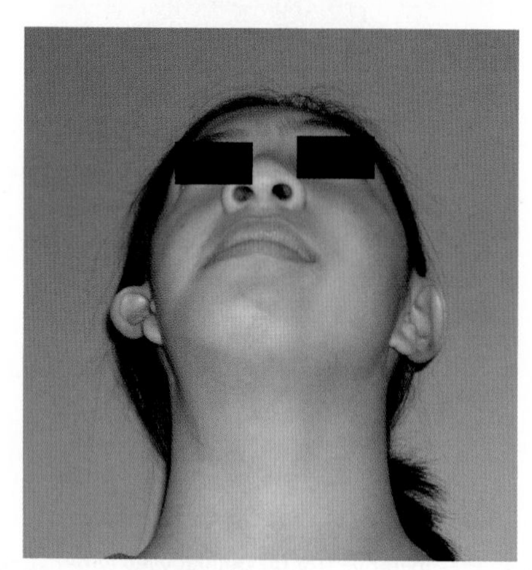

10.6.3 Pre-operative submental view demonstrating the extreme rotation of the chin point and deficiency of the right facial soft tissues.

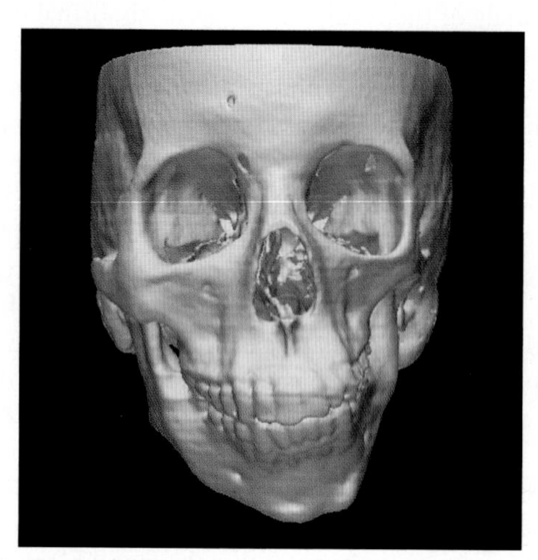

10.6.4 Pre-operative 3D reformatted CT showing the frontal view of a patient with left dominant hemifacial microsomia and type IIb mandible. From the 3D images it is clear that hemifacial microsomia is not a unilateral condition but a condition that ultimately affects growth bilaterally.

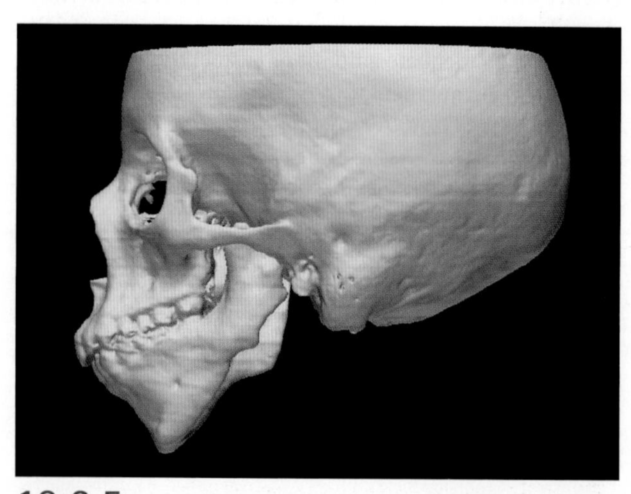

10.6.5 Pre-operative 3D reformatted CT of the lateral view of the same patient as in Figure 10.6.4.

fulcrum in the anterior maxilla on the unaffected side. The affected side often requires even further lengthening to correct the cant, thus, the surgical movements on the affected side become greater than 10 mm in most cases. The maxilla is often advanced and rotated to the facial midline (Figure 10.6.6). The mandible is then positioned to the maxilla. The muscle attachments and structures, such as the inferior alveolar neurovascular bundle, may limit the ease of moving the mandible into an ideal position. If necessary, the unaffected side is shortened.

Conventional model surgery is then performed on plaster models of the patient mounted in a semi-adjustable articulator.

The following points should be considered:

- Slight over-rotation of the maxilla (1–2 mm beyond the midline) is helpful.
- Intermediate splint is often bulky and demonstrates the significant change in position of the maxilla.
- The final splint can be fabricated in a non-adjustable articulator with the models in ideal maximal intercuspal position and then opened 2 mm at the molars on the affected side in anticipation for costochondral graft settling and remodelling.
- The maxillary occlusal plane is obtained with the face-bow parallel to the projected horizontal facial plane without placing the ear rod in the external auditory canal on the affected side if it is abnormally positioned.
- It may take multiple attempts to establish the CR of the mandible due to the absence of the GCR unit.

SURGICAL MANAGEMENT

Once the patient is nasally intubated and positioned as if for an orthognathic procedure, a small area is shaved over the affected side to allow for a temporal extension of a preauricular incision (Figure 10.6.7). Pre-operative antibiotics, such as clindamycin, and corticosteroids, such as dexamethasone, are provided. A shoulder roll is placed for extension of the neck with the head resting in a jelly doughnut. The patient is prepared and draped in the standard fashion for an orthognathic procedure. A kirshner rod (k-rod) is sterilely placed between nasion and glabella to establish the pre-operative vertical position of the maxillary canines and central incisor and the alar base width. A throat pack is placed. Local anaesthetic, typically 1 per cent lidocaine with 1:100 000 epinephrine, is injected along the unaffected ramus and in the maxillary vestibule. As with a two-jaw orthognathic surgical procedure, the unaffected side sagittal split osteotomy is initiated but not completed (see Chapter 10.2 Orthognathic surgery of the mandible).

Epinephrine-soaked neuropaddies are placed in the incision site for haemostasis. Attention is then directed to the maxilla where a LeFort I osteotomy is performed (see Chapter 10.3 Orthognathic surgery – maxilla (Le Fort I, II and III)). Mobilization of the maxilla with Rowe disimpaction forceps is critical. Both descending palatine arteries are routinely preserved. The intermediate splint is then secured between the mobile maxilla and the mandible using 26 gauge wires. With the mandible carefully placed in centric relation, the maxilla

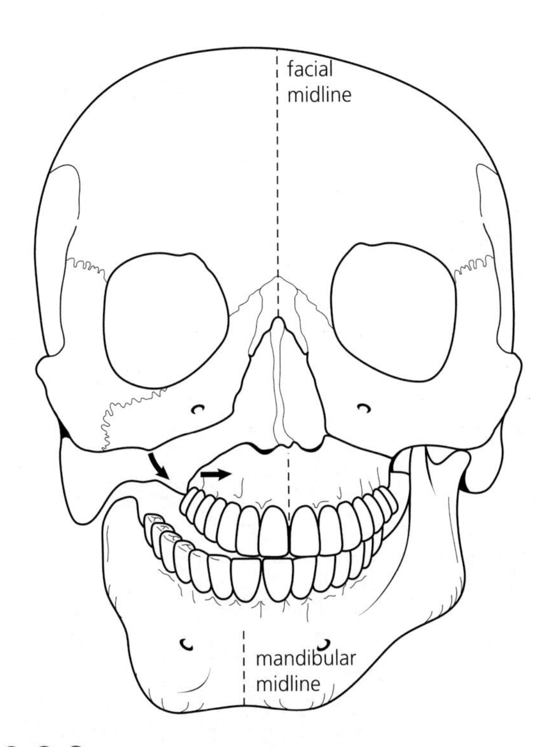

10.6.6 Model surgery on the anatomical model demonstrates the significant changes in the position of the maxilla and the expected rotation of the mandible in the intermediate phase.

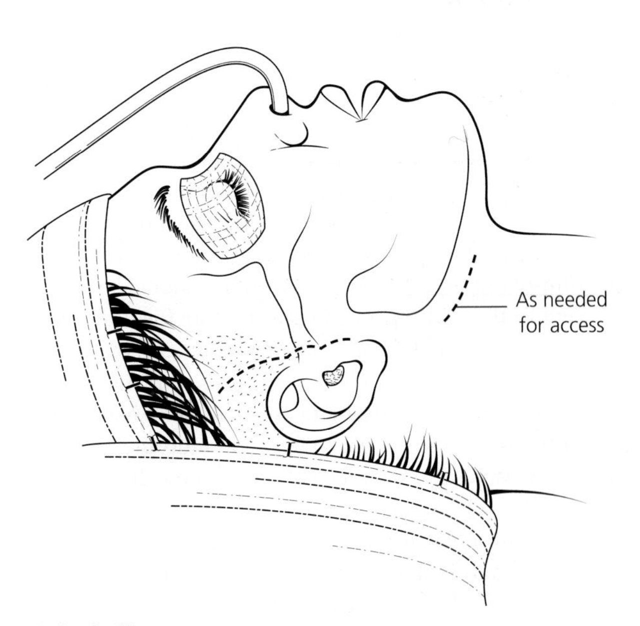

10.6.7 The skeletal structures and landmarks are identified and the preauricular incision with the temporal extension is mapped.

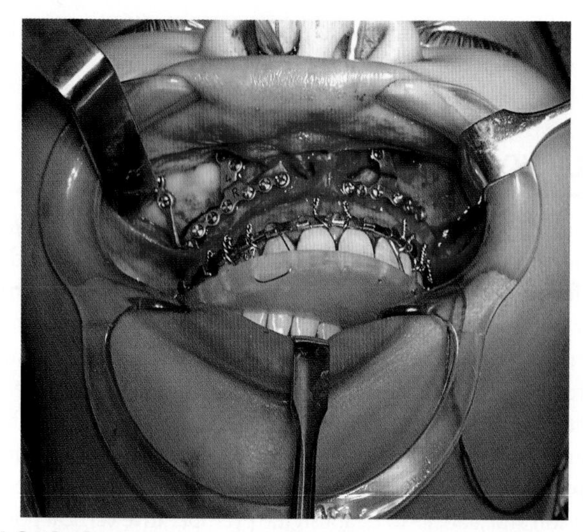

10.6.8 The maxilla is mobilized and rigidly fixed. Note the large intermediate splint and the intermediate position of the mandible.

is rigidly fixed using 2.0 plates at the piriform rims and buttresses (a total of four plates), starting with placement of the plates on the unaffected side (Figure 10.6.8). A laminar spreader is often used to stent down the maxilla on the affected side while the plates are placed. Measurements are taken from the k-rod to the canines and central incisor to confirm that the cant is corrected according to the planned movements. The sagittal split osteotomy is completed on the unaffected side and epinephrine-soaked neuropaddies are placed for haemostasis. Hypotensive anaesthesia is requested during the orthognathic procedures.

EXTRAORAL APPROACH

Sterile preparation and draping of the patient is necessary for the extraoral approach to the remnant joint and ramus on the affected side and the harvesting of the costochondral bone grafts. The patient is positioned with the affected side exposed including the temporal, preauricular and submandibular incision sites. A soft roll is placed under the chest, preferably the contralateral chest to take advantage of the favourable anatomy of the rib. A sterile adhesive drape should be placed adjacent to the oral commissure to separate the oral cavity from the sterile field. Draping should be done such that access to the mouth is possible without contaminating the field. A two-team approach is ideal and efficient (see Chapter 3.4, Reconstructive surgery – harvesting, skin mucosa and cartilage, and Chapter 8.3, Treatment of temporomandibular joint ankylosis).

The preauricular incision is made anterior to the constructed ear and in the vicinity of the zygomatic root of the temporal bone. It is not unusual to find the constructed ear over the future site of the constructed condyle since the abnormal ear is often anterior and inferior in position. Care must be taken not to disrupt the soft tissue overlying the cartilage of the constructed ear. The site is anaesthetized with local anaesthetic. The preauricular incision extends to the constructed earlobe inferiorly and has a temporal extension that allows for greater anterior flap release and access to the temporalis myofascia if needed to line the constructed glenoid fossa. Despite the hypoplasia or agenesis of the local skeletal structures, there is some remnant of the anterior component of the temporalis muscle. Additionally, identifying the temporalis myofascial plane provides orientation, access to the zygomatic arch (if present) and allows for protection of the facial nerve if dissection is kept deep to this plane. Nerve stimulation is performed throughout the dissection to preserve the facial nerve. Once at the zygomatic arch, the dissection is carried out to the potential superior joint space. Medial dissection is kept minimal due to the potential vasculature that resides medially and due to the goal of positioning the constructed condyle laterally and posteriorly. A 2–3 cm submandibular incision is made approximately 2 cm below the rudimentary ramus and mandibular angle. This allows the incision to be below the final position of the angle and constructed ramus. Dissection is carried down to the affected mandible using nerve stimulation. Subperiosteal dissection is continued along the vestigial ramus to its most superior aspect. Muscle detachment, including the medial attachments, is necessary around the vestigial ramus to allow lengthening of the affected side. If a remnant disc is present, it can be seen around the rudimentary condyle. It typically cannot be used. Blunt dissection is used to create a throughway from the mandible to the superior incision in the region of the zygomatic root where the glenoid fossa will be constructed. Gentle enlargement of this throughway is possible with blunt finger dissection to accommodate the costochondral graft. If there is an elongated coronoid process, it is resected through either incisions. At this point, one person can access the oral cavity without con-

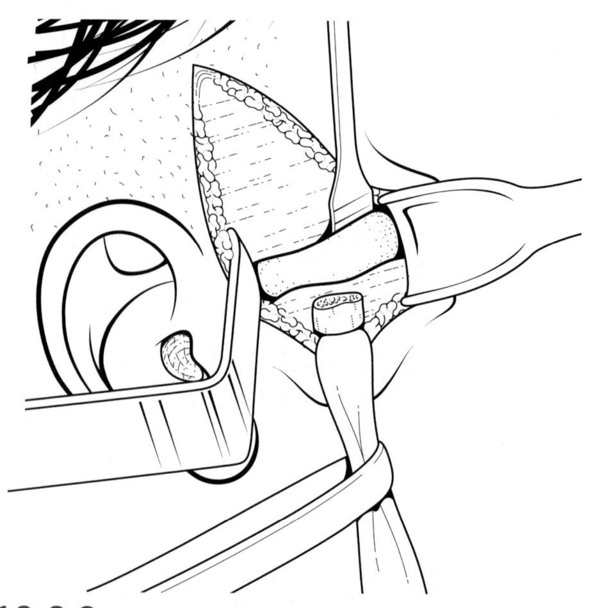

10.6.9 The costochondral graft is positioned superiorly and laterally.

taminating the preauricular field and secure the final splint to the maxilla and place the patient in intermaxillary fixation (IMF) using 26 gauge wires.

One of two rib grafts, the costochondral bone graft with a 3–5 mm cartilage cap, is positioned from the vestigial ramus to the superior joint space (Figure 10.6.9). A 6–7 cm costochondral graft is often required and positioned posteriorly and as far laterally as possible. A second 6–7 cm rib graft without a cartilage cap is cut into two shorter grafts; one graft is set aside for the maxilla and one is used to construct the glenoid fossa and deficient or missing zygomatic arch, thus functioning as a posterior and lateral stop (Figure 10.6.10). This bone graft is secured to the deficient zygomatic arch or temporal bone with washers and 10–12-mm 2.0 screws. Prior to constructing the condyle, a temporalis myofascial flap is elevated and wrapped over the zygomatic arch and secured to the medial tissues with 4/0 interrupted vicryl sutures. This interpositional flap lines the newly constructed glenoid fossa and appears to prevent ankylosis of the joint. The costochondral bone graft is then secured to the native mandible (vestigial ramus) using three washers and 10–12 mm 2.0 screws (Figure 10.6.11). All sites are irrigated and a butterfly drain is placed in the area of the constructed condyle which exits in the submandibular region. The incisions are closed in layers with 4/0 vicryl with staples for the superficial layer of the scalp and 5/0 nylon for the superficial layer of the preauricular and submandibular incisions.

Attention is then turned to the oral cavity. The IMF is released and the mandible is gently opened and closed to determine the stability of the posterior/superior/lateral stop and mobility as a unit. Once confirmed, attention is then turned to the chin to complete the sliding genioplasty (see Chapter 10.2 Orthognathic surgery of the mandible). The chin is often advanced, lengthened and rotated.

With the remaining rib graft, the lengthened maxilla on the affected side is stabilized with the interpositional bone graft. It is secured with a plate or sutured to one of the fixation plates. All intraoral sites are irrigated and closed with running 4/0 vicryl sutures. The patient is place in IMF elastics for 3–4 weeks.

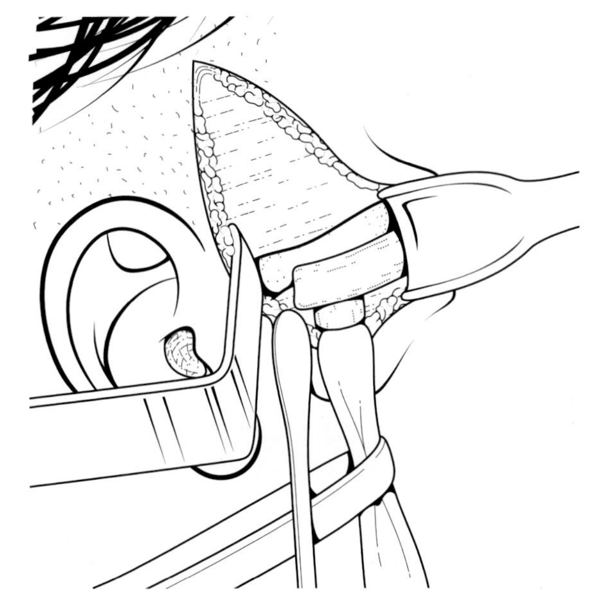

10.6.10 The second rib graft is used as a lateral stop and augments the deficient zygomatic arch.

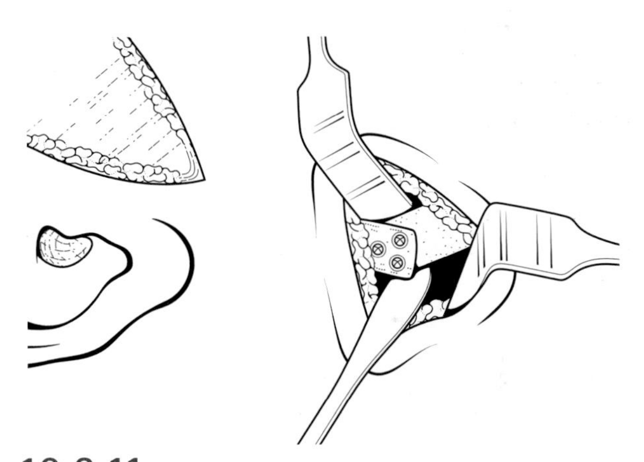

10.6.11 The costochondral graft is secured to the native mandible with screws and washers.

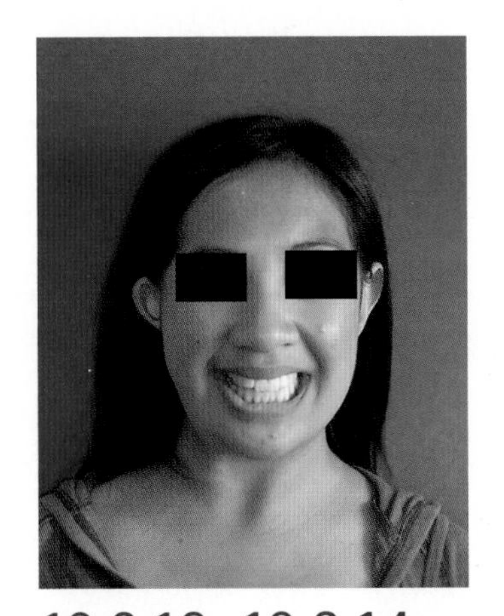

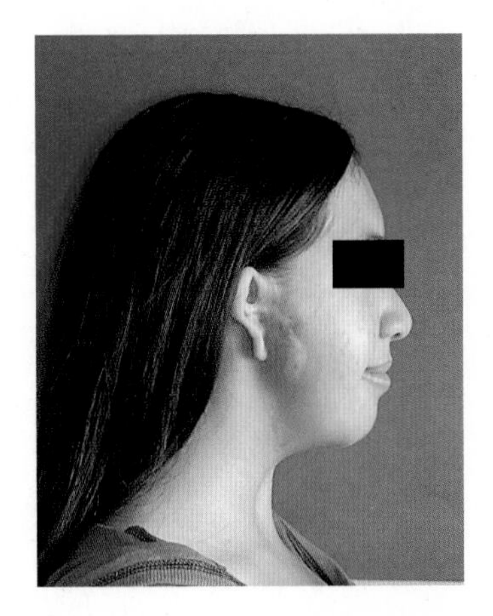

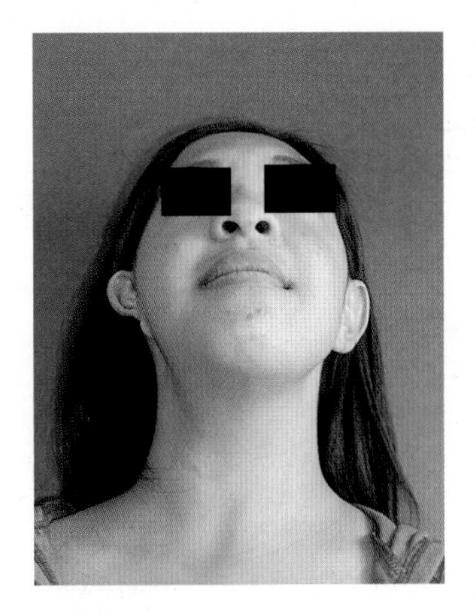

10.6.12–10.6.14 Three years post-operative assessment demonstrating good facial symmetry and a stable occlusion. The patient had fat injections of the right face for soft tissue augmentation one year after the skeletal surgery.

Post-operative points include:

- maintain guiding elastics once out of IMF for 4 more weeks with maxillary splint in place; encourage gentle opening exercise;
- resume orthodontics once maxillary splint is removed (at 7–8 weeks after surgery);
- soft tissue augmentation after six months, may include free flap or fat injections;
- prior to soft tissue augmentation and as patient's oedema decreases, soft tissue asymmetry becomes marked, skeletal symmetry is stable.

Top tips

- Preparation and work-up of the hemifacial patient is the most critical step.
- Diagnostic imaging, particularly 3D imaging, and anatomic models are critical for treatment planning in patients with severe facial asymmetry.
- Basic orthognathic surgery principles apply.
- Anatomic limitations may restrict complete mobilization and ideal positioning of either the maxilla or mandible.

FURTHER READING

Brent B. Technical advances in ear reconstruction with autogenous rib cartilage grafts: personal experience with 1200 cases. *Plastic and Reconstructive Surgery* 1999; **104**: 319–34; discussion 335–8.

Inigo F, Jimenez-Murat Y, Arrovo O *et al.* Restoration of facial contour in Romberg's disease and hemifacial microsomia: experience with 118 cases. *Microsurgery* 2000; **20**: 167–72.

Kaban LB, Moses MH, Mulliken JB. Surgical correction of hemifacial microsomia in the growing child. *Plastic and Reconstructive Surgery* 1988; **82**: 9–19.

Kaban, LB, Padwa BL, Mulliken JB. Surgical correction of mandibular hypoplasia in hemifacial microsomia: the case for treatment in early childhood. *Journal of Oral and Maxillofacial Surgery* 1998; **56**: 628–38.

Kearns GJ, Padwa BL, Mulliken JB, Kaban LB. Progression of facial asymmetry in hemifacial microsomia. *Plastic and Reconstructive Surgery* 2000 **105**: 492–8.

Longaker MT, Siebert JW. Microsurgical correction of facial contour in congenital craniofacial malformations: the marriage of hard and soft tissue. *Plastic and Reconstructive Surgery* 1996; **98**: 942–50.

Polley JW, Figueroa AA, Liou EJ, Cohen M. Longitudinal analysis of mandibular asymmetry in hemifacial microsomia. *Plastic and Reconstructive Surgery* 1997; **99**: 328–39.

Posnick JC. Surgical correction of mandibular hypoplasia in hemifacial microsomia: a personal perspective. *Journal of Oral and Maxillofacial Surgery* 1998; **56**: 639–50.

Pruzansky S. Not all dwarfed mandibles are alike. *Birth Defects* 1969; **1**: 120.

Rune B, Selvik G, Sarnas KV, Jacobsson S. Growth in hemifacial microsomia studied with the aid of roentgen stereophotogrammetry and metallic implants. *Cleft Palate Journal* 1981; **18**: 128–46.

Werler MM, Sheehan JE, Hayes C *et al.* Demographic and reproductive factors associated with hemifacial microsomia. *Cleft Palate-Craniofacial Journal* 2004; **41**: 494–50.

10.7

Sleep apnoea and snoring, including non-surgical techniques

JOSEPH R DEATHERAGE, PETER D WAITE

DEFINITION

Obstructive sleep apnoea syndrome refers to the condition of complete or partial airway obstruction during sleep which disrupts sleep architecture. It also results in excessive daytime somnolence.

Snoring is noisy breathing during sleep and represents partial airway obstruction. If loud enough, snoring can disrupt sleep architecture.

ETIOLOGY

Obesity related cranio-maxillofacial syndrome, skeletal abnormalities, nasopharyngeal obstruction, macroglossia.

INDICATIONS FOR INTERVENTION

- Excessive daytime somnolence (EDS)
- Respiratory distress index (RDI) > 20
- O_2 – Desaturation >90% during sleep
- Hypertension
- Dysthythmias.

INDICATIONS FOR SURGICAL INTERVENTION

- Failure of non-surgical management
- Maxillofacial skeletal-anatomic airway abnormalities.

CONTRADICTIONS TO SURGERY

- Gross obesity
- Unstable cardiovascular disease
- Severe pulmonary disease
- Alcoholism or drug abuse
- Elderly.

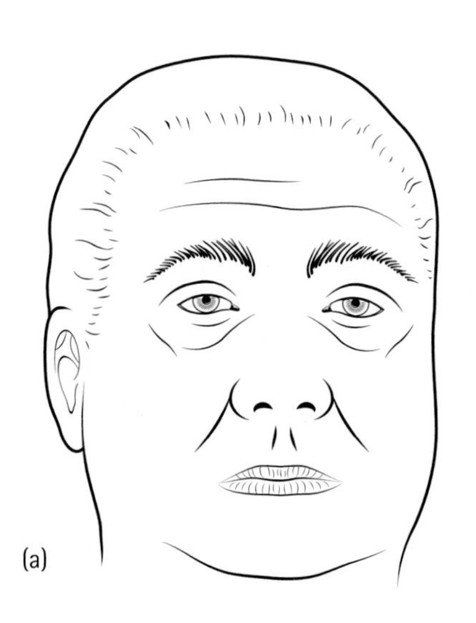

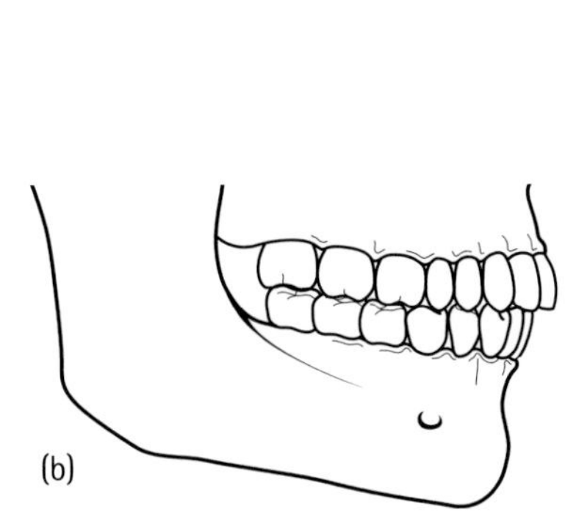

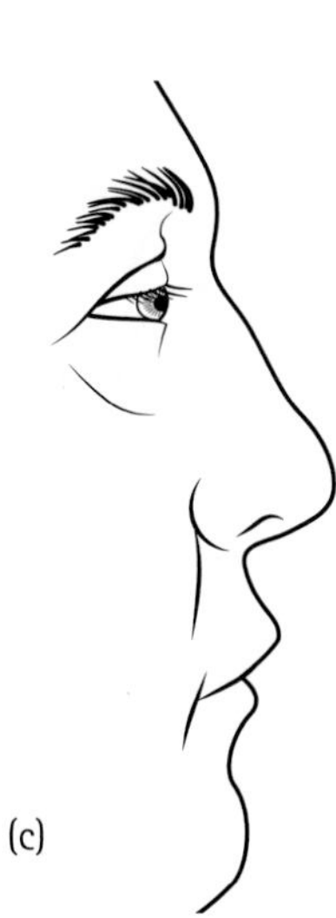

10.7.1 Obese, retognathic male, lateral cephalometric film.

EVALUATION

- Medical and sleep history
- Polysomnogram
- Head and neck evaluation, neck circumference
- Body habitus
- Fiber optic nasopharyngoscopy Muller manoeuvre
- Nose: septum, turbinates, nasal valve
- Intranasal examination via fiberoptic nasopharyngoscopy.

INTRAORAL: OROPHARYNX, UVULA, TONSILS, BASE OF TONGUE

- Fujita Classification of Obstructive Regions:
  - Type I Palate (normal base of tongue)
  - Type II Palate and Base of Tongue
  - Type III Base of Tongue (normal palate)
- Radiographic evaluation: lateral cephalometric film – radiographic analysis.

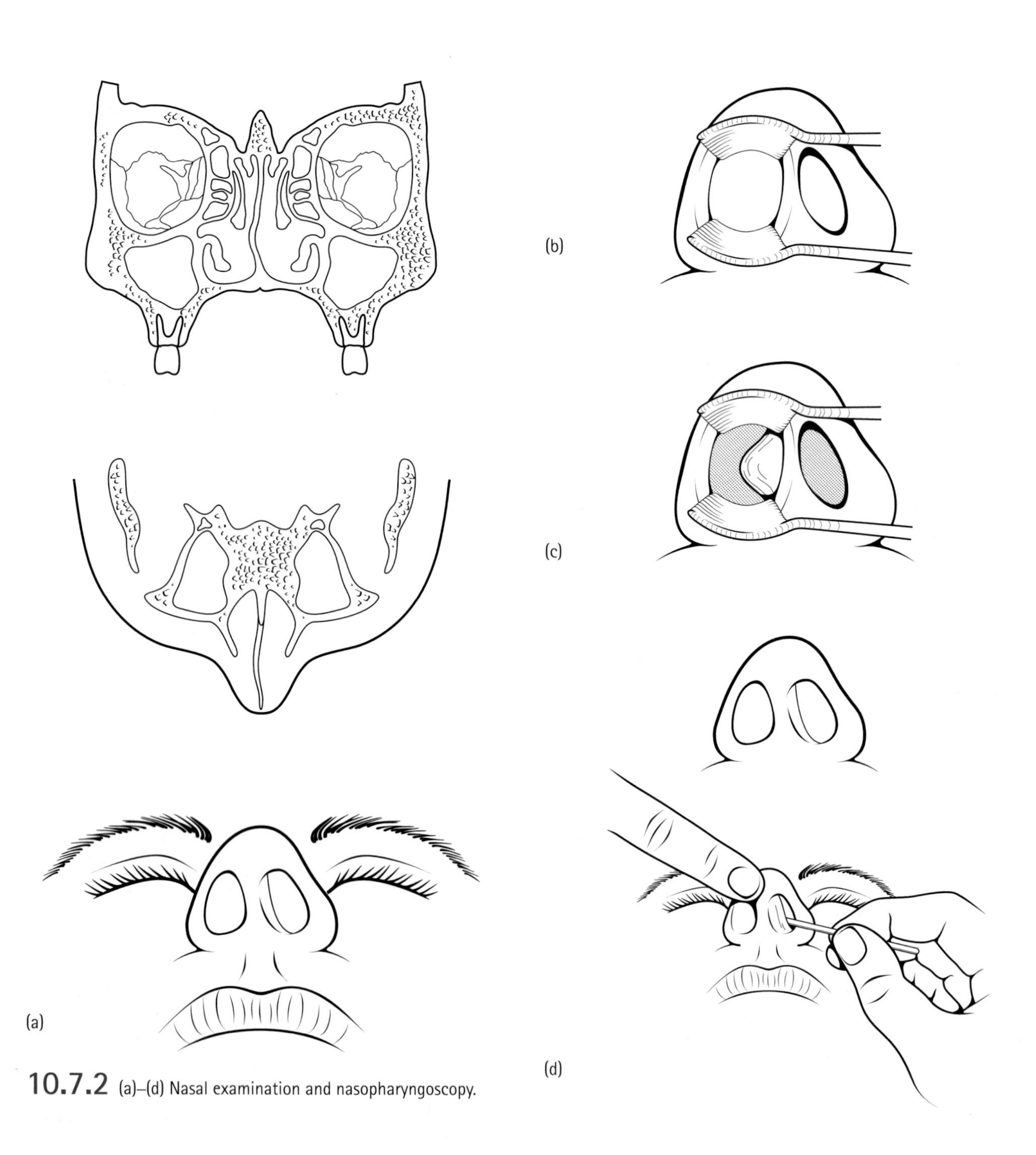

10.7.2 (a)–(d) Nasal examination and nasopharyngoscopy.

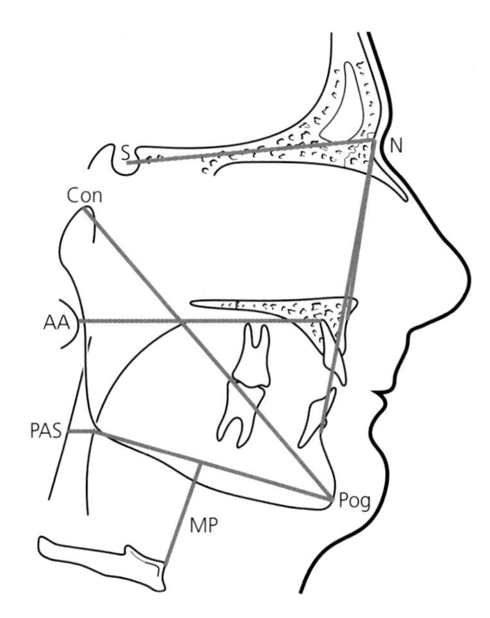

10.7.3 Lateral cephalometric film.

NORMAL CEPHALOMETRIC VALUES

- SNA: 82
- SNB: 80
- PAS: 11
- PNS: -P-35 mm
- MP: -hyoid 15 mm

NON-SURGICAL MANAGEMENT

- Weight loss
- Sleep hygiene: elimination of caffeine late in the day.
- Avoidance of excessive exercise prior to sleep.
- Sleeping with the head elevated reduces upper airway closure.
- Sleeping in the lateral recumbent or prone position is helpful.
- Safety pinning a tennis ball in a sock to the sleep garment is helpful in preventing sleep in the supine position.
- Avoidance of alcohol prior to sleep lessens obstructive events.
- Sedative agents can worsen obstruction.
- Smoking increases upper airway resistance through increased mucosal oedema.
- Pharmacologic supplemental O_2 is of questionable benefit. Apnoea may be prolonged in hypercapneic individuals with supplement O_2.
- Proptriptyline may reduce obstructive events by diminishing REM sleep.
- Supportive airway muscle tone may be increased.
- Protriptyline reduces subjective daytime somnolence.
- Multiple side-effects related to anticholinergic properties limit protriptyline use.
- Serotonin uptake inhibitors may increase upper airway muscle tone, particularly in REM sleep.

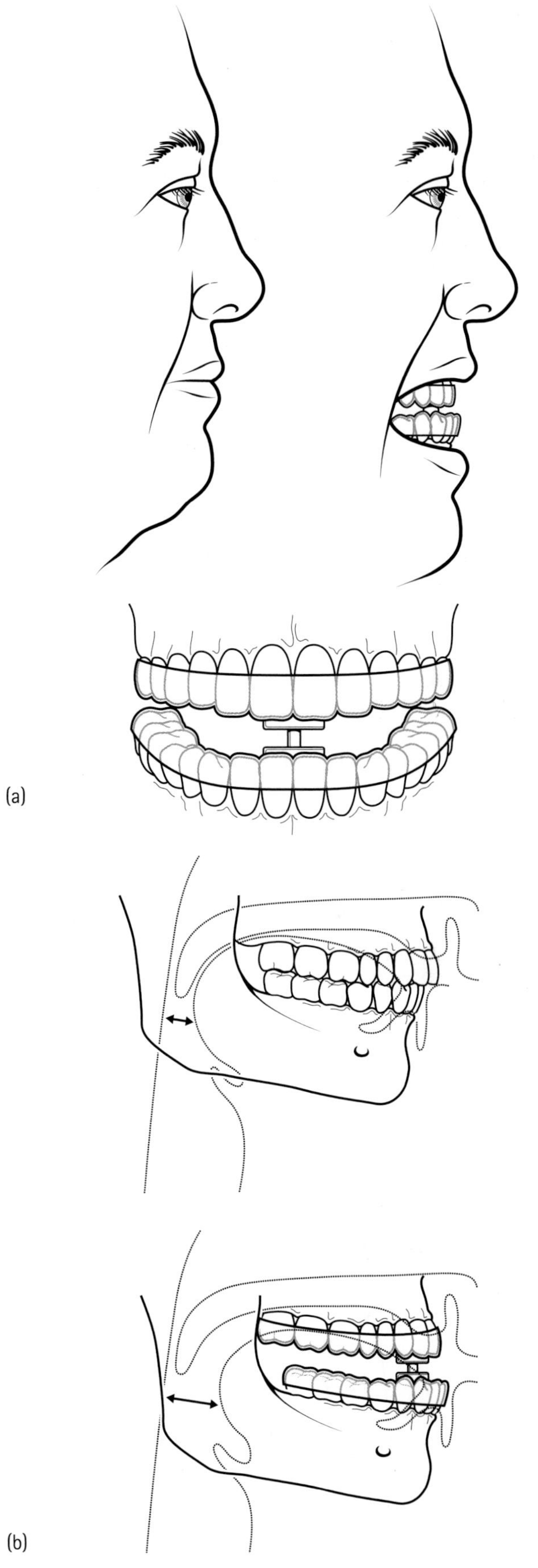

10.7.4 (a,b) Mandibular repositioning device, lateral film of dental device in place.

MECHANICAL DEVICES

Nasal dilators may decrease upper airway resistance. Intra- and extra-nasal dilators only help a few select patients with nasal airway issues. Nasopharyngeal airways have limited utility because of poor tolerance.

Mandibular repositioning devices are helpful in mild to moderate cases.

Continuous positive airway pressure devices: Nasal CPAP remains the first line of treatment of obstructive sleep apnoea.

MODE OF ACTION

Nasal CPAP pneumatically stents the airway open during sleep.

GENERAL CONSIDERATIONS REGARDING CPAP MANAGEMENT

Initiation of CPAP therapy should commence within a sleep lab, monitored during polysomnography. Airway pressures should be increased to the level necessary to overcome obstruction. Proper instruction is critical to proper utilization. Compliance is also critical. The device must be worn all night to correct the ill effects of obstructive sleep apnoea on sleep architecture.

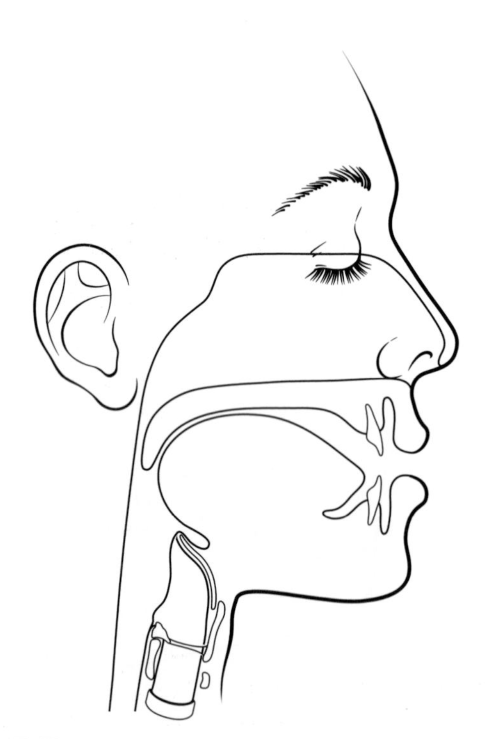

10.7.5 Lateral view of airway while asleep with airway collapse.

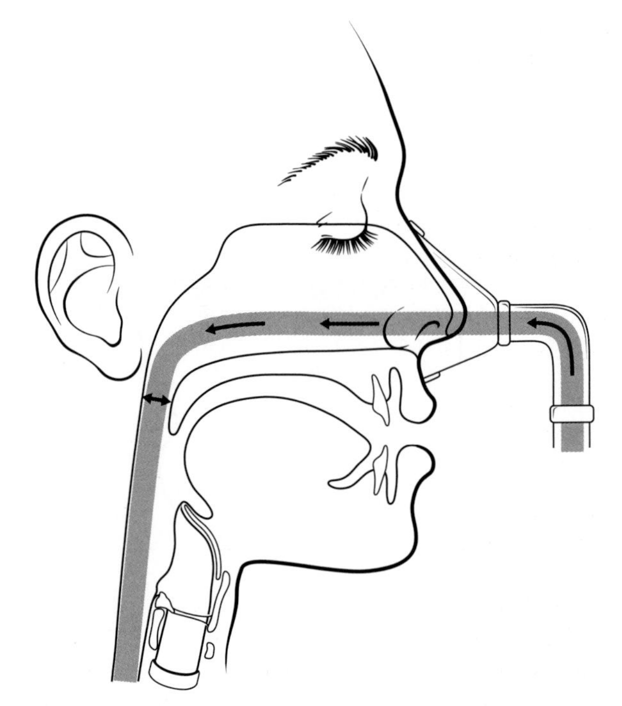

10.7.6 Lateral view with CPAP device and airway pneumatically stented open.

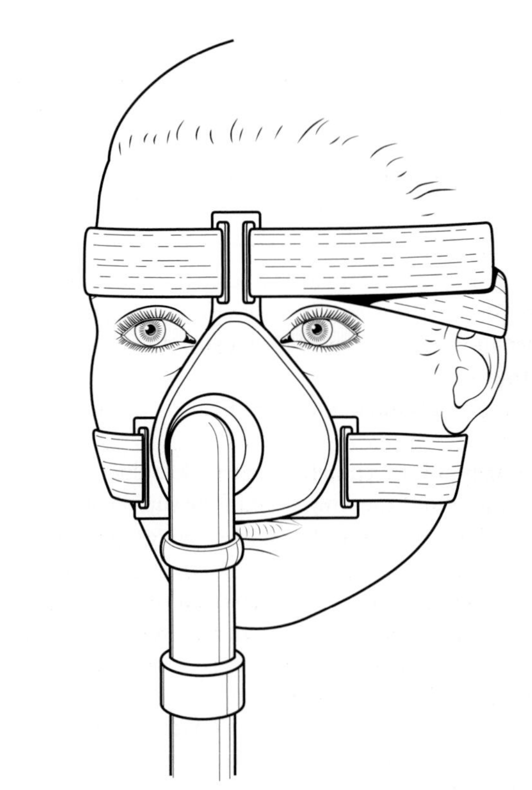

10.7.7 CPAP device in place on a patient.

COMPLIANCE WITH CPAP THERAPY

Studies have shown that refusal rates for prescribed CPAP therapy range from 58 to 80 per cent. Objective evaluation for compliance shows that only 40 per cent of patients use nasal CPAP for at least 4 hours for 7 nights out of 10. Poor compliance can usually be attributed to intolerance of the device.

SURGICAL MANAGEMENT OF OBSTRUCTIVE SLEEP APNOEA

Indications for surgical intervention failure of non-surgical measures include:

- Intolerance of nasal CPAP
- Excessively high CPAP pressures
- Rationale and surgical goals.

The goal of surgery should be a cure of the disease. The particular surgery should be directed at the site of obstruction.

Powell–Riley advocate a staged approach to surgery.

Phase I therapy is directed towards the upper airway. The simplest and most conservative option is considered at a specific anatomic region only when obstruction exists there.

- Nasal regions: Correction of nasal obstruction directed at the specific deformity: nasal valve deformities, septum, turbinates.
- Pharynx: UPPP, tonsillectomy, chemical sclerosis.
- Hypopharynx: Advancement of tongue base through genioglossus advancement, infra-hyoid myotomy and suspension.
- Tongue reduction through partial glossectomy, laser reduction and temperature-controlled radiofrequency reduction.

Phase II Therapy utilizes maxillofacial skeletal advancement referred to as mandibulo-maxillary advancement.

Presurgical preparation involves obtaining accurate dentofacial records through plaster casts of the jaws. The denatal models must be mounted on an articulator.

In the pre-surgical planning the mandible is advanced maximally. This is usually about 10–12 mm depending on the patient and bony morphology of the mandible. The maxilla is then advanced to achieve the original maxillary-mandibular dental relationship. Cephalometric evaluation of the genial region is considered to allow maximal advancement with facial aesthetics in mind. An acrylic dental splint is fabricated to allow the desired repositioning of the mandibular dental model.

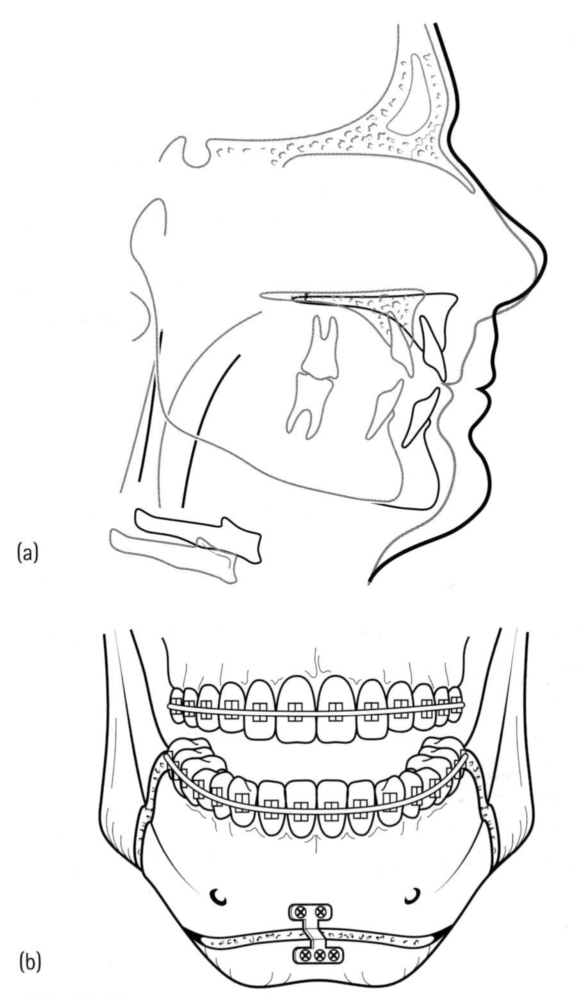

10.7.8 (a) Lateral view of pre- and post-MMA diagram. (b) Post-operative panoramic view. Note increase is posterior airway space (PAS).

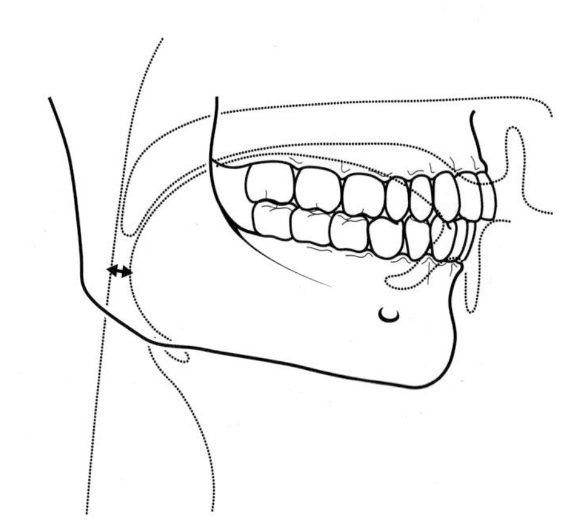

10.7.9 Lateral ceph and tracing.

SURGERY

General nasal endotracheal anaesthesia is required. A hypotensive anaesthetic technique reduces blood loss. Patients with obstructive sleep apnoea syndrome have airways which can present challenges to intubation. Consequently, jet ventilation equipment must be available. An awake fiberoptic intubation may be necessary to secure the airway. It is critical that the anaesthesiology team be competent in the management of the difficult airway.

After securing the endotracheal tube, the patient must be padded, the arms tucked and pneumatic compression devices placed on the lower extremities to prevent deep

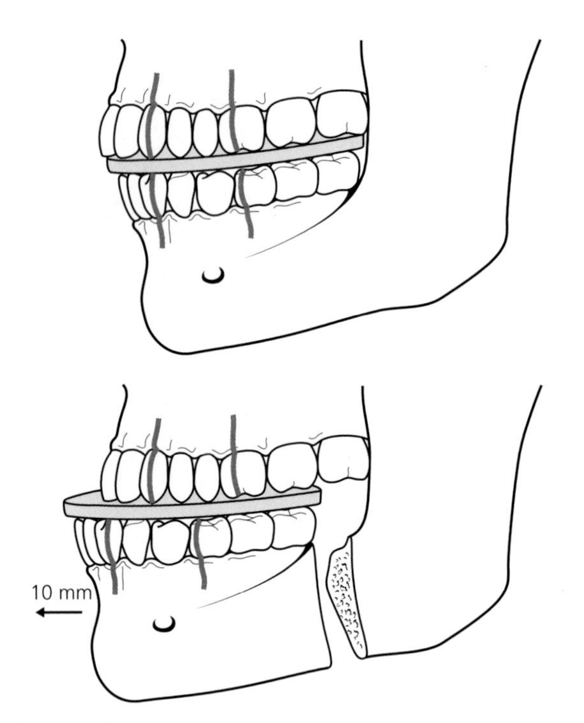

10.7.10 Dental models and surgical splint.

venous thrombosis. Surgery is directed to the mandible first. Local anaesthetic with epinephrine is injected along the anterior ramus in a standard fashion. The incision extends laterally along the mandibular body region and terminates in the molar region. A full thickness mucoperiosteal flap is elevated exposing the lateral ramus and body region. Dissection is then directed along the medial ramus region taking care to protect the inferior alveolar neurovascular bundle. A forked retractor is extended up the anterior ramus to the coronoid. A clamp is then used to retract the tissues. A horizontal osteotomy is then made through the medial coretex. The osteotomy then is continued anteriorly to the body of the mandible, staying medial to the external oblique ridge. It terminates in the1st or 2nd molar region depending on the amount of anterior movement required. A vertical osteotomy is then made in lateral body. A sagittal split is then made and the segments freely mobilized. The inferior alveolar nerve is gently mobilized from the proximal segment.

The acrylic splint is then affixed to the teeth and the jaws are wired shut and into the new desired occlusion.

The mandibular condyles are then seated into the most posterior-superior portion of the glenoid fossa. The bony segments are then clamped together and rigidly fixed together with titatnium bone plates and/or screws.

The jaws are then released and the occlusion and bony segments are checked for accuracy and stability with the condyles seated.

Attention is then directed to the maxilla. Once again, local anaesthetic with epinephrine is injected in the area of planned surgery.

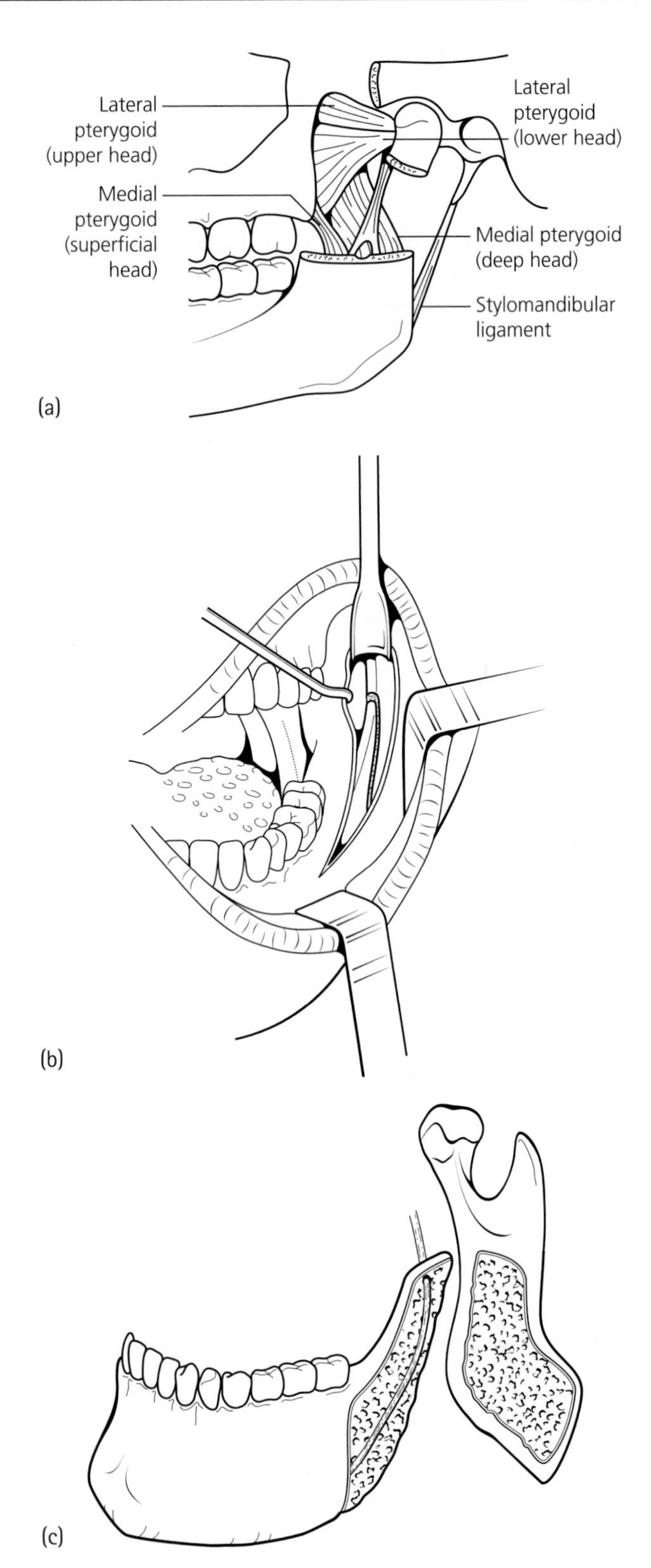

10.7.11 (a–c) Sagittal split advancement of the mandible, manually mobilise segments.

A modified incision is then made in the anterior maxillary vestibule with the electrocautery unit from the anterior maxilla and terminating in the zygomatic buttress region. A full thickness mucoperiosteal flap is elevated

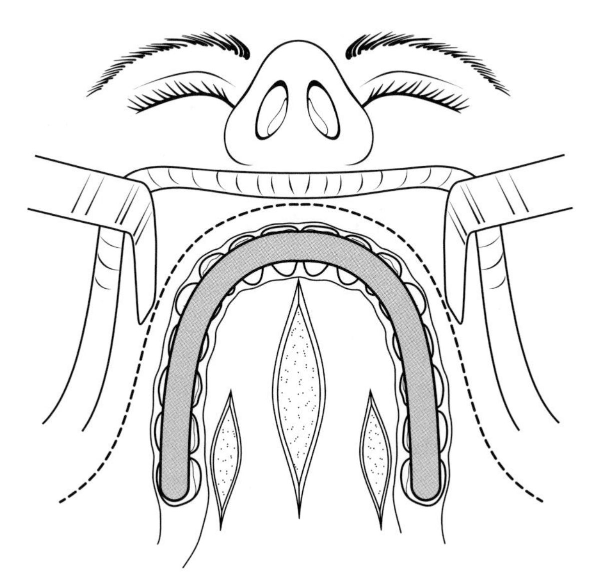

10.7.12 Attention is then directed to the maxilla. Once again, local anaesthetic with epinephrine is injected in the area if surgery is planned.

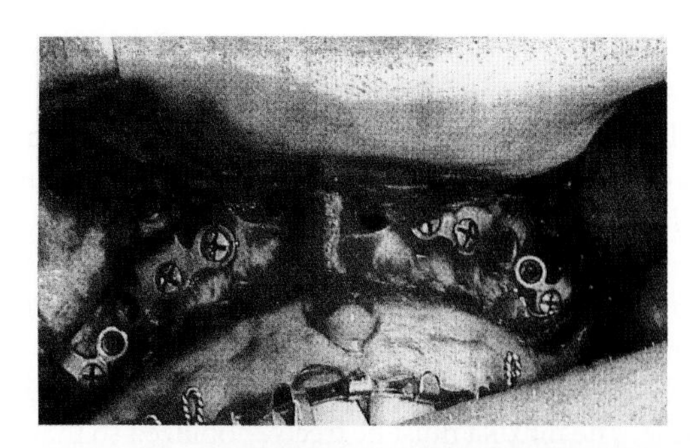

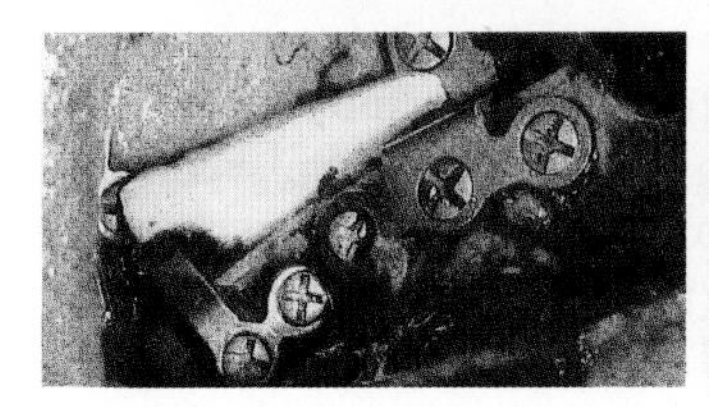

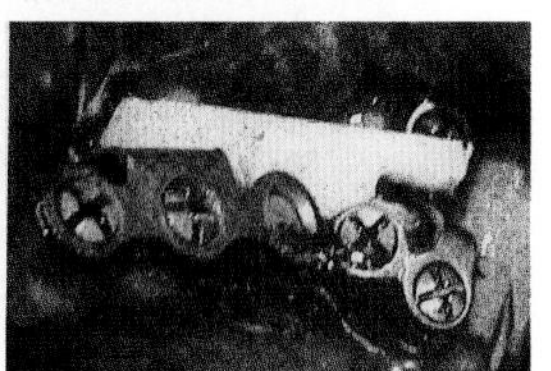

10.7.13 Maxilla with bone graft in place.

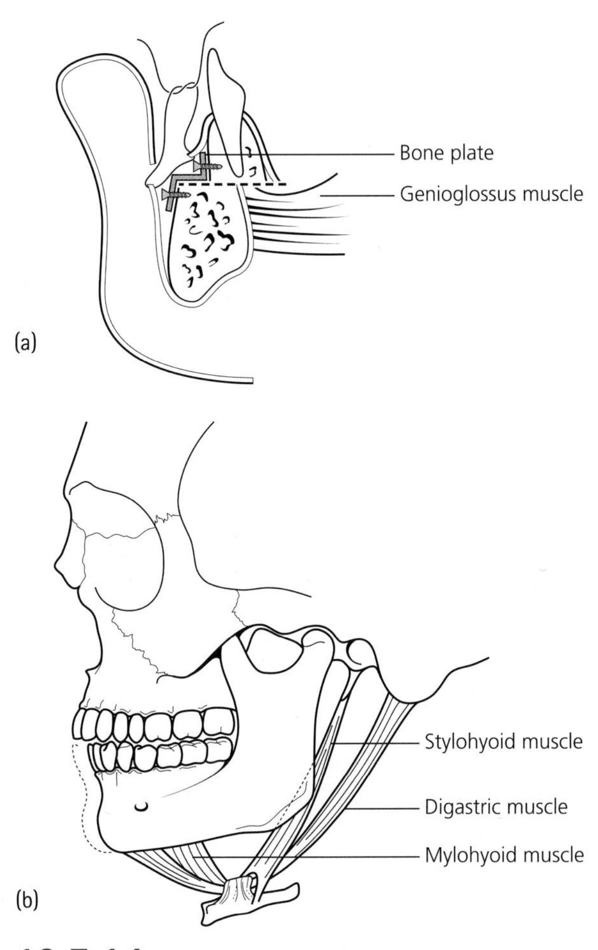

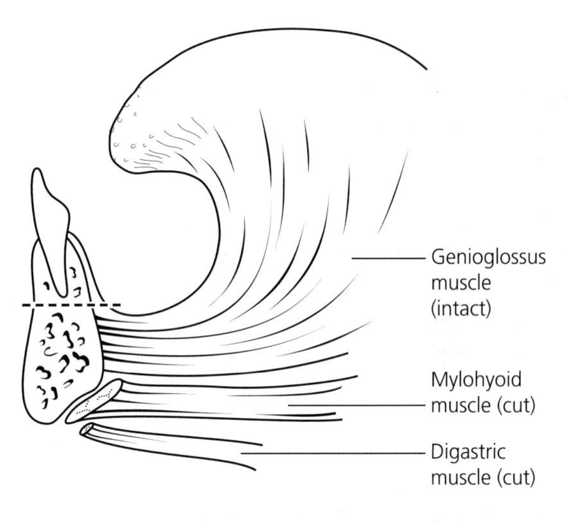

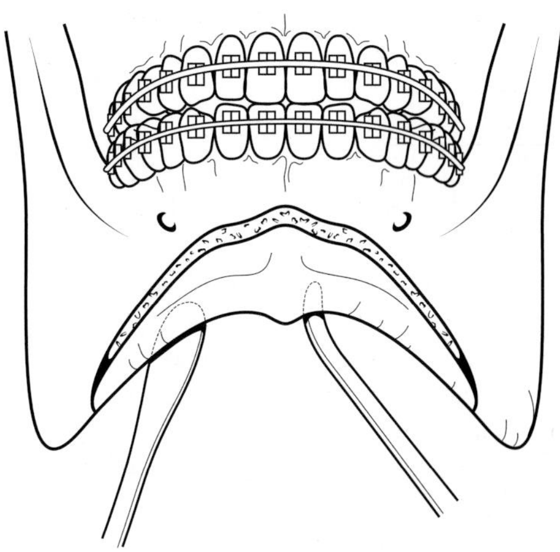

10.7.14 Geniotomy.

exposing the anterior maxilla. The anterior nasal spine is exposed and the nasal floor mucosa is elevated.

A horizontal osteotomy is made from the lateral pyriform rims extending posteriorly to the malar region. Osteotomes are then used to osteomotize the lateral nasal bony walls. A guarded osteotome is then used to achieve nasomaxillary separation. Finally a curved osteotome is used to achieve pterygomaxillary separation.

Disimpaction forceps are then used to downfracture the maxilla. The maxilla must be freely mobilized so that it will passively advance to its new anterior position.

The jaws are then brought back into the original occlusion taking great care to seat the mandibular condyles again. The jaws are wired together again. The advancement of the maxilla is such there is little bony overlap and this can result in poor stability. This can be addressed with the mortizing of a piece of cadaveric cortical bone between the segments.

Rigid fixation is then used in the pyriform rim and malar buttress regions with titanium plates and screws.

A demineralized bone matrix can be applied to the osteotomy sites along with a restorable membrane. This modification can result in a more rapid bony healing and lessens sinusitis issues from a large gap in the bony segments.

While the jaws are still wired together, attention is directed to the genial region. Once again, local anaesthetic with epinephrine is injected in the planned area of surgery.

An incision is then made in the labial mucosa and then advanced in a stepped fashion to the anterior genial region. The genial region is degloved. A horizontal osteotomy can be performed in the standard fashion or just the segment containing the genial tubercles.

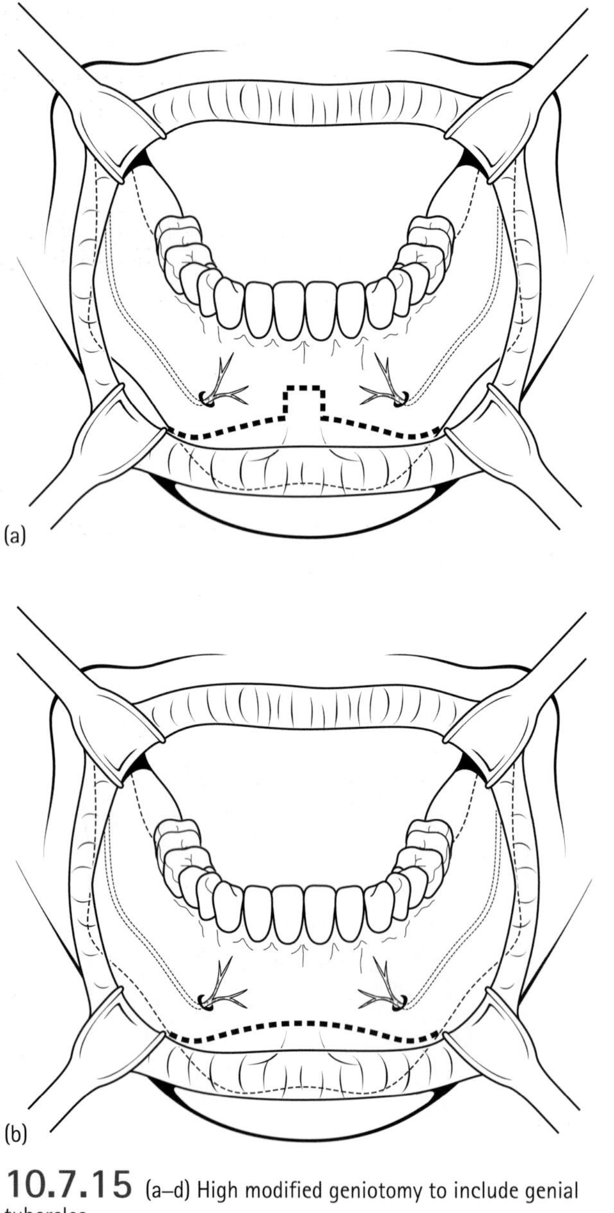

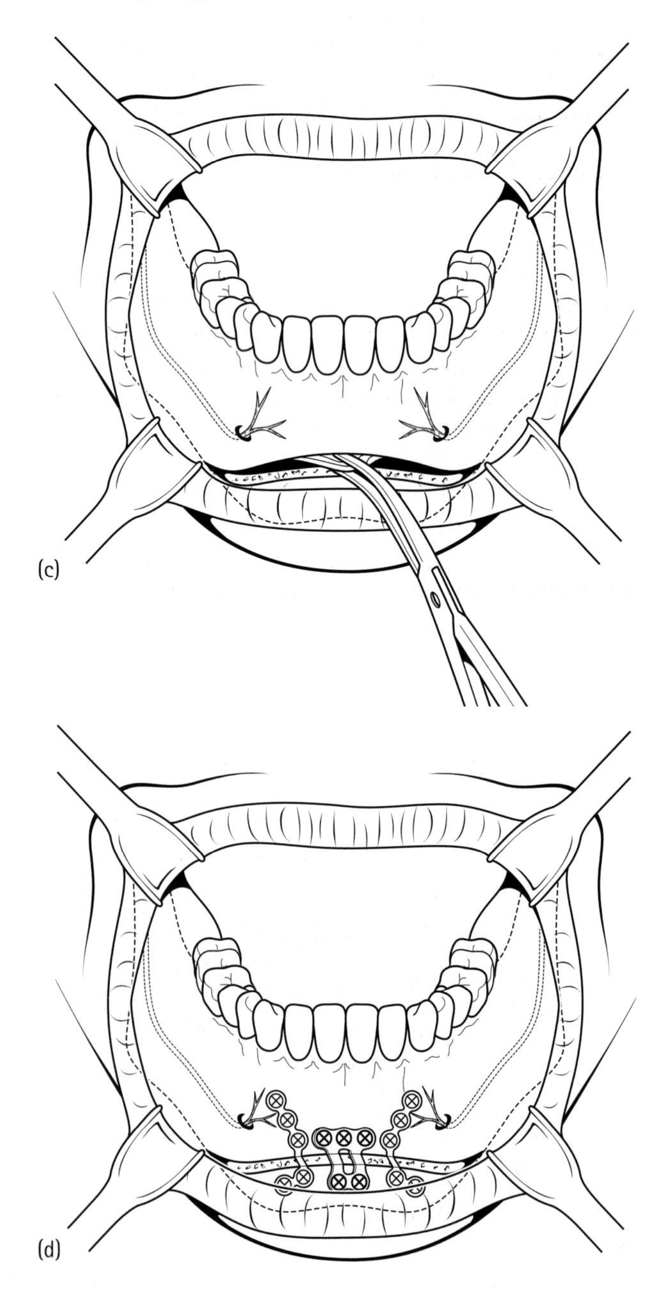

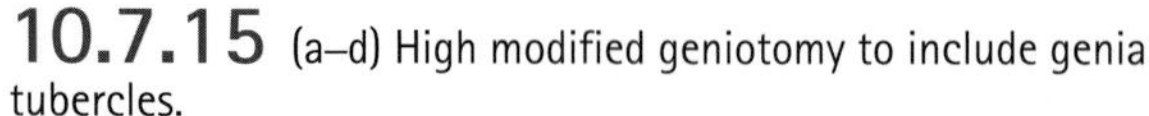

10.7.15 (a–d) High modified geniotomy to include genial tubercles.

It is critical that with each technique the genial tubercles be included in the mobilized segments.

The segment including the genial tubercles is advanced and secured with rigid fixation.

Attention is then directed to the hyoid region. The area of planned incision directly overlying the hyoid bone is marked with a pen. An incision is then made in the skin with the scalpel. Hemostasis is obtained. Blunt dissection is continued until the hyoid is encountered. The hyoid bone is exposed. Then, infra-hyoid muscles are released. Two permanent braided synthetic nonresorbable sutures are then passed around and under the hyoid laterally and passed subcutaneously up into the genial region. Two holes in the mobilized genial segment are made with the drill and the sutures passed through them. The sutures are then passed around and under the hyoid laterally and passed subcutaneously up into the genial region. Two holes in the mobilized genial segment are made with the drill and the sutures passed through them. The sutures are then tightened to the desired level of hyoid suspension and tied securely.

A modification of the hyoid suspension procedure shows promise.

In this technique the inferior body of the hyoid is stripped of muscle and then advanced over the thyroid cartilage and sutured to its superior aspect. The superior hyoid musculature is left intact.

Wound closure of the mandibular and hyoid regions can be accomplished in a standard fashion. However, closure of the maxillary wounds merits some elaboration. The standard technique using an alar cinch suture in the lateral nasal region to prevent unaesthetic widening of the nose should be used with caution. Since this surgery is for an airway problem, the alar cinch should not be so tight as to narrow the nasal airway.

The maxillary mucosa closure should incorporate a V-Y advancement to prevent wound contracture and undesired shortening of the upper lip.

After wound closure, a pressure dressing should be adapted to the mandibular regions.

Closure of the incision of the hyoid region is performed in a standard fashion after haemostasis has been obtained.

It is prudent to keep these patients intubated and in the intensive care unit overnight. As their clinical status dictates, they can usually be weaned and extubated on post-op day one. It is also wise to keep them in the intensive care unit one additional night after extubation.

The post-surgical management of the sleep apnoea patient is similar to other orthognathic patients, with a few exceptions. Their airways will hopefully be greatly improved after surgical intervention. Nonetheless, postsurgical oedema will impact their airway in a negative fashion until it resolves. In most cases the airway is so greatly improved that nasal CPAP is not necessary, even in the presence of post-surgical oedema.

In the personal experience of the authors, the post-surgical management of sleep apnoea surgery patients has been remarkably trouble-free. This supports the concept that once the airway is open for normal respiration during sleep, the associated co-morbidities are often ameliorated.

Top Tips

- Freely mobilize the osteotomized segments for passive advancement.
- Use bone grafts in the maxilla along with demineralized bone matrix and resorbable membranes to aid in complete bony union.
- Advance the hyoid so far to allow for some relapse, and still stent the airway open.
- Keep the patient sedated and on the ventilator for the first post-operative night.

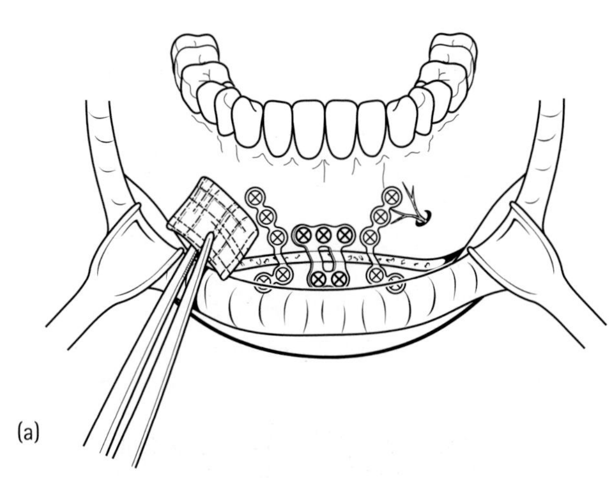

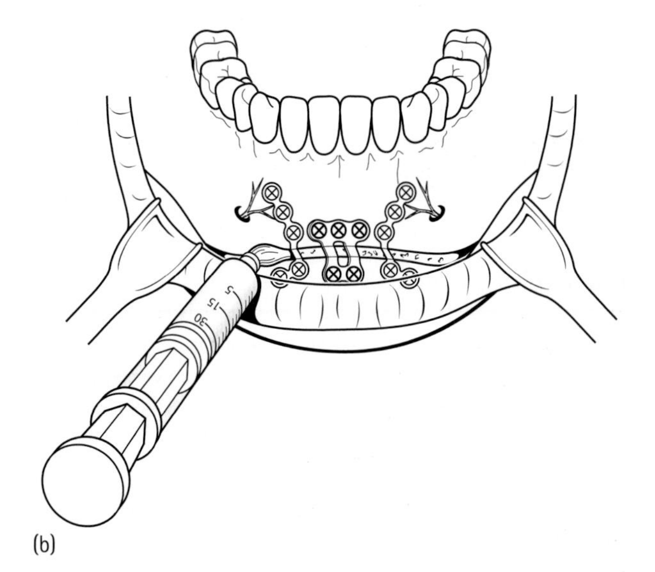

10.7.16 (a,b) Demineralized bone matrix to fill osteotomy gap.

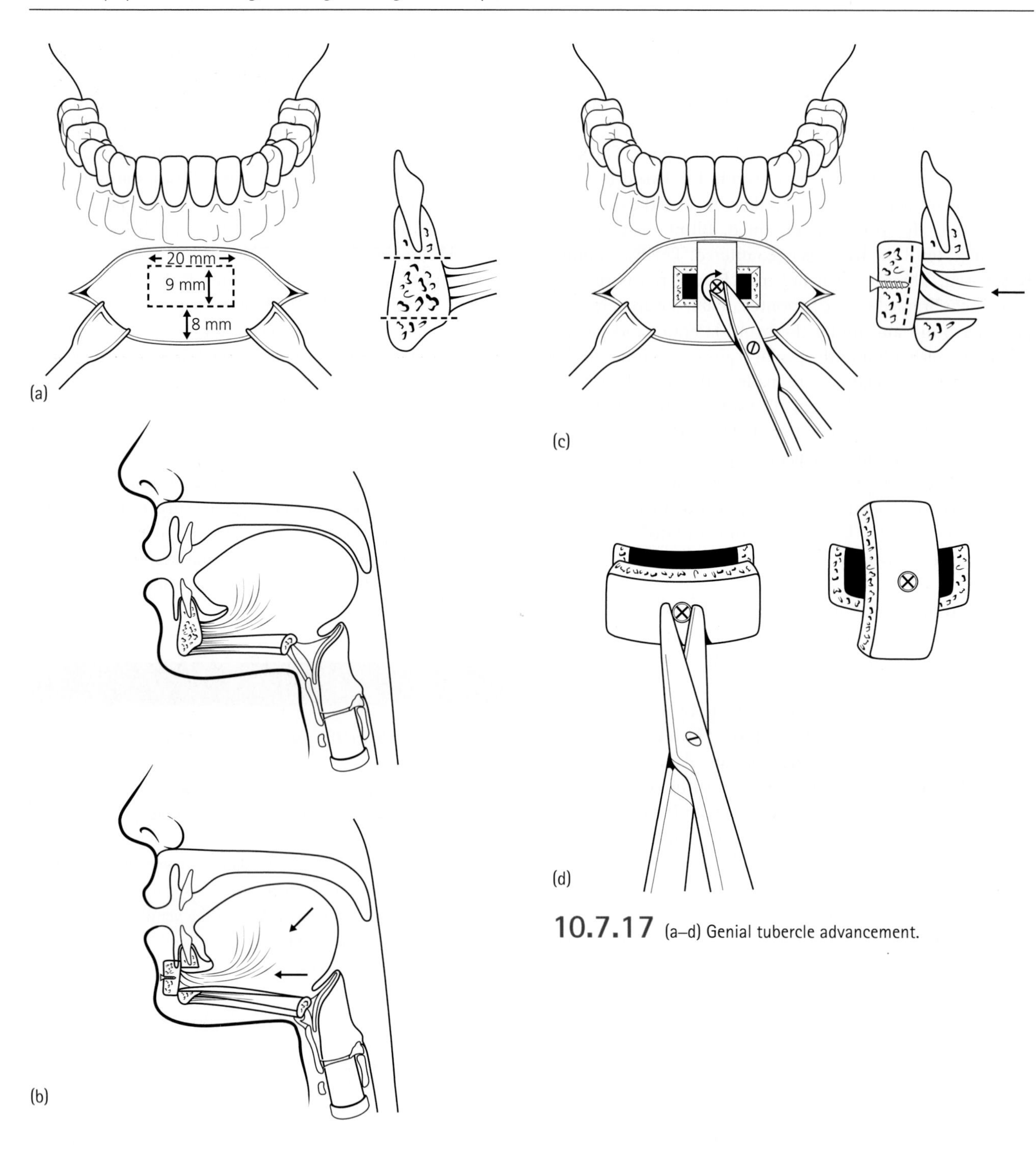

10.7.17 (a–d) Genial tubercle advancement.

FURTHER READING

Kribbs NB, Pack AI, Kline LR et al. Objective measurement of patterns of nasal CPAP by patients with obstructive sleep apnea. American Review of Respiratory Disease 1993; 149: 287–8.

Powell N, Riley RW, Guilleminault C, Murcia GN. Obstructive sleep apnea, continuous positive airway pressure and surgery. Otolaryngology–Head and Neck Surgery 1988; 99: 362–9.

Riley R, Powell N, Guilleminault C. Cephalometric roentgenograms and computerised tomographic scans in obstructive sleep apnea. Sleep 1986; 9: 514–15.

Riley R, Guilleminault C, Powell N, Derman S. Mandibular osteotomy and hyoid bone advancement for obstructive sleep apnea: a case report. Sleep 1984; 7: 79–82.

PART 11

FACIAL AESTHETIC SURGERY

11.1

Nonsurgical techniques: Botox, fillers

N RAVINDRANATHAN

INTRODUCTION

Methods of restoring facial aesthetics in a noninvasive or minimally invasive way are now well established. The armamentarium of the modern cosmetic surgeon includes Botox, fillers, commonly used peels, lasers and radiofrequency wave application. The skin is a major indicator of a person's age and health. With ageing, the dermis becomes thinner and the epidermis becomes thicker or thinner. There is, in addition, bone resorption, the appearance of furrows, wrinkles, crow's feet and platysmal bands in the neck. One of the main reasons why patients seek treatment for age changes is to restore soft tissue volume, contour and absorption or reduction of wrinkles and with the aim to restore a youthful appearance.

INDICATIONS

- Soft tissue atrophy, e.g. thinning of the lips.
- Appearance of crow's feet, glabella furrows.
- Lipoatrophy of the face, e.g. cheeks.
- Presence of all the features of ageing in the face and neck.
- Pigmentary dyscrasia of the skin associated with ageing.
- Bony resorption leading to reduction of facial bony contour, loss of facial height.

CASE SELECTION AND PRE-PROCEDURE PREPARATION (GENERAL PRINCIPLES)

- Any patient who wishes to look younger is a potential candidate for rejuvenation by noninvasive methods provided he or she fully understands what it is realistically possible to achieve and the known complications.
- In general, smokers and those who indulge in heavy or regular consumption of alcohol are not good candidates.
- Patients with adverse medical histories, for example uncontrolled diabetes, those on warfarin, abnormal bleeding disorders and those prone to developing frequent herpetic infections in the peri-oral region, etc., are not good candidates.

Medications containing aspirin and nonsteroidal anti-inflammatory agents should be discontinued at least 5–7 days before any minimally invasive surgical procedure. Likewise herbal formulations, gingko biloba, ginseng, garlic and ginger should also be discontinued. Minimally invasive procedures such as injection of fillers intradermally should be avoided during active acne eruptions.

Patients should be given a detailed explanation regarding the likely outcome of the procedure and techniques involved, materials being used and their known adverse effects before any procedure is undertaken.

FILLERS

Soft tissue augmentation may be accomplished by surgery or intradermal injection of synthetic implants or biologic implants. Soft tissue augmentation using various filler materials has gained enormous popularity as there is no recovery time and can be conveniently undertaken at the end of a week to allow recovery during a weekend.

IDEAL PROPERTIES OF A FILLER

Ideally, it should be of non-animal origin, biocompatible, biodegradable, low risk of allergic reaction, easy to use and have minimal side effects such as bruising, infection, migration and tissue reaction.

An injectable filler should be able to restore facial contour. There are several fillers available and they include:

- autogenous fat;
- autogenous dermis;
- synthetic poly L-lactic acid;
- liquid silicone;
- collagen, polymethylmethacrylate microspheres/collagen;

- hyaluronic acid derivatives;
- expanded polytetrafluoroethylene.

PRINCIPLES OF AUTOGENOUS FAT INJECTION AS FILLERS

- Autologous fat is harvested with an open tipped blunt cannula under tumescent anaesthesia.
- Harvested fat is transferred to 1 mL syringes for injection into the areas concerned.
- Injection of fat into the deep tissues of the face is carried out using a small bore blunt cannula.
- Any patient who wishes to restore their facial contour to their youthful appearance would be a good candidate for pan facial fat augmentation.
- Any patient who has a recent history of deep venous thrombosis, pulmonary embolism, compromised liver function, allergy to lignocaine, coagulopathy or inability to stop anticoagulant drugs is contraindicated for fat augmentation.

TECHNIQUES OF FAT HARVESTING AND TRANSFER

1. Pre-operative assessment using photographs. Discuss with the patient areas for augmentation. If adjunctive microliposuction is planned, e.g. neck, jowls, indicate on photograph. An A4 photograph permits a large image for discussion. Take frontal, lateral and inferior oblique views.
2. Laboratory work-up includes urine pregnancy test if premenopausal, clotting profile, full blood count, renal and liver profiles.
3. An antibiotic is administered orally or intravenously 1 hour before the procedure. A first generation cephalosporin is preferred.
4. Tumescent anesthesia solution is prepared using 500 mL Ringer's Lactate, 0.5 mg of epinephrine, 1 per cent lignocaine 25 mL. Anaesthetic solution is administered into the prospective donor site for fat harvest (Figure 11.1.1). I prefer the anterior abdominal wall (Figure 11.1.2) or lateral outer thigh. When local anaesthetic has taken effect, make an incision with size 11 blade as a stab and introduce a curved haemostat to create a subcutaneous tunnel (Figure 11.1.3). Other areas which can be used are hips or posterior waist. Subsequently, the tumescent solution is infiltrated (Figure 11.1.4). After injection wait 15–20 minutes.
5. A low negative pressure is created in a 10 mL syringe. An open tipped cannula (Figure 11.1.5) is attached to the syringe and is inserted into the donor site through the same small stab incision. The cannula is moved back and forth within the donor site 1 cm below the skin surface. This will help to avoid surface irregularities.

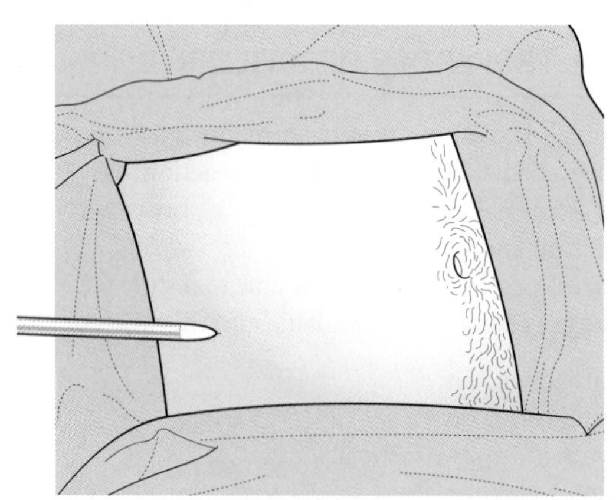

11.1.1 Infiltrating local anaesthesia.

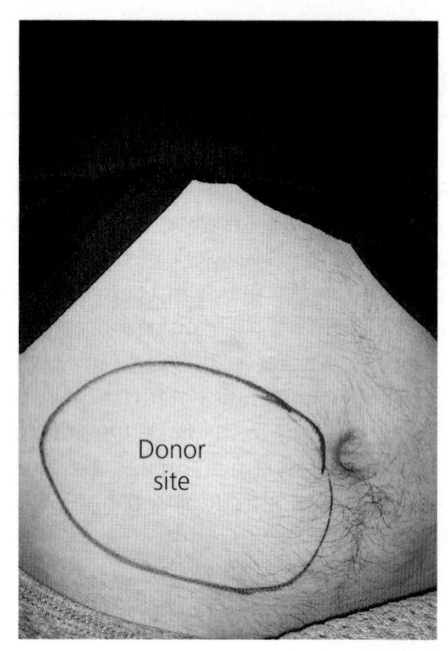

11.1.2 Anterior abdominal wall donor site.

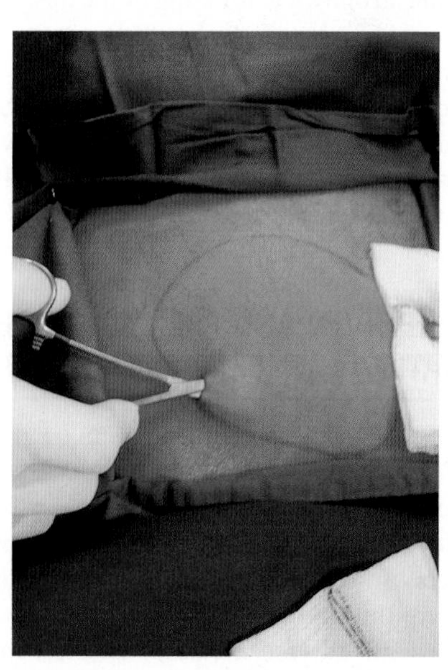

11.1.3 Creating a subcutaneous tunnel to inject tumescent solution.

The plunger of the syringe containing the harvested fat is pushed, the cannula removed and the syringe is capped (Figure 11.1.6) and allowed to stand in a test tube. Centrifuge the collected fat in 10 mL syringes placed in a centrifuging machine at 3400 rpm for 20 seconds. The centrifuged fat will separate from an infranatant. The infranatant consists of, at the top, liquid triglyceride, blood and tumescent fluid, and below, the fat (Figure 11.1.7). Carefully decant off the top layer. Transfer the fat from the 10 mL syringes into 2 mL syringes using a connector (Figure 11.1.8). From these syringes, using special cannulas, fat is injected into the recipient sites which have been marked at the commencement of the procedure (Figure 11.1.9).

6 Injection of fat is carried out with blunt cannulas and the injection is done as a 'layering' technique (Figures 11.1.10–11.1.12). If injection is done in the forehead, small incisions are made at the hairline. Injection is done in a plane above the galea. Fat can be transferred to the glabella, forehead, upper eyelids and brow. Fat can also be injected into the lower eyelid, for example when too much fat had been removed during blepharoplasty or tear trough deformities seen in ageing. In this area, fat is injected in a subcutaneous plane.
7 Fat augmentation of the buccal area is via a stab incision made anterior to the upper end of the ear and is in a superficial plane making radial fan-like

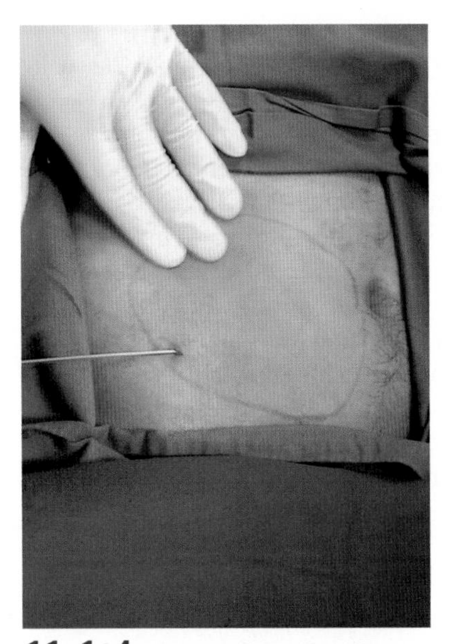

11.1.4 Infiltration of tumescent solution.

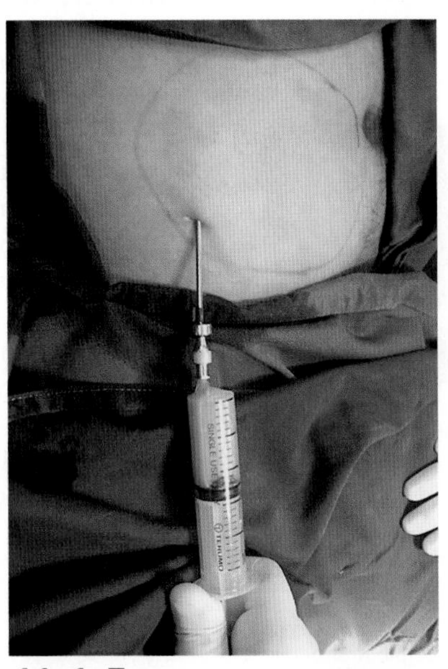

11.1.5 Aspiration of fat using 10 mL syringe from anterior abdominal wall.

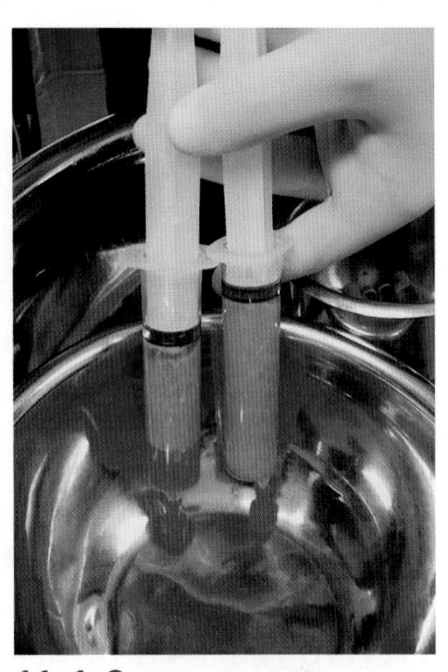

11.1.6 Fat in harvested syringes.

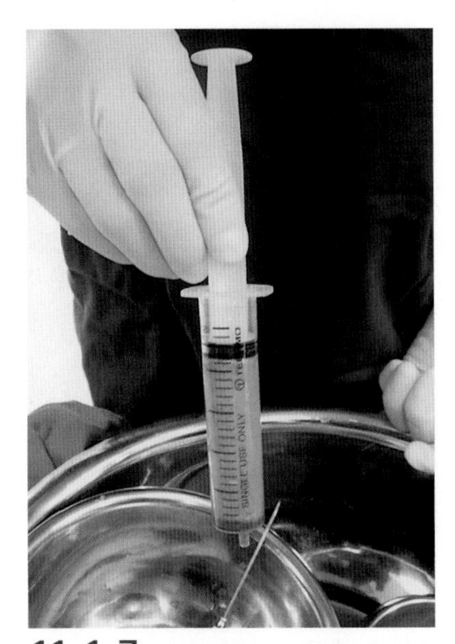

11.1.7 Harvested fat in 10 mL syringe allowed to stand vertically, supernatant fluid is injected.

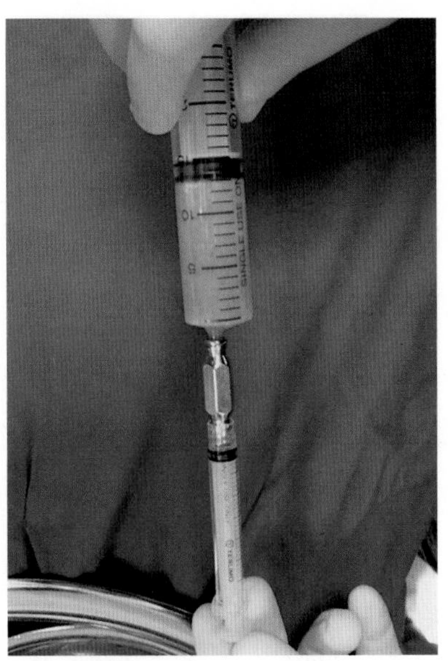

11.1.8 Harvested fat in 10 mL syringe being transferred from 10 mL syringe to 2 mL syringe via a connector.

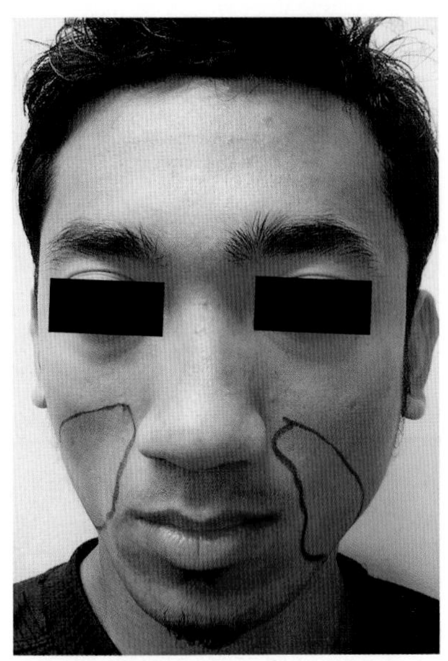

11.1.9 Recipient sites – bilateral nasolabial folds, subcutaneous atrophy (variant of Romberg's disease).

movements. Fat augmentation can also be carried out to enhance the lower jaw border, chin prominence, cheek prominence by infiltration in a deep plane and layering in a plane superficial to this. In the peri-oral area, vertical ageing lines and lips can be augmented. Prior to introduction of the fat, to augment the lips, carry out an incision between the muscle and the skin and introduce fat into this plane. The vermillion of the lips can also be enhanced and for this purpose use a 20 gauge needle. Typically, the author uses approximately 3 mL for the upper and 2–3 mL for the lower lip.

8 Fat augmentation can also be successfully used in the nasolabial creases and labiomental creases (Figure 11.1.13).

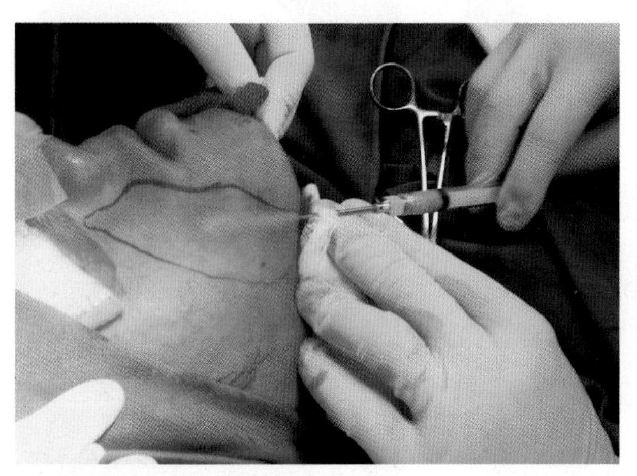

11.1.10 Harvested fat being injected into recipient site.

POST-OPERATIVE INSTRUCTIONS AND CARE AFTER FAT TRANSFER

- As oedema after fat transfer by blunt infiltration can be profound, prescribe oral steroids in a dose of 40 mg prednisolone 1 hour before the procedure and a daily dose post-operatively for 2 days.
- Ice packs for 48 hours for at least 20 minutes per hour.
- Medications such as aspirin, plavix, blood thinning supplements or vitamin E should be avoided for 72 hours.
- No active physical exercise, such as jogging, weight training or swimming, should be undertaken for 1 week.

COMPLICATIONS

- Oedema, contour irregularities, echymosis (usually temporary).
- Infection and submandibular lymphadenitis.
- Fat embolism resulting in cerebral infarction and or sudden blindness (a rare complication).
- Fat cysts or hard nodules. These are treated initially by an injection of triamcinolone. If this does not resolve after two injections, a direct excision is carried out.
- Post-inflammatory pigmentation is sometimes seen and it is best treated upon recognition with hydroquinone 4 per cent for 4–12 weeks. If there is no response, intensity pulse light (IPL) can be used and, with two or three sessions, it should resolve.

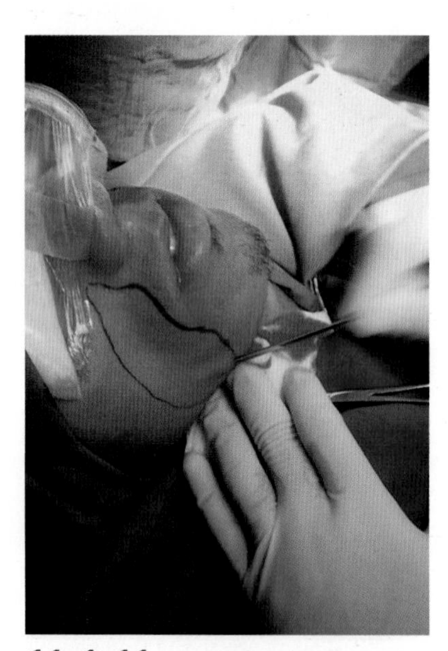

11.1.11 Harvested fat being injected into recipient site.

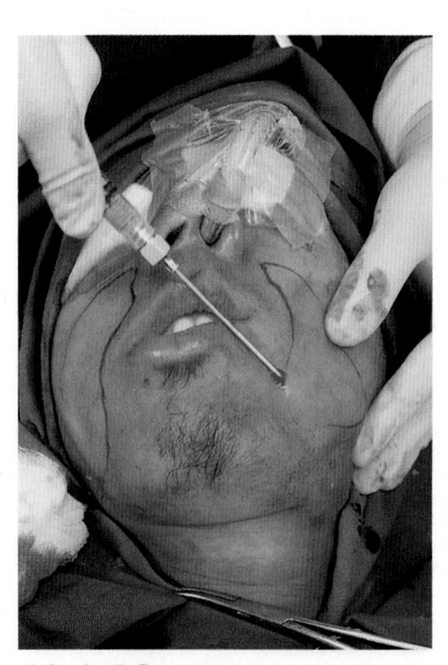

11.1.12 Injection of harvested fat into recipient area.

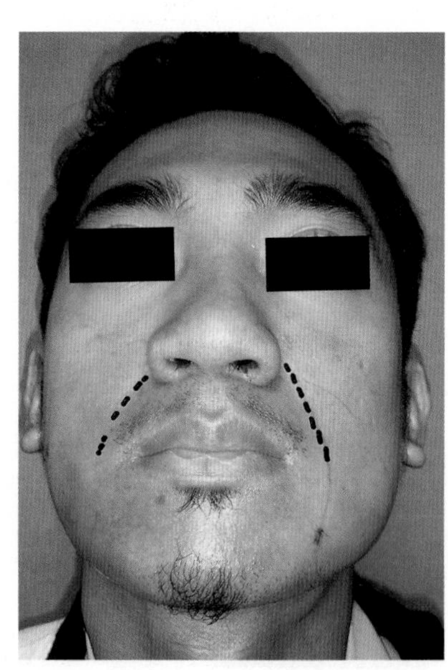

11.1.13 Appearance after injection of fat into recipient areas (4 weeks after injection).

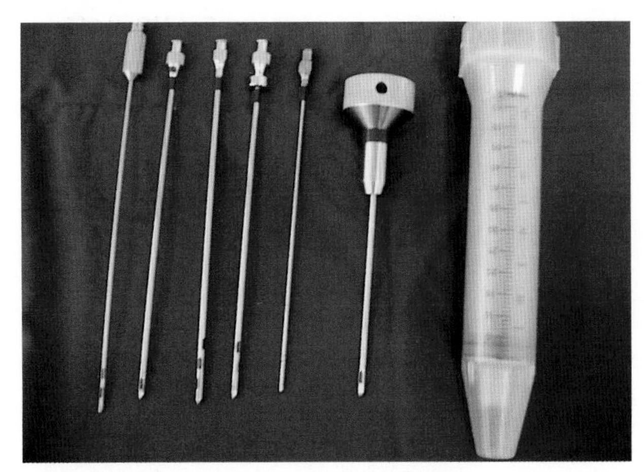

11.1.14 Illustrates 60 mL Tulip syringe and various aspiration cannulas useful for harvesting fat from donor site.

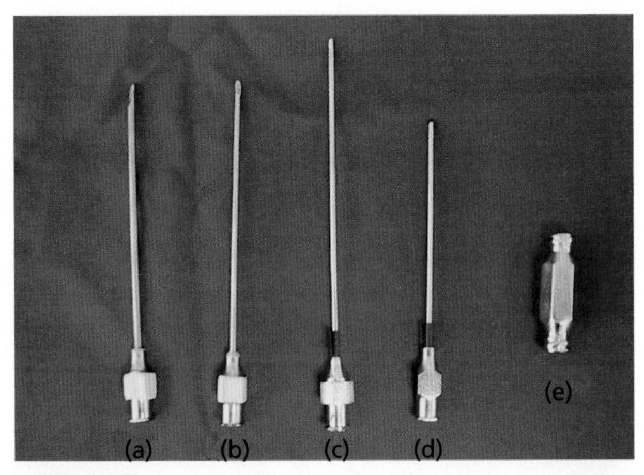

11.1.15 (a)–(d) Cannulas for injection of fat. (e) Connector used to transfer fat from 10 mL syringe to 3 mL syringe.

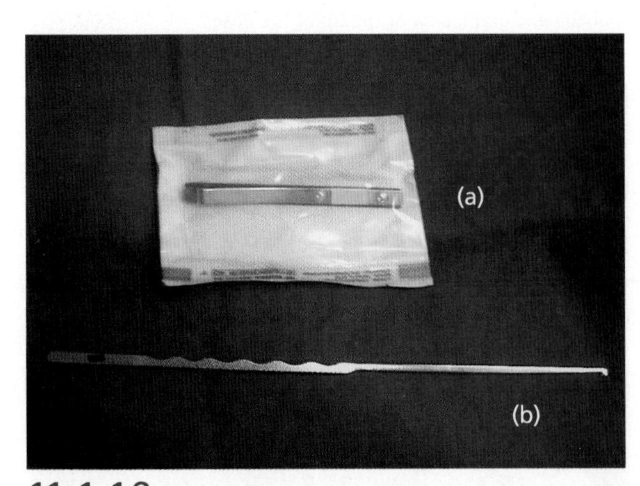

11.1.16 (a) Plunger to be fitted into syringe to maintain negative pressure. (b) Wilkinson dissector to create subcutaneous tunnel by sharp dissection.

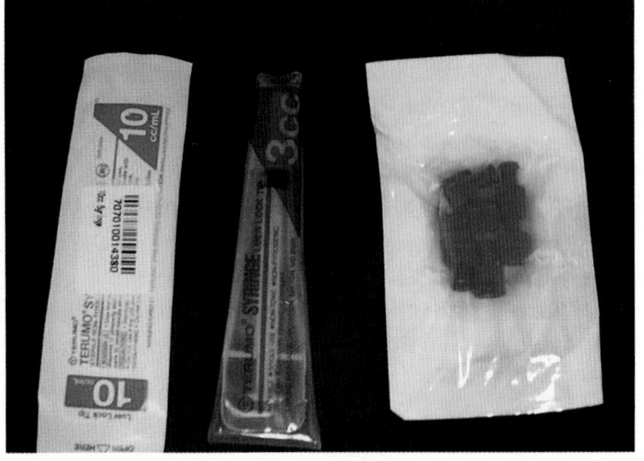

11.1.17 Three mL, 10 mL syringe (luer-lock) and stops (sterile) to insert onto the syringe to contain the harvested fat.

SYNTHETIC FILLERS

Polymers of lactic acid are currently available commercially as injectable poly-L-lactic acid, a biodegradable polymer. They are in the same family of aliphatic polyesters as glycolic and citric acid. They are available as microparticles measuring 40–63 microns in diameter suspended in sodium carboxymethylcellulose. Upon injection into the subcutaneous tissue or deep intradermal space, it undergoes gradual degradation over a period of years and there is increased collagen fibre formation around the microparticles with the passage of time.

It is available as a lyophilized powder and reconstituted with 3–5 mL sterile water. The powder is mixed thoroughly with water to achieve a homogenous mix and the preparation is carried out preferably 2 hours before the injection. The author prefers to use 5 mL dilution except in cases where there is marked lipoatrophy when 3 mL dilution is used. I usually apply EMLA cream topically 45 minutes before injection or give a local anaesthesia. Upon injection, a sculpting massage is carried out for approximately 2–3 minutes. The injection can be repeated at 4-weekly intervals.

The author has used this product as a filler for deep nasolabial folds, as a subperiosteal injection over the dorsum of the nose for subtle augmentation and subperiosteally in the lower orbital rim for teartrough deformities. Granuloma formation has been encountered in two of ten patients. The granuloma was difficult to treat and hyaluronic acid derivatives are now used instead.

For several years, bovine collagen was the gold standard as a soft tissue augmentation material. However, it is only short lived and serious hypersensivity reactions have been reported. To overcome this, human based collagen has been used. Hyaluronic acid based fillers are ideal because they are less immunogenic and have a longer duration effect than collagen. Patient tolerability is good. Hyaluronic acid in smaller particles are marketed by Q-Med Uppsala as Restylane and larger particles as Perlane. Restylane usually lasts approximately six months and Perlane can last 6–12 months. The same company is about to launch hyaluronic acid of even greater size (Macrolane). The hyaluronic acid injections can be repeated at 4–6 monthly intervals. These fillers are a useful adjunct in facial cosmetic procedures. They very rarely cause allergic reaction. The US Food and Drug Administration (FDA) has approved hyaluronic acid (Restylane) as a filler for nasolabial fold augmentation. Injection-related side effects include bruising, erythema, pruritis and discolouration. Sometimes granulomas occur and they respond well to injection of corticosteroids followed by massage.

TECHNIQUE FOR NASOLABIAL FOLD

Prior to injection, the area is cleaned with an antiseptic solution. A local anaesthetic is used. The filler of hyaluronic acid origin is injected into the deep and mid dermis with Perlane and subsequently Restylane is used for surface feathering. The material is injected while withdrawing the needle. Complications include bruising, bleeding, swelling and uneven surface irregularities (rarely), discolouration of skin, pruritus and delayed skin reactions.

SILICONE OIL

Silicone oil has been used in its injectable form for filling defects of the facial soft tissue in HIV positive patients who develop lipodystrophy. Use of silicone in its liquid form as a filler is controversial. Currently, the FDA has approved liquid silicone for retinal tamponade (a viscous compound of 5000 centistokes) manufactured by Bausch & Lomb, CA, USA. The duration is longer according to particle size. Silicone liquid of 1000 centistokes manufactured by Alcon Labs, Fortworth, TX, USA is also useful for soft tissue augmentation. It is inexpensive, can be sterilized, does not permit bacterial growth and it can be stored without refrigeration. Currently, there are multicentre trials in progress using liquid silicone oil for soft tissue augmentation. Silicone is best used without complication only in small amounts.

Indications for using silicone oil

- Contour defects.
- Photoageing resulting in rhytides.
- Atrophy of skin following corticosteroid injections.
- Linear sclerodema.

Contraindications

- Do not inject large volumes, risk of embolism.
- Patients with autoimmune disorders.
- Patients with multiple allergies.
- Patients who have complications due to silicone injection by another practitioner.

Technique of injection

1 Inject as microdroplet technique using very small amounts into deep dermis.
2 Treatment can be repeated after 6 weeks.

Complications

- Migration of injected silicone.
- Facial skin necrosis, granuloma formation, formation of nodules (Figure 11.1.18, showing granuloma formation over dorsum of nose).
- When injected superficially, it produces erythema over the overlying skin and recurrent inflammatory oedema (Figure 11.1.19, showing erythema over dorsum of nose).
- Over the injected area, a definite demarcation appears.
- The only way to prevent complications is strictly use only small amounts of pure silicone oil.
- Delayed reactions such as rosacea and rosacea-like syndromes can develop years after injection. Likewise, granulomas can develop years later.

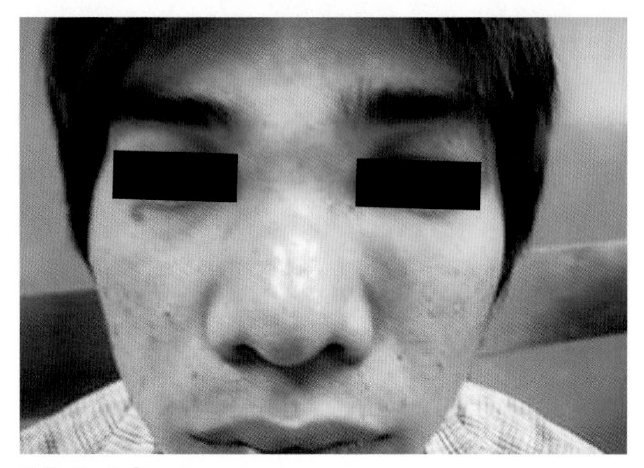

11.1.18 Injected silicone producing nodule over the glabella and granuloma at the tip of the nose.

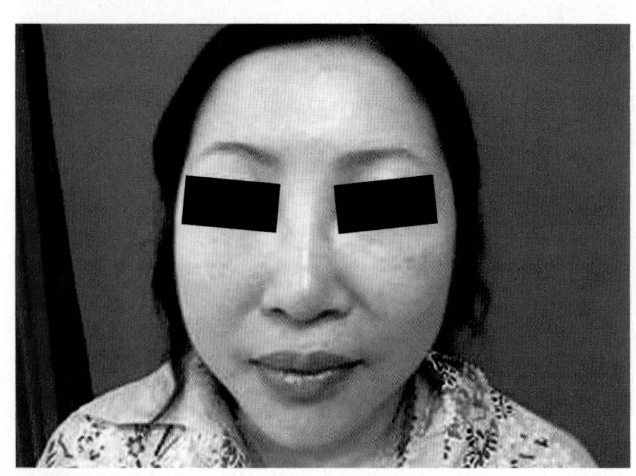

11.1.19 Injected silicone producing erythema.

Treatment of silicone-induced granulomas

- Oral prednisolone starting with 40 mg per day and tapering over 10 days.
- Intralesional corticosteroid injection starting at 5 mg/cc and increasing up to 30 mg/cc every 3 weeks.
- Minocycline simultaneously 100–200 mg per day for up to 2–4 weeks.

POLYMETHYLMETHACRYLATE MICROSPHERES (ARTEFILL, ARTECOLL)

This product has been approved by the FDA as a soft tissue augmentation material. It is a suspension of polymethylmethacrylate microspheres in 3.5 per cent bovine collagen. It is useful to fill subcutaneous atrophy and atrophy of the buccal fat pad. It is best to inject small amounts each visit in incremental doses 4–6 weeks apart as it is a permanent filler.

Complications

- Beading, ridging, formation of nodules.
- Granulomas and nodule formation can occur after years. The author has encountered this in a patient who had it injected three years previously. If the nodule does not respond to corticosteroid injection, excision would be the choice.
- Artecoll should not be used in areas of thin skin, e.g. lower eyelid.

Technique

- Artecoll should not be injected intradermally. It should only be injected subdermally.
- It is best to inject it in very small amounts incrementally.

Contraindications

- Allergy to bovine collagen.
- Those prone to develop keloids.

Note: As bovine collagen is the vehicle for the microsphere particles, allergy testing must be carried out prior to use.

POLYACRYLAMIDE HYDROGEL (AQUAMID)

In the last few years, the author has used this product as the preferred choice. It is supplied in 1 mL syringes as an injectable form containing 97.5 per cent non-pyrogenic water. It is long lasting, biocompatible and does not migrate from the site of injection. It contains no animal extracts and has been authorized for sale in Europe since March 2001 and requires no prior testing.

Indications

- Cheek remodelling.
- Treatment of perioral wrinkles.
- Lip augmentation (Figures 11.1.20 and 11.1.21).
- For elimination of nasolabial folds.
- For correction of depressed scars (Figures 11.1.22 and 11.1.23).
- Treatment of deep wrinkles.
- For subtle dorsal nasal augmentation.

Technique

- It is best injected under local anaesthesia by an appropriate nerve block. It is best to use 27G needle for injection.
- Injection must be carried out under sterile conditions.
- Inject while withdrawing the needle in a retrograde manner.
- After injection, perform gentle massaging.
- Do not overcorrect.

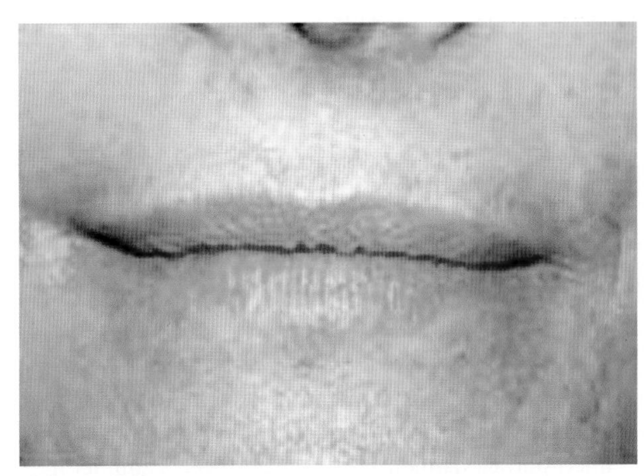

11.1.20 Pre-operative – pre lip augmentation.

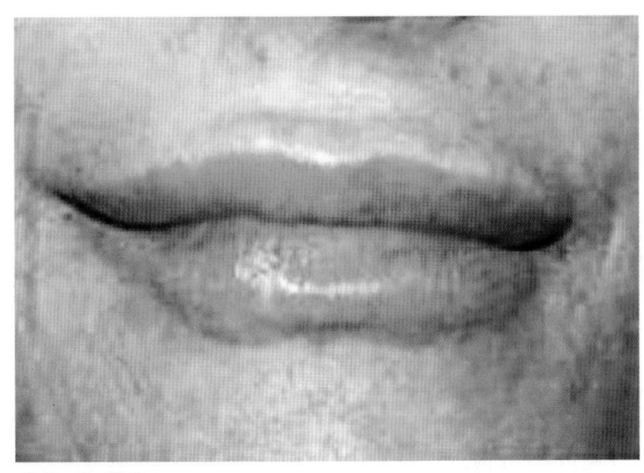

11.1.21 Six months after lip augmentation with 'Aquamid' (Polyacrylamide).

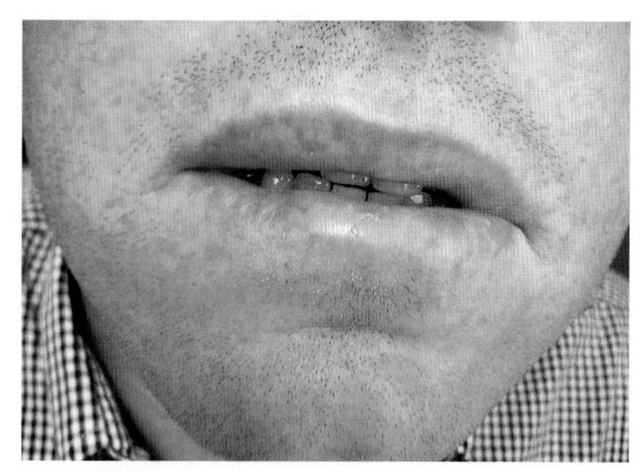

11.1.22 Lower right myomucosal deformity following traumatic injury.

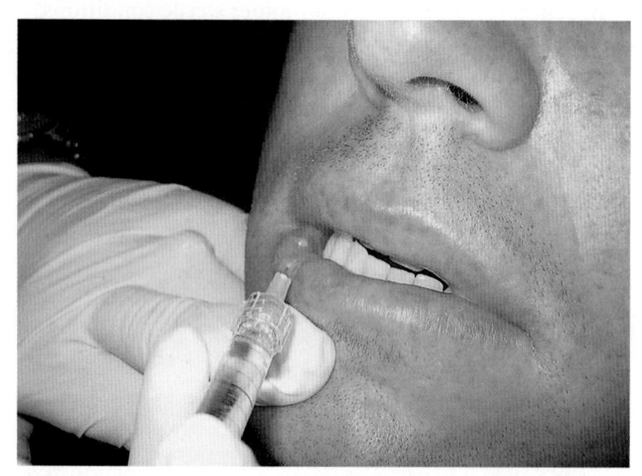

11.1.23 Injection of 'Perlane' (hyaluronic acid) into the lip deformity – submucosally.

- If in doubt, add in increments as a touch up a week later.
- The gel should not be injected intradermally. Do not inject polyacrylamide gel into an area where another filler has been injected previously until absorption has been complete.

Contraindications

- Do not inject sites where there is active skin disease or inflammation.
- Do not inject in lactating mothers or during pregnancy.
- Injection when herpes labialis is present should not be carried out.

Post-operative instruction after injection

- Ice pack application locally for 48 hours for at least 20 minutes per hour for 12 hours.
- Avoid direct sun exposure for 24 hours.

Complications

- Bruising and oedema.
- In very few instances, allergic reactions have been reported.

Adverse reaction to dermal fillers and implications

In general, injectable fillers can result in adverse reactions and complications and are summarized below:

- reactions at the site of injection – pain, bruising, oedema, erythema, itchiness;
- infection;
- hypersensitivity reactions – erythema, nodules, formation of granulomas resulting in lumps;
- discolouration may be as redness or hyperpigmentation;
- necrosis of the skin overlying the injected site;
- migration of injected implant;
- embolism;
- blindness.

BOTULINUM TOXIN TYPE A (BOTOX)

Facial enhancement using Botox (Alergan Inc, Irvine, CA, USA) is a safe and effective procedure for the abolition of lines and wrinkles on the face. Lines typically occur due to muscular contractions of the facial muscles (Figure 11.1.24, showing facial muscles). Botulinum toxin type A can temporarily eliminate these lines and enhance the effect of laser resurfacing procedures. It is now well accepted by cosmetic surgeons that pretreatment of wrinkles and lines due to hyperfunctioning of the muscles with Botox followed by laser resurfacing gives optimal results.

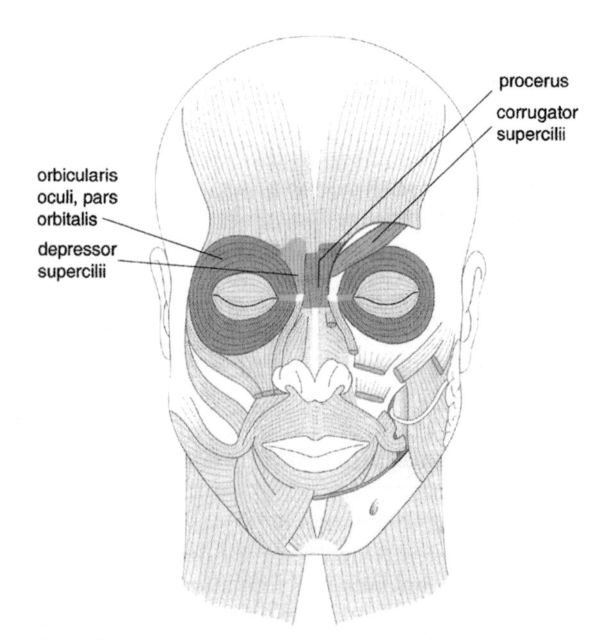

11.1.24 Showing facial muscles six months after Botox injected into the forehead and glabella complex (forehead 12 units, glabella 20 units).

It has been observed that, in Asians, resurfacing results in troublesome pigmentary complications and hence it is not a good option for elimination of wrinkles and lines. Botox is the best primary line of treatment for abolition of these lines. In Caucasians, where skin resurfacing is undertaken for facial rejuvenation, rhytides can reappear after resurfacing, particularly in the glabella and crow's feet area.

PREPARATION AND RECOMMENDED METHOD FOR USAGE

Botox is supplied in a vial which contains 100 units of vacuum dried complex of neurotoxin (Figure 11.1.25). Dilute this with 2 or 2.5 mL of 0.9 per cent preservative free saline to a concentration of either five or four units per 0.1 mL dilution. In most instances, use 2 ml dilution as it minimizes diffusion of the solution to neighbouring muscle groups. Upon reconstitution with preservative-free saline, it can be stored at 4°C and be used with no decrease in efficacy for up to 2 weeks.

Technique of mixing

1 Open the bottle of Botox (botulinum toxin A) by removing the cap.
2 The rubber cover is sterile and does not need to be wiped with spirit swab.
3 Two or 2.5 mL of saline, either preservative free, is drawn up in a 2.5 mL syringe with a size 25-Gauge needle with no air bubbles.
4 The syringe containing saline is held vertically and the needle pierces through the rubber bung of the freeze-dried Botox vial. There is no necessity to inject as the negative pressure in the bottle will suck in the saline. The bottle should not be shaken but gently rolled between the palms of the hands to ensure a good, even mix.
5 The mixed Botox solution is now drawn through the 25-Gauge needle into insulin syringes. Use either a 30-Gauge half-inch or 32-Gauge half-inch needle attached to the insulin syringe to inject the Botox.

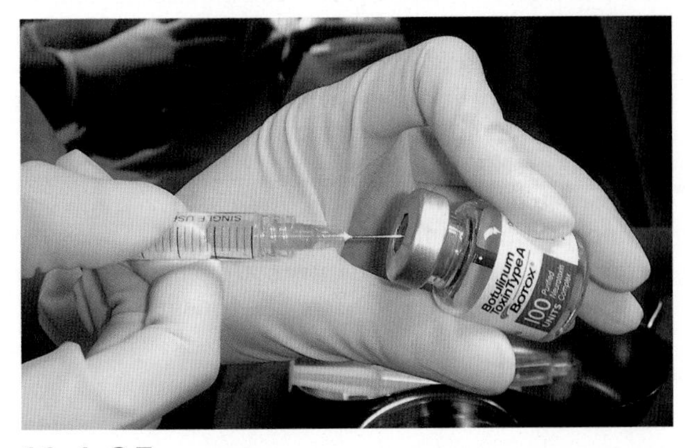

11.1.25 Showing Botox vial (100 units) 2 cc of preservative free saline is being injected.

Injection technique and dosing for various sites

In order to reduce pain, always use ice application to the area concerned for at least 10 minutes and after injection for another 5–10 minutes. Upon injection, it should not be massaged as this will result in rapid diffusion producing undesired side effects.

The number of units to be injected depends on:

- the specific region;
- muscle mass (gender dependent);
- skin thickness (thicker skin in some Asians will require a higher dose).

Table 11.1.1 illustrates the units used for the various applications in facial rejuvenation.

The following illustrates the various sites for injection:

- Glabella complex (Figure 11.1.26);
- Forehead horizontal lines (Figure 11.1.27);
- Crow's feet (Figure 11.1.28);
- Bunny lines (Figure 11.1.29);
- Dimpled chin (Figure 11.2.30).

When injecting into the muscle mass, the injection needle should be perpendicular to the skin and into the muscle. In areas where skin is thin, for example periocular, the injection needle should be in a subcutaneous plane.

Table 11.1.1 Units used for various applications in facial rejuvenation.

Sites	No. units (average)
Corrugators – glabella complex	Women 20
Procerus – glabella complex	Men 30
Orbiculars oculi – crow's feet	Per side 12–14
Horizontal lines on the forehead	Women 15, men 24
Brow rejuvenation	4 units per side
Masseteric hypertrophy	Women 30, men 35
Bunny lines on the nose	3
Lines along the lateral wall of the nose	4
Poppy chin	Women 5, men 8

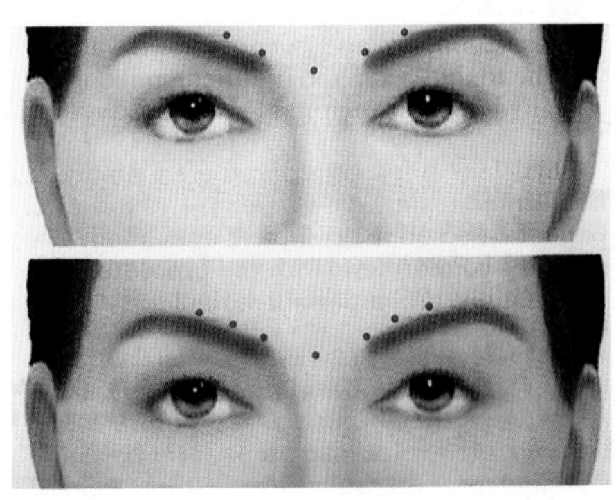

11.1.26 The points for injecting Botox in treating the glabella complex.

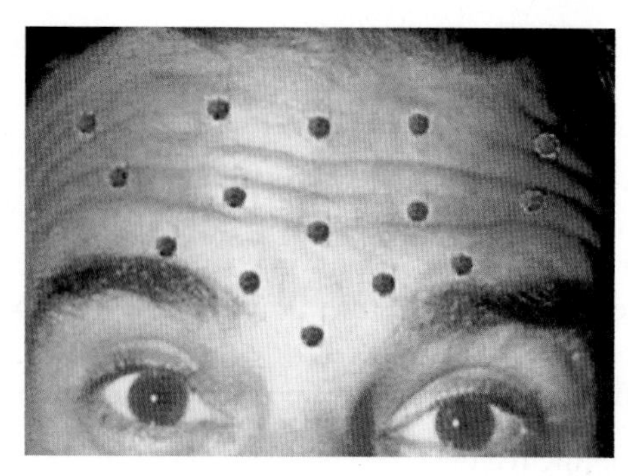

11.1.27 The points at which Botox is injected typically for forehead horizontal lines and the glabella complex.

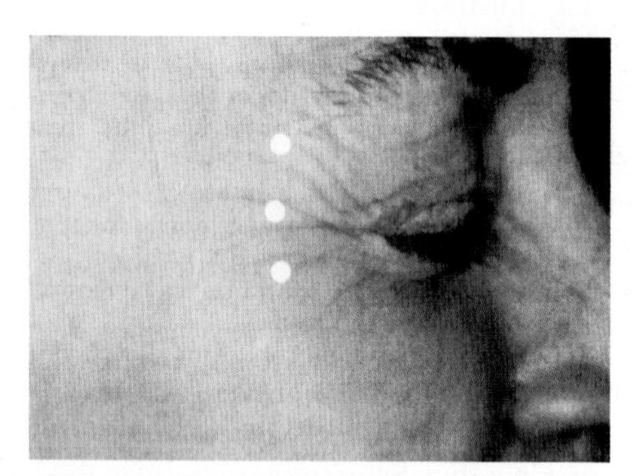

11.1.28 The injection sites for crow's feet. It should be a minimum of 1 cm lateral to the orbital bony rim.

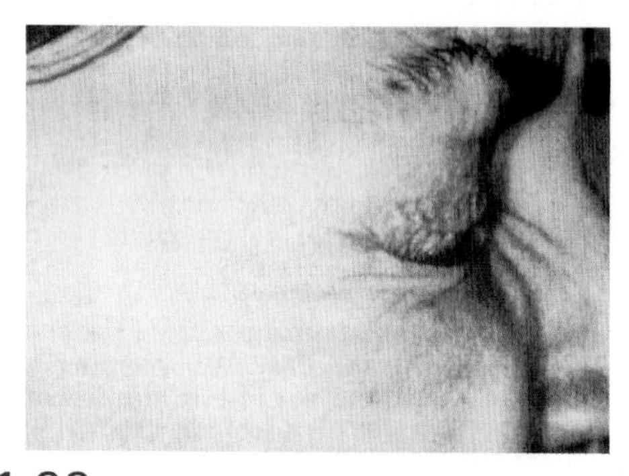

11.1.29 Sites for injection to rid of bunny lines.

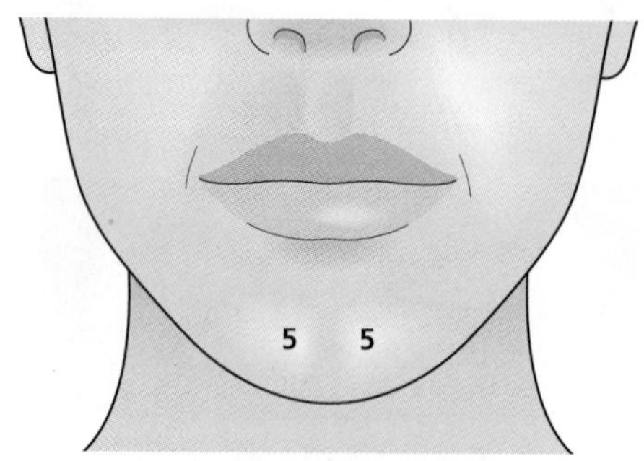

11.1.30 Site for injection to treat dimpled chin.

PATIENT SELECTION, COUNSELLING AND INFORMED CONSENT

The initial consultation is critical in understanding the patient's expectations of the treatment if unhappy patients are to be avoided. A medical and drug history is essential. Patients on aspirin, nonsteroidal anti-inflammatory drugs or vitamin E should be stopped 7–10 days before treatment to avoid bruising. Likewise, anticoagulants should be adjusted appropriately by the treating physician to bring the INR to around two or if there is no contraindication to stop the warfarin at least 72 hours before the procedure.

In the initial examination, document the wrinkles and lines seen in a static position and in a dynamic setting. Most patients would like to know the safety of Botox, particularly if they are having the treatment for the first time. There is adequate evidence to support the fact that botulinum toxin A used in facial areas has long-term safety. It is important to discuss known adverse effects reported such as ptosis, headache, pain at injection site, bruising, unexpected results such as brow asymmetry, drooling of saliva and asymmetry at the angle of the mouth. Botulinum toxin A should not be given in the following conditions:

- during lactation;
- inflammatory skin conditions;
- patients with myaesthesia gravis or Eaton Lambert syndrome.

Some of the specific uses at certain anatomic locations are listed below.

Glabellar complex

The musculature responsible for producing the deep furrows in the glabella complex are corrugator supercili, procerus and depressor supercili (Figure 11.1.31). The fibres of ocularis oculi and frontalis interdigitate with the corrugator. The corrugators move the eyebrow medially inwards and depress the brow. Procerus is also a depressor of the medial eyebrow. Orbicularis oculi also depresses the medial eyebrow. Injection sites for the glabellar complex are shown in Figure 11.1.26. In general, for the glabella complex an average of 20–25 units of Botox at 2 mL dilution is used. Men require a greater dosage (approximately 30–35 units). In oriental women with epicanthal folds, a lower dose is used and the author does not exceed 15 units. Patients are seen at 2 weeks and another 5–10 units reinjected, if necessary accordingly. Use four or five units at each injection point depending on the depth of the furrows. Always see these patients at 2 weeks and carry out 'top ups'. If this area has to be retreated, the author waits 4–6 months.

Horizontal lines of the forehead

The hyperactivity of the large vertically oriented frontalis muscle is responsible for the horizontal lines. The frontalis elevates the brow. It is very important while injecting Botox into the frontalis that the needle should be 2 cm above the orbital rim to prevent brow ptosis. Do not inject the horizontal lines at the same sitting as the vertical furrows of the glabellar complex. The author usually defers it by 2 weeks. Inject the first horizontal line and ensure that you are 2 cm above the orbital rim. Three injection sites are generally used on either side of the midline for each line for men and two sites for women. Use a total of approximately 20 units for women and 30 units for men. If brow elevation in a female patient has been discussed as part of the treatment, use 2–4 units into the lateral orbicularis oculi so that the frontalis is unopposed.

Recall all patients after 2 weeks and carry out 'top ups'. One important aspect of injecting Botox into horizontal lines is to assess brow asymmetry at the initial visit and show this to the patient.

Crow's feet

These result from hyperactivity of the orbicularis oculi muscles. Prior to injection of this area, assess for lower eyelid laxity and lid retraction. The orbicularis oculi encircles the eye as a sphincter. In treating crow's feet, an injection is made into the lateral orbital component of the orbicularis oculi. Depending on the lines, typically use 3–5 injections. The injection site should be 1.5 cm from the orbital rim. The author would normally use four or five units per site. Recall patients in 2 weeks and top up if necessary. Prior to injection, ice application is used to minimize bruising as the injection is made subcutaneously. Injection should not be carried out for at least 4 weeks following a blepharoplasty or a rhytidectomy or laser assisted *in situ* keratomileusis (Lasik).

Bunny lines

They are seen on the sides of the nose and result from contraction and hyperactivity of the transverse portion of the nasalis. Into each line no more than two units is necessary and another two units in the midline into the procerus (dilution 2.5 mL).

The use of Botox in the perioral area should be avoided and instead use fillers. Dimpled chin is due to hyperactivity of the mentalis muscle. Typically the author uses five units per injection into two sites (usually 10 units in total) and top up 2 weeks later (Figure 11.1.30). Platysma bands can also be treated by Botox (see Figure 11.1.24). They appear as vertical bands. Typically for a vertical band, use 5–6 injection sites (25–30 units in total) and top up 2 weeks later. One of the complications of injecting into the platysma bands is dysphonia, dysphagia and neck weakness.

(a) 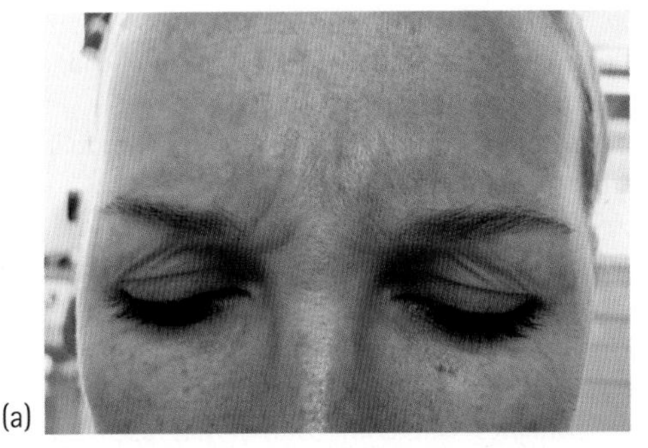

(b) 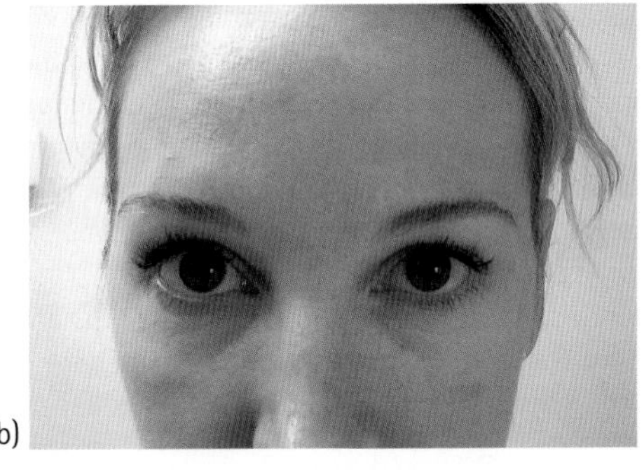

11.1.31 (a) Pre-Botox injection – 40 year old female. (b) Post-Botox injection (four months later) – 40-year-old female showing abolition of furrows in glabella complex and brow elevation. Brow plasty done with Botox injection four units on each side.

(a) 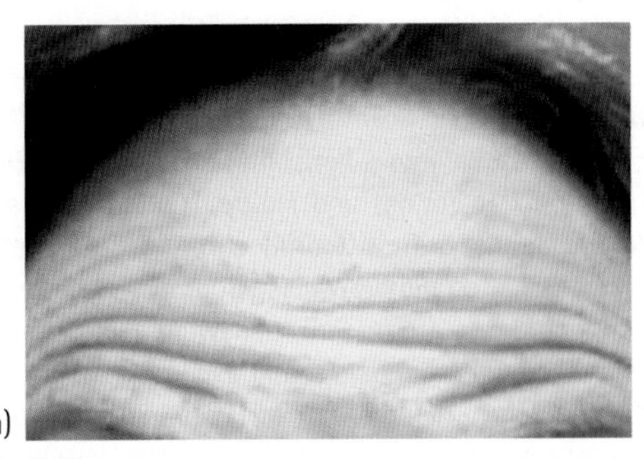

(b) 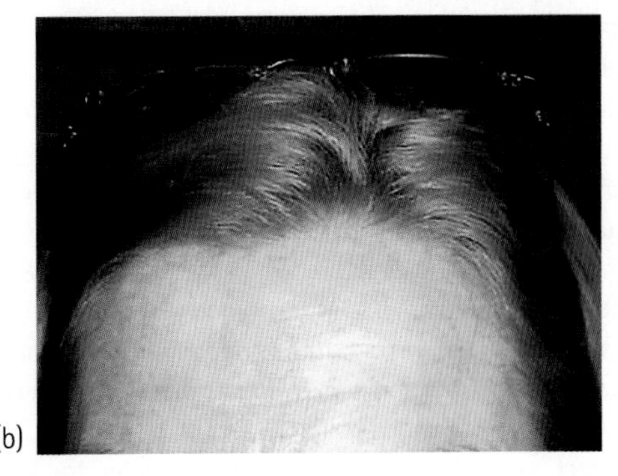

11.1.32 (a) Horizontal lines in the forehead. (b) Four months after injection of 12 units of Botox in each side into the horizontal line followed by 20 per cent trichloroacetic acid peel 4 weeks later.

Top tips

Fillers

- Harvested fat can be stored long term at -20°C for up to two years.
- Fat can be reinjected at 6 weeks to 12-weekly intervals by rapid thawing.
- When fat is stored, it is best saved in labelled 10 mL syringes. The infranatant should be decanted, but keep the triglyceride layer intact.
- While injecting fat, use only blunt needles (a Coleman needle).
- In the first post-operative visit a week later, fat protrusions may exist. Use a Coleman cannula to 'feather' this using a negative suction in a 10 mL luer lock syringe (liposculpturing).
- Fat injected into cheek and the eyelids lasts well.
- Fat injected into the lips disappears rapidly and is not the ideal choice as a filler for the lips.
- Injected fat undergoes fibrosis, progenitor cells differentiate into mature adipocytes.
- It is an excellent adjunctive technique for facial volumetric rejuvenation.
- Figure 11.1.3 illustrates a subcutaneous tunnel being made after a stab incision.
- Figure 11.1.4 illustrates infiltration of tumescent solution through the entry site.
- Figure 11.1.14 illustrates the various cannulas used for aspiration of fat.
- Figure 11.1.15 illustrates the cannulas used for injection of fat and the connector used to transfer the fat from the 10 mL syringe to the 3 mL syringe used for injecting the fat.
- Figure 11.1.16a shows the suction maintaining 'lock' inserted into the plunger of the syringe to maintain the negative suction. Figure 11.1.16b shows the Wilkinson dissector used for creating a subcutaneous tunnel prior to injecting the fat.
- Figure 11.1.17 shows the 10 mL syringe used to harvest the fat, the 3 mL syringe used to inject the fat and the stopper fitted to the syringe to contain the harvested fat.

Synthetic fillers

- Give as much information as possible to your patient regarding the filler you propose to use. In particular, discuss all complications and your reasons for recommending the particular fillers.
- Obtain an informed consent.
- Avoid using them in patients taking medications likely to promote bleeding and bruising e.g. aspirin, plavix, anticoagulants. Stop these medications including supplements, e.g. gingko biloba, for at least 5–7 days before the procedure and do not recommence until after 48 hours.
- Be very atraumatic in your technique.
- Each agent requires a different technique and when you begin, learn from someone who has used the material for some time and attend a course.
- Select your filler according to your wish for a more permanent, semi-permanent or temporary result. If a permanent filler is to be used, over-correction should be avoided. Inject permanent fillers in a much deeper plane. Liquid silicone is notorious in producing fibrosis if injected subcutaneously.
- Apply ice packs for 24–48 hours.
- If swelling is severe, use oral corticosteroids.
- Avoid fillers in patients with autoimmune disorders.
- In general I advise against the use of collagen or collagen containing fillers .
- The safest are hyaluronic acid derivatives of synthetic origin and polyacrylamide gel.
- Inject fillers, when possible, under local anaesthetic block to avoid pain.
- Ask your patient to report immediately if any adverse reaction is noted.

Botulinum toxin type A (Botox)

- Carry out a careful assessment of the wrinkles and lines at rest and in function.
- Understand the patient's desires and if unrealistic do not accept.
- Give a detailed explanation of the underlying problems, your proposed treatment plans, known complications and contact details of the clinic should any complications arises.
- Give precise post-Botox instructions in a written leaflet.
- The patient must understand that the effect of Botox is temporary and further treatments will be necessary.
- It is essential to have an informed consent signed.
- Stop all medications such as vitamin E, aspirin, anticoagulants, supplements, e.g. gingko biloba, at least 7 days before the procedure.
- Apply an ice pack for at least 10 minutes prior to injection and another 5 minutes after injection.
- After injection, the area should not be massaged.
- Carefully inspect the lower eyelids for any lid laxity.
- Do not inject Botox into lactating mothers.
- No injection of Botox should be given into areas where there is skin infection.
- Case examples where the author has used Botox are illustrated:
  - Figure 11.1.31a shows furrows in glabella complex and Figure 11.1.31b shows glabella complex four months after injection of 20 units of Botox (2 mL dilution for 100 units).
  - Figure 11.1.32a shows horizontal lines in the forehead and Figure 11.1.32b shows forehead after injection of Botox and a 20 per cent trichloroacetic acid peel.
  - Figure 11.1.33a shows horizontal lines in the forehead (pre-Botox injection) and Figure 11.1.33b shows the forehead and brow after injection of Botox to the horizontal lines and brow plasty four months later.
  - Figure 11.1.34a pre-operative showing deep nasolabial fold and platysma bands and Figure 11.1.34b post-operative three months later, injection of polyacrylamide gel into nasolabial folds and Botox into the platysma bands (total 28 units)

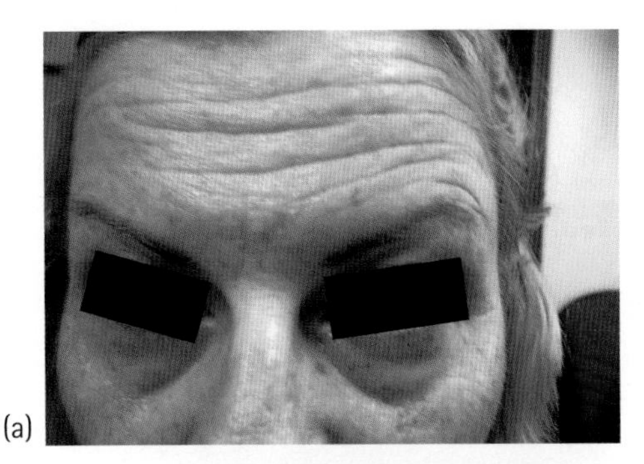

(a)

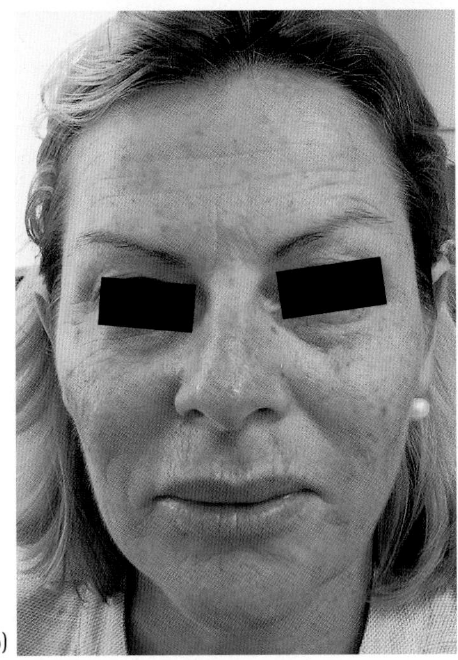

(b)

11.1.33 (a) Pre-Botox injection – horizontal lines in the forehead. Note the brow position. (b) Post-Botox injection to the horizontal lines and brow plasty. Note the brow position (chemical brow plasty).

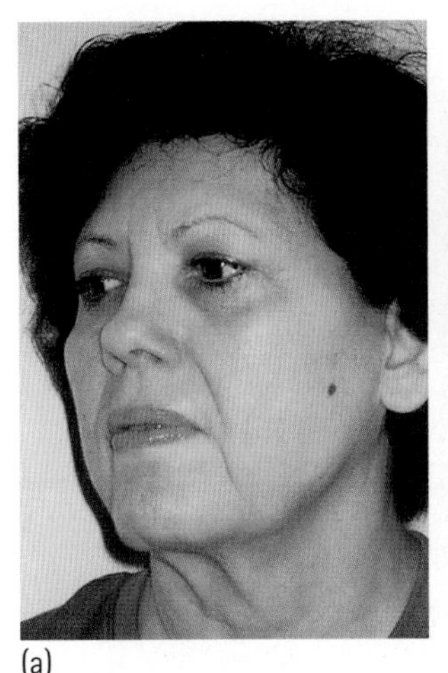

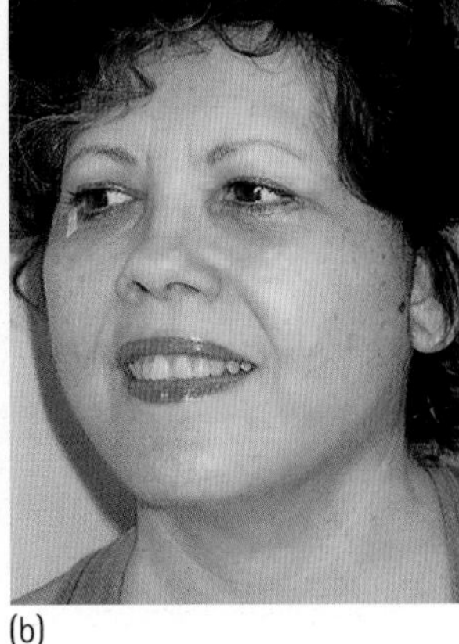

(a) (b)

11.1.34 (a) Pre-operative showing deep nasolabial fold and platysma bands. (b) Post-operative three months later injection of polyacrylamide gel into nasolabial folds and Botox into the platysma bands (total 28 units).

FURTHER READING

Aronsohn RB. A 22-year experience with the use of silicone injection. *American Journal of Cosmetic Surgery* 1984; **1**: 21–8.

Barnett JG, Barnett CR. Treatment of acne scars with liquid silicone injections: 30-year perspective. *Dermatologic Surgery* 2005; **31**: 1542–49.

Butterwick KJ. Fat autograft muscle injection (FAMI): new technique for facial volume restoration. *Dermatologic Surgery* 2005; **31**: 1487–95.

Carruthers A, Carruthers JDA. Polymethylmethacrylate microspheres/collagen as a tissue augmenting agent: personal experience over 5 years. *Dermatologic Surgery* 2005; **31**: 1561–5.

Carruthers A, Carey W, De Lorenzi C *et al.* Ramdomized, double-blind comparison of the efficacy of two hyaluronic acid derivatives, restylane perlane and hylaform, in the treatment of nasolabial folds. *Dermatologic Surgery* 2005; **31**: 1591–8.

Danesh-Meyer HV, Savino PJ, Sergott RC. Case reports and a small case series; ocular and cerebral ischemia following facial injection of autologous fat. *Archives of Ophthalmology* 2001; **119**: 777–8.

Dreizen NG, Framm L. Sudden unilateral visual loss after autologous fat injection into the glabellar area. *American Journal of Ophthalmology* 1989; **107**: 85–7.

Duffy DM. Tissue injectable liquid silicone: new perspectives. In: Klein A (ed.). *Augmentation in clinical practice: procedures and techniques.* New York: Marcel Dekker, 1998: 237–63.

Duffy DM. Liquid silicone for soft tissue augmentation. *Dermatologic Surgery* 2005; **31**: 1530–41.

Duffy DM. Complications of fillers: overview. *Dermatologic Surgery* 2005; **31**: 1626–33.

Egido JA, Arroyo R, Marcos A, Jimenez-Alfaro I. Middle cerebral artery embolism and unilateral visual loss after autologous fat injection into the glabellar area. *Stroke* 1993; **24**: 615–16.

Feinendegen DL, Baumgartner RW, Schroth G *et al.* Middle cerebral artery occlusion and ocular fat embolism after autologous fat injection in the face. *Journal of Neurology* 1988; **245**: 53–4.

Feinendegen DL, Baumgartner RW, Vaudens P *et al.* Autologous fat injections for soft tissue augmentation in the face; a safe procedure? *Aesthetic Plastic Surgery* 1998; **22**: 163–7.

Klein AW, Rish DC. Substances for soft tissue augmentation: collagen and silicone. *Journal of Dermatologic Surgery and Oncology* 1985; **11**: 337–9.

Le AT. Rhinoplasty using injectable polyacrylamide gel – a patient study. *Australasian Journal of Cosmetic Surgery* 2005; **1**: 1.

Lee DH, Yang HN, Kim JC, Shyn KH. Sudden unilateral visual loss and brain infarction after autologous fat injection into the nasolabial groove. *British Journal of Ophthalmology* 1996; **80**: 1026–7.

Orentreich D. Liquid injectable silicone. *Clinics in Plastic Surgery* 2000; **27**: 595–612.

Orentreich DS, Orentreich NO. Injectable fluid silicone: principles of dermatologic surgery. In: Roenigk RK, Roenigk HH (eds). *Dermatologic surgery: principles and practice.* New York: Marcel Dekker, 1989: 1349–95.

Teimourian B. Blindness following fat injections. *Plastic and Reconstructive Surgery* 1988; **82**: 361.

Thaler MP, Ubogy ZI. Artecoll: the arizona experience and lessons learned. *Dermatologic Surgery* 2005; **31**: 1566–76.

Vleggaar D. Facial volumetric correction with injectable poly-L-lactic acid. *Dermatologic Surgery* 2005; **31**: 1511–18.

11.2

Hair transplantation

N RAVINDRANATHAN, E ANTONIO MANGUBAT

INTRODUCTION

Modern hair restoration surgery (HRS) has evolved significantly since its original introduction in the USA in 1959. HRS includes many different techniques including hair transplantation (HT), scalp reduction, scalp flaps and tissue expansion. The most common hair loss aetiology is androgenetic alopecia (AGA), more commonly known as male pattern baldness. Other processes that lead to hair loss are trauma, diseases, such as alopecia areata and lichenplanopilaris, and iatrogenic causes, most commonly prior surgery.

HAIR RESTORATION SURGERY TECHNIQUES

The modern surgical treatment of AGA was introduced in the USA by Norman Orentreich with the publication of his landmark article hypothesizing his theory of donor dominance. He postulated that autografted hair follicles grew in bald scalp because the donor hair bearing tissue retained its dominant expression despite being transplanted into bald scalp. Thus, the modern HT was born.

The essence of HT is the movement of hair bearing donor tissue from the 'permanent' occipital scalp to the balding frontal scalp in the same patient. This is simply rotation of current hair inventory; more hair is not produced, just simply rearranged. Orentreich originally accomplished this by taking 4 mm round punch biopsies of occipital scalp and placing it in the bald frontal scalp. The skin graft would take and hair would grow in previously barren scalp. For most balding men and women, this was a miracle and an answer to their hair loss concerns. For Orentreich's patients at the time, any hair was good hair regardless of its unnatural appearance.

HAIR TRANSPLANTATION

Factors affecting the success of a hair transplantation procedure are numerous and must be considered in the treatment of any hair deformity. Natural cosmetic results are highly dependent on these factors, which include:

- Extent of hair loss. This determines the amount of work required to cover the defect.
- Age of the patient. Bear in mind that the extent of hair loss increases with age. Young men with AGA will have less hair to transplant and more bald area to cover as they grow older.
- Adequate donor tissue. There must be sufficient donor hair density and tissue to provide enough grafts to cover the hair defect. Hair transplantation does not produce more hair but rather relocates existing hair on the patient's scalp. Unfortunately for most patients, the more hair they need, the less donor tissue they have.
- Hair colour affects perceived coverage. The darker the colour, the greater the apparent coverage per graft; however, dark hair also tends to create a more unnatural appearance.
- Hair curl increases the apparent volume of hair present in that curly hair covers more area as it bunches up on itself.
- Hair contrast plays an important role in naturalness. The greater the contrast, e.g. black hair on white skin, the more unnatural the appearance. Care must be taken to use the finest single hair grafts in the most exposed area, i.e. the hairline.
- Hair shaft diameter is an important determinant in how much hair is moved in a graft. The thicker the diameter, the more prominent the hair and the more contrast it provides. Thick hair shaft diameters make producing a fine natural hair line challenging.
- Hair direction of the grafted hair must be matched to the existing naturally occurring hair follicles of area being transplanted.
- Hairline considerations. A natural hairline is actually a misnomer. A natural hairline is actually a zone of fine irregular hairs that create the feathering zone as the bald scalp gradually yields to hair bearing scalp.
- Ethnic differences are wide and varied and usually can be described as a combination of the above characteristics.

For example, Asian hair is less dense than Caucasian hair, but the hair shaft diameters are typically thicker. The converse is also true that Caucasians typically have greater density (hair follicles/mm^2) but smaller shaft diameters.

HAIRLINE DESIGN

The most important area of presenting the greatest challenge to HRS surgeons is the hairline, which is the transition from bald skin to hair-bearing skin. Hairline is actually a misnomer as it is not a line at all. The natural hairline is more of a zone at the bald skin–hair perimeter that exhibits the characteristics of an uneven undulation of the hairs along the border of the bald skin–hairline interface as well as a gradually increasing hair density gradient. Figure 11.2.1a demonstrates a 17-year-old male with no hair loss. Note the large numbers of fine vellus hairs present in the anterior border that will eventually be lost as he ages. Figure 11.2.1b is a 15-year-old who lacks any vellus hairs but note the strikingly nomadic hairline. Figure 11.2.1c is the hairline of a 50-year-old man. Note the loss in density in the hairline with a more gradual density gradient. These examples are not transplanted hairlines and they all exhibit an uneven undulating zone of hair.

Also note the important variations in hair direction. The vellus hair gives clues as to the true natural hair direction that the transplant must simulate in order to achieve a natural result. In general, frontal scalp hair point forward, parietal scalp hair point lateral and inferior, occipital scalp hair is oriented posteriorly and inferiorly.

When designing a hairline for transplantation, the surgeon must be aware of these subtleties in order to avoid drawing attention to the transplantation. Most lay people do not understand what a natural hairline is but they can usually detect an unnatural hairline. The results produced with contemporary techniques go virtually undetected (Figure 11.2.2a–d). Unfortunately, the old pluggy results (Figure 11.2.3) still exist as a constant reminder of our struggle to perfect the technique and of why the lay public hesitate to seek out a surgical treatment for hair loss until they have exhausted all other possibilities.

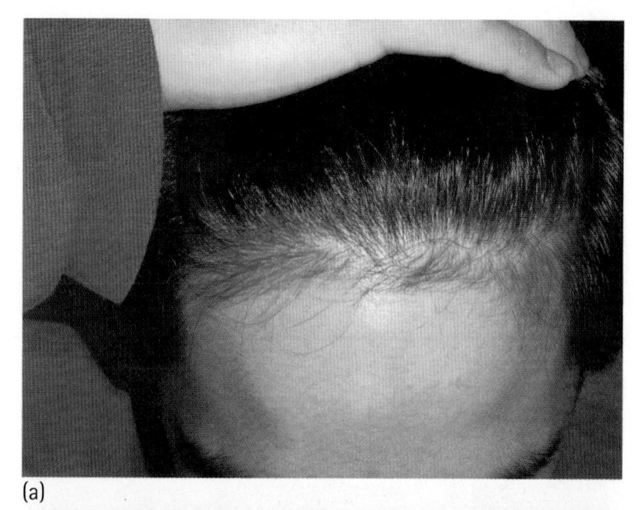

(a)

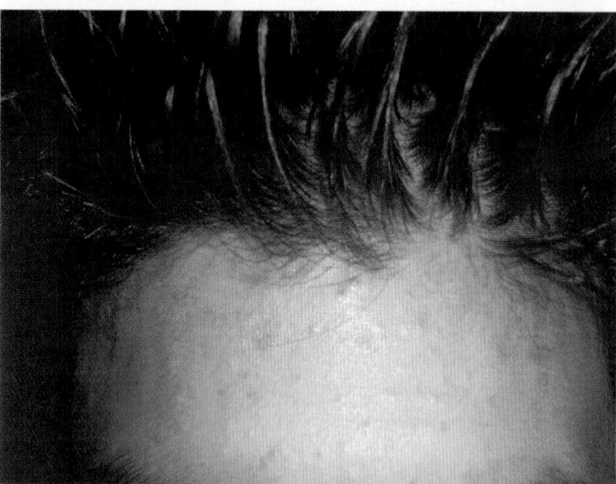

(b)

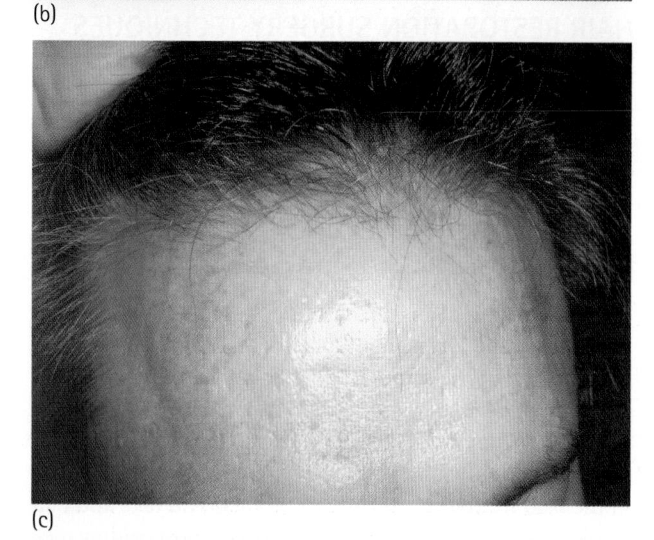

(c)

11.2.1 (a) A 17-year-old male with no hair loss. (b) A 15-year-old who lacks any vellus hairs but note the strikingly nomadic hairline. (c) The hairline of a 50-year-old man.

FOLLICULAR UNIT TRANSPLANTATION

In the last two decades, the trend has been to transplant very small grafts using 1–4 hair follicles. Now termed 'follicular unit transplantation' (FUT), modern technological advances have increased the number of follicle units transplanted in each session from an average of 1000 up to 3500.

Indications in males

- Androgenetic alopecia (hereditary baldness or male pattern hair loss).
- Loss of scalp hair in selected cases following burns and accidents.
- To cover surgical scars.
  - Mustache creation to camouflage bilateral cleft lip scars.
  - Bicoronal scalp scars associated with loss of hair.

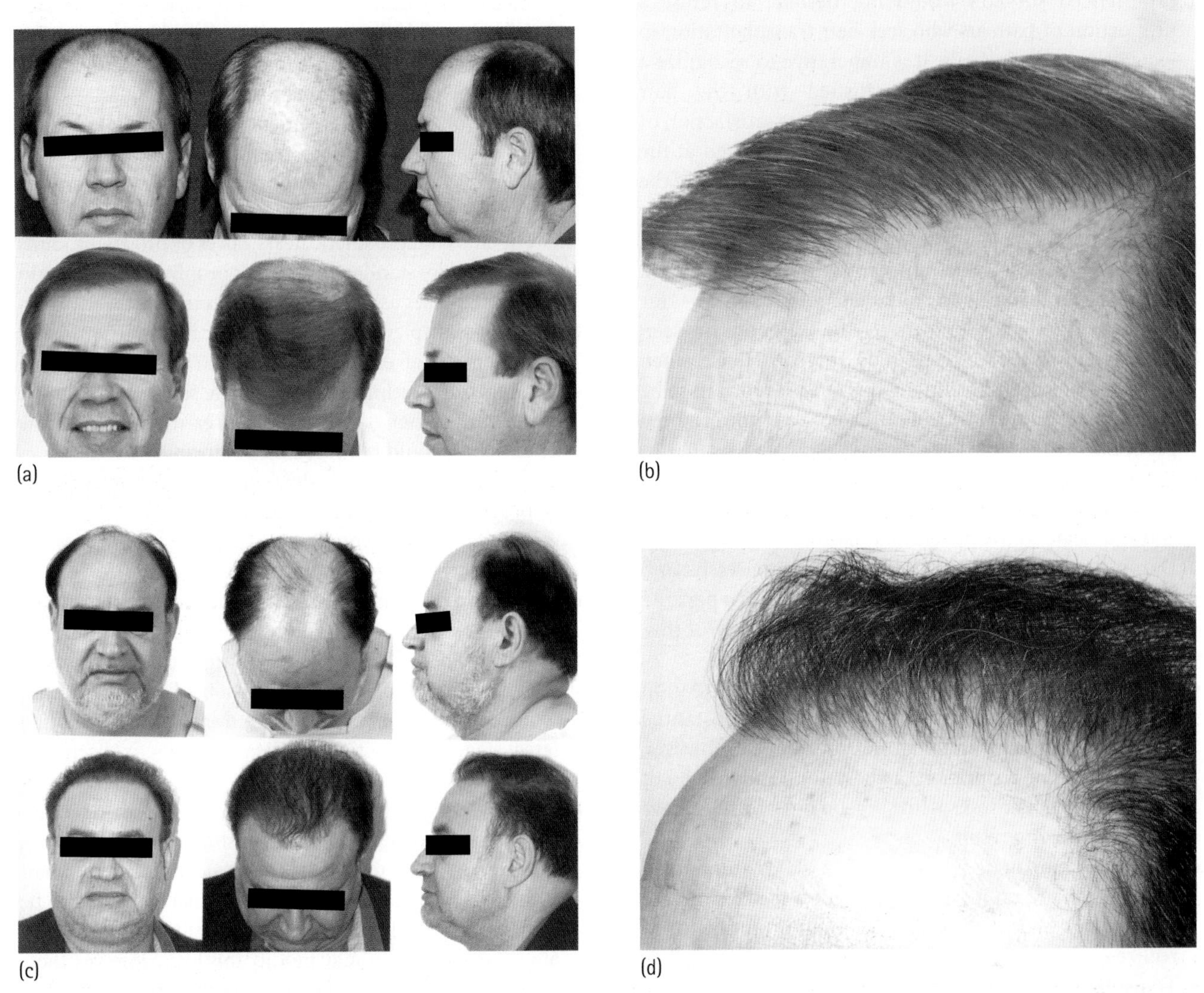

11.2.2 (a) Hair transplant. (b) Close up transplanted hairline. (c) Hair transplant. (d) Close up hair transplant.

- Loss of eyebrow hair.
  - Alopecia areata.
  - Lichenplanopilaris.

The consultation

The process of consultation is an interactive decision of ascertaining the goals of the patient and assess if these are achievable. The key points are:

- The ascertainment of patient goals. An experienced surgeon must exercise the power of judgement in eliciting patient's goals. A specific question needs to be asked on what area of hair loss is most bothersome to the patient and understand the motivating factor for seeking hair transplantation. Upon understanding the patient's goals, analyse if these are achievable or unrealistic. An

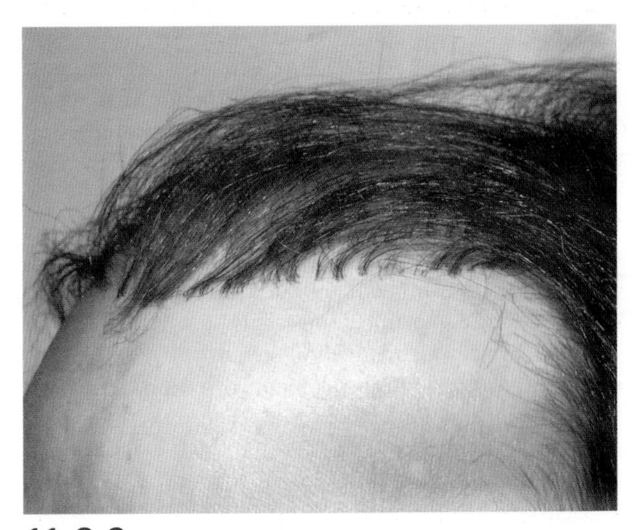

11.2.3 Unnatural hairline.

experienced surgeon would not hesitate to refuse a proportion of patients who seek hair transplantation in view of unrealistic goals. It is imperative to recognize a patient who will not be satisfied with the hair transplantation procedure. The long-term satisfaction of the patient depends largely on decisions arrived at the initial consultation rather than the technical ability of the surgeon. It is customary for most patients who seek hair transplant to have tried medical treatment, herbal therapies, previous hair transplants but dissatisfied with the result and may have obtained referral from your patients, physicians known to the surgeon or seen photographs in the web page of the surgeon. Hence, when such a patient seeks treatment, it is most important to be honest in revealing what you can achieve and the required process to achieve the goals.

- Explanation regarding the progressive nature of hair loss. In the process of consultation, the surgeon must communicate to the patient that hair loss is progressive. Despite transplantation, hair loss may be progressive and at present we are unable to predict the extent of a person's baldness. It must also be made clear that in view of this, the long-term result is unpredictable.
- Requests for transplantation into vertex. Transplantation into the vertex is accompanied by progressive substantial hair loss resulting in an unnatural appearance. However, anterior hairline restoration can be natural and the aim of any practising hair transplant surgeon must be to achieve a natural looking result.
- Hair restoration in a bald patient returns the natural facial appearance and unquestionably restores the central face as the focus of attention. This is an important factor to realize in the initial consultation.
- Transplanted hairline. This is initially permanent. Upon restoring the hairline, there is an appreciable difference in facial appearance. As hair loss is progressive, the created hairline must be acceptable throughout the lifetime. A young person seeking hair transplant may address only the frontotemporal troughs. However, in an older person, it would be an unrealistic expectation if bald in the hairline.
- At the very onset, elicit if the patient is seeking hair restoration only by medical treatment. If hairline restoration is being requested by only medical therapy, this would not be a possible option. Likewise, if the hair loss and associated baldness cannot be restored by medical treatment alone, the surgeon should clearly explain that this would not be possible. If the patient accepts the recommendation of surgical restoration, at this juncture explain the necessity to be treated with supportive adjunctive medical therapy.
- If a surgical option is being planned, a detailed medical and drug history is important. The most pertinent questions to be asked are:
  - previous bleeding problems;
  - current hair loss medication;
  - history of drug allergies;
  - intake of medicines such as aspirin, warfarin, clopidogrel. When possible these medications should be stopped. It is customary to stop aspirin for 1–2 weeks and Clopidogrel 5 days before hair transplantation
  - Intake of dietary supplements, such as gingko biloba, vitamin E, garlic and ginseng, increase tendency to bleed. They should be stopped for a week before the procedure.
  - Patients with prosthetic heart valves or prosthetic joints may require standard antibiotic prophylaxis regimes in selected cases as guided by the physician.
- In a hair transplantation practice, we highly recommend employment of either a full- or part-time counsellor. Patients often feel more comfortable speaking about the procedure other than to the treating doctor. The counsellor should reinforce the following:
  - explanation regarding the patient's status of hair loss;
  - progressive nature of balding;
  - reiterate the treatment plan;
  - explain the likely complications.
- Discussion of limitations. Convey at the very outset that the hair loss is not static and further transplantation may become necessary. Do not give a time frame. A patient who has understood very clearly that balding is progressive would easily accept maintenance transplant sessions at a later stage. Adjunctive medical therapy is useful in preventing continued hair loss.
- Explain very clearly that in the immediate post-operative period there would be hair loss (post-operative effluvium). It is believed to occur due to local tissue trauma. Vellus hair is the most susceptible although terminal hair can also be affected. Some believe prescribing finasteride immediately after transplantation may modify this loss. However, there are no double-blind studies to prove this observation. The surgeon and the counsellor should emphasize that there would be an interval of approximately six to nine months between the transplantation and the expected result of new hair growth.
- Selection of the appropriate patient. This is governed by (a) degree of baldness, (b) patient expectations, (c) calibre of the hair shaft, (d) donor hair availability and its quality, (e) age of patient. In general, it is best to avoid young patients in the group 20–25 years. Young men in this age group usually consult to explore transplantation to restore the areas of baldness due to frontotemporal recession (Norwood stages 1 and 2). In these patients, if facial framing is intact, there is no benefit in transplantation. Calibre of the hair can vary from fine to coarse hair. The larger the diameter, the better the result. Patients with fine hair have a diameter of less than 60 microns. Fine hair covers less surface area and hence yields poor results. Some would refuse to carry out transplantation in these individuals.
- Donor hair quality determines surgical outcome. In general, men require 40 follicular units per cm^2 in the occiput for successful transplants. In general, Caucasians have more follicular unit counts than Asians.

- The ultimate determining factor for the success of hair transplantation depends on the patient's expectations. If the patient's expectations are unreal and, through the process of consultation and use of the counsellor, cannot be modified, the patient should not be accepted for transplantation. For patients with fine hair, a limited donor site source cannot be provided with transplanted hairs of satisfactory density. In such patients, time spent in detailed explanation is very worthwhile. Patients who seek vertex transplantation should be warned of significant future loss. Likewise, patients who request transplantation from vertex to frontal scalp should be discouraged.

  Thereafter the main steps are:

- Establishment of hairline. This is often an area for misunderstanding. An unrealistic request to make the hairline too low which would be unnatural must be pointed out clearly in the discussion. A good method to adopt is to seat the patient in front of a mirror and draw the proposed hairline.
- Assessment of the state of baldness and assigning the patient to the Norwood classification (Figure 11.2.4). At this stage, bring it to the attention of the patient that baldness is progressive and this should be considered in the discussion.
- Once the discussions have been completed and the decision for transplantation has been made, discuss other surgical options such as scalp reduction and the reasons why as a procedure this is no longer popular.
- No consultation is complete without a discussion of risks and complications and obtaining an informed consent (Table 11.2.1 showing sample of consent form).
- Photographs – the following views are required.
  - frontal view;
  - lateral views (right and left);
  - vertex view;
  - posterior view;
  - hairline close up.

It is important for the transplant surgeon to be aware of medico-legal issues in this practice. This surgery is not dealing with 'life and death issues' and therefore litigation is more common.

Principles of hair transplantation

The following principles and guidelines must be adhered to in achieving success in hair transplantation surgery.

Donor site

- Harvesting hair from the occiput should be from within a margin of clearance of about 2.5 cm from the lateral and inferior fringes of the occipital hairline (Figure 11.2.5 – donor site).

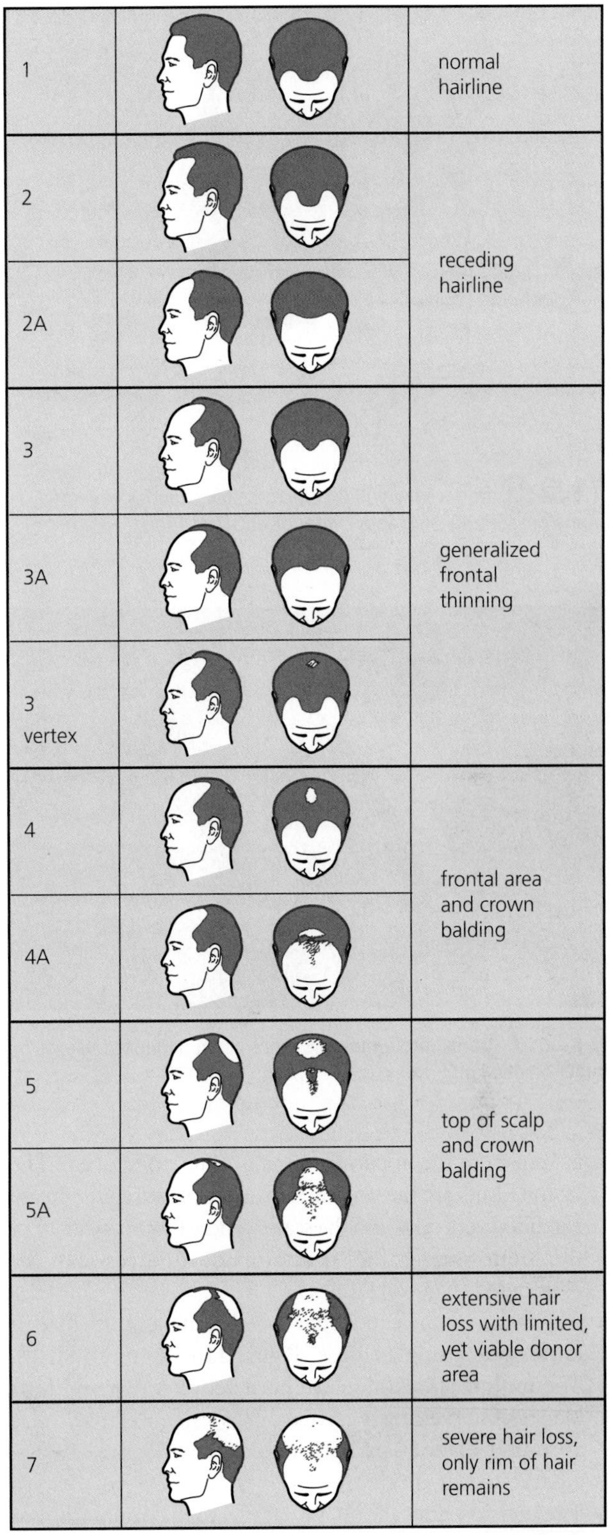

Class		Description
1		normal hairline
2		receding hairline
2A		
3		generalized frontal thinning
3A		
3 vertex		
4		frontal area and crown balding
4A		
5		top of scalp and crown balding
5A		
6		extensive hair loss with limited, yet viable donor area
7		severe hair loss, only rim of hair remains

11.2.4 Hair loss classifications (Norwood classifications).

- Avoid harvesting above and medial to the mastoid area.
- The lateral limit of harvesting should not extend beyond a vertical line extending into the scalp from the preauricular line. Harvesting performed anterior to this line can result in visible scar formation. The upper limit of the donor site

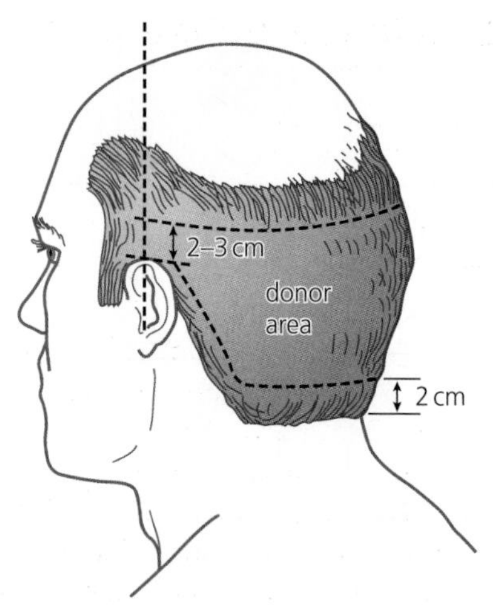

11.2.5 Donor area will be 2.5 cm below superior edge of fringe border and 2 cm above inferior occipital fringe.

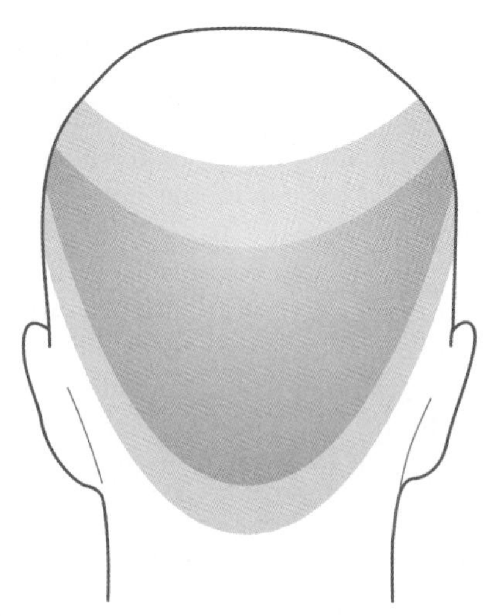

11.2.6 Donor area.

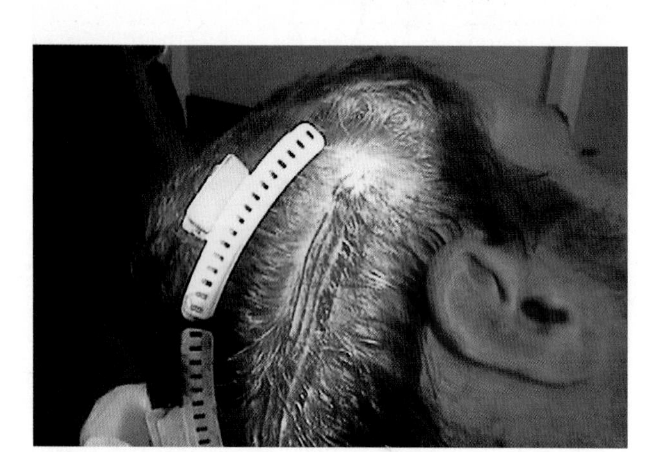

11.2.7 Donor site – multiple strips being harvested using multi-bladed knife.

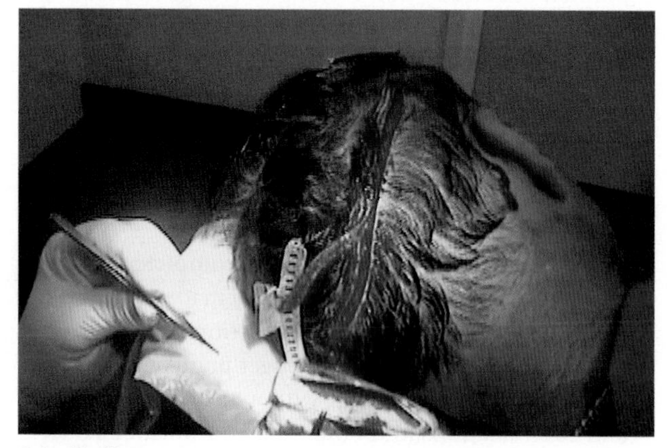

11.2.8 An elliptical strip being harvested from occipitoparietal donor site.

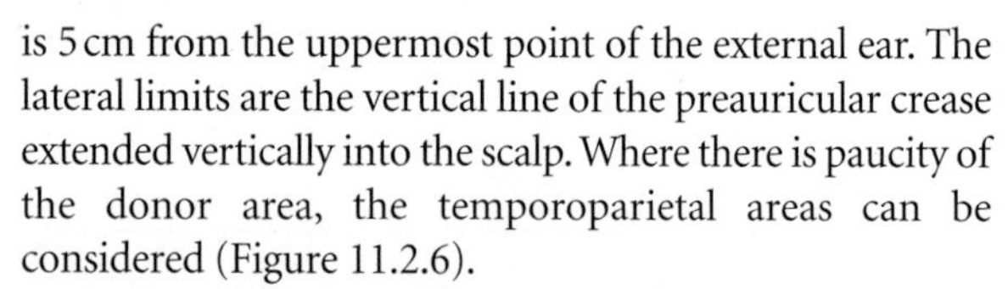

is 5 cm from the uppermost point of the external ear. The lateral limits are the vertical line of the preauricular crease extended vertically into the scalp. Where there is paucity of the donor area, the temporoparietal areas can be considered (Figure 11.2.6).

- The donor tissue can be harvested using a multi-bladed knife or as a single ellipse (Figure 11.2.7 – multi-strip). The multi-bladed knife can have between two and four blades. If harvesting is carried out as a single ellipse, a size 10 scalpel blade (Bard Parker) is utilized (Figure 11.2.8 – a harvested single ellipse).
- The incision lines should be parallel to the orientation of the hair follicles to avoid transection and parallel to the lines of minimum tension (Figure 11.2.9 – harvesting graft strip). Use local anaesthesia in the strength of 1 per cent xylocaine with 1:100 000 epinephrine (adrenaline) when using the tumescent technique. If using a multi-bladed knife to harvest multiple strips, use the tumescent technique to achieve tissue turgor. Subsequently, 100 mL of normal saline is injected into the donor site for tumescence to build up the turgor pressure.

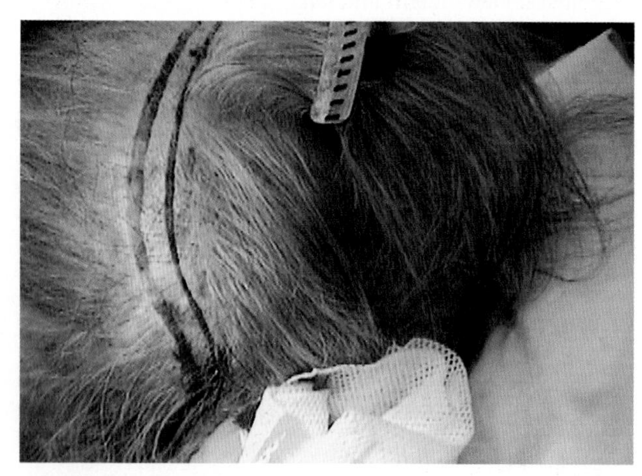

11.2.9 An elliptical strip after incision ready for excision.

Table 11.2.1 Consent for hair transplantation.

The procedure of hair transplantation has been explained to me. The area to be transplanted and the areas of anticipated coverage have been discussed and mutually agreed upon. I am aware that hair transplantation is to be completed over several sessions and a final appraisal of the results cannot be adequately done until the procedure is complete.

I am aware of the following complications associated with hair transplantation:

1. Pain, tingling, 'pins and needles' sensation
2. Bleeding, crusting and scab formation
3. Swelling around the forehead and occasionally the tissue around the donor area, nose, cheeks and eyes
4. Numbness or loss of sensation on the scalp
5. Infection
6. Dizziness or fainting (either from bleeding, medications or anxiety)
7. Allergic reaction to medications
8. Scar formation (depressions or bumps)
9. Insufficient growth of hair requiring more than anticipated transplantation procedures to provide expected results
10. Irregular, uneven or delayed hair growth. Many transplanted hairs will shed after each session. Generally, 3–4 months after the transplantation new hair growth begins. The new hair will sometimes grow in with a variation in texture (coarser, finer, darker or lighter) until it normalizes

I give permission to perform the hair transplantation on me and agree to follow up as directed by the hair transplant surgeon.

For harvesting the donor tissue as a single ellipse, the author used 2 per cent lignocaine with 1:80 000 epinephrine (adrenaline) up to three vials or 1 per cent lignocaine with 1:100 000 epinephrine (adrenaline) and inject up to a maximum of 15 cc.

If the tumescence technique is used, use 100 cc of cold normal saline solution for harvesting a strip of 12 cm long and 1 cm wide. Debate continues as to whether tumescence is essential. However, if tumescence is used, multi-strip harvesting is easier. If a single strip is to be harvested utilizing a single blade, it is not necessary to inject tumescent solution. If a tumescent solution is to be injected, it must be done slowly, 2 cm per time.

Positioning of patient during the procedure

There are two options:

1. Option 1 – Patient is placed in prone position with the head down on a head rest for harvesting of the donor graft and once this is completed, the patient sits on a comfortable dental chair in a partially reclined position.
2. Option 2 – The patient sits on a reclined dental chair for the entire procedure.

TECHNIQUES OF HARVESTING THE GRAFTS

Multi-blade technique

A multi-blade scalpel is utilized. The type most commonly used is an Arnold multi-blade knife. According to the number of strips required, the number of blades used varies. For each 2 mm strip, one blade is required. The width between each blade can be adjusted by utilizing the appropriate spacer. Spacers come as 1.25, 1.5 or 2 mm (Figure 11.2.10). Multi-blade harvesting may increases follicular transection. Most prefer a single blade technique. However, the disadvantage is that the strips have to be cut and prepared from the main elliptical harvest and is more time consuming. However, the transection rate is less.

Technique of harvesting

- The donor area which has been identified is trimmed. The incision is made along the lines marked parallel to the hair follicles and deepened through below the follicular bases but above the deep vasculature. It is necessary to maintain a small amount of subcutaneous fat at the base of the hair follicles. While the strip is being elevated, the surgeon should be careful to ensure that the depth is correct, follicles are not being transected and there is subcutaneous fat at the base of follicles. Use a 4× magnifier when harvesting (Figure 11.2.11 – harvesting). Use of cautery must be avoided and hence only pressure is applied to control bleeding. During closure, carry out minimal undermining (Figure 11.2.12). Apply tension clamps across the edges to approximate and use a few deep dermis sutures of 2.0 polydioxonane (PDS) at least 5 mm away from the wound edges (Figure 11.2.13 – closure). The preferred choice for skin closure is staples as it gives the best scar. However, if using a suture, use a continuous 4/0 nylon suture. Remove the staples or

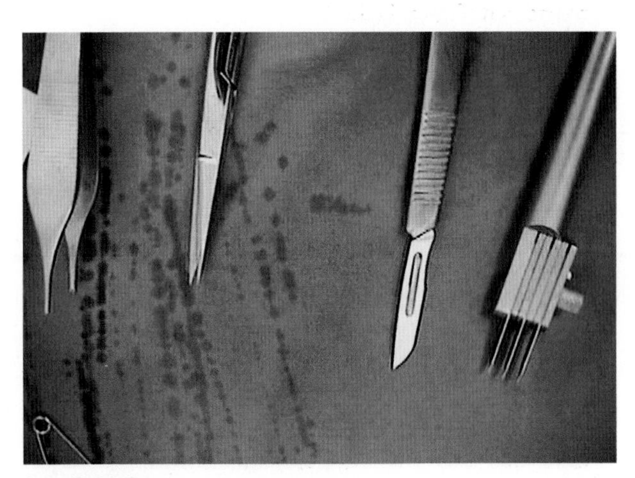

11.2.10 Multi-bladed knife for harvesting multi-strips and single blade for harvesting an ellipse.

sutures on the tenth day. See the patient on the following day and apply hair gel, the hair is washed and the wound is inspected to ensure that there is no blood collection.

- The preparation of grafts from the harvested multi-blade strip or ellipse (Figure 11.2.14).
  - Once the graft has been harvested, either as an ellipse or multi-strip, it should be placed in cold saline.
  - Hair technologists working on a well-lit bench and wearing magnifiers start to prepare the micro or minigrafts (2–4 follicles). If single follicular unit transplantation has been envisaged, microscopes are used for dissection of follicular units.
  - The strips or sectioned ellipses are placed on a spatula (Figure 11.2.15a) and using a Persanna blade 10, the hair technologist will start sectioning them carefully leaving some subcutaneous fat below the follicles either as mini or micrografts (Figure 11.2.15b, showing grafts on spatula being cut). When prepared, the grafts must be placed in a separate dish with cold saline and they should be placed into the recipient sites within 4 hours to give maximum viability of the grafts. During the preparation, the surgeon should oversee the team preparing the grafts to ensure there is no transection of the follicles and there is atraumatic tissue handling. At the commencement of the procedure, a calculation would have been done to estimate the number of mini and micrografts needed for the planned restoration.
- Techniques of recipient site preparation and graft insertion.
  - Local anaesthesia is administered as a nerve block or ring block with 1 or 2 per cent lignocaine containing 1:100 000 epinephrine. If recipient sites are to be created in the frontal hairline, bilateral supraorbital nerve blocks would be adequate. Similarly, if posterior scalp is the recipient area, occipital ring block can be used.
  - When anaesthesia is established, the recipient sites are created as follows: for single graft use 19 gauge needle (Figure 11.2.16); for mini grafts use 15C blade (Figure 11.2.17).

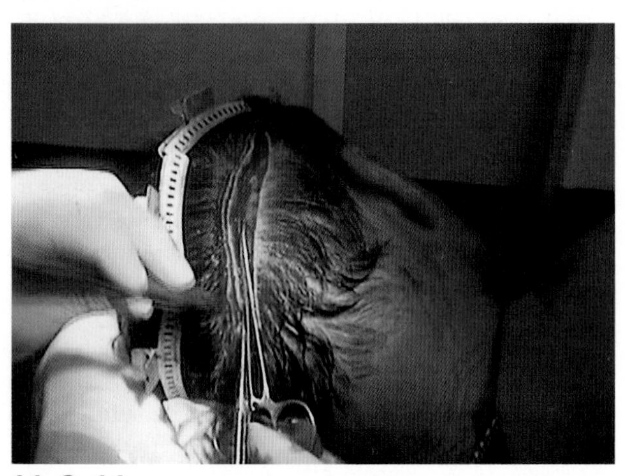

11.2.11 Multi-strip harvesting.

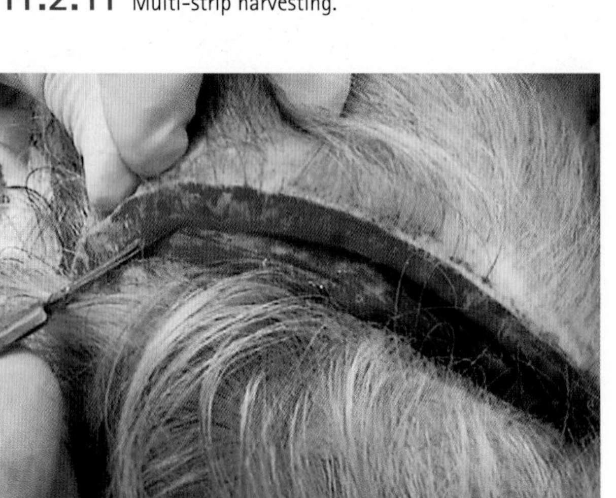

11.2.12 Minimal undermining of the donor site prior to closure.

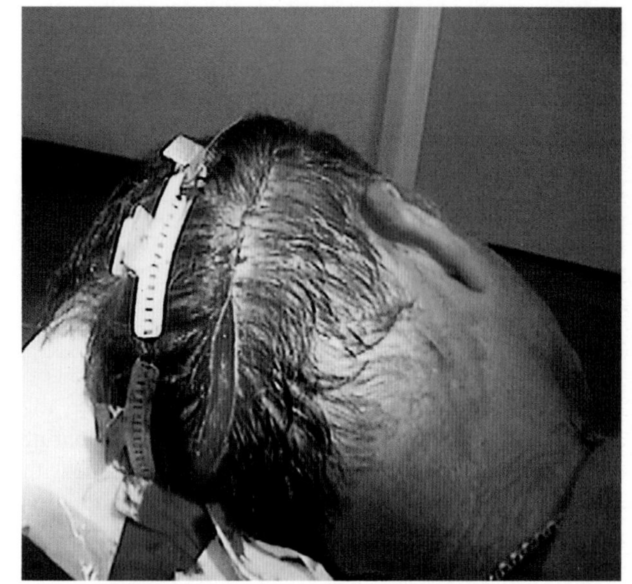

11.2.13 Donor site being closed with continuous suture.

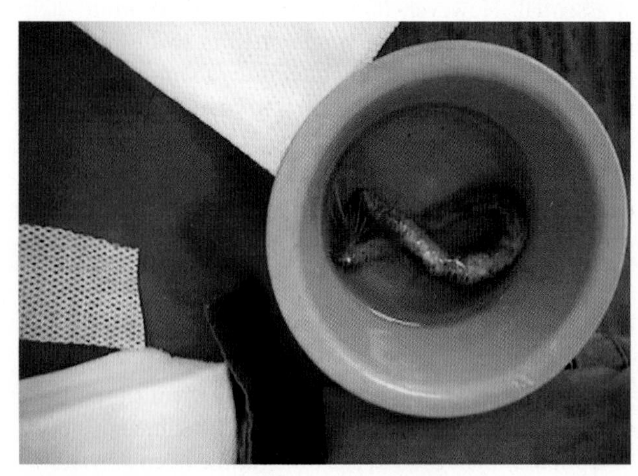

11.2.14 Harvested ellipse in cold saline.

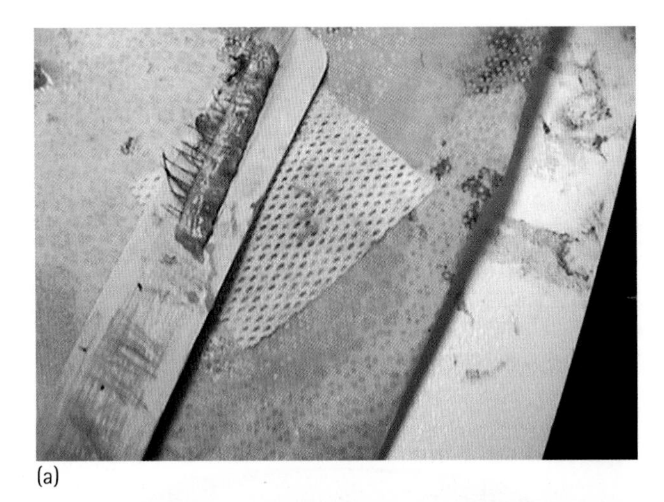

(a)

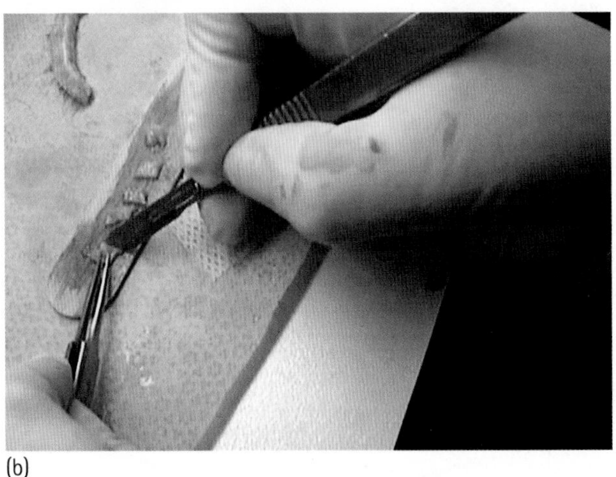

(b)

11.2.15 (a) Harvested ellipse cut into a strip. (b) Strips being cut into further smaller strips on a spatula.

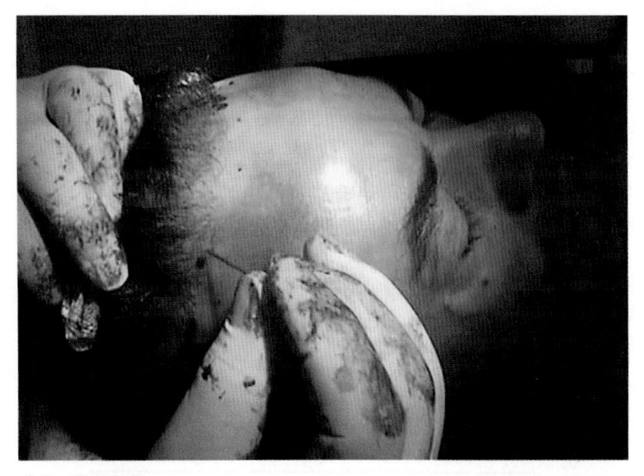

11.2.16 Recipient site being created for restoring hairline.

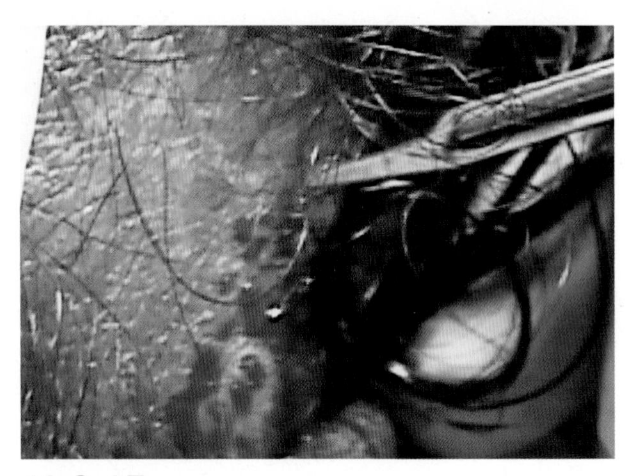

11.2.17 Making slits using 15C blade.

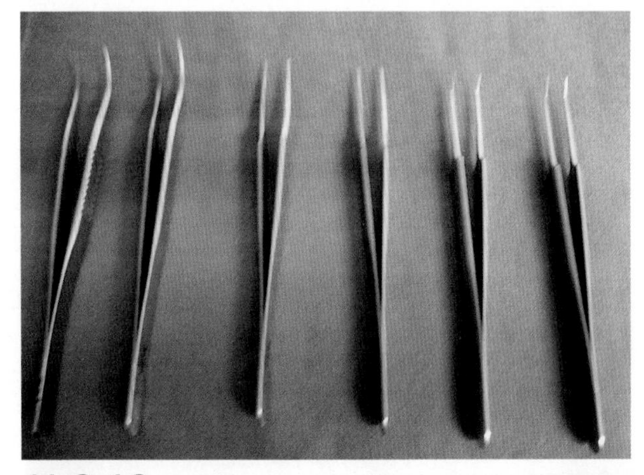

11.2.18 Curve and straight jewellers' forceps.

Slits are made as single stab incisions and can be made in large numbers. Some use 19G Nokor needles. With each slit there may be brisk bleeding. Usually it stops after the application of pressure for a few minutes with gauze. Sometimes dilators are necessary to facilitate closer placement of grafts. However, dilators take more time. Nevertheless, it is an important surgical tool in the armamentarium of a transplant surgeon.

Insertion of grafts at the recipient site is carried out using jewellers' forceps (Figure 11.2.18 showing curved and straight jewellers' forceps). Use the finer version of jewellers' forceps. It is only with considerable patience and effort that the skill of graft placement is mastered. If the grafts are placed too close, adjacent grafts will 'pop out'. This can be controlled by gentle pressure with moist gauze or a graft stick. Regular spraying with saline is done to keep the grafts moist.

Creation of hairlines

When hairline restoration has been planned, in deciding on the hairline, the rule of thirds of the face is followed. The lower third, mid third and upper third of the face are in equal proportions. It is most important NOT to place the hairline too low. The line is usually 8–10 cm above the glabella (Figure 11.2.19). In patients suffering from severe hair loss, the hairline can be raised higher by 1–2 cm.

However, in some patients the line is elevated higher by 1–2 cm, creating a 'widow's peak' (Figure 11.2.20 – widow's peak) giving a camouflaging effect to create a lower hairline.

The aim of hairline restoration is to create a most natural hairline which cannot be detected. The hairline consists of an anterior portion (transition zone) and a posterior portion (defused zone) (Figure 11.2.21). The transition zone is usually 0.5–1 cm and is irregular. Variation of hair density in this zone is normal (Figure 11.2.22 – hairline). In this zone (0.5–1 cm) only single hair follicular units or micrografts must be used to ensure the result appears natural.

The defused zone is usually 2–3 cm in width and should have a higher density of hair. In this zone, minigrafts containing two to four follicles or two to three follicular units are placed (Figure 11.2.23).

Creating the lateral border of the hairline and the frontotemporal angle

In all males, the frontal hairline meets the temporal hairline at the frontotemporal angle (Figure 11.2.24a–c). The angle

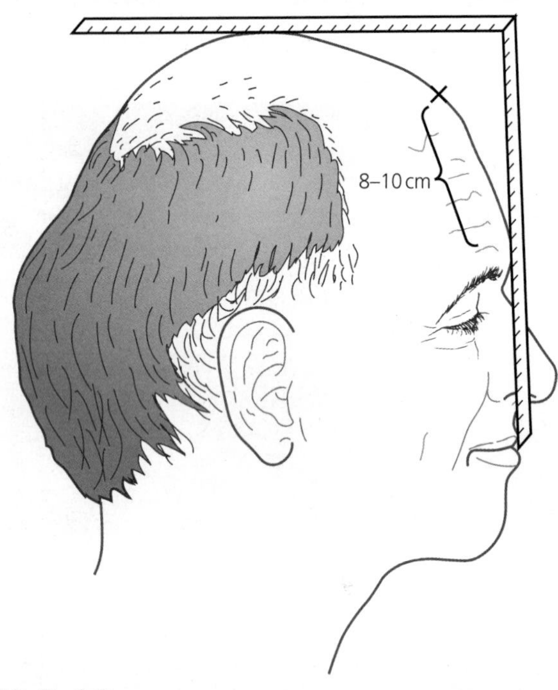

11.2.19 Proper placement of the anterior border of the hairline. Common guidelines for locating the anterior border of the hairline include: (1) 4 finger-breadths above the glabella; (2) 8–10 cm above the glabella; (3) the point where the horizontal plane of the scalp meets the vertical plane of the face.

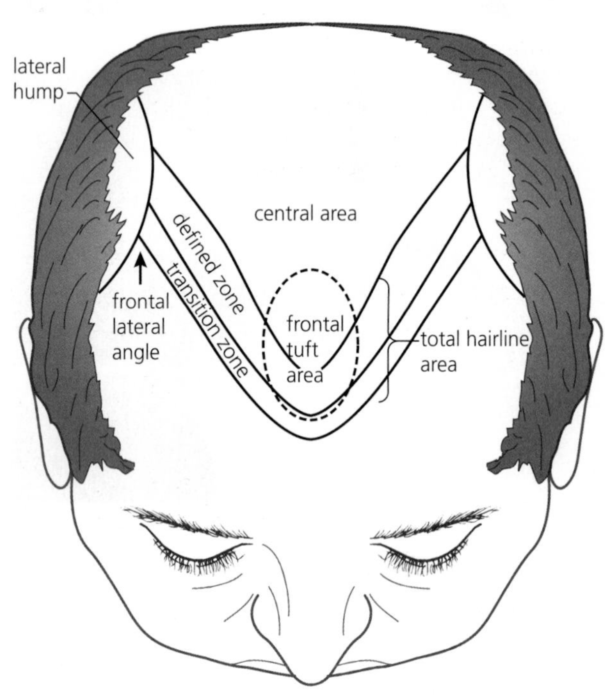

11.2.21 Hairline zones: The hairline consisting of two zones: the anterior portion ('transition zone') and the posterior portion ('defined zone'). The transition zone should be soft and irregular, and the defined zone should be more defined and dense. Both these zones are important to the overall appearance of the hairline.

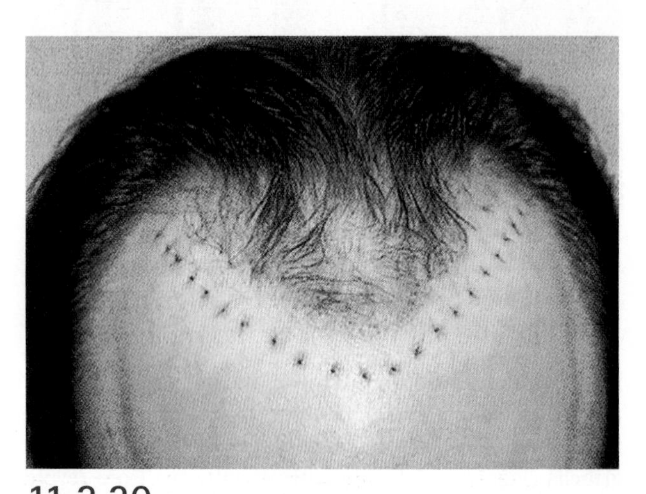

11.2.20 Creating a 'widow's peak'.

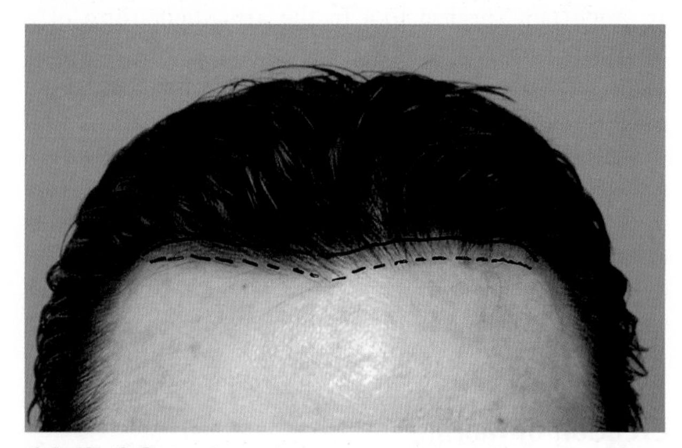

11.2.22 Note the hair between the dotted line and the line denotes transition zone. Line demarcates posteriorly the 'defined zone'. Variation of hair density in transition zone is normal.

at its union between the frontal and temporal line is called the apex (Figure 11.2.25 – diagram of frontal line, apex and temporal line).

- Do not create this angle too low.
- Do not blunt this angle.
- It must appear natural as far as possible.
- In achieving this point, draw a line from the lateral epicanthus to where it meets the existing temporal hair.
- The hairline should be best parallel or slope upward.

Figure 11.2.26 illustrates the placement of frontotemporal angle in severe hair loss.

Summary of creating hairlines

- Mark the anterior border of hairline, the transition zone and the defined zone.
- Mark the frontotemporal angle.
- Draw the widow's peak if it has been planned.

If no hairline restoration was planned:

- Mark out the area of baldness over the occiput or vertex. Draw the intended lines along which the minigrafts are to be placed (four to five hair follicles).

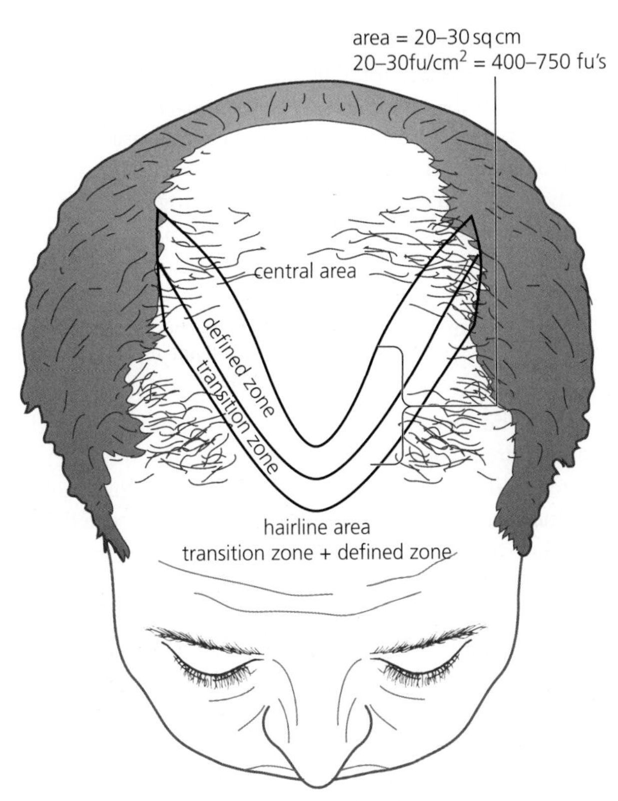

11.2.23 Estimated area of the hairline area: the total hairline area is the combination of the transition zone (TZ) the defined zone (DZ). The average size of the total hairline area ranges from 20–30 cm^2. At 25–30 fu/cm^2 it takes about 600–750 follicular units for this area.

- Transplant in each row, placing the follicles at least 2 mm apart and 1 mm between each row. If the follicles are placed too close during the placement, the hair follicles will 'pop out'.
- Preparing the recipient sites:
  - for restoring the anterior and temporal hairline;

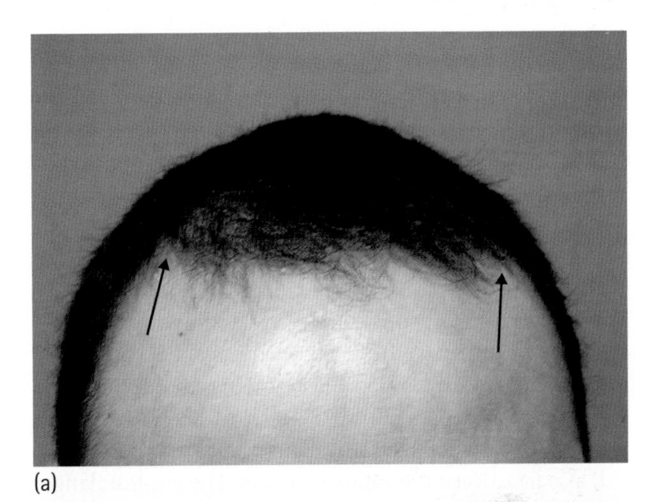
(a)

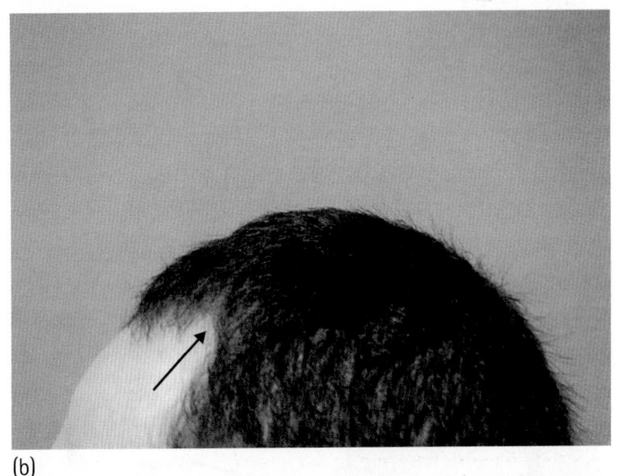
(b)

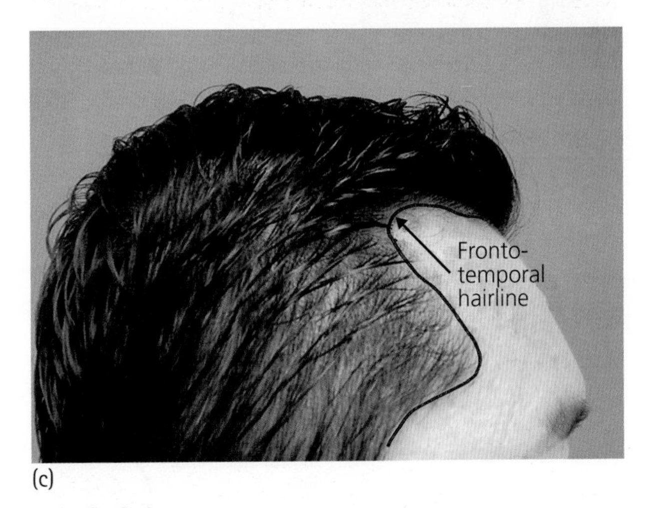

(c)

11.2.24 (a) Frontotemporal angle. (b) Frontotemporal angle. (c) The frontotemporal hairline in a 24-year-old Asian male.

- supraorbital and supratrochlear nerve blocks are given using 2 per cent lignocaine with 1:80 000 epinephrine (adrenaline) in a dental syringe containing 2.2 mL cartridges. Usually, 4–5 cc would suffice and anaesthesia can be obtained up to mid scalp;
- for posterior occipital area, occipital ring block is given;
- for eyebrow restoration, supraorbital block is given;
- for mustache creation, bilateral infraorbital nerve block is given.

Important notes

- If oral or intravenous sedation is used, continuous oxygen saturation and blood pressure monitoring is mandatory. The most preferred sedative agent is midazolam.
- Prior to the administration of local anaesthesia in an anxious patient, conscious sedation can be used (relative analgesia using nitrous oxide oxygen combination).
- The most preferred local anaesthetic agent is lignocaine. Some prefer bupivacaine. Bupivacaine is four times more potent than lignocaine. Therefore, 0.25 per cent bupivacaine would be equivalent to 1 per cent lignocaine. It also has a longer duration of action. The greatest danger of using bupivacaine is its property to induce arrythmia resulting in ventricular tachycardia resistant to treatment.
  - The maximum recommended dose for lignocaine with epinephrine is 7 mg/kg or 0.7 mL/kg of 1 per cent lignocaine. One per cent lignocaine has 10 mg/mL.
  - For an average 70 kg man, the maximum dose would be 50 mL of 1 per cent lignocaine with epinephrine.
  - The maximum recommended dose for 0.25 per cent bupivacaine with 1:100 000 epinephrine is 90 mL or 225 mg.

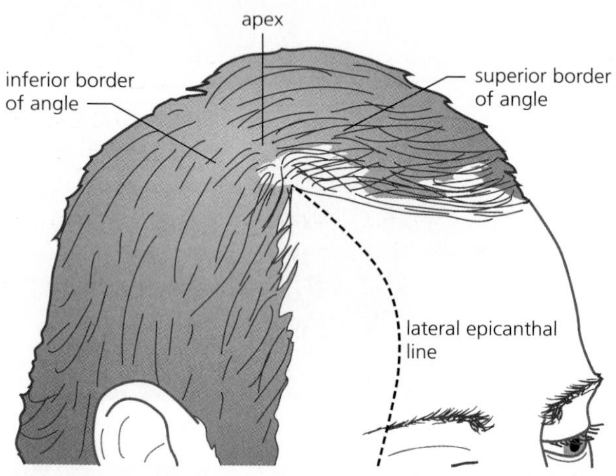

11.2.25 Placement of fronto temporal hairline when there is moderate hair loss.

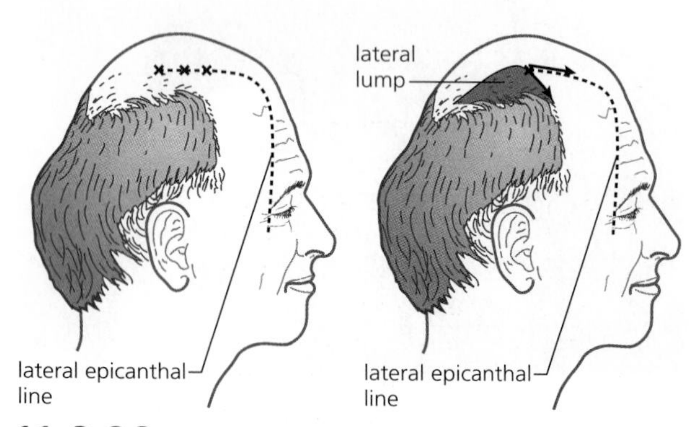

11.2.26 Placement of frontotemporal hairline in severe hair loss.

Giving detailed information and obtaining informed consent

- After hair transplantation, the hair is shed within 3–4 weeks. New hair growth will only be seen after 12 weeks and should grow at approximately 1 cm per month. After the transplantation procedure, there may be a temporary increase in natural hair loss but this will regrow within 3–6 months.
- Every hair follicle has a life cycle. Therefore, when transplanted into a new site it will produce pairs which are of a more permanent nature.
- The newly transplanted hair will grow, but with time it will become thin and undergo greying.
- Harvesting of donor hair will not damage the remaining hair.
- Information regarding creation of the front hairline and temporal hairline should be given. Ideally, they should be drawn and the consensus obtained and, if agreement is reached, photos should be taken. Personal preference of the patient is an important consideration.
- Advise to stop supplements such as gingko biloba and vitamin E 7 days before surgery. Aspirin should be stopped 5 days before the surgery. Alcohol should be forbidden for 24 hours before the surgery.
- An approximate estimate of time to be taken for the procedure should be given. The patient should be accompanied by another person and arrangements should be made to stay for at least 2 hours after the procedure is completed.
- There will be a bandage applied over the forehead to reduce oedema if a frontal hairline has been created. The patient is instructed to wear a theatre cap loosely if required. No shower is to be taken for 24 hours until after the first review.
- Instruction regarding pain at the donor site and recipient site should be given. Before leaving the surgical suite, analgesics should be prescribed. The patient should be instructed to sleep on their side. To avoid post-operative oedema, steroids are prescribed at the commencement of the transplantation and continued 8-hourly for 3–5 days. Instructions are also given to take the analgesics regularly with antacids to avoid gastric irritation by the steroids and the analgesics.
- Generally, there is only a faint scar at the donor site.

Likely post-operative complications are:

- Bruising around the forehead and eyelids usually on the third day, which may last up to a week.
- Scalp may ooze from the donor and recipient sites for 24 hours.
- The scalp may be numb.
- There may be headaches for 24–48 hours.
- It is unusual to develop infection.
- Recommend to be off work for 2–3 days if necessary. No active sports should be undertaken for 1 week.

Adjunctive medical therapy in hair transplantation

Currently, the US Food and Drug Administration approved agents that promote hair regrowth are:

- Topical minoxidil solution which comes in strength 2 per cent for females and 5 per cent for males. Women may use 5 per cent minoxidil; however, it has been associated with greater side effects, most notably scalp irritation and increased growth of facial hair.
- Oral finasteride tablets (1 mg daily) for men only. The above two agents will increase hair density, spread of regrowth of transplanted follicles and slow or stop hair loss in areas of active alopecia.

Hair growth is a dynamic process which consists of repeated cycles of active growth (anagen 2–6 years), involution (catagen 2–3 weeks) and rest (telogen 2–3 months). Approximately 90 per cent of all scalp follicles are in the anagen phase. Androgenetic hair loss in males and female pattern hair loss is induced by androgens in genetically susceptible hair follicles. Under the influence of dihydrotestosterone, the hair follicles shrink in size and the anagen phase becomes shorter.

The majority of hair transplant surgeons recommend the use of minoxidil and finasteride after the initial consultation for hair loss. These two medications have a synergistic effect. However, when finasteride is given, patients must be warned that there may be side effects during treatment, such as loss of libido, ejaculation disorder and erectile dysfunction. These effects are reversible and affect 2 per cent of men. It usually takes 3–4 months to see demonstrable effects with minoxidil treatment.

The advantages of using minoxidil prior to surgery are:

- increased number of hairs in anagen phase;
- increased hair density and hair weight;
- decreased post-surgical telogen shedding;
- the primary benefit of using minoxidil is within and surrounding the areas of hair loss;
- in the donor area, they may transform telogen follicles into the anagen phase and thereby these grafts would be more visible during the transplantation.

The benefits of using minoxidil after transplantation are:

- increase in number of hairs in the anagen phase;
- promotion of growth in the transplanted follicles and surrounding areas, reduction of post surgical 'shock' and telogen effluvium. It also enhances the diameter of the hair shaft, increases hair density and thereby enhances the result. In particular, the following two categories of patients require minoxidil after transplantation:
  - young male patients with diffuse hair thinning;
  - females with diffuse hair thinning.

Minoxidil should be stopped 5 days prior to transplantation as it may cause increased intra-operative bleeding and it can sometimes cause scalp irritation. After transplantation, minoxidil is started 5–14 days after surgery to avoid damage to the transplanted hair follicles. This delay also allows time for the healing of the epithelium. Finasteride, however, can be continued until the day of the surgery and immediately after surgery.

Use minoxidil 5 per cent as the author has noted greater density than when 2 per cent is used. One of the complications of using 5 per cent minoxidil is scalp irritation and facial hair appearance in women, but it is reversible when stopped. There is uniform consensus among most hair transplant surgeons to use finasteride and minoxidil pre-operatively and post-operatively in males and minoxidil in females. There is now emerging new evidence that finasteride can also be used in female patients.

Post-operative instructions (Table 11.2.2)

- Preferred option – use Graftcyte (manufactured by Procyte, Montgomeryville, PA, USA) for the first 48 hours as a spray over the grafted sites to prevent crusting.
- Patient is seen 24 hours later and a hair wash given. The forehead bandage is removed.
- Daily hair wash is permitted, but no scrubbing of the scalp is allowed.
- Staples over the donor site are removed on the 10th to 12th day.

COMPLICATIONS

Peri-operative complications and side effects are uncommon but may include:

- post-operative oedema over the frontal and periorbital region;
- haemorrhage from recipient sites;
- post-operative haematoma at donor site;
- after 48 hours, itchiness of the scalp;
- discrepancy between recipient slit size and donor grafts resulting in dropping out of the grafts;
- stretching of the donor site scar;
- poor growth – grafts were not kept as desired in storage solution (saline) and the follicles were dehydrated;
- overly dense packing of grafts resulting in ischaemia and poor growth;
- wound infection.

Table 11.2.2 Post-operative instructions for hair transplant

1. Do not take any medications (other than prescribed), vitamin E or alcohol for 48 hours after hair transplant
2. No dental work 72 hours following surgery
3. If at any time should any graft begin to bleed or pull out, simply apply direct pressure to the site for a minimum of 15 minutes. If that does not stop the bleeding, continue to apply pressure and immediately call the hair transplant surgeon
4. You will come back to the office in approximately 10 days to have your staples removed

Care of grafts after surgery:

You may start washing your hair on the third day after your surgery. You will want to wash it twice a day and we recommend using a mild shampoo. You must be very gentle with the grafts during shampooing, pat the area gently with your fingertips only, rinse thoroughly with low-pressure water flow and gently blow the grafts dry.

Swelling is a normal and harmless occurrence following the transplant and usually occurs 2–4 days from the date of surgery. In order to avoid swelling around the eyes when doing the hair transplant in the frontal area, lie down with your head elevated as much as possible. If swelling comes down the forehead, work the swelling to the side with your fingers so that it will go down the temples rather than down the bridge of your nose. Use ice packs or frozen peas to decrease swelling, but do not put them on top of the grafts.

DO NOT PICK THE SCABS, LET THEM FALL OFF!

Extreme care must be exerted so that your comb or brush does not catch on the scabs or staples during the healing process.

Refrain from any strenuous physical activities for at least 5 days.

Guidelines for deciding the width and length of donor strip to harvest

1 Make a decision of how many grafts are required, e.g. 1450.
2 Measure the circumference of the back of the head, e.g. 22 cm.

One graft per mm length is the rule of thumb. Therefore, in a 22 cm long strip, 220 grafts can be obtained. Hence, to harvest 1450 grafts, six strips would be required. If a 1.75 and 1.25 mm spacer is used in a multi-bladed knife, you could accordingly obtain micro and minigrafts.

Recipient sites

- Proper depth control in site creation is critical (Figure 11.2.27 illustrates recipient sites).
- If the sites are too deep, damage is done to the deeper vascular plexus. Likewise, if the sites are too shallow, graft loss can occur. If the site created is too small, excessive manipulation is required to plant the graft and this would cause damaging pressure on the graft.
- Patience and flexibility in preparation of recipient sites is the key for success. Sometimes, during recipient site creation, bleeding occurs with the slightest manipulation and the adjacent grafts pop up with each new graft insertion. Patience is the virtue. Do not rush the creation of recipient sites. Depth control, angulation and direction of the grafts govern success in a transplant procedure.
- Figures 11.2.28, 11.2.29 and 11.2.30 illustrate grafts in recipient sites.

Hair transplantation in Asians

The following are key important facts to be taken into consideration for hair transplant in Asians.

- Usually hair density is lower when compared to Caucasians. The hair is coarse and straight. Hair is darker.
- Asians have a much greater tendency to form hypertrophic scars and keloids. Hence, scalp reduction is a poor option. Likewise, donor site scars may also become hypertrophic. At the earliest detection, intradermal steroids should be injected.

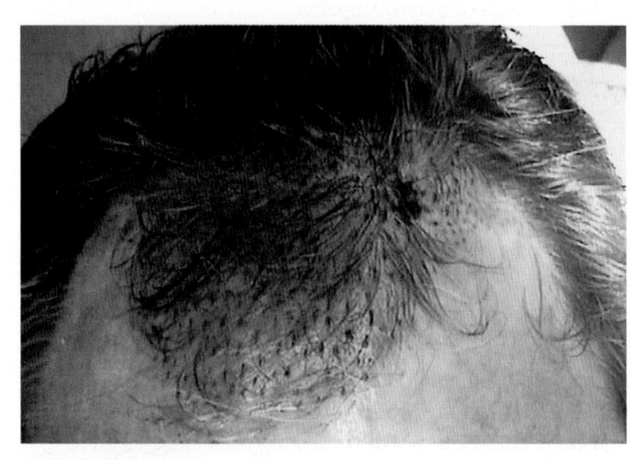

11.2.27 Recipient sites after creation.

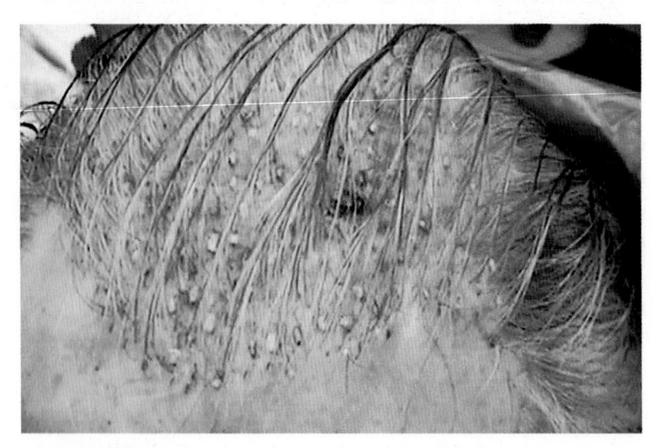

11.2.28 Grafts in sites after placement into slits.

- Asians like to have a low hairline and this request should be resisted and the hairline should only be chosen according to facial proportions and what is most natural.
- Figure 11.2.31 illustrates a pre-operative view of an anterior hairline in an Asian patient. Figure 11.2.32 illustrates the hairline after restoration with micro and minigrafts.

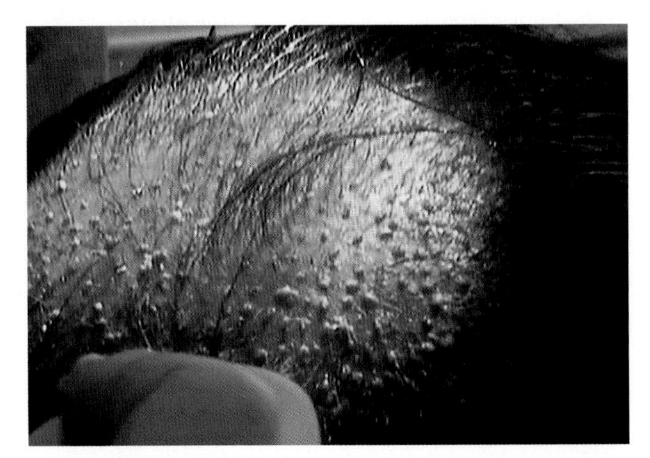

11.2.29 Grafts in place in the recipient sites.

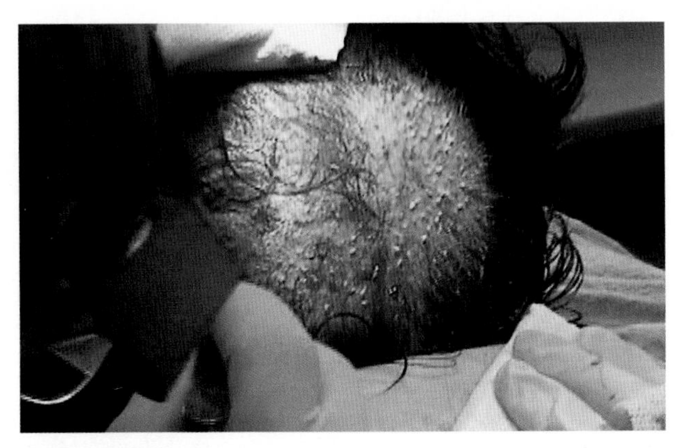

11.2.30 Grafts in place at the recipient sites.

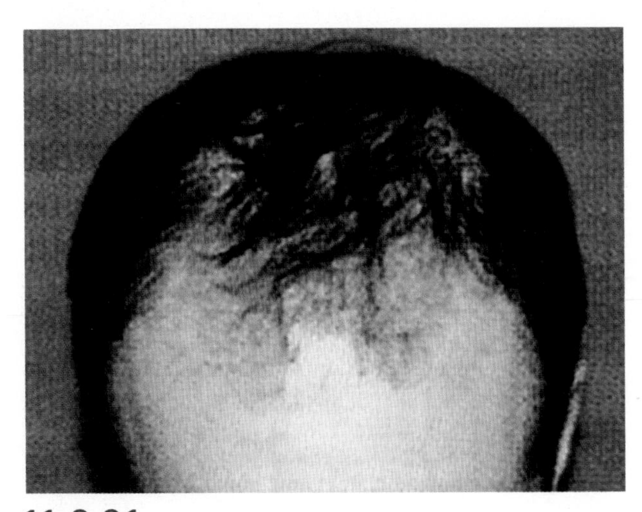

11.2.31 Pre-operative photo for restoration of anterior hairline and anterior scalp.

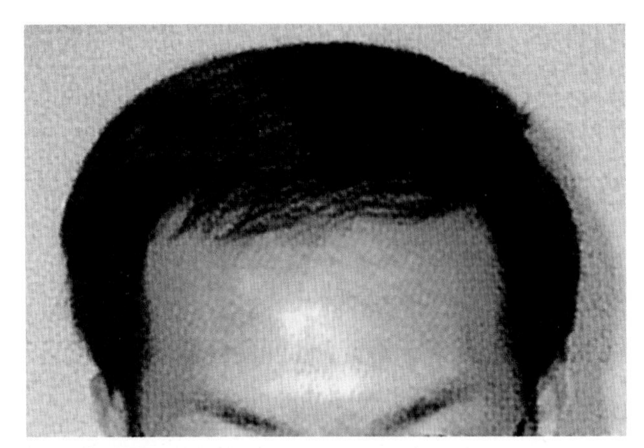

11.2.32 Post-operative photo.

Top tips

- Harvesting of grafts (donor site – occipital scalp)
  - Maximum length 25 cm and width 10 mm.
  - If a multi-bladed knife is used, spacers between the blades come as 2 or 1 mm spacers. If a previous scar is incorporated into the graft, a 4 mm spacer is used so that in such cases two strips can be obtained. The hair follicles can be dissected from these two strips. To harvest the follicles from these strips, the author uses the 15C blade for monografts and a Persanna size 10 blade in the multi-bladed knife between the spacers.
  - If the donor graft is to be harvested as a single ellipse, a conventional scalpel is used with a size 10 blade. Prior to harvesting, trim the hair to a plane where you can just see the hair direction as you would alter the direction of the scalpel with the direction of the hair follicles. From the harvested strip, small strips are made by slicing into small pieces. From each small piece, single, two and three hair grafts are dissected either with or without the use of a ×10 stereoscopic microscope. Each follicular unit may have three hairs, two hairs or one hair. Close the donor site as a single layer with staples as this gives the best scar.
  - At no time should the harvested hair follicles be allowed to dehydrate. The grafts must be kept moist throughout the procedure. The best solution in use is either cold Ringer's lactate or cold saline.
  - Warning: while preparing the grafts, DO NOT cause damage to the pilosebaceous unit and transection to the follicles.
- Creating recipient sites in the bald areas or areas to be transplanted:
  - for micrografts – 19G needle;
  - for minigrafts – 15C blade.

Good rules:

- Aim for 30–25 grafts/cm^2.
- Place the grafts 3 mm apart laterally and 1 mm apart posteriorly.

FURTHER READING

American Society of Hair Restoration Surgery. Available from: www.cosmeticsurgery.org

Ayres S. Prevention and correction of unaesthetic results of hair transplantation for male pattern baldness. *Cutis* 1977; **19**: 117–21.

Bernstein RM, Rassman WR. Follicular transplantation. Patient evaluation and surgical planning. *Dermatologic Surgery* 1997; **23**: 771–84; discussion 801–5.

International Society of Hair Restoration Surgery. Available from: www.ISHRS.org

Limmer BL. Elliptical donor stereoscopically assisted micrografting as an approach to further refinement in hair transplantation. *Journal of Dermatologic Surgery and Oncology* 1994; **20**: 789–93.

Marritt E. Transplantation of single hairs from the scalp as eyelashes. Review of the literature and a case report. *Journal of Dermatologic Surgery and Oncology* 1980; **6**: 271–3.

Marritt E. Single-hair transplantation for hairline refinement: a practical solution. *Journal of Dermatologic Surgery and Oncology* 1984; **10**: 962–6.

Marritt E. Follimmerlicular transplantation. Giving credit where credit is due. *Dermatologic Surgery* 1998; **24**: 925–9; discussion 929–32.

Nordstrom RE. Methods to improve old results of punch hair grafting. *Plastic and Reconstructive Surgery* 1983; **72**: 803–9.

Orentreich N. Autografts in alopecias and other selected dermatological conditions. *Annals of the New York Academy of Sciences* 1959; **83**: 463–79.

Shapiro R. Creating a natural hairline in one session using a systematic approach and modern principles of hairline design. *International Journal of Cosmetic Surgery and Aesthetic Dermatology* 2001; **3**: 89–99.

Stough D. Presentation at International Society of Hair Restoration Surgery Live Surgery Workshop, Orlando, FL. Feb 21, 2001.

Unger WP (ed). *Hair transplantation*, 4th edn. New York: Informa Healthcare, 2004.

11.3

Brow lift and face lift, including endoscopic surgery

TIRBOD FATTAHI

INTRODUCTION

Brow lifts and face lifts are commonly performed aesthetic procedures of the facial region. Hallmarks of the ageing process include descent of the brows, redundant tissue in the upper lids, rounding of the lower lids, ptosis of the mid face and the superficial musculoaponeurotic system (SMAS), fullness of the nasolabial fold, loss of the jaw line, dermatochalasia of the facial region, formation of jowls, platysmal redundancy and submental fullness. Goals of any facial aesthetic surgery must include repositioning of ptotic tissues to their original position, reversal of the vector of the ageing process from an inferior and medial direction to a superior and posterior direction, and obtaining a natural appearing 'unoperated' final result. It is imperative to remember that total facial rejuvenation requires addressing three distinct regions: forehead and brows, face and neck. Each region requires a separate operation; each procedure can be carried out simultaneously with the other two or, in some instances, some can be performed independently. A brow lift will address the forehead, brows and, to a lesser extent, the upper eye lids. A face lift will address the central and lateral portions of the face, jowls and the posterior neck. A cervicoplasty (with platysmaplasty and open submental liposuction) addresses the anterior or central portion of the neck. The most consistent method to obtain a long-lasting total facial rejuvenation involves a brow lift (endoscopic), a deep plane face lift and a cervicoplasty. The purpose of this chapter is to discuss pre-operative assessment and patient selection, surgical execution and potential complications of each surgical procedure used in facial rejuvenation.

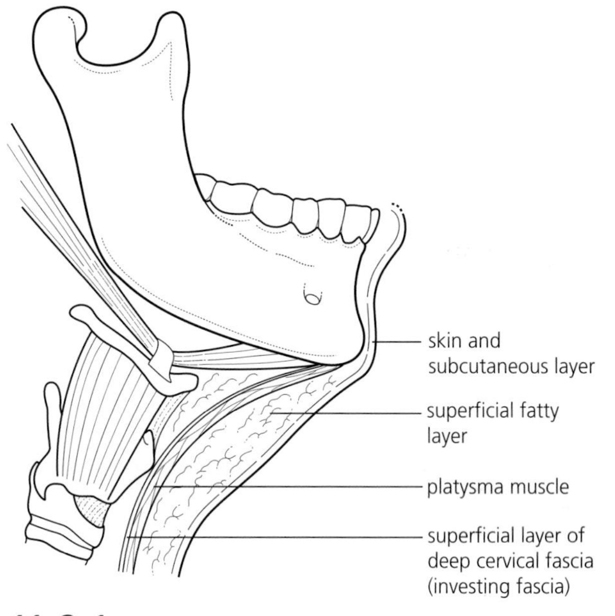

11.3.1 Anatomy of the central neck where a cervicoplasty is performed (from T. Fattahi, Management of isolated neck deformity. *Atlas Oral Maxillofac Surg Clin N Am* 2004; **12**: 263.)

CERVICOPLASTY

PRE-OPERATIVE ASSESSMENT

Pre-operative assessment for the patient seeking a cervicoplasty must include evaluation of the following structures (Figure 11.3.1):

- cervicomental angle;
- platysmal appearance – presence of bands or redundancy of the muscle in its central region;
- submental lipomatosis;
- position of the hyoid bone;
- position of the mandible and chin and assessment of the occlusion;
- presence of jowling and facial dermatochalasia;
- position of the submandibular glands.

Ideal neck appearance should include smooth neck skin, lack of submental lipomatosis, presence of defined jaw line, subtle inframandibular concavities anterior to the sternocleidomastoid (SCM) muscles, a small thyroid cartilage and a cervicomental angle of 110°. It is important to remember that an isolated cervicoplasty will not dramatically improve jowling; this deformity is mainly addressed by a deep plane face lift. Since many patients (over the age of 40) who desire a face lift also have jowlings, the author always performs a cervicoplasty at the time of a face lift. Isolated cervicoplasty is indicated in patients who have submental lipomatosis and platysmal redundancy in the absence of jowls.

SURGICAL PROCEDURE

The patient should be marked in the pre-operative room while sitting up. The inferior border of the mandible, anterior borders of the SCM muscles, inferior extent of the submental lipomatosis and any existing cervicomental crease are marked with ink (Figure 11.3.2). A 2–2.5 cm incision (slight curved) is marked just posterior to any existing cervicomental crease, since placing the incision within the crease can create an exaggerated and deep crease post-operatively. The procedure is carried out under general anaesthesia with intubation. After administration of local anaesthetic with a vasoconstrictor, the incision is made through the skin and subcutaneous fascia (cervical fascia). Any existing cervicomental crease (anterior to the incision) is sharply incised in the subcutaneous plane. Next, using curved face lift scissors, a skin flap with 3–4 mm of subcutaneous fat on its deep side is elevated from the centre portion of the neck all the way to the anterior borders of the SCM bilaterally. It is imperative to keep 3–4 mm of fat on this skin flap in order to prevent excessive scar contracture post-operatively. Once the skin flap is elevated and free of any ligamentous attachments to the underlying tissues, open liposuction is performed via liposuction cannulas (2–3 mm ports) in the central and lateral aspects of the neck in between the SCM muscles (Figure 11.3.3). Care is taken not to perform any liposuction above the inferior border of the mandible to prevent damage to the marginal mandibular branch of the facial nerve. Liposuction is completed when the investing layer of the deep cervical fascia is clearly visible atop the platysma muscle. Next, a subplatysmal flap is elevated and the central portion of the platysma (the redundant portion or the aponeurosis) is sharply excised starting at the genial tubercles and extending inferiorly to the thyroid cartilage. This is carried out with caution since the anterior jugular veins run just deep to the muscle in this region. The resected portion of the platysma should have a diamond or oval shape to it (Figure 11.3.4). The two edges of the muscle are then brought together in the midline and imbricated using 3/0 PDS sutures in a continuous locking fashion in a cephalo-caudal direction. During the imbrication of the muscle, it is important to close the patient's mouth and establish occlusion; this ensures the most posterior (deep) placement of the muscle flap. After muscle closure, the author uses a fibrin sealant (spray) under the skin flap to decrease the chances of haematoma formation; no surgical drains are ever used in cervicoplasty, face lift or endoscopic brow lift as long as fibrin sealants have been used prior to skin closure (Figure 11.3.5). No skin is excised around the incision since skin contracture and shrinkage over the next few weeks obviate the need for this manoeuver. The incision is closed in a two-layered fashion and dressed with Steri-strips. A pressure dressing is applied over the patient's head and is maintained for 24–48 hours.

POST-OPERATIVE MANAGEMENT

The patient is seen in the office within 24 hours post-operatively to ensure that no haematoma formation has

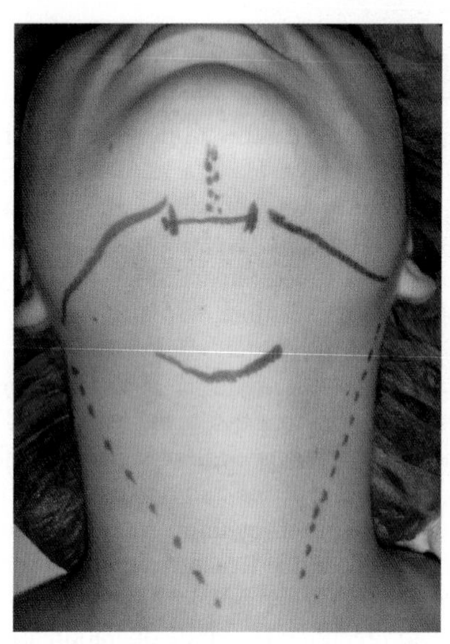

11.3.2 Typical markings for a cervicoplasty. The anterior borders of the SCM, the inferior border of the mandible and the proposed incision are marked in the pre-operative area.

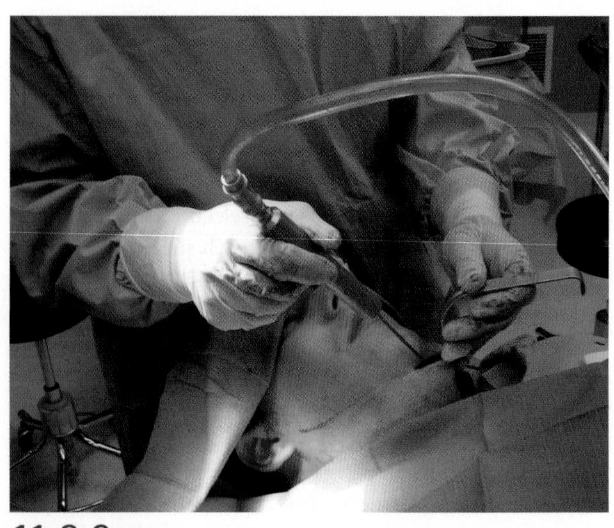

11.3.3 Open liposuction of the submental region following elevation of a skin flap.

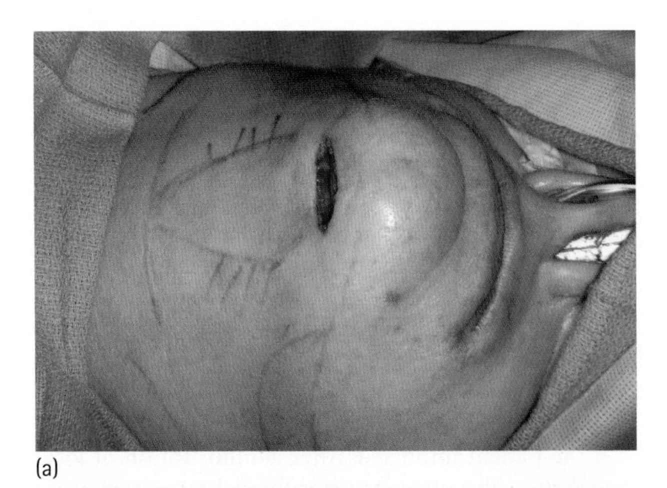

(a)

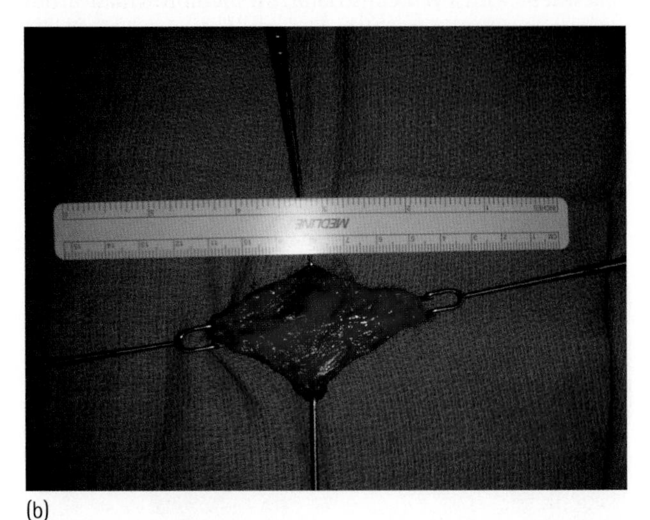

(b)

11.3.4 (a and b) Appearance following excision of redundant platysma. The two edges of platysma are then imbricated together.

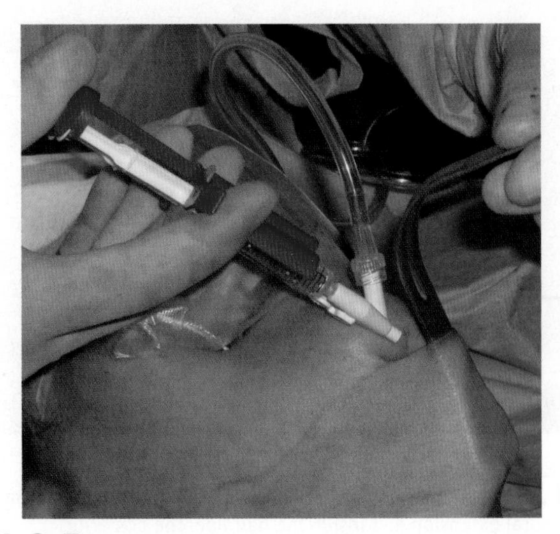

11.3.5 Application of fibrin sealant into the surgical site in place of surgical drains.

occurred. The pressure dressing can be removed in 24–48 hours according to surgeon preference. The patient is restricted from any strenuous physical activity for 2–3 weeks to prevent dehiscence of the platysmal closure. The patient is also asked not to turn his/her head during the same period; rather it is advised that patient turns his/her entire shoulder/body. This is also to prevent dehiscence of the platysmal closure. Perioperative antibiotics are administered for 24–48 hours according to surgeon preference.

COMPLICATIONS

Complications associated with cervicoplasty are rare. The most commonly encountered risks include haematoma formation, skin asymmetry or dimpling, damage to the marginal mandibular branch of the facial nerve and a 'cobra neck deformity'. Risk of haematoma formation is significantly reduced by the use of fibrin sealants; some surgeons advocate use of surgical drains, although it is the opinion of the author that surgical drains are unnecessary as long as a fibrin sealant is used. Skin asymmetries and dimpling can occur as the skin flap contracts and re-adheres to the underlying muscle. Minor asymmetries are easily managed by massage. If persistent, scar revision and/or lysis of adhesions may be required. Marginal mandibular nerve injuries can easily be avoided by adhering to sound surgical techniques; skin flap elevation and liposuction should not be performed superior to the inferior border of the mandible. The marginal mandibular branch can cross the inferior border of the mandible in an inferior–superior direction to reach the depressors of the lower lip and can be injured if the dissection or liposuction is performed above the inferior border of the mandible. The 'cobra neck deformity' can occur when excessive and injudicious liposuction has been carried out. Also, if an adequate amount of subcutaneous fat (3–4 mm) has not been maintained on the skin flap, damage to the subdermal vascular layer can occur which can lead to excessive scarring and a 'skeletonized' look.

DEEP PLANE FACE LIFT

PRE-OPERATIVE ASSESSMENT

It is once again important to mention that a face lift only addresses the central and lateral portions of the face, the jowls and the posterior neck. Rejuvenation of the central or anterior aspect of the neck requires a cervicoplasty which, as stated previously, is always performed simultaneously with the face lift (when a face lift is indicted) by the author. The patient desiring a face lift should be counselled on the following:

- degree of ptosis of the midface;
- dermatochalasia of the facial skin and subcutaneous tissues;

- laxity of the facial skin;
- loss of volume (especially in thin patients along the prezygomatic space anterior to the masseter muscle);
- presence of jowls;
- loss of definition of the jaw line;
- presence of rhytids;
- fullness of the nasolabial fold.

The youthful face exhibits no redundancy or ptosis of the facial skin and its subcutaneous tissues. Hallmarks of an attractive and youthful face also include a triangular shaped face, high cheek bones, mild depression in the prezygomatic space anterior to the masseter muscles, absence of nasolabial fullness or a crease, a well-defined jaw line and no jowling. A face lift, when performed properly, can reposition the ptotic facial tissues back to their original position. Since the vector of descent in the aged face is in an anterior and medial direction, redundant tissues should be redraped in a posterior and superior direction. It is important to establish pre-operatively if the patient can benefit from bony volume augmentation, such as cheek, chin or mandibular angle implants. If the patient has lost volume in the face due to the ageing process or congenital hypoplasia of the facial skeleton, simultaneous placement of the implants at the time of face lift surgery can significantly improve the final outcome.

The main benefit of a deep plane (SMAS flap) face lift is the ability to reposition the SMAS, which in turn reduces the amount of tension placed on the skin flap. It is easy to recognize patients who have had a 'skin'-only face lift by the 'pulled' appearance of the face, which can be quite unnatural. Since the ageing process is not simply limited to the skin, it is logical to address all of the tissues of the aged face during a face lift by performing a deep plane face lift.

SURGICAL PROCEDURE

The patient is marked in the pre-operative area while sitting up. The incision is composed of temporal, preauricular and postauricular components (Figure 11.3.6). The vertical portion of the temporal incision is marked just inside the temporal hairline. This is only about 1–1.5 cm in length. The horizontal component is also just inside the most inferior aspect of the side burn (usually at the level of the top of the helix). This portion of the incision must be beveled about 20° for cosmesis and future hair growth. The posterior aspect of this incision is hidden behind the superior helix for about 1 cm. The preauricular aspect of the incision is marked from the posterior aspect of the temporal incision inferiorly following a natural skin crease anterior to the ear to just above the tragus. The incision must not be in a straight line; rather curling the incision to just above the tragus provides a much more aesthetic result. From the superior aspect of the tragus, the incision can be again made preauricularly or retrotragally, depending on surgeon's preference. The preauricular incision must also be made with a 20° bevel for a more aesthetic closure. The marking for the postauricular component begins from the most inferior aspect of the preauricular incision, curls around the ear lobe, extends cephalad on the posterior ear skin, 1–2 mm from the junction of the mastoid skin and ear skin, and then gently curves posteriorly and inferiorly along the posterior hair line. The height of the postauricular incision is at the level of the widest portion of the ear. The inferior aspect of the marking along the posterior hair line is determined by the amount of lateral pull necessary to define the jaw line. The more inferior the incision, the more posterior and lateral the vector of the flap will be.

The procedure is performed under general anaesthesia with the patient intubated. After administration of local anaesthetic with a vasoconstrictor, the incision is made from the temporal aspect with a No. 15 blade, paying special attention to the areas which require a bevel. Once the entire incision is made, attention is directed towards the preauricular area. While applying counter traction on the cheek (assistant's hand on the cheek), a skin flap is elevated leaving

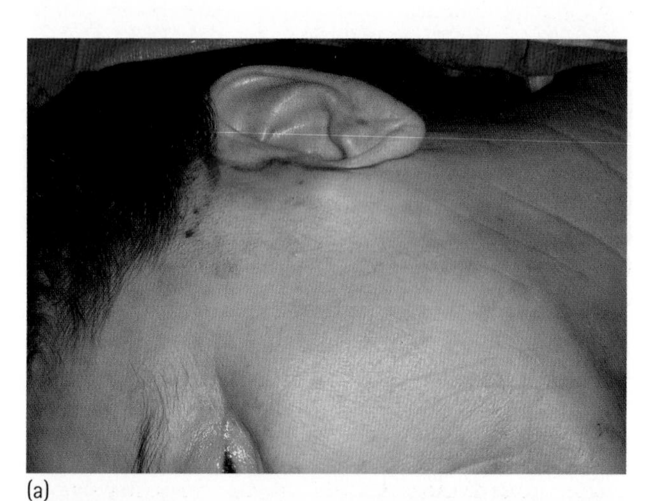

(a)

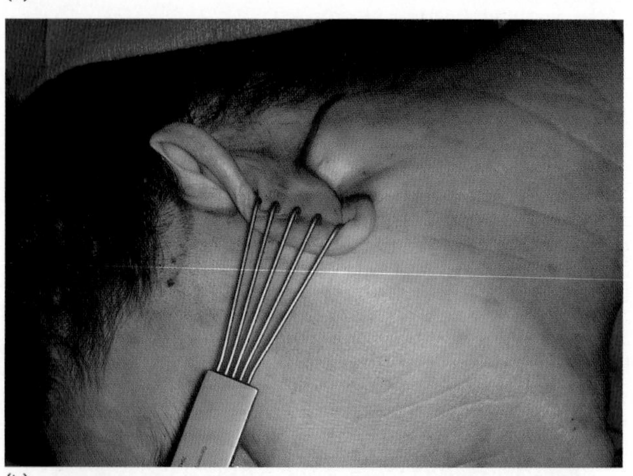

(b)

11.3.6 (a and b) Proposed incision for a face lift. Note the temporal extension just inside the hair line, the posterior extension of the temporal incision, the preauricular and postauricualar markings.

adequate amount of fat on its under side (3–4 mm). This is initially done with a blade and can be advanced using face lift scissors. The anterior aspect of this flap is only about 5–6 cm (Figure 11.3.7). This skin flap is easily elevated in supra-SMAS plane. The postauricular skin flap is more difficult to elevate due to the fusion of multiple fascias in the area. Care is taken not to enter the SCM muscle while elevating this skin flap. Once an adequate skin flap is elevated circumferentially, a SMAS flap is outlined extending from the temporal side burn down on to the neck. This marking is about 1 cm anterior to the skin flap incision (Figure 11.3.8). Local anaesthesia with a vasoconstrictor is administered into the SMAS. Next, using a No. 15 blade the SMAS is incised in a vertical fashion. There should be little concern with the facial nerve at this point since the underlying parotid capsule (which protects the nerve) is never incised. Once the SMAS incision has been made, blunt dissection under good visualization of the SMAS flap is undertaken in an anterior direction over the parotid gland between the zygomatic arch superiorly and 2 cm below the jaw line inferiorly (Figure 11.3.9). The anterior (medial) extent of the SMAS flap is dependent on the amount of posterior and superior repositioning necessary to efface the nasolabial fold and redundant skin. However, once the zygomaticus major muscle is encountered, the sub-SMAS dissection must be converted into a supra-SMAS dissection to prevent injury to the branches of the facial nerve since almost all of the muscles of the facial expression are innervated on the deep side. The deep plane (SMAS) dissection also allows for sharp dissection of several osteo-cutaneous retaining ligaments of the face such as the McGregor's patch (Figure 11.3.10). Release of these ligaments allows significant elevation of the SMAS flap and allows for a much more aesthetic final result. If the submandibular glands are ptotic, they can be elevated through the SMAS flap.

Once the SMAS flap is elevated, it is placed on tension and pulled in a superior and posterior vector along its entire length. Excess SMAS is incised (Figure 11.3.11). Key sutures using 2/0 PDS are placed within the SMAS and anchored on

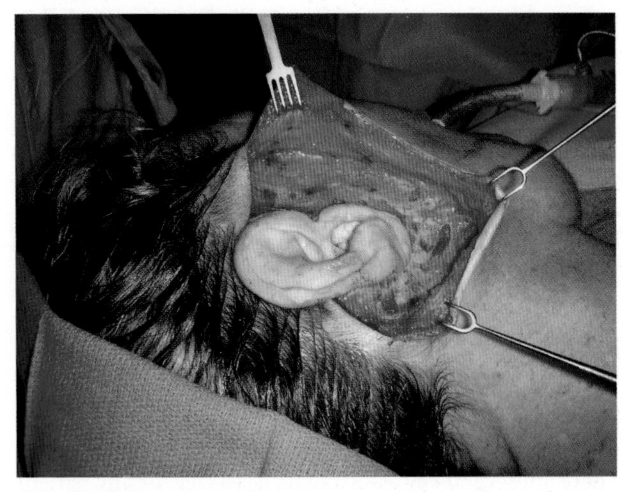

11.3.7 Elevation of a skin flap.

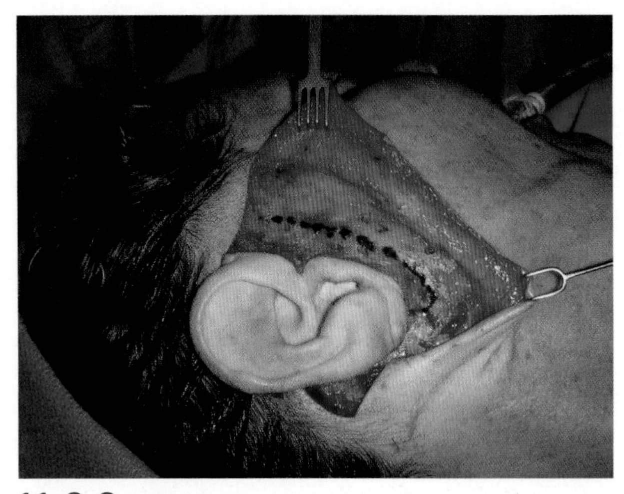

11.3.8 Marking of SMAS incision approximately 1 cm anterior to the preauricular incision.

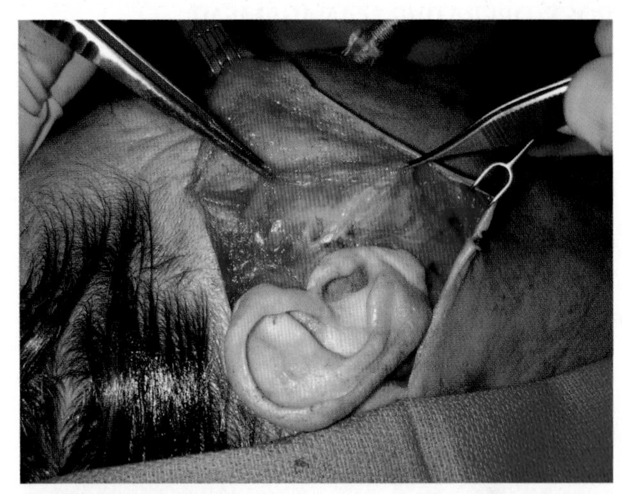

11.3.9 Elevation of a SMAS flap. Note retaining ligaments attached to parotid capsule deep to the SMAS.

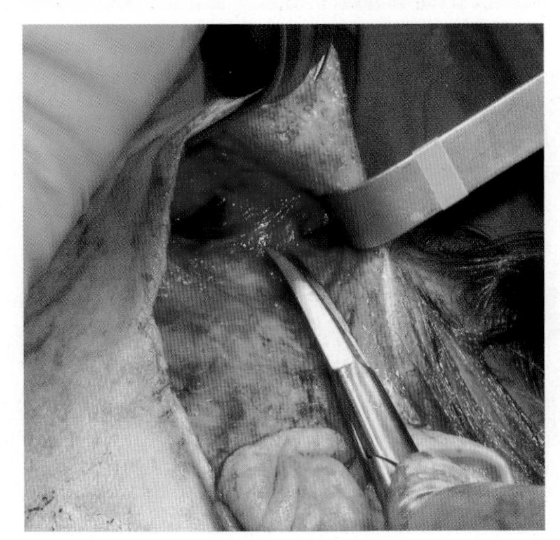

11.3.10 Scissors pointing to the McGregor's osteocutaneous ligaments.

the deep temporal fascia, preauricular perichondrium and mastoid fascia posteriorly. This should allow for a well-defined jaw line. The SMAS flap is essentially acting as a carrier for the skin flap. Once the SMAS flap has been sutured properly, there should be almost no tension on the skin flap above it. The skin flap is then redraped; excess skin is incised. Care is taken to incise the skin flap in a beveled fashion as well in order to align the skin flap bevel with the preauricular bevel. The skin is closed in two layers using 5/0 vicryl sutures (deep) and 6/0 resorbable sutures on the skin. The author routinely used skin adhesives (DermaBond) on the preauricular aspect of the closure. The postauricular aspect is closed in two layers as well, using 5/0 vicryl and 5/0 skin sutures. Prior to closure of the skin flap, fibrin sealant is sprayed on the field (between the SMAS flap and skin flap). This obviates the need for placement of surgical drains. A compression dressing is then applied to the patient head.

POST-OPERATIVE MANAGEMENT

The patient is seen in 24 hours. The pressure dressing is removed to determine skin flap viability and the presence of any haematomas. The pressure dressing is reapplied for another 24–48 hours. The patient is instructed to avoid strenuous physical activities and to apply ice packs to the face to help with post-operative oedema. The patient's head must stay elevated compared to his/her body to reduce swelling. Perioperative antibiotics can be discontinued in 24–48 hours. Any permanent suture is removed in 5 days.

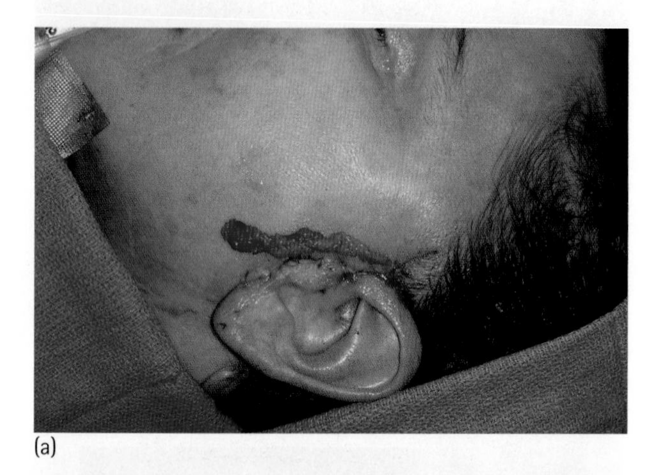

(a)

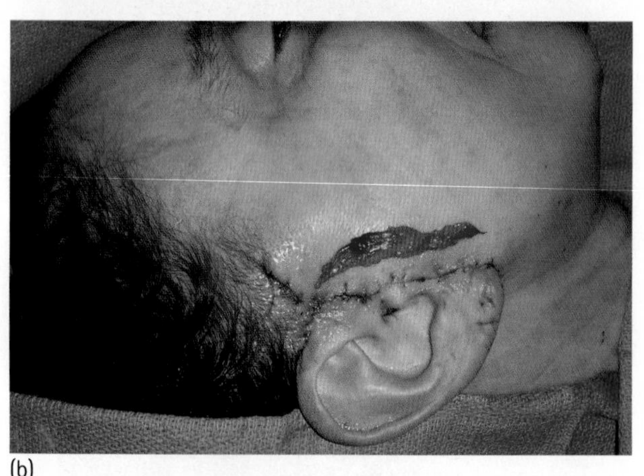

(b)

11.3.11 (a and b). Excised SMAS from left and right following skin closure.

COMPLICATIONS

The most common and feared complication of a face lift is haematoma formation post-operatively. For this reason, surgical haemostasis intraoperatively and use of fibrin sealants is mandatory. No surgical drains are used when the author performs a deep plane face lift, although many surgeons continue to advocate their utility. If a haematoma is present post-operatively, it must be drained in order to prevent skin flap necrosis and significant post-operative scarring. When performing a deep plane face lift, damage to the branches of the facial nerve is a possibility. It is imperative to elevate the SMAS flap in a blunt fashion and use good visualization (surgical head lights). Neuropraxia of the facial nerve branches usually resolves in a few weeks post-operatively. Other complications include asymmetries between the right and the left sides, hypertrophic scars, inadequate repositioning of the redundant skin flap, malposition of the hair line and a pixie ear deformity. Mild asymmetries between the two sides of the face may not be noticeable to the patient and usually do not require any treatment. Obviously, it is important to 'pull' equally on both sides to ensure symmetrical repositioning of the skin flap on both sides. Hypertrophic scars can be avoided if no tension is placed on the skin flap at closing. If they are present, intradermal steroid injection and constant massaging may improve their appearance. In order to avoid malposition of the hair lines, the skin flap must be adapted properly. If a dog ear is created (usually around the anterior aspect of the side burns and at the postauricular area), it must be excised carefully. Face lift incisions that are carried superiorly on to the temple from the superior helix usually lead to malpositioning of the hair line. Pixie ear deformities occur when the ear lobe is reattached to the facial skin improperly and no longer has mobility to it. This is problematic, especially when earrings are attached to the ear lobe. Ear lobe deformities can be avoided by reattaching the most superior portion of the ear lobe to the facial skin flap. It is also important to recall the position of the earlobes pre-operatively when performing this manoeuver (patient photos in the operating room is quite helpful).

ENDOSCOPIC BROW LIFT

PRE-OPERATIVE ASSESSMENT

There are several key assessments necessary for any patient undergoing an endoscopic brow lift. These include:

- position of the eye brows;
- presence of dermatochalasia of the upper lids;
- forehead rhytids;
- position of the frontal hairline;
- slope and length of the forehead;
- status of the corrugator muscles.

An endoscopic brow lift is intended to elevate the ptotic brows and brow (galea) fat pads to a more normal position. The ideal eyebrow in a male is a straight brow that is 0–2 mm above the supraorbital rims. The ideal female brow should be arched with the medial head 0–2 mm above the supraorbital rim, apex 10–12 mm above the supraorbital rim, and the tail sloping slightly inferior (Figure 11.3.12). The amount of brow ptosis is determined by measuring the distance in millimetres from the inferior aspect of the brow to the supraorbital rim. Dermatochalasia of the upper lids may actually resolve once the brows are placed into their normal positions. Often, patients will seek aesthetic rejuvenation of the upper lids when it is the ptotic brows which is the actual culprit. Forehead rhytids, especially deep rhytids, are improved with an endoscopic brow lift. Superficial and shallow rhytids usually require a laser resurfacing. The position of the hair line, slope and length of the forehead are also important parameters to assess. The patient with a receding hair line will certainly require modification of incisions which can make the surgical procedure difficult. Similarly, a forehead that is sloped too acutely will also present special challenges during an endoscopic brow lift. Some surgeons will not use an endoscopic brow lift if the forehead is too long; rather, a pretrichial forehead lift is used in order to shorten an excessively long forehead. If the corrugator muscles are too active and have caused formation of vertical rhytids in the naso-frontal area, then a myectomy of the corrugator is necessary to efface such rhytids.

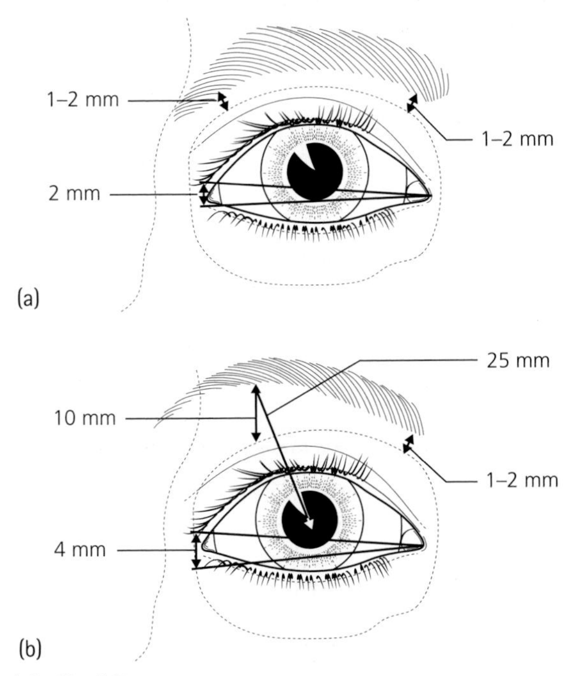

11.3.12 (a and b). Ideal brow positions in male(a) and female (b) (from T Evans, Brow lift. *Atlas of the Oral and Maxillofacial Surgery Clinics of North America* 1998; **6**: 118–119).

SURGICAL PROCEDURE

The patient is marked in the pre-operative area while sitting. Most clinicians use five ports for an endoscopic brow lift including two temporal ports, two lateral (paramedian) ports and a central (median) port. The median and paramedian ports are marked 1 cm inside the hair line. Each of these incisions is 1–1.5 cm in length in a cranio-caudal direction. The central port is marked in the middle of the frontal hairline; the two paramedian ports are parallel to the lateral limbus/canthus region. The two temporal markings are made after drawing a line that intersects the ala of the nose and the lateral canthus and extends on to the temple. The temporal port is tangent to this line, is 2 cm in length and is obliquely directed (Figure 11.3.13).

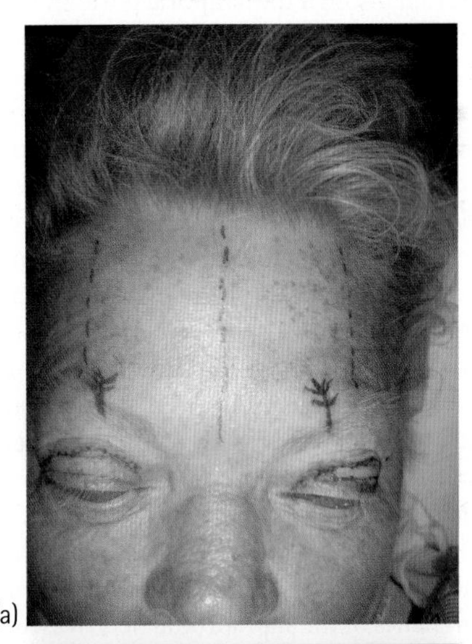

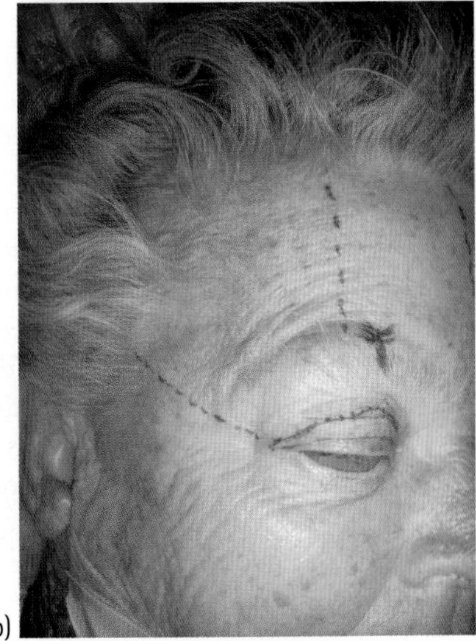

11.3.13 (a and b). Typical markings for an endoscopic brow lift.

The procedure is performed under general anaesthesia with the patient intubated. After administration of a local anaesthetic with a vasoconstrictor, the central and paramedian incisions are made with a No. 15 blade through all five layers of the scalp onto the bone (Figure 11.3.14). The two temporal incisions are then made with a No. 15 blade through skin, subcutaneous layer and temporoparietal fascia. The incision stops at the superficial layer of the deep temporal fascia. All incisions should be beveled along the length of hair follicles to reduce alopecia. A subperiosteal dissection is then performed through the median and paramedian ports. The dissection should extend posteriorly to the vertex of the skull to allow dissipation of the forehead flap in a superior and posterior direction. The anterior aspect of the dissection is visualized using a 30°, 4 mm endoscope inserted through any of the three ports. An endoscopic sheath can facilitate insertion of endoscope instruments (Figure 11.3.15). The dissection proceeds all the way anteriorly until the supraorbital rims and the supraorbital neurovascular bundles are visualized. A periosteal elevator is inserted through the temporal ports and is advanced medially until the temporal fusion line is reached. Also known as the condensation zone, this is the location of fusion of the deep temporal fascia, temporoparietal fascia and the pericranium. While the endoscope is in the paramedian ports, the fusion line is released under endoscopic visualization using a periosteal elevator (Figure 11.3.16). The fusion line must be released all the way down inferiorly until the zygomatic process of the frontal bone is reached. This causes release of the orbital retaining ligaments which in turn allows elevation of the forehead and the brows. Once the entire forehead has been dissected, the periosteum must be released at the supraorbital rim/frontal bar region. This is accomplished under endoscopic visualization using an endoscopic dissector. Release of this periosteum will reveal the underlying brow fat pad (galeal fat pad, portion of the retro-orbicularis fat – ROOF), the corrugator muscle and the deep branches of the supraorbital neurovascular bundle (Figure 11.3.17). This is a critical portion of the operation; failure to release the periosteum in this area will not allow sufficient elevation of the forehead. In patients who need to have elevation of the lateral canthus region and even the midface, the endoscopic elevator can be advanced down the fronto-zygomatic region onto the zygoma to elevate the entire region (Figure 11.3.18). If the corrugator muscles need a myectomy, using endoscopic alligator clamps, small pieces of the corrugator are grasped and removed.

After the periosteum has been released, the forehead flap must be elevated and fixated. Several methods exist to fixate the forehead flap. The author routinely uses titanium miniplates or resorbable plates to anchor the forehead flap and fixate the flap in an elevated fashion. The amount of elevation depends on the amount of brow ptosis measured pre-operatively. Using calipers, the amount of brow ptosis is added to the most inferior aspect of the two paramedian incisions. One mm is added to each measurement to allow for relapse. For example, if there is 5 mm of brow ptosis at the apex, the calipers are set at 6 mm, inserted into the paramedian incisions and the fixation device is placed exactly at 6 mm. Then, using a 2/0 PDS suture, the flap is elevated and secured to the fixation device. Usually two points of fixation is sufficient unless severe medial brow ptosis is present at which time three points of fixation (median, two paramedian) will be necessary. The two temporal incisions are closed while the assistant elevates the lateral brow region and the inferior limb of the incision is elevated and anchored to the deep temporal fascia superior to the initial incision using 2/0 PDS. This allows temporal elevation of the lateral brow. Next, to obviate the need for a surgical drain, fibrin sealant is sprayed into the surgical field. Next, the three forehead incisions are closed in two layers. Staples are used on the scalp. A pressure dressing is applied to the forehead.

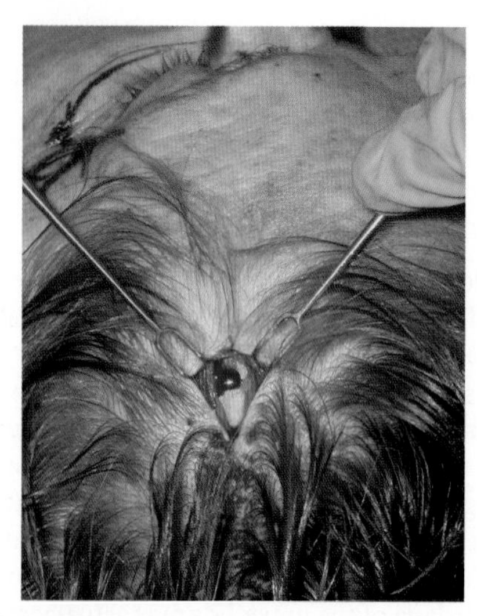

11.3.14 Appearance of a midline central/median incision. Note full thickness nature of the incision.

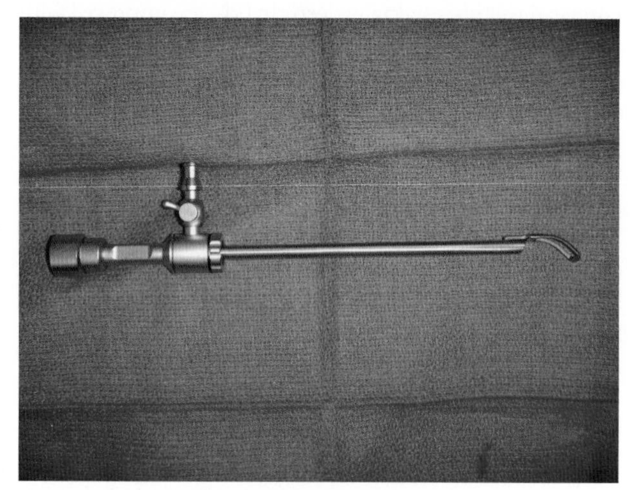

11.3.15 An endoscopic sheath with a curved tip. The curved tip retracts the scalp flap away from the field and allows for unimpaired visualization and dissection.

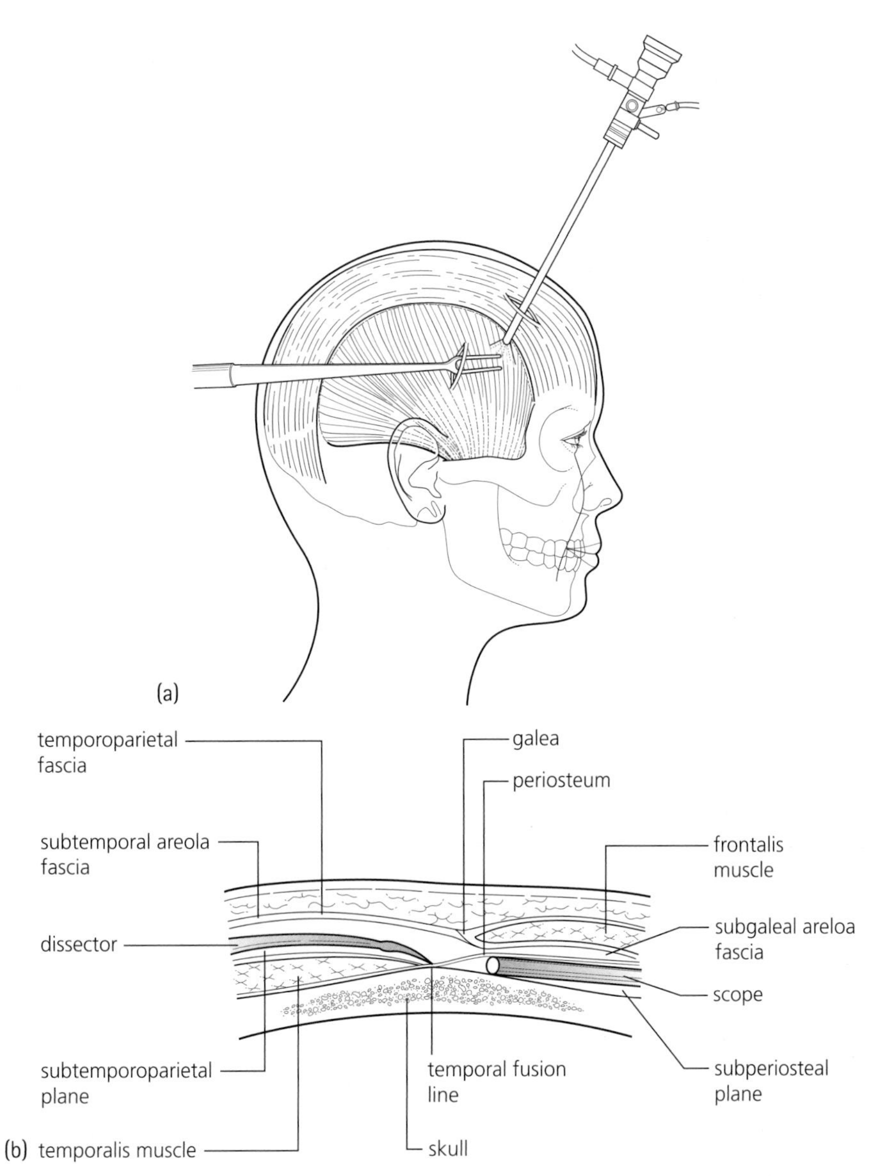

11.3.16 (a and b). Location of the endoscope and dissector over the temporal crest (from T Evans, Brow lift. *Atlas of the Oral and Maxillofacial Surgery Clinics of North America* 1998; **6**: 125).

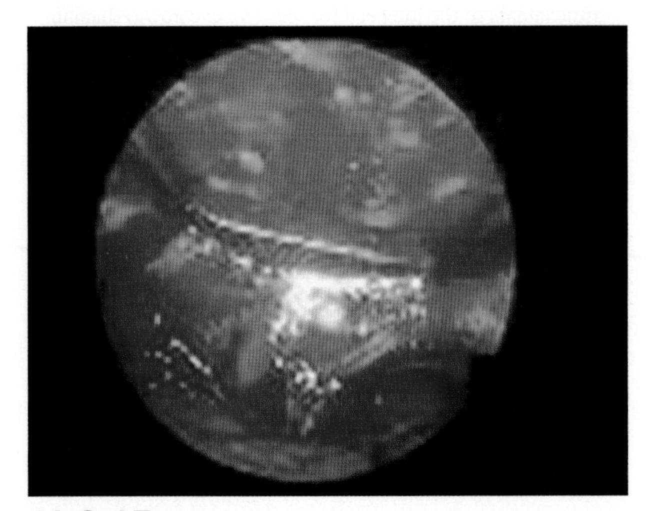

11.3.17 Endoscopic appearance of the supraorbital neurovascular bundle at the supra orbital rim.

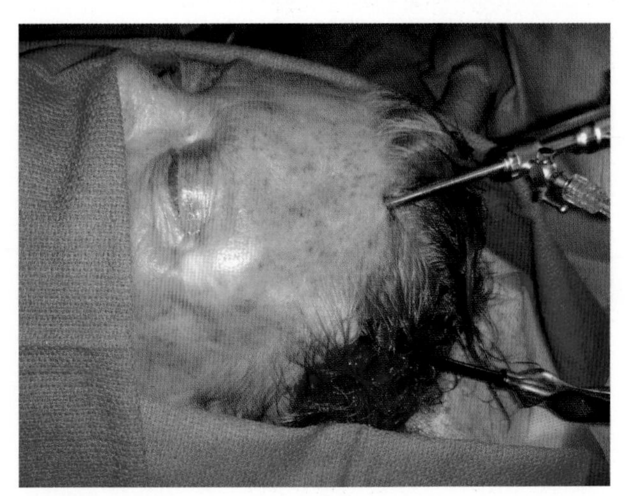

11.3.18 Dissection over the zygomatico-frontal area to elevate the lateral canthus and mid face.

POST-OPERATIVE MANAGEMENT

The patient is seen in 24 hours to remove the pressure dressing and assess any haematoma formation. If a haematoma is present, it needs to be evacuated. Most patients will experience transitory headaches following an endoscopic brow lift; the author always tells the patient of this possibility preoperatively. The patient is instructed to refrain from strenuous exercise. The scalp stapes are removed in 10 days. Perioperative antibiotics are discontinued in 24–48 hours as per the surgeon's discretion.

COMPLICATIONS

Complications following an endoscopic brow lift are minimal. The most common complications are paraesthesia of the forehead and scalp, mild alopecia along the incisions, inadequate brow elevation, damage to the frontal branches of the facial nerve and haematoma formation. Paraesthesia of the forehead occurs due to neuropraxia of the supraorbital nerve; this usually resolves with time. Alopecia can be reduced if the incisions are made parallel to hair follicles. Inadequate brow elevation usually occurs due to improper release of the orbital ligaments and the periosteum along the supraorbital region. Damage to the frontal branches of the facial nerve should not occur as long as proper adherence to the different planes of dissection has occurred during surgery. It is imperative that the forehead elevation is under subperiosteally while the temporal dissection is atop the deep temporal fascia. This will allow protection of the nerve in the temporoparietal fascia superior to the surgical field. Mild neuropraxia usually resolves within weeks. Haematoma formation is very rare; the author routinely uses fibrin sealants in place of surgical drains to prevent haematoma formation.

Top tips

Cervicoplasty

- Do not place incision in the cervicomental crease; place it posterior to it and then obliterate the crease with scissors or knife.
- Liposuction should be performed until the investing fascia of the platysma muscle is clearly visible.
- Do not perform any liposuction superior to the jaw line.

Deep plane face lift

- Proper pre-operative markings are essential.
- Elevation of the SMAS will significantly improve final results.
- Key sutures of the SMAS to the temporal fascia, perichondrium and mastoid fascia are critical.
- Use of fibrin sealants in place of surgical drains is advised.

Endoscopic brow lift

- Subperiosteal dissection over the forehead and atop the deep temporal fascia temporally is essential to minimize damage to the facial nerve.
- Releasing the periosteum and orbital retaining ligaments to ensure adequate elevation of the flap is necessary to allow proper forehead elevation.

FURTHER READING

Behmand RA, Guyuron B. Endoscopic forehead rejuvenation: II. Long-term results. *Plastic and Reconstructive Surgery* 2006; **117**: 1137–43.

Evans TW, Stepanyan M. Isolated cervicoplasty. *American Journal of Cosmetic Surgery* 2002; **19**: 91–113.

Evans TW. A case for deeper plane facelifts. *Journal of Oral and Maxillofacial Surgery* 1998; **56**: 352–8.

Fattahi T. Management of isolated neck deformities. *Atlas of the Oral and Maxillofacial Surgery Clinics of North America* 2004; **12**: 261–70.

Fattahi T, Mohan M, Caldwell G. Clinical applications of fibrin sealants. *Journal of Oral and Maxillofacial Surgery* 2004; **62**: 218–24.

Feldman JJ. Corset platysmaplasty. *Plastic and Reconstructive Surgery* 1990; **85**: 333–43.

Guyuron B. Endoscopic forehead rejuvenation: I. Limitations, flaws, and rewards. *Plastic and Reconstructive Surgery* 2006; **117**: 1121–33.

Hamra ST. Composite rhytidectomy. *Plastic and Reconstructive Surgery* 1992; **90**: 1–11.

Knize DM. The importance of the retaining ligamentous attachments of the forehead for selective eyebrow reshaping and forehead rejuvenation. *Plastic and Reconstructive Surgery* 2007; **119**: 1119–20.

Mitz V, Peyronie M. The superficial musculo-aponeurotic system in the parotid and cheek area. *Plastic and Reconstructive Surgery* 1976; **38**: 80–88.

Perkins SW. Achieving the 'natural look' in rhytidectomy. *Facial and Plastic Surgery* 2000; **16**: 269–82.

Sykes JM. Surgical rejuvenation of the brow and forehead. *Facial Plastic Surgery* 1999; **15**: 183–91.

11.4

Aesthetic blepharoplasty

LEO FA STASSEN

INTRODUCTION

Aesthetic blepharoplasty is frequently requested by patients to restore their youthful looks. The term blepharoplasty was first introduced by van Graefe in 1818. The patient group is usually the 40–50 year age group, but this age is getting lower. Females request the procedure more frequently than males, but male requests are increasing. The indications are excess eyelid skin, excess eyelid skin and muscle, fat prolapse through a weakened orbital septum and muscle hypertrophy of lower lid orbicularis. The usual cause is one of the following: ageing, obesity, post-thyroid eye disease decompression, oriental eyelid and familial. Occasionally, excess skin in the upper lids can present as decreased superior vision detected by our ophthalmology colleagues.

PRE-OPERATIVE ASSESSMENT

The patient needs to be screened very carefully and the surgeon must pay meticulous attention to detail in recording findings (Figure 11.4.1) and in assessment:

- patient's general health;
- cigarette consumption (ask patient to stop);
- alcohol intake;
- patient's goals and attitudes (obsessiveness, unrealistic aims, psychiatric history, etc.);
- visual acuity, gross visual fields, especially superior field;
- tear production (dry, normal, excessive);
- brow level/ptosis (real and pseudoptosis);
- vertical and horizontal glabellar lines;
- upper lid in relation to iris;
- upper lid crease/levator superioris action;
- amount of excess upper skin, skin and muscle;
- fat prolapse medial, middle and lateral;
- lacrimal gland prolapse;
- other upper lid pathology;
- canthal areas medial and lateral;
- lower lid level in relation to iris (measure scleral show);
- nasojugal groove deformity;
- amount of excess lower lid skin, skin and muscle, festoons and muscle hypertrophy;
- eyelid margin laxity assessed by manual distraction test or inferior traction test;
- fat prolapse medial, middle and lateral (ask patient to look up);
- other facial signs of ageing (wrinkles, deep nasolabial fold, loss of neck angularity, a break in the straight jawline (jowling), a witch's chin indicating the need for more extensive procedure);
- cranial nerves II, III, IV, VI, VII and ensure a positive Bell's phenomenon;
- photographs (frontal, oblique, lateral facial views and close-up eyelid views).

Ensure that your perspective and that of the patient are at one. It is worth a number of visits before surgery, examining, explaining and discussing the procedure. The support of a beauty therapist, counsellor and post-operative make-up facility is a great advantage. When the assessment is finished and the analysis of the cause of the problem completed, the surgery itself is relatively easy. Each patient requires an individualized plan based on the type and severity of the problem.

PRE-OPERATIVE MARKING

The procedure can be undertaken on a day-case basis. The author advises all patients to have a very thorough facial wash, including hair washing with a medicated shampoo the night before and morning of surgery. The patient is asked to avoid applying make up on the morning of surgery. All markings are normally made in the patient's room with the patient sitting up prior to going to theatre. Ensure that the eyebrows are in their correct position (simulate brow-lift): the supraorbital rim for males and just above for females.

Occasionally, a brow-lift may be more appropriate than an upper blepharoplasty or may be required as an adjunctive procedure. Mark out the exact amount of skin and/or muscle planned for excision from the upper lids and outline the areas of prolapsed fat from the fat pads (Figure 11.4.2).

The inferior incision is sited in the natural tarsal fold or at a minimum of 10 mm from the ciliary margin in the vertical mid-pupillary line, 5 mm above a proposed lower crowfoot incision in the lateral canthal area and 5 mm above the punctum medially. The skin above this is picked up and gently pinched, with more and more skin taken until the upper lid just begins to pull away from the lower lid. With a second forceps, the marking is continued laterally and then medially (Figure 11.4.3).

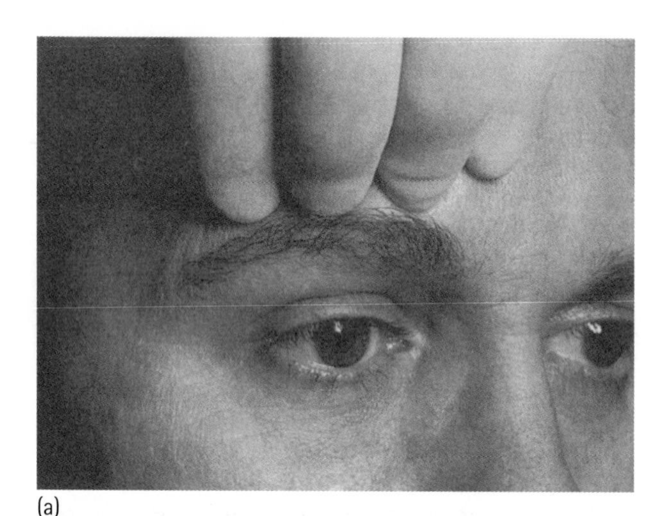

(a)

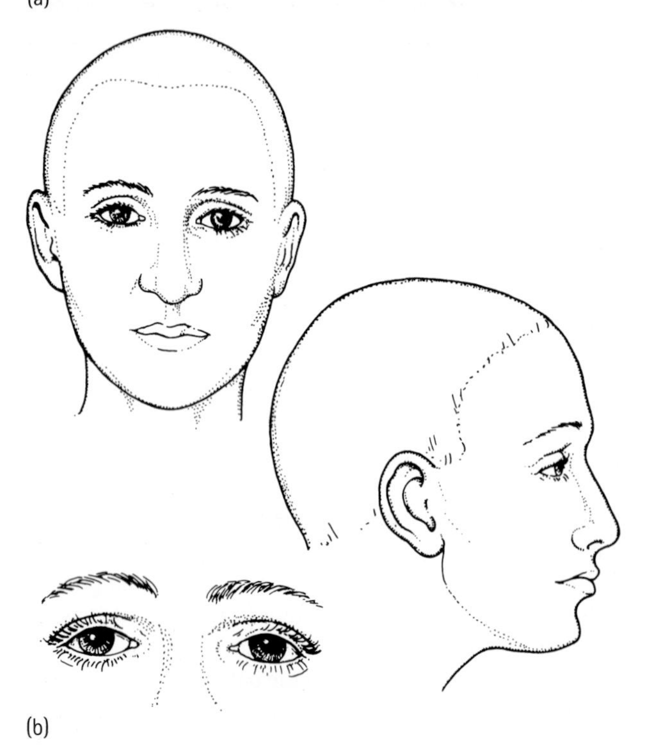

(b)

11.4.1 (a and b) Assessment and recording findings.

Mark out the lower blepharoplasty incision with its crowfoot extension and again plan the ideal amount of skin and muscle to be excised (Figure 11.4.4). The medial extent is the inferior lacrimal punctum. Outline the areas of prolapsed fat from the fat pads and the nasojugal fold (Figure 11.4.5).

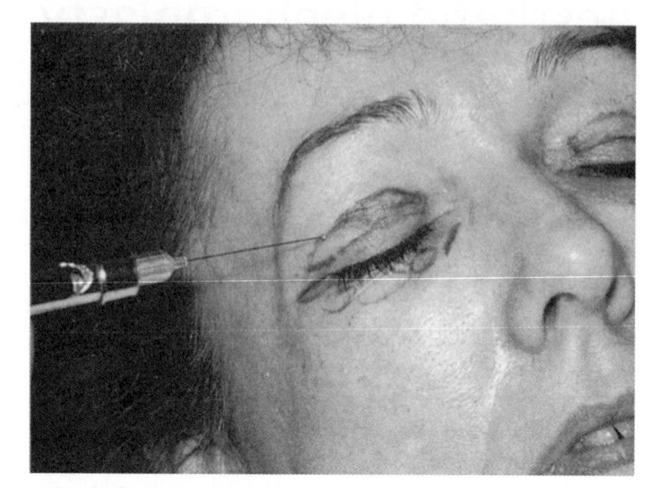

11.4.2 Skin markings.

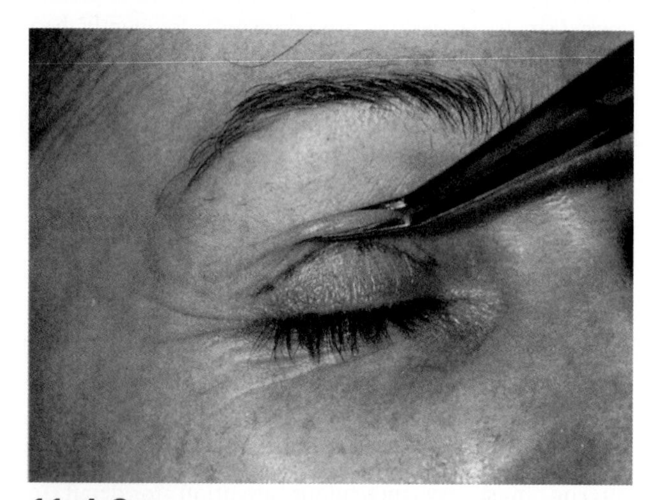

11.4.3 Marking out the upper eyelid incision.

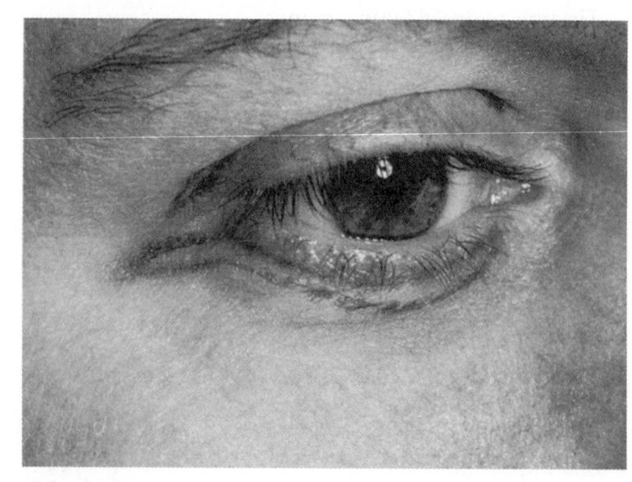

11.4.4 Lower blepharoplasty incision.

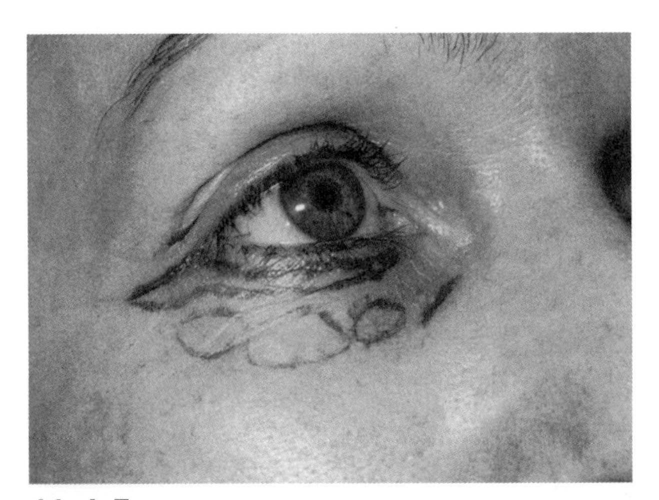

11.4.5 Prolapsed fat.

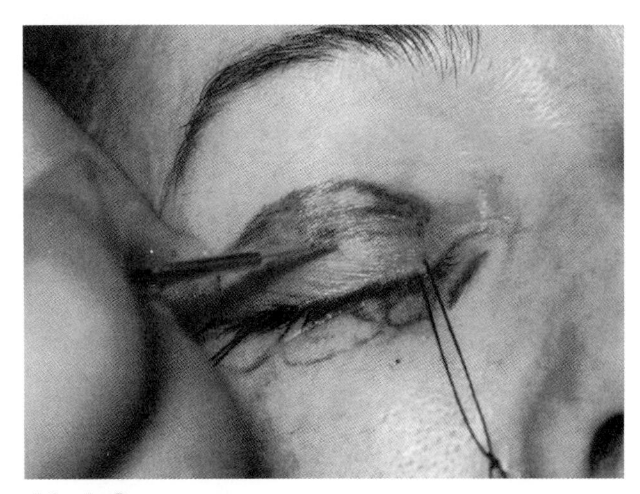

11.4.6 Lid under tension.

Festoons are marked but are more difficult to treat and may indicate the need for a more extensive facelift procedure or inferolateral orbicularis resection. Remember that the amount of skin to be removed may be slightly different for each eye.

CHOICE OF ANAESTHETIC

The procedure can be easily carried out on an outpatient basis under local anaesthetic (2 per cent lignocaine with epinephrine (adrenaline) 1:80 000) and intravenous sedation (usually midazolam). You must remember to infiltrate the fat pads before manipulating them to prevent pain and an acute bradycardia secondary to an occulocardiac stimulus. If other surgery such as a face lift or brow lift is contemplated, general anaesthesia with local anaesthetic and epinephrine infiltration is best. Topical anaesthetic eye drops are applied.

Patients receive intravenous steroids perioperatively (methylprednisolone 250 mg). Prophylactic antibiotics are unnecessary.

The time required for upper and lower blepharoplasties is 60–120 minutes. The patient is placed in a head-up position. The face needs to be exposed from upper lip to hairline and ear to ear. The area is cleaned with an aqueous chlorhexidine solution; ensure that the pre-operative marks are not removed.

TECHNIQUE

Tension sutures are placed in the medial and lateral aspects of the upper and lower eyelids; avoid the punctae medially and allow the skin to be stretched and cut cleanly with a No. 15 blade at right angles to the skin (Figure 11.4.6).

The upper blepharoplasty is completed first. The skin is removed and this is all that may be required in patients with thin skin. Haemostasis is secured. A strip of orbicularis occuli is usually excised, with care taken to lift the muscle only and to work from medial to lateral. Just before the muscle is divided laterally a polyglactin 5/0 colourless holding suture is placed in the lateral superior and inferior orbicularis muscle margins. This allows the muscle to be lifted and the orbital septum, with the levator palpebrae superioris aponeurosis beneath it, inspected and protected (Figure 11.4.7).

Haemostasis is secured with bipolar electrocoagulation. If fat is to be removed, the full extent of the fat pads are identified, infiltrated and then gently opened with knife dissection. The fat is teased free from the compartments, cross-clamped and the stumps coagulated with the bipolar electrocoagulator and the excised fat measured (Figure 11.4.8). Haemostasis is now secured. The levator superioris is inspected to ensure no damage. The muscle layer is repaired with polyglactin 5/0 colourless, buried interrupted sutures so that the muscle margins are gently apposed. If

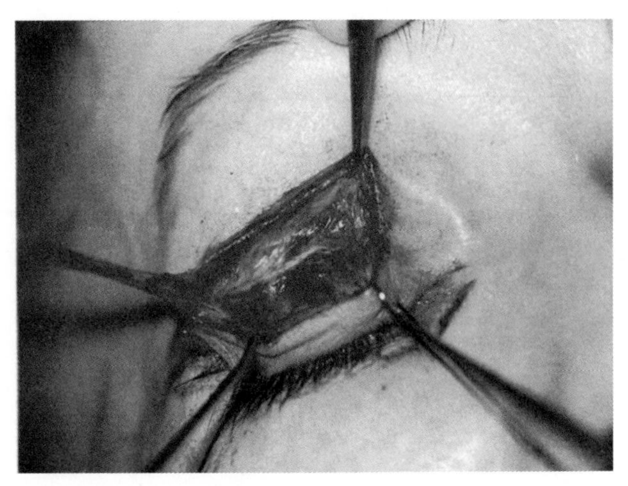

11.4.7 Orbital septum and levator superioris aponeurosis.

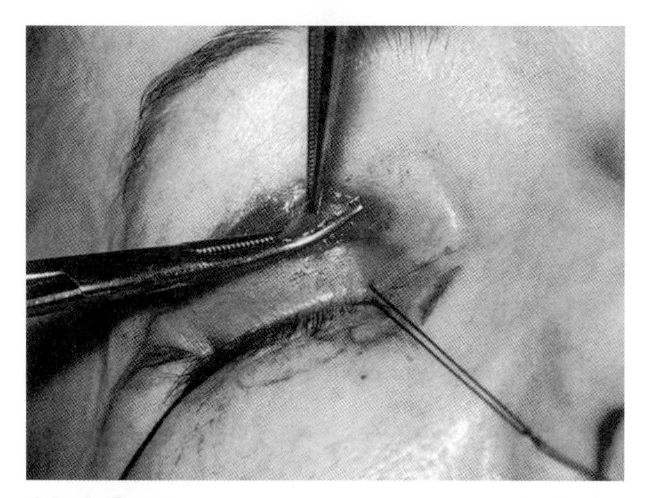

11.4.8 Fat cross-clamped.

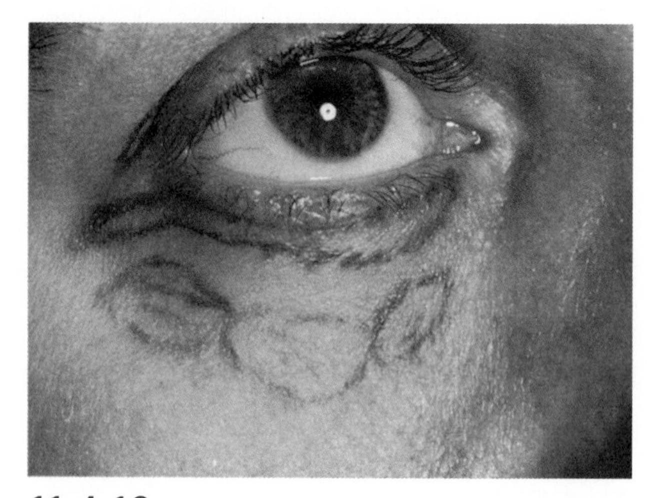

11.4.10 Lower blepharoplasty incision.

further definition of the tarsal fold is required, some of the latter sutures pick up the submuscular levator aponureurosis layer. If the lacrimal gland is prolapsing, it is supported under the supraorbital rim by hammock-type sutures between the gland and periosteum. The skin is closed with interrupted 5/0 Ethilon sutures (Figure 11.4.9).

The final scar should be the ideal supratarsal crease. When both upper blepharoplasties are complete, the lower ones are done. The author prefers to use knife dissection. The incision is 2 mm below the ciliary line and extends medially from the level of the inferior punctum to the lateral canthal area and then into an appropriate crowfoot crease (Figure 11.4.10).

The skin is maintained under tension by the holding sutures and skin hooks. A submusculocutaneous dissection is followed down to the level of the orbital rim. This should then leave the three fat pads exposed superficial to the orbital septum (Figure 11.4.11).

If fat is to be removed or redraped, the fat pads are opened, the fat allowed to prolapse and either cross-clamped and excised or mobilized to augment the nasojugal area or soften the orbital rim by the fat draped evenly over the rim. If fat is removed, the amount is measured and recorded by placing it in a syringe (Figure 11.4.12).

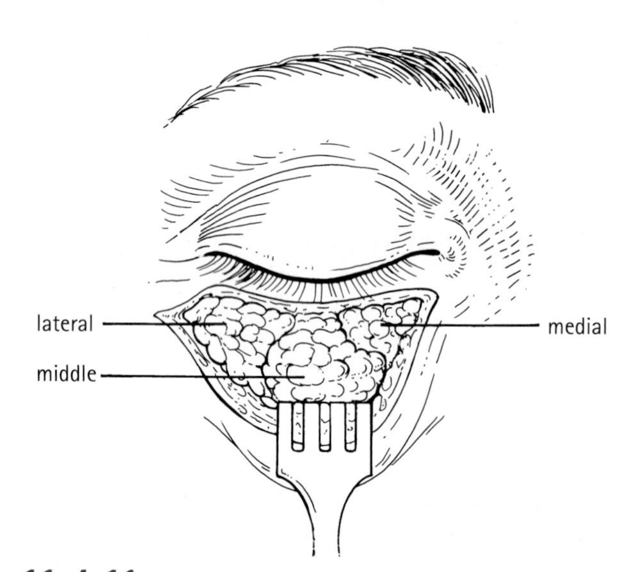

11.4.11 Exposed lower lid fat pads.

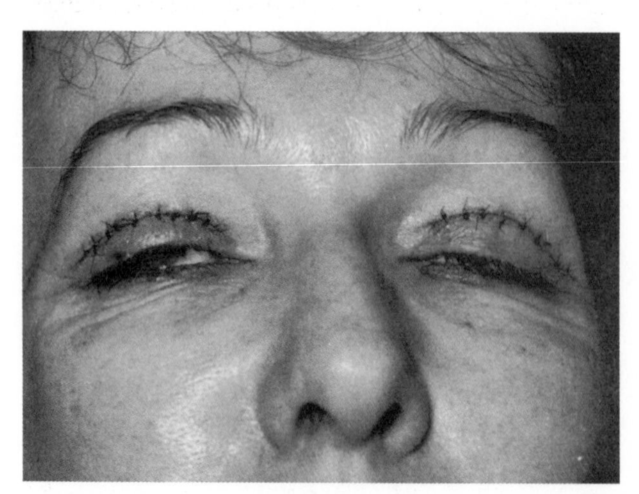

11.4.9 Skin closure.

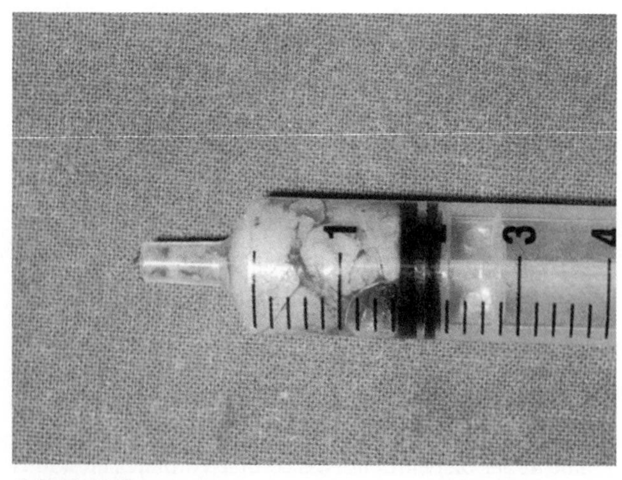

11.4.12 Excess fat in syringe.

Haemostasis is secured. The lower skin flap is redraped over the wound and gently pulled in a cephalad direction, and excess skin and muscle excised (Figure 11.4.13) to allow the skin margins to fit together gently and snugly.

The first and most important suture is the lateral canthal supporting suture. A 5/0 polyglactin colourless, buried suture is used to ensure close, tension-free adaptation. The muscle layer is then repaired with interrupted sutures and the skin repaired with interrupted sutures to ensure well everted margins.

The eyes are lavaged with normal saline and chlormycetin eye ointment applied to the conjunctival and blepharoplasty incisions.

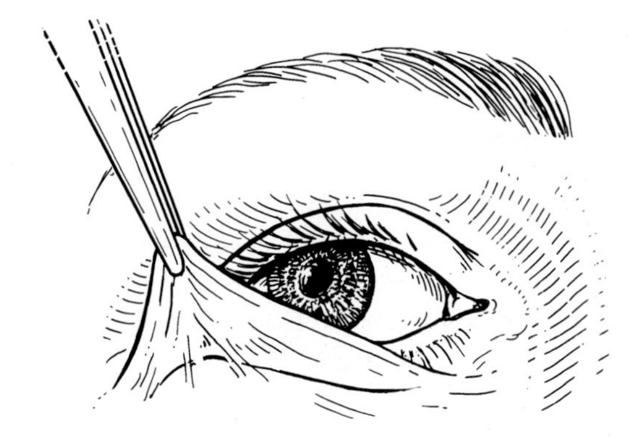

11.4.13 Excess skin draped prior to excision.

POST-OPERATIVE CARE

The patient returns to the recovery area in a sitting-up position. Ice-cold compresses (Figure 11.4.14) in the form of cooled gel are placed over damp gauze to decrease the swelling. The patient's vision is recorded every 30 minutes for 2 hours and then the patient is discharged. The patient should continue with the cold compresses for 24–36 hours, sleep propped up and avoid exercise. Simple ambulation is encouraged. Sutures should be removed at 2–4 days. The patient can wash the day following surgery and can return to normal activities 2 weeks following the surgery. Some swelling and bruising is likely to remain for 2–3 weeks and the patient should have been warned about this pre-operatively.

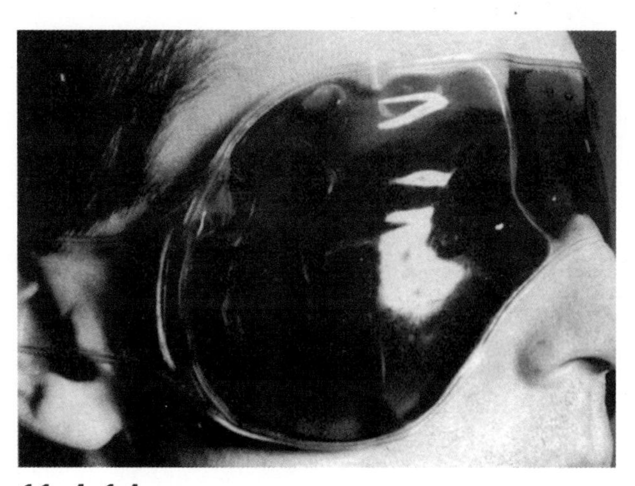

11.4.14 Ice-cold compress in place.

COMPLICATIONS

Visual loss is the most serious consequence of blepharoplasty surgery. Its incidence is hard to ascertain but is quoted as 0.04 per cent and the usual cause is a retrobulbar haemorrhage. This complication can be decreased by careful, deft surgery with careful haemostasis and by nursing the patient upright with cold compresses in place. Patients are advised to avoid alcohol, exercise and smoking and to report any changes in visual acuity, severe pain or swelling.

Transient diplopia occasionally occurs secondary to local anaesthesia of the ocular muscles, oedema or a small haematoma. Injudicious dissection may lead to damage to the inferior oblique, inferior rectus or the superior oblique muscle during fat resection.

Ptosis owing to upper lid oedema is common and resolves rapidly, but beware the situation where the levator aponeurosis has been damaged. The latter requires immediate repair.

Ectropion of the lower lid is usually due to excessive skin resection (never >6 mm), a missed diagnosis of lower lid laxity or poor position of sutures. This is best prevented by secure support of the tension on the stable lateral canthal area.

Round eye deformity is an opening of the lateral canthal angle due to excessive tension on the lateral canthus. It requires a lateral canthopexy to support the lower eyelid to the periosteum.

Incomplete fat removal will show up as persistent deformities and usually involves the lateral fat pads. Excessive fat removal leads to very deep sulcus and the appearance of an enophthalmic eye in the upper eyelid; this is very difficult to treat. Excessive fat removal in the lower lid leads to prominence of the inferior orbital rim.

Infection is very rare because of the excellent blood supply.

Skin asymmetry occurs if the upper skin crease is not planned in an equal position on both sides, if an excessive amount of skin or fat is removed from one side or if a unilateral ptosis is missed.

Occasionally, a pseudoepicanthal fold may result from excessive skin excision in the medial upper eyelid, or a curved incision or an incision too close to the lid margin.

Epiphora may be a problem for a few weeks, usually because of lower lid margin oedema leading to temporary occlusion of the punctum. Occasionally, dry eyes become evident post-operatively because of a small increase in the palpebral width; this usually settles with time.

FURTHER READING

DeMere M, Wood T, Austin W. Eye complications with blepharoplasty or other eyelid surgery. *Plastic Reconstructive Surgery* 1974; **53**, 634–7.

Gradinger GR Preoperative considerations in blepharoplasty. In: Peck GC (ed.), *Symposium on problems and complications in aesthetic surgery of the face.* St Louis: Mosby, 1984: 195–207.

Hamra ST. Concepts and elements of composite rhytidectomy. In: *Composite rhytidectomy.* St Louis, MI: Quality Medical Publishing, 1993: 23, 24, 56.

Harley RD, Nelson LB, Flanagan JC *et al.* Ocular motility disturbance following cosmetic blepharoplasty. *Archives of Ophthalmology* 1986; **104**: 542–4.

Hill JC. Treatment of epiphora owing to flaccid eyelids. *Archives of Ophthalmology* 1979; **97**: 323–4.

Kaye BL. The forehead lift: a useful adjunct to facelift and blepharoplasty. *Plastic and Reconstructive Surgery,* 1977; **60**: 161–71.

Langdon JD, Patel MF (eds). *Operative maxillofacial surgery.* London: Chapman and Hall, 1998.

Lloyd WC, Leone CR. Transient bilateral blindness following blepharoplasty. *Ophthalmic Plastic and Reconstructive Surgery* 1985; **1**: 29–34.

Matarasso A. The oculocardiac reflex in blepharoplasty surgery. *Plastic and Reconstructive Surgery* 1989; **83**: 243–50.

Sheen JH. A change in the technique of supratarsal fixation in upper blepharoplasty. *Plastic and Reconstructive Surgery,* 1977; **59**: 831–4.

11.5

Aesthetic otoplasty (bat ear correction)

LEO FA STASSEN

INTRODUCTION

Patients frequently present, or their parents or friends advise them to come, complaining of 'not liking their ears'. Their ears are too prominent, too big, too small, unusual shapes, unusual positions and, because of them, they are being called names. The problem is made worse for the child because the ears approach adult size early in the growing face. The psychological problems associated with this deformity are significant and often only come to light after discussion (Figure 11.5.1).

These defects are very common (3–5 per cent) and relatively easily corrected. The usual problem is lack of definition of the antihelical fold and/or conchal overdevelopment. A choice of techniques is necessary. There is not one technique for all cases although it is best to rely mainly on one technique to begin with. There are so far over 100 methods described. Ely, in 1881, was the first to describe a technique for correction of prominent ears.

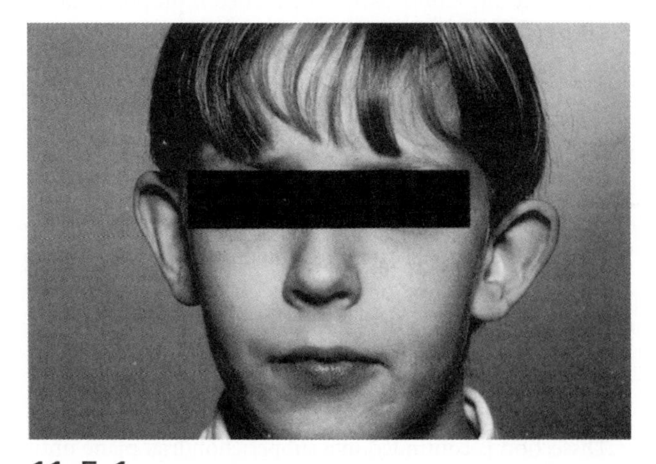

11.5.1 Patient with prominent ears.

PRE-OPERATIVE ASSESSMENT

The most important aspect in management is assessment. Compare left with right and with normal population (*n*) for racial group from in front, behind and above:

- level of ear (*n* = level with eyebrow): high, normal, low;
- angle between ear and mastoid process >30° is prominent;
- Distance between helical rim and skull (*n* = 1–2 cm);
- vertical axis: 20–30° posteriorly (lobule to dome);
- vertical height: approximately 5–6.5 cm (males > females and right slightly > left);
- width = 55 per cent of length;
- conchal size and depth;
- helix and antihelix form: poor, deficient, normal, excessive;
- scapha: size and form;
- cartilage: quality, thickness and firmness;
- presence or absence of Darwinian tubercles, sinuses and preauricular tags;
- photographs front, rear and individual ear ± models for difficult cases.

The surgeon should know and understand the anatomy of the normal ear (Figure 11.5.2) and its three-dimensional position (Figure 11.5.3).

The ear has a very rich blood supply via the superficial temporal, the posterior auricular and the occipital vessels. The sensory nerve supply is via the auriculotemporal, the lesser occipital and the greater auricular nerves, and the concha also receives sensory innervation via the vagus nerve. The vascular supply and innervation are such that the procedures can easily be carried out under local anaesthetic, local anaesthetic and sedation or general anaesthesia (which should be used only for children <14 years). The aim is to achieve ears of equal and normal prominence and shape with a soft gentle appearance and no evidence of breaks or pinch effects. Ideally, size should be equal, but not necessarily so. It is prominence that is more obvious to the on-looker rather than size (Figure 11.5.4).

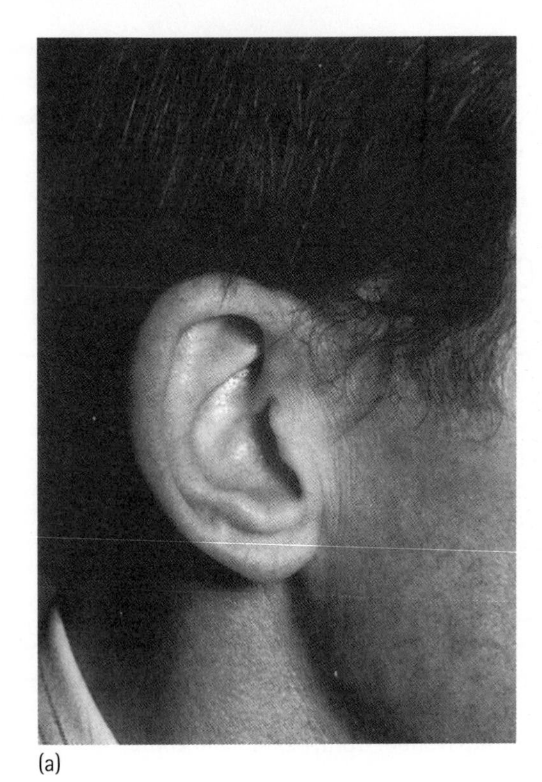

(a)

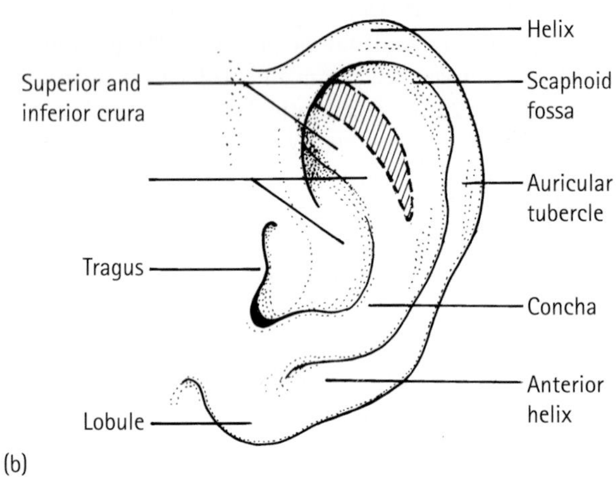

(b)

11.5.2 (a and b) Normal ear.

TIMING OF CORRECTION

There is evidence now that, if the deformity is obvious in a child at birth, it can be corrected by the application of ear moulds held in place for a month. The cartilage can be moulded significantly and permanently at this stage. Most prominent ears are not detected, however, until later.

The next best time to correct the deformity is when the child is older (>14 years), under local anaesthetic and sedation, unless the deformity is obvious and causing psychological problems and then the ears should be corrected at the age of five years before the child starts school. There is no indication to correct the deformity surgically before the age of five years.

TECHNIQUES

There are multiple techniques: they must eliminate tension and left and right ears should be exposed and symmetry obtained.

Mustarde technique

This is a very simple, efficient and reliable technique for the inexperienced, but does not address concha or scapha problems and often gives an unnatural and poorly defined appearance.

Converse technique

This is a fairly complicated but excellent aesthetic technique involving incising, mobilizing and deforming cartilage with sutures to develop an antihelical rim with prominent superior and inferior crura.

Furnas technique

This technique involves creating space posterior to the concha to allow the concha to be pinned back without the cartilage bulging forward and occluding the external auditory meatus. It requires two stitches of non-resorbable material to be placed between the perichondrium of the concha and periosteum of the mastoid.

Stark and Saunders technique

This technique is the mainstay of the author's treatment supported by the Furnas conchal mastoid suture.

Both ears are prepared with an antiseptic and exposed (Figure 11.5.8). The proposed antihelix and superior and inferior crura and their junction are tattooed with the use of a 22G green needle (Figure 11.5.9).

A dumb-bell ellipse of skin is outlined in the postauricular area; the amount of skin to be excised is proportional to the prominence of the ears and can be judged by folding back the ear to simulate the proposed ear position. This should be excised mainly from the ear aspect (Figure 11.5.10).

When the ear is folded back in its proposed position, feel the maximum area of resistance and look to see if the external acoustic meatus has been closed by the conchal cartilage bulging forward. Outline the areas of excess tension. If the conchal cartilage is bulging forward, a Furnas suturing technique is required.

Infiltrate the postauricular area with 2 per cent lignocaine and 1:80 000 epinephrine (adrenaline). The dumb-bell ellipse is excised and the postauricular muscle identified and preserved (Figure 11.5.11).

Dissection is continued in a subperichondrial plane until the tattoo marks plus 5 mm are visible. The proposed

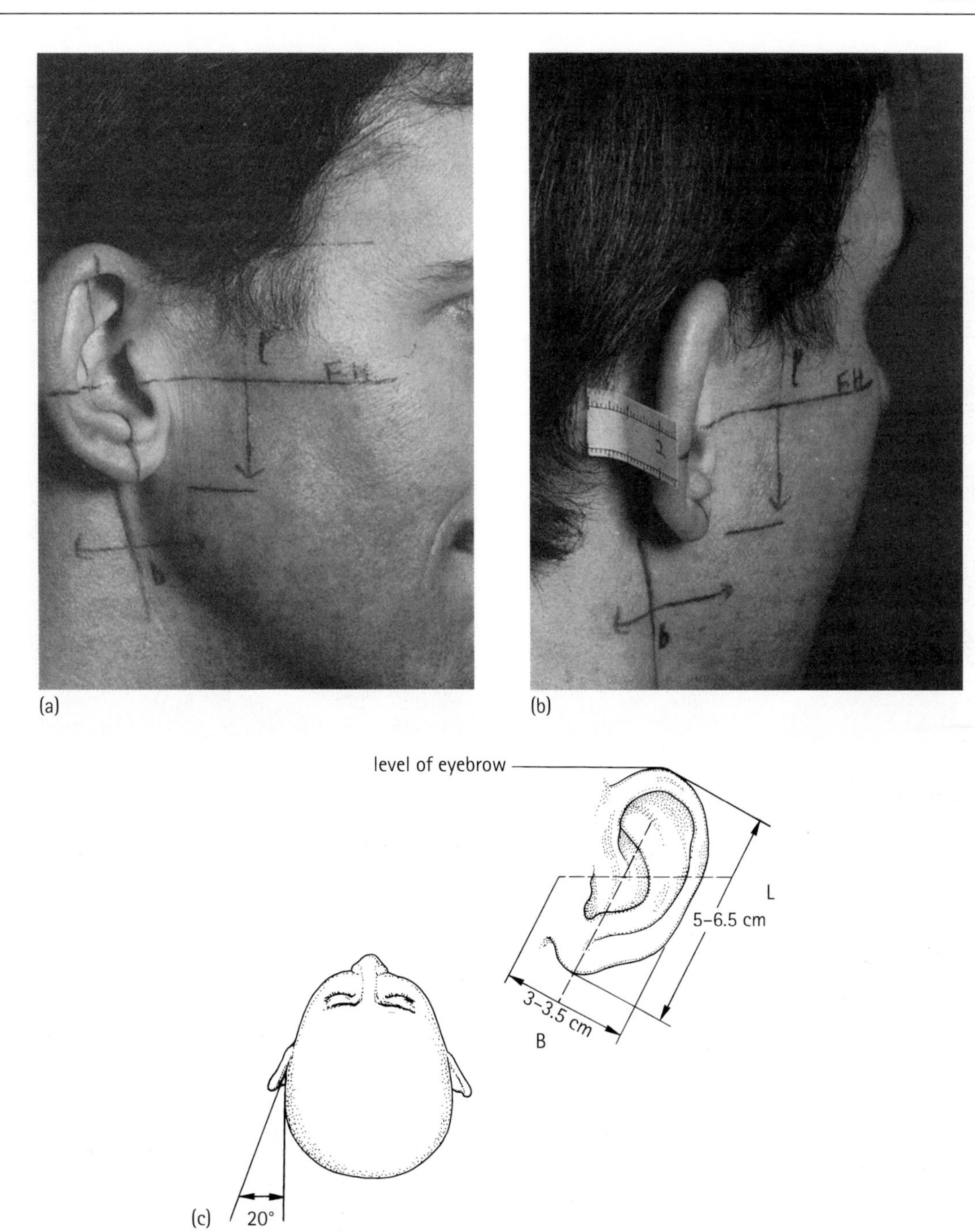

11.5.3 (a–c) Three-dimensional ear position.

antihelix and superior and inferior crura are drawn on the cartilage. An acrylic or diamond burr is used to weaken a 1 cm area simulating the crura and the antihelix (Figure 11.5.12).

The cartilage is weakened until the ear can be easily bent back with no tension and no sharp ridge. Attention needs to be paid especially to the helical tail and antitragus which may require further trimming (drill or knife) to prevent the lobule protruding (Figure 11.6.13).

The ear is allowed to lie freely and then gently placed in its new position to allow the surgeon to decide the most advantageous position for the two to four holding sutures. The number of sutures is dependent on the extent of the original deformity. The proposed holding suture sites are outlined on the anterior ear lateral to the proposed antihelix. A 2–3 mm incision with a No. 15 blade is made down to the cartilage and then, with scissors, the cartilage is gently cleaned (Figure 11.5.14).

For each external incision, a 3/0 clear nylon suture is then passed from the retroauricular dissection through the cartilage and then back again, with a millimetre bite of

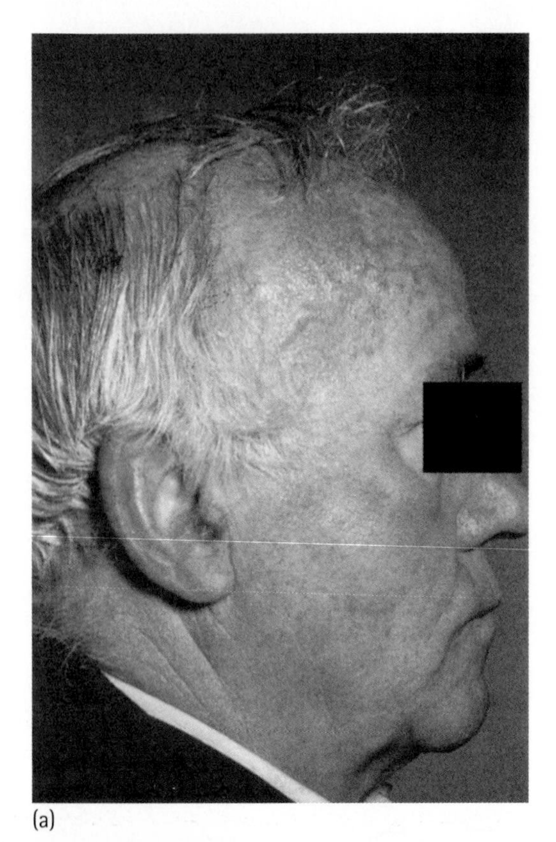

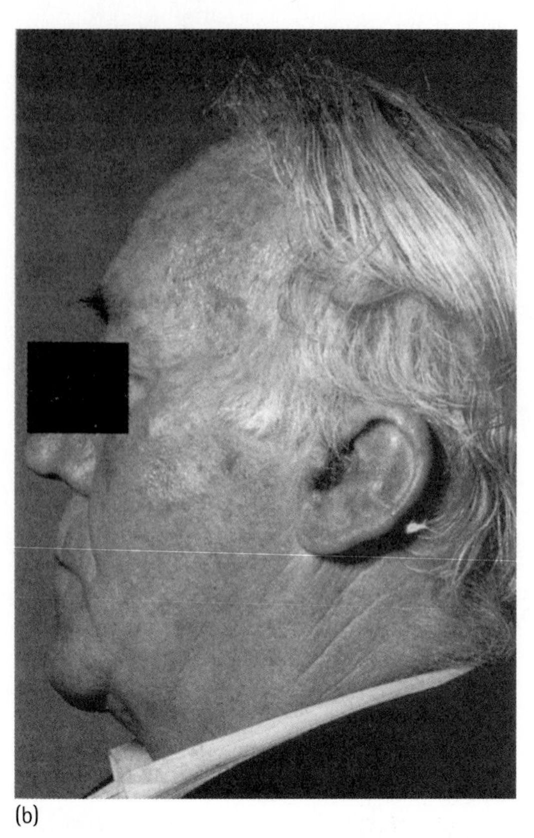

(a) (b)

11.5.4 (a) Right normal ear; (b) left ear following excision of lesion 3×3 cm.

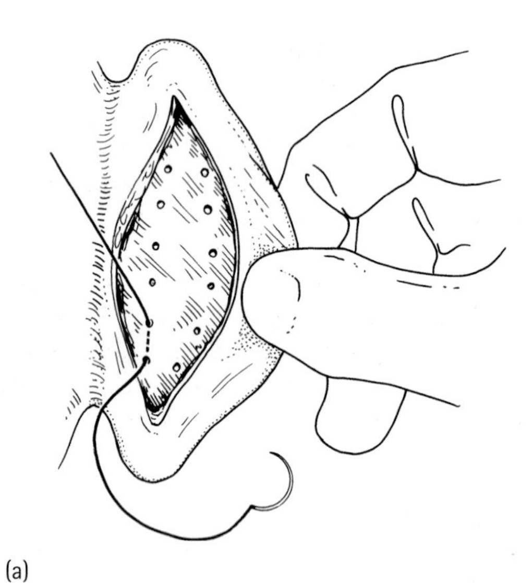

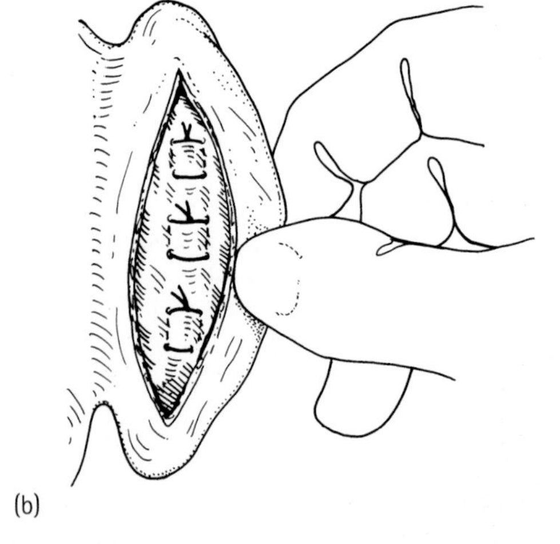

(a) (b)

11.5.5 (a and b) Mustarde technique.

cartilage. This technique avoids fixation to the overlying skin.

The need for a mastoid conchal stitch is now decided. It is best to place at least one of these and, if placed, it will involve dissecting the posterior auricular muscle free from its auricular attachment to create space for the conchal retropositioning. The ear is held in its proposed position and the mastoid fascia marked to allow the holding stitches to get the best purchase and best direction of support. The holding stitches are used to pick up mastoid fascia (and periosteum). The attachment to the fascia should be tested by traction on the suture before the final position is accepted (Figure 11.5.15).

The sutures are then clipped and the other ear prepared. In unilateral cases, the holding sutures are tightened until

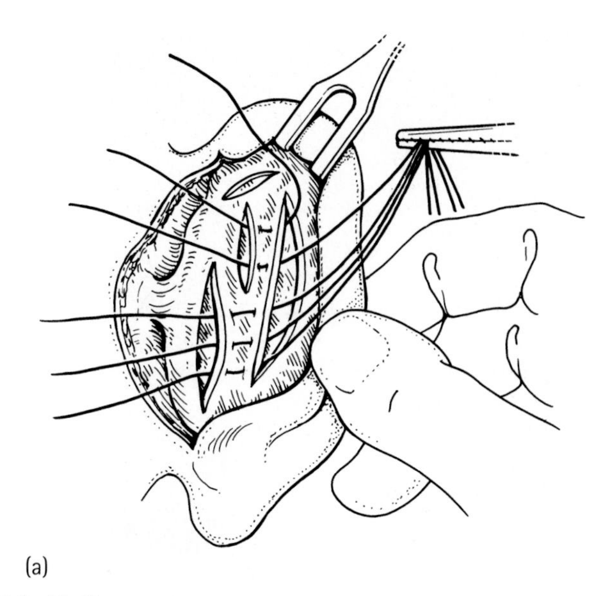
(a)

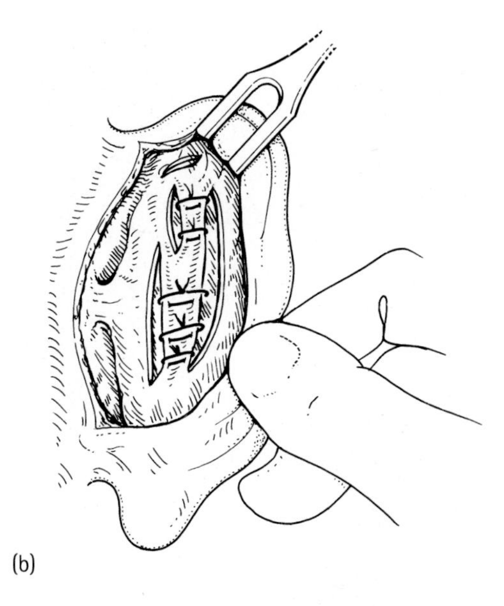
(b)

11.5.6 (a and b) Converse technique.

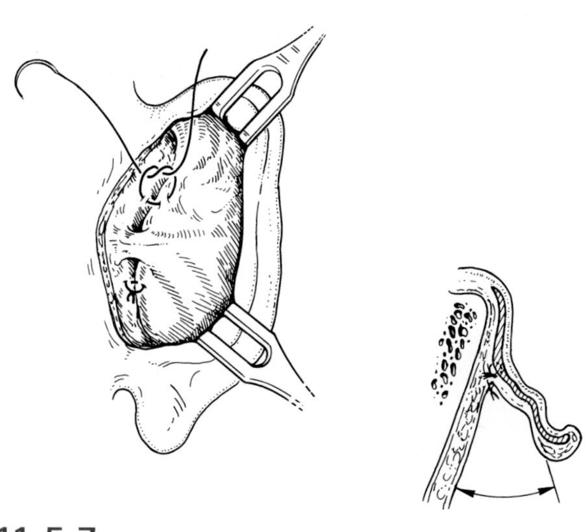

11.5.7 Furnas technique.

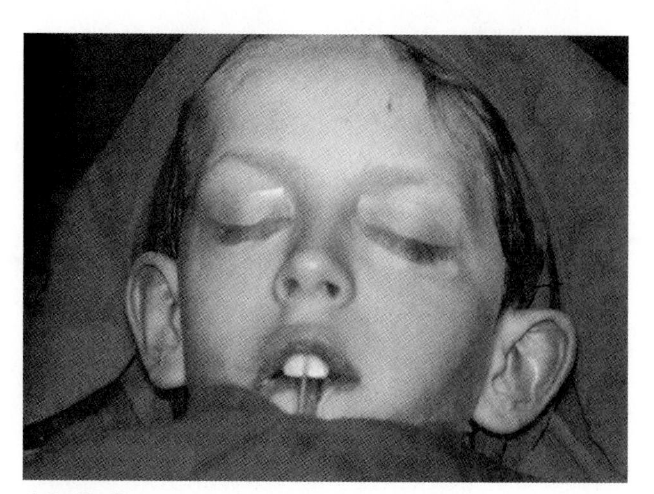

11.5.8 Both ears exposed.

the ear is slightly over-reduced. In bilateral cases both ears are reduced, one suture at a time and again slightly over-reduced (Figure 11.5.16).

The postauricular incision is closed with an interrupted subcuticular resorbable suture, the skin with interrupted (or continuous) 4/0 nylon. Bupivacaine 0.5% (2 mL) is infiltrated into the retro-auricular area.

POST-OPERATIVE CARE

The wound and the three stab wounds are liberally dressed with chloramphericol eye ointment. A proflavine wool dressing is applied just to support the posterior of the ear and also to cover and shape the lateral surface of the ear. A crepe dressing in the form of a mastoid-like bandage is applied which is kept *in situ* for 7 days (Figure 11.5.17).

Analgesics are prescribed and the patient told to attend if moderate pain is experienced. A support dressing, such as a hairband or a knitted hat, is then worn at night for a further 2–3 weeks. The final result is shown in Figure 11.5.18.

COMPLICATIONS

The most common complication is relapse, usually owing to an inappropriate technique or suture slippage. This warrants recorrection. Inappropriate placement of sutures can lead to the deformity known as telephone ear, with the mid portion of the ear pinned back and prominence of the superior and inferior aspects of the ear. The most serious complications are chondritis, haematoma and infection. Haematomas require immediate drainage. Infection requires drainage and antibiotics. Haematoma and infection can lead to severe destruction and distortion of auricular cartilage, correction of which can be very difficult.

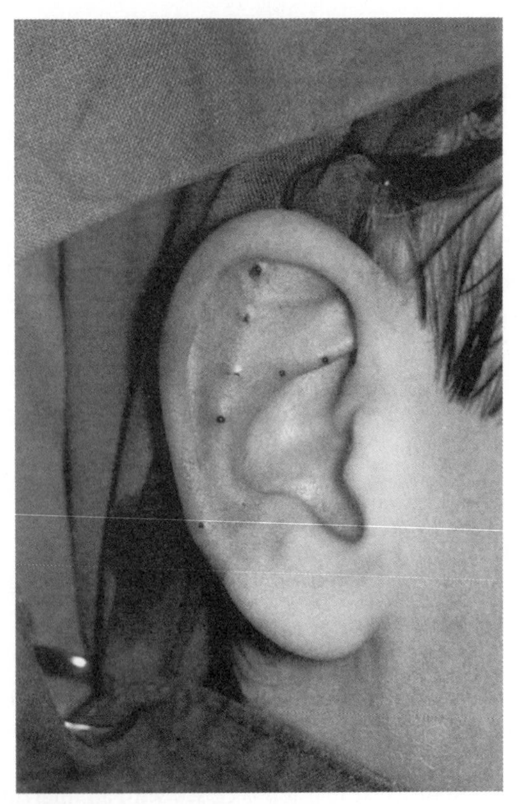

11.5.9 Ear markings.

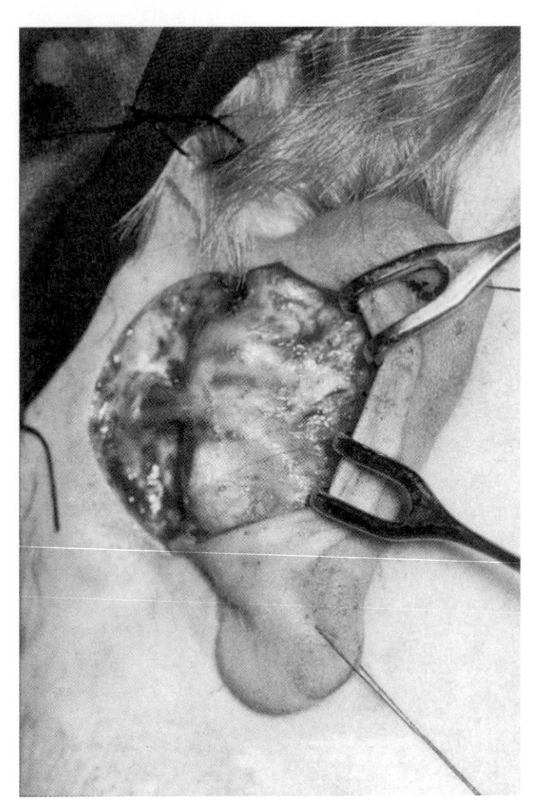

11.5.11 Postauricular dissection.

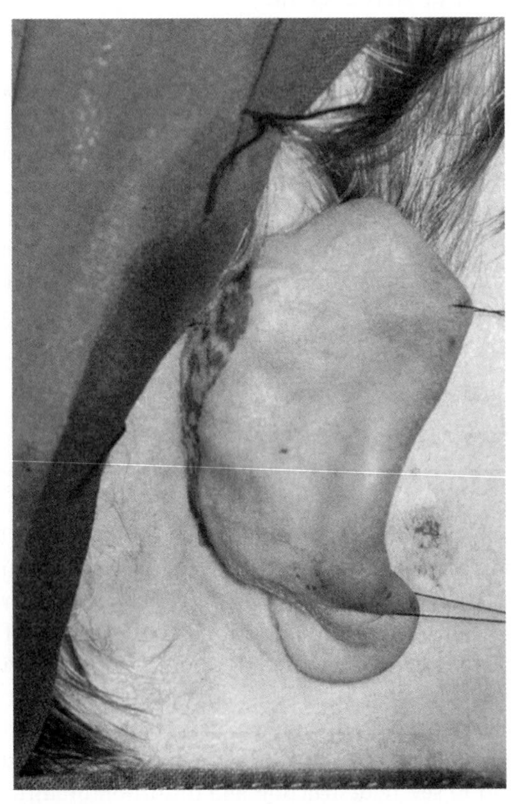

11.5.10 Dumb-bell skin excision.

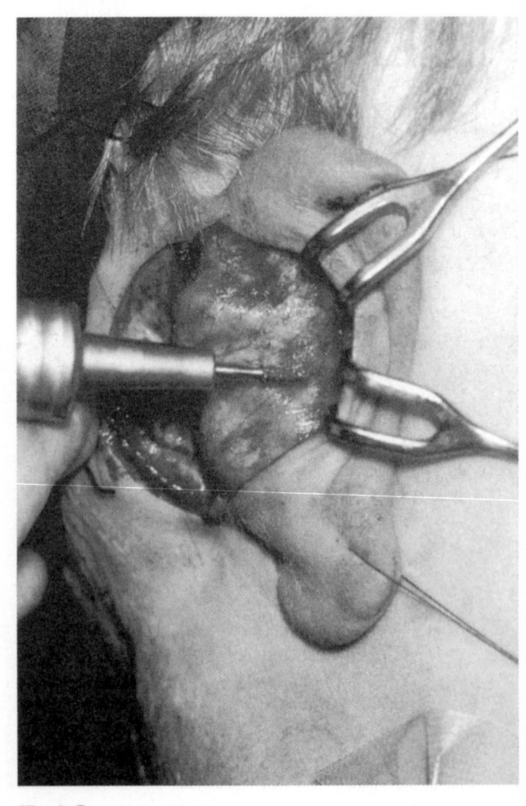

11.5.12 Burr to weaken cartilage.

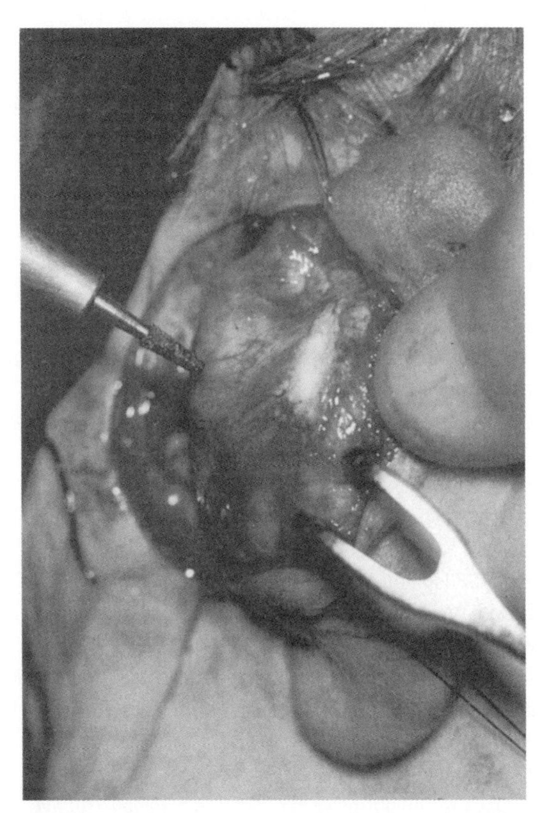

11.5.13 Weakening of cartilage to allow a tension-free ear position.

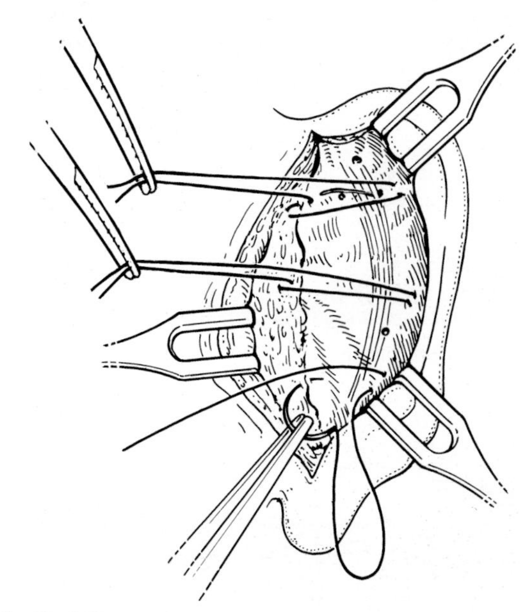

11.5.15 Mastoid cartilage sutures.

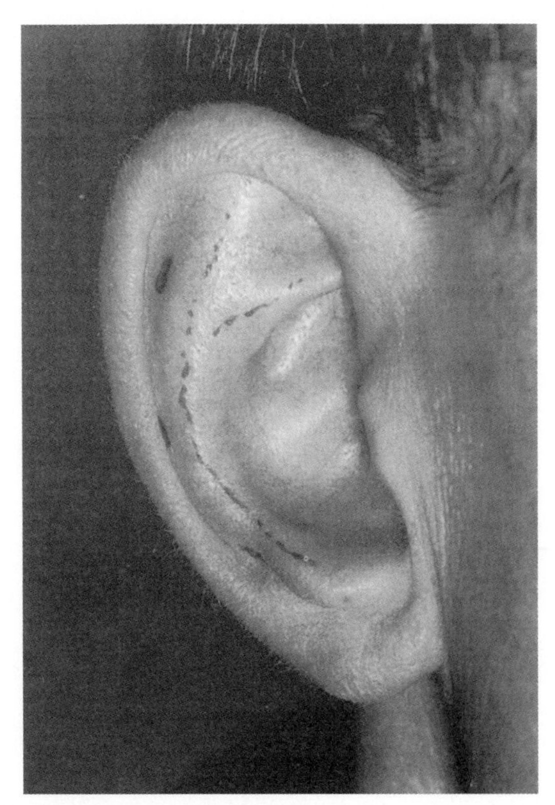

11.5.14 External ear incisions.

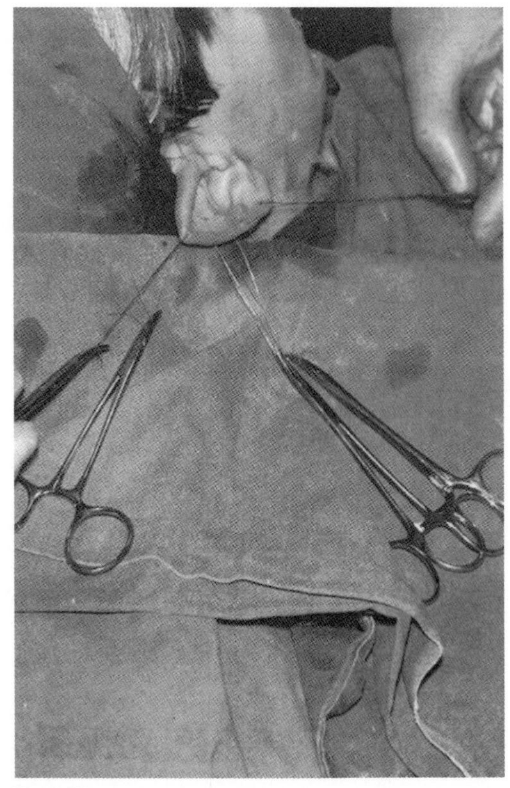

11.5.16 Holding sutures in place.

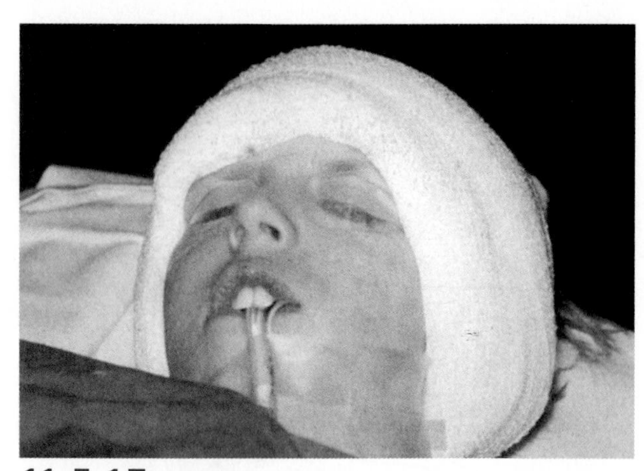

11.5.17 Dressing in place.

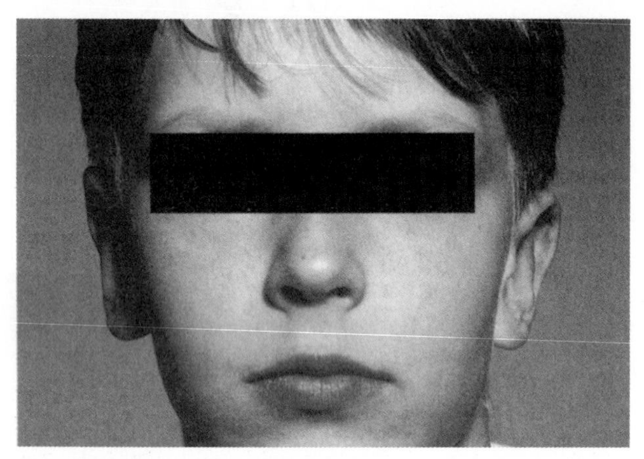

11.5.18 Final post-operative result.

FURTHER READING

Bradbury ET, Hewison J, Timmons MJ. Psychological and social outcome of prominent ear correction in children. *British Journal of Plastic Surgery* 1992; **45**: 97–100.

Brent B. Auricular repair with autogenous rib cartilage grafts: two decades of experience with 600 cases. *Plastic and Reconstructive Surgery* 1992; **90**: 355–74.

Converse JM. A technique for correction of lop ears. *Plastic Surgery* 1955; **15**: 411–18.

Ely ET. An operation for prominence of the auricles. *Archives of Otolaryngology* 1884; **10**: 97.

Farkas LG. Anthropometry of the normal and defective ear. *Clinics in Plastic Surgery* 1990; **17**: 213–21.

Furnas D. Correction of prominent ears by concha-mastoid sutures. *Plastic and Reconstructive Surgery* 1968; **42**: 189–93.

Langdon JD, Patel MF (eds). *Operative maxillofacial surgery.* London: Chapman and Hall: London, 1998

MacDowell AP Goals in otoplasty for protruding ears. *Plastic and Reconstructive Surgery* 1968; **41**: 17–27.

Mustarde JC. The correction of prominent ears by using simple mattress sutures. *British Journal of Plastic Surgery* 1963; **16**: 170–78.

Rubin LR, Bromberg BE, Walden RH, Adams A. An anatomic approach to the obtrusive ear. *Plastic and Reconstructive Surgery* 1962; **29**: 360–70.

Stark RB, Saunders DE. Natural appearance restored to unduly prominent ears. *British Journal of Plastic Surgery* 1962; **15**: 385–97.

11.6

Rhinoplasty and septoplasty: Closed and open rhinoplasty techniques and the Oriental nose

LUC CESTELEYN, N RAVINDRANATHAN, CORAZON COLLANTES-JOSE

CLOSED AND OPEN RHINOPLASTIC TECHNIQUES (Luc Cesteleyn)

PRINCIPLES AND JUSTIFICATION

Rhinoplasty is the most frequently requested aesthetic procedure usually directed towards reduction, augmentation or subtle refinement of the bony-cartilaginous skeleton. The skin soft tissue envelope (SSTE) redrapes to its new foundation. Many components of the operation can be variably affected by the healing process. The philosophy is preservation, reconstruction and cartilaginous grafting, providing tip-support and creating a strong, high profile that provides and maintains the shape to the overlying SSTE by opposing the distorting scar contracture, and preserving or correcting the nasal airway.

PRE-OPERATIVE

Surgical anatomy

THE BONY PYRAMID: UPPER THIRD

The nasal vault:

1 Paired nasal bones, thick at the frontal bone junction (no osteotomies!).
2 Nasal processes of the maxilla overlap the upper lateral cartilages (ULC) (no downward rasping!).

THE CARTILAGINOUS VAULT (NASAL BRIDGE): MIDDLE THIRD

The quadrangular septal cartilage acts as a supporting strut and contributes to the convex dorsum (nasal hump). It extends anteriorly as the posterior septal angle (PSA) from the anterior nasal spine (ANS) as a cantilever, to support the nasal tip at the anterior septal angle (ASA), and posteriorly articulates with the vomer and perpendicular plate of the ethmoid.

Superiorly, it connects deep to the nasal bones and the paired ULC to form the cartilaginous vault. The septum's most caudal mobile aspect articulates with the medial aspect of the lower lateral cartilages (LLC), supporting the tip, and facilitates LLC movements during respiration.

Inferiorly, the ULC are folded back on themselves at the plica nasi, where they articulate with the overlying superior border of the LLC, and their inferior border makes an angle of 10 to 15° with the septum at the valve area. The integrity of this angle is important for nasal airway patency and may be disrupted by disarticulation of the ULC from the nasal bone, rupture of the connection with the LLC and disconnection with the SSTE.

THE TIP: MOBILE AND SUPPLE LOWER THIRD

The LLC are composed of a medial (MC^{3b}) and a lateral crus (LC^{3a}) to form an arch with domes at the level of their connection by an intermediate crus (ImC^{3c}). The straight and thin MC are connected by the interdomal ligament and by the suspensory ligament to the ASA at the soft medial triangle of Converse. They come together in the midline to be part of the columella where they strongly articulate with the septum by ligaments in the mobile membranous septum. They end posteriorly in the MC foot plates around the ANS, and superiorly diverge (angle of divergence) as ImC, also making an angle of rotation (infra-tip break) to form the dome and then the quadrangular and convex LC. At the dome and LC the lower border of the cartilage is some distance from the nostril border; the space of superposition of skin and vestibular skin is the soft triangle of Converse or facet, to be respected by the marginal incision which follows the caudal LC margin. The LC extend down to the pyriform orifice and are connected with the ULC by fibrous and musculoaponeurotic tissue or SMAS. The weak triangle of Webster is located between the ULC, the LLC and the pyriform aperture (osteotomies can disrupt the triangle and result in airway obstruction!).

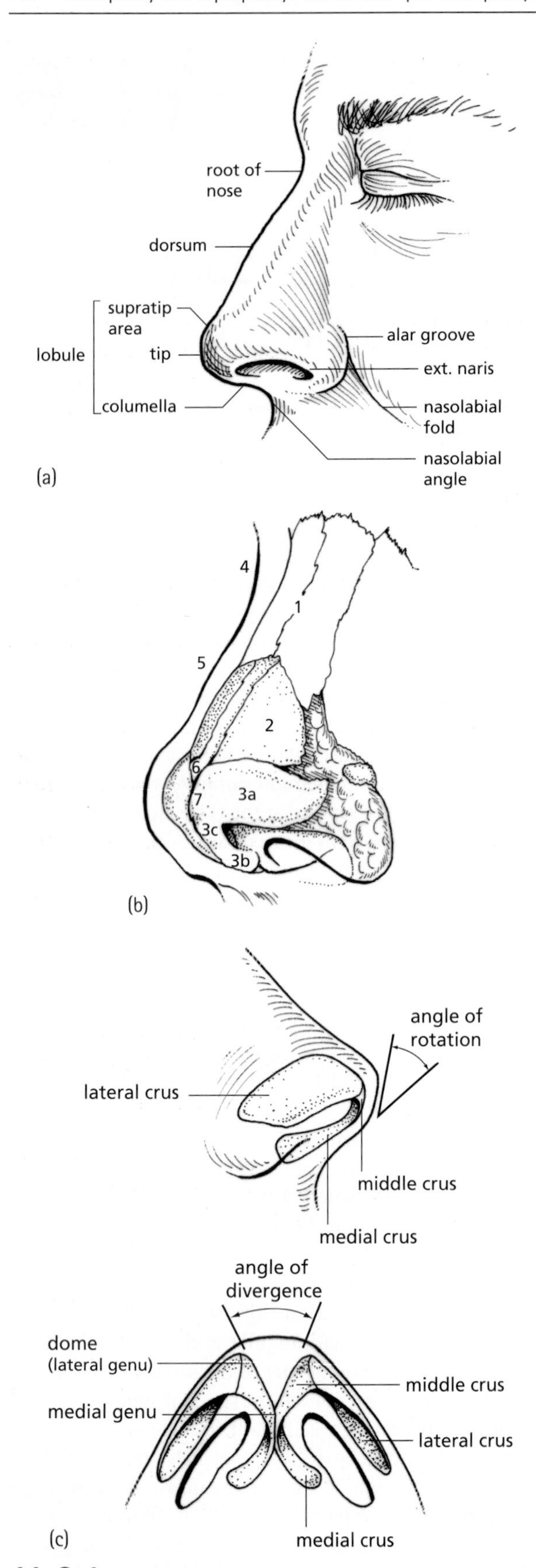

11.6.1 Surgical anatomy of the nose. (a) Soft tissues. (b) Osseocartilaginous structures and landmarks: (1) nasal bone, (2) ULC, (3) LLC: 3a LC, 3b MC, 3c ImC, (4) nasion, (5) rhinion, (6) ASA, (7) dome. (c) Alar cartilages and tip-structures (Tardy – Sheen)

The support of the nasal tip

Support mechanisms are divided into major and minor components (Figure 11.6.3). The nasal pyramid is a tripod concept consisting of the lower lateral cartilages (Anderson). The LC represent the upper legs and the linked MC the lower leg of the tripod. Tip-characteristics (TP, TR, nasal length) may be adjusted by alteration of the tripod limbs and the tip supporting structures.

The superficial muscoloaponeurotic system (SMAS) and the skin-soft tissue envelope (SSTE)

The superficial muscoloaponeurotic system (SMAS) covers the nasal pyramid in a continuous sheet of mimetic muscles

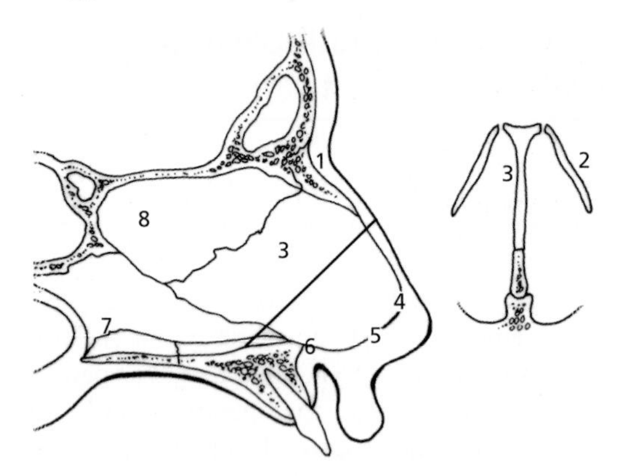

11.6.2 Surgical anatomy of the septum: (1) nasal bone, (2) ULC, (3) quadrangular septal cartilage, (4) ASA, (5) middle septal angle, (6) PSA-ANS, (7) maxillary crest, (8) perpendicular ethmoid plate.

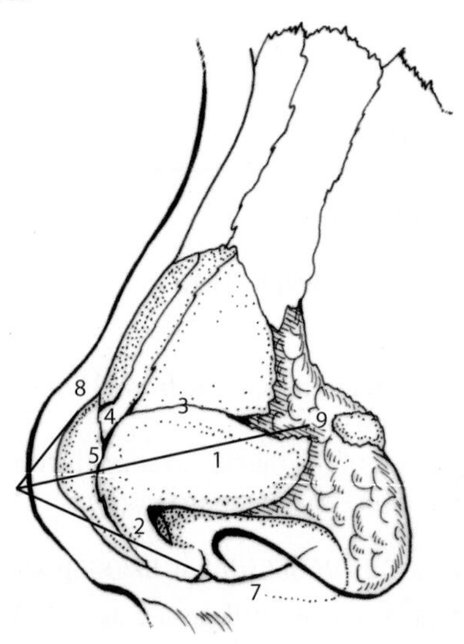

11.6.3 Tripod concept and elements of structural tip-support (TS): (1) major, (2) and (3) minor; (1) size, shape and strength of LLC (major TS), (2) medial crural-septal ligament, (3) intercartilaginous ligament, (4) SSA and cartilaginous dorsum, (5) interdomal – suspensory ligament to ASA, (–) attachment LLC and ULC to SMAS, (7) ANS and membranous septum, (–) thickness skin and SMAS, (9) alar sidewalls.

interconnected by a tendon-like aponeurosis. The SSTE is elevated in the plane just deep to the SMAS, above the perichondrium and beneath the nasal bone periosteum to which it is adherent. The SSTE overlying the nose varies in thickness, mobility and pliability; thickest at the nasion, the supratip and at the NLA, thinnest at the rhinion and the domes (Figure 11.6.1b). The mimic muscles of nasal animation can influence long-term healing with regard to the position of the tip, the upper lip or NLA and can be individually and synergistic overactive. A 'plunging tip' deformity can be due due to overactivity of levator labii alaeque nasi (LLAN) and depressor septi nasi (DSN) muscles.

EXAMINATION

Facial analysis for the rhinoplasty patient

Besides the classical divisions in thirds and fifths, examination should include: the curved unbroken aesthetic line from the eyebrow or supraciliary ridge over the nasal root to the lateral wall of the dorsum till the tip-defining (highlight) point, the width of the dorsum, the base of the bony pyramid, the ULC and the alar base (no larger than the intercanthal distance), nasofrontal angle (NFA) and soft tissue nasion or sellion (deepest portion of NFA): normally positioned horizontally 12 mm anterior to the corneal plate and vertically between upper eyelash and supratarsal fold.

Nasal analysis

MORPHOLOGY (DEFINITION) OF THE TIP

Double break (lateral view, Figure 11.6.4): STB (supra tip break) and CLA (columellar-lobular angle or infra tip break) defining transition from mesial to intermediate crus. The tip position is determined by tip projection TP and tip rotation TR. TP = CB (Figure 11.6.4), overprojection if CB >60 per cent of AB. TR is reflected in the nasio-labial angle (90–120°).

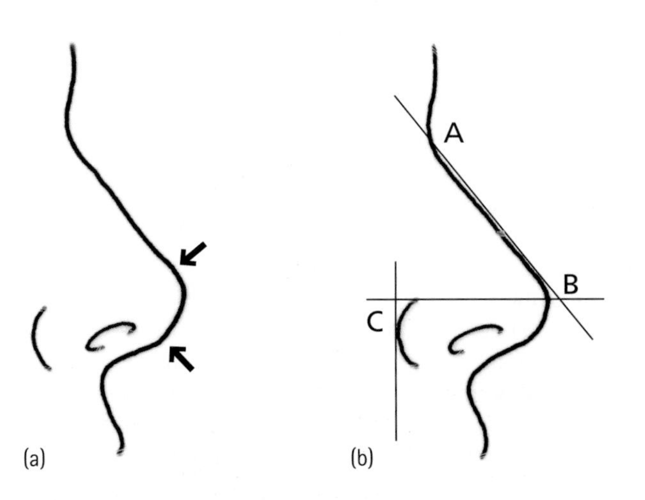

11.6.4 Nasal analysis: (a) morphology; (b) projection (AB: nasal length, CB: tip-base distance).

ALAR COLUMELLAR RELATIONSHIP

The columella should be visible and project 2–3 mm below the alar rim, as 'columellar show'. Overprojection of the columella and retracted alar rim exposes the columella and membranous septum in a 'true and pseudo hanging columella'. A hypertrophic ala is a hanging ala. Retraction of the septum in drooping tips with acute NLA diminishes the columellar show in a 'retracted' columella (Figure 11.6.5).

Pre-operative photographs in a frontal, lateral, oblique and base view, and smiling to check the synergic muscle activity for plunging tip and gum smile, are essential. Differences in anatomical shape of the LLC, thickness, strength and recoil or 'spring' of the anterior septal angle and the LLC are assessed by palpation as well as skin thickness and quality. Oily thick skin limits post rhinoplasty tip definition because of lack of contractility even after defatting. Thin skin shows all post-operative irregularities and may necessitate interpositioning of temporoparietal fascia.

Evaluation of the airway is critical (see Chapter 11.7, Post-traumatic rhinoplasty).

OPERATION

Approach to the nasal skeleton: closed endomucosal versus open extramucosal

The choice is based on the anatomical deformity and the training and experience of the surgeon. The closed or endonasal access combines an intersepto-columellar (transfixion) incision with lateral intra- or inter-cartilaginous incisions.

In the transcartilaginous approach (cartilage splitting technique), the amount of cephalic resection of the LLC is determinated pre-operatively, before the through nasal skin and cartilage incision. The transfixion incision (TI) (Figure 11.6.6c) is initiated over the SSA, continues between cartilaginous and membranous septum and extends variably from SSA to the ANS. The complete TI divides the septo-crural ligaments with potential loss of TP. The cephalic strip of cartilage is removed. The incision does not interrupt the plica nasi. A low incision, 3–6 mm from the lower border of the LC, with resection of one piece of LLC that can be reinserted if required (Millard and Peck) gives, even in thick skin noses with narrow nostrils, good access for scalpel dissection on the dorsum.

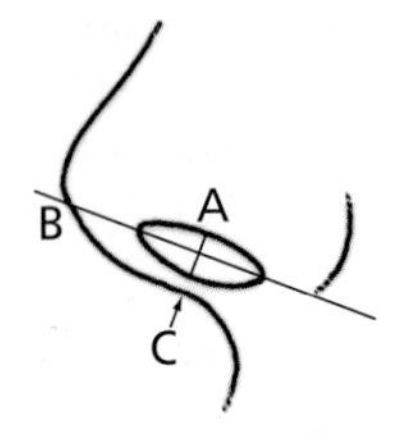

Normal
Normal alar rim, AB=1-2mm
Normal columella, BC=1-2mm

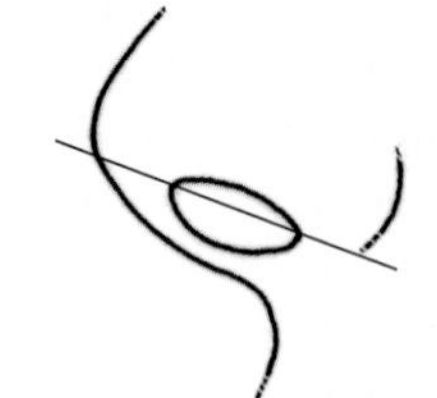

True hanging columella
Normal alar rim, AB=1-2mm
Prominent columella, >2mm

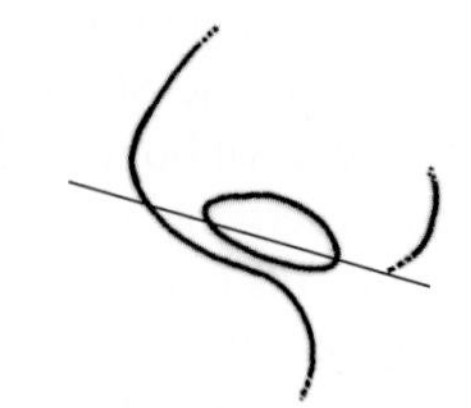

Pseudo hanging columella
Retracted alar rim, >2mm
Normal columella, 1-2mm

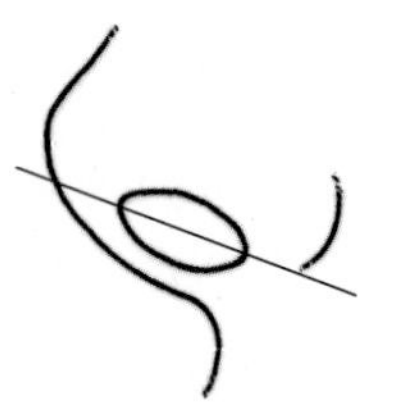

Combination
Retracted alar rim, >2mm
Prominent columella, >2mm

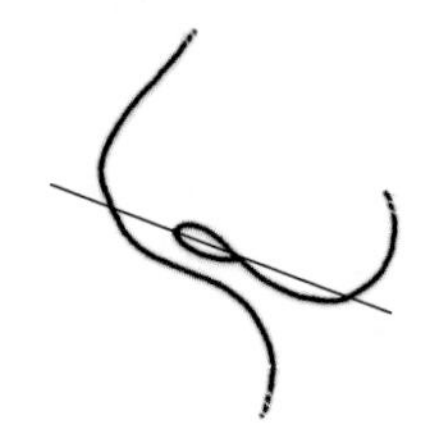

Hanging alar
Hanging alar rim, <1mm
Normal columella, 1-2mm

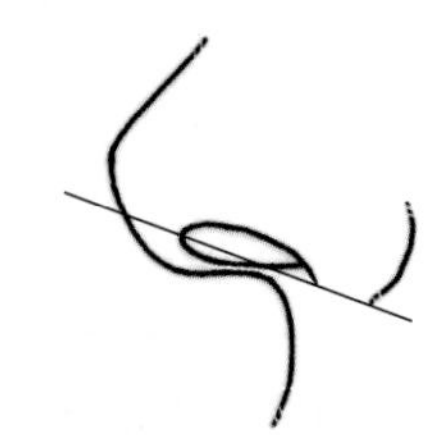

Retracted columella
Normal alar rim, 1-2mm
Retracted columella, <1mm

11.6.5 Alar–columellar relationship.

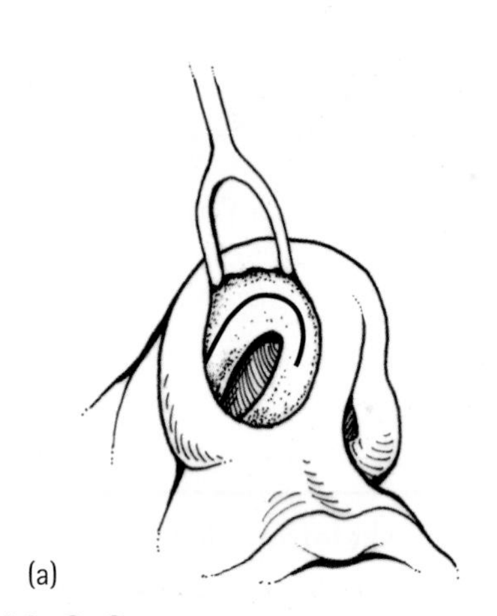

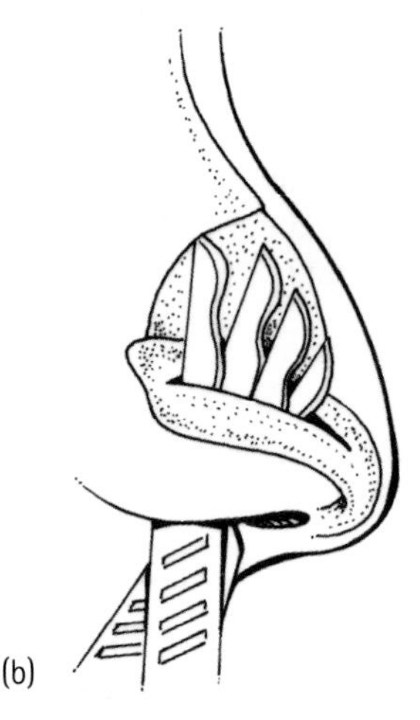

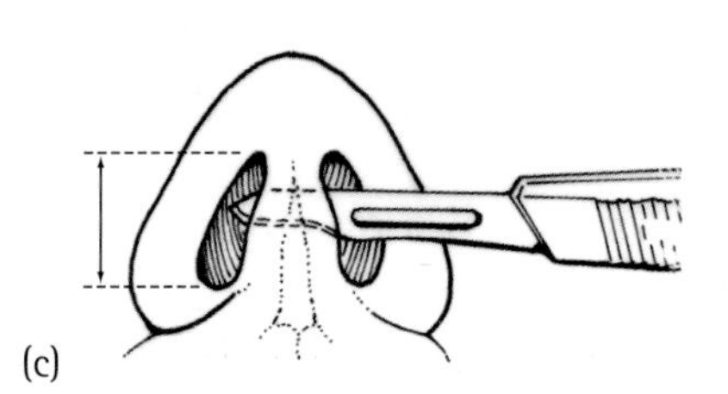

11.6.6 Transcartilaginous approach: (a) the cartilage splitting incision through the vestibular skin; (b) and through the LC; (c) transfixion incision: the partial transfixion incision stops short of the ANS. The complete transfixion incision divides the septo-crural ligaments with potential loss of TP.

Non-delivery techniques are conservative with stable healing and minimal tip numbness only indicated for minimal tip refinements (minimal volume reduction), little tip rotation, in thin skin noses with symmetric strong LLC needing maximal cartilage preservation.

In the intercartilaginous approach (delivery-technique) (Figure 11.6.7), bilateral intercartilaginous incisions are combined with marginal incisions following the lower border of the alar cartilages, respecting the soft triangle of Converse. The LLC are delivered as chondrocutaneous bipedicled flaps, allowing for direct inspection and appropriate tip modifications, dome sutures and asymmetry correction. The intercartilagenous incision can disturb the valve and interruption of the interdomal ligament can lead to decreased nasal tip support and TP loss.

The open approach or external rhinoplasty technique (Figure 11.6.8) combines marginal incisions, 1 mm behind the columellar border, with a mid-transcolumellar connection. The SSTE is then dissected off the nasal skeleton under direct vision.

1. Advantage: perfect visualization of the cartilages, better diagnosis, an intact valve, easier and precise grafting.
2. Indications: severe post-traumatic deformities, secondary rhinoplasties, difficult and cleft noses, simultaneously maxillary orthognathic surgery to reconstruct tip support and a strong profile.
3. Disadvantages: increased scarring by dissection of the skin from the cartilages, potential trauma to the tip and dorsal skin by manipulation and retraction.

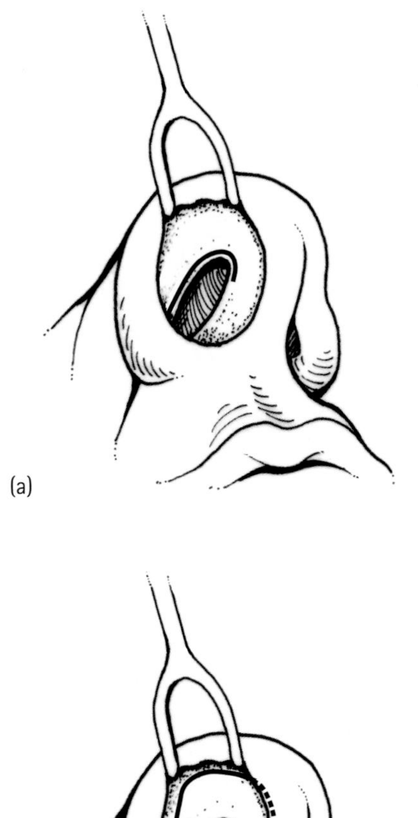

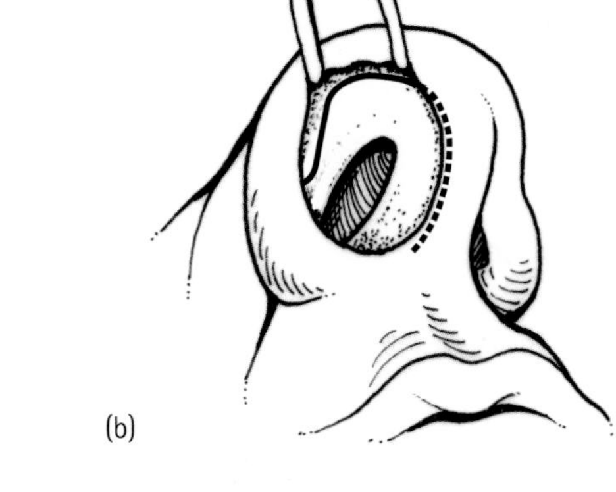

11.6.7 Intercartilaginous access or delivery technique: (a) intercartilaginous and (b) marginal incisions.

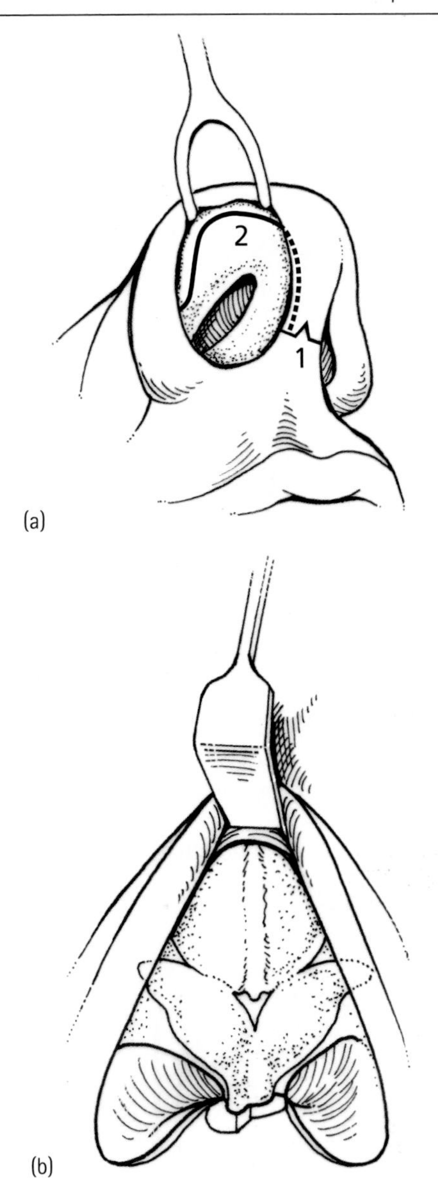

11.6.8 The open/external approach: (a) (1) transcolumellar, (2) bilateral vertical columellar and marginal incision; (b) elevation of the SSTE offering a direct view on the tip and middle vault.

Surgery of the dorsum

Exposure of the osseocartilaginous vault requires sharp dissection as close as possible to the cartilages and subperiostally at the nasal bones keeping the SMAS intact; in thick skin noses de-fatting or resection of the SMAS is possible (Figure 11.6.9). For hump resection, an extramucosal dissection is utilized elevating the mucosa of the ULC and the nasal bones periosteum starting from the submucoperichondial layer of the septum. to prevent mucosal tearing during hump reduction and endonasal mucosal retraction. Cartilage grafting has less risk of infection, elimination or rejection in a closed compartment (Figure 11.6.9b).

Hump resection is performed with a scalpel for the cartilage as a single unit (ULC and septum) and with a Rubin guided osteotome, introduced in the 'fish mouth' created, for the bony hump. Bony irregularities are corrected with bone scissors or upward rasping. An 'open roof deformity' results after hump resection.

Overresection of the bony hump and underresection of the cartilaginous hump causes a 'pollybeak or surgical look'.

A slight residual convexity should be preserved at the rhinion after hump resection as straight line removal of the skeletal hump can result in a concave, over-reduced bridge. This can be corrected by cartilage onlay grafting, or reintroduction of a reduced resected hump (Skoog).

Narrowing the nose: osteotomy techniques

The primary indication for narrowing the nose by lateral osteotomies is to close the open roof deformity following hump resection (Figure 11.6.10).

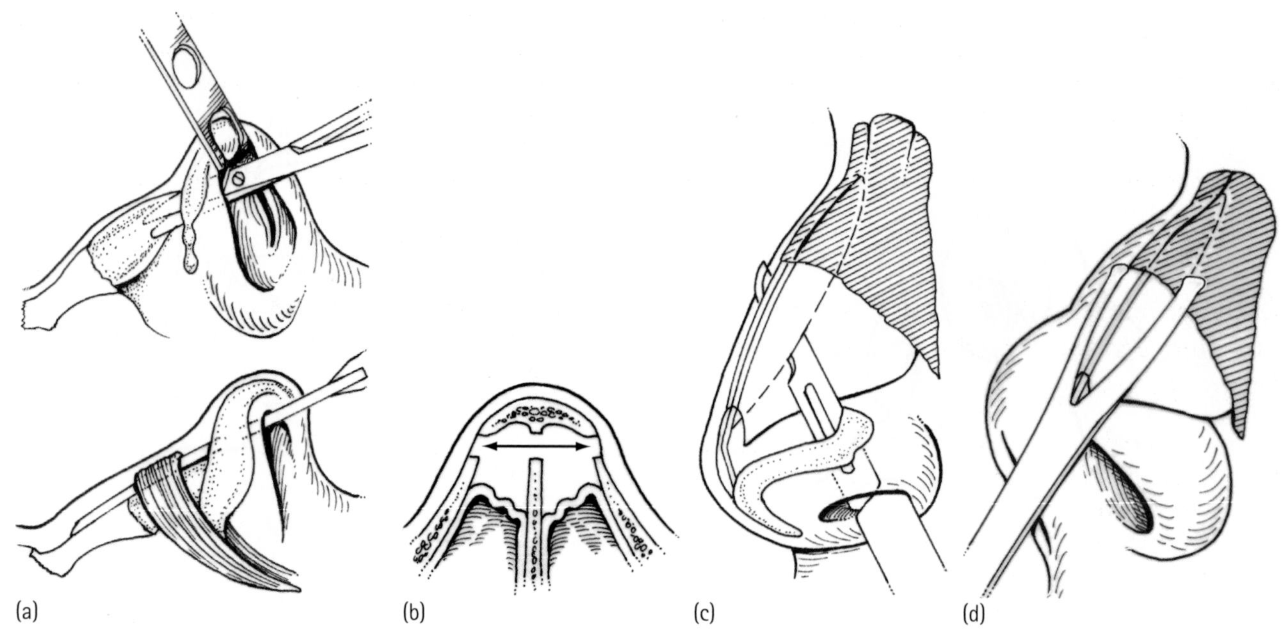

11.6.9 Dorsal hump surgery: (a) dissection below the SMAS and exactly on the perichondrium and ideally below the periosteum at the bridge leaving the lateral side of the nasal bones attached to the SSTE; (b) separation of the nasal mucosa away from the ULC and septum; (c) hump resection initiated with scalpel on cartilaginous portions of hump (Peck); (d) hump resection completed with rounded edges osteotome (Rubin) on the bony portions of hump.

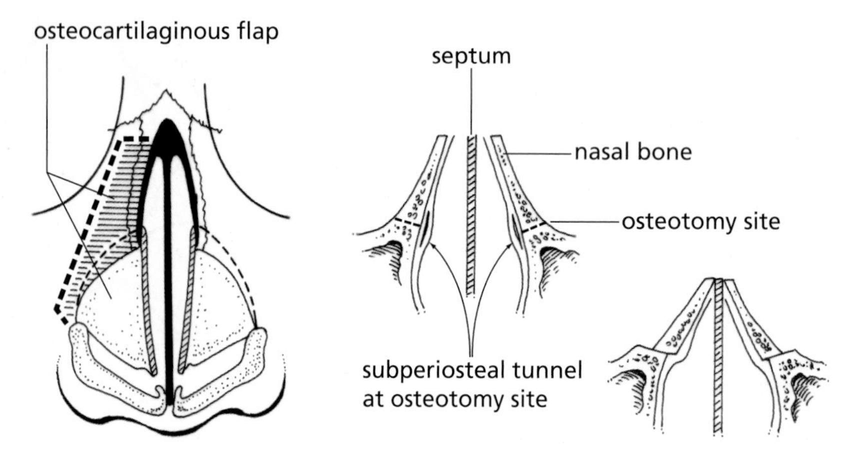

11.6.10 Nasal osteotomies. The 'open roof' is corrected by lateral osteotomies to mobilize the pedicled osteocartilaginous flap.

The standard approach is intranasal after stab incision and tunneling, or directly through the mucosa, at the pyriform rim just superior to the inferior turbinate, respecting the valve area at Websters triangle. The lateral osteotomy runs low in the nasofacial groove to below the medial canthus, where it is angled towards the midline. In primary rhinoplasties, the lateral osteotomy alone is sufficient, because, by twisting the osteotome and finger pressure, a back fracture creates superior and medial fractures. If not, transnasal medial osteotomies with an osteotome placed laterally along the septum and driven upwards till the sound change indicates thick bone, and transcutaneous superior osteotomies are performed.

For more predictable and precise osteotomies, a transcutaneous approach, lateral to the nasofacial groove, with a 2 mm osteotome, leaving no visible scar, is preferred. The superior transverse osteotomy, as well as an osteotomy of a deviated bony septum, can be carried out through the glabellar skin.

Common problems: 'rocker' formation (osteotomy too high), lateral depression (too low), stair step deformity (too medial) and recoil of bony flap or drop into the nasal fossa (too wide underming or too thin maxilla).

NASAL TIP SURGERY

Generalities and tip dynamics

TIP PROJECTION AND TIP ROTATION

As described earlier, the nasal tip can be likened to a tripod (Figure 11.6.3) with the LC representing two legs and the conjoined MC a third. Selective increase or decrease in the length of the tripod legs can be used to attain the desired TP and/or TR, for example by shortening the two superior legs of the tripod, one can increase TR and decrease TP, or by shortening the conjoined MC, one decreases TP and TR. It is nearly impossible to alter tip projection without changing tip rotation (Anderson and Webster).

Cephalic volume reduction: complete and interrupted strip, rim strip and lateral crural flap procedures

In tip refinement, the complete strip (Figure 11.6.11), leaving behind a 6 mm caudal LC for alar support, is a basic and conservative technique, for mild increase in tip definition with slight decrease in TP and increase in TR. The complete strip will resist upward rotation and refinement, unless additional manoeuvres as incomplete incisions, cross-hatching or morselization are added. Sectioning the lateral parts of the LC will also increase TR. The amount of upward rotation and decrease in TP is more important with more developed ULC.

In more aberrant anatomy, interrupted strip procedures with vertical lateral excisions are indicated; they require suture reconstruction and need supportive struts or contouring grafts to stabilize and prevent loss of projection, alar collapse, notching, pinching and asymmetry.

The rim strip (Figure 11.6.12) and lateral crural flap (Webster) (Figure 11.6.12) are useful in thick skin noses, strong enough to support the alae and prevent them from collapsing, needing tip repositioning: increased TR and decreased TP.

Dome suture techniques

Complementing complete strip techniques, interdomal sutures and transdomal horizontal mattress sutures are indicated for greater tip-narrowing in broad-boxy or bifid tips with excess divergence of intermediate crura. After removing the soft tissue occupying the interdomal space, a more triangular lobule and improved support are obtained. If obliteration of the external soft triangle occurs due to medialization of the LC, the cartilage has to be trimmed.

SEPTAL SHORTENING

Essential in correction of a long nose, performed through a (high) transfixion incision or directly in the open technique. The shortening encroaches on the ANS and can be modified as illustrated in Figure 11.6.14.

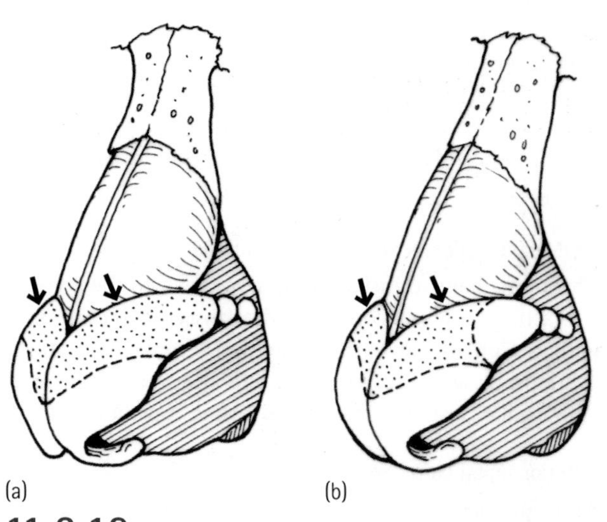

11.6.12 Cephalic volume reduction: (a) rim strip technique; (b) lateral crural flap (Webster) technique.

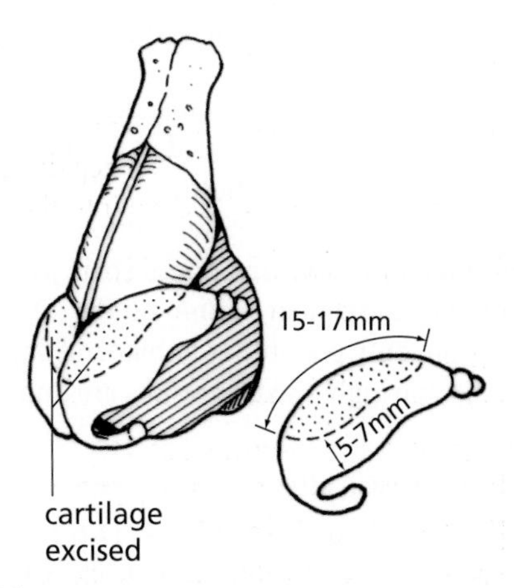

11.6.11 Complete strip technique.

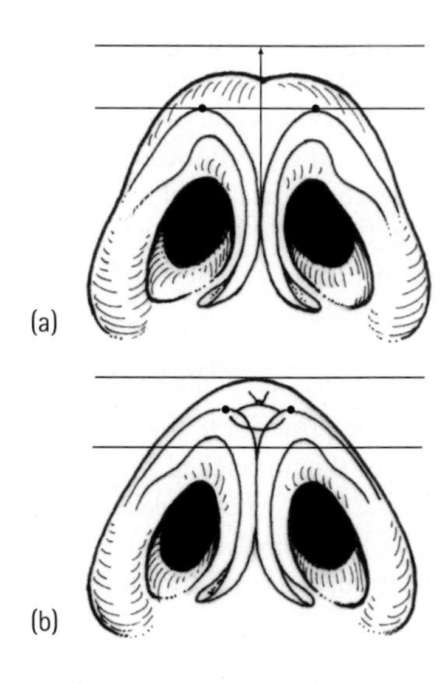

11.6.13 Interdomal sutures technique.

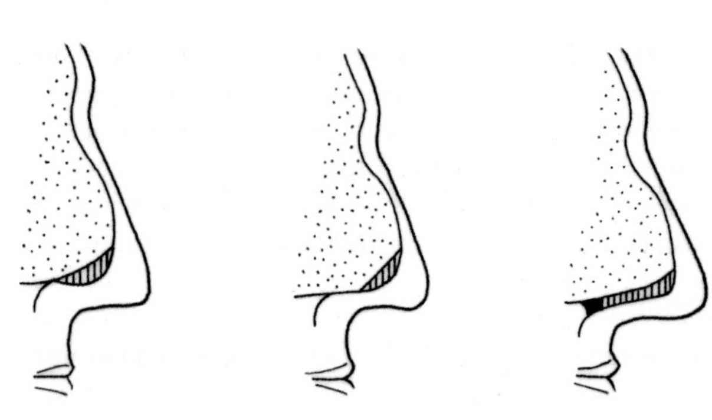

11.6.14 Septal shortening (Aiach).

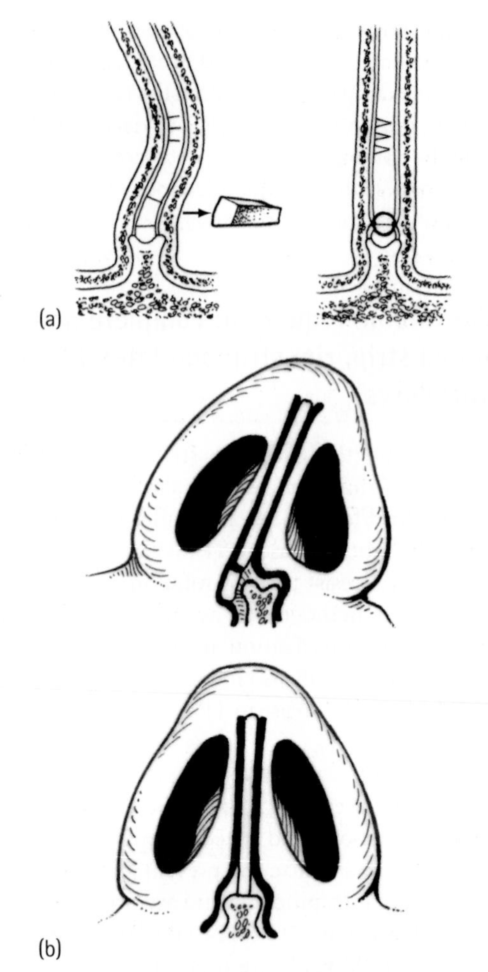

11.6.15 Anterior septal corrections through a hemitransfixion incision and unilateral flap elevation: (a) incision on the concave side and partial resection; (b) repositioning of caudal deflections with displacement from bony groove, resection of cartilaginous spur, osteotomy of palatal/vomeral crest offending medial reposition of caudal septum.

Adjunctive procedures

SEPTOPLASTY, SEPTAL GRAFT HARVESTING

Septal surgery is performed to correct septal deviations with airway obstruction or aesthetic problems due to anterior deflections, and to harvest (osseo) cartilaginous grafts. All displaced structures should be exposed with limited mucoperichondrial detachment and maintaining 1 cm of dorsal and caudal structure to prevent dorsal saddling, tip drooping, columellar retraction and septal flaccidity.

Septo-columellar (hemi)transfixion incision

Through a hemi-transfixion incision down to the spine to the cartilage, a submucoperichondral dissection is performed with a Cottle's elevator. If fracture adhesions, cartilage overlaps, or severe scarring interfere, the area is infiltrated with local anaesthesia to facilitate further elevation.

Anterior septal corrections

Anterior cartilaginous thickenings can be thinned by shaving, concave cartilaginous deviations are corrected by resection of excess inferior cartilaginous combined with full thickness incisions on the concave side of the contralateral pedicled cartilage to break the spring (memory) (Figure 11.6.15). The swinging-door technique is used to reposition a displaced caudal septum. After unilateral elevation of the mucoperichondrial flap, the septal cartilage is excised along the floor of the nose and repositioned on the premaxillary crest, and fixated on the contralateral mucoperichondrium by a bur hole in the ANS. Bony spurs and angulated deformities (see Chapter 11.7, Post-traumatic rhinoplasty) need resection or osteotomy.

Posterior septal corrections and for graft harvesting

Cartilage incision 1 cm posterior to the border of the caudal septum. Elevation of the untouched mucoperichondrium on the contralateral side where needed, mostly at the junction of the cartilage–maxillary crest.

Septal modifications, after positioning of a long small speculum, by:

1. Resection/osteotomies: most common method for septal correction and graft harvesting. Deviations limited to the posterior septum are treated by endonasal submucous resection after bilateral mucoperichondrial flap elevation. A 1 cm caudal and dorsal L-shaped strut is left attached to the perpendicular ethmoidal plate and maxillary crest–ANS area to maintain support. Cartilage and bone for grafting can be harvested.
2. Segmental scoring/weakening.
3. Swinging-door flaps, indicated in angular deviations of the dorsal strut, which are incised at the angle to 2 mm of the dorsal border. Repositioning in the midline and splinting for stabilization before multiple cartilage incisions interrupt a twisting dorsal strut, as well as stabilization of the caudal septum on the ANS.
4. Morselization, only possible after bilateral flap elevation, is sparingly used, as results are unpredictable.

Tardy's modified incision after Killian

In Tardy's modified method (Figure 11.6.16): a vertical sinuous incision sited just cephalically to the caudal end of the septum and proximal to the mucocutaneous junction, avoiding scar formation or retraction in the cutaneous portion of the caudal septum allows full septal exposure through retrograde dissection to and around the caudal septum while maintaining the vital medial crural footplate attachment to the septum.

After unilateral flap elevation, and if osseocartilagenous grafts are not needed, disarticulation with slight pressure with the elevator at the chondro-osseous junction or in previous fracture lines, exposing the contralateral perichondrium permitting contralateral submucoperiosteal dissection. This often allows the deviated cartilage to return to the midline as a 'swinging door', sometimes after resection of fibrous tissue bands, subluxated cartilage or bone along the nasal floor. Correction of bony obstructions is performed with a biting forceps. Cartilaginous obstructions are corrected by incisions in different directions through the cartilage but not into the opposite mucoperichondrium, to create multiple cartilage islands, supported and nourished by the opposite intact mucoperichondrial flap.

Transoral sublabial approach

Use

- Children with caudal subluxation. An intact caudal septum is important for the development of the columellar–labial complex.
- In secondary septoplasties and potstraumatic rhinoplasties for anterior bony crest (re)sections or graft offers the possibility of separate elevation of the flaps to reduce the chances of perforation.

Open or external approach

The open rhinoplasty technique offers a remarkable exposure for anterior and infero-anterior septal corrections, secondary septoplasties and graft harvesting from the ASA and caudal septal border to correct caudal deviations.

Separation of the domes and the MC to the ANS, with submucoperichondral dissection cranially to the ethmoid. Caudally, separate elevation of the periosteum by tunnelling from the ANS on the floor of the nose. By semicircular sweeping motions both tunnels are connected over the chondro-osseous junction area to prevent lacerations. Bilateral dissection is possible but in angulated deformities, a unilateral attachment is preferred for stabilization. The medial crural support is re-established by suturing the MC together post-septoplasty.

From the anterior septal border to correct anterior deviations in secondary septoplasties, where the dissection from the caudal border is impossible due to scar formation, and has to be dissected from anteriorly at the middle third after section of the ULC at their septal junction; modification and graft harvesting can then be carried out behind the area of adherences.

At the end of the procedure redundant bony-cartilaginous fragments can be repositioned as free grafts between the septal flaps, to prevent a flaccid septum (floating during inspiration and expiration). Through-and-through mattress resorbable sutures reapproximate the septal flaps and stabilize the repositioned fragments. Inadvertent perforations of the mucoperichondrium are meticulously closed if they are opposing each other. Incisions are closed and disrupted supporting ligaments: interdomal and medial crural–septal attachments are restored. Bilateral soft silastic stenting is placed for 5–7 days (Figure 11.6.17).

Nasal grafting

Grafting provides shape and definition, establishes solid tip support, opposes scar contracture and distortion of the SSTE and functionally grafting is used to improve and maintain an open nasal airway.

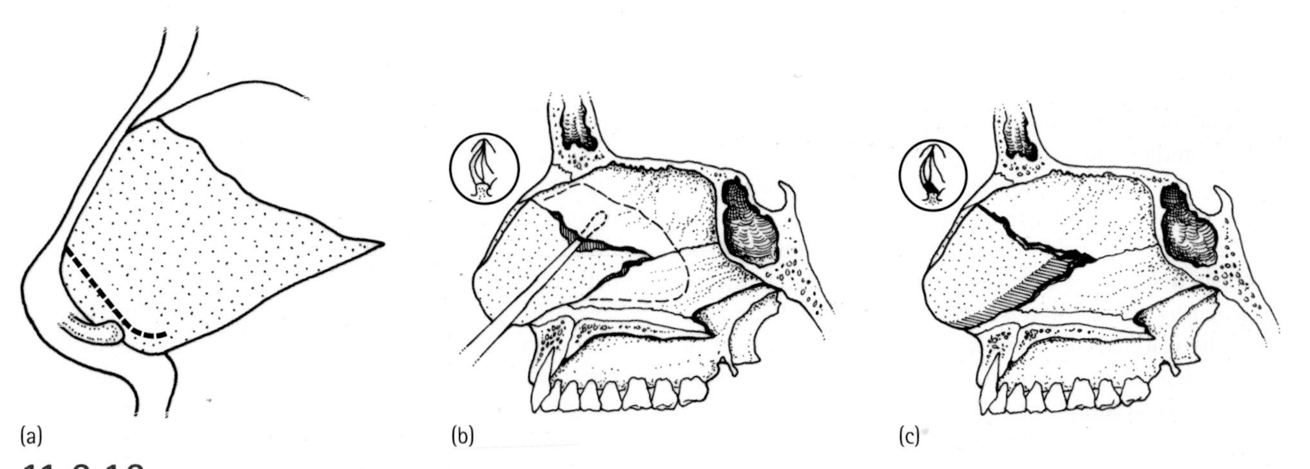

11.6.16 Tardy's septoplasty technique: (a) serpentine mucoperichondral incision 2-3 mm above caudal septum border; (b) unilateral mucoperichondrial flap, disarticulation of the cartilaginous septum and contralateral subperiosteal dissection; (c) resection of subluxated cartilage (and bone) along the floor of the nose and replacement of the anteriorly pedicled septum as a 'swinging door' to the midline.

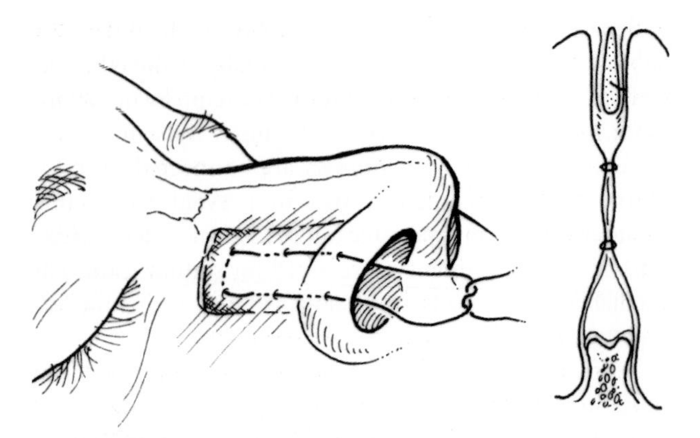

11.6.17 Reapproximating the mucoperichondrial septal flaps and stabilizing the septal remnants.

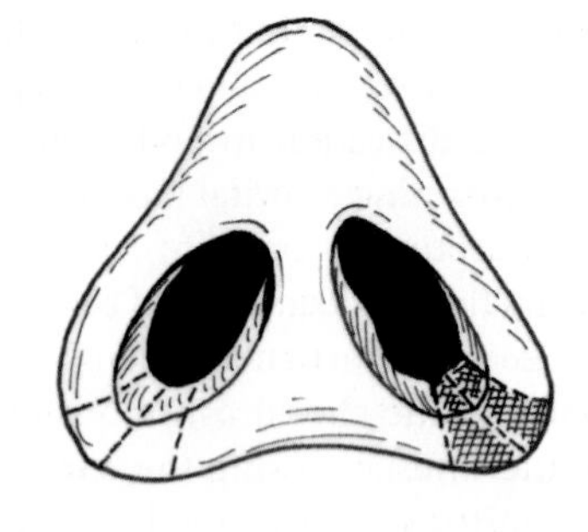

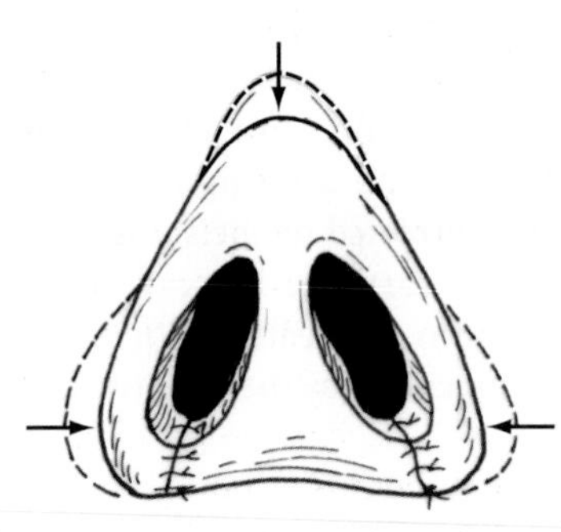

11.6.18 Alar base surgery: Alar resection in combined vertical and horizontal part.

Septal cartilage is the preferred source of grafting material. Other excellent sources include remnants of the resected osseocartilagenous dorsal hump and the cartilage obtained from the cephalic trim of strong LLCs. Conchal ear cartilage can also be used. Thin bony plates from the perpendicular ethmoid and vomerine septum may be used where a more rigid graft is needed. Description of all grafting techniques is beyond the scope of this section, they include columellar struts, tip onlays, infratip lobular grafts, etc. In addition to these tip grafts, contouring grafts are frequently required.

Alar base surgery

Aesthetic narrowing of the nasal skeleton and tip must be balanced by concomitant reduction of the alar base. Alar surgery is one of the final steps in aesthetic rhinoplasty in a conservative and symmetric manner (Figure 11.6.18).

SURGICAL TECHNIQUES

- Internal nostril floor reduction preserving the nostril sill provides subtle improvement in repositioned nasal tips without visable scar.
- Alar lobule excision at the nostril floor and sill results in reduction of flare as well as in slight reduction of the alar bulk, and provides medial alar repositioning.
- In reduction of overprojecting tips, alar wedge excisions reduce the overall length of the alar sidewalls.
- Maximal alar reduction with medial repositioning will be effected from the alar sliding flap technique, with a generous incision in the alar–facial junction. Reduction of the volume, curve and flare will result, the extent of each dependent on the angulation of the excision. Skin repair is accomplished with inradermal absorbable suture. Skin sutures are placed 1 mm above the alar–facial groove to avoid sebaceous glands located in the junction. The repair can be further supported and enhanced with the use of an alar cinch suture of 3/0 PDS.

HOW I DO IT: A MODIFIED OPEN STRUCTURE RHINOPLASTY TECHNIQUE

General anesthesia with orotracheal intubation is preferred. The nose is packed with neurosurgical cottonoids in a cocaine–epinephrine (adrenaline) solution for vasoconstriction and shrinkage of the mucosae; local anesthesia (0.5 per cent xylocaine- 1:100 000 epinephrine) is infiltrated between the skin and the skeleton and submucosally.

The mid-columellar incision (inverted V) to the level of the medial crura at a site just anterior to and above the flare of the medial footplates is made with a No. 15 blade. The transcolumellar incision is connected to bilateral columellar marginal incisions running 1 mm behind and parallel to the rim of the columella. The lateral part of the marginal incision is placed along the caudal margin of the lateral crura. The back of the scalpel is used to palpate the edge of the cartilage to identify the correct position for the lateral incision. A double skin hook retracts the alar margin while simultaneously applying finger pressure over the LLC to evert the caudal margin. Then the hook is placed between the lateral portion of the marginal incision and the columellar portion, with simultaneous traction on the nasal skin with a single hook to make the connecting incision, respecting the facet or soft triangle of Converse, which should be preserved; incisions too close to the nostril rim can result in alar notching or distortion of the facet.

Using small pointed serrated scissors or a scalpel, the SSTE overlying the medial crura is dissected without injuring the underlying cartilage. By using three-point counter-traction, sharp dissection along the medial crurae and LLC is performed in the avascular immediate supraperichondrial plane, preserving the subdermal plexus and avoiding flap breakdown. Flap elevation is carried laterally to the point of attachement of the lateral crura with soft tissue. The interdomal ligament is not disturbed.

The loose connective tissue (Pitanguy's ligament) overlying the anterior septal angle at the soft supratip triangle is resected and an avascular supraperichondrial plane is identified over the lower dorsum. At the rhinion, the remainder of the dissection of the nasal bones is performed subperiosteally, using sharp dissection. An Aufricht retractor is placed and lateral bands between the SSTE and the osseocartilaginous structure are divided bluntly, until the entire nasal skeleton can be clearly observed.

For septoplasty and cartilage harvesting for later grafting a hemitransfixion incision is used. In difficult septoplasties or in asymmetric tips, the interdomal ligament is cut and the medial crura separated. Using a speculum the caudal edge of the septal cartilage is visualized. The subperichondrial plane is established using the tips of pointed scissors or Cottle's elevator and the mucoperichondrium is elevated using sweeping motions. Incisions are made in the cartilaginous septum at 1 cm parallel to the caudal septum and dorsum, leaving in an inverted L-shape support, allowing the maximal amount of cartilage to be harvested. Deviated cartilagenous fragments are disarticulated and removed.

Turbinate surgery further corrects airway obstruction.

Routinely, the author prefers to address the osseo-cartilaginous vault before the tip and lower third with alar base correction as the last step.

Under direct visualization, reduction of the cartilagenous dorsum is performed with a No. 15 blade, the cartilage is maintained in continuity with the nasal bone. Sharpened Rubin osteotomes are used to resect the bony hump to nasion in continuity with the cartilaginous resection. Initially, a 16 mm osteotome is placed in the 'fish-mouth' created by the cartilage resection, then a 14 mm Rubin as the line of resection approaches the narrower naso-frontal angle. In the glabellar area, the hump is sharply separated from the attaching soft tissues, before being removed and preserved together with the harvested cartilage in a physiologic solution. Irregularities are removed with sharp resection to avoid disruption of the osseous-cartilagenous junction.

The dorsum appears to be broadened and the 'open roof' aspect shows through the overlying skin.

Closure of the open roof deformity is through the use of osteotomies, under direct vision using a 3 mm micro-osteotome, creating a laterally fading line for controlled back-fracture created by the lateral osteotomies. Only in broad strong noses are medial osteotomies utilized. If these are especially thick then triangular wedges are removed along the medial osteotomy.

The lines of the lateral osteotomies are low to the face, respecting Webster's triangle and directed towards the highest thin part of the nasal bones. No infiltration, stab incision or periosteal raising is carried out to prepare the lateral osteotomies. The same 3 mm osteotome is immediately engaged on the pyriform aperture just superior to the inferior turbinate's origin. The osteotome is initially engaged in a plane perpendicular to the pyriform aperture. Once a triangle of bone is preserved at Websters area, the osteotome is directed up the lateral bony wall under finger control. Just below the level of the medial canthus, the cut is directed more anteriorly to meet the medial osteotomy when required. The back fracture is completed with rotation of the osteotome and finger pressure. The inward fractures can be performed with greater accuracy and precision transcutaneously at the lateral mid portion of the osteotomy and through the glabella if necessary with a 2 mm micro-osteotome and without stab incision.

The mobility of the nasal bones can be palpated through the skin and controlled under direct vision. The dorsum is palpated and visually checked to make sure that no irregularities or projections of bone or cartilage exist. Small bony fragments can be resected with bone scissors and cartilaginous protrusions can be trimmed by blade.

The concept of the open-structure rhinoplasty supports reconstitution of disrupted support mechanisms by suturing and grafting which will resist the effects of scarring and contracture of the soft tissue envelope. The elevation of the SSTE during rhinoplasty violates a minor support mechanism. Therefore, the medial crura are generally strengthened with a septal cartilage graft or the resected osseocartilagenous hump, sandwiched between them as a supporting strut. A pocket to receive the graft is dissected between the medial crura towards, but not to, the nasal spine. The strut not extending above the ASA is fixated with through and through Vicryl™ 4.0 from the level of the medial footplates. Care is taken not to distort or rotate the nasal tip area by malpositioned sutures. The strut increases support and stability and maintains symmetry of the nasal tip. It can also serve as a foundation for a tip graft.

The medial crural/columellar strut complex is sutured to the caudal septum. This will effectively reconstruct the medial crural–septal ligaments sectioned when a transfixion incision is used.

If tip narrowing and upward tip rotation is desired, cephalic trim of the LLC is performed. Care is taken not to weaken the lateral crura, by leaving a symmetrical strip of cartilage at least 6 mm in width. Over-resection can weaken the lateral legs of the nasal tripod, resulting in external valve collapse on inspiration and retraction of the nostril rim from scar contracture on the LLCs. This is remedied during surgery with alar batten grafts.

The recurvature of the ULC contributing to intercrural width is resected together with the cephalic edge of the lower lateral cartilage. The cartilage is removed while leaving the nasal skin intact at all times.

Aesthetic adjustments to the position of rhinion to create a more natural dorsum are often accomplished using Skoog's technique of replacing the resected dorsal hump after sculpting to the desired shape and size, into the dorsal pocket thereby avoiding irregular edges, asymmetry and the 'open roof deformity'.

Modification of the caudal aspect of the medial crura can be carried out for such abnormalities as a hanging columella deformity.

Opening up an obtuse nasofrontal angle or widening the root of the nose can be done by cartilaginous grafts.

Debulking of the undersurface of thick sebaceous tissue of the nasal tip is accomplished under direct visualization. Care is taken not to injure the dermis. The effects of debulking the tip skin can be seen in the redraping of the skin-soft tissue envelope providing superior tip definition.

A widely arched dome may be narrowed and lowered by excising triangles of LLC cartilage, leaving the skin intact. The free ends of the lateral crura are reconstructed into a continuous strip by suturing the ends with 5/0 resorbable sutures to maintain the strength of the tip tripod. Irregularities can be trimmed. The interdomal ligament is restored by an interdomal mucosal apposition mattress suture, lying just below the domes, acting to restore reattachments between the lower lateral cartilages and the anterior septal angle, thus contributing to tip support.

A septal cartilage graft sculpted into a three-dimensional shield-like tip lobular graft with bevelled contours is placed over the stable nasal tip structure. This establishes the desired projection, angle of the infratip region, a double break and the bidomal shape. This graft is usually thickest at its dorsal aspect and gradually tapers to the ventral. Resorbable 5/0 sutures can secure the graft to the underlying septal crural foundation. An elongated tip graft extending along the greater part of the columella is used to provide greater stability for increased projection. In general, this graft is not fixated so, after initial wound closure, it can be displaced to the desired position, creating a more pleasing tip definition.

After careful inspection of the reconstructed skeleton, the skin incisions are meticulously closed with 6/0 nylon sutures. With Rees and Skoog we believe that no amount of post-operative splinting, clamping or other forms of pushing and pulling, nor healing, will provide a better outcome.

The skin-soft-tissue envelope is taped to the nasal skeleton, especially in the supratip region, thus eliminating dead space. An additional adhesive strip is placed along the nasal tip for support.

A plaster of Paris with forehead extension, avoiding any movement, is used (Tessier). A generous amount of antibiotic ointment is placed in both nares.

A reinforced Silastic™ sheet is used as a septal splint at the right side where functional surgery has been performed. Although through-and-through sutures readapt the mucoperichondral flaps, nasal packing is frequently used. Unless contraindicated, intraoperative steroids and antibiotics are given routinely. A gauze is taped over the nostrils to function as a drip pad.

The patient receives facial ice packing and a position of at least 45° is advised for up to 24 hours. Antibiotics are given for 3–4 days till the packing is removed. Upon follow-up in 7 days, the splint and the Silastic sheet(s) is removed, as well as the sutures.

THE ORIENTAL NOSE (N RAVINDRANATHAN AND C COLLANTES JOSE)

INTRODUCTION

Since the early 1960s, the demand for oriental rhinoplasty has increased in countries such as Japan, Thailand, Taiwan, Philippines, Malaysia and Singapore. At one time, injection of silicone and paraffin was a cheap popular method. As complications associated with the latter became known, the demand for augmentation rhinoplasty with solid silicone became popular. The use of medical grade silicone manufactured by companies such as Dow Corning were used by companies like Nagashima, Koken, Allied Medical, McGahn and Implantech to produce several different length, designs and sizes of nasal implants and the demand for augmentation rhinoplasty increased.

HOW DOES AN ORIENTAL NOSE DIFFER FROM A CAUCASIAN NOSE?

1. The oriental nose is smaller and lower than that of Caucasians.
2. The lobule (lower third of the nose) is lower and wider than the Caucasian nose.
3. The tip is round compared to the Caucasian nose.
4. The distance between the sides of the alar base is large, alae are round and extrude laterally.
5. Lack of dorsal projection.
6. Retracted or hidden columella. (Figure 11.6.19 illustrates the features).
7. Recessive pyriform fossae.
8. The overlying 'skin envelope' is thick (Figures 11.6.19–21 illustrate features 1 to 8).
9. The lower lateral cartilages – both lateral and medial crurae are weak and attenuated (Figure 11.6.22).

COMMON INDICATIONS FOR ORIENTAL RHINOPLASTY

1. For 'Westernization' – elevating the dorsum, refining the tip, narrowing the alar bases, correcting the overhanging alar margins and the hidden columella (entirely cosmetic reasons).
2. To improve airway and appearance (functional rhinoplasty).
3. Improvement of cleft nasal deformities in orientals.

This section will cover exclusively cosmetic oriental rhinoplasty.

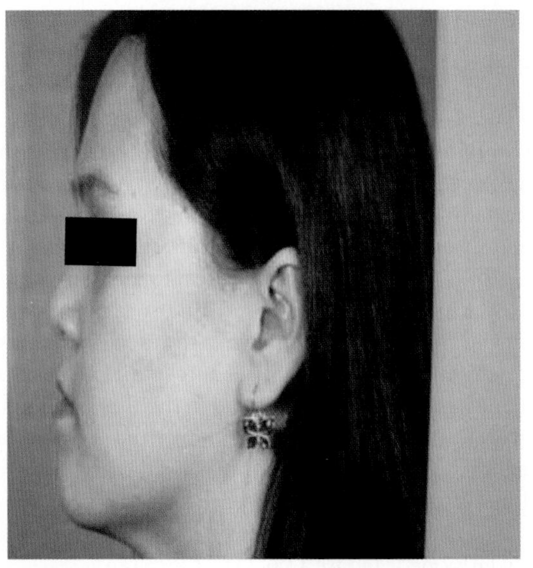

11.6.19 Side view of an oriental nose showing overhanging ala and short columella.

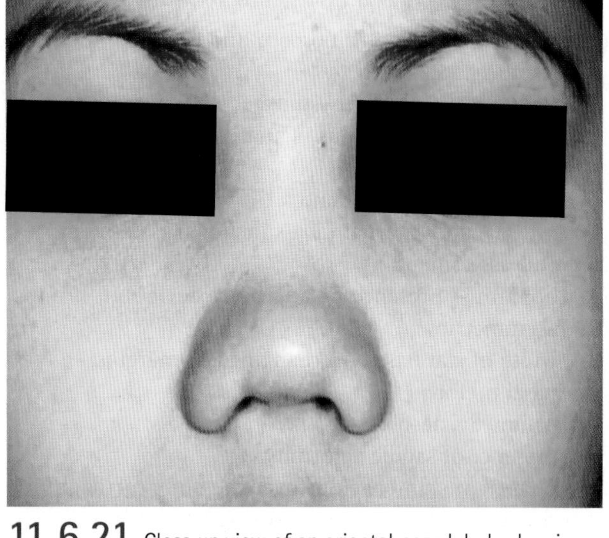

11.6.21 Close up view of an oriental nose lobule showing thick skin over the tip, wide, overhanging alar bases and short columella.

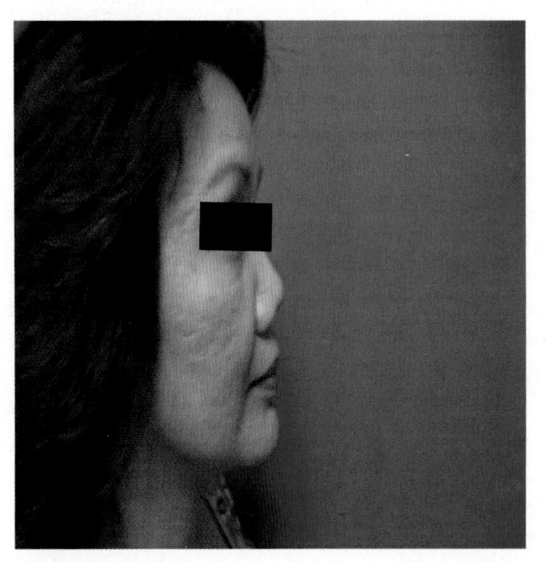

11.6.20 Side view of an oriental nose from the opposite side showing hidden columella.

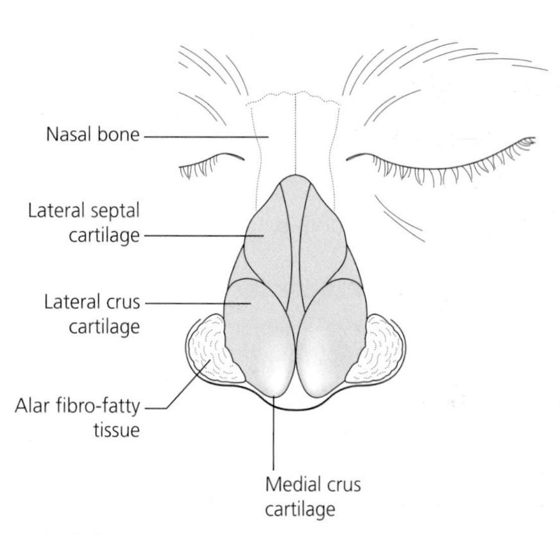

11.6.22 In an oriental nose, both lateral and medial crurae are weak and attenuated.

INITIAL CONSULTATION AND PRE-OPERATIVE ASSESSMENT

1. Exclude any dysmorphism.
2. Obtain a history of all previous rhinoplasty procedures, if any were carried out:
3. A detailed medical and drug history.
4. Defer proposed surgery if patient has any of the following:
   - untreated sinusitis, vasomotor rhinitis;
   - prolonged intake of blood thinners such as vitamin E, aspirin, anti-cholesterol drugs, herbal supplements such as gingko biloba, oral anticoagulants. These medications must be stopped for at least 5 days before surgery, except anticoagulants which require coordination with the appropriate prescribing physician;
   - history of bleeding tendencies – may require further investigations;
   - they are smokers.
5. Listen carefully to the patient's main concerns and the desired changes.

Take close up photographs of the following:

- full face;
- frontal view of the nasal complex from root of nose to the lips;
- side profile;

- basal view of the lobule.

6 Airway assessment – rhinoscopy and flexible nasoendoscopy:
   - note septal deflections, spurs;
   - evidence of previous septal surgery, any septal perforation;
   - hypertrophy of turbinates;
   - internal and external valve functional assessment.

7 Profile assessment:
   - dorsum – presence of any bony deviation, humps, asymmetries;
   - width of alar bases, overhanging alar margins;
   - nasal tip form;
   - columella, nasolabial angle;
   - presence of saddle deformity;
   - quality of skin envelope over the bony cartilaginous skeleton;
   - presence of any previous operative scars.

CONCLUSIONS TO BE REACHED AT THE END OF INITIAL CONSULTATION AND DISCUSSION OF THE PROPOSED TREATMENT PLAN

1. Dorsal augmentation to improve projection – discuss regarding choices of material to be used, complications both short and long term.
2. Narrowing of the width of alar bases – discuss possibility of conspicuous scars, either external or vestibular.
3. Correcting the overhanging alar margins – surgical excision may result in conspicuous scarring and may sometimes result in notching due to scar contracture.
4. Discussion of costs involved as it is a potential area for dispute.

MATERIALS AVAILABLE FOR AUGMENTATION RHINOPLASTY

The most important factor for any material to be used for augmentation is biocompatibility. An ideal material should be non-absorbable, easily modified and shaped. They should elicit no inflammatory response and have no potential to transmit infections. They can be classified as autogenous, synthetic or homologous. The commonly used synthetic materials are:

- silicone (medical grade);
- expanded polytetra fluoroethylene (Gore-Tex);
- Medpor – porous polyethylene implant;
- vicryl mesh;
- Mersilene.

The commonly used sources of autogenous materials are:

- bone – iliac crest, olecranon;
- cartilage – costochondral, auricular, septal.

Available homologous graft materials are:

- bank bone;
- bank cartilage.

Homologous materials are not used by most cosmetic surgeons as it is not a preferred choice of most orientals.

Initially, mostly bone and cartilage grafts were used. Patients were not satisfied and the author was unhappy with the results and was sceptical of silicone as a material. However, silicone has been used almost exclusively for 18 years and the author is happy with the excellent results one can achieve and which will ensure patient satisfaction. Silicone has been widely criticized in the Western literature. However, it is the most commonly used material in Thailand, China, Japan, Korea, Malaysia, Singapore, Indonesia and the Philippines. Silicone is easy to carve, is available in various shapes and sizes in carved forms and is easily fashioned (Figure 11.6.23).

In orientals, the volume of material needed for dorsal augmentation is much more than that needed for Caucasians for whom septal cartilage is the most commonly used material followed by auricular cartilage. The soft tissue envelope for oriental noses is different to that of Caucasians. It consists of dense fibromuscular and fatty layers offering greater tissue protection.

The author has used Gore-Tex and Mersilene only in secondary augmentation rhinoplasty where the silicone was removed owing to infection or extrusion. In such instances, Gore-Tex and/or Mersilene were used six months after removal of the implant. In the last few years, it has been used to correct dorsal irregularities. Lately, injectable fillers have been used subperiosteally, for example polyacrylamide (Aquamid) for dorsal augmentation.

TECHNIQUE OF AUGMENTATION RHINOPLASTY USING SILICONE

Most often, the procedure is carried out under local anaesthesia.

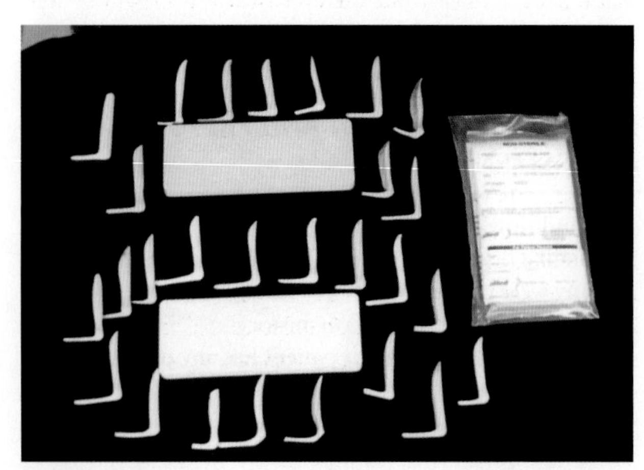

11.6.23 Various shapes of available pre-carved silicone implants which can be fashioned as required.

Incision

OPTIONS

- Transcolumella incision (Figure 11.6.24a–c), insertion of implant through a columella approach).
- Bilateral rim incision (Figure 11.6.25).

Creating the pocket

Using blunt curved scissors, the plane for entry is above the lower lateral cartilages toward the periosteum over the dorsum of the nose (Figure 11.6.26). Subsequently, a subperiosteal pocket is created using a small Joseph periosteal elevator.

The periosteum should be respected by not tearing it carelessly as the implant is best placed below the periosteal covering.

The pocket size should be created just adequately to accommodate the implant. The implant should be carefully carved to the planned size according to the measurements taken from the root of the nose to the tip. Accordingly, the width in the dorsum and the columella length should be carved accordingly. Upon careful placement, ensure it is in the midline (Figure 11.6.24a).

Closure is carried out by approximating wound edges with 5/0 nylon or 5/0 monofilament resorbable suture (e.g. PDS or Monocryl).

APPLICATION OF SPLINT OVER THE DORSUM

Clean the dorsum of the nose with a spirit swab. Pat dry and apply a coating of tincture benzoin as an adhesive using a cotton bud. There are several splints on the market. The splint of the author's choice is Denver. It consists of a self-contained pack with skin-coloured one inch steristrips and the mouldable splint in two halves. The tapes are applied along the length of the dorsum transversely overlapping each other. At the upper end, the tape length should be such that it should not irritate the eyelashes and should be well away from them. Over the tapes, the inner adhesive component of the splint is applied. The adaptable aluminum outer half of the splint is moulded over the adhesive inner half. The splint is left *in situ* for 7 days (Figure 11.6.27).

In patients who require tip refinement, via the bilateral rim incision, the lower lateral cartilages can be reached easily and transdomal suturing using 5/0 non-resorbable monofilament nylon can be used. The effect of transdomal suturing in Caucasians is easily reflected in achieving a more definable tip. However, this may not be the case in orientals owing to the thickness of the skin. In patients with a thick skin envelope, transdomal suturing would not seem to alter tip definition.

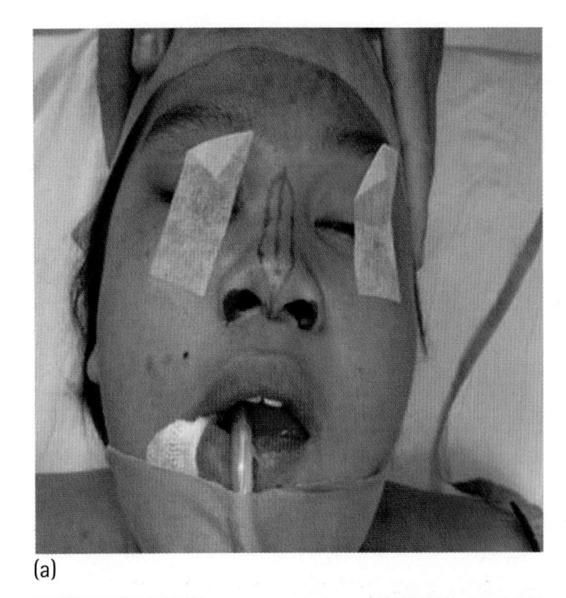

(a)

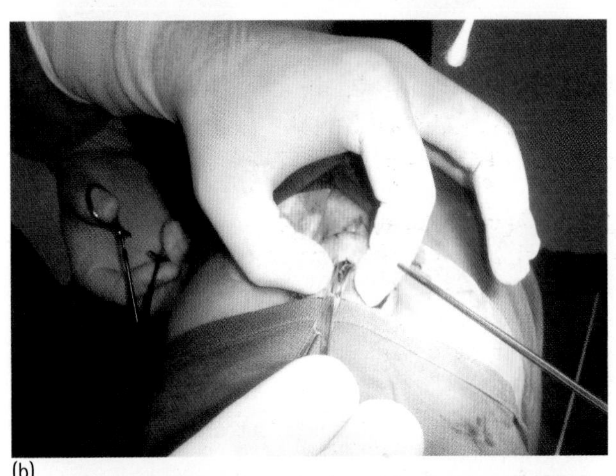

(b)

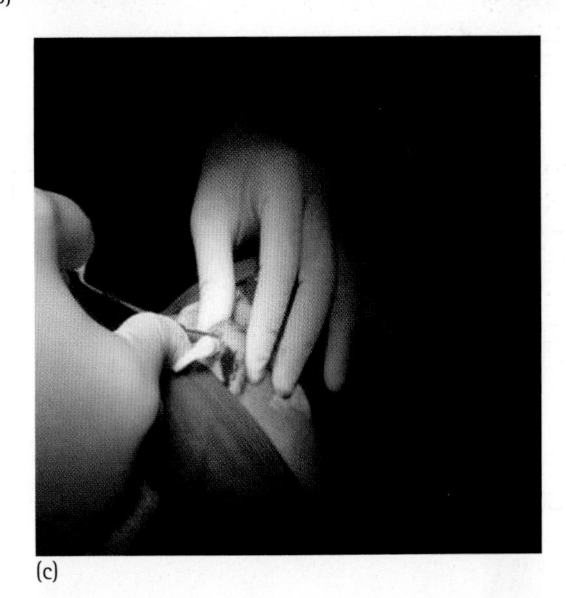

(c)

11.6.24 (a) Dorsal augmentation: vertical incision along the columella marked. Dorsal outline of proposed implant marked. (b) Dorsal augmentation: a pocket being created through the columella above the medial crura. (c) Dorsal augmentation: implant being inserted through the pocket created subperiosteally over the dorsum of the nose.

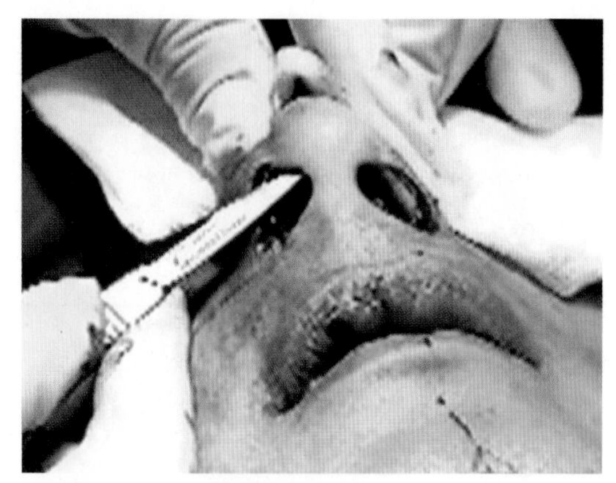

11.6.25 Rim incision.

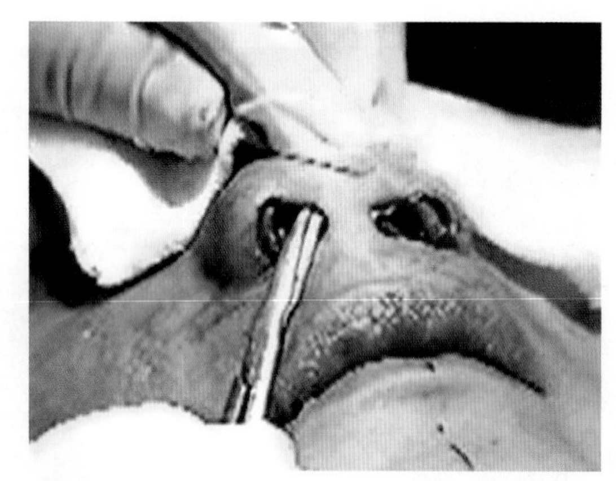

11.6.26 Blunt dissection in the subcutaneous tunnel with blunt scissors towards the dorsum.

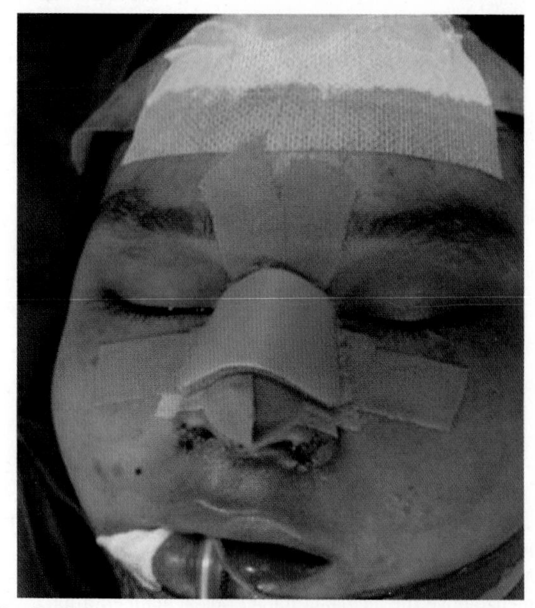

11.6.27 Denver nasal splint *in situ*, placed over the adhesive tapes.

COMBINING AUGMENTATION RHINOPLASTY WITH ALAR BASE MODIFICATION

In orientals, the distance between the alae may be large. The basal view of a nose resembles an isosceles triangle consisting of the nasal tip, the columella and the alae surrounding the nostril. When the alae are large, the nostril shape cannot be seen as beautiful and patients seek modification to improve the appearance of the lobule. Two methods in use are popular, i.e. that described by Weir and the other by Millard. These two methods may leave external scars. In 1994, Watanabe described a method of using incisions inside the ala and grafting to avoid external scarring.

The shape of the basal view can be changed as described in the following.

1. Elongation of the columella increases nasal tip projection (increases the height of the isosceles triangle) (Figure 11.6.28). Excessive augmentation will result in perforation of the skin.
2. Partial resection of the ala base will correct lateral extrusion of the ala and the breadth. This method is effective when alae are long and extruding laterally.

TECHNIQUE OF ALAR BASE REDUCTION AND CORRECTION OF OVERHANGING ALAR MARGINS

- Inject local anaesthesia 2 per cent lignocaine with 1:80 000 epinephrine (adrenaline) to the alae.
- Excise the overhanging ala which should have been marked by using a size 11 blade on a scalpel perpendicular to the alae (Figure 11.6.29a).
- Excise an elliptical strip of 3–4 mm symmetrically on both alae to avoid discrepancy (Figure 11.6.30).
- Reduction of increased alar base width (Figure 11.6.29b). For reduction of increased alar base width, local anaesthesia is injected into the alar base. Once the local anaesthesia has taken effect, a predetermined amount of the alar base medial to the alar curve is excised as a v-shaped wedge in a manner similar to cutting a slice of a 'pie'. Similar procedure is repeated on the opposite ala

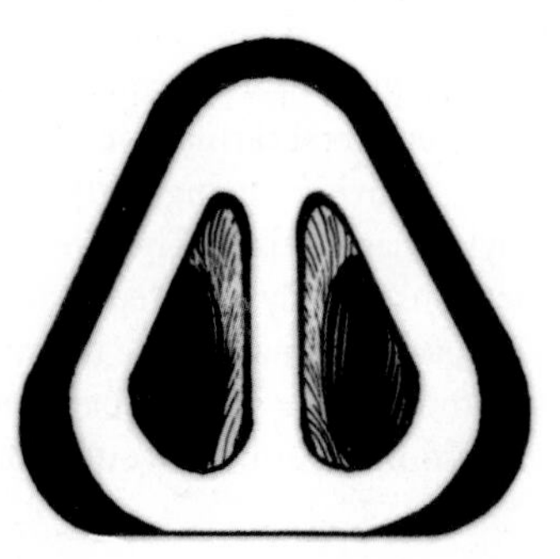

11.6.28 Base of the nose is an isosceles triangle.

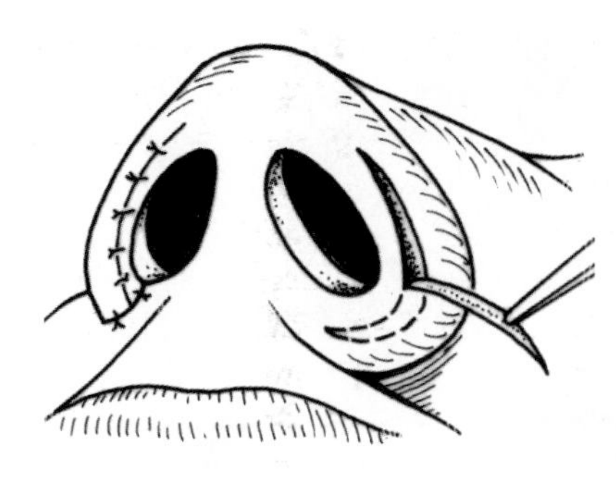

(a)

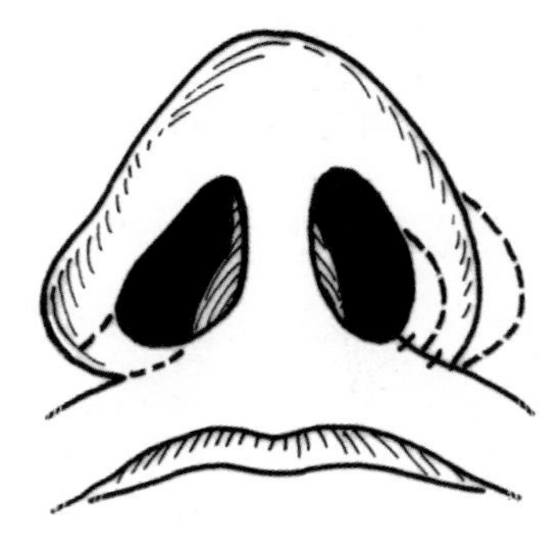

(b)

11.6.29 (a) Correction of overhanging alar margins. (b) Shows excision of wedge at the alar base.

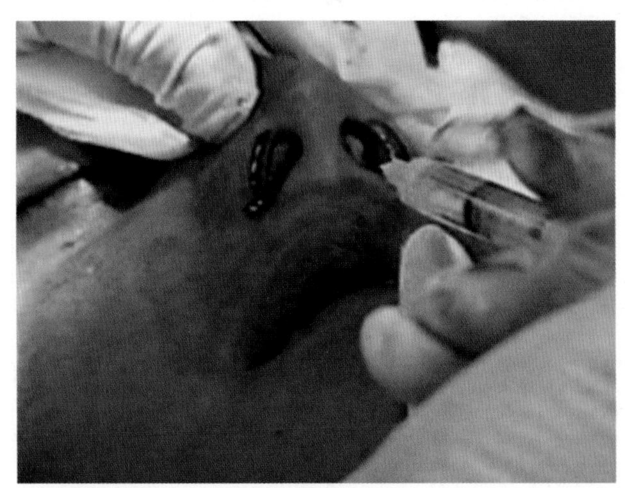

11.6.30 Excision of overhanging alar margins.

(Figure 11.6.31a–e). We carry out an 'ala cinch' to reinforce the reduction as follows:

- A straight needle with 4.0 Nylon is passed at the base of the ala from one side and transverse through the subcutaneous tissue below the skin and exits through the opposite alar base. A 'bite' is taken through the soft tissue and the needle reversed back through the same route to emerge at the same entry point. The suture needle is removed and the suture is tied (Figure 11.6.32).
- Finally, the incision margins are closed with 6.0 Nylon.

- Figures 11.6.30–11.6.37 illustrate the operative technique of correction of overhanging alar margins and dorsal augmentation.
- Figures 11.6.38–11.6.41 illustrate operative steps of correcting overhanging alar margins, alar base reduction without dorsal augmentation.

CLINICAL EXAMPLES TO ILLUSTRATE ORIENTAL RHINOPLASTY

Case 1

- Pre-operative view prior to alar base reduction in a 35-year-old female (Figure 11.6.41).
- Immediate post-operative view after alar base reduction, correction of overhanging alar margins and dorsal augmentation. Note the immediate change in shape of lobule in a 35-year-old female.

Case 2

- Pre-operative view of a 28-year-old female (frontal view) (Figure 11.6.42).
- Post-operative view of a 28-year-old female (front view) after dorsal augmentation and alar base reduction.

Case 3

- Frontal view of a 28 year old female (Figure 11.6.43).
- Frontal view 1 year after dorsal augmentation.
- Side view preoperative.
- Side view post-operative 1 year later – only dorsal augmentation.

COMPLICATIONS

1 Extrusion of implants. This can happen at the tip or at the columella (Figure 11.6.44a, b). This is the most common complication. The main reason for this is because the implant size chosen was too large. When this happens, the implant should be removed and the wound allowed to heal. A new well-carved implant to

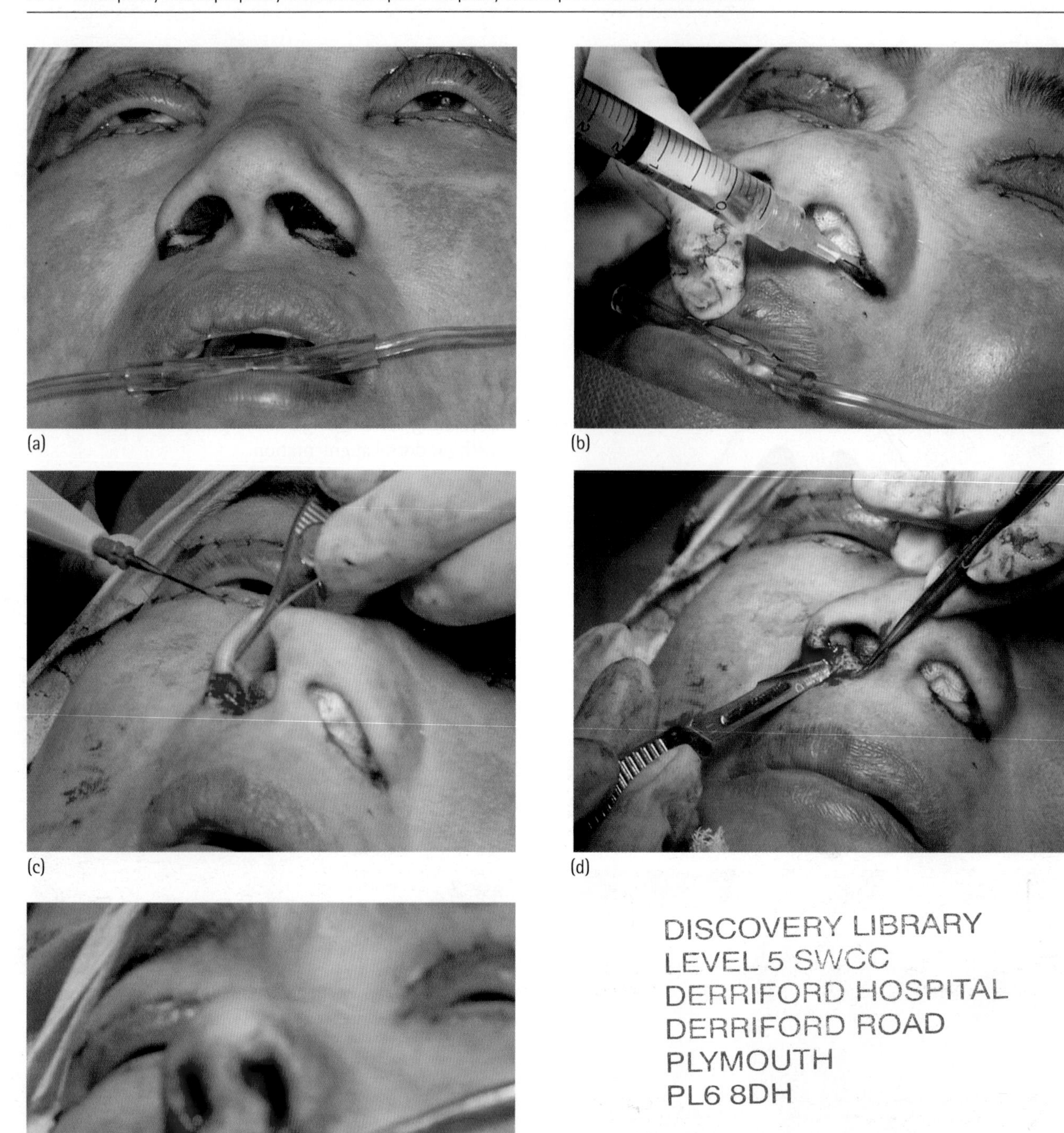

11.6.31 (a) Alar base reduction: markings of wedge to be excised. (b) Alar base reduction: the 'wedge' to be excise is marked. Local anaesthesia is injected. (c) Alar base reduction: wedge excised. (d) Alar base reduction: wedge being excised using a size 11 blade. (e) Alar base reduction: after excision of alar base, edges approximated.

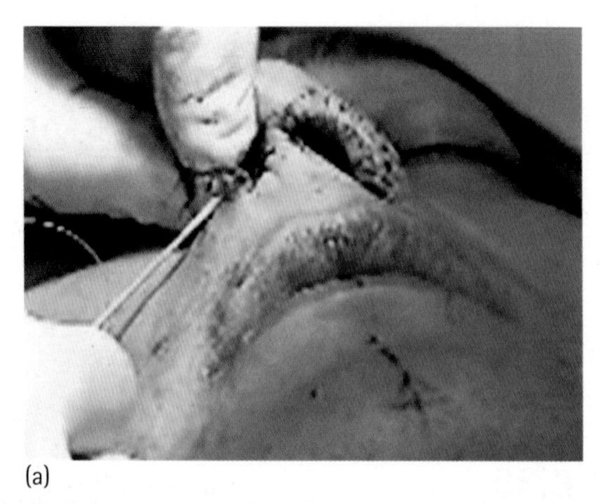

(a)

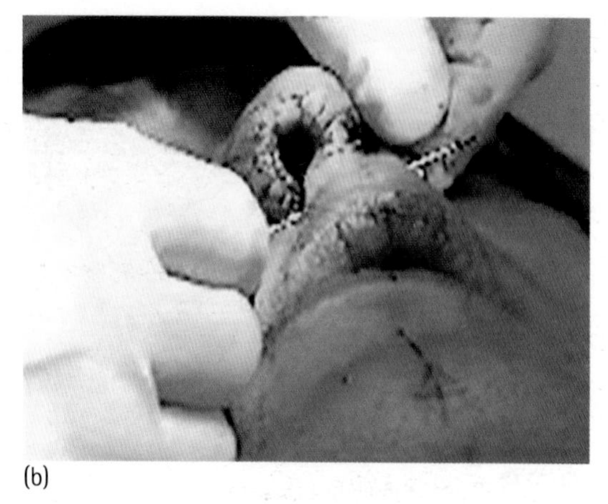

(b)

11.6.32 (a, b) After completion of alar base reduction, 'alar cinch' being carried out using a straight needle with 4.0 monofilament nylon.

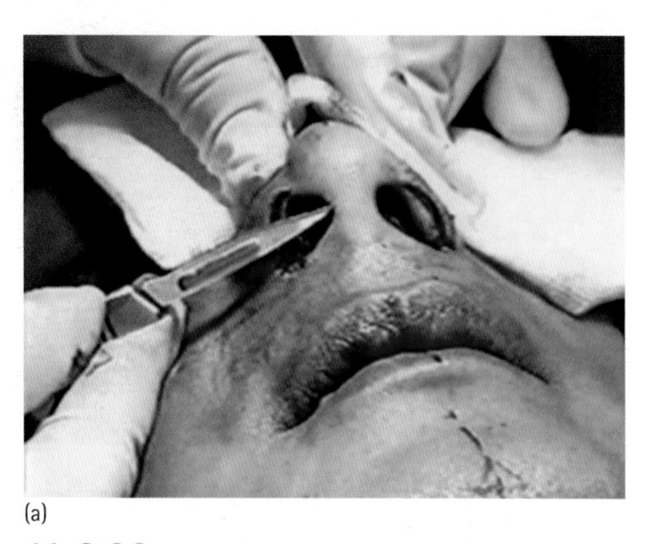

(a)

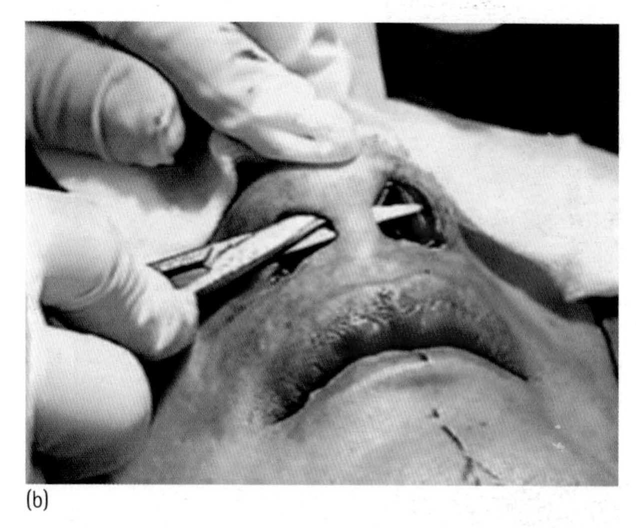

(b)

11.6.33 (a) Rim incision within the columella being made, overhanging alar margins excised, alar base wedges excised. (b) Through the rim incision within the columella, transcolumellar blunt dissection being performed.

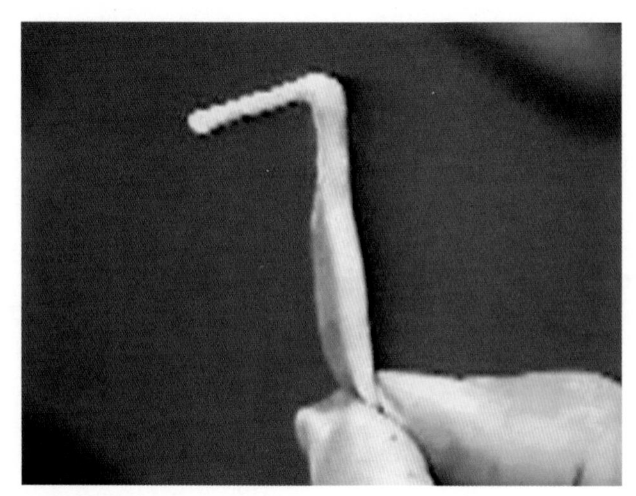

11.6.34 Pre-carved implant chosen according to dissections.

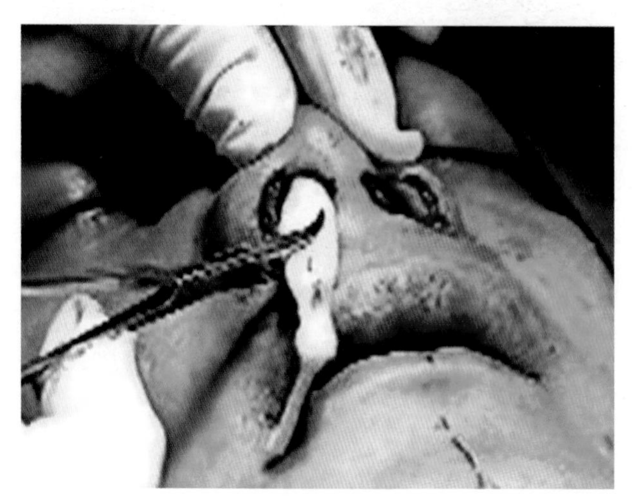

11.6.35 Implant being inserted through a rim incision within the columella.

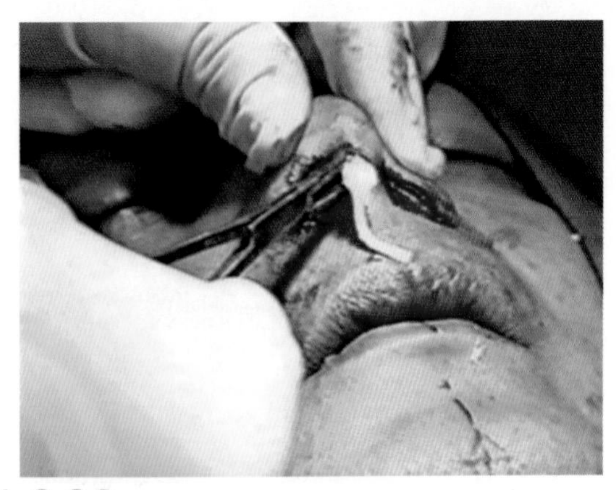

11.6.36 Silicone implant being inserted through the columella into the subperiosteal pocket.

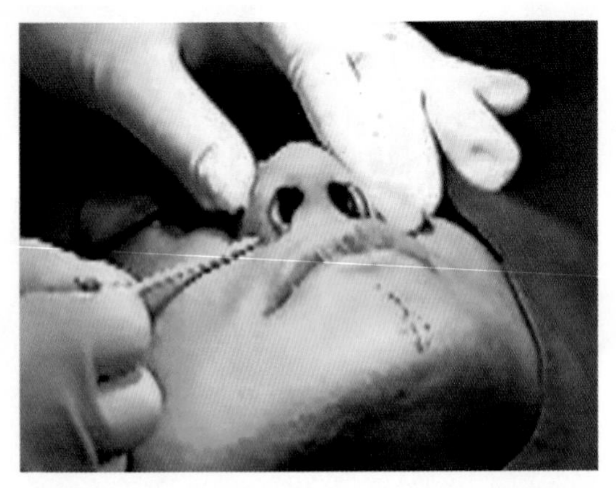

11.6.37 Pre-operative basal view in a 35-year-old female.

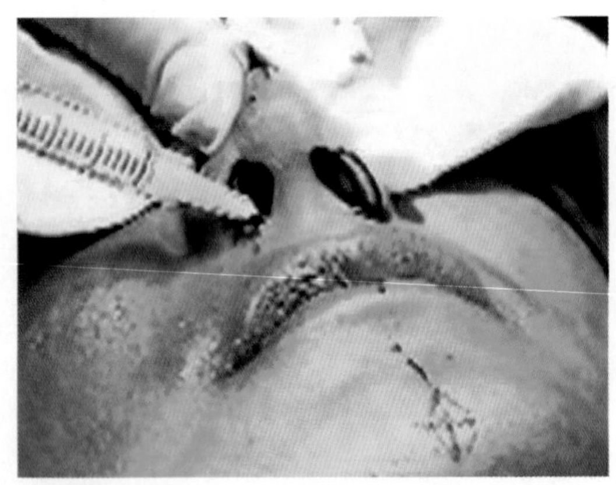

11.6.38 Injecting local anaesthesia into alar bases.

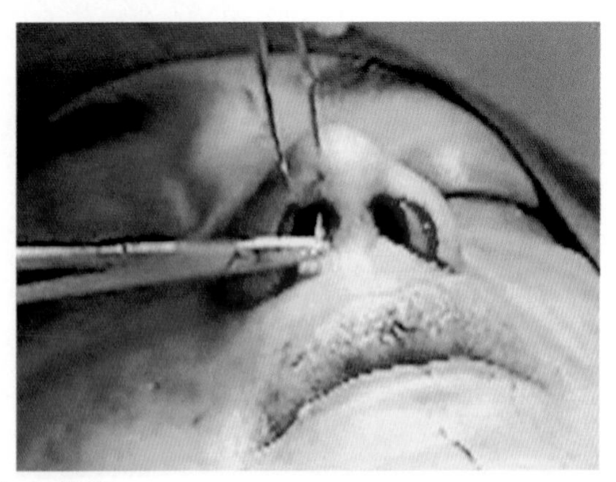

11.6.39 Basal view after alar base reduction as a wedge and correction of overhanging alar margins.

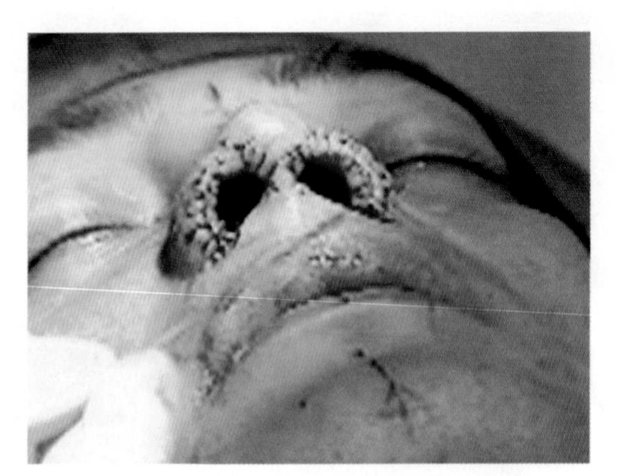

11.6.40 Immediate post-operative basal view after alar base reduction, correction of overhanging alar margins. Note change of lobule shape.

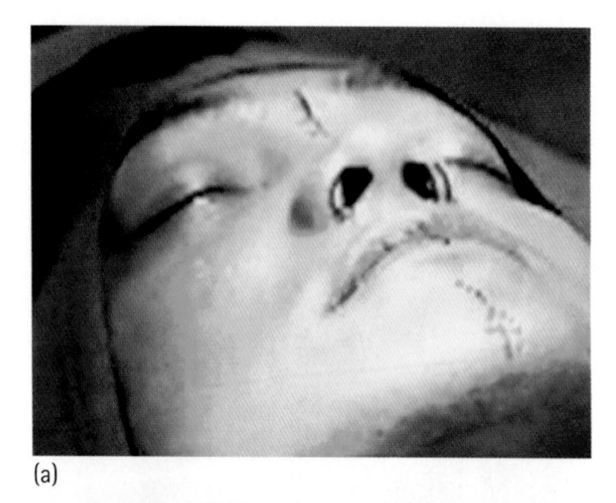

(a)

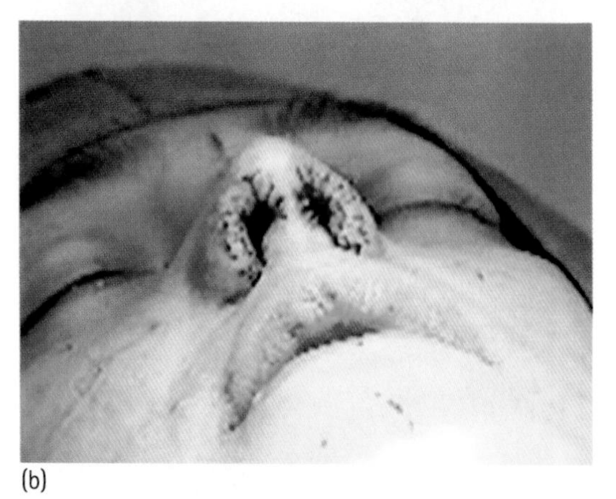

(b)

11.6.41 (a) Pre-operative view prior to correction of alar base and overhanging alar margins. (b) Post-operative view after alar base reduction and correction of overhanging alar margins.

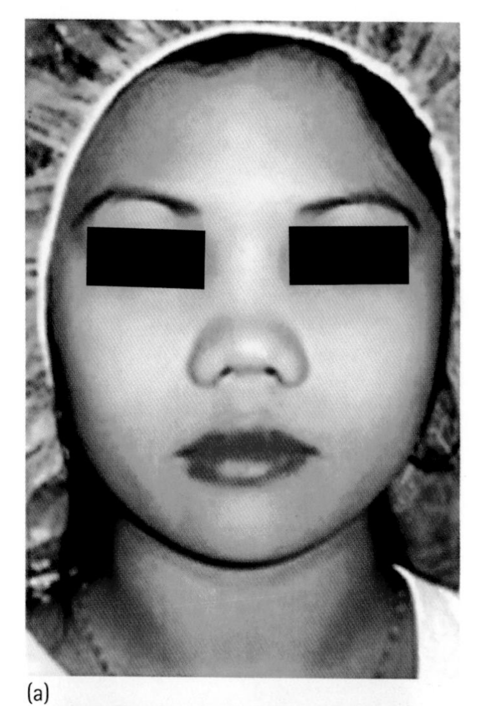

(a)

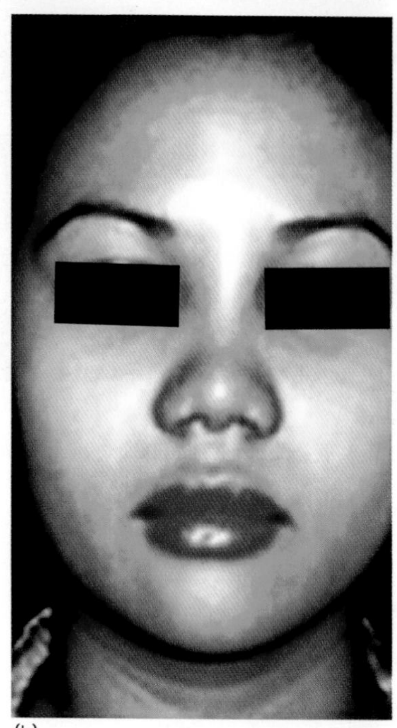

(b)

11.6.42 (a) Pre-operative view of a 28-year-old female oriental. (b) Post-operative – after alar base reduction and augmentation.

the appropriate size can be inserted again after six months. In instances where the patient has requested a greater degree of augmentation than what is realistically possible within the skin 'envelope', this should not be done as extrusion of the implant would occur (Figure 11.6.44c shows several implants we have removed as a result of extrusion in the last ten years).

2 Infection. This may present as oedematous tip, overlying skin of the dorsum of the nose being erythematous and patients complain of pain and sometimes referred headache. To avoid infections, the implants for use must be autoclaved. During the operative procedure, ensure there is minimal handling of the implant and use unpowdered sterile gloves. If polytetrafluoroethylene implants (Gore-Tex) are used, soak the implant in ampicillin solution for 5 minutes to reduce the incidence of infection.

3 Drift of the implant leading to a deviation. This can happen due to a longer implant being used or a traumatic injury. This will require removal if obvious. Allow the wounds to heal and redo the augmentation rhinoplasty. Misdirected implants can cause distressing facial disfigurement to patients. The most common cause is due to incision being placed on only one side of the vestibule or the upper edge of the nostrils. This can result in increased asymmetric scarring. Scar contracture results in implant deviation.

4 Step-like deformity at the bridge of the nose (at the nasal root). The severity of the step deformity can vary. This can be due to the tunnel in which the silicone implant

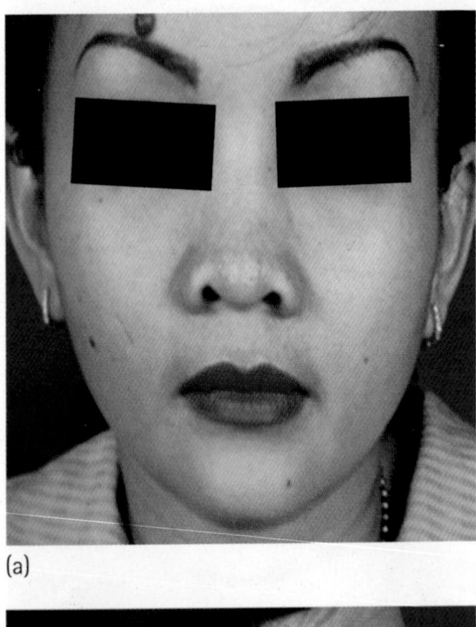

(a)

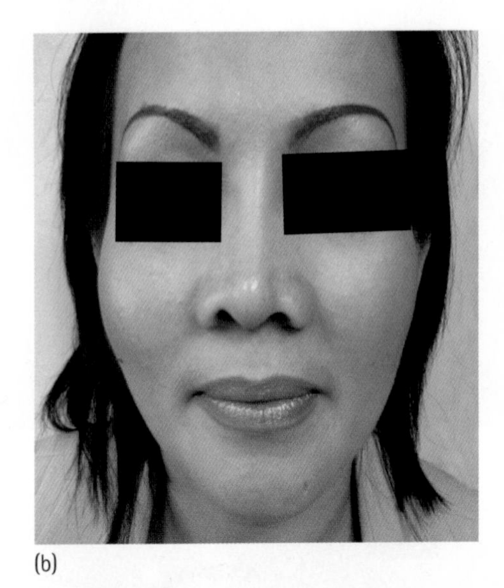

(b)

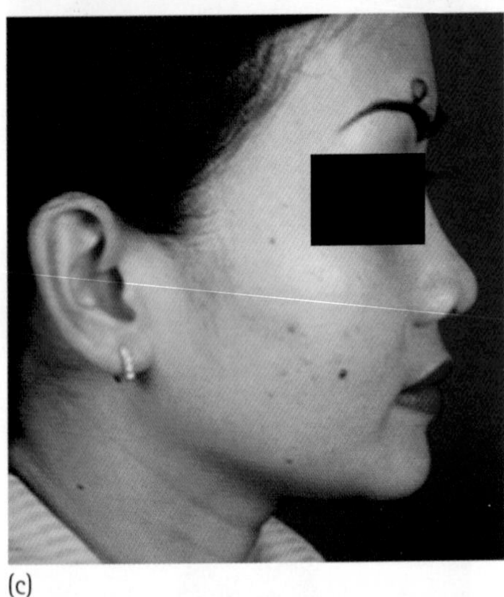

(c)

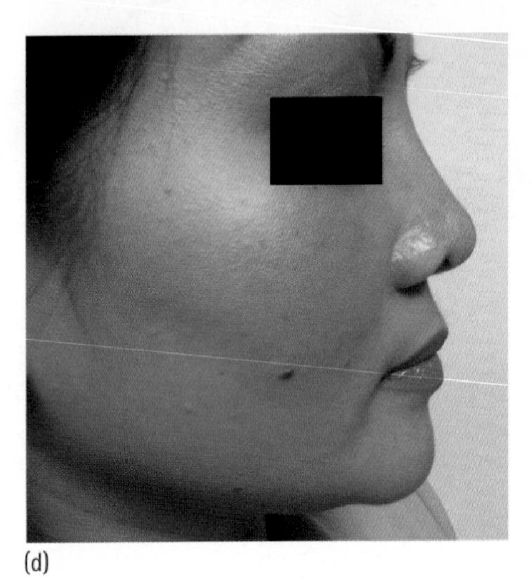

(d)

11.6.43 (a) Pre-operative frontal view of a 28 year old female. (b) Frontal view of a 28 year old female, 1 year after augmentation. (c) Pre-operative side view of a 28 year old female. (d) Post-operative side view of a 28 year old female, 1 year after augmentation.

placed was shallow and this resulted in the upper end of the silicone implant being attached to the skin closely. Another reason is due to inadequate nasal columella elongation following implantation. If this was of concern to the patient, it would require removal and a repeat procedure after four to six months is carried out.

5 Change in skin colour. This can be a distressing complication. If the implant is placed too close to the skin, tension on the skin increase leads to a poor blood supply to the nasal skin. In patients with thin skin, such pigmentary changes can be long lasting. If persistent, the implant should be removed if the skin changes are distressing to the patient.

6 In a small group of patients, numbness, itchiness and abnormal sensation along the dorsum of the nose is experienced. These symptoms usually disappear within a year.

7 In patients who have undergone alar base reduction:
   - Scars may become conspicuous. Scars can be external depending on the method used and when vestibular mucosal plasties are carried out, in some exceptional cases vestibular hypertrophic or keloid scar may occur. They are rare but can occur. Triamcinolone should be injected into the scar as soon as it is visible.
   - There may be irregularity of nostril openings due to asymmetric reduction (Figure 11.6.45). This is a very difficult condition to correct and can be very distressing to the patient and is an area for potential dispute between the surgeon and the patient.

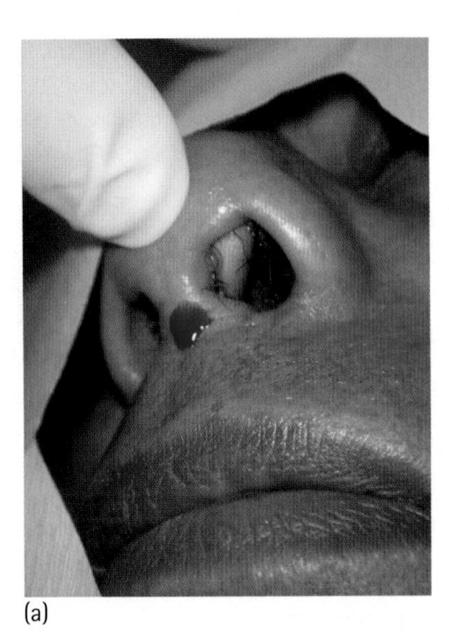

(a)

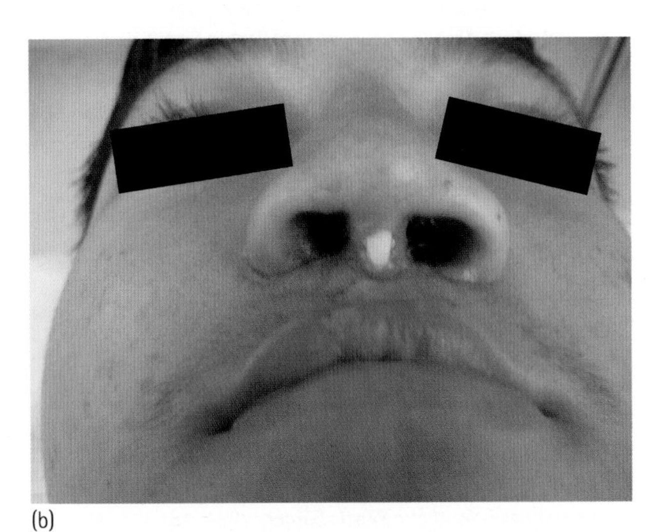

(b)

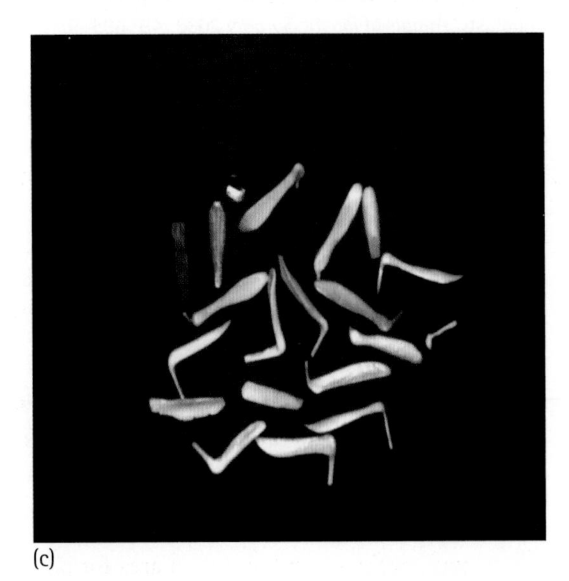

(c)

11.6.44 (a) Extruded implant in columella. (b) Extruded implant which requires removal. (c) Extruded implants which were removed.

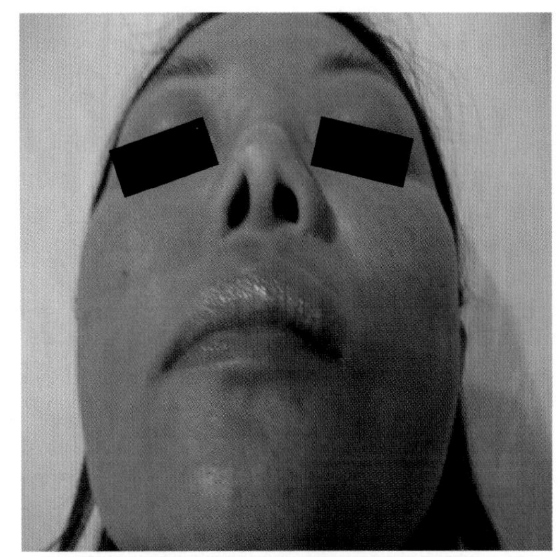

11.6.45 Complication right nostril opening narrower than left owing to asymmetric reduction of alar base.

Top Tips

Rhinoplasty and septoplasty: Closed and open rhinoplasty techniques

The oriental nose

- At initial consultation, exclude dysmorphism.
- Discuss in detail with your patient the desired changes requested by the patient. Assess if these changes are possible and would fit in with their facial proportions and racial phenotype.
- Give a list of likely complications and obtain informed consent.
- If a previous rhinoplasty had been carried out, make a good assessment of why it was unsuccessful and in what areas, for example patient may say the implant size was too large and it was so obvious, the skin over the nose was red since the implant was inserted (skin reaction). Listening carefully to these complaints would help you to take greater caution in planning your procedure.
- Incisions to place the implants can be performed either along the rim or paracolumella. If rim incisions are made, the author recommends bilateral incisions to allow more symmetrical positioning of the implant.
- If transdomal suturing is planned to achieve better tip definition, this should be carried out first before inserting the implant.
- The subperiosteal pocket to place the implant should be just enough to accommodate the implant. If the pocket is too large, the implant will undergo displacement easily.
- When you are beginning to carry out this procedure, the author highly recommends you to observe and assist a senior colleague as there is a 'learning curve' in how to choose your implant size, handling the implant atraumatically and in a sterile manner (minimum handling). Like all surgical techniques, this procedure is no exception.

- If alar base reduction is being planned, explain clearly regarding the likelihood of formation of hypertrophic or keloid scar within the vestibule.
- Discuss all available materials for augmentation and respect patient's wishes if they choose their own bone or cartilage as a substitute for religious reasons. Nevertheless, you should clearly indicate the donor site morbidity, difficulty in carving to the desired shape.
- Give clear post-operative instructions. The nasal splint should not get wet or be dislodged preferably for 5–7 days. Sutures are usually removed on the 7th day. If septal procedures were carried out for correcting septal deformities, usual care after septoplasty is followed.
- Give post-operative antibiotics for 7 days and analgesics are usually required only for 24 hours.

FURTHER READING

RHINOPLASTY AND SEPTOPLASTY: CLOSED AND OPEN RHINOPLASTY

Aiach G, Levignac J. *Aesthetic rhinoplasty*. Edinburgh: Churchill Livingstone, 1991.

Aiach G. *Atlas de rhinoplastie et ad la voie d'abord externe*. Paris: Mason, 1993.

Cheney M. *Facial surgery, plastic and reconstructive surgery*, Chapters 44, 45, 46 and 47, pp. 803–866. Baltimore: Williams & Wilkins, 1997.

Gonzalez-Ulloa MR, Smith JW, Zaoli G. *Aesthetic plastic surgery, Vol 3: Rhinoplasty septoplasty*. Piccin Nuova Libraria. St Louis: CV Mosby, 1988.

Johnson C, Turiumi D. *Open structure rhinoplasty*. Philadelphia: WB Saunders, 1990.

Kennedy B, Kinnebrew M. Indications and techniques for rhinoplasty. In: Peterson L, Indresano T, Marciani, Roser S (eds). *Principles of oral and maxillofacial surgery*, vol. III, Chapter 62, pp. 1719–1776. Philadelphia: Lipinicott-Raven, 1997.

Peck GC. *Techniques in aesthetic rhinoplasty*. New York: Thieme-Stratton, 1984.

Rees T. *Aesthetic plastic surgery*. Philadelphia: WB Saunders, 1980.

Rohrich R, Sheen J, Burget G, Burget D. *Secondary rhinoplasty and nasal reconstruction*. St Louis: Quality Medical Publishing, 1996.

Sheen J, Sheen A. *Aesthetic rhinoplasty*. St Louis: CV Mosby, 1987.

Tardy E Jr. *Rhinoplasty. The art and science*. Philadelphia: WB Saunders, 1997.

Werthere J, Tanner J. *Basic rhinoplasty*. OMS Knowledge update. Home study program. Vol. 1, Part II, Nov 1995.

Werther J. *Post-traumatic rhinoplasty*. OMS Knowledge Updates, Home study Program. Vol. 1, Part II, Nov 1995.

ORIENTAL RHINOPLASTY

Deva AK, Merten S, Chang L. Silicone in nasal augmentation rhinoplasty: a decade of clinical experience. *Plastic and Reconstructive Surgery* 1998; **102**: 1230–37.

Inanli S, Sari M, Baylancicek S. The use of expanded polytetrafluoroethylene (Gore-Tex) in rhinoplasty. *Aesthetic Plastic Surgery* 2007; **31**: 345–8.

Khoo BC. Augmentation rhinoplasty in the orientals. *Plastic and Reconstructive Surgery* 1964; **34**: 81.

Oritz-Monasterio F, Olmedo A. Rhinoplasty on the Mestizo nose. *Clinics in Plastic Surgery* 1977; **4**: 89–102.

Shirakabe Y, Shirakabe T, Kishimoto T. The classification of complications after augmentation rhinoplasty. *Aesthetic Plastic Surgery* 1985; **9**: 185–92.

Watanabe K. Rhinoplasty in orientals. In: *Plastic surgery*, vol. 1, Lecture and panels. Amsterdam: Excerpta Medica 1992; 405.

Watanabe K. New ideas to improve the shape of the ala of the oriental nose. *Aesthetic Plastic Surgery* 1994; **18**: 337–44.

Zeng Y, Wu W, Yu H *et al.* Silicone implant in augmentation rhinoplasty. *Annals of Plastic Surgery* 2002; **49**: 495–9.

11.7

Post-traumatic rhinoplasty

LUC CESTELEYN

PRINCIPLES, JUSTIFICATION AND INDICATIONS

Post-traumatic deformities

Nasal trauma is the most frequent facial injury, usually from vehicle accidents and interpersonal violence.

In many cases, functional airway obstruction and external deformities make the patient seek treatment.

The post-traumatic situation creates a significant disharmony of proportion: twisted and angulated noses upset the flowing line from the supraorbital rim to the tip of the nose, as does an avulsed or depressed upper lateral cartilage, a deviated dorsal cartilaginous septum, or an asymmetric alar–cartilage complex.

Those patients who sustain sufficient nasal trauma and require relatively acute nasal reconstruction and rhinoplasty compose a different category of patients presenting for nasal cosmetic surgery. Many would have never considered surgery if acute trauma had not produced a deformity or an airway insufficiency. Their motivations are often different from the patient troubled by a long-standing nasal deformity, since they essentially wish the nose be restored to its former pre-injury appearance and function. Others will wish to correct a pre-existing deformity under the justification of the recent nasal injury. Generally, trauma patients are clearly well motivated as a result of the nasal injury.

EXAMINATION

Inspection and photographic documentation should pay special attention to external deviation and contour deformities. Even more important than assessing objective criteria, which are utilized in profile planning, is the study of standardized photographs, since the aesthetic appearance predominates.

The width of nose and the alar base should be compared with the intercanthal distance: in noses with traumatically lowered dorsum, an illusion of widening must be controlled. Manual palpation is necessary for the length and symmetry of the bones, dorsal projection and the superior septal angle. Palpation of the caudal septum and tip cartilages can yield valuable information regarding the underlying deformities or deviations.

The rhinoscope is necessary for inspection of the nasal mucosae, the septum, the turbinates and the nasal valve. External deformations should be correlated with internal changes of the bony-cartilaginous septum and the lateral sidewalls with the effect on the nasal tip. Airway evaluation calls for anterior rhinoscopy before and after vasoconstrictive shrinkage, palpation of subtle abnormalities of the septal cartilage, ANS and floor of the nose.

Transillumination of the septum allows assessement of trauma and residual cartilage in operated noses.

Cephalometric and lateral 'soft tissue' RX examination is used to measure tip rotation (TR by the NLA) and tip-projection (TP by angle sella-nasion and sellion to tip). The nasofrontal angle (125–135°) and the CLA or 'double break' (45°) should also be measured on lateral cephalograms.

We found the Cottle test and the cotton-tip applicator technique useful (Figure 11.7.1). By pulling the cheek laterally, the contribution of the vestibular portion (nostril, ULC and alar rim) of the valve to airway obstruction can be tested. If there is a positive response to the cotton-tip applicator lifting the caudal end of the ULC, the indication for spreader grafting is obvious; similarly lifting of the LLC can diagnose alar collapse with the indication for alar reinforcement by batton or lateral crural grafts.

OPERATION

Post-traumatic nasal reconstruction

Primary post-traumatic surgery is limited to symptomatic treatment of haemorrhage and reduction of major dislocations. In general, the reconstruction is planned 6–12

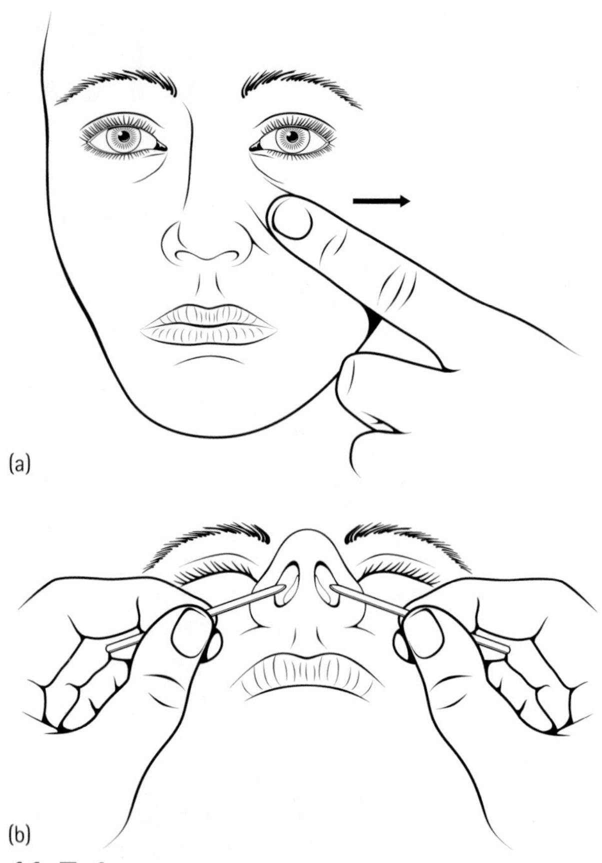

11.7.1 Airway Examination: (a) Cottle Test and (b) Cotton-tip Applicator technique.

months after the injury or the primary repair, at the time of maturation of scar tissue and stable deformity.

After blunt trauma, a twisted saddle deformity with broad and flattened pyramid and loss of septal height with columellar retraction and acute NLA must be corrected. The open approach is preferred, but sometimes a direct or endonasal approach in combination with a transoral access to a displaced ANS and caudal septum are chosen.

SADDLE NOSE DEFORMITY

Saddle nose deformity is the most common sequelae of direct nasal injury with displacement of fractured nasal bones and cartilage into the pyriform aperture, rarely as a result of loss of tissue, or unrecognized septal haematoma. For correction only, homologous material is used (Figure 11.7.2). Septal cartilage, stacked or layered, is the material of choice for dorsal onlay. Septal bone from the maxillary crest and the vomer can be used in the deep layers. Autografts of bone or cartilage from the nose seem to survive almost *in toto* in contrast with iliac bone or costal cartilage. If not available in quality or quantity, conchal ear cartilage is used. Dorsal graft of rolled ear cartilage filled with scarps of cartilage and bone were used successfully. For severe deformities, we tend to use reliable calvarial bone, covered with cartilage and/or temporoparietal fascia, harvested through the same hemicoronal approach. In total collapse, a bony strut is fixated in or at the ANS to support a dorsal graft fixated in or at the glabella. Iliac bone grafts are rarely used by us because of the morbidity, the second operation field and variable resorption over time. Exceptionally, in young children, rib-cartilage is used because harvesting of

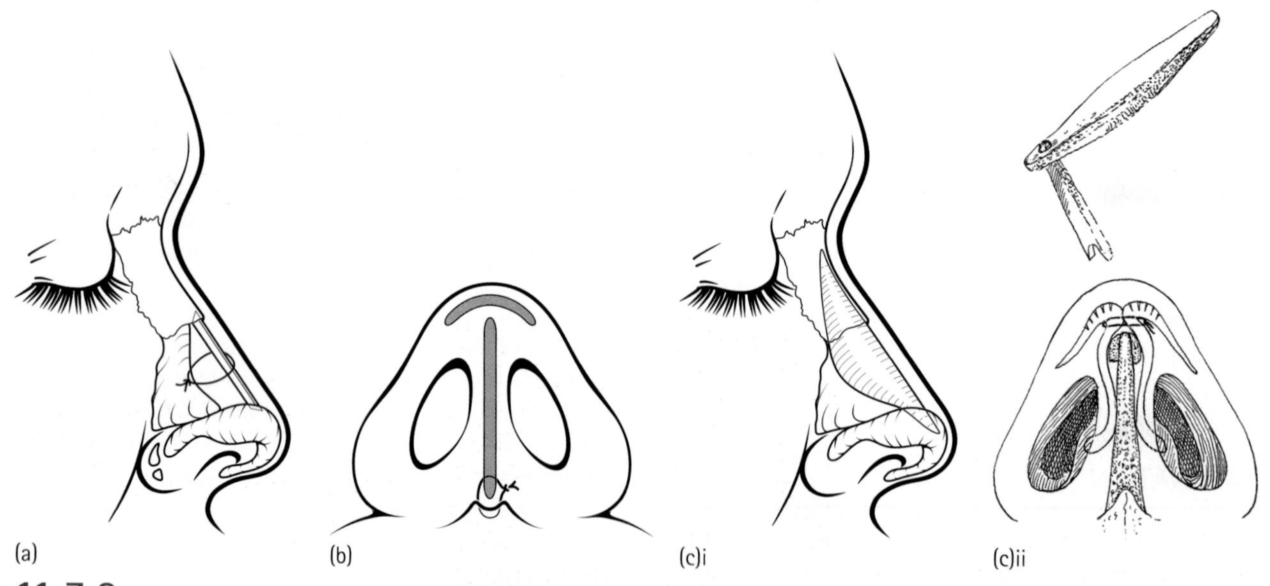

11.7.2 (a) Cartilaginous grafts (sutured together or not) for depression of cartilaginous dorsum. (b) (Osseo)cartilaginous grafts for dorsal augmentation or camouflaging a deviation by asymmetrical placing. (c) Bony grafts can be wired at the ANS in total loss of tip support, for prevention of pinching tip onlay grafts are used. (d) Bone grafts to reconstruct severe saddling: subperiosteally at the nasal bones, below the sutured domes at the tip. Important saddle corrected by osteosynthesized osseous strut on the ANS, dorsal layered calvareal bone graft covered with temporoparietal fascia and modified long tip-columellar graft. (e) Early posttraumatic septorhinoplasty for total nasal destruction, septal collapse, saddle deformity and loss of tip support with calvarial bone grafts for tip support and covered with fascia grafts for dorsal reconstruction, the bone grafts in postoperative radiography and the residual coronal scar.

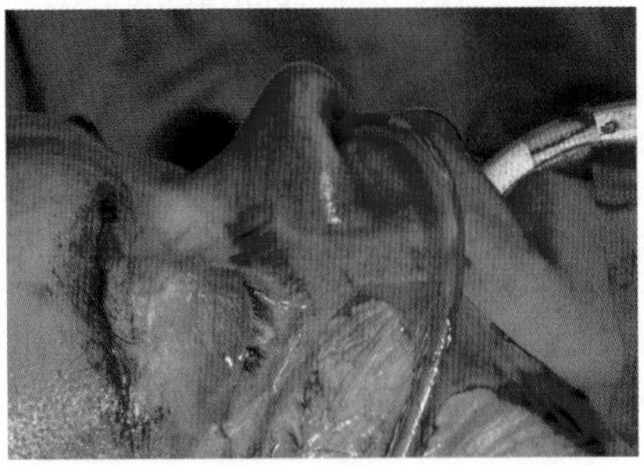

(d)i

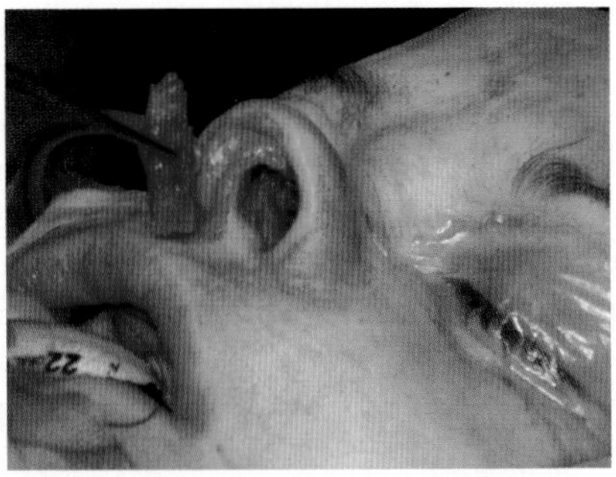

(d)ii

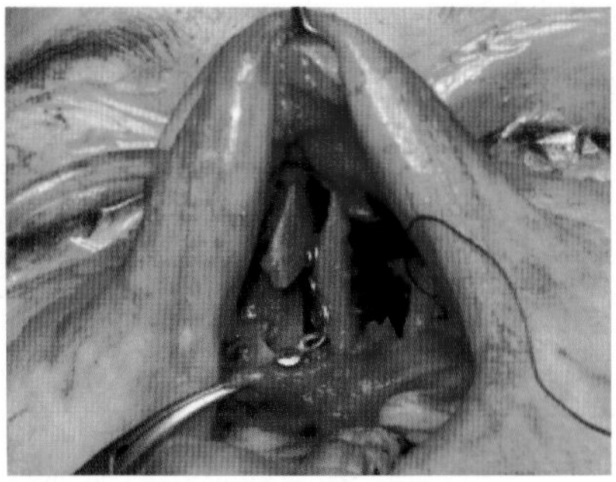

(d)iii

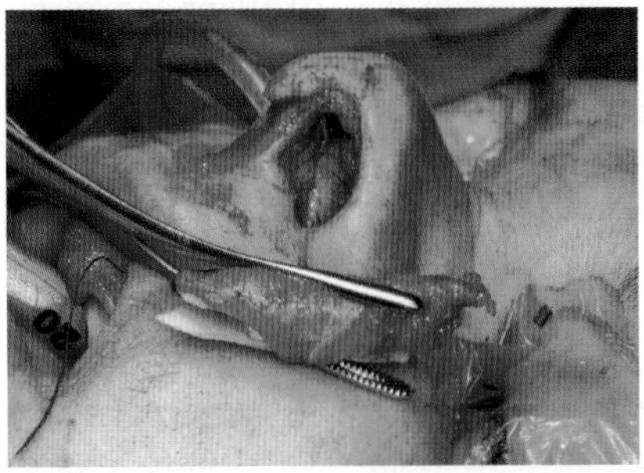

(d)iv

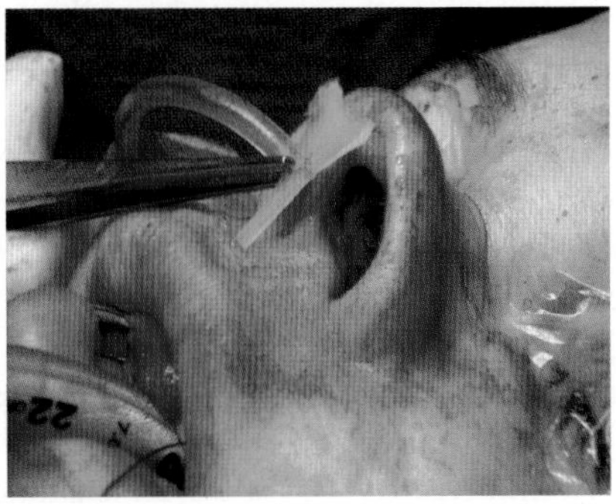

(d)v

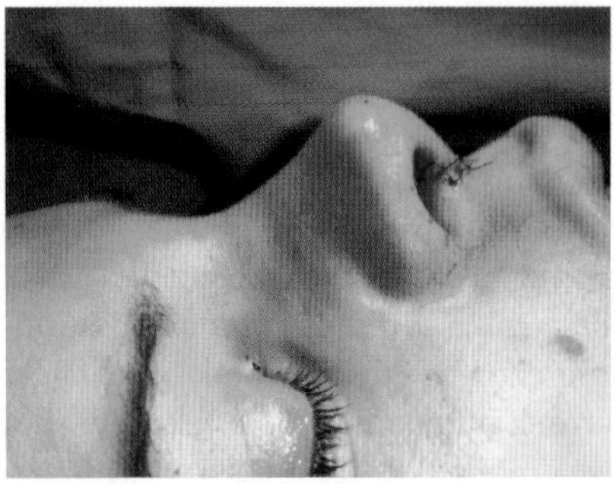

(d)vi

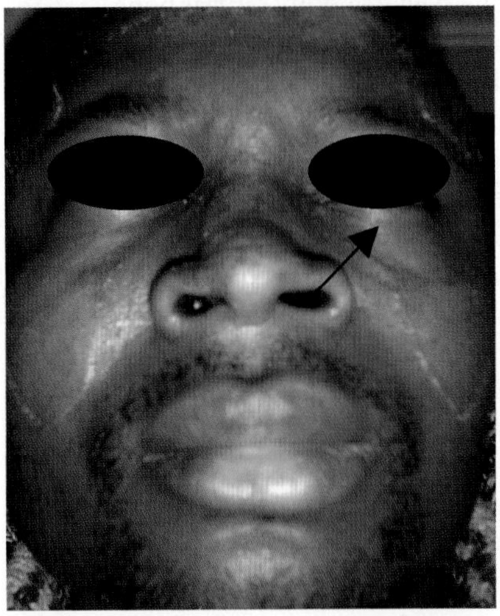

(e)i

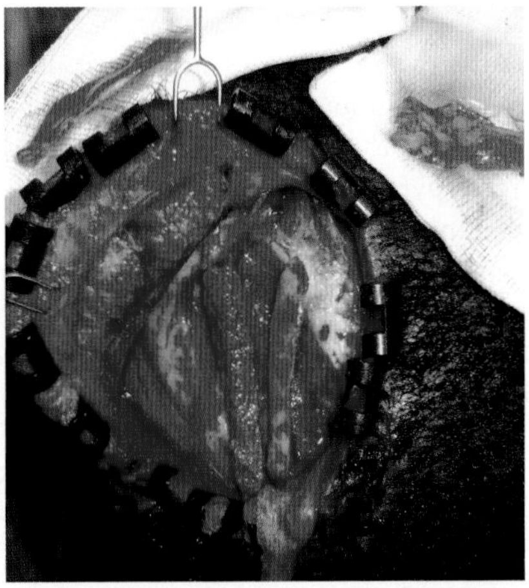

(e)ii

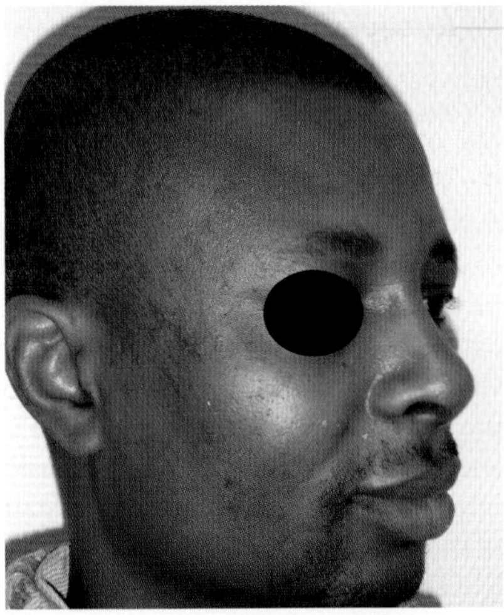

(e)iii

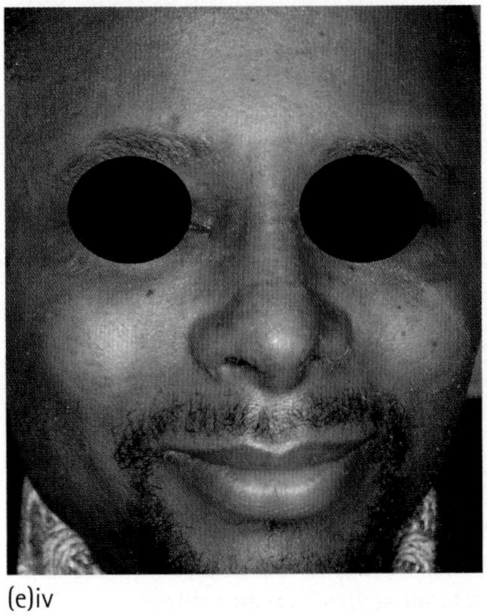

(e)iv

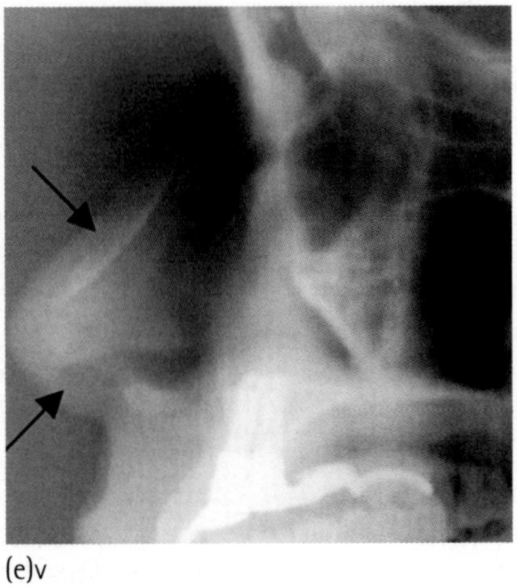

(e)v

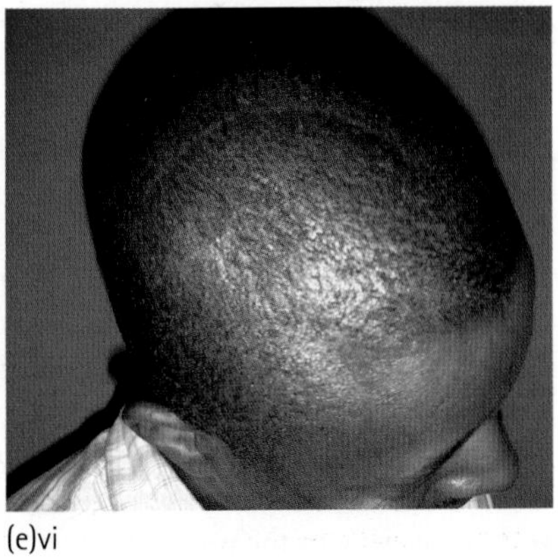

(e)vi

unicortical calvarial bone is problematic and resection on the septum condemned. Ideally, the grafts should be placed in a subperiosteal pocket at the cephalic dorsum and underneath the tip cartilages at the caudal end. To prevent pointed tips they should be onlay grafted. In total reconstructions, the glabellar region and the lateral walls have to be grafted: crushed cartilage, plumping bony fragments and thin bone plates are useful.

SEPTAL DEFORMITY

Major septal deviations, from trauma, sometimes an occult injury in childhood, and usually in combination with deviated pyramids and compensatory hypertrophic inferior turbinates, cause functional airway obstruction with mild symptoms to obstructive sleep apnoea. Septal deviation can cause major asymmetry of the cartilaginous vault and the tip, creating a tension tip. Therefore, a septoplasty must be performed with the rhinoplasty (usually before), which by narrowing can cause decompensation of marginal airway problems due to deflections or septal thickening in the valve area. If hump resection is needed it should be osteotomized as a monobloc, if nescessary asymmetrically, immediately after the extramucosal dissection, permitting a better dorsal access to the septal deformity and saving a one piece hump for repositioning or as a grafting material.

If there is no need for bridge reduction, the ULC are sectioned at the junction with the septum. After the lateral osteotomies, a medial osteotomy frees the osteocartilaginous flaps and permits luxation of the bony septum to the midline. High deviations may cause recurrent pyramidal deviation as the roof is uncapped by lowering the dorsum; in such noses lateral, sometimes also an intermediate, osteotomy is indispensable. In 'tension' tips, the septoplasty will release the tip and influence its position. Accordingly, the septoplasty should be performed before the tip-plasty, and total septorhinoplastic reconstruction is necessary to improve the nasal airway and maintain long-term success of the rhinoplasty.

Cartilaginous septal deflections result from traumatic fracture lines, creating angulations up to 90° and spurs. Vertical, oblique or horizontal septal angulations, the sites of old fractures, may be excised with conservative wedges, removing a small amount of normal adjacent cartilage or bone. The remaining cartilage is left attached to the contralateral mucoperichondrium for strength and support after realignment by suturing through an endonasal approach (Figure 11.7.3a).

In marked angulations of the septum, responsible for external deformations at the middle third, the columella and the aesthetic aspect of the NLA, as saddling of the middle third in case of loss of height (horizontal fractures), and columellar retraction in case of loss of length (vertical fractures), an open approach is preferred.

Vertical fractures may create a lateral deviation of the nose and may be associated with a bulbous ULC impacted between the septum and the pyriform aperture, as well as with a lowering of the nostril sill.

Horizontal angulations perpendicular to the anterior crest will create a saddle deformity of the middle vault, which can not be treated with dorsal augmention, leaving the airway obstruction untouched; the total height of the septum has to be restored (Figure 11.7.3b). Fractures with combinated angulations can result in an impaction of the dorsum on the cranioanterior part of the inferior turbinate. The ULC can be carried with the deviated septum.

Through the open approach, L-strut fractures or multiple incisions for straightening can be bridged or reinforced with cartilaginous or thin bony grafts to straighten and strengthen the crooked portions of dorsal or caudal septum.

Total endomucosal excision of the cartilaginous septum and replacement as a straightend free graft, if needed, with additional support by grafts can be carried out; according to Rees, follow-up did not reveal chondromalacia in cases of bony/cartilaginous septal reconstruction.

Complications

- Septal haematomas and infection.
- CSF leak, due to disturbance of the cribriform plate after high osteotomy of a deviated bony septum.
- Septal perforations (Figure 11.7.4) with symptoms, for example whistling or crusting and epistaxis can theoretically be repaired by sliding mucosal flaps advanced anteriorly and posteriorly on the ipsi- and contralateral side. Inadequate blood supply and scarred host bed can lead to recurrence or larger perforations. The authors always prefer a more reliable closure with a horizontal myomucosal flap derived from the undersurface of the upper lip that can be performed with minimal discomfort for the patient.

TWISTED NOSE

A significant post-traumatic deviation of the external pyramid is practically always accompanied by a deviated septum. After septoplasty, correction of the deviated bony pyramid through an open technique with modified osteotomies: narrowing broad or asymmetric noses can be performed with a combination of medial, intermediate and low lateral osteotomies, and camouflage grafting. A sequential osteotomy technique begins with an intermediate osteotomy on the long side (1) sequentially classic lateral (2) and fading medial osteotomy (3) on the long side, and medial (4) and lateral osteotomies (5) on the short side with full mobilization of the bony fragments to reform the pyramid in the midline (Figure 11.7.5).

Visual correction can be accomplished by asymmetrical shaping of the dorsal hump and inward fractures in the absence of high septal deviation that eventually can be lowered together with that portion of the cartilaginous septum associated with the ULC, so that upon infracture, the dorsal border of the nose lies in the midline.

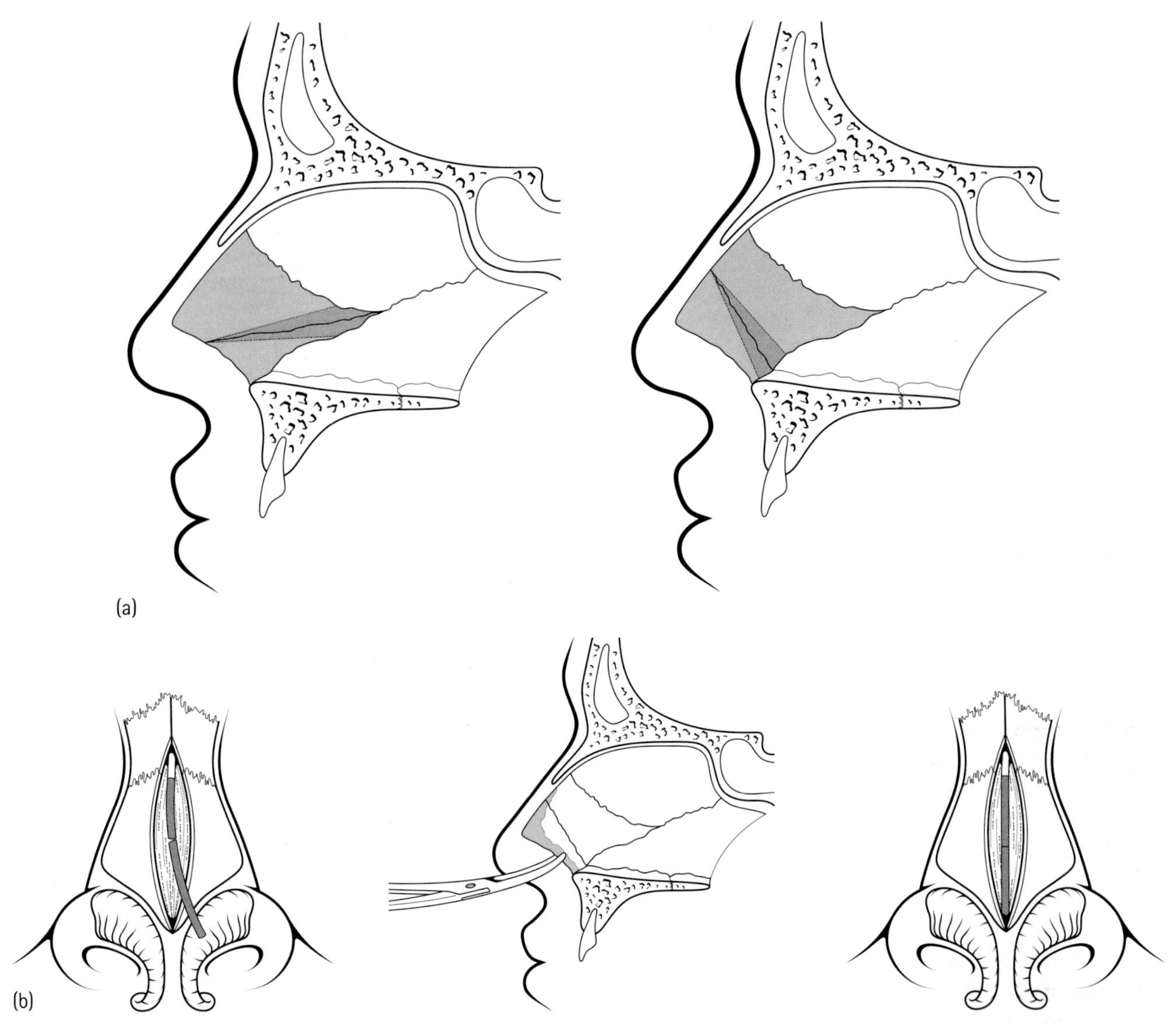

11.7.3 Septal Surgery. (a) Excision of of septal angulation at old fracture sites through endonasal approach (Tardy). (b) 'Swinging-Door' technique to reposition lower septum. If bony septum is straight after sectioning of septum at point of maximal deviation. Disarticulation at the osseocartilaginous junction. Freeing the septum along the floor of the nose and swinging it to the midline with the opposing lining intact.

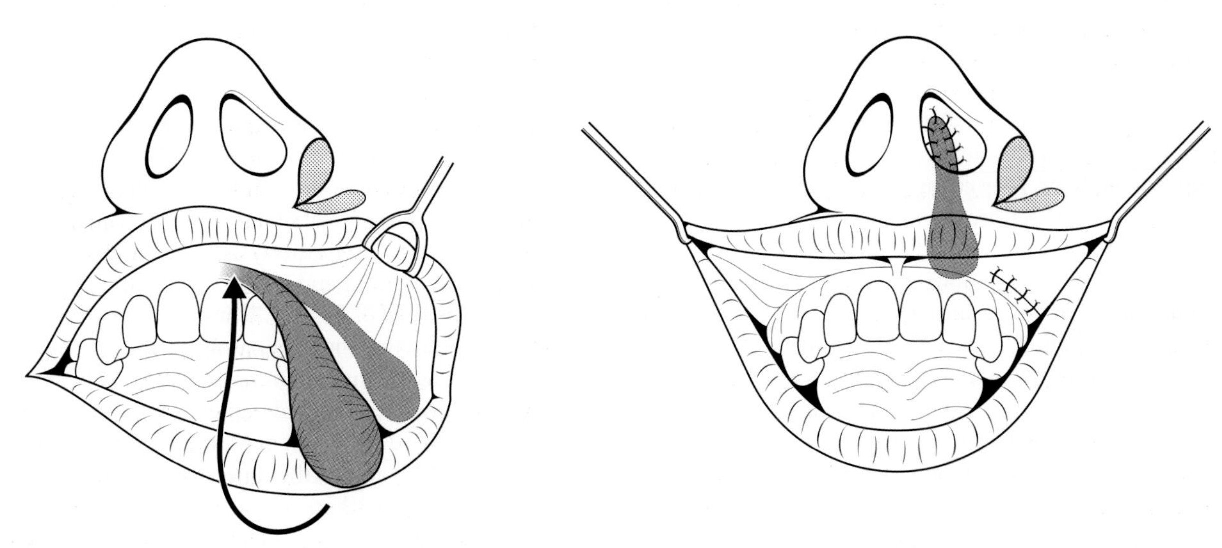

11.7.4 Septal perforation. Closure of septal perforations: myomucosal vestibular lip flap.

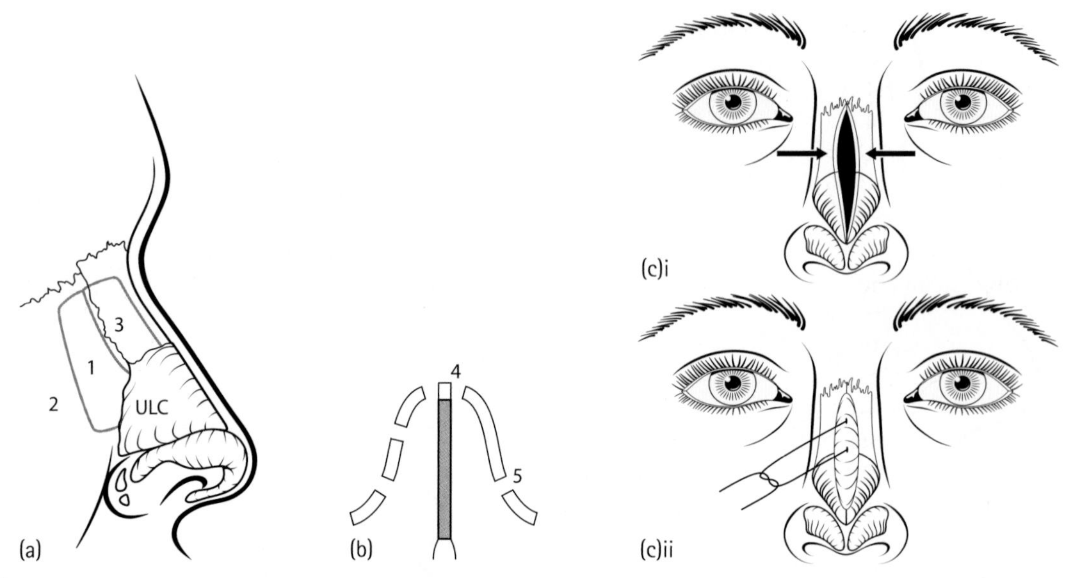

11.7.5 Correction of twisted nose. (a, b) Sequential osteotomy technique: intermediate osteotomy on the long side (1) and sequential classic lateral (2) and medial (3) on the long side and medial (4) and lateral osteotomies (5) with full mobilization of the bony fragments. (c)(i) Crooked noses with dorsal deviations uncorrectable by standard rhinoplasty are treated with camouflaging techniques including (ii) dorsal septal grafting.

Osteotomies are transcutaneously performed with a 2 mm micro-osteotome and without stab incision or any subperiosteal elevation. Endonasal osteotomies are more aggressive and disrupt the soft tissues more, are less precise and may dive into an undesired path of an old fracture site with possible shattering of the lateral nasal wall. Webster's triangle and the triangular bone at the pyriform rim cranially to the inferior turbinate are respected to prevent airway impingement. Spontaneous back-fractures can occur in prefractured, sometimes thickened, bony structures. To control such and to prevent 'rocker' formation, transcutaneous superomedial and superolateral osteotomies are performed through the the glabellar region. The same route is followed for the mobilizing osteotomy of a deviated perpendicular plate of the ethmoid, a possible reason for persistent deviation.

Deviations of the dorsum that are uncorrectable by standard approaches can often be camouflaged by various techniques such as septal and ULC overlap and grafts of nasal septum, which are beyond the scope of this chapter. Camouflaging an imperfectly straightened nose can be carried out with autografts removed during the septorhinoplasty. They can mask a high septal deviation or augment a depressed area on one side by insertion off center to improve the contour (Figure 11.7.5c).

In conclusion, the author strongly believes that the best results over time are obtained by the open approach and that lateral osteotomies are virtually always necessary for complete mobilization of the nasal bones and avoiding post-operative 'drift'. The osteotomies must be performed transcutaneously with a micro-osteotome without periosteal underming for preservation of periosteal attachment and a supportive sling or internal splint for the mobile bones avoiding collapse into the pyriform aperture. Particularly in twisted noses, a Webster's triangle should be respected with preservation of a triangle of bone not being narrowed and remaining lateral along the floor of the nose, thus preserving the full airway which is vital for patient comfort. Remembering the importance of camouflage grafting and strive for a high dorsum and a super strong tip, autografts of cartilage, bone and fascia grafts are primordial to improve the overall aesthetic outcome.

NASAL AIRWAY OBSTRUCTION

After confirmation of the patient's complaint of nasal obstruction, functional tests (Cottle manoeuvre and cotton-tip applicator test) before and after vasoconstriction, CT scan and inspection can diagnose.

Collapse of the middle vault

Evidenced by a pinched middle vault or oblique furrow, confirmed by a positive cotton-tip applicator test at the caudal end of the ULC, can be corrected with spreader grafts. Through the open approach, a thick septal graft is harvested at the maxillary crest. The graft should be at least 15 by 2 mm to fit passively in an intramucosal pocket between the septum and the ULC from the rhinion to the caudomedial end of the ULC. The graft opens the nasal valve angle by moving the ULC away from the septum and decreases the resistance to nasal breathing. In bilateral cases, the grafts can cause a broadening of the dorsum, which can be camouflaged by augmentation grafting of the dorsum, lifting the SSTE and further opening the valve.

Pinching can aesthetically be corrected by onlay grafting of crushed or morselized cartilage or by thin bone plates, acting as a batten being supported by the nasal bones.

In cases of ULC-valve collapse with a horizontal deformity of the lateral wall due to disruption of the osseo-cartilaginous junction, a thin bony septal graft can be placed from a subperiosteal pocket of the nasal bone to underneath the ULC through an intercartilaginous incision after extramucosal dissection

Airway narrowing at the alar margin

Cartilage buckling and fracture with concomitant airway narrowing at the alar margin, due to blunt trauma, can be corrected by batten grafts from the ear, placed with the concave side down. If simultaneous alar retraction is present, composite chondrocutaneous grafts are needed. These grafts are usually harvested from the contralateral cymba concha, because of approximating shape, with the skin component oversized to allow for contraction.

Inferior turbinate hypertrophy

Hypertrophic inferior turbinates, commonly on the concave side of the septal deviation, may cause airway obstruction and may interfere with septal repositioning. Outfracturing and lateralizing with Boise instrument can be a conservative therapy in noses with large inferior meatus. Additional conservative submucosal bony resection, mostly of the anterior part, can be performed through an incision along the length of the turbinate and submucoperiosteal elevation of the soft tissue. The redundant soft tissue is resected after redraping.

Our personal preference is resection of the anterior part after infracture with Cottle's elevator. Articulated scissors are placed above the anterior tip of the turbinate and angled inferior and posterior at 45°. The cut is through mucosa and bone. With the exception of mulberriform degeneration, the posterior part of the turbinate is left untouched.

POST-OPERATIVE CARE IN COMBINED SEPTOPLASTY – TURBINATE SURGERY: SEPTAL SPLINTING – NASAL PACKING

Although continuous suturing of the septum provides stability, we believe supplemental intranasal splinting is useful with extensive surgery in post-traumatic septal collapse. Soft 1 mm thick reinforced Silastic sheets (Dow Corning, Midland, MI) cut to line the septum, are always placed at both sides of the septum for 1 week, allowing the mucoperichondrial septal flaps to remain reapproximated in the midline, protecting lacerations and avoiding adhesions or synechiae. Nasal packing with Merocel™ (laminated nasal dressing, Medtronic Xomed, Jacksonville, FL) in antibiotic ointment, in slight over-correction of the former septal deviation, support the Silastic and prevent dorsal collapse. Antibiotic protection is preferred during the period of routine nasal packing, 3–5 days. After removal of the septal splints, routinely at day 7, but sometimes longer if the epithelial surfaces are not yet healed and synechiae formation should be prevented, the patient is advised to 'mechanically' apply ointments for several weeks post-operatively to prevent crusting and adhesions and to support the recuperation of the mucosae.

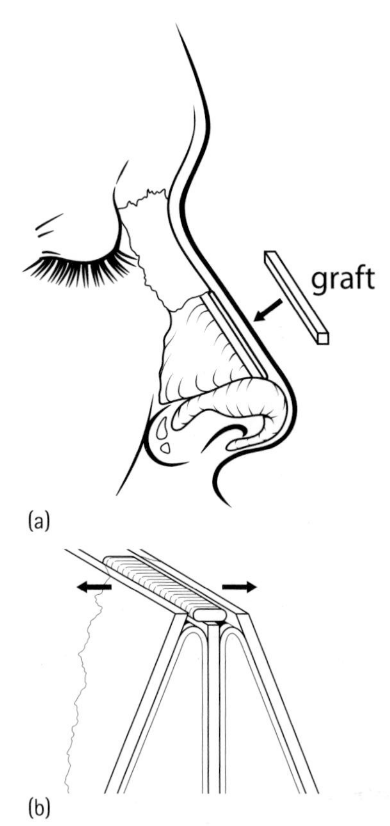

11.7.6 Correction of valve collapse – nasal obstruction: Spreader graft placed intramucosally through an open approach; in bilateral collapse two separate spreader grafts can be placed, or one broader graft can be used as an 'inlay' between the ULC (Sheen's spreader technique to correct a collapse of the middle third of the nose).

SOFT-TISSUE DEFICIENCY

Replacing traumatic loss of soft tissues or loss of total fragments of the nose calls for local flaps. The median forehead flap is the workhorse, sometimes in combination with nasolabial and advancement flaps, but this will not be discussed in this chapter.

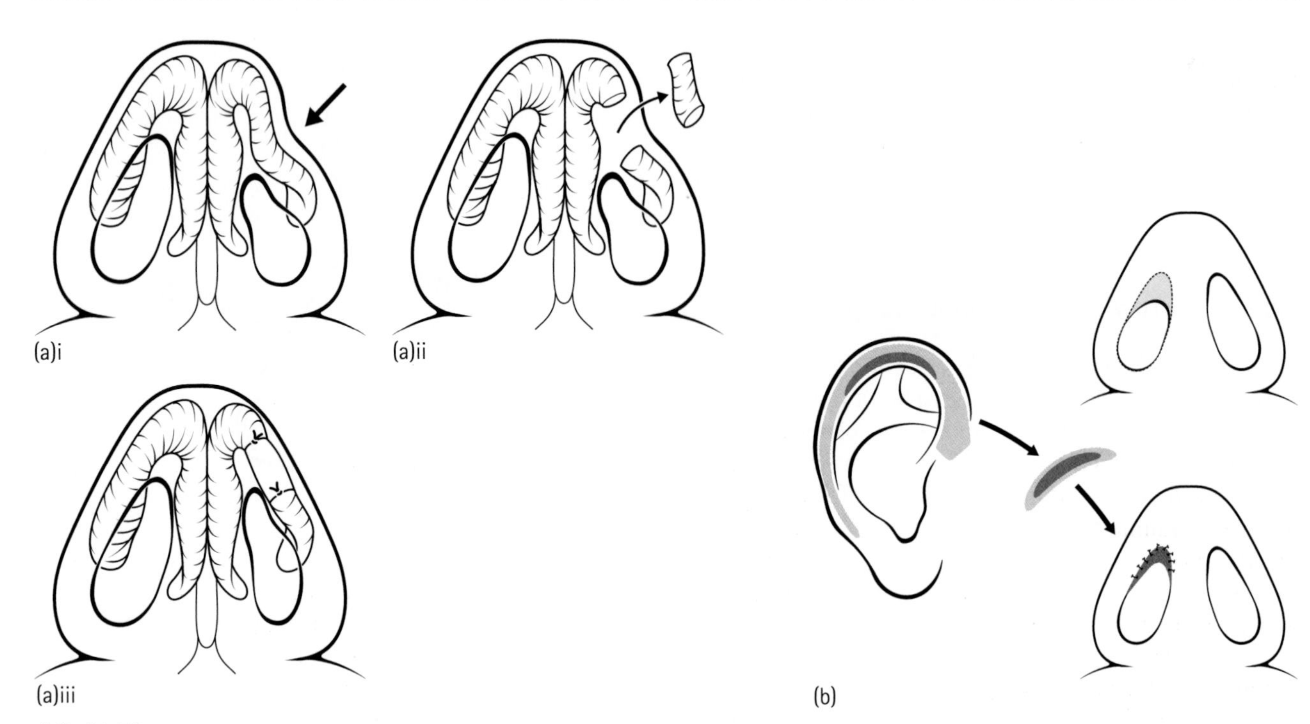

11.7.7 Alar collapse – nasal obstruction resulting from (a)(i) abnormal LC and corrected with (a)(ii, iii) cartilaginous grafts from the ear as batten grafts for abnormal LC. (b) Chondrocutaneous graft for alar retraction with soft tissue deficiency and correction/expansion of collapsed/scarred lateral vestibular wall (composite graft from inner side of crus helicis).

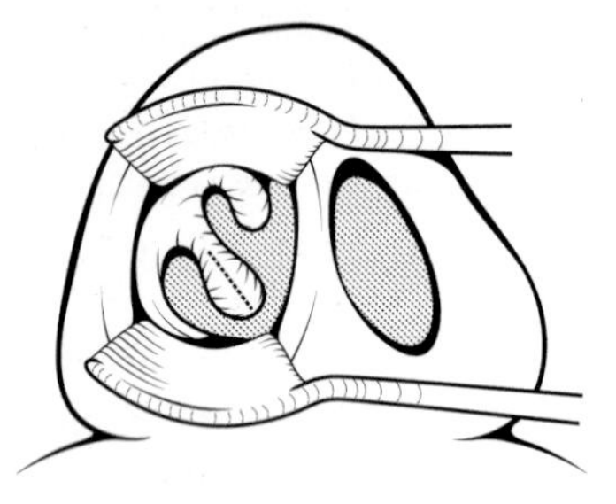

11.7.8 Resection of inferior turbinate: submucous conservative resection.

Top tips

- Create high smooth dorsum and over-supported tip.
- Harvest calvarial bone, fascia grafts and conchal cartilage.
- Open technique respecting integrity of the SSTE.
- Transcutaneous atraumatic micro-osteotomies for precision.
- Minimal resectioning, realistic repositioning and camouflage grafting.
- Reconstruct airway by septal and valve reconstruction, splinting and tamponade.
- Alar base surgery with alar cinch and perialar readaptation on ANS.
- Plaster of Paris with forehead extension for immobilization.

Index